TEXTBOOK OF GENERAL MEDICINE

TEXTBOOK OF GENERAL MEDICINE

Edited by

MAHENDR S. KOCHAR, M.D., M.S., M.R.C.P. (London), F.R.C.P.(C), F.A.C.P., F.A.C.C.P., F.A.A.F.P.

Associate Professor of Medicine and Pharmacology
The Medical College of Wisconsin
Associate Chief of Staff for Education and Chief, Hypertension Section
Wood Veterans Administration Medical Center
Co-Director, Dialysis Unit
St. Michael Hospital
Attending Physician
Froedtert Memorial Lutheran Hospital,
Milwaukee County Medical Complex
and St. Joseph's Hospital
Consultant in Nephrology and Hypertension
Elmbrook Memorial Hospital
Milwaukee, Wisconsin

With a Foreword by

DANIEL J. McCARTY, M.D.

Professor and Chairman
Department of Medicine
The Medical College of Wisconsin
Milwaukee, Wisconsin

A WILEY MEDICAL PUBLICATION
JOHN WILEY & SONS
New York • Chichester • Brisbane • Toronto • Singapore

Cover design by Wanda Lubelska

Dosage Notice

Care has been taken to ensure that dosage recommendations are in accordance with current medical practice. However, dosage schedules are subject to change in light of research and experience. It is recommended that the physician consult the latest issue of *Physicans Desk Reference* (PDR) or the package insert before prescribing an unfamiliar drug.

The editor's royalities from this edition will go to the All India Institute of Medical Sciences, New Delhi, India, and to the Medical College of Wisconsin Student Loan Fund.

Library of Congress Cataloging in Publication Data:

Kochar, Mahendr S., 1943-
Textbook of general medicine.

Includes index.
1. Internal medicine. I. Title. [DNLM: 1. Medicine.

WB 100 T3537]
RC46.K65 1982 616 82-8437
ISBN 0-471-09645-8 AACR2

Printed in the United States of America

10 9 8 7 6 5 4 3 2 1

To my mother and guide, Mrs. Chanan Kaur Kochar

CONTRIBUTORS

Carlos A. Agudelo, M.D.
Assistant Professor of Medicine
Bowman Gray School of Medicine
Wake Forest University
Winston-Salem, North Carolina

John A. Arkins, M.D.
Professor of Medicine
Allergy-Immunology Section
The Medical College of Wisconsin
Milwaukee, Wisconsin

James C. Arseneau, M.D.
Associate Professor of Oncology in Medicine
University of Rochester Cancer Center
Medical Oncology Unit
Rochester General Hospital
Rochester, New York

Virinderjit S. Bamrah, M.D.
Associate Professor of Medicine
The Medical College of Wisconsin
Chief, Cardiovascular Section
Wood Veterans Administration Medical Center
Milwaukee, Wisconsin

Anthony A. Da Costa, M.D.
Consultant, Neurophysiologist
St. James' Hospital, Leeds and
Bootham Park Hospital, York
Yorkshire, England

Edmuond H. Duthie, M.D.
Assistant Professor of Medicine
The Medical College of Wisconsin
Chief, Nursing Home Care Unit
Wood Veterans Administration Medical Center
Milwaukee, Wisconsin

Steven R. Gambert, M.D.
Associate Professor of Medicine and Physiology
The Medical College of Wisconsin
Chief, Geriatrics and Gerontology Section
Wood Veterans Administration Medical Center
Milwaukee, Wisconsin

Ved V. Gossain, M.D.
Professor of Medicine
Michigan State University
East Lansing, Michigan

Harry N. Hoffman II, M.D.
Professor of Medicine
The Mayo Medical School
Consultant in Gastroenterology and Internal Medicine
The Mayo Clinic
Rochester, Minnesota

Mahendr S. Kochar, M.D.
Associate Professor of Medicine and Pharmacology
The Medical College of Wisconsin
Associate Chief of Staff for Education
and Chief, Hypertension Section
Wood Veterans Administration Medical Center
Co-Director, Dialysis Unit
St. Michael Hospital
Attending Physician
Froedtert Memorial Lutheran Hospital,
Milwaukee County Medical Complex
and St. Joseph's Hospital
Consultant in Nephrology and Hypertension
Elmbrook Memorial Hospital
Milwaukee, Wisconsin

Kesavan Kutty, M.D.
Assistant Professor of Medicine
The Medical College of Wisconsin
Associate Academic Chairman of Medicine
St. Joseph's Hospital
Staff Physician, Pulmonary Section
Wood Veterans Administration Medical Center
Milwaukee, Wisconsin

Assa Mayersdorf, M.D.
Associate Professor of Neurology
The Medical College of Wisconsin
Chief, Neurology Service
Wood Veterans Administration Medical Center
Milwaukee, Wisconsin

Ashok R. Patel, M.D.
Chairman, Division of Hematology and Oncology
Cook County Hospital and the Hektoen Institute
for Medical Research
Chicago, Illinois

Edward J. Pisko, M.D.
Associate Professor of Medicine
Rheumatology Section
Bowman Gray School of Medicine
Wake Forest University
Winston-Salem, North Carolina

Susan N. Rosenthal, M.D.
Associate Professor of Oncology in Medicine
University of Rochester Cancer Center
Medical Oncology Unit
Rochester General Hospital
Rochester, New York

Philip W. Smith, M.D.
Assistant Professor of Medicine
University of Nebraska College of Medicine
Hospital Epidemiologist
Bishop Clarkson Memorial Hospital
Consultant to Nebraska State Health Department for
Infectious Diseases and Hospital Epidemiology
Omaha, Nebraska

Richard D. Stewart, M.D., M.P.H.
Clinical Professor of Pharmacology and Toxicology
The Medical College of Wisconsin
Milwaukee, Wisconsin
Corporate Medical Director
S. C. Johnson & Son, Inc.
Racine, Wisconsin

Robert A. Turner, M.D.
Chief of Rheumatology
Professor of Medicine
Bowman Gray School of Medicine
Wake Forest University
Winston-Salem, North Carolina

Basil Varkey, M.D.
Associate Professor of Medicine
The Medical College of Wisconsin
Chief, Pulmonary Diseases Section
Wood Veterans Administration Medical Center
Milwaukee, Wisconsin

R. Mala Vohra, M.D.
Attending Physician
Division of Hematology and Oncology
Cook County Hospital and the Hektoen
Institute for Medical Research
Chicago, Illinois

L. Samuel Wann, M.D.
Associate Professor of Medicine
The Medical College of Wisconsin
Chief, Echocardiography
Wood Veterans Administration Medical Center
and Milwaukee County Medical Complex
Milwaukee, Wisconsin

Charles Zugerman, M.D.
Assistant Professor of Dermatology
Chief, Section on Industrial and Contact Dermatitis
Northwestern University Medical School
Chicago, Illinois

FOREWORD

The methodical assimilation of medical knowledge is a problem for all physicians, even for internists, most of whom enjoy reading. Most medical schools wisely emphasize teaching in small groups using available case material. While this format serves to focus discussion on the reality of an existing problem, it presupposes a broad background knowledge of internal medicine and the basic medical sciences. Such knowledge is absolutely essential for differential diagnosis and rational therapeutics.

Most existing internal medicine textbooks are encyclopedic works by multiple authors. All are biased in various ways. Their quality of scholarship is uneven, and they are quickly out of date as new information is published or presented at meetings during the interval of 2 or more years between the writing and publication of a textbook. But such books remain important because they provide rapid, authoritative reference to specific clinical problems and a comprehensive, coherent overview of internal medicine.

I am impressed that, for numerous reasons, the teaching of medicine in medical schools has suffered a decline that nearly parallels that of the teaching of grammar in grammar school. Thinking, especially rigorous, integrative thinking, has been displaced inexorably by procedural technology. Many physicians engaged in the operation and supervision of these admittedly marvelous advances have themselves become highly competent, highly compensated technicians. Narrow subspecialization frequently supplants broad professional scholarship. It is unlikely that either contemporary medical students or these medical technocrats have ever read a comprehensive textbook of medicine cover to cover.

It is to this audience that this condensed overview of internal medicine is directed. Its virtues are brevity and readability. Both qualities reflect the judgment of its editor; this effort should broaden the base of medical knowledge of medical students and physicians. The self-assessment questions built in to each chapter should reinforce their grasp of essential information.

Daniel J. McCarty, M.D.
Professor and Chairman
Department of Medicine
The Medical College of Wisconsin
Milwaukee, Wisconsin

PREFACE

"To study the phenomena of disease without books is to sail an uncharted sea; while to study books without patients is not to go to sea at all," wrote Sir William Osler in 1901.*

There is only one way to learn clinical medicine, and that is at the bedside participating in diagnosis and treatment of the patient's illness; however, no one can expect to acquire even the essential knowledge of internal medicine without books. With intensive biomedical research, there has been a knowledge explosion in medicine in the last three decades; there is too much to learn in a limited amount of time. It is impossible for a medical student to read the standard textbooks of medicine from beginning to end, but the student must acquire knowledge of the essentials of internal medicine in order to become a Doctor of Medicine.

The purpose of this book is to provide the student with a course in internal medicine that can be read from cover to cover during an 8- to 12-week rotation in medicine; it contains the essentials of internal medicine that the student must know before graduating. The book will also serve as a source of concise information for family practice and internal medicine residents desiring a rapid review of internal medicine. Allied health professionals, particularly nurse practitioners and physicians' assistants, will find the book readable and understandable.

Each chapter begins with an outline that defines the scope of the subject matter that one needs to learn and ends with multiple-choice questions, which should help in recapitulating what has been learned. Liberal use of headings and use of simple yet precise language should make the reading of this book an enjoyable experience.

This text has been written by specialists who are among today's leading teachers of internal medicine. All of the authors are board certified in both internal medicine and their subspecialties and have written their chapters with the objective of presenting all relevant information in the most lucid manner. The use of references has been deliberately avoided, but a selected bibliography is provided at the end of each chapter for further reading.

I would like to take this opportunity to thank Daniel J. McCarty, M.D., Professor and Chairman of the Department of Medicine at the Medical College of Wisconsin, Milwaukee, for writing the foreword to this book.

Mahendr S. Kochar

*Osler W: Books and men. *Boston Med Surg J* 144:60-62, 1901.

ACKNOWLEDGMENTS

It is almost impossible to list the names and contributions of all individuals who have assisted in the preparation and publication of this book. Without their assistance this book would have never seen the light of day. First and foremost I express my gratitude to each and every one of these individuals. During my professional career, I have been associated with some of the finest physicans who have contributed immensely to my own education; I remain indebted to all my teachers and colleagues. I am grateful to Mrs. Elaine Otto, Mrs. Susan Holtz, and Ms. Linda Corrao for their excellent secretarial support. The services of the medical media production department, the library, the copy center, and the editorial assistant of the Wood Veterans Administration Medical Center are gratefully acknowledged. I also express my appreciation to the contributors and their secretaries, who have displayed immense patience and worked hard to bring this book to fruition. The reviewers deserve a special vote of thanks. Their constructive criticisms were most helpful. The staff of John Wiley & Sons, Inc., was marvelous to work with during publication of this book. Last, but not least, I am indebted to my wife, Arvind, and our children, Baj and Jay, for their selfless devotion and love.

Mahendr S. Kochar

CONTENTS

TEXTBOOK OF GENERAL MEDICINE

CHAPTER 1
THE ART AND SCIENCE OF MEDICINE

Mahendr S. Kochar

THE ART AND SCIENCE OF MEDICINE

Medicine is both an art and a science. Diagnosis of illness is based on clinical methods and laboratory tests, sometimes requiring the application of the most modern technology. Eliciting a good history, performing an appropriate physical examination, and selecting the most crucial laboratory tests without subjecting the patient to undue risk or expense require skill. Laboratory tests, x-ray, and electrophysiologic tests constitute the application of science in medicine; however, extracting the relevant information from a mass of conflicting physical signs and laboratory data to arrive at a correct diagnosis requires application of the art of medicine. Similarly, whereas pharmaceutical modalities and surgical procedures are highly developed from the scientific standpoint, the decisions on when or how to use them require experience and judgment.

PRIMARY CARE PHYSICIAN

Internists, family practitioners, and pediatricians are often referred to as primary care physicians. Such physicians are usually the first health care professionals consulted when a patient enters the health care system. These physicians are able to take care of as many as 80 percent of all illnesses, usually in an outpatient setting. A primary care physician also acts, if need be, as the patient's spokesperson and adviser in health and medical matters, and coordinates the work of specialists and consultants in the event the patient is afflicted by a serious illness requiring such expertise. Once health is restored and the patient leaves the hospital and returns home and to work, the primary care physician provides follow-up care, referring the patient back to the specialist only if necessary.

Approach to the Patient—Special Situations

Physicians must be tactful, sympathetic, and understanding in their approach to patients. The patient should never be regarded as a case with a collection of symptoms, signs, damaged organs, and disturbed emotions but as a fellow human being seeking relief, cure, and reassurance. The physician is expected to be humble, courageous, and wise. Today's patient is more intelligent and better informed than in earlier generations; often the patient is technologically oriented, busier, and sometimes skeptical. Since any departure from good health involves a potential threat of dependence, disability, or death, even the most intelligent and best-informed patients are often more concerned about these eventualities than about their diseases. The physician should therefore establish good communication with patients, be truthful, and attempt to allay anxiety.

Certain patients require special attention and skills. A few examples follow.

Adolescent Patients

The adolescent patient needs special attention, emotional support, and understanding. The physician can act as a confidant and an adviser. The physician should encourage adolescent patients to ask questions and provide them with detailed and relevant information. Information regarding the use of contraceptives and prevention of venereal diseases is extremely important in this age group.

Alcoholic Patients

As many as 15 percent of the American population is estimated to consume an excessive amount of alcohol. Working aocholics are not easy patients to deal with because they exhibit a great deal of denial of alcoholism. Although many of these patients are successful in their professions, they are destined to experience emotional, social, and physical complications unless they can be convinced to reduce or give up drinking. The alcoholic patient not only is susceptible to the complications of alcoholism but also has low resistance to various infections.

Drug-Dependent Patients
The drug of dependence can vary from nicotine and caffeine to narcotic analgesics or opiates. Dependence on central nervous system depressants, such as diazepam (Valium), and central nervous system stimulants, such as amphetamines and their congeners, is much more common than opiate dependence. Opiate-dependent patients are extremely manipulative, and are often criminals. In dealing with drug-dependent patients, physicians should be sympathetic and understanding; however, they also need to be firm and should not allow themselves to be manipulated by the patient.

Homosexual Patients
Homosexual men are more often exposed to various types of venereal disease and serious systemic disorders, such as viral heptatitis, than are heterosexual men. Physicians should not impose their own moral and social values on such patients; they should offer counseling and psychiatric referral for changing to heterosexual behavior only if so requested by the patient.

Geriatric Patients
Although old age is often associated with illness and greater dependency, the elderly, like the young, wish to be well regarded, listened to, and respected as worthwhile people. The effects of aging on the body must be differentiated from illness. Subjecting the elderly to expensive and invasive diagnostic tests in an effort to find a curable disease is often fruitless. The physician's attitude toward the aged should be humane and supportive.

Terminally Ill Patients
Among the most difficult tasks of the physician is that of dealing with a terminally ill patient. A sustaining, supportive relationship between the patient, the family, and the physician is of crucial importance to all three. Good physicians do not attempt to preserve life regardless of pain, misery, and expense. Modern techniques of maintaining respiration and circulation can prolong the length of a terminal illness and therefore should be used with caution and discretion.

Approach to the Patient's Family

The structure and importance of the family are undergoing major changes. Divorce and cohabitation are common and are increasingly acceptable to society. As in the case of the homosexual patient, physicians must avoid imposing their own values on the patient. The physician should find out the names and relationships of the "significant others" in the patient's life, include them in communicating with the patient, and seek their support in restoring the patient to health. When a patient is seriously ill, the physician should comfort the family and allay any guilt that the family members may feel. When a patient dies, the physician must inform the family gently, offering such comfort as may be possible. If an autopsy is contemplated, the physician should tactfully seek the family's permission, explaining the reasons for the autopsy.

Maintenance of Health and Prevention of Disease—Health Education

Few areas of medicine are of greater benefit to any one person or to the community than health maintenance and preventive medicine. Social, economic, and geographic factors are all important in maintaining the health of the population. More skill is required to recognize the early signs of ill health than to diagnose an illness after it is well established. The discovery and cure of potentially serious disease represent a service of paramount importance to the patient. Regular and frequent recording of blood pressure, breast examination, and the Pap smear for detection of cervical cancer are examples of preventive care. It is not always easy to persuade asymptomatic persons to accept the diagnosis of illness and follow medical advice that may require changes in life style and diet. Health education wherein the patient and the family are informed of preventive health measures conducive to a beneficial modification of behavior can be effective in preventing illness and prolonging life.

Physician as a Healer—Iatrogenic Disorders

With advances in therapeutics, potent medications are now available for the treatment of many illnesses for which in the past only symptomatic relief could be offered. These drugs, however, have a potential for harm and can produce iatrogenic disorders. The physician must take precautions to minimize the dangers of therapy. Drugs or surgery alone can seldom provide maximal benefit. Physicians must learn to treat the patient as a person who is ill, and not the illness for which the patient seeks relief. Patients must be encouraged to feel that their individuality is respected and appreciated. The caring attitude of the physician should supplement and complement the drugs and/or surgical procedure in restoring the patient to health and happiness.

ROLE OF A CONSULTANT

When not sure of a diagnosis or the prognosis, the physician should say so honestly and seek consultation with a specialist. No physician loses respect or confidence by admitting ignorance and seeking help. The primary care physician must select the best consultant available, depending on what the patient's problem may be and, with the help of the consultant, take appropriate measures to make a diagnosis and provide treatment. The primary care physician should also make use of this opportunity to learn from the consultant about the latest advances in treating the illness in question, and related matters. Whenever the patient desires another opinion, the physician should respect the patient's wishes and assist in obtaining a second opinion without hesitation.

When called on as a consultant by another physician, the consultant should serve both the physician and the patient.

Consultants should be both honest and tactful. They must display confidence without conveying the inference of superiority over the physician who consulted them. They should answer all the patient's questions. If the primary care physician made errors in diagnosis and treatment, consultants must courteously point these out to the primary care physician and suggest corrective measures. If the patient persists in asking questions whose answers may be embarrassing to the primary care physician, consultants should answer them honestly and tactfully, keeping the primary care physician fully informed.

ROLE OF ALLIED HEALTH CARE PROFESSIONALS IN MEDICAL PRACTICE

Because of increasing demands from patients and society at large, as well as technologic advances and social changes, a variety of trained professionals other than physicians and nurses are involved in the treatment of patients. These professionals include physician's assistants, dietitians, physical therapists, inhalation therapists, biochemists, psychologists, and other health care personnel. Both the patient and the primary care physician can greatly benefit from such collaboration, but the physician must maintain responsibility as the team leader, be familiar with the techniques, skills, and objectives of the allied health care professionals, and oversee the total care delivered to the patient.

MULTISPECIALTY CLINICS AND HEALTH MAINTENANCE ORGANIZATIONS

Increasing numbers of patients are being cared for by groups of physicians, clinics, hospitals, and health maintenance organizations (HMOs), rather than by solo practitioners. Even if patient care is rendered in a clinic setting, the identity of the physician who is primarily and continuously responsible for each patient must be clearly defined. The responsibility of overseeing the patient's total care rests with the primary care physician. The patient's cooperation in this regard is essential; the patient must understand the shortcomings of a multispecialty organization and make every effort to stay with the primary care physician, giving this physician the opportunity to deliver continuity of care.

MEDICAL RECORDS

It is imperative that the physician promptly and accurately commit all pertinent data relating to the patient's clinical and laboratory examinations and treatment to the patient's permanent medical record. This is particularly important in the present-day practice of medicine in that, at any one time, several physicians and allied health care professionals may contribute to the care of a particular patient; also, patients as well as physicians are becoming increasingly mobile. Furthermore, medical records are good indicators of the quality of care and are presently being used for recertification of family practitioners.

To enhance communication, education, and rapid retrieval of stored information, the system of problem-oriented medical records (POMR) has been devised. The problems as stated by the patient or identified by the physician are central to its formulation. As the diagnosis emerges, current problems are replaced by the former ones on the problem list. The progress notes are recorded under the subheadings of subjective complaints (S), objective findings (O), assessment (A), and plan (P), or "SOAP," for each problem. The criticisms of the POMR system are that it is time-consuming and may cause the medical record rather than the patient to become the primary focus of attention.

ROLE OF COMPUTERS IN MEDICINE

The uses of the computer in managing the economics of medical practice are well established. Computers are also being increasingly used in the clinical laboratory for processing automated chemical and microbiologic data. Automated information systems are also being used in pharmacies and for maintaining patients' hospital and outpatient records. Computers are available at several large centers to facilitate differential diagnosis and to evaluate clinical decision making. Computers can save much time and effort; they can quickly supply accurate and reliable information to use for the benefit of the patient. Many physicians, however, express concern that computers may destroy whatever is left of the patient-physician relationship and also play havoc with the patient's right to confidentiality. Their concern is valid, and present and future physicians must guard against the misuse of computers while encouraging their use to enhance patient care.

ACCOUNTABILITY IN MEDICAL PRACTICE

Physicians are being held increasingly accountable for their actions in terms of the quality and cost-effectiveness of care. Review of medical records, mandatory continuing education for relicensure, and recertification by examination are examples of government measures and voluntary efforts by physicians to demonstrate competence. For the patient, it has become essential to reduce costly hospital admissions as much as possible, and to keep the cost of medical care affordable. In the last analysis, the public must look to the medical profession for leadership and guidance in matters of health-related legislation. While maintaining concern for the welfare of their patients, physicians must make every possible effort to alleviate the socioeconomic problems involved in health care delivery.

HUMAN RESEARCH

If the science of medicine is to progress, research must be performed on human beings. It is incumbent upon the physician engaged in human research to explain to the patient, in clear and understandable language, the nature, risks, and benefits of all diagnostic and therapeutic procedures that are not well established or are considered experimental, and obtain the patient's informed consent. When performing research, the physician must take extraordinary precautions to protect the patient's interests and to minimize risks. Only by using these safeguards can human research be undertaken for the progress of medicine without jeopardizing the patient's health.

PHYSICIANS' RESPONSIBILITIES TO THEMSELVES, THEIR FAMILIES, AND THE COMMUNITY

Physicians lead stressful lives, often despite the amassing of material wealth. The suicide rate among physicians is one of the highest compared to that of other professions. Every physician must devote time to recreation and family, and engage regularly in physical exercise.

The physician's responsibility does not end with the care of patients. As an outstanding and respected member of society, the physician must participate to some extent in civic affairs and politics for the benefit of the community and the nation.

CLINICAL METHODS

Clinical information is obtained from the patient by taking a history, by observation of the patient through physical examination, and from investigations such as laboratory tests, radiographic examinations, and other procedures. The whole body of clinical information enables the physician to make a diagnosis, to decide on the best therapy, and to give a prognosis. The term *clinical methods* encompasses all the ways of obtaining clinical information.

HISTORY

Obtaining an accurate and comprehensive history is the most fruitful of all the techniques used in the appraisal of a clinical problem; the patient's history is the key to diagnosis. The history records the patient's story and describes symptoms, suggesting certain diagnostic possibilities, excluding others, and pointing to investigations that should be considered. The history may, at times, provide the only clue to a diagnosis. All data must be as accurate and specific as possible.

It is essential that the physician adopt a form and style to use in writing down the history of patients, adhering to this pattern until it becomes a habit. The advantages are that no intellectual effort is devoted to taking the history itself, and full attention can be devoted to interpreting the meaning of each response. In addition, it is much less likely that a topic will be overlooked. The following outline for taking a history is used by most physicians.

Demographic Information

Demographic information includes the patient's name, age, race, sex, marital status, address, hospital number, date of examination, and source and reliability of the informant.

Presenting Complaints and Their Durations

Information on the patient's complaints includes the answer to the question, "What prompted you to seek medical attention?" The complaints are usually listed, each on a separate line, followed by their approximate duration. The patient's symptoms provide clues to the differential diagnosis, and the list also reminds the physician that these are the symptoms that most concern the patient.

Present Illness

Information on the patient's present illness should be written as an orderly and chronologic account. It should be a lucid and succinct narrative. If the patient is not sure when the illness began, the physician should ask, "When did you last feel well or normal." Each symptom should be described in detail, including specifics about intensity and location, accompanying symptoms, factors that relieve or aggravate the symptom, and the course (progression or regression). When a symptom suggests several conditions, statements about the lack of concomitant symptoms that often accompany the original symptom should be included. If the present illness has progressed in attacks separated by symptom-free intervals, a typical attack should be described in terms of onset, duration, and associated symptoms. In both acute and chronic illnesses, the date that the patient stopped work or assumed bedrest should be noted. When there is a conspicuous disturbance of a particular organ or system, direct questions should be asked about all possible symptoms referable to the particular organ system. The patient's previous treatment should be noted, including over-the-counter medications that the patient may have taken. Inquiry should also be made about general abnormalities, such as pain, chills, fever, night sweats, and loss of weight. Finally, mention should be made of the patient's level of activity at work and during leisure time.

Past History

The patient's past history includes a description of previous illnesses, general health, operations, injuries, hospitalizations, and allergies.

Family History

The family history includes a statement on similar illness or symptoms in the family, or the lack thereof; it notes the age and state of health of parents, siblings, and children, or the cause of their death and the age at death. It also includes the family history of common heritable diseases, such as diabetes, hypertension, heart disease, kidney disease, cancer, allergy, and mental illness. A family tree is helpful if the same illness has appeared in several members of the family.

Personal and Social History

Personal and social history includes information on diet and nutrition, smoking, alcohol consumption, sleep and exercise habits, education and occupation, marital status and sex life, and home and environmental conditions.

Review of Systems

The patient should be asked about salient symptoms pertaining to each organ system. All the symptoms reported by the patient should be described, and the lack of significant symptoms noted.

PHYSICAL EXAMINATION

The physical examination is conducted by means of the four basic methods of inspection, palpation, percussion, and auscultation. Often there are aspects of the patient's illness that are revealed only by physical examination. Thoroughness in the routine examination is therefore essential. Physical examination is indispensable in obtaining the following information about a patient: general appearance, including mental status; vital signs (temperature, pulse rate, respiration rate, blood pressure); visible lesions on the body; palpable lesions, such as masses, local tenderness, deformities, and pulsations; signs of respiratory difficulty; auscultatory findings, such as murmurs, friction rubs, and alteration in bowel sounds; and neurologic signs.

The environment in which the patient is examined should be quiet and well lighted, preferably by daylight. The physician should be considerate in examining the patient, paying heed to the patient's need for privacy and avoiding discomfort to the patient as much as possible. A systematic approach is desirable. The physician's aim is to maintain objectivity and record observations instead of interpreting them. For the routine physical examination, a full complement of equipment includes stethoscope, penlight, tongue blades, otophthalmoscope, reflex hammer, sphygmomanometer, tuning fork, gloves, lubricating jelly, guaiac test reagents, and a pelvic speculum.

The following is an outline for performing the physical examination and recording the finds.

General Appearance

The physical examination begins with observations on the patient's nutritional state, habitus, apparent age, state of health, comfort, emotional state, and ability to cooperate; obvious mental disease, or striking findings, such as pallor, constant coughing, respiratory distress, voice abnormality, or cyanosis are noted. Temperature, pulse rate, respiration rate, height, weight, and blood pressure are recorded (describe the patient's position and where the blood pressure is taken, and if abnormal, check in other positions and limbs).

Skin

Note the skin color, texture, moisture, temperature, and scars. Describe in detail any eruption, abnormal pigmentation, skin tumors, or Raynaud's phenomenon. Note the condition of the nails and hair.

Lymph Nodes

Check for enlargement, consistency, mobility, and tenderness of the lymph nodes. If enlarged, record the approximate size of nodes in centimeters.

Head

Determine the size, shape, and contour of the head; note asymmetry, tenderness over the sinuses or mastoids, the facial expression, and any abnormal movements.

Eyes

Check the conjunctivae, the sclerae, and the pupillary size and reaction. Note any protrusion, ptosis, arcus senilis, nystagmus, lid lag, or icterus. Use finger tension for introcular pressure; check extraocular movements and gross visual fields. Do an ophthalmoscopic examination.

Ears

Note any tophi or discharge; describe the eardrums and hearing acuity.

Nose

Check for septal deviation, airway obstruction, and nasal discharge; note the condition of the mucosa, turbinates, and polyps. Transillumination of the sinuses should be performed if indicated.

Mouth and Throat

Note the odor of the breath, and the color and appearance of the lips, tongue, and gums. Check the condition of the teeth, or dentures, and the appearance of the mucosa. Describe the palate, uvula, tonsils, and posterior pharynx.

Neck

Check the neck for rigidity or limitation of motion, abnormal pulsations, scars, masses, and enlarged salivary glands or lymph nodes. Describe the thyroid gland (size, consistency, tenderness, nodules). Note the position of the trachea. Also note any vascular thrills, bruits, or abnormal pulsations of veins.

Back

The back should be checked for mobility, kyphosis, lordosis, and scoliosis. Note any tenderness on palpation or percussion.

Thorax

Check the thorax for configuration, symmetry, and respiratory movements. Estimate tactile fremitus. Note chest tenderness; percuss the chest, front and back, and excursion of the diaphragm. On auscultation, characterize breath sounds and voice sounds, and note any rales, rhonchi, or friction rubs. Describe the character of the rales, location, type, and part of respiratory cycle.

Breasts

Note the size, consistency, symmetry, and tenderness of the breasts. Describe any palpable masses or discharge from the nipples.

Heart

Inspect the precordium and describe any abnormal pulsations, bulging, or heaving. Carefully localize the apical impulse.

Palpate the entire precordium systematically for impulses, thrills, and rubs, noting the location and timing. Define the area of cardiac dullness by percussion. Auscultate over the entire precordium systematically, especially at the valve areas, characterizing rate, rhythm, quality of sounds, splitting, extra sounds, murmurs, or rubs. Note the effect of position or respiration on heart sounds or murmurs.

Abdomen

Check the abdomen for appearance, distention, retraction, symmetry, and local prominences; describe any intrinsic movements. Note dilated vessels, or pulsations. Palpate, noting tenderness, rigidity, hyperesthesia, guarding, masses, and fluid. Palpate and note the size of the liver and its upper and lower margins in the midclavicular line. Palpate for the kidneys, spleen, and other organs. Use percussion and auscultation for bowel sounds, bruits, and shifting dullness.

Genitalia

Men: inspect the penis, and palpate the testes. If the scrotum is enlarged, transilluminate. Examine the urethral orifice and epididymides; check for hernia.

Women: perform a pelvic examination, checking the perineum, vulva, vagina, cervix and fundus, and adnexa. Note any discharge and tenderness.

Rectum

Check the rectum for sphincter tone, hemorrhoids, and masses. In men, describe the size and consistency of the prostate and any nodules present. In women, a rectal examination is done at the time of the pelvic examination.

Limbs and Musculoskeletal Examination

Check for clubbing, cyanosis, edema, the character and volume of all peripheral pulses, and calf tenderness. Record any trophic changes or ulcerations. Examine the joints for swelling, tenderness, redness, temperature, deformity, and range of motion. Note any limitation of motion of joints.

Neurologic Examination

Check cranial nerve function, muscular bulk, strength, and tone. Check reflexes and sensory function. Proceed to a more detailed neurologic examination if indicated.

LABORATORY DIAGNOSIS

Laboratory tests cannot be substituted for a careful history and physical examination, but tests do provide diagnostic information not obtainable by other means. Skills in making effective use of the laboratory are developed through training and experience. Physicians must acquire the ability to integrate laboratory data with other clinical information.

Uses of Laboratory Tests

Laboratory data can be useful for a number of purposes.

Screening

The usefulness of the laboratory tests in screening is limited; tests usually include urinalysis, complete blood count, and multiphasic screening.

Diagnosis

The most common and important use of laboratory tests is diagnostic. Physicians use them as aids in selecting the most likely diagnosis from a list of several possibilities that may have been suggested by the history and physical examination, that is, in making the differential diagnosis. Further laboratory testing can help the physician to reach a precise diagnosis.

Selection of Therapy

Laboratory studies can be useful to the physician in selecting the appropriate mode of therapy. Antimicrobial susceptibility tests used in selecting the most effective antibiotic for bacterial infections are the prime example. Other examples are blood grouping and crossmatching before blood transfusion, and tissue typing before tissue transplantation.

Follow-up

Inasmuch as many laboratory tests are much more objective than the history and physical examination, and because they provide quantitative information, they have proved useful in following the course of a disease and determining the effectiveness of the therapy. One such test monitors serum complement to detect activity of systemic lupus erythematosus.

Prevention

Tests used in genetic counseling to detect carrier states are an excellent example of using the laboratory in the prevention of diseases.

Medicolegal Uses

Legal evidence is collected, for example, by examining fingerprints or dried blood on clothing, by examining body fluids of rape victims, and by performing autopsies. These are examples of the medicolegal uses of the laboratory.

Environmental Protection

Microbiologic and toxicologic surveillance is commonly used by environmental protection specialists.

Qualitative Versus Quantitative Testing

Qualitative data are descriptive and include information on the presence or absence of a partricular finding. For example, qualitative data include a statement on the presence or absence of sugar in the urine. Qualitative data are often expressed in semiquantitative terms. On the other hand, quantitative data are expressed in numbers, such as blood sugar levels and blood counts.

Sensitivity Versus Specificity

Sensitivity indicates that the result of the test is positive in the presence of disease, whereas specificity indicates that it is negative in healthy persons. An ideally sensitive test is one in which all patients with a disease show positive results. A highly sensitive test is used to exclude a diagnosis, whereas a specific test is used to confirm it. For example, in the diagnosis of tuberculosis, the tuberculin test is highly sensitive and the result is positive in almost all patients with tuberculosis. Although negative tuberculin test result excludes the diagnosis of tuberculosis, a positive test result does not prove the diagnosis of active tuberculosis; it only indicates exposure to tubercle bacilli. On the other hand, sputum examination for acid-fast bacilli is a highly specific test, and a positive result indicates active tuberculosis. In general, as the specificity of a test rises, the sensitivity diminishes, and as the sensitivity rises, the specificity diminishes.

Precision Versus Accuracy

A precise test is one that is highly reproducible, and an accurate test is one that gives a true measurement of the tested variable. A precise test need not be accurate. Accuracy in clinical laboratories is continually monitored by regional and national laboratory proficiency surveys.

Normal Ranges for Laboratory Values

Normal ranges for quantitative test results allow for both the biologic variability in the normal population and the analytic imprecision of the method. Imprecise methods produce wider normal ranges. Nearly all clinical laboratories have a list of normal values that are established by doing the tests on a large number of healthy persons.

Errors in Laboratory Testing

Errors can occur in clinical laboratories at any one or more of three steps: during the collection of specimens, during performance of the tests, and in the interpretation of the test results. The physician has to appreciate the inherent limitations of laboratory tests and must be aware that misleading or diagnostically useless information may be obtained if inappropriate tests are ordered. Incorrect handling of the specimen often leads to errors, an example being incorrect use of anticoagulants in tubes used for collecting blood. Improperly handled or inadequate specimens are not an uncommon problem. Technical and clerical errors in the laboratory are additional sources of errors. Although laboratory errors are common, one should not routinely attribute unanticipated results to laboratory error. The test in certain instances should be repeated and, if the results are the same as before, they should not be ignored. Medications can interfere with laboratory tests; however, this is not a common occurrence despite combination drug therapy.

The ultimate value of the laboratory test is dependent on the physician's appreciation of the limitations and capabilities of the clinical laboratory.

DIAGNOSTIC IMAGING

Imaging using x-rays, sound waves, and radioactive isotopes has an increasingly important role in diagnosis today.

Diagnostic Roentgenography

Diagnostic roentgenography supplements the physical examination. For example, whereas wheezing in an asthmatic and a murmur of a diseased heart valve can best be detected by physical examination, lung cancer in its early stages is best detected by a chest x-ray examination. Since prolonged or frequent exposure to x-rays can be a health hazard, only essential diagnostic radiographic examinations should be performed. X-ray examination of the chest is the commonest radiographic examination. Plain x-ray films (without the use of radiopaque contrast material) are also widely used in evaluating bones and detecting radiodensities in soft tissues.

Contrast radiography is used to delineate soft tissue organs, to study the function of certain organs, such as the kidneys, and to observe blood flow patterns using angiography. The most commonly employed contrast agents are compounds of iodine and barium, which absorb more x-rays than do soft tissues. Iodine-containing contrast materials are usually injected intravenously; when ingested orally, they are absorbed into the blood stream through the gastrointestinal tract. Barium, on the other hand, is used only for gastrointestinal examinations and is not absorbed through the gastrointestinal tract. Contrast materials can be used to study almost all the organ systems of the body.

The request for a radiographic study should always be accompanied by a brief clinical summary and the reason for requesting the procedure. The radiologist uses this information to determine the best procedure to provide the required information and also takes it into account in interpreting the x-ray films. In many instances, direct communication between the clinician and the radiologist before the x-ray study is done not only helps the radiologist to provide the maximumal information but also can minimize the radiation exposure of the patient since the radiologist then performs only necessary procedures. The clinician must make it a practice to review the radiographs also, and not be satisfied simply by reading the radiologist's report. Consultation with a radiologist in interpreting the films is often beneficial in patient care, and also the exchange of information is educational for both the clinician and the radiologist.

Computed axial tomography (CAT scanning) has added a new dimension to radiographic diagnosis. Organs that could not previously be visualized on x-ray examination can now be studied using this technique. CAT scanning with or without contrast enhancement can help in making an early diagnosis with the least amount of discomfort and risk to the patient. Because of the cost and the radiation exposure, this technique should be reserved for conditions in which plain x-ray films and routine contrast studies do not reveal sufficient information for a diagnosis. The advent of CAT scanning has greatly reduced the need for angiographic examinations and exploratory surgery.

Diagnostic Ultrasound

Ultrasonography is a noninvasive technique that has no known harmful effects, and the examination is painless. A pulse of high-frequency sound waves (1 to 20 million hertz, which is well above 20,000 hertz, the upper limit of human hearing) is emitted from a transducer placed on the body surface over the organs that are to be studied. The sound waves are reflected in the form of echoes that are converted electronically into a display on a cathode ray oscilloscope. Acoustic interfaces occur whenever a substance changes in acoustic density. Larger reflections occur when the acoustic density difference is greater. Because the sound is well transmitted through fluid, a large reflection occurs when sound passes from fluid to soft tissues.

The greatest usefulness of ultrasound examination lies in the detection of fluid as it occurs in pseudopancreatic cysts, renal cysts, and pericardial effusions. Echocardiography has proven to be a useful test in the diagnosis of heart disease; it is described in greater detail in the chapter on cardiology.

Nuclear Imaging

With the widespread use of sonography and the availability of CAT scanning, nuclear scans are now performed less frequently. However, lung, liver, spleen, and bone scans are still performed quite often. Cardiac imaging with radioisotopes is being increasingly used to detect myocardial ischemia and infarction.

OTHER DIAGNOSTIC MODALITIES

In the last two decades, numerous other diagnostic modalities have emerged. Fiberoptic endoscopy, for example, permits visualization of areas of the gastrointestinal tract and bronchi that were previously inaccessible for inspection. Through endoscopes it is now possible to take biopsy specimens for histopathologic evaluation.

Electrocardiography and electroencephalography are examples of diagnostic electrophysiologic procedures that have been used for decades.

Radioimmunoassay techniques now permit measurement of hormone levels in picogram quantities. They have proved immensely helpful in understanding the physiology of various organs, and they allow a precise diagnosis to be made.

BIBLIOGRAPHY

Bates B: *A Guide to Physical Examination*, ed 2. Philadelphia, JB Lippincott, 1979.

DeGowin EL, DeGowin RL: *Bedside Diagnostic Examination*, ed 3. New York, Macmillan, 1976.

Freitag JJ, Miller LW (eds): *Manual of Medical Therapeutics*, ed 23. Boston, Little, Brown, 1980.

Halpern SL (ed): *Clinical Nutrition*. Philadelphia, JB Lippincott, 1979.

Harvey AM, Johns RJ, Owens AH, et al (eds): *The Principles and Practice of Medicine*, ed 20. New York, Appleton-Century-Crofts, 1976.

Hunter D, Bomford RR, Pennington DG: *Hutchinson's Clinical Methods*, ed 16. Philadelphia, JB Lippincott, 1975.

Isselbacher KJ, Adams RD, Braunwald E, et al (eds): *Harrison's Principles of Internal Medicine*, ed 9. New York, McGraw-Hill, 1980.

Wyngaarden JB, Smith LH (eds): *Cecil Textbook of Medicine*, ed 16. Philadelphia, WB Saunders, 1982.

CHAPTER 2
ALLERGY AND CLINICAL IMMUNOLOGY

John A. Arkins

Allergic disease accounts for approximately 9 percent of patients seeking medical care. Childhood asthma is the most frequent cause of school absenteeism for chronic illnesses. It has been estimated that 35 million people in the United States, or about 17 percent of the population, have allergic disease. Of these people, 8.9 million (4 percent) have asthma, and 14.7 million (7 percent) have hay fever alone. Another 11.8 million have eczema, urticaria, food, drug, or insect sting allergy; this comprises another 6 percent of the population.

BASIC MECHANISMS

ANTIGENS

For the most part, the antigens that cause clinical allergic responses are naturally occurring, are usually macromolecules with a molecular weight equal to or greater than 5,000, and are proteins. Exposure to these antigens can occur by various routes. These routes may include inhalation, injection, dermal contacts, or ingestion.

ANTIBODY RESPONSE

Classically, there are two distinct routes for antibody response. One involves the development of a humoral antibody, which is called the B cell (bursal system), and the other is the cellular antibody, or T cell (thymus system). Both of these cell types are lymphocytes. They do not operate completely independently in that the T-cell system has a regulatory function over the B-cell system. The B cells produce immunoglobulins whose characteristics are represented in Table 1. It can be seen from this table that the concentrations of the immunoglobulins vary from 12 mg/ml of IgG to 0.001 mg/ml of IgE. The T cells act as helper cells to aid antibody function, are cytotoxic, produce soluble mediators (lymphokines), and are immunoregulatory (suppressor cells).

OTHER INVOLVED SYSTEMS

The complement system is a group of plasma proteins that act sequentially to mediate inflammatory effects. The actions of these proteins include chemotaxis, cell lysis, and cell-to-cell interactions. Complement has an important role in the defense mechanisms of the body and is also a useful indicator in determining the activity of various immune complex diseases in

Table 1. Structural and Biologic Features of Human Immunoglobulins

Class	Constituent Chains	Weight (× 10^3) Whole Molecule	Heavy Chain	Combining Sites/ Molecule	Concentration in Serum (mg/ml)	Complement Fixation: Classical	Complement Fixation: Alternative	Sensitizing Activity	Half-life in Serum (days)	Synthetic Rate (mg/kg/day)
IgG[a]	$\kappa_2\gamma_2$ or $\lambda_2\gamma_2$	150	52-54	2	12.1	+[b]	+	–	23[c]	33
IgM	$(\kappa_2\mu_2)_5$ J or $(\lambda_2\mu_2)_5$J	900	65-70	10	0.93	+	–	–	5.1	6.7
IgA[a]	$\kappa_2\alpha_2\lambda_2\alpha_2$ (S,J)	160[d]	57	2.4[d]	2.6	–	+	–	5.8	24
IgD	$\kappa_2\delta_2,\lambda_2\delta_2$	175	60-65	2	0.02	–	–	–	2.8	0.4
IgE	$\kappa_2\epsilon_2,\lambda_2\epsilon_2$	190	71-73	2	0.001	–	+	+	2.3	0.02

[a]IgG has four subclasses and IgA has two subclasses: IgG-1 50%, IgG-2 24%, IgG-3 8% in Caucasians.

[b]IgG-4 lacks the activity.

[c]IgG-3 has a half-life of 6.6-7.7 days.

[d]Dimers of IgA in serum and in secretions have molecular weights of 318 and 370, respectively. Dimers contain J. chain. Secretory IgA contains secretory piece.

which complement is being actively utilized. This is reflected by a reduced complement level in the serum.

The mediators of immediate hypersensitivity are listed in Table 2 with their effects. The major mediators that play a role in human allergic disease are histamine, eosinophilic chemotactic factor A, or ECF-A, and slow-reacting substance of anaphylaxis (SRS-A). Histamine is responsible for the immediate effects, namely, smooth muscle contraction, capillary dilatation, and edema, whereas SRS-A has a delayed effect with a more prolonged action on smooth muscle. The most common roles of the mediators are in the IgE-mediated diseases. In these conditions, histamine is released from the granules of basophils and mast cells after the interaction of antibody and IgE on their surface. The other group of mediators that are related to T-cell function consists of an extensive array of factors and their actions. They have been classified as migration inhibitory factors (MIF), factors stimulating macrophage function, chemotactic factor, mitogenic factor, cytotoxic factor, and factors stimulating B-lymphocyte maturation and antibody production.

RESPIRATORY ALLERGIES

Most of the respiratory allergies discussed in this section are IgE mediated, and are often called atopic diseases. These

Table 2. Primary Mediators of Immediate Hypersensitivity

Mediator	Physiocochemical Characteristics	Effects
Histamine	β- imidazol ethylamine MW = 111	Via H_1 receptor: Bronchoconstriction; increase of vascular permeability. Via H_2 receptor: Gastric acid secretion; modulation of granulocyte chemotaxis, lymphocyte functions, and mast cell reactivity.
ECF-A	Low mol wt peptides MW = 360-390	Chemotactic attraction of eosinophils and neutrophils; eosinophil and neutrophil deactivation.
NCF-A	Protein MW > 750,000	Chemotactic attraction of neutrophils and eosinophils; neutrophil and eosinophil deactivation.
SRS-A	Leukotrienes	Bronchoconstriction; increase of vascular permeability.
PAF	? mixture of phospholipids and free fatty acids	Platelet aggregation; platelet degranulation.

diseases are a form of the anaphylactic diseases that are genetically transmitted.

HISTORY

The single most important step in making an accurate diagnosis is a careful history. Questions asked are not the usual type of inquiries the physician seeks in a standard history. The patient should describe the symptoms; descriptions like hay fever and asthma are not sufficient and may be misleading lay diagnoses. In terms of specific symptoms relating to nasal allergy, the patient must be asked whether there are bouts of sneezing, nasal itching associated with itching of the soft palate, conjunctiva, and occasionally of the ears, profuse clear, watery nasal discharge, and nasal stuffiness. In terms of respiratory symptoms simulating asthma, questions concerning dyspnea, cough (productive or nonproductive), type of sputum, wheezing, and a sensation of tightness of the chest are important. In addition to these specific symptoms, specific information should be obtained about following:

- *Seasonal variation:* It is often difficult for a patient to recall specific days or even weeks that symptoms occur. It is not advisable to accept such terms as spring or fall, as this will vary not only in the individual's mind but actually in various areas of the country. It is important to obtain the specific months, weeks, or even days involved. Often it is necessary to correlate symptoms with specific events such as vacation, school recess in June, Fourth of July, Labor Day, start of school, and Thanksgiving. In the case of children, often a birthday party or family event can be clearly identified by date, leading to recall of specific symptoms during that period.
- *Other time relationships:* Do symptoms occur primarily in the morning upon arising, do they occur at night, waking the patient from sleep, or do they occur over the entire 24 hour day? This may also give a clue as to the type of exposure the patient is having. Are the symptoms worse while the patient is at work or at home? Are they relieved while the patient is on vacation or away from home? Are they worse when the patient is visiting someone who may have a pet?
- *Progression:* It is also important to note whether the symptoms are progressive in nature since this will influence therapy. Is this year worse than last year? Are symptoms stable over the last few years? In terms of progression, it would be worthwhile to know what medications controlled symptoms in the past. Do these same medications control symptoms now or does the patient need stronger medications to get the same degree of relief?
- *Other precipitating variables:* In addition to seasonal variations, do other variables such as smoke, odors, respiratory infections, anxiety, and humidity affect the symptoms?

Such diseases as cardiovascular disease, peptic ulcer disease, and hypertension have important implications in drug therapy for asthma. A positive family history adds additional evidence in favor of atopic disease.

PHYSICAL EXAMINATION

Although less important than the history, the physical examination is a necessary portion of the work-up. Examination of the eyes may reveal lacrimation and edema of the conjunctiva. It is important to examine the nasal mucosa to determine if there are classic findings of allergic rhinitis. These findings consist of a boggy, pale, and edematous mucous membrane with a clear, watery discharge. The degree of obstruction and the presence of polyps should also be noted. Examination of the oropharynx is usually not very revealing; however, there may be a similar appearance of the mucosa and evidence of some postnasal drainage. The sinuses should be palpated to determine if there is any tenderness. Examination of the ears, although usually normal, may reveal evidence of serous otitis that may accompany severe allergic rhinitis. Evidence of dyspnea associated with the use of accessory muscles of respiration and cyanosis may be present. Examination of the chest generally reveals the classic wheezing, which should be diffuse and both inspiratory and expiratory in nature with a prolonged expiratory phase. The absence of wheezing does not rule out asthma but may reveal only a quiescent episode. In a patient with asthma, wheezing may often be elicited by having the patient forcefully exhale several times.

LABORATORY

The following findings are useful in the work-up and support an allergic disorder as the cause of the patient's complaints:

- An elevated eosinophil count. Total white blood cell (WBC) count may or may not be elevated.
- Eosinophils in nasal secretions, demonstrated by Wright's or Hansel's stain.
- A chest radiograph, which may help rule out other causes for the respiratory symptoms.
- Positive skin tests manifested by immediate wheal and flare reactions occurring within 10 to 15 minutes after application of the antigen.

It is important to remember that skin tests do not establish a diagnosis, but must be correlated with the history. The skin tests are therefore confirmatory; patients should not be specifically treated merely on the basis of positive skin tests. This applies both to inhalants and foods. Asthma may also be nonatopic, in which skin tests are negative and IgE levels are normal. These patients are frequently less than 2 or more than 40 years of age. This type of asthma is frequently perennial and often precipitated by upper respiratory infections.

Other tests that may be performed on certain individuals include sinus x-rays, IgE levels, and pulmonary function tests. Pulmonary function tests are useful in assessing the degree of reversibility of the bronchospasm. Diagnosis of airway obstruction by spirometry needs to be collaborated with other clinical features in arriving at a diagnosis of asthma. If spirometry is normal, it may be useful to challenge the patient with beta methacholine (Mecholyl) inhalation. This cholinergic stimulation will result in a greater than 20 percent drop in 1.0-second forced expiratory volume ($FEV_{1.0}$) in patients with asthma. A positive Mecholyl test does not in itself indicate atopic asthma. Positive responses may be seen with all bronchospastic diseases, as well as after viral respiratory infections (up to 8-12 weeks after an episode), indicating hyperreactive airways.

ALLERGIC RHINITIS

Allergic rhinitis is a disease manifested by intermittent, reversible edema of the nasal mucosa associated with sneezing, itching, and obstruction on an allergic basis. The pathophysiology of this disease is characteristic of the classic IgE-mediated reaction. Prior sensitization to antigen leads to production of specific IgE, which attaches to the mast cells and basophils. Upon reexposure to the antigen, there is union of the antigen with IgE on the cell surface resulting in the release of mediators. In allergic rhinitis, there is vasodilatation and edema involving the nasal mucosa. This gives rise to the classic symptoms. The diagnosis is usually easy, but occasionally must be differentiated from several other diseases.

One of the common diseases that an allergist sees is *vasomotor rhinitis*. This disease has a similar appearance to allergic rhinitis and its exact etiology is unknown. Eosinophils are not often present in the nasal mucosa, the patients do not have a typical seasonal story, and there is no family history of allergic disease. These patients' response to antihistamines and decongestants are frequently not as dramatic as in those with allergic rhinitis.

Another common disorder is *rhinitis medicamentosa*. This disease is due to the constant application of vasoconstrictor nose drops or spray over a long period. This results in a high degree of nasal obstruction associated with rhinorrhea. These patients may or may not also have underlying allergic disease. Sinusitis may be associated with a nasal obstruction, and may or may not be on an allergic basis. An injected mucosa is seen, and often there may be a purulent discharge. In addition, the patient has facial pain and tenderness over the involved sinuses and has a positive x-ray study demonstrating sinusitis. Complications associated with allergic rhinitis, in addition to the degree of irritation and discomfort that interferes with normal functions, include recurrent respiratory tract infections, often viral in nature, and nasal polyps.

THERAPY

The therapy for allergic rhinitis falls under two categories: specific and symptomatic therapy.

Specific therapy includes:

1. Avoidance: Obviously, if the patient is allergic to certain danders, foods, or other substances that can be avoided in the environment, this should be attempted. Maintenance of a dust- and allergen-free environment is important and may be achieved by use of air-filtration devices, although no guarantee can be given regarding relief of symptoms by this method. In addition, if the patient is sensitive to pollens or molds, he should stay away from areas where pollen and mold counts are high. Examples of this are driving through the country with the windows open, playing golf, picnicking, and so on. In the case of mold sensitivity, spending time on farms and in barns should be avioided. Last but not least, change of occupation may be needed if exposure to inhaled allergens at work is responsible for the symptoms.
2. Hyposensitization: This is a time-honored procedure that has proved efficacious if done properly and includes repeated injections in increasing doses of antigen over several years. The basic principle is the production of a blocking antibody that inhibits union of IgE with the allergen, resulting in a reduction of mediator release and therefore a reduction in symptoms. The tolerance of the individual is also raised so that it takes more exposure to considerably higher concentrations of antigens to produce symptoms. This form of therapy of allergic rhinitis should be reserved for individuals in whom rhinitis is poorly responsive to symptomatic therapy or in whom the rhinitis is associated with bronchial asthma.
3. Symptomatic Therapy: It consists of medications that only relieve the symptoms. The mainstay of this therapy is the anti-histamines. There are a large group of antihstamines on the market; the patient may have to try several different forms to accomplish symptomatic relief. Side reactions, mainly drowsiness, may preclude its use in certain patients. In general, the antihistamines come in short-acting and long-acting forms. In the more complicated cases it may be advisable to give the patient a long-acting antihistamine combined with a decongestant such as pseudoephedrine on an 8- to 12-hour basis, and supplement this with a short-acting antihistamine plus decongestant. Pediatric preparations are also available. Because the effects of antihistamines are not known during the first trimester of pregnancy, there is some reluctance on the part of physicians to administer them during this time. In addition, drowsiness may interfere with certain functions: the patient should be warned about this. In addition to the antihistamines and decongestants, topical corticosteroids are also occasionally used. The newer topical steroids, such as beclomethasone, have minimal systemic absorption, and are proving useful for nasal application in addition to their use in asthma. Other drugs will be available for intranasal application in the future; one of these is cromolyn sodium. This drug is available for asthma, and is used in other countries as a topical drug on the nasal and conjunctival mucosa. Topical decongestants in the nose should be avoided or used for very short courses since patients tend to become

chronic users of these preparations and may subsequently develop rhinitis medicamentosa.

BRONCHIAL ASTHMA

This is defined as an extraordinary sensitivity of the airways to a variety of stimuli manifested by reversible airway obstruction. The obstruction may be chronic or intermittent, manifested by wheezing, cough, and dyspnea; reversibility may be spontaneous or in response to drug therapy.

PATHOPHYSIOLOGIC FEATURES

The alterations found in bronchial asthma are as follows:

1. All asthmatics, whether symptomatic or not, show evidence of increased airway resistance. When patients are totally free of symptoms, expiratory flow rates may be normal but they are generally decreased. These manifestations represent the effects of increased bronchial smooth muscle tone, mucosal edema, and the tenacious intrabronchial mucus.
2. Generally the forced vital capacity (FVC) is normal, but may be decreased. The $FEV_{1.0}$ is generally reduced, with a subnormal $FEV_{1.0}$/FVC ratio. Asthmatics are generally symptom free when the $FEV_{1.0}$ exceeds 60 percent predicted.
3. There may be elevations of functional residual capacity and residual volume, particularly during acute episodes. The total lung capacity increases during an acute episode but is generally normal during quiscent periods.
4. In a severe asthmatic attack, increase in pulmonary artery pressures relative to pleural pressures may be encountered, manifested by electrocardiographic evidence of right ventricular strain or P pulmonale. Similarly, increased negative pleural pressure resulting in marked respiratory variations in arterial pressure, or pulsus paradoxus, may also be seen in a severe attack when $FEV_{1.0}$ is less than 1.25 L.
5. Arterial oxygenation may be subnormal, reflecting ventilation-perfusion (V/Q) mismatch. Pa_{CO_2} is normal, generally below 37 mm Hg. In the initial phase of an acute attack Pa_{CO_2} is reduced but with worsening obstruction may gradually increase. In general, such increases are not seen as long as the $FEV_{1.0}$ is greater than 35 percent predicted.

DIFFERENTIAL DIAGNOSIS

The conditions considered in the differential diagnosis are as follows:

1. Conditions with acute onset, short duration, and severe dypsnea
   (a) Acute respiratory infections
   (b) Acute caridac failure
   (c) Aspiration
   (d) Foreign body in the bronchi
   (e) Hyperventilation
   (f) Metabolic disorders (e.g., acute salicylism, acidosis)
   (g) Obstruction of the larynx, trachea, or major bronchi (by internal or external pressure)
   (h) Pneumothorax
   (i) Pulmonary embolism
   (j) Toxic inhalation (e.g., smoke, nitrous oxide)
2. Chronic and/or recurrent conditions with moderate dyspnea
   (a) Aspiration
   (b) Carcinoid syndrome
   (c) Chronic obstructive pulmonary diseases (e.g., bronchitis, bronchiectasis, bronchostenosis, emphysema)
   (d) Foreign body
   (e) Inherited metabolic disorders with pulmonary manifestations (e.g., α_1-antitrypsin deficiency, cystic fibrosis) fibrosis)
   (f) Obstruction of the larynx, trachea, or major bronchi (by internal or external pressure)

COMPLICATIONS

The following list are conditions that may occur as complications of asthma.

1. Infection
   (a) Bronchitis
   (b) Pneumonia
2. Atelectasis
3. Allergic bronchopulmonary aspergillosis
4. Mucoid impaction
5. Bronchiectasis
6. Pneumothorax
7. Pneumomediastinum
8. Rib fracture
9. Status asthmaticus
10. Death

THERAPY

The specific treatment of asthma is identical to that of allergic rhinitis. This includes avoidance, partial avoidance, and hyposensitization.

Avoidance includes not only specific antigens but a variety of substances that increase irritability of the airway. These include smoke (particularly cigarette smoke), fumes, strong odors, pollution, and sudden changes in humidity and temperature.

Symptomatic Therapy

- *Environmental control:* Patients should not only avoid smoking, but should also avoid a smoky or dusty environment.
- *Management of infections:* Most infectious episodes that precipitate asthma are viral and antibiotics therefore are not indicated. When bacterial infections are present and characterized by pulmonary infiltrations, purulent sputum, or purulent sinusitis, an appropriate antibiotic should be used.
- *Physical activity:* Asthmatics should maintain physical fitness. Children should not be restircted in their activities unless it precipitates disabling asthma. Prophylactic bronchodilators may be helpful when asthmatic symptoms are induced by exercise. Swimming is the least asthmogenic exercise.
- *Psychologic management:* Anxiety and other forms of emotional stress can precipitate asthma, and in some cases may be the major precipitating factor. Appropriate counseling is indicated in severe cases. This is also true for parents of asthmatic children who may react adversely to acute attacks.

Drug Therapy

This is directed at relieving bronchial smooth muscle contraction, relieving edema of the mucosa, and reducing the production of mucoid sputum. Other factors such as hypoxia, dyspnea, anxiety, and hyperventilation will respond when the above measures are accomplished.

Specific therapy for asthma is based on severity: mild, moderate, or severe (status asthmaticus).

Mild asthma is usually seasonal, IgE mediated, and easily controlled with a minimum of medication on an intermittent basis. Specific therapy is important here and may result in complete relief of the disease. There may be important precipitating factors such as exercise, cold air, and anxiety. Specific therapy requires only a dose of oral sympathomimetic amines, such as ephedrine sulfate (25 mg), terbutaline (5 mg), or metaproterenol (20 mg). Combination drugs containing theophylline offer no advantage. Inhaled sympathomimetic amines are dramatic in their effect, but patients tend to overuse them; hence, they are generally not recommended on a continuous basis. Isoproterenol is a major offender in this regard. Sympathomimetic agents such as isoetharine (Bronkosol) or metaproterenol (Alupent, Metaprel) may be used, but on an infrequent basis. Refills of these agents must be regulated to ensure that the patient is not overusing them.

Moderate asthma is a more severe form of seasonal asthma, or may occur on a perennial basis. It may or may not be IgE mediated, and is often precipitated by upper respiratory tract infections. Specific therapy is also important to these patients; however, symptomatic therapy is of utmost importance. These patients are frequent visitors to the emergency room unless their asthma is controlled. An organized approach to these patients is as follows:

Theophylline Preparations

Numerous preparations are on the market. The active ingredient is anhydrous theophylline. A starting dose of 3 mg/kg (usually 200 mg in the average adult) orally every 6 hours is used. Because of marked individual variation in metabolism of this drug, each patient will require different doses, ranging from 800-1600 mg daily. Theophylline blood level measurements are available at many institutions. A level of between 10-20 μg/ml is ideal. Toxic reactions occur in most patients at levels above 20 μg/ml. Blood should be drawn 4-6 hours after the last dose. Sustained-release preparations are also available.

Sympathomimetic Amines

Oral drugs in this category are almost the same as theophylline. These drugs, ephedrine (25 mg), terbutaline (5 mg), metaproterenol, (20 mg) or albuterol (2 mg), must be taken on a regular basis around the clock at 4- to 6-hour intervals. Many combination drugs containing theophylline are available but offer no advantage over the single drug. The aerosol drugs also fall in this category· the warning regarding their use in mild asthma applies here also.

Mediator Inhibitors

The only available drug in this category is cromolyn sodium (Aarane, Intal). Cromolyn is not a bronchodilator but does inhibit mediator release from mast cells. It is useful in atopic (IgE mediated) and exercise-induced asthma. The drug is administered by inhalation from a Spinhaler in a dosage of 1 capsule (20 mg) four times daily. This drug may reduce the requirements for sympathomimetic amines and lessen the need for corticosteroids. Patients should be specifically instructed that this drug should not be used during an acute asthmatic attack.

Corticosteroids

If the aforementioned methods are unsuccessful in controlling asthma, corticosteroids are indicated. A starting dose of prednisone, 40-60 mg per day, is usually satisfactory. This dose is maintained until there is a definite clinical response, and then is tapered to the minimal tolerated daily dose or, better yet, alternate-day doses. Other forms of corticosteroids may be used; however, prednisone is effective in most patients. There is little advantage in administering parenteral corticosteroids or adrenocorticotropic hormone (ACTH). Pulmonary function studies may be useful in finding the optimal steroid dosage.

Expectorants

Fluids are probably the best expectorants; however, potassium iodide, 10 drops four times daily, and glyceryl guaiacolate, 200 mg four times daily, are used empirically by many physicians although there is no evidence that they are of any benefit. A good mucolytic agent is acetylcysteine (Mucomyst), but it should be given in a 10 percent solution with a bronchodilator. It may aggravate asthma if used in a higher concentration or if used alone.

Antibiotics

Because most respiratory infections are due to viruses, the indiscriminate use of antibiotics should be avoided. If the signs of bacterial infection are present—i.e., purulent sputum with many polymorphonuclear cells and bacteria, fever, chills, leukocytosis, and pulmonary infiltrates—antibiotics should be administered after cultures are taken. Even though purulent sputum is the hallmark of bacterial infection, sputum laden with eosinophils in an acute exacerbation of asthma may appear yellow on gross examination. If the patient is not allergic to penicillin, ampicillin, 1 g/day for 10 days, is used. Tetracycline, 1 g/day for 10 days, is a good alternative.

Toxicity

With the use of the above drugs the following toxic manifestations can occur:

Theophylline: gastrointestinal upset, arrhythmias, convulsions.

Sympathomimetic amines: cardiac stimulation, adrenergic stimulation, muscular tremor, and cramps.

Cromolyn: very few—local irritation, dermatitis, and, rarely, granuloma formation in the lung.

Corticosteroids: all the effects of hypercortisolism.

Beclomethasone: monilia overgrowth.

SEVERE ASTHMA (STATUS ASTHMATICUS)

This is the most severe form of asthma and is life threatening. The patient must be hospitalized. A team approach is advisable, including the primary care physician, allergist, pulmonary specialist, and anesthesiologist.

In the past, status asthmaticus was defined as an episode of asthma that fails to respond to epinephrine and/or aminophylline. This definition needs to be rewritten since arterial blood gas measurements have revolutionized the concept of this entity. Status asthmaticus, when manifest, generally represents an attack that has gone unabated for over 24 hours, manifested by extreme dyspnea and wheezing, retraction of the sternocleidomastoids, and pulsus paradoxus. Physiologically, the $FEV_{1.0}$ is less than 1.0 L, peak expiratory flow rates are less than 80 L/min and the Pa_{O_2} generally around 70. In the early phases, the Pa_{CO_2} is less than 35 (stage 3A); between 35 and 45 in moderately advanced cases (stage 3B) and exceeds 45 in extremely severe status (stage 3C). In the latter, there is invariably cyanosis, wheezing may not be heard since the patient moves very little air, and disturbed sensorium is usual. A paradoxic pulse of greater than 10 mm Hg always indicates an $FEV_{1.0}$ of less than 1.25 L and is useful in staging the severity of illness and response following therapy. Similarly, retraction of the sternocleidomastoids indicates an $FEV_{1.0}$ less than 1.0 L. Apart from arterial blood gas analysis and Gram's stains of sputum, the other useful bedside tests are spirometry, measurement of peak expiratory airflow, and a roentgenogram of the chest. It should be mentioned, however, that one should not await results of these tests in initiating therapy.

Therapy

1. Oxygen is administered first, in doses of 2-4 L/min.
2. Corticosteroids are given intravenously. Hydrocortisone hemisuccinate is given in a loading dose of 4 mg/kg followed by 0.5 mg/kg/h. Dexamethasone or methylprednisone may also be used in equivalent dose.
3. Intravenous administration of bronchodilator drugs should be started promptly. A careful history of any recent drug therapy is important. Epinephrine or terbutaline may be given subcutaneously if these have not been given recently. Intravenous aminophylline may also be started. For those who have not recieved theophylline-containing medications within the past 24-48 hours, a loading intravenous dose of 6 mg/kg is given in 30-40 minutes. In patients who have received theophylline recently the loading dose is omitted, and only maintenance doses are given. There is a wide range for the maintenance dose, varying between 0.2 and 0.6 mg/kg/h, the lower doses being applicable for patients with renal/hepatic/cardiac failure, and higher doses for smokers or those receiving phenobarbital. Serum theophylline levels are extremely useful in this setting in determining an efficacious dose.
4. Other ancillary measures include correction of severe acidosis if present (pH less than 7.2, but is seldom seen in nonacute respiratory acidosis), correction of dehydration, and initiation of antibiotic therapy if Gram's stain findings warrant this. Improvement in status from corticosteroid administration is rarely apparent before 6 hours have elapsed; hence, the role of bronchodilator medications cannot be overemphasized.

The patient shoud be managed in an intensive care unit and should be frequently reassessed clinically, probably every 4 hours or more frequently if needed, by arterial blood gas analysis. The Pa_{CO_2} is an ideal indicator of the adequacy of respiratory gas exchange and is one of the major factors in deciding in favor of mechanical ventilation, if this is needed. It should be stressed that a rising Pa_{CO_2} is the major determinant rather than any single isolated level of Pa_{CO_2}. An uncooperative patient, with a disordered sensorium, who develops fatigue and retention of carbon dioxide is a candidate for mechanical ventilation. Before instituting endotracheal intubation and ventilatory assistance, the physician should ensure that other less invasive alternatives have been tried.

In patients who show response, oral corticosteroids are substituted for intravenous agents, generally by the third day (prednisone, 60 mg/day) and tapered gradually. Similarly, oral bronchodilators are also introduced appropriately. The final regimen is a matter of trial and adjustment.

EXERCISE-INDUCED ASTHMA

Exercise intolerance occurs to a variable degree in all asthmatics, but the term exercise-induced asthma must be limited to episodes of bronchospasm precipitated only by exercise.

Several theories have been proposed to explain the tendency of these patients to develop wheezing during exercise. These include lactic acidosis, hyperpnea, hypocapnia, and exposure to cold air. Recent data suggest that abnormal heat exchange in the airways may be responsible for these episodes of bronchospasm. Normally, inhaled air is warmed to body temperature in the airways and humidified before it enters the alveoli. This process of vaporization of the inhaled air leads to cooling of the respiratory mucosa by the principle of latent heat of vaporization. During exhalation, part of this heat is returned to the mucosa, but this amount falls significantly in the presence of hyperventilation because of the rapidity of airflow. During the phase of hyperpnea that accompanies exercise, excessive cooling of the airways takes place that leads to episodes of bronchospasm. Such bronchoconstriction is preventable by pretreatment with cromolyn sodium.

FOOD ALLERGY

Food allergy is more common in children. Allergies to fish, shellfish, nuts, and cottonseed meal often persist into adult life. Conversely, egg, milk, grain, fruit, vegetable, beef, pork, and poultry sensitivities frequently disappear during adolescence. Skin testing with foods is not as reliable as with inhalants. There are false positives and false negatives. The only proven in vitro study is the radioallergosorbent test (RAST), a measurement of specific IgE by means of radioimmunoassay. Cytotoxic tests and sublingual challenges have not been scientifically proven. The treatment is avoidance of the offending foods. Food allergy has been suspect in many conditions, including behavior disorders and migraine, but these also have not been proven.

HYPERSENSITIVITY PNEUMONITIS

There are a group of allergic lung disorders known as hypersensitivity pneumonitides that result from sensitization and recurrent exposure to inhaled organic dusts. Hypersensitivity pneumonitis is a diffuse, predominantly mononuclear reaction of the lung parenchyma involving predominantly the terminal bronchioles and alveoli. This reaction may progress to granulomata that may in turn progress to fibrosis. There are a large group of dusts that cause this disease; they are listed in Table 3. It is interesting that the majority of these cases follow occupational exposure. There is increasing evidence to indicate that this conditions is a result of contamination in home heating and air-conditioning systems.

Table 3. Etiologic Agents of Hypersensitivity Pneumonitis

Disease	*Exposure*	*Specific Inhalant*
Farmer's lung	Moldy hay and other fodder	*Micropolyspora faeni* *Thermoactinomyces vulgaris*
Bagassosis	Moldy sugarcane	*Thermoactinomyces vulgaris*
Mushroom worker's disease	Mushroom compost	*Micropolyspora faeni* *Thermoactinomyces vulgaris*
Humidifier lung	Contaminated System	*Thermophilic actinomycetes* Other?
Air conditioner lung	Contaminated System	*Thermophilic actinomycetes* Other?
Malt worker's disease	Moldy malt	*Aspergillus clavatus* *Aspergillus fumigatus*
Sauna taker's disease	Contaminated applicance	*Pullularia*
Bird fancier's disease	Pigeon, budgerigar, parrot, hen, turkey droppings	Avian serum proteins
Maple bark stripper's disease	Moldy maple logs	*Cryptostroma corticale*
Sequoiosis	Moldy redwood sawdust	*Graphium* *Aureobasidium pullulans*
Wood pulp worker's disease	Moldy logs	*Alternaria*
Pituitary snuff taker's disease	Desiccated pituitary	Bovine and porcine proteins
Suberosis	Moldy cork dust	*Penicillium frequetans*
Cheesewasher's disease	Cheese mold	*Penicillium caseii*
Wheat weevil disease	Wheat flour	*Sitophilis granarius*
Furrier's lung	Hair dust	Animal proteins?
Coffee worker's lung	Coffee dust	?
New Guinea lung	Thatched roof dust	?

ETIOLOGY

The organic dusts responsible for this disease are derived from fungal, bacterial, or serum protein sources. The particles are usually less than 5 μm in diameter; because of the large surface area of the lungs, a large quantity of antigenic material can be deposited in the airways and alveoli. The disease is divided into three forms.

The acute form is characterized by chills, fever, cough, dyspnea, and malaise occurring 4-10 hours after exposure. Wheezing is notably absent in this form. There is a correlation between severity of the episode and magnitude of the antigenic challenge. Usually the episode ceases within 24 hours. The pulmonary function changes that occur are predominantly restrictive, with a fall in forced vital capacity and the $FEV_{1.0}$ with little change in flow. There is also a decrease in the static compliance. There is nonuniform ventilation giving rise to a disturbance in ventilation-perfusion relationships. Furthermore, hypoxemia and a fall in the diffusing capacity also occur. In atopic individuals, an acute asthmatic attack may occur initially that subsides with or without treatment; however, 4-10 hours later the typical reaction of hypersensitivity pneumonitis occurs.

The subacute form is a more insidious form of the disease that resembles progressive chronic bronchitis with a productive cough, dyspnea, fatigue, and weight loss. In this situation, both restrictive and obstructive defects may occur; hypoxemia also occurs that becomes markedly aggravated by exercise.

In the chronic form disabling respiratory symptoms with irreversible changes may occur after prolonged exposure. Pulmonary fibrosis develops along with progressive restrictive disease, diffusion defect, hypoxemia, and decreased lung compliance.

Both the acute and subacute forms respond to long-term avoidance and the administration of corticosteroids. However, the chronic form may progress in spite of these treatments.

DIAGNOSIS

A careful environmental history is tantamount to making a diagnosis. It is not uncommon for these patients to remain undiagnosed for many months and treated as though they had viral or bacterial infections. The laboratory is of considerable use: during the acute febrile episodes, there is frequently an elevation of the white blood cell count to a level of 15,000-25,000/cu mm. There is often an elevation of gamma globulins and the rheumatoid factor may be present. X-ray of the chest reveals a diffuse interstitial micronodular infiltration that occasionally may become confluent and present as a patchy infiltrate; the x-ray may also be normal during these episodes. Pulmonary function tests may show decreased lung volumes along with a decreased diffusing capacity without airway obstruction. Blood gases show a fall in PO_2 either with slight respiratory alkalosis or normal pH.

Immunologic Tests

Skin tests with various organic dusts are not widely available. If skin tests are performed, there may be a dual-phase positive skin test consisting of an immediate wheal and flare followed in 3-8 hours by development of induration. The most useful test is the precipitin test that is performed in agar gel. Although a positive test may not necessarily indicate clinical sensitivity, there is a high degree of correlation in patients with the disease and positive precipitin tests.

Occasionally, a lung biopsy is necessary to establish the diagnosis of hypersensitivity pneumonitis. The characteristic histology will differentiate this disorder from other interstitial lung diseases. In special centers, diagnostic challenges are performed by aerosolizing the antigen under controlled conditions. Within 4 to 6 hours the patient develops fever, rales, and a drop in diffusing capacity.

One type of hypersensitivity pneumonitis that should receive special attention is allergic bronchopulmonary aspergillosis. This is a hypersensitivity reaction to the fungus *Aspergillus fumigatus*, but other aspergilli may also be responsible. The disease is commonly seen in patients who have severe allergic asthma and is manifested by recurring pulmonary infiltrations, mucoid impaction, eosinophilia, elevated IgE levels, and central saccular bronchiectasis. This disease, although historically considered unusual in the United States, is recognized with increasing frequency; there are now several hundred cases reported in the literature, and it is felt that there may be approximately 10,000 cases of hypersensitivity pneumonitis in the United States. Since this disease progresses to fibrosis and bronchiectasis, it is important to make the diagnosis and treat it early. The following outline should be an approach to the diagnosis of this disease:

Suspect the diagnosis: In patients with asthma and pulmonary infiltrates with eosinophilia (particularly if infiltrates are in the upper lobes or hilar areas).

Confirm the diagnosis by

1. Positive immediate and late skin test reactions with intradermal aspergillus antigen
2. Positive aspergillus precipitins
3. Elevated serum IgE level
4. Positive *A fumigatus* sputum cultures,

or with bronchograms or tomograms demonstrating proximal saccular bronchiectasis.

Pitfalls

1. Sputum cultures are not always reliable
2. Sufficient doses and duration of corticosteroid therapy may suppress laboratory abnormalities and the late skin test reaction, and
3. Aspergillus antigen may produce false-negative skin or precipitins results.

The therapy is oral corticosteroids in sufficient doses to suppress the asthma. A dose of 15-20 mg every other day is usually effective. A variety of other drugs have been used including amphotericin B and cromolyn sodium as well as aerosolized steroids; however, these have not proved to be beneficial.

ANAPHYLAXIS

Anaphylaxis is an immune response due to an agent to which the person has been previously sensitized. This results in a generalized reaction affecting the respiratory tract, skin, cardiovascular system, and gastrointestinal tract. Symptoms include generalized erythema followed by urticaria, severe progressive respiratory distress resulting from bronchospasm or angioedema of the larynx, gastrointestinal symptoms of vomiting, abdominal cramps, diarrhea, and vascular collapse. The reaction has a rapid onset and may be fatal within a short period. A reaction indistinguishable from anaphylaxis may occur, in which no immune mechanism can be determined.

A variety of substances including drugs, pollens, foreign sera, and foods may be responsible for this reaction. Most reactions in man are mediated by IgE. The mediators that cause the symptoms are histamine, slow-reacting substance of anaphylaxis (SRS-A), and eosinophil chemotactic factor of anaphylaxis (ECF-A). Platelet activating factor (PAF), and prostaglandins may also be involved. The anaphylactoid reactions that are not immunologically mediated are precipitated by such substances as iodinated radiographic contrast media and aspirin. The mechanism for these reactions is not clear; however, complement seems to be involved.

The diagnosis of anaphylaxis is not difficult; however, the specific etiology can on occasion be elusive. Obviously, in a patient who is penicillin sensitive and has just recieved an injection of penicillin, the diagnosis is obvious. The same is true of a patient who was just stung by an insect. On the other hand, if the reaction occurred after the ingestion of food or if the patient has taken a variety of medications, the diagnosis may not be apparent. In the case of foods and penicillin, skin testing will be helpful. However, it should be pointed out that skin testing must not be performed for 1-2 weeks after anaphylaxis since the entire amount of IgE may have been bound during the reaction, and a false negative skin test might result. Skin testing should be done carefully, starting with a scratch or prick test, since the test itself may precipitate a reaction in a very sensitive individual. A reaction may also occur following immunotherapy for atopic disease if there has been administration of too large a dose of antigen or an inadvertent intravenous injection. The treatment of anaphylaxis is outlined in Table 4.

If laryngeal edema is present, the treatment outlined in Table 5 should be followed.

After the patient responds successfully to treatment, it is imperative that the patient be instructed to avoid the offending substances. It would be wise to have the patient wear a tag (Medic Alert) indicating the allergies. In addition, if there is danger of exposure to similar substances in the future such as stinging insects, the patient should carry an emergency kit containing a syringe with epinephrine and be taught how to administer it.

Table 4 Treatment of Anaphylaxis[a]

1. When applicable, place tourniquet near site of injection or sting to obstruct venous return or stop the administration of the causative agent. Remove tourniquet temporarily every 10 to 15 minutes.
2. Place patient in recumbent position and elevate lower extremeties.
3. Administer aqueous epinephrine 1:1,000, 0.3-0.5 cc subcutaneously or intramuscularly (or if necessary 0.1 cc in 10 cc saline solution given intravenously over several minutes) and repeat as necessary.
4. Inject aqueous epinephrine 1:1,000, 0.1-0.3 cc at the site of the injection.
5. Establish and maintain airway, first with oral airway. If necessary, use endotracheal tube.
6. Give oxygen as needed.
7. Monitor vital signs frequently.
8. If patient is not responding, give diphenhydramine hydrochloride (Benadryl), 60-80 mg intravenously over 3 minutes (maximum, 5 mg per kg in 24 hours).
9. If blood pressure cannot be obtained, give normal saline intravenously and maintain blood pressure with levarternol bitartrate (Levophed), 1 or 2 ampules (8-16 mg) in 500 cc 5 percent glucose in water, or metaraminol bitartrate (Aramine), 100-200 mg in 500 cc 5 percent glucose in water. Titrate to blood pressure.
10. In severe asthma without shock give aminophylline, 500 mg intravenously over 10-20 minutes.
11. While corticosteroids will not be helpful for acute anaphylaxis, they may prevent protracted anaphylaxis.

[a]Adjust drug dosages to weight in children.

Table 5. Treatment of Laryngeal Edema[a]

1. Aqueous epinephrine 1:1,000, 0.3-0.5 cc every 15-20 minutes or as often as necessary.
2. Diphenhydramine hydrochloride (Benadryl) 60-80 mg. intramuscularly or intravenously, depending on severity (maximum, 5 mg per kg in 24 hours).
3. Maintain airway with oral airway or, if necessary, insert endotracheal tube or perform tracheotomy.
4. Corticosteroids will not be helpful for acute laryngeal edema, but will prevent protracted laryngeal edema.

[a]Adjust drug dosages to weight in children.

DRUG ALLERGY

True drug allergy must be differentiated from the more common side reactions that are often related to dose. Drug allergy may take many forms and includes the following:

1. Anaphylaxis
2. Serum sickness
3. Drug fever
4. Cutaneous reactions
5. Hematologic reactions
   (a) Hemolysis

   (b) Thrombocytopenia
   (c) Granulocytopenia
6. Pulmonary reactions
7. Hepatic reactions
8. Gastrointestinal reactions
9. Vasculitis
10. Lymphadenopathy

One must also be aware of certain cross-reacting antigens. Examples of these are penicillin and cephalothin, sulfonamides and certain local anesthetics, and acetylsalicylic acid, which cross reacts with indomethacin and tartrazine (FD & C Yellow No. 5). The following is a list of reactions with examples of drugs that may cause them.

1. Anaphylactic reaction—these have been previously described.
2. Serum sickness—penicillin, sulfonamides, thiouracil, phenytoin, and heterologous antisera.
3. Drug fever—this frequently occurs after 7-10 days of treatment; the drugs involved here include penicillin, streptomycin, para-amino-salicyclic acid, quinidine, barbiturates, phenytoin, and methyldopa.
4. Cutaneous reactions—there is a high incidence of cutaneous reactions with a wide variety of drugs. Some examples are as follows:
   (a) Urticaria and angioedema—penicillin
   (b) Diffuse morbilliform lesions—penicillin, barbiturates, sulfonamides
   (c) Cutaneous purpura—penicillin, quinidine, chlorothiazides, sulfonamides
   (d) Contact dermatitis—penicillin, local anesthetics, antihistamines
   (e) Fixed eruptions—phenolphthalein, barbiturates, sulfonamides
   (f) Exfoliative dermatitis—arsenicals, barbiturates, penicillin, phenothiazines

There is a further description of these entities in the Dermatology section (Chapter 4).

DIAGNOSIS

For the most part, the accurate diagnosis of drug allergy is based on a careful history. A determination of all drug exposures during a reasonable time before the onset of symptoms must be carefully elicited. This not only includes prescribed medications but also over-the-counter drugs and household remedies. A patient must be asked specific questions such as: What do you take for headaches (?), What do you take for an upset stomach (?), What do you take for your bowels (?), Are you taking vitamins (?), and, Are you on birth control pills (?). The time relationships of each drug and prior exposure to these drugs are also important information. In addition to the drug itself, the reaction may also be a result of other ingredients such as binders in the medication or even contaminants. A case of urticaria secondary to the ingestion of a digitalis preparation was due to penicillin contamination of the digitalis during its manufacturing process. The acid yellow dyes (FD & C yellow No. 5, tartrazine) are examples of nontherapeutic constituents of medications. This substance may give rise to urticaria and, in certain asthmatics, may exacerbate their asthma. Skin testing for drug sensitivity is relatively ineffective due to the vast number of drugs. Exception to this are penicillin and the biologicals such as insulin. Most of the other drugs act as haptens and may combine with serum proteins to form the antigenic structure. Therefore, skin testing is applicable in only a few situations. There are other assays that are being developed such as the radio-allergo-absorbent test (RAST) for penicillin but, as of yet, they are of no practical value. On occasion, when a patient has a fairly minor reaction and is on a variety of medications, it may be necessary to rechallenge the patient with one drug at a time over a period of weeks. This is particularly important in patients for whom the medications are necessary for maintenance of health This form of challenge should be reserved for reactions that are not life threatening.

THERAPY

First and foremost, of course, is prevention. Indiscriminate use of drugs is one of the common causes of drug reactions. In addition, a careful history must be elicited from patients to determine whether they have previously had drug reactions. In the case of insulin, an allergic reaction is much more common in patients who are on intermittent insulin therapy. When insulin is readministered after a period of time, the patient may develop generalized urticaria or more serious reactions.

In the case of penicillin sensitivity, tests with major and minor determinants should be performed on patients in whom penicillin allergy is suspected. The major determinants are available commercially in the form of penicilloyl-polylysine. Although the minor determinants are not yet available commercially, penicillin G can be used. In patients who have had previous generalized reactions to the radio contrast dyes, it is strongly advised to pretreat these patients with antihistamines and steroids for 24 hours prior to the x-ray study. This will substantially reduce, although not completely eliminate, the incidence of reactions. Patients who have had prior reactions must be screened carefully as to the need for the x-ray study. Desensitization is possible under certain circumstances. In the case of penicillin sensitivity, desensitization is occasionally done in an individual in whom penicillin is the only drug to be used for the treatment of their disease. It is also used in the case of insulin allergy and can be effectively accomplished over a period of several days. In addition to the above mentioned specific prophylactic treatments, it is imperative, of course, to treat the reactions symptomatically when they occur.

HYMENOPTERA SENSITIVITY

Individual insects responsible for this sensitivity include the bee, wasp, yellow jacket, hornet, and fire ant. In the case of the bee, wasp, yellow jacket, and hornet, about 40 deaths per year are reported. Reactions can occur at any age, and rates in males outnumber females by two to one. Reactions that may occur range from a severe local reaction to generalized anaphylaxis and death. This condition constitutes a medical emergency. As a rule, the patient is not aware of the specific type of insect involved. The bee leaves the stinger in place and this may be a clue, since other insects do not. The diagnosis is confirmed not only by history but by two tests. One is the skin test, which is performed using the specific venoms. These venoms are available commercially and the procedure for skin testing must be followed very closely. Reactions may occur from the skin testing, and they should be performed by experienced individuals. In addition, the RAST test can also be performed as an in vitro test in which specific IgE antibody can be determined against the individual venoms.

Therapy for insect stings includes the immediate treatment of anaphylaxis or generalized urticaria, and long-term therapy. The long-term therapy consits of careful education of the patient on how to identify and avoid the offending insects. Such things as the proper clothing, the avoidance of strong perfumes and bright colors, and avoiding known habitats should be emphasized to the patient. The patient should also be provided with an emergency kit consisting of injectable epinephrine and an antihistamine, and should be taught how to administer the epinephrine. Hyposensitization should also be considered, although this form of therapy must be performed by an individual experienced in the use of venom immunotherapy since serious reactions may occur. After the diagnosis is established and the patient has had serious skin reactions to the stinging insect, hyposensitization therapy with specific venoms should be tried. This is an expensive form of therapy and the diagnosis should be firmly established before subjecting the patient to this form of treatment.

FIRE ANT

The fire ant is prevelant in the southeast and south central areas of the United States. Its reactions consist of severe local involvement with secondary infections, and anaphylaxis may also occur. The treatment of fire ant sensitivity is basically avoidance of the areas where they reside. There is an extract for hyposensitization that is made from the whole body of the fire ant; however, its efficacy is still not certain. When and if venom becomes available, this will probably be more effective.

IMMUNE DEFICIENCY STATES

These are disorders that represent an impairment in one or more of the immune mechanisms. They involve impairment of:

1. Various surfaces including
   (a) Skin
   (b) Mucous membrane of the GI tract
   (c) Mucous membrane of the respiratory tract
2. Bactericidal activity and phagocytosis
3. Inflammatory response, including complement
4. Humoral antibody responses and production (B cells)
5. Cell-mediated immunity (T cells)

These diseases may occur as primary disorders or they may be secondary to other diseases or injury states. Primary immunodeficiency diseases can be classified as:

1. Stem cell defects
   (a) Reticular dysgenesis
   (b) Severe combined immunodeficiency
      (1) With thymic Alymphoplasia
      (2) Swiss type
      (3) With Adenosine deaminase deficiency
      (4) With Ectodermal dysplasis and dwarfism
      (5) Sporadic
2. Predominantly B-cell defects
   (a) Congenital hypogammaglobulinemia (Bruton type, X-linked)
   (b) Congenital hypogammaglobulinemia (autosomal recessive)
   (c) Common variable immunodeficiency
   (d) IgA deficiency
   (e) IgM deficiency
   (f) IgG subclass deficiency
   (g) Immunodeficiency with elevated IgM
   (h) X-linked immunodeficiency with
      (1) normal globulin
      (2) hyperglobulinemia
   (i) Hypogammaglobulinemia with thymoma
3. Predominantly T-cell defects
   (a) Thymus hypoplasia (Nezelof's syndrome)
   (b) DiGeorge's Syndrome
   (c) Nucleoside Phosphorylase Deficiency
   (d) Chronic Mucocutaneous Candidiasis with endocrinopathy.
4. Complex immunodeficiencies
   (a) Wiskott-Aldrich syndrome
   (b) Ataxia-telangiectasia
   (c) Hyper-IgE syndrome
   (d) Cartilage-hair dysplasia

Most of these are clearly genetic diseases. Some of the secondary host-related diseases are listed below.

1. Integumental disorders—burns
2. Malnutrition

3. Neoplasia–lymphomas
4. Congenital defects–congenital heart disease
5. Congenital Infections–rubella
6. Metabolic disease–diabetes

Since many of the diseases listed above are rare, only the more common ones will be discussed.

PRIMARY DISORDERS OF THE B-CELL SYSTEM

These diseases result in an impairment of the secretion of immuniglobulins.

Congenital Hypogammaglobulinemia

This is the first of the immunodeficiency diseases to be recognized and usually occurs in infants during the first few months of life. After the transplacental immunoglobulins are catabolized, the child begins to develop recurrent infections. The most common infections include those caused by pyogenic organisms such as *Micrococcus pyogenes, Hemophilus influenzae, Diplococcus pneumoniae,* and *Streptococcus pyogenes.* There does not appear to be any impairment of the response to viral infections but these infants do have a predisposition to the autoimmune diseases such as rheumatoid arthritis and dermatomyositis. The disease is diagnosed by the absence of immunoglobulins, or at least a very low IgG level of less than 2 mg/ml per deciliter. These patients also fail to respond to certain antigenic stimuli. The treatment of this disease is intramuscular injections of commercial gamma globulin in a dose of 0.025 g/kg every 3-4 weeks. This treatment is not without risk and some patients may develop serious allergic reactions. There is also the danger of hepatitis.

Common Variable Immunodeficiency

This disease occurs most commonly in adult life without prior history of any unusual susceptibility to infections during childhood. It is manifested by recurrent pyogenic infections, particularly of the sinuses and respiratory tract. These patients also may develop a malabsorption syndrome associated with hyperplasia of the lymphoid tissues of the small bowel and infestation with giardia. This disease is also diagnosed by the absence or a deficiency of gamma globulins, particularly IgG, which may not be as low as in congenital hypogammaglobulinemia. The therapy for this disease is the same as that for congenital hypogammaglobulinemia.

Dysgammaglobulinemias

This is a group of diseases in which there are selected deficiencies of one or more, but not all, of the immunoglobulin classes. The patient may not be able to synthesize or secrete immunoglobulins, or may have immunoglobulins that are functionally deficient. Examples of the dysgammaglobulinemias include IgA deficiency and selective IgM deficiency.

IgA Deficiency

This is the most common of the dysgammaglobulinemias, reportedly occurring in approximately one in 500 to one in 700 patients. There are also a number of patients with IgA deficiency who are asymptomatic. The patients with clinically significant IgA deficiency are at risk for repeated infections, autoimmune diseases, and developing malignant neoplasms. The clinical manifestations of this disease are recurrent pneumonia, bronchitis, and sinusitis. In some patients, allergic symptoms are common since increased amounts of IgE are produced; they are therefore subject to atopic diseases. The diagnosis of this disease is confirmed by the absence or extremely low levels of IgA. The treatment of this disease is not satisfactory. Gamma globulin therapy is of little value because it contains almost no IgA. Furthermore, a number of these patients have IgA antibodies in their sera and may react to the administration of gamma globulin. They are also at risk if they receive blood transfusions. All their bacterial infections must be treated aggressively and as early as possible.

Selective IgM Deficiency

This is the second most common of the dysgammaglobulinemias and is usually manifested by a sudden overwhelming sepsis. These patients may also have atopic disease, hemolytic anemia, and splenomegaly. This may be confused with the Wiskott-Aldrich syndrome; however, they lack the characteristic eczema and thrombocytopenia. The treatment for this disease also is inadequate and only acute episodes of infection require prompt and enthusiastic therapy.

T-CELL DEFICIENCIES

Di George's Syndrome

This is an unusual syndrome characterized by neonatal hypocalcemia with tetany and aplasia of the thymus. A number of other abnormalities of the midline structures of the face may also occur. These patients usually develop candidiasis of the oral cavity (thrush), chronic diarrhea, and failure to thrive in the first year of life. The treatment of this disease consists of either injections of thymosin or thymus transplantation. Spontaneous remissions of this disease have been reported.

Chronic Mucocutaneous Candidiasis

In this disease, there may be a specific deficit limited to the lack of response to candida, or the patient may develop total anergy with a failure to respond to any of the test antigens. These patients develop severe candidiasis, often starting in the perineal and circumoral areas and spreading over the limbs, scalp, face, and nails. There is also a subgroup of these patients in whom endocrine failure occurs. This may involve the adrenals, parathyroids, thyroid, or gonads. The treatment of this disease includes thymus or bone marrow transplants, the use of transfer factor, and also the use of ketoconazole.

COMPLEX IMMUNODEFICIENCIES

Wiskott-Aldrich Syndrome

This is an X-linked disease that is manifested by thrombocytopenia with a hemorrhagic tendency, eczema, and immunodeficiency with recurrent infections. The disease may present during infancy with a bleeding tendency secondary to thrombocytopenia. Eczema often appears later and cannot be differentiated from typical atopic eczema. These patients have an increased incidence of lymphoma, especially of the central nervous system. Examination of the serum reveals a low level of IgM, normal or elevated levels of IgA and IgG, and extremely high levels of IgE. These patients have a variable response to antigenic stimulation and abnormal T cells, with an absolute reduction in the E-rosette-forming T cells. The treatment of this disease consists of topical steroid therapy and local skin care. Platelet transfusions may be necessary to correct severe thrombocytopenia but splenectomy should be avoided since it may precipitate overwhelming sepsis. There have been some successful results with thymus or bone marrow transplants, as well as the use of transfer factor.

Ataxia-Telangiectasia

This is an autosomal recessive disease that is manifested by severe cerebellar ataxia, multiple telangiectases involving the skin and ocular mucosa, recurrent sinopulmonary infections, and endocrine abnormalities. This disease may not become manifest until the child starts to walk. Infections of the lung, bronchi, and sinuses also occur but they do not develop diseases of the central nervous system or bone, nor do they develop sepsis. The growing child may develop endocrine abnormalities such as juvenile diabetes or gonadal dysgenesis, or liver abnormalities. These patients also are more prone to develop lymphomas, and this is a common cause of death. The treatment of this disease is unsatisfactory. Attempts at the use of bone marrow and thymus transplantation, thymosin, and transfer factor have met with little success.

Deficiencies of the Complement System

There have been increasing reports of diseases involving abnormalities in the complement system that present as systemic diseases.

Hereditary Angioedema

In this disease, there is a deficiency of activity of an α_2-globulin that normally inhibits C_1 esterase. The deficiency may result from lack of production of the globulin, or production of an abnormal nonfunctional protein. This disease can occur at any age and is manifested by recurring attacks of nonpitting, nonpruritic edema confined to the skin, gastrointestinal tract, or respiratory mucosa. These episodes may last for 2-3 days; involvement of the larynx may be life threatening. Acute episodes are often precipitated by oral pharyngeal trauma such as dental work. However, these patients do not develop urticaria. The diagnosis is established by the quantitative measurement of C_1 C_2, or C_4 esterase inhibitors, all of which may be depressed. There is also an acquired form of this disease that is seen in conjunction with lymphomas or epithelioid tumors. A number of drugs have been used in the treatment of this disease; however, once an episode occurs there is very little that will stop its progression. An adequate airway is of prime concern. Drugs such as ϵ-aminocaproic acid (EACA) and tranexamic acid are used because of their antifibrinolytic activity and efficacy in reducing the frequency of attacks. More recently, danazol, a derivative of ethinyltestosterone, also has been shown to be effective in preventing acute episodes.

Other complement deficiencies have been described; however, since they are extremely rare they will not be discussed here.

ABNORMALITIES OF LEUKOCYTE FUNCTION

This category includes acquired neutropenias, inherited neutropenias, chronic granulomatous disease, Chédiak-Higashi syndrome, neutrophilic chemotaxic deficiency, and deficient phagocytosis.

Acquired Neutropenias

These may be caused by infections, radiation, pollutants, drugs, hypersensitivity states, malignancies, and splenic disorders. It also may occur in association with various autoimmune diseases such as lupus erythematosus.

Inherited Neutropenias

These may occur as part of a congenital disease or as an isolated defect, and may be cylic or noncylic. The cylic neutropenias are often manifested by fever and malaise, with an aphthous stomatitis occurring approximately at 3-week intervals. The noncyclic form may be a benign disease with spontaneous cure in childhood, or it may be associated with more severe infections, and children may die in the first year of life. The clinical features of both forms are infections caused by the same organisms that are found in hypogammaglobulinemia. There is no therapy except in the case of drug-induced disease. Treatment is directed at preventing infections through the use of long-term prophylaxis and aggressive therapy for infections when they are present.

Chronic Granulomatous Disease

This is a rare disease in which there is defective bactericidal activity within the leukocytes. The defect is the impaired generation of hydrogen peroxide and the metabolism of oxygen resulting from a deficiency of the enzyme NADPH oxidase. This disease usually occurs about the first year of life and is manifested by recurrent episodes of sepsis and disseminated abscesses. The agents responsible for infections in this disease are usually agents found on the skin and are often organisms of low-grade virulence that are catalase-positive or peroxide-negative. These include the staphylococci, *Escherichia coli, Klebsiella, Serratia marcescens,* enterobacter, *Proteus vulgaris,* and *Actinomyces* species. The treatment of this disease is based on early intervention with high doses of bactericidal antibiotics.

Chédiak-Higashi Syndrome

This is an autosomal recessive disorder characterized by oculocutaneous albinism, neurologic abnormalities, recurrent pyogenic infections, and high incidence of lymphoma. There is deficient bactericidal activity in the neutrophils and delayed degranulation following stimulation of phagocytosis.

Deficiencies of Neutrophil Chemotaxis

These deficiencies may be due to a defect extrinsic to the neutrophils such as the fifth component of complement dysfunction, or there may be an intrinsic cellular defect. The intrinsic defect is sometimes called the lazy leukocyte syndrome.

Deficient Phagocytosis

This may be manifested by a deficient number of phagocytes or qualitative defects in their function. This also results in deficient killing of bacteria by the neutrophils.

QUESTIONS

1. The major mediators in IgE mediated diseases are (one answer)
   A. histamine, SRS-A, lymphokines
   B. histamine, SRS-A, ECF-A
   C. histamine, serotonin, prostaglandins
   D. histamine, MIF, ECF-A
   E. histamine, SRS-A, MIF
2. The single most important modality in making a diagnosis of atopic disease is
   A. history
   B. physical examination
   C. RAST
   D. skin tests
   E. response to medication
3. Hyposensitization is recommended in allergic rhinitis in all except
   A. skin test positive individual
   B. presence of asthma
   C. poor control with antihistamines
   D. progressive disease
4. The most common infectious agent that is a precipitating factor in asthma is
   A. bacteria
   B. viruses
   C. fungi
   D. rickettsiae
5. The drugs of choice in chronic moderate asthma are
   A. sympathomimetic amines
   B. corticosteroids
   C. cromolyn sodium
   D. theophylline
6. The least effective drug in anaphylaxis is
   A. epinephrine
   B. antihistamines
   C. corticosteroids
   D. oxygen
7. Skin testing in drug allergy is only useful with
   A. acetylsalicylic acid
   B. iodides
   C. sulfonamides
   D. hydrochlorothiazide
   E. penicillin
8. Immunoglobulin deficiency is associated with (one answer)
   A. increased fungal infection
   B. increased bacterial infection
   C. increased viral infection
   D. T-lymphocyte deficiency

ANSWERS

1. B	5. D
2. A	6. C
3. A	7. E
4. B	8. B

BIBLIOGRAPHY

TEXTBOOKS AND MONOGRAPHS

Bellanti JA: *Immunology*. Philadelphia: W B Saunders Co, 1978.

Middleton E, Reed CE, Ellis EF (eds): *Allergy: Principles and Practice*. St. Louis: The C V Mosby Co, 1978.

Patterson R (ed): *Allergic Diseases: Diagnosis and Management*, ed. 2. Philadelphia: J B Lippincott Co, 1980.

Task Force on Asthma and the Other Allergic Diseases, National Institutes of Allergy and Infectious Diseases: *Asthma and the Other Allergic Diseases*. NIH Publication No. 79-387/G. Bethesda: National Institutes of Health, 1979.

ARTICLES

Bronchial Asthma

Godfrey S: The relative merits of cromolyn sodium and high-dose theophylline therapy in childhood asthma. *J Allergy Clin Immunol* 65: 97-104, 1980.

Hogg JC, Paré PD, Boucher RC, Michoud MC: The pathophysiology of asthma. *Can Med Assoc J* 121:409-14, 1979.

Kuzemko JA: Natural history of childhood asthma. *J Pediatr* 97:886-892, 1980.

Leffert F: The management of chronic asthma. *J Pediatr* 97:875-885, 1980.

McFadden ER Jr, Ingram RH Jr: Exercise-induced asthma: Observations on the initiating stimulus. N Engl J Med 301:763-769, 1979.

Turner ES, Greenberger PA, Patterson R: Management of the pregnant asthmatic patient. Ann Intern Med 93:905-918, 1980.

Hypersensitivity Pneumonitis

Pennington JE: Aspergillus lung disease. *Med Clin North Am* 64:475-490, 1980.

Salvaggio JE: Immunological mechanisms in pulmonary diseases. *Clin Allergy* 9:659-668, 1979.

Anaphylaxis

Beaven MA: Anaphylactoid reactions to anesthetic drugs (editorial). *Anesthesiology* 55:3-5, 1981.

Jacobs RL, Rake GW Jr, Fournier DC, Chilton RJ, Culver WG, Beckmann CH: Potentiated anaphylaxis in patients with drug-induced beta-adrenergic blockade. *J Allergy Clin Immunol* 68:125-127, 1981.

Kellerman R: Reactions to radiographic contrast media. *Am Fam Physician* 23:149-152, 1981.

Immune Deficiency States

Denman AM: Immunodeficiency and general medicine. Br Med J 281: 1376-1378, 1980.

Hong R, Schulte-Wissermann H, Horowitz SD: Thymic transplantation for relief of immunodeficiency diseases. *Surg Clin North Am* 59: 299-312, 1979.

Mitchell BS, Kelley WN: Purinogenic immunodeficiency diseases: Clinical features and molecular mechanisms. *Ann Intern Med* 92:826-831, 1980.

CHAPTER 3
CARDIOLOGY

Virinderjit S. Bamrah

L. Samuel Wann

HISTORY

A detailed and accurate history in a cardiac patient is extremely helpful in reaching the correct diagnosis, in assessing functional status, and in deciding the proper time for referring a patient for further tests or surgical therapy. Hence, the value of a good history cannot be overemphasized. The common symptoms encountered in cardiac patients are described in this chapter.

CHEST PAIN

Angina pectoris is defined as an episodic discomfort in the chest precipitated by exertion or emotion that is relieved by rest and/or nitroglycerin. Angina has the deep, achy character of a visceral pain that is usually described as tightness, heavy pressure, or a choking or burning sensation in the chest. Occasionally it is described as indigestion that may be somewhat relieved after belching. The episode may be accompanied by heavy breathing and acute anxiety. The most common location of the discomfort is either substernal or across the anterior chest and is felt deep in the chest. Occasionally it may be located in the precordial area, but pain in the region of the cardiac apex is not usually angina. The discomfort usually radiates to one or more of the following regions: left arm, right arm, shoulders, neck, throat, jaw, cheeks, teeth, upper abdomen, and sometiems the interscapular area. Angina is precipitated by physical activity, especially if it is performed in a hurried manner and the patient is unaccustomed to it. Sexual intercourse, walking (especially going uphill, exposure to cold wind, following a heavy meal), arm work overhead, hurrying to answer a phone call, and an emotional buildup (anger, fright, or excitement) are some of the common situations precipitating angina. The intensity of the pain is variable. Most often the discomfort builds up quickly with activity, forcing the patient to stop and rest. Occasionally it builds up to a tolerable intensity and lasts till the end of activity. There is rarely spontaneous relief of angina during continued activity and the patient can continue exerting at an even greater level afterward without stopping. This is termed walk-through angina or second-wind angina in the literature. Most angina episodes last 3-5 minutes, and may abort after use of nitroglycerin and/or rest. The very intense attacks of angina may last anywhere from 5-30 minutes.

A patient should be asked about history of chest discomfort rather than chest pain, since many patients deny having pain during their episodes of angina. Not uncommonly, discomfort in the secondary regions of radiation, for example, the arms and neck, may be more intense than in the chest. Moreover, discomfort in the chest may be totally absent. The most helpful diagnostic feature of angina is its precipitation by exertion and relief with rest. Any type of discomfort located between the nose and the umbilicus and having a characteristic exercise-rest relationship should be seriously investigated. Sometimes the attacks of angina occur during recumbency (angina decubitus) or at night (nocturnal angina). These episodes generally indicate an advanced degree of coronary artery disease and maybe a manifestation of left heart failure. Increased sympathetic activity during dreams may be responsible for nocturnal angina.

The following questions are extremely important and the responses to these should be recorded: total duration since inception of attacks; frequency of attacks; typical daily activities leading to angina; and changes in the pattern of angina, that is, changes in the duration of each attack, intensity of pain, activity threshold, relief with nitroglycerin and so on.

Pericardial pain is of variable intensity and is more often felt in the precordial area rather than in the substernal area. It has a sharp character and may be felt either deeply or superficially in the chest. The pain is aggravated by recumbency, especially in the left lateral position, cough, deep inspiration, and swallowing. It is relieved by sitting up when the patient leans forward. It may radiate to the neck, left shoulder, left arm, and upper back.

DYSPNEA

Dyspnea is a subjective sensation of difficult or uncomfortable breathing. Patients may describe it as feeling breathless, short-winded, or not getting enough air. Besides heart disease, dyspnea may be due to a variety of lung diseases, diseases of the chest wall, anemia, obesity, and anxiety states. The following remarks refer to dyspnea secondary to heart disease: It is one of the most common symptoms of heart disease and usually indicates pulmonary venous hypertension secondary to left heart failure or mitral stenosis. With a mild degree of left ventricular failure, dyspnea occurs only on exertion. However, with progressive heart failure the activity threshold for dyspnea decreases. In addition, the patient starts experiencing orthopnea, paroxysmal nocturnal dyspnea, or full-blown attacks of acute pulmonary edema.

Orthopnea means dyspnea during recumbency with relief on sitting up. Orthopnea occurs in diseases of heart and lungs.

Paroxysmal nocturnal dyspnea (PND) is a specific feature of heart disease. Typically the patient goes to bed and sleeps comfortably for one to two hours. At that point, the patient wakes up acutely short of breath with a feeling of suffocation, sits upright at the edge of the bed gasping for breath, walks for a few minutes, or may open a window for fresh air. The shortness of breath may be accompanied by cough, sweating, pallor, cyanosis, and cold extremities. Approximately 10-30 minutes after the start of this episode, the patient experiences spontaneous relief of dyspnea and sleeps comfortably through the rest of the night. When an acute episode of breathlessness secondary to left heart failure is associated with wheezing, it is referred to as cardiac asthma. Sometimes patients present with nocturnal coughing spasms that are due to pulmonary edema and can be confused with bronchitis.

Acute pulmonary edema indicates sudden and severe decompensation of the left ventricle or severe mitral stenosis. The episode starts with extreme shortness of breath and persistent cough productive of white or pink frothy sputum. The accessory muscles of respiration are used. The extreme degree of anxiety and agony is obvious. The patient prefers to sit up and often leans forward. The skin is cold, pale, and gray with profuse sweating. The severity of pulmonary edema varies from mild to severe. Usually the attack subsides spontaneously or with treatment after a few minutes to a few hours. However, severe pulmonary edema may result in death.

EDEMA

Edema is a late feature of heart failure. It is due to sodium and water retention. Patients may gain weight up to approximately 10 lb without apparent edema. Others may notice swelling of the ankles and feet toward the end of the day, experience nocturia, and by morning the swelling has disappeared. With progressive heart failure, swelling of the ankles and feet becomes persistent. In addition, the edema slowly ascends to the legs, external genital organs, trunk, and even the face. The edema in heart failure is dependent and is therefore located in the feet, ankles, and legs in those patients who are upright most of the time. On the other hand, in recumbent patients it is located in the sacral region. Edema also occurs due to cirrhosis of the liver, nephrotic syndrome, malnutrition, and venous and lymphatic diseases.

FATIGUE

Patients with heart disease often complain of weakness and exhaustion on mild exertion. This is usually attributed to low cardiac output and generally occurs in patients with advanced cardiac disease and congestive heart failure. Fatigue is, however, a nonspecific symptom; besides heart disease, it occurs in many other chronic illnesses as well as in anxiety states.

DIZZINESS AND SYNCOPE

History of syncope (transient loss of consciousness) may be volunteered by the patient or family members. A large number of patients with heart disease may feel light-headed, weak, and unsteady on their legs (dizzy) but may not experience total loss of consciousness. The majority of attacks of dizziness and syncope are brief and occur in an upright posture. Dizziness and syncope in cardiac disease are due to low cardiac output (heart failure and/or arrhythmias) resulting in decreased perfusion to the brain. Other common causes of syncope are cerebrovascular, inner ear, and metabolic diseases (e.g., hypoglycemia). The determination of the etiology of syncope is by no means an easy task, especially in the elderly who constitute the majority of patients with this symptom. Difficulties in eliciting a good history in this age group as well as coexistence of cerebrovascular and cardiac diseases in the same patient often preclude a precise diagnosis on a clinical basis, necessitating greater reliance on laboratory tests.

PALPITATION

Palpitation indicates unpleasant awareness of one's heart beat. Patients describe it as pounding, thumping, fluttering, throbbing, or skipping of the heart beat. Normal persons may experience palpitation under certain circumstances such as physical exertion, emotional excitement, acute anxiety, fright, or while laying on the left side. Excessive use of tea, coffee, tobacco, or alcohol may also give rise to palpitation. Palpitation occurs in the following cardiac conditions: hyperkinetic states such as anemia, thyrotoxicosis, fever, pregnancy, and idiopathic hyperkinetic heart syndrome; hyperadrenergic states such as pheochromocytoma, hypoglycemia, and postural hypotension; volume overload of the heart, as in aortic insufficiency, mitral insufficiency, atrial septal defect, ventricular septal defect, and patent ductus arteriosis; and arrhythmias such as paroxysmal atrial tachycardia, atrial fibrillation, and premature beats. A premature beat may be felt as an uncomfortable, out-of-time contraction of the heart, followed by a more powerful beat. Patients should be asked about the onset and termination of rapid heart action, that is, whether the episode starts and terminates suddenly or gradually and also whether the heart beat is regular or irregular during the episode.

In the above situations, unusual motion of the heart in the thorax, enhanced force of contraction, or increased stroke volume may be the underlying mechanism producing the feeling of palpitation.

CYANOSIS

Cyanosis indicates a blue-tinged discoloration of the skin and mucous membranes. It occurs due to the presence of at least 5 gm of reduced hemoglobin per 100 ml of capillary blood. Smaller concentrations of methemoglobin and sulfmethemoglobin (1.5 and 0.5 g/dl, respectively) also give rise to cyanosis. Cyanosis is conventionally divided into central and peripheral types. Central cyanosis is due to arterial desaturation. Arterial blood in normal subjects shows $\geqslant$95 percent oxygen saturation. Central cyanosis is associated with $\leqslant$85 percent oxygen saturation. Central cyanosis is recognized by a blue tinge of the tongue, conjunctivae, lips, nose, ears, and nail beds. Central cyanosis occurs in lung diseases, congenital heart diseases with right to left shunt, methemoglobinemia and sulfmethemoglobinemia.

In peripheral cyanosis the arterial oxygenation is normal; however, due to sluggish blood flow there is an increased extraction of oxygen peripherally by the sinuses, resulting in an increased amount of reduced hemoglobin. Peripheral cyanosis is seen in the ears, nose, lips, nails, and fingertips but not in the tongue or conjunctivae. Peripheral cyanosis occurs with low cardiac output states, exposure to cold, and arterial and venous obstruction.

MISCELLANEOUS

A variety of other symptoms described below may occur in patients with heart disease and must be recorded. Hemoptysis or coughing of blood in mitral stenosis, pulmonary infarction, or acute pulmonary edema, oliguria during the day and polyuria at night, insomnia, anorexia, and cachexia in heart failure; nausea, anorexia, and vomiting in digitalis toxicity; fever and chills in infective endocarditis; epistaxis in hypertension; and repeated chest infections in large left-to-right shunts. In addition, a past history of rheumatic fever, scarlet fever, an awareness of heart murmur during childhood or adolescence, and history of dental work or surgery in a patient presenting with a febrile illness should be recorded.

PHYSICAL EXAMINATION

ARTERIAL PULSE

Rate and rhythm should be examined from the radial artery. The abnormalities of rate and rhythm are discussed in the section on cardiac arrhythmias. Amplitude or volume of various peripheral pulses, that is, radial, brachial, carotid, femoral, popliteal, posterior tibial, and dorsalis pedis, should be compared on both sides to detect any differences. The femoral pulse is normally stronger than the radial pulse; however, the two pulses occur simultaneously in normal subjects. In patients with coarctation of the aorta, the femoral pulse is weaker than the radial pulse and is delayed. A careful examination of the carotid pulse provides important information about left ventricular ejection, stroke volume, and aortic valve function. Only one carotid pulse should be examined at a time. In normal subjects, a rapid upstroke followed by a gentle downslope is perceived. The downslope is suddenly interrupted by a dicrotic notch (incisura) that occurs at the time of aortic valve closure. The following abnormalities of arterial pulse occur in various heart diseases.

Large-amplitude (volume) pulse, or bounding pulse, corresponds to increased pulse pressure (systolic minus diastolic pressure) that occurs when the increased stroke volume is ejected rapidly and systemic vascular resistance is low. A high-volume pulse is palpable in hyperkinetic states (fever, anemia, anxiety, thyrotoxicosis) and arterial runoff (aortic regurgitation, mitral regurgitation, ventricular septal defect, patent ductus arteriosus, arteriovenous fistula). An extreme degree of a large amplitude pulse is described as a waterhammer or collapsing pulse and is observed in severe aortic regurgitation.

Small-amplitude (volume) pulse corresponds to the decreased pulse pressure that occurs when a normal or decreased stroke volume is ejected slowly and/or systemic vascular resistance is high. A weak and thready pulse is felt in left heart failure and shock. In severe aortic valvular stenosis, the pulse is typically low in volume with a slowly rising upstroke and a delayed peak. This has been variously described as pulsus parvus, pulsus tardus, anacrotic pulse, or plateau pulse.

Pulsus bisferiens has two peaks produced by percussion and tidal waves before the dicrotic notch. This occurs in idiopathic hypertrophic subaortic stenosis, severe aortic regurgitation, and in combined stenosis and regurgitation of the aortic valve.

In a dicrotic pulse, the second palpable wave is produced by an unusually prominent dicrotic wave after the dicrotic notch. It occurs when diastolic pressure and systemic vascular resistance are low as in febrile states. A dicrotic pulse may also be observed in cardiac tamponade, severe heart failure, and hypovolemic shock.

Pulsus alternans indicates alternately strong and weak pulses, even though they occur at regular intervals. It is best detected by sphygmomanometer, even though it can be palpated over the peripheral arteries. Pulsus alternans is produced as high and low stroke volumes are ejected alternately from larger and smaller enddiastolic volumes of the left ventricle. It has also been suggested that a different number of myocardial fibers are recruited in alternate beats, resulting in stronger and weaker myocardial contractions. Pulsus alternans indicates severe myocardial failure.

Pulsus paradoxus is defined as an excessive ($>$10 mm Hg) fall of systolic pressure during inspiration. In normal subjects, there is a 3-10 mm Hg inspiratory fall of systolic pressure. Even though the respiratory variation of pulse amplitude is perceptible on palpation, the degree of paradox can be measured best with a sphygmomanometer. The mercury column should be lowered slowly with systolic pressure being noted during quiet inspiration and expiration over several cycles. When the inspiratory fall is $\geq$20 mm Hg, it is specific for cardiac tamponade due to pericardial effusion. In cardiac tamponade due to effusion, increased right ventricular filling during inspiration occurs; the increased right ventricular volume hampers the filling of the left ventricle, which ejects a smaller stroke volume and results in a lower pulse amplitude during inspiration. Pulsus paradoxus is uncommon in constrictive pericarditis. A mild paradoxical pulse (10-20 mm Hg) is commonly present in chronic obstructive lung disease, severe congestive heart failure, pulmonary embolism, and superior vena cava syndrome.

JUGULAR VENOUS PULSE

Physiologic events occurring in the right heart chambers can be assessed by a careful bedside examination of the jugular venous pulse. The neck veins should be observed under adequate light, the patient should be recumbent with the trunk elevated enough so that the venous pulse becomes visible, and the neck should be relaxed. Examination of the right internal (deep) jugular vein is better for pulse wave analysis since it is in line with the superior vena cava and reflects right heart events better than the external jugular vein. Examination of the external jugular vein may yield false information since it pierces the deep fascia and may also have various anomalies. The internal jugular venous pulse can be differentiated from carotid pulsation by its more undulating and wavy pattern, the ease with which it can be abolished with light pressure, and by the elevation of venous pressure during expiration, cough, or abdominal pressure. Moreover, the venous pulse is located under the posterior part of the sternocleidomastoid muscle, whereas the carotid pulse is located anteriorly.

The normal jugular venous pulse has two positive a and v waves, and two troughs, or x and y descents. The a wave is produced by right atrial contraction, and the x descent is caused by relaxation of the right atrium. The x descent is interrupted by an abrupt small positive c wave produced by ascent of the closed tricuspid valve in early systole. The v wave is produced by continuous filling of the right atrium during ventricular systole. A y descent results from rapid blood flow into the right ventricle as the tricuspid valve opens. At the bedside, the a and v waves can be distinguished by correlation with the carotid pulse. The a wave precedes the carotid pulse and the v wave follows it. The a wave and x descent disappear during atrial fibrillation. A prominent a wave occurs with a forceful right atrial contraction (tricuspid stenosis or atresia, right atrial myxoma, and right ventricular hypertrophy due to pulmonary stenosis or pulmonary hypertension). Contraction of the right atrium against a closed tricuspid valve also results in a prominent a wave usually referred to as a cannon wave. This occurs regularly in junctional rhythm and irregularly in atrioventricular dissociation. The x descent (systolic collapse) becomes rapid in cardiac tamponade due to pericardial effusion. A prominent v wave occurs in tricuspid regurgitation and also in marked right heart failure. In severe tricuspid regurgitation, the v wave also occurs early, replacing the c wave and x descent. An unusually rapid x descent or systolic collapse with a deep y trough is typically seen in constrictive pericarditis. The y descent is also rapid in tricuspid regurgitation and right heart failure. On the other hand, the y descent is very slow in tricuspid stenosis or atresia and right atrial myxoma.

Jugular venous pressure reflects the mean right atrial pressure. It can be estimated at the bedside if the patient is recumbent and the trunk is elevated so that the upper level of venous pulsation becomes visible. Vertical distance between the sternal angle and the average level of venous pulsation is measured in centimeters. If this distance is more than 3 cm it is considered abnormal. The distance between the center of the right atrium and the sternal angle is constant at 5 cm irrespective of body position. This 5 cm distance, plus the measured vertical distance between the level of venous pulsation and stennal angle in centimeters, should match the central venous pressure measured with an intravenous catheter. Abnormally elevated jugular venous pressure is indicative of right heart failure and pericardial compression. In superior vena cava obstruction, the venous pressure is also elevated; however, the waves are absent. In incipient or early right heart failure when venous pressure is normal at rest, a positive hepatojugular reflux may be elicited. After observing the upper level of venous pulsations, steady pressure is applied to the right upper quadrant of the abdomen and maintained for 60 seconds. The level of venous pulsations rises and stays at a higher level (positive reflux). In healthy persons, the level of pulsations rises transiently and falls to the control level despite continued abdominal pressure (negative reflux).

INSPECTION AND PALPATION OF THE PRECORDIUM

The apical impulse is located normally in the fourth or fifth left intercostal space medial to the midclavicular line. It should be located by inspection and palpation in the supine patient. A left lateral posture may facilitate palpation of the apical impulse. If the apical impulse is displaced downward and outward from the normal location, it indicates cardiomegaly. Pectum excavatum, scoliosis, and pleural adhesions may also displace the apical impulse. In dextrocardia, the apical impulse is palpated on the right side of the chest.

In addition to the location of the apical impulse, its character is important in determining the type of workload on the heart. Normally the apical impulse is felt as a tapping outward motion of 2-3 cm of chest wall during the first one-third of systole. This is produced by low-frequency vibrations as a result of counterclockwise rotation of the heart and recoil of the ventricles during ejection of blood. The apical impulse is normally produced by the left ventricle since the right ventricle underlies the left parasternal area. In conditions with marked right ventricular enlargement, the apical impulse may come from the right ventricle. The following types of abnornal precordial impulses are encountered in heart diseases.

A heaving apical impulse occurs in pressure overload of the left ventricle as in aortic stenosis, hypertension, and coarctation of the aorta. Outward motion of the chest wall in the apical region is exaggerated and is sustained through most of the systole (> first one-third of systole).

A hyperkinetic apical impulse occurs in volume overload of the left ventricle as in aortic or mitral regurgitation and other hyperkinetic states such as anemia and thyrotoxicosis. The apical impulse is located over a larger area (>3 cm of chest wall) and the outward motion is exaggerated in its amplitude; however, it is not sustained. It is perceived as a tumultuous or rocking motion of the chest wall.

A heaving left parasternal impulse is the sustained outward motion of the left middle and lower parasternal regions. It occurs in pressure overwork of the right ventricle (right ventricular hypertrophy) due to pulmonary stenosis or pulmonary hypertension. A heaving right ventricle impulse may also be palpated under the xiphisternum. Left parasternal lift may also be produced by expansion of the left atrium in severe mitral regurgitation.

A hyperkinetic left parasternal impulse is the exaggerated outward motion of this region. It occurs in volume overwork of the right ventricle such as in an atrial septal defect.

Midprecordial heave is the abnormal systolic outward motion in the midprecordium that is produced by left ventricular aneurysms following myocardial infarction. Rarely, one can perceive a similar impulse during attacks of angina.

A rapid left ventricular distension during early and late diastole may produce distinctly visible and palpable impulses. These impulses correspond in timing to ventricular and atrial gallops, respectively.

The aortic impulse can be seen and palpated in the right upper parasternal region in an aneurysm of the ascending aorta.

The pulmonary artery impulse becomes visible in dilatation of the pulmonary trunk. It is located in the left upper parasternal area.

Sometimes the accentuated heart sounds may also become palpable. An apical tap in mitral stenosis is the palpable first heart sound. In pulmonary hypertension, the pulmonary component of the second heart sound may be palpable in the left upper parasternal region. Loud and low frequency murmurs may also be palpated and are described as thrills.

AUSCULTATION

Auscultation should be performed in a systematic fashion, for example, listening over the cardiac apex; the left lower, middle, and upper sternal border, and then the right upper sternal border. One should listen over the carotid arteries for bruits and radiation of a systolic murmur of the aortic valve. Depending on the findings, the right sternal border, left axilla, interscapular area, and chest should be carefully auscultated for heart murmurs. It is extremely important to focus attention on one auscultatory event in the cardiac cycle at a time. In patients with severe emphysema, heart sounds and murmurs are easier to hear over the xiphisternum or epigastrium rather than over the standard areas mentioned above. High frequency sounds and murmurs (S_1, S_2, murmur of aortic regurgitation) are heard best with the diaphragm of the stethoscope, whereas low frequency sounds and murmurs (S_3, S_4, mitral stenosis) are more audible with the bell of the stethoscope.

Heart Sounds

In healthy adults, two heart sounds are audible over the precordium (S_1 and S_2) during each cardiac cycle.

First Heart Sound (S_1)

The first heart sound (S_1) signals the beginning of ventricular systole. It is audible over the entire precordium, but is loudest over the apical area and left lower sternal border. The audible portion of S_1 consists of two high frequency components. The precise mechanism of the production of S_1 is still controversial. However, the first component coincides with full closure of the mitral valve leaflets and the second component coincides with full closure of the tricuspid valve leaflets. Rapid changes in intracardiac pressures, and sudden acceleration and then deceleration of the blood column produced by ventricular systole, set up vibrations in the mitral and tricuspid valves, as well as the whole cardiohemic system, resulting in the S_1. Some investigators have recently attributed the second component of S_1 to opening of the aortic valve leaflets and the acceleration of blood into the aorta. The two components are normally 10-30 milliseconds apart and, in the majority of subjects, are distinctly audible over the left lower sternal border.

There are three important factors that determine the intensity of the first heart sound: the position of mitral and tricuspid valve leaflets at the onset of ventricular systole, the force of ventricular contraction, and the distance between the heart and the anterior chest wall. The S_1 is greatly accentuated in instances where the atrioventricular valves are wide open at the onset of ventricular systole, such as in mitral stenosis, a short P-R interval, tachycardia, and increased diastolic flow rates. Examples of the latter include an atrial septal defect, ventricular septal defect, and hyperkinetic states. In addition, greater force of ventricular contraction results in a loud S_1. On the other hand, the S_1 is soft in instances where the atrioventricular valves are in a partly closed position at the onset of ventricular systole as in a long P-R interval, aortic incompetence, and decreased flow rates (low cardiac output). Decreased force of contraction, such as in acute myocardial infarction, and increased distance between the heart and the chest wall as seen in obesity or emphysema, also result in a soft S_1.

Delayed onset of right ventricular systole in right bundle-branch block produces a late tricuspid component resulting in a widely split S_1.

Second Heart Sound (S_2)

The second heart sound (S_2) is most audible over the base of the heart, especially the left upper sternal border. It signals the end of systole and the beginning of diastole. S_2 has two distinctly audible components: aortic (A_2), and pulmonary (P_2). It is convenient to relate A_2 and P_2 to the aortic and pulmonary valves, respectively. The production of A_2 is attributed to a sudden deceleration of blood, setting up vibrations in the closed aortic valve leaflets, aortic wall, and blood column in the aorta. Similar events in the pulmonary artery are believed to produce P_2. A_2 normally precedes P_2.

The splitting of S_2 varies with the phases of respiration. The split widens during inspiration and narrows during expiration. During inspiration, there is more negative intrathoracic pressure and venous return to the right heart increases, resulting in greater stroke volume of the right ventricle. Since the right ventricle requires a longer time to eject this increased stroke volume, P_2 is delayed, resulting in a wide separation of A_2 and P_2. Three to four heart beats later, during expiration, the increased stroke volume of the right ventricle is delivered to the left heart. This results in a greater stroke volume of the left ventricle, which results in delay of A_2. Concomitantly P_2 occurs earlier, since during expiration venous return to the right heart decreases, resulting in smaller right ventricular stroke volume. This sequence of events causes an almost complete overlap of A_2 and P_2 during expiration. In some individuals an S_2 split persists even during expiration, especially in a recumbent posture. On assuming an upright posture, expiratory splitting of S_2 disappears. Persistence of a split S_2 in the upright posture is highly abnormal and requires an evaluation for the presence of cardiac disease.

A_2 is the louder component and is audible over the entire precordium, including the apex. On the other hand, P_2 in normal subjects is audible only over the upper left sternal border. It is not audible over the apex under normal circumstances.

Fixed splitting of S_2, or absence of normal respiratory variation of splitting of S_2, occurs in an atrial septal defect and advanced right heart failure. In an atrial septal defect, right ventricular stroke volume exceeds that of the left ventricle, resulting in a delayed P_2. Furthermore, due to the communication between the right and left atria, inspiratory increase and expiratory decrease of systemic venous return affect equally the filling, and hence the stroke volumes, of the two sides of the heart. This eliminates the respiratory variation of an S_2 split. In advanced right heart failure, the right ventricle operates at a flat and depressed Starling's function curve, causing the stroke volume to vary little despite augmented filling during inspiration and decreased filling during expiration. These hemodynamic alterations cause the interval between A_2 and P_2 to remain relatively fixed in the presence of severe right heart failure.

Wide splitting of S_2 during expiration with further widening during inspiration occurs in right bundle-branch block (RBBB), pulmonary valve stenosis with intact ventricular septum, ventricular septal defect (VSD), and mitral regurgitation. Right bundle-branch block causes a delay in the onset of right ventricular systole, resulting in a late P_2. In pulmonary stenosis, the right ventricle requires a longer than normal time to complete ejection of blood across the obstructed valve and thus delays the P_2. Furthermore, the degree of pulmonary stenosis has a direct correlation with delay in the P_2. A left-to-right shunt in VSD causes right ventricular stroke volume to exceed that of the left ventricle, resulting in a late P_2. In mitral regurgitation, left ventricular ejection is completed relatively early since it ejects into the aorta as well as the left atrium simultaneously; thus, A_2 also occurs relatively early.

Paradoxical splitting of S_2 occurs characteristically in conditions that cause delayed onset of left ventricular ejection such as in left bundle-branch block (LBBB), or a prolonged left ventricular ejection time as seen in aortic stenosis. Splitting of S_2 narrows during inspiration and widens during expiration. In LBBB, A_2 occurs late and actually follows the P_2 sound. As previously described, there is an inspiratory delay of P_2 while A_2 occurs earlier, causing a narrow split or even a single S_2 during isnpiration. On the other hand, during expiration the right ventricular stroke volume decreases (earlier P_2) and left ventricular stroke volume increases (later A_2). Thus, P_2 and A_2 develop a wider split.

Increased intensity of A_2 and P_2 is due to elevated pressure and/or flow in the aorta and pulmonary artery, respectively. A loud A_2 is often observed in systemic hypertension. It should be emphasized again that, even in normal subjects, A_2 is the louder component and audible over the entire precordium, whereas P_2 is not transmitted to the apex. However, in pulmonary hypertension, P_2 is accentuated and is transmitted to the apex.

A decreased or absent A_2 occurs when the aortic valve leaflets become immobile due to thickening and calcification, as seen in calcific aortic stenosis. A decreased or absent P_2 occurs in severe pulmonary stenosis or atresia. Intensity of P_2 decreases with an increase in age. Loud murmurs may conceal one or both of the components of S_2, for example, masking of A_2 with a mitral regurgitation murmur. Emphysema, obesity, and pericardial effusion also dampen the intensity of heart sounds in general.

Diastolic Sounds

A ventricular gallop (S_3) sound occurs in early diastole, 140-160 milliseconds following S_2. It is a low-frequency dull sound, best heard with the bell of the stethoscope lightly applied to the apex (left ventricular S_3), or left lower sternal border (right ventricular S_3). Auscultation in the left lateral position and during expiration may be required to elicit ventricular gallop. The S_3 results from ventricular vibrations produced by deceleration of blood flow when the rate of ventricular filling exceeds the ventricular distensibility during early diastole. Ventricular gallop occurs under the following circumstances:

- *Physiologic S_3:* This sound is commonly audible in children and young adults. It usually disappears after age 40.
- *Increased diastolic flow:* Ventricular septal defect, patent ductus arteriosus, and mitral regurgitation increase diastolic flow into the left ventricle, resulting in an audible S_3 over the apex. In an atrial septal defect, however, augmented diastolic flow into the right ventricle causes an audible S_3 over the left lower sternal border. In hyperkinetic states like thyrotoxicosis and pregnancy, S_3 usually becomes audible.
- *Early sign of heart failure:* An audible S_3 is frequently an early sign of heart failure. It correlates with an abnormally high filling pressure, low cardiac output, and ventricular dilatation. It also provides important prognostic information. A loud and persistent S_3 indicates a poor prognosis. On the other hand, a soft S_3 disappearing spontaneously or with treatment implies a good prognosis.

Pericardial knock is commonly heard in patients with constrictive pericarditis. Its mechanism of production is similar to that of an S_3 sound. However, it has a higher frequency and occurs earlier than S_3.

Atrial gallop (S_4) is a dull low-frequency sound that precedes S_1 and is most audible over the cardiac apex (left sided), or left lower sternal border (right sided). The techniques useful to elicit an S_3 sound also apply for S_4. The S_4 is attributed to forceful atrial contraction to fill a noncompliant or stiff ventricle. It correlates with a prominent presystolic impulse of an apex cardiogram and prominent a wave of atrial and ventricular pressure curves. The S_4 becomes audible under the following situations:

- *Decreased ventricular compliance:* Decreased compliance of the ventricles occurs in ventricular hypertrophy such as in systemic and pulmonary hypertension, aortic and pulmonary stenosis, idiopathic hypertrophic subaortic stenosis, cardiomyopathy, myocardial ischemia and infarction, or an over-filled ventricle (acute mitral or aortic regurgitation).

- *Atrioventricular (AV) block:* In first degree AV block, S_4 is frequently audible and the S_4-S_1 interval is directly proportional to the P-R interval. In second and third degree AV block, S_4 is also audible and corresponds to the P waves in the ECG. It should be noted that the S_4-S_1 interval also depends on the status of ventricular function independent of the P-R interval on the ECG. Improvement of ventricular function shortens and deterioration prolongs this interval.
- *Hyperkinetic states:* The S_4 becomes audible in hyperkinetic states like thyrotoxicosis and anemia.

The S_4 disappears in atrial fibrillation.

Summation gallop occurs in the presence of tachycardia in a patient who has both S_4 and S_3. During tachycardia the diastolic phase becomes short causing the S_4 and S_3 to fuse into a loud, single diastolic sound. This is referred to as a summation gallop.

Mitral opening snap (OS) is a sharp, high-frequency sound heard best over the left lower sternal border in patients with mitral valve stenosis. Mitral OS is transmitted throughout the precordium. This sound is attributed to a sudden arrest of the rapidly opening motion of a stenotic but pliable mitral valve. When the mitral valve leaflets become calcified and immobile, the OS becomes soft or may disappear. The A_2-OS interval correlates inversely with the severity of mitral stenosis. Since left atrial pressure rises with the increase in severity of mitral stenosis, OS occurs earlier, resulting in a narrow A_2-OS interval. Tricuspid stenosis also produces a tricuspid opening snap; however, it is seldom detected on auscultation.

Systolic Sounds

Ejection clicks (EC), or sounds, are very sharp, high-frequency sounds audible immediately after S_1. Ejection clicks occur in aortic and pulmonary valvular stenosis as well as in dilatation of the ascending aorta and pulmonary artery. Aortic EC are audible over the entire precordium and are transmitted to the carotid vessels as well. They show little variation with respiration. On the other hand, pulmonary EC are most audible along the left upper sternal border and become louder during expiration. They may become soft or even disappear altogether during inspiration. The EC occur due to abrupt cessation of the systolic motion of the dome-shaped, stenotic aortic and pulmonary valves. In aortic stenosis, EC coincide with the anacrotic notch of the aortic pressure curve. In aortic and pulmonary valvular stenosis, as the valves become stiff, calcified, and immobile, EC tend to disappear. Ejection clicks also occur in conditions causing dilatation of the ascending aorta (aneurysm, coarctation, hypertension, aortic regurgitation, tetralogy of Fallot) and the pulmonary artery (pulmonary hypertension, idiopathic dilatation of the pulmonary artery).

Nonejection clicks (midsystolic clicks) (MSC) are abnormal, high-frequency sharp clicks occurring in early, middle, or late systole. They are loudest over the apex or left lower sternal border. These sounds may be an isolated finding or may be followed by a late systolic murmur. Sometimes MSC is heard only in the left lateral position. Squatting and hand grip move the MSC toward S_2, whereas standing and Valsalva's maneuver move the MSC toward S_1. A midsystolic click arises from the sudden tension on the chordae tendinae or sudden halt of the prolapsing mitral valve leaflet during ventricular systole.

Sounds of an Artificial Valve Prosthesis

A ball valve prosthesis such as a Starr-Edwards valve produces loud, crisp opening and closing sounds. For example, in the mitral position it will give rise to a closing sound that comprises the loudest component of S_1 and an opening sound that follows the A_2. On the other hand, a Bjork-Shiley valve prosthesis, the most commonly used disk type prosthesis, produces an extremely soft opening sound and a loud closing sound. One should become familiar with the characteristics of these sounds, since a change in the timing or intensity of these sounds indicates prosthesic malfunction.

Pacemaker Sound

In some patients with electronic pacemakers, an extra sound just preceding S_1 may be heard. This sound occurs about 3.5 milliseconds following pacemaker spike and is presumably due to stimulation of the intercostal muscles.

Heart Murmurs

A prolonged series of audible vibrations constitutes a heart murmur. It results from vibrations set up in the cardiohemic system, that is, the blood stream, valve structures, and walls of the cardiac chambers and great vessels. Heart murmurs have been attributed to one or more of the following factors:

1. Augmented flow through normal or obstructed valves
2. Antegrade flow through narrow and/or irregular valve openings
3. Retrograde or regurgitant flow through incompetent valves
4. Blood flow through septal defects or arteriovenous communications

While listening to a murmur, the following features should be defined: timing in cardiac cycle, intensity, frequency (pitch), radiation, duration, and quality. Heart murmurs are traditionally classified as systolic, diastolic, and continuous murmurs. The intensity and frequency of a murmur are determined by the velocity of flow across the valve or septal defect; the higher the velocity, the greater the loudness and pitch. Decreased velocity due to congestive heart failure results in a softening of all heart murmurs except for a murmur of papillary muscle dysfunction. Freeman and Levine arbitrarily divided the intensity of murmurs into six grades. A grade 1 murmur is extremely faint and heart only after the examiner has auscultated for a while. A grade 2 murmur is faint, but is easily heart immediately after placing the diaphragm of a stethoscope on the chest wall. Grade 3 is moderately loud but is not associated with a thrill. Grade 4 is a loud murmur generally associated with a thrill, which is the palpatory counterpart of the murmur. Grade 5 is a very loud murmur that is audible when the edge of the diaphragm is in contact with the skin, and a grade 6 murmur is heard even when the diaphragm is removed from, but close to, the chest wall. The radiation, quality, and duration will be described for each individual murmur.

Systolic Murmurs

Systolic murmurs are further categorized according to their duration and relationship to S_1 and S_2.

Pansystolic or holosystolic murmurs occupy the entire systole, usually masking S_1 and S_2. This type of murmur is characteristically audible in rheumatic mitral regurgitation, ventricular septal defect, and tricuspid regurgitation associated with pulmonary hypertension. In these conditions, since the pressure difference between the two chambers is established very early in systole, the murmur covers S_1. Also, since the pressure difference persists until after the A_2, the murmur also masks A_2. A large pressure difference between these two chambers causes a high velocity regurgitant stream (or left-to-right shunt in a ventricular septal defect) throughout systole; the resultant murmur, therefore, is loud, high frequency and blowing in quality with a plateau-like configuration.

A mid-systolic ejection murmur occupies only the ejection portion of the systole. Ejection starts with opening of the semilunar valves following S_1; there is a distinct gap between S_1 and the start of the ejection murmur. This murmur is typically diamond shaped (crescendo-decrescendo) and ends before the semilunar valve closure. The midsystolic murmurs are heard in the following conditions: left ventricular outflow obstruction (valvular, supravalvular, subvalvular); right ventricular outflow obstruction (valvular, infundibular); increased systolic flow through the semilunar valves, for example, augmented systolic flow across the pulmonary valve in an atrial septal defect, increased systolic flow across the aortic valve in aortic incompetence, and across both the aortic and pulmonary valves in various hyperkinetic states such as thyrotoxicosis, anemia, and pregnancy. As already mentioned, a vast majority of midsystolic murmurs originate at the semilunar valves. In some cases, mitral regurgitation due to papillary muscle dysfunction may give rise to a midsystolic murmur.

Early systolic murmurs start with S_1 and end by midsystole due to a marked decrease or cessation of flow. Early systolic murmurs are audible in the following conditions:

- Small ventricular septal defect in the muscular septum. The murmur ends as the defect closes in mid or late systole.
- Large ventricular septal defect with pulmonary hypertension.
- Acute mitral regurgitation, which occurs when the left atrial pressure rises rapidly, limiting the velocity of regurgitation in the latter part of systole; the murmur is confined to early systole.
- Mild mitral regurgitation due to papillary muscle dysfunction is usually seen in patients with coronary artery disease.
- Tricuspid regurgitation without pulmonary hypertension as is seen in infective endocarditis of the tricuspid valve in drug addicts.

Late systolic murmurs occur in the later part of systole, well after the onset of ejection and end in A_2. These murmurs may or may not be preceded by a midsystolic click. Late systolic murmurs are most audible over the apex and indicate late systolic mitral regurgitation due to mitral valve leaflet prolapse or papillary muscle dysfunction. A late systolic murmur tends to become louder and longer with Valsalva's maneuver or during upright posture. On the other hand, a squatting posture or hand grip make the murmur shorter.

Peculiar muscle sounds described occasionally as systolic whoops or honks are audible over the apex in mid or late systole. These sounds also have been attributed to abnormalities of mitral valve apparatus.

Diastolic Murmurs

The diastolic murmurs are categorized as early, middle, or late (presystolic).

Early diastolic regurgitant murmurs are present typically in aortic and pulmonary incompetence with pulmonary hypertension. As soon as the ventricular pressure falls below the aortic or pulmonary pressure, regurgitation starts through the closed but incompetent semilunar valves. This explains the beginning of these murmurs with A_2 or P_2 without any delay. Since the pressure difference between the aorta and the left ventricle (or pulmonary artery and right ventricle) progressively decreases as the diastole proceeds, causing a reduced rate of regurgitation, these murmurs are typically decrescendo in nature. These murmurs have an unusually high frequency and extra effort may be required to detect them. Listening with a rigid diaphragm firmly applied on the mid-left sternal border in a patient sitting and leaning forward, the breath held in full expiration, will elicit an aortic regurgitation murmur. The murmur of rheumatic aortic regurgitation is heard best over the mid-left sternal border. On the other hand, in aortic regurgitation due to lesions, which cause marked dilatation of the aortic root (aneurysm, dissection, ankylosing spondylitis), the murmur is most audible over the right sternal border. Increase in systemic vascular resistance (hand grip, squatting, or phenylephrine) accentuates the aortic regurgitation flow and the murmur. Decrease in systemic vascular resistance (amyl nitrite, nitroglycerine, nitroprusside infusion, hydralazine) decreases the aortic regurgitant flow and the intensity of the murmur. The murmur of pulmonary regurgitation due to pulmonary hypertension (Graham Steell's murmur) is similar with the exception that a pulmonary regurgitation murmur becomes louder during inspiration and is heard best in the left upper sternal border.

Mid and late diastolic filling murmurs are caused by increased diastolic flow across normal mitral and tricuspid valves, or normal diastolic flow across stenosed or distorted mitral and tricuspid valves. Rapid ventricular filling occurs in two phases during diastole, that is, shortly after the mitral and tricuspid valves open (protodiastole) and during late diastole (presystole) due to atrial contraction; filling murmurs tend to be prominent during these phases. After closure of the aortic and pulmonary valves, the mitral and tricuspid valves must open before rapid filling starts; there is a considerable period of silence between A_2 and P_2 and start of the middiastolic flow rumble. Middiastolic flow rumbles are low frequency and are heard best with the bell of the stethoscope applied lightly to the chest wall. The middiastolic filling rumbles due to increased flow across normal atrioventricular valves have a short duration and are usually preceded by an S_3. In a large ventricular septal defect, patent ductus arteriosus, and mitral regurgitation, increased diastolic flow across a normal mitral orifice gives rise to an audible diastolic rumble over the apex. On the other hand, in a large atrial septal defect or tricuspid regurgitation, augmented diastolic flow across the tricuspid valve results in a middiastolic rumble over the left lower sternal edge. A right-sided diastolic filling murmur becomes louder during inspiration.

In acute rheumatic fever, mitral valve leaflets become edematous and distorted due to valvulitis. Diastolic flow across the distorted but wide open mitral orifice may cause a short middiastolic rumble, which is called a Carey-Coombs murmur.

A long mid and late diastolic (presystolic) rumble occurs in mitral stenosis. This murmur is low frequency, is usually preceded by an opening snap, and does not radiate widely. A left lateral position and light application of the stethoscope's bell to the region of apical impulse will facilitate the detection of this murmur. Minimal exercise like five or six deep coughs may increase its intensity. The duration of the rumble has a direct relationship to the severity of mitral stenosis: in mild stenosis the rumble is short, whereas in severe stenosis the murmur occupies practically the total diastole. Also, the murmur becomes louder in late diastole, reaching its peak intensity at the time of a loud S_1. This presystolic accentuation of the mitral stenosis murmur is ascribed to forceful atrial contraction. When atrial fibrillation develops, this presystolic accentuation of the murmur disappears. Enhanced diastolic flow across the mitral valve during amyl nitrite inhalation or exercise accentuates the rumble of mitral stenosis.

The murmur of tricuspid stenosis is audible at the left lower sternal border, and is accentuated during inspiration. Other features of the murmur resemble those of a mitral stenosis rumble.

A left or right atrial myxoma may obstruct the mitral or tricuspid valve orifice, respectively, giving rise to a mid and/or late diastolic rumble simulating that of mitral stenosis.

An Austin Flint murmur is a low frequency middiastolic or presystolic rumble audible in some patients with wide open aortic regurgitation. A third sound may initiate this murmur, which has been ascribed to vibrations of the anterior mitral valve leaflet sandwiched between the aortic regurgitant stream on one side and blood flowing across the mitral valve orifice on the other side.

Continuous Murmurs

Continuous murmurs occur when there is a large and persistent pressure difference throughout the cardiac cycle, which may occur in the following instances: between two communicating chambers or vessels with no intervening valve or across a severely stenosed segment of an artery. Typically, a continuous murmur begins in systole and continues without any interruption or change in character into diastole. These murmurs usually peak at the occurrence of S_2. A continous murmur is a hallmark of patent ductus arteriosus. The diastolic portion of the murmur disappears after the development of pulmonary hypertension. Other common examples of continuous murmurs are rupture of a Valsalva's sinus aneurysm into the right heart chambers, bronchial collaterals, severe coarctation of the aorta, and systemic, pulmonary, and coronary arteriovenous fistulae. It is important to differentiate a continuous murmur from coexistent systolic and diastolic murmurs, which are present in a ventricular septal defect with aortic regurgitation, and mitral and aortic regurgitation. In the latter examples, the systolic and diastolic murmurs sound to and fro because of their different character. There is also a silent gap between the end of the systolic murmur and the beginning of the diastolic murmur. On the other hand, as mentioned earlier, a continuous murmur is uninterrupted and possesses the same character throughout.

Cervical venous hum is a continous murmur audible over the right supraclavicular region in children and in adults with hyperkinetic circulation. The diastolic component of the venous hum is the loudest component. A venous hum is abolished by digital compression of the internal jugular vein on the same side and is accentuated by turning the head leftward and upward in a sitting position. This murmur is innocent by itself; however, at times it may radiate below the clavicle and simulate the murmur of patent ductus arteriosus.

Pericardial Friction Rub

A pericardial friction rub is a superficial scratching noise heard over the precordium in acute pericarditis. Faint rubs are heard best in a patient sitting up and leaning forward. It may have systolic, early diastolic and/or late diastolic (presystolic) components.

Effects of Vasoactive Maneuvers and Drugs on Cardiac Murmurs

Certain physical maneuvers and drugs profoundly change the intensity of murmurs by their vasoactive effects. These physical maneuvers should be exploited at the bedside in the differential diagnosis of various heart murmurs. The use of vasoactive drugs is reserved for the phonocardiographic laboratory.

Valsalva's Maneuver. During the straining phase the venous return to the heart decreases, causing shrinkage of the right and left ventricles and diminished stroke volumes. The smaller left ventricular cavity produces greater obstruction of the outflow tract in idiopathic hypertrophic subaortic stenosis (IHSS) leading to a louder systolic murmur. In mitral valve prolapse syndrome (MVP), the smaller left ventricular cavity causes earlier and greater slackening of the chordae. This allows a greater degree of mitral valve prolapse and hence a greater degree of regurgitation. This will result in a louder murmur with an earlier start in systole. All other murmurs decrease with Valsalva's maneuver.

Sustained Hand Grip (Isometric Exercise). Elevated arterial pressure during sustained hand grip offers greater resistance (impedance) to ventricular emptying during systole. This results in an accentuation of the murmur of a ventricular septal defect, aortic regurgitation, and rheumatic mitral regurgitation. On the other hand, murmurs due to IHSS and aortic stenosis decrease.

Dynamic Exercise. This maneuver increases the cardiac output. Augmented flow results in increased intensity of murmurs caused by stenosis of the mitral, aortic, tricuspid, and pulmonic valves.

Change in Posture. Slightly increased heart rate and flow rate across the mitral orifice when turning from a supine to the left lateral position accentuates the rumble of mitral stenosis. This position also favors left atrial myxoma obstruction of the mitral valve orifice, which results in a diastolic rumble. Sometimes the midsystolic click related to mitral valve prolapse can also be heard better in this position.

Lying flat with passive leg raising increases suddenly the venous return to the heart, resulting in greater stroke volume. Murmurs of aortic and pulmonary stenosis and ventricular gallops become louder with this maneuver.

Squatting suddenly from a standing posture results in greater venous return and elevated systemic vascular resistance with an increase of arterial pressure. Both factors result in an enlarged left ventricular chamber size. Murmurs of the IHSS and MVP type decrease, whereas murmurs of aortic regurgitation, rheumatic mitral regurgitation, and a ventricualr septal defect become loud. An aortic stenosis murmur is variably affected.

Assumption of upright posutre from squatting causes venous pooling in the legs. The left ventricular cavity size becomes smaller. This leads to accentuation of IHSS and MVP murmurs, and softening of murmurs of aortic and pulmonary stenosis.

The effect of phases of respiration and ectopic beats on the murmurs should also be determined. Right heart murmurs such as tricuspid stenosis, tricuspid regurgitation, and pulmonic regurgitation, increase during inspiration. Midsystolic ejection murmurs from the semilunar valves show a significant increase during the postectopic beat or after a long pause in atrial fibrillation. On the other hand, a mitral regurgitation murmur does not vary with different cycle lengths in atrial fibrillation or during a postectopic beat. This difference is very helpful in deciding the origin of a systolic murmur that is audible over the cardaic apex.

The effects of vasopressor and vasodilator agents on various murmurs is described in Table 1.

Table 1. Effect of Vasoactive Agents on Heart Murmurs

Murmur	*Vasodilator (amyl nitrite)*	*Vasopressor (phenylephrine)*
Rheumatic mitral regurgitation	↓	↑
Aortic regurgitation	↓	↑
Ventricular septal defect	↓	↑
Tetralogy of Fallot	↓	↑
Idiopathic hypertrophic subaortic stenosis	↑	↓
Mitral valve prolapse	↑	↓
Mitral stenosis	↑	-
Tricuspid stenosis	↑	-
Aortic stenosis	↑	↓ or -
Pulmonic stenosis	↑	-

↓ = Decrease; ↑ = Increase; - = No change

ELECTROCARDIOGRAPHY

Electrocardiography is the most widely used diagnostic test in cardiology. The electrocardiograph records electrical changes occurring in the heart, and the resulting graph is called an electrocardiogram (ECG). For a better understanding of the ECG changes in various heart diseases, it is important to be familiar with basic electrophysiology and the sequence of depolarization and repolarization of the entire heart.

BASIC ELECTROPHYSIOLOGY

In the resting or polarized state, the inside of the myocardial cell is electrically negative by −92 mV as compared to the outside. This is called resting membrane potential (RMP) and is due to 20-fold concentration of K^+ inside the cell as compared to the outside. On stimulation (activation or depolarization), the inside of the cell rapidly becomes positive (+ 20 mV) (Fig. 1). This initial phase of action potential is called phase 0, which results from a sudden influx of Na^+ into the cell through a specific Na^+ channel (fast channel) in the cell membrane. Phase 0 is followed by phase 1 (initial repolarization), during which the potential falls from +20 to +0 mV; that, in turn is followed by phase 2, or the plateau phase. Phase 2 indicates slow repolarization and is attributable predominantly to a Ca^{2+} influx. It is followed by phase 3, indicating rapid repolarization that occurs due to the efflux of K^+ from the cell enabling the potential to return to RMP. During phase 4, the sodium pump actively causes an efflux of Na^+ and influx of K^+ maintaining the cell in its resting, or polarized, state. It is now ready for the next depolarization. During the time interval from the initiation of depolarization (phase 0) to midway of phase 3, the cell is unexcitable (absolute refractory period). During the latter part of phase 3, the cell can be depolarized or excited by a suprathreshold stimulus (relative refractory period). These are typical features of an action potential of working myocardial cells. Normally, these myocardial cells do not generate an impulse. Pacemaker cells, on the other hand, spontaneously generate an electric impulse and are present in the sinus node, atrioventricular junction (AVJ), and His-Purkinje system. The action potential of these cells is different from that of working myocardial cells. In pacemaker cells, during phase 4 the resting membrane potential slowly drifts upward and, as soon as the threshold (−60 mV) is reached, the action potential results. This slowly rising potential during phase 4 is called spontaneous diastolic depolarization and is characteristic of all pacemaker or automatic cells. Normally,

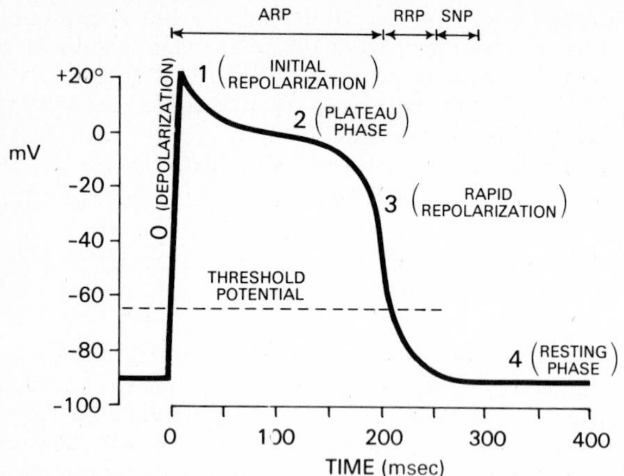

Figure 1. Idealized transmembrane action potential of a myocardial cell. It is characterized by a resting transmembrane potential (phase 4) at −92 mV. On excitation, the transmembrane potential is lowered to threshold potential resulting in depolarization (phase 0). This is followed by repolarization, which has three phases: initial repolarization (phase 1), plateau phase (phase 2), and rapid repolarization (phase 3), which returns the cell to resting transmembrane potential (phase 4). During phases 1, 2, and early phase 3, the myocardial cell is completely unexcitable (ARP = absolute refractory period). During late phase 3, the cell is excitable by a strong stimulus (RRP = relative refractory period). During the last portion of phase 3, a subthreshold stimulus can excite the cell (SNP = supernormal period).

the action potential arising from a sinus node sets up a chain reaction and depolarizes the entire heart.

Normally, the cardiac impulse arises in the sinus node that is located in the right atrium near its junction with the superior vena cava. The impulse travels through the anterior, middle, and posterior internodal tracts, connecting the sinus and atrioventricular (AV) nodes. The anterior internodal tract sends a branch to the left atrium. Whether the impulse travels only through these tracts or over the atrial musculature as well is still controversial. The AV node is located in the right atrium between the opening of the coronary sinus and attachment of the septal leaflet of the tricuspid valve. The impulse transmission through the AV node is slow (50 mm/s) and complex. Upon reaching this structure, the impulse undergoes sudden slowing (decremental conduction) and, after approximately 60-100 ms, enters the His-Purkinje system. The depolarization of sinus and AV nodal cells is dependent predominantly on Ca^{2+} influx during phase 0 (slow channel). The AV node is continuous with the His bundle that is present on the right side of the membranous ventricular septum. As it reaches the muscular portion of the ventricular septum, the His bundle continues as a slender right bundle following the right side of the ventricular septum to the apex of the right ventricle and then enters the moderator band. A large number of branches (left bundle) from the His bundle penetrate the membranous ventricular septum below the aortic ring to enter the left ventricle, where they are grouped into anterior and posterior fascicles of the left bundle. All three fascicles, that is, the right-bundle and anterior and posterior left-bundle fascicles, break into numerous Purkinje fibers that are distributed over the endocardial surfaces of the two ventricles. From the AV node, the impulse travels rapidly (2,000-3,000 mm/s) over the His-Purkinje system; thereafter, conduction from the endocardium to the epicardium is relatively slow (200-500 mm/s). The middle portion of the ventricular septum is activated from left to right, followed sequentially by the lower septum, right ventricular apex, right ventricular free wall, left ventricular free wall, and bases of both the ventricles. The outflow tract of the right ventricle, or crista supraventricularis, is the last portion of the heart to be activated.

Repolarization follows the same pathway as depolarization with the exception of the ventricular wall. In the ventricular wall, the sequence of repolarization is from the epicardium to the endocardium, which is opposite to the depolarization sequence. Exposure of the endocardium to high intraventricular pressure and differences in blood supply of the subendocardial and subepicardial muscle layers are probably responsible for this difference in sequence of depolarization and repolarization.

The normal rate of impulse formation in the sinus node is 60-100 beats/min. The sinus node is controlled by the sympathetic and parasympathetic nervous system. If there is no impulse from the sinus node, the AV junction depolarizes the heart at a rate of 40-60 beats/min. If both the sinus node and AV junction fail, the cells in the His-Purkinje system will respond automatically and drive the heart at 20-40 beats/min.

Electrocardiographic Leads

The electrocardiogram is recorded by connecting electrodes from the electrocardiograph to standard parts of the body. Einthoven proposed that the body acts as a volume conductor for the electrical changes produced by the heart, which is located at the center. He popularized three standard bipolar leads: lead I records the potential difference between the left arm (LA) and right arm (RA), *lead II* between the left leg (LL) and RA, and *lead III* between LL and LA. The positive and negative sides of the leads were devised to record upright complexes in all three leads in normal subjects. The electrode connected to the right leg acts as an inactive ground. Wilson later devised the unipolar leads: in this system, RA, LA, and LL are connected through high resistance to a single central terminal that has roughly 0 potential and acts as an indifferent electrode. The second electrode, the exploring electrode, is attached to RA and records V_R, LA records V_L, and LL records V_F leads. To augment the amplitude of various ECG waves, Goldberg temporarily disconnected its indifferent electrode from the limb being recorded. These augmented leads are referred to as aV_R, aV_L, and aV_F. The three augmented leads and three standard limb leads make a hexa-axial system. The precordial leads are recorded by placing the exploring electrode over the anterior chest wall. The exploring electrode is positioned in the fourth intercostal space at the right parasternal line for lead V_1, and the left parasternal line for lead V_2; the fifth left intercostal space at the midclavicular line for V_4; between positions V_2 and V_4 for V_3; at the anterior axillary line for V_5; and midaxillary line for V_6 in a horizontal line from V_4. The three standard bipolar leads I, II, and III, and three augmented unipolar leads aV_R, aV_L, and aV_F, give frontal plane representation; six unipolar precordial leads give horizontal or transverse representation.

The direction and spatial orientation of the electrical force has a profound effect on the configuration of the ECG waveforms in a given lead. Conventionally, an electrical force coming toward a lead is recorded as positive in that lead, and one directed away from the lead is recorded as negative. In addition, if the electrical force is parallel to the lead, the recorded wave will show maximal amplitude; whereas an electrical force that is perpendicular to the lead may show no voltage deflection.

Electrical Axis

Since the millions of myocardial cells are depolarized in all directions, most of the electrical activity is canceled out; the surface ECG records only the net resultant electrical force. Since the entire heart is depolarized in sequence, the direction (axis) of depolarization changes from moment to moment. The overall, or mean, axis of the total depolarization of atria (mean P axis), ventricles (mean QRS axis), and ventricular repolarization (mean T axis) in the frontal plan can be calculated from the standard six leads, that is, I, II, III, aV_R, aV_L, and aV_F. In clinical electrocardiography, the mean QRS axis is more important than the P and T axes. The method of computing the mean QRS axis in the frontal plane is described below: The resultant positive or negative values from leads I and aV_F are plotted appropriately on the leads. The perpendiculars defines the mean axis of QRS (Fig. 2).

The mean QRS axis in a normal subject lies between -30° and $+110^\circ$. The axis in a -30° to -90° range is described as an abnormal left axis deviation. An abnormal right axis deviation is from $+110^\circ$ to $+180^\circ$. The axis in the right upper quadrant, that is, from -90° to $+180^\circ$, could represent an abnormal right or left axis deviation.

During the first year of life, the mean QRS axis is usually between $+90^\circ$ and $+150^\circ$. With increasing age, the axis shifts leftward. Thus, in an older person, an axis of $+100^\circ$ is probably abnormal, even though it is still within the arbitrary normal range. By contrast, an axis of 0° in a child is abnormal. A left axis deviation occurs in inferior myocardial infarction and left anterior hemiblock. A right axis deviation is found in right ventricular hypertrophy, lateral wall infarction, and left posterior hemiblock.

Normal Electrocardiogram

A normal ECG consists of a sequence of P, QRS, and T waves. The ECG is recorded on graph paper for rapid measurements of time intervals and amplitudes. The thin lines are 1 mm apart and the thick lines are 5 mm apart. At a standard speed of 25

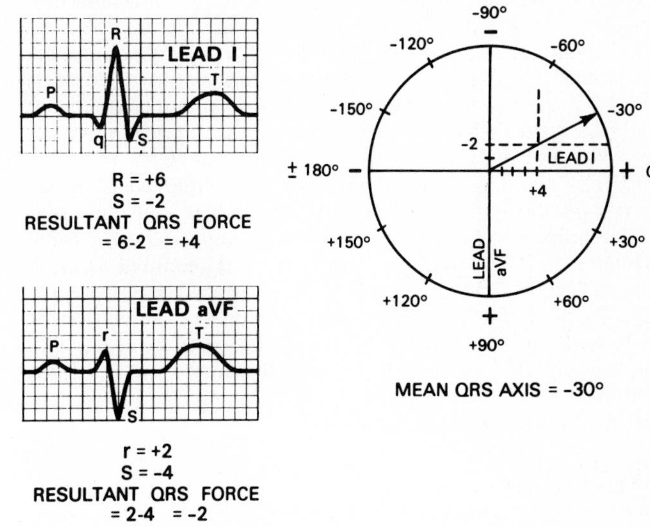

Figure 2. Method of calculating mean QRS axis. The resultant positive or negative forces from leads I and aV_F are plotted on the respective lead axes. Perpendiculars are drawn as shown by dotted lines. The line connecting the center with the point where the perpendiculars intersect represents the mean QRS axis.

mm/s, the interval between vertical thin lines is 0.04 seconds. At standard calibration, a 1 mm height is equal to 0.1 mV.

P Wave

Depolarization of the atrial musculature results in a P wave. As the impulse from the sinus node travels inferiorly and leftward, leads I, II, III, aV_L, and aV_F usually record an upright P wave. Lead aV_R records a negative P wave since the impulse is traveling away from this lead. In the precordial leads, the P wave is positive except for V_1, which may be positive, negative, or biphasic. A normal P wave is <2.5 mm in amplitude and <0.10 in width. The initial portion of the P wave represents right atrial and the terminal portion represents left atrial depolarization.

P-R Interval

The P-R interval is measured from the start of the P wave to the beginning of the QRS complex. It indicates the time from start of atrial depolarization to the beginning of ventricular activation. Normally, the P-R interval is 0.12-0.20 seconds. Most of the conduction delay occurs in the AV node. The P-R interval is affected by heart rate: At slower heart rates, it is longer; at rapid rates, it is shorter within the normal range.

QRS Complex

The first negative wave after a P wave is the Q wave, and the first positive wave after a P wave is the R wave. An S wave is the first negative wave after the R wave. The QRS complex represents depolarization of the ventricular musculature. Configuration of the QRS complex is variable in different leads. The initial portion of the QRS complex reflects depolarization of the left midseptum; this electrical force is directed to the right and anteriorly. It is recorded as a small R wave (<5 mm) in V_1 and a small Q wave (<2 mm) in leads I, aV_L, V_5, and V_6. The main portion of the QRS complex represents depolarization of the free ventricular walls. Since the left ventricular muscle mass is greater than the right ventricular muscle mass, the main resultant depolarization force is oriented leftward and posteriorly. This is recorded as an R wave in leads I, aV_L, V_5, and V_6, and as an S wave in leads aV_R, V_1, and V_2. The terminal S wave reflects activation of the base of the heart and right ventricular outflow tract. The duration of QRS complex is 0.06-0.10 seconds and indicates the time period between initiation and completion of ventricular depolarization.

ST Segment

The ST segment is the isoelectric portion between the S and T waves. This segment denotes the period of time that the ventricles are partially depolarized, corresponding to phase 2 of the action potential.

T and U Waves

The T wave reflects rapid repolarization of the ventricles. After the T wave, another positive wave (U) is sometimes seen, especially in the midprecordial leads. Some investigators have attributed the U wave to repolarization of the papillary muscles. The repolarization of the atria produces a negative T wave that is difficult to identify because it is hidden by the QRS complex.

ELECTROCARDIOGRAPHIC DIAGNOSIS

Myocardial Ischemia, Injury, and Infarction

Decreased coronary perfusion results in regional myocardial ischemia. If this perfusion deficiency is severe and prolonged, the affected myocardium progresses from a stage of reversible ischemia to a stage of reversible injury and then to infarction, which is reversible at a very early stage but soon becomes irreversible. The terms ischemia, injury, and infarction are used here in the electrical sense. Generally, there are no histologic changes during ischemia, injury, and early myocardial infarction (MI). As ischemia persists, the central portion of the affected region, which is most deprived of a blood supply, becomes necrotic. This necrotic region is surrounded by injured tissue that, in turn, is surrounded by ischemic tissue.

The earliest ECG change during the evolution of a transmural MI is in the T wave. In the leads facing the infarcting region, the T wave becomes tall and spiked (hyperacute T wave), probably due to ischemia at the subendocardial layer of the myocardium. This change is very early and short-lived, and is therefore overlooked in most patients.

The next ECG change that occurs after the hyperacute T-wave change is elevation of of the ST segment in leads facing the infarcting region. Reciprocal depression of the ST segment , recorded in the opposite leads. An electrical gradient between the injured myocardial cells and the adjoining healthy cells develops in the subepicardial layers, and is responsible for ST segment elevation. At this stage, the T wave is usually obscured by the elevated ST segment. ST segment elevation lasts from a few hours to a week or more, becoming isoelectric by 2 weeks at the most.

A few hours to a few days after the onset of ST segment elevation, a pathologic Q wave appears in the leads facing the infarcted zone. Since the infarcted muscle is electrically inert, the initial QRS vector is directed away from it and is recorded as a negative Q wave. The Q wave persists for months, years, or indefinitely, and serves as an ECG sign of an old scar.

As the ST segment regresses toward the isoelectric line, a symmetrically inverted T wave becomes more clear. The T-wave inversion reflects transmural ischemia. This change persists for several months to years. Thus, ST segment elevation is the only ECG sign of acute myocardial injury and, when accompanied by the development of a new Q wave, indicates an acute transmural MI. The ECG may not show any changes during very early stages of an MI and should be repeated daily for at least 3 days to determine if the evolutionary changes described above develop in patients with a history compatible with an acute MI.

Standard 12-lead ECG permits approximate localization of an infarction. Infarction changes in leads V_1 and V_2 indicate an anteroseptal MI; in V_3 and V_4, a midanterior MI; in leads I, aV_L, V_5, and V_6, an anterolateral MI; in leads I, av_L, and V_1 through V_6, an extensive anterior MI; and in leads II, III, and aV_F, an inferior or diaphragmatic MI. In cases of a true posterior MI, leads V_1 and V_2 register a tall and broad R wave and an upright T wave, since these leads are separated from the infarcted region by the healthy anterior wall. Subendocardial infarction produces ST segment depression and T inversion without pathologic Q waves.

There are several limitations in the ECG diagnosis of an MI. ECG changes occur in approximately 80 percent of patients with an MI. In the presence of conduction defects like LBBB and Wolff-Parkinson-White (WPW) syndrome, MI changes are not apparent. In patients with multiple infarcts in the past, electrical forces may counterbalance one another and a new infarct may not produce any ECG changes. An ECG may show no changes with infarction of the left ventricular apex, high lateral wall, or a small infarction anywhere in the myocardium.

It is important to recognize a pattern of early repolarization that occurs in some young healthy subjects. It is more common in blacks. It consists of ST segment elevation, mostly in leads I, aV_L, and V_4 through V_6. The ST segment is concave upward and starts from the descending limb of the R wave before it reaches the baseline. By contrast, an elevated ST segment representing injury is convex upward.

Hypertrophy of Heart Chambers

Left Atrial Hypertrophy

The P wave becomes >2.5 mm wide and shows double peaks, the second peak representing left atrial depolarization. As the

P axis shifts leftward (−30 to +45°), a double-peaked P wave is best seen in leads I, II, aV_L, and V_4 through V_6. In lead V_1, the P wave is biphasic and the terminal negative component is deep and wide (>0.04 mm-s). Electrocardiographic changes of left atrial hypertrophy are commonly seen in conditions with impaired left ventricular compliance such as aortic stenosis, hypertension, coronary heart disease, and cardiomyopathy, as well as in mitral valve disease.

Right Atrial Hypertrophy
The P waves become tall (>2.5 mm) and spiked usually in leads II, III, aV_F, and V_1. The P axis shifts to the right (> +75°). Right atrial hypertrophy most commonly occurs secondary to right ventricular hypertrophy (pulmonary stenosis, pulmonary hypertension, cor pulmonale) and tricuspid stenosis.

Left Ventricular Hypertrophy (LVH)
Increased left ventricular mass results in greater amplitude of QRS complex. However, voltage criteria alone may give false positive result for LVH especially in thin chested individuals. Estes has, therefore, described a point scoring system to diagnose LVH as follows:

- Three points for:

  R and/or S > 20 mm in any one or more of the six limb leads

  or

  S in V_1, V_2, or V_3 > 25 mm

  or

  R in V_4, V_5, or V_6 > 25 mm
- Three points for ST segment deviation opposite to main QRS complex, provided the patient is not taking digitalis. If patient is on digitalis, ST segment change counts for one point.
- Two points for left axis deviation > −15°
- One point for QRS duration > 0.09 second
- One point for ventricular activation time > 0.04 second

A sum of 4 points indicates probable LVH and 5 or more points is considered diagnostic of LVH.

Right Ventricular Hypertrophy (RVH)
RVH is diagnosed on the basis of one or more of the following features:

Right axis deviation (>+110°)

R/S ratio in lead V_1 of >1 (provided R in V_1 is >5 mm)

R in V_1 ⩾7 mm

R in V_1 plus in V_5 or V_6 ⩾10.5 mm

Secondary ST depression and T inversion in leads V_1 and V_2 (RV strain)

Clockwise rotation, that is, persistence of a prominent S in V_5 and V_6.

In infants less than 6 months of age, the ECG normally shows RVH; however, this pattern gradually regresses with increasing age.

Acute Pericarditis

In this condition, both layers of the pericardium and the adjacent subepicardial layer of the myocardium become inflamed. Since virtually all the leads face the injured subepicardium, occurrence of injury (ST elevation) is recorded in all leads except aV_R and V_1. As the inflammation subsides several days later, the ST segments return to baseline and the T waves then become inverted. It is extremely important to differentiate these changes from those of infarction. In infarction, an elevated ST is convex upward; there is reciprocal ST depression in some leads; ST elevation and inverted T coexist, and evolution is somewhat rapid. In acute pericarditis elevated ST is concave upward, there is no reciprocal ST depression, T becomes inverted only after ST returns to baseline, and evolutionary changes are slow.

Electrolyte Disturbances and Drug Effects

In hyperkalemia, the T waves become tall and spiked. With an increasing degree of hyperkalemia, the P waves become less distinct and may totally disappear, the QRS complex widens, and ultimately QRS-T assumes the configuration of a sine wave.

Hypokalemia produces depression of the ST segment, T flattening, and prominence of U and P waves. As T becomes less distinct, it merges into the U wave, and the Q-T interval (actually Q-U) is prolonged. In severe hypokalemia, widening of the QRS occurs.

In hypocalcemia, the QRS and T appear normal, but the ST segment is prolonged. On the other hand, hypercalcemia shortens the ST segment.

Digitalis produces a sagging or hammock-shaped depression of the ST segment, flattening or inversion of the T wave, and shortening of the Q-T interval. These changes may be seen even with a therapeutic dose and constitute the digitalis effect.

Pronestyl and quinidine prolong the Q-T interval and cause flattening or inversion of the T wave and widening of the QRS.

In neurologic conditions like head trauma and subarachnoid hemorrhage, an ECG may show bizarre, wide and tall, or deeply inverted T waves with Q-T prolongation.

OTHER NONINVASIVE TECHNIQUES OF CARDIAC DIAGNOSIS

ROENTGENOGRAPHIC EXAMINATION

A standard chest roentgenogram, recorded in posteroanterior (PA) projection, 2 m or 6 ft from the x-ray tube, in an upright posture and during deep inspiration, permits a fairly accurate assessment of cardiac size and configuration as well as pulmonary vascularity. The cardiac size is expressed as a cardiothoracic ratio that is derived by dividing maximal transverse cardiac width (distance from outermost point of the right heart border to midline plus a similar distance from the left heart border) by maximal internal width of the thorax above the diaphragm. In normal subjects, the cardiothoracic ratio is less than 0.5. To assess the enlargement of individual cardiac chambers additional views, that is, left lateral (LL), right anterior oblique (RAO), and left anterior oblique (LAO) are needed. All four views are obtained after outlining the esophagus with barium (cardiac series). Various organ structures that border the cardiac silhouette in different projections and location of the cardiac valves are shown in Figure 3.

Left ventricular enlargement (LVE) is best judged from the PA, LAO, and LL views. In the PA view, the left heart border becomes more convex and the apex moves leftward and downward below the diaphragm. In the LAO and LL projections, the LV shadow overlays the spine. In addition, a greater than 2 cm distance between the inferior vena cava and posterior LV border in the LL view indicates LVE.

Right ventricular enlargement (RVE) is best visualized in the RAO, LAO, and LL views. Encroachment of retrosternal space by anterior bulging of the RV outflow tract in these views indicates RVE. In the PA view, RVE may cause upward tipping of the cardiac apex.

A modest degree of left atrial enlargement (LAE) is best seen in the RAO and LL views. In these views, the enlarged left atrium makes a definite dent in the barium-filled esophagus. Greater magnitude of LAE may result in one or more additional radiographic features: double shadows of the right atrium and LA in the PA view, appearance of an enlarged LA appendix just below the pulmonary trunk shadow on the left heart border in the PA view, widening of the carina and elevation of the left bronchus, which is visualized best in LAO and PA projections.

Right atrial enlargement (RAE) is suggested by the rightward extension of the right heart border in a PA projection.

It must be emphasized that because of overlap of these chambers, the reliability of determining individual chamber enlargement on chest x-ray is at best fair, especially when there is multiple chamber enlargement.

Dilatation of the pulmonary artery accentuates the shadow of the pulmonary artery segment seen on the left heart border in a PA view. This segment becomes prominent in the following conditions: increased pulmonary blood flow as seen in left-to-right shunts, pulmonary arterial hypertension, idiopathic dilatation of the pulmonary artery, and poststenotic dilatation in pulmonary valvular stenosis. A decrease in the pulmonary artery segment is recognized by increased concavity at its location on the left heart border in a PA view. This is seen in the tetralogy of Fallot, tricuspid atresia, and Ebstein's anomaly.

The thoracic aorta is customarily divided into three parts: the ascending aorta, the arch, and the descending aorta. The aorta may become dilated, tortuous, or frankly aneurysmal. In a PA projection, dilatation of the ascending aorta causes a prominent convexity of the right upper cardiac shadow above the right atrial shadow. This is seen in aortic valvular stenosis and aneurysms of the ascending aorta. Dilatation, elongation, and tortuosity of the aortic arch cause a prominent aortic

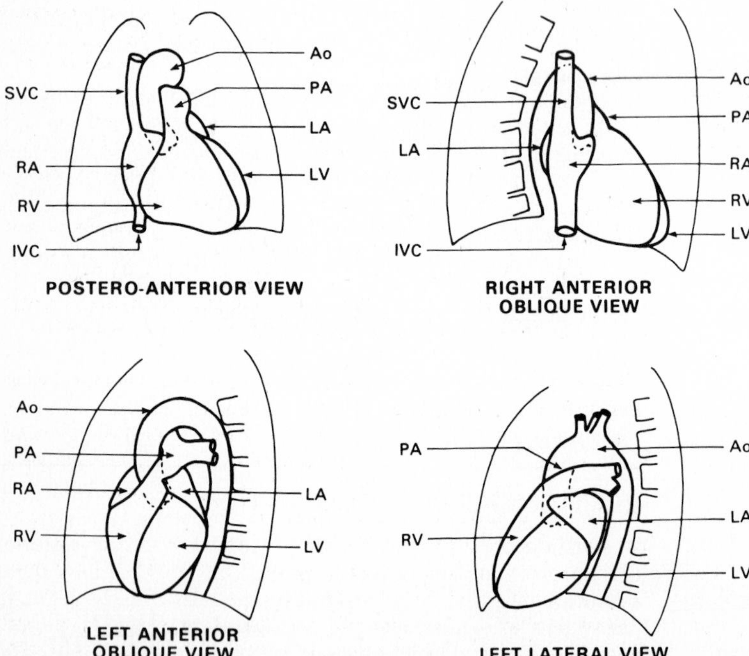

Figure 3. Appearance of various cardiac chambers and great vessels in posteroanterior, right anterior oblique, left anterior oblique, and left lateral views, SVC: superior vena cava; RA: right atrium; RV: right ventricular; IVC: inferior vena cava; AO: aorta; PA: pulmonary artery; LA: left atrium; LV: left ventricle.

knob shadow. The thoracic descending aorta is usually visualized through the cardiac silhouette, partially covering the vertebral column in a PA projection. Dilatation and tortuosity of the descending thoracic aorta results in a more leftward extension of this shadow. In an LAO projection, all three sections of the aorta may be visualized. Hypertension, arteriosclerosis, and aortic insufficiency produce dilatation of the aorta. The aorta is also enlarged in patent ductus arteriosus, tetralogy of Fallot, and tricuspid atresia.

A careful examination of lung fields in a chest x-ray is important in determining the status of pulmonary vascularity. The vascular shadows are produced by pulmonary arteries and veins. The differentiation of pulmonary arteries from veins in a chest x-ray is difficult, although it is somewhat easier in the right lung field. In general, upper lobe veins are lateral to the corresponding arteries. The lower lobe veins are medial to the arteries although they are more horizontal than the arteries.

The pulmonary veins in the lower lung fields are more prominent normally than in the upper lung fields. In left heart failure and mitral stenosis, as pulmonary venous hypertension develops the veins in the upper lung fields become more prominent than veins in the lower lung fields. This is usually described as redistribution of the pulmonary blood flow. When the pulmonary wedge pressure approaches 25-30 mm Hg, it exceeds the oncotic pressure of plasma proteins leading to exudation of fluid into the interstitial spaces of the lungs. The lung fields appear cloudy and the small pulmonary vascular markings are indistinct. In addition, Kerley's B lines appear: these are 1-2 cm thin horizontal lines present in the lower lung fields near the costophrenic angles. These lines are attributed to thickened interlobular septa due to edema or fibrosis. Fuzziness of the small pulmonary vascular markings, Kerley's B lines, and redistribution of the pulmonary blood flow are important early signs of left heart failure and pulmonary venous hypertension in mitral stenosis. With advance in the degree of left heart failure or increasing severity of mitral stenosis, fluid exudes into the alveoli and causes confluent opacities in the central lung fields resembling wings of a butterfly that is typical of pulmonary edema. With persistent heart failure, fluid accumulates in the interlobar fissures and/or causes pleural effusions.

Enlargement of the large central pulmonary arteries with abrupt tapering of their size peripherally indicates pulmonary arterial hypertension with increased pulmonary arterial resistance. This occurs in cor pulmonale, Eisenmenger's syndrome, and primary pulmonary hypertension. When severe pulmonary hypertension develops secondary to left heart disease, pulmonary veins as well as pulmonary arteries are prominent.

Increased pulmonary blood flow occurs in large left-to-right shunts, and both the pulmonary arteries and veins become prominent; however, both the central and peripheral arteries become enlarged and there is no sudden tapering in size of the peripheral arteries. Normally, the outer one-third of the lung fields do not show any vascular markings. However, in large left-to-right shunts, even these outer regions start showing prominent vascular markings.

Both the pulmonary arteries and the veins decrease in size when pulmonary blood flow is reduced. This occurs most commonly in conditions such as Fallot's tetralogy, in which there is right ventricular outflow tract obstruction and right-to-left shunt.

Various cardiac structures can undergo calcification. Fluoroscopy using image intensification is more sensitive in detecting calcification than a conventional chest x-ray. Calcification of the mitral valve is an important finding because it indicates prior rheumatic disease. On the other hand, calcification can occur in a congenitally biscuspid aortic valve as well as in a normal tricuspid valve damaged by rheumatic disease. Calcification of the pericardium occurs in approximately 50 percent of patients with constrictive pericarditis. Calcification may also occur in the wall of ventricular aneurysms, atrial myxoma, intracardiac blood clots, and walls of the coronary arteries.

ECHOCARDIOGRAPHY

Echocardiography is a diagnostic technique that employs pulsations of high frequency ultrasound to image directly the internal structures of the heart. Short bursts or pulses of high-frequency sound are produced by an electrically excited piezoelectric crystal that is applied to the chest wall. These sound waves pass through the chest wall and the underlying heart. As the sound encounters acoustic interfaces within the heart, such as the junction between the heart muscle and blood, part of the sound passes through the interface and part is reflected back toward the piezoelectric crystal or transducer. This sound is converted back into electrical energy for display.

M-mode, or motion-mode, echocardiography uses a single pencil-like beam of ultrasound to examine the heart. Since the speed of sound transmission through the heart is constant, the distance between reflecting structures within the heart and the transducer can be calibrated by measuring the time taken for a pulsation of sound to travel from the transducer to that structure and return. Thus, intracardiac structures such as valves are displayed on an oscilloscope or on a strip chart recording. Their motion over time can be accurately determined, but structure size is seen only in one dimension. Some appreciation of the shape and lateral relationships of intracardiac structures can be gained by manually moving the transducer during recording (Fig. 4), but true spatial orientation is not possible with M-mode echocardiography.

Two-dimensional echocardiography provides distance information about the location of structures in the lateral as well as vertical dimensions. This is accomplished by rapidly steering the same pencil-like beam of ultrasound used in M-mode echocardiography through an arc or sector. Reflecting structures within the path of this arc of sound are displayed on a cathode ray tube and recorded on television videotape for later analysis. Two-dimensional echocardiography provides accurate real-time visualization of the intracardiac structures.

Both M-mode and two-dimensional echocardiography are quite useful in elucidating the structural abnormalities under-

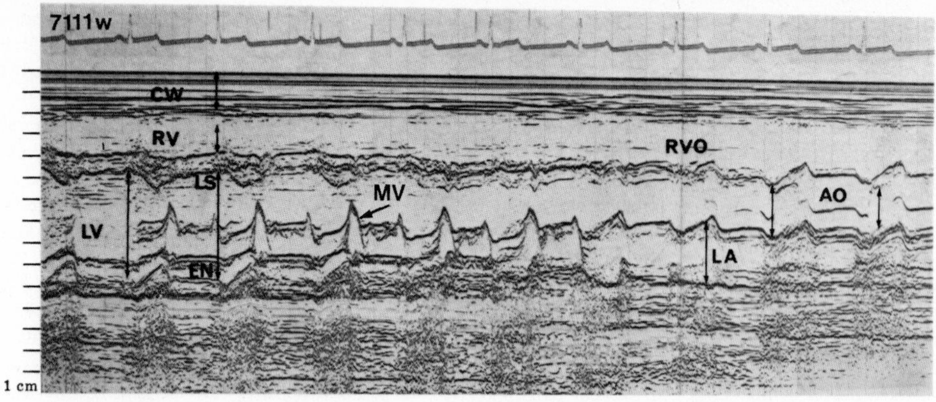

Figure 4. Normal M-mode echocardiogram. The transducer is directed through the left ventricle (LV) at the left hand side of the illustration, and is gradually steered through the region of the mitral valve (MV) to the aorta (AO) and aortic valve at the right hand side of the picture. CW: chest wall; RV: right ventricular cavity; LS: left side of septum; EN: endocardium of posterior wall; RVO: right ventricular outflow; LA: left atrium.

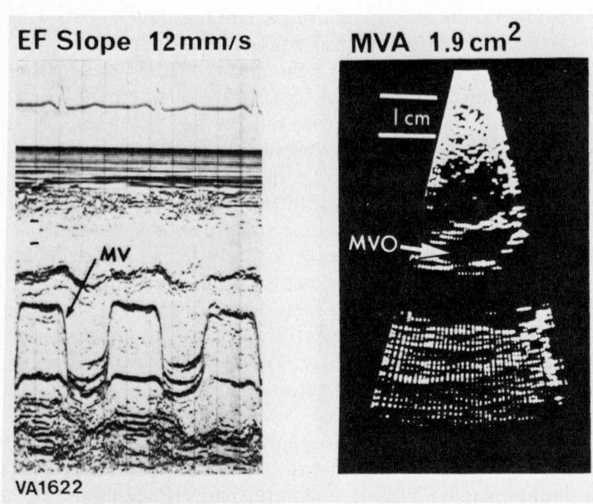

Figure 5. M-mode and two-dimensional echocardiograms of a stenotic mitral valve. The M-mode echocardiogram at the left shows classic features of mitral stenosis, including thickening of the valve leaflets, anterior diastolic motion of the posterior leaflet, and slowing of the diastolic closing slope of the anterior leaflet (EF slope). The EF slope is roughly correlated with the severity of stenosis but true mitral valve area (MVA) can be measured with two-dimensional echocardiography as shown in the short-axis view of the mitral orifice at the right. MVO: mitral valve orifice.

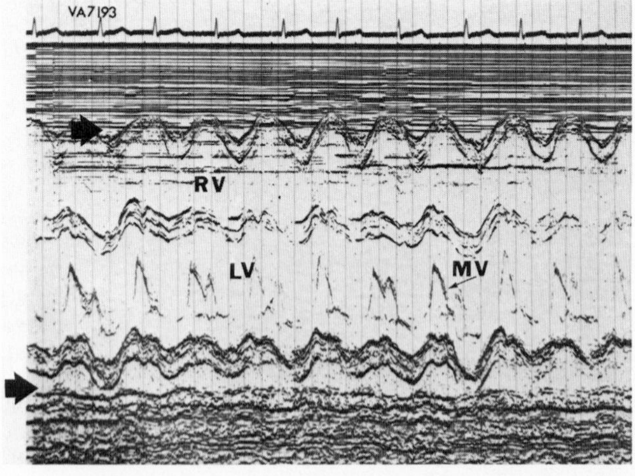

Figure 6. M-mode echocardiogram of pericardial effusion. Large arrows indicate an echo-free space anterior and posterior to the heart that is characteristic of a moderate sized pericardial effusion. Other abbreviations as in Figure 4.

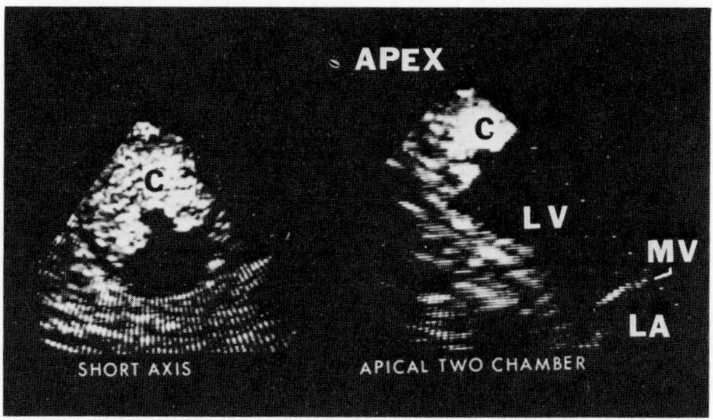

Figure 7. Two-dimensional echocardiogram of a left ventricular thrombus. At the left, a short-axis view of the cardiac apex shows a crescent shaped clot (C) within the circular left ventricle. At right, an apical two chamber view shows the clot in the apex of the heart. The mitral valve can also be seen.

lying several different cardiac diseases. In general, echocardiography is most helpful in the diagnosis and evaluation of valvular heart disease. Thickening and calcification of the aortic valve are readily detected in older patients with aortic sclerosis or aortic stenosis. Congenital bicuspid aortic valves can be recognized. The diagnosis of mitral stenosis is readily made by echocardiography, and the mitral valve area can be reliably determined using two-dimensional echocardiography (Fig. 5). The evaluation of patients suspected of having mitral valve prolapse usually includes echocardiography. Two-dimensional echocardiography is especially helpful in demonstrating anatomic displacement of the mitral valve leaflets into the left atrium. Aortic regurgitation can be detected as a rapid high-frequency fluttering of the anterior mitral valve leaflet caused by a jet of regurgitation. Causes of mitral regurgitation, including flail mitral valve leaflets and papillary muscle dysfunction, can be evaluated. Echocardiography is also quite useful in examining valvular vegetations due to endocarditis.

Echocardiography is the procedure of choice for demonstrating pericardial effusion (Fig. 6). The amount and exact location of pericardial effusion can be readily determined using the two-dimensional technique. While clues to indicate cardiac tamponade and constrictive pericarditis are seen on the echocardiogram, it cannot be used to exclude their presence.

Both M-mode and two-dimensional echocardiography are quite useful in the examination of left ventricular function. In patients with symmetrically contracting left ventricles, M-mode echocardiographic dimensions can be used to calculate an accurate ejection fraction and cardiac output, and sophisticated parameters of left ventricular thickening and fractional shortening can be reliably measured. Two-dimensional echocardiography is more helpful in the identification of regional segmental wall motion abnormalities due to cornary artery disease. The diagnosis of left ventricular aneurysm and intracardiac thrombus is readily made with two-dimensional echocardiography (Fig. 7). An estimate of the functional size of a myocardial infarction can also be made. Complications such as intracardiac thrombi can be directly visualized. Right ventricular infarctions can also be recognized, and complications such as rupture of the interventricular septum and pseudoaneurysm formation can be demonstrated.

Echocardiography is also useful in diagnosing a variety of congenital heart diseases, especially such entities as an atrial septal defect, a ventricular septal defect, tetralogy of Fallot, and other complex congenital anomolies. Echocardiography is the procedure of choice for diagnosing hypertrophic cardiomyopathy and left atrial myxoma.

Since it is a noninvasive, harmless, and reasonably inexpensive test, echocardiography is widely employed in diagnosing many different types of heart disease. The major limitations of echocardiography are inability to record a technically adequate study in approximately 10 percent of patients due to body habitus, primarily those with barrel chests and chronic obstructive lung disease. In addition, it is difficult to quantitate many of the two-dimensional echocardiographic findings because of the tomographic nature of the study. Thus, a precise measurement of ejection fraction or left ventricular volume may not be feasible using this technique, whereas qualitative visualization of very small areas of abnormal wall motion may be easily accomplished.

RADIONUCLIDE IMAGING

Nuclear cardiology is at present a rapidly growing field in cardiology. Recent development of new radionuclides, high-resolution scintillation cameras, and computers have furnished new diagnostic tools in cardiovascular diseases. The ability of these techniques to measure various physiologic parameters and their nontraumatic nature make them particularly attractive to the practicing physician. Three types of radionuclide imaging procedures appear to be especially promising.

Radionuclide Angiocardiography

The most commonly used radionuclide for this technique is technetium 99m (^{99m}Tc) tagged to human serum albumin (HSA) or the patient's own red blood cells. Radionuclide angiocardiography allows determination of left and right ventricular function and intracardiac shunts.

Left Ventricular Function

With the first-pass method, after injection of a radionuclide bolus into a peripheral or central vein, the scintillation camera records the activity as the bolus travels for the first time through various cardiac chambers and blood vessels. This activity is stored for later computer analysis.

Since ^{99m}Tc tagged to albumin or red cells stays in the intravascular space for approximately 4 hours after intravenous injection, an equilibrium method can also be employed to determine ventricular function. With this method, several minutes after radionuclide administration blood pool images of the heart are recorded over several hundred cardiac cycles and stored for later analysis. A computer allows exact superimposition of these images to generate a technically superior composite image.

Both of these methods possess advantages as well as disadvantages, discussions of which are beyond the scope of this book. With either method, enddiastolic and endsystolic counts are determined with the help of a simultaneously recorded ECG. From these data, the left ventricular ejection fraction (LVEF) can be easily calculated as follows:

$$\text{LVEF} = \frac{\text{(end-diastolic counts)} - \text{(end-systolic counts)}}{\text{(end-diastolic counts)}}$$

Correlation of the ejection fraction calculated by contrast angiography and radionuclide ventriculography has been excellent. The multiple-gated acquisition technique (MUGA) allows the display of ventricular images throughout the cardiac cycle in a ciné format, greatly facilitating the detection of segmental wall motion abnormalities. In most patients with coronary heart disease who have normal LVEF and normal segmental wall motion at rest, radionuclide ventriculography demonstrates a decreased ejection fraction and segmental wall motion abnormalities during maximal exercise.

The chamber size and ejection fraction of the right ventricle can also be reliably assessed by radionuclide ventriculography. The current clinical applications of radionuclide ventriculography may be listed as follows:

1. Rest and exercise radionuclide ventriculography to detect coronary heart disease in patients with chest pain and an abnormal resting ECG, atypical chest pain, and in asymptomatic patients with a positive exercise ECG.
2. To determine left ventricular function in a patient suspected to have an acute myocardial infarction. It can confirm the diagnosis, indicate the extent of infarction, and is therefore helpful in determining the prognosis. It can also demonstrate the efficacy of various interventions.
3. To determine whether right ventricular dysfunction is responsible for a low output state in a patient with acute inferior wall myocardial infarction.
4. To determine whether a discrete left ventricular aneurysm or generalized poor left ventricular contraction is responsible for congestive heart failure.
5. By demonstrating left ventricular dysfunction in patients with aortic regurgitation, it may be helpful in determining the timing for cardiac catheterization and surgical intervention.
6. To determine right and left ventricular function in patients with chronic obstructive lung disease.
7. To detect and quantitate intracardiac shunts.
8. To monitor left ventricular function in patients taking cardiotoxic drugs such as Adriamycin.

Myocardial Perfusion Imaging

Thallium-201 (^{201}Tl) is currently the most suitable radionuclide available for myocardial perfusion imaging. It is rapidly extracted from the blood stream by normally functioning myocardial cells. The amount of initial ^{201}Tl extraction depends on two factors, that is, cell viability, since the extraction is Na^+, K^+-ATPase dependent, and regional blood flow. Myocardial regions deprived of adequate blood flow (ischemic) as well as necrotic or scarred regions (acute or remote infarction) accumulate little ^{201}Tl and appear as cold spots.

Thallium-201 is usually injected into a peripheral vein at peak exercise (treadmill/bicycle) and imaging is begun immediately after termination of exercise (immediate postexercise images). Images are obtained in the anterior, 45°, and 70° left anterior views. Images in identical projections are repeated 3-4 hours later (delayed images). The majority of transient ischemic myocardial regions show cold defects in the immediate postexercise images and normal perfusion in delayed images. On the other hand, infarcted regions reveal persistent cold defects both in immediate postexercise and delayed images. The ^{201}Tl stress test enhances the sensitivity of the standard treadmill stress test by approximately 20 percent for the detection of coronary heart disease. Moreover, a ^{201}Tl stress test identifies patients with a false-positive exercise ECG. The major limitations of ^{201}Tl imaging are cost and considerable interobserver and intraobserver error of interpretation. Furthermore, it underestimates the extent of coronary artery disease. The technique is clinically useful in patients with abnormal resting ECGs in whom an exercise ECG would be unreliable. The current clinical applications of ^{201}Tl imaging are summarized below:

1. Detection of coronary heart disease in patients with chest pain and ST-T abnormalities or left bundle-branch block on resting ECG or digitalis therapy, atypical chest pain, and asymptomatic patients with a positive exercise ECG.
2. Confirmation of coronary heart disease in patients with chest pain and a negative exercise ECG.
3. Determination of graft patency following coronary artery bypass surgery.
4. Localization and approximate sizing of areas of old and new myocardial infarctions.

Radionuclide ventriculography aids ^{201}Tl imaging in this respect by demonstrating the location and extent of any wall motion abnormality. Both techniques are superior to the standard 12-lead ECG for assessment of approximate infarct size.

Infarct Imaging with Technetium-99M Stannous Pyrophosphate (^{99M}Tc-PPi)

Imaging with ^{99m}Tc-PPi is also a form of perfusion imaging. The radionuclide concentrates in the acutely damaged myocardial region and appears as a hot spot. Unlike ^{201}Tl imaging, which shows cold defects for both acute and remote infarcts, ^{99m}Tc-PPi delineates only the acutely necrotic myocardial tissue. Imaging with PPi is positive from 24 hours to 6 days after the onset of acute infarction. The sensitivity and specificity are excellent for transmural myocardial infarction, but the technique is less reliable for detecting subendocardial infarction. Positive images may also be obtained in some patients with ventricular aneurysms, calcified heart valves, and some patients undergoing electrical defibrillation. The main clinical utility of this technique is to confirm, localize, and evaluate the size of acute myocardial infarction in patients in whom serial ECGs are negative or difficult to interpret as in the presence of LBBB, WPW syndrome, pacemaker rhythm, or in patients with equivocal ECG and cardiac enzyme changes as seen during the immediate postoperative period.

The measurement of regional coronary blood flow can be performed by injecting ^{133}Xenon or radioactively labeled microspheres selectively into individual coronary arteries. These are research tools that are not suitable for clinical use. The combined use of blood pool cardiac imaging and posterioanterior chest x-ray permits detection of pericardial effusion. However, echocardiography has proved more sensitive for detection and rough quantification of pericardial effusion and has largely replaced the blood pool imaging technique.

CARDIAC CATHETERIZATION

Cardiac catheterization is a powerful diagnostic tool that provides precise assessment of anatomic and physiologic changes in many cardiovascular diseases. Since this technique provides direct and definitive information, it is considered to be the gold standard for various noninvasive tests. In general, this technique permits measurement of:

1. Pressures in various cardiac chambers and blood vessels
2. Pressure gradients across stenotic cardiac valves
3. Cardiac output
4. Systemic and pulmonary vascular resistances
5. Hemodynamics during stress (e.g., supine exercise)
6. Shunts between systemic and pulmonary circulations

A selective injection of contrast material during catheterization is helpful in defining the anatomy of cornary arteries and various congenital heart diseases, quantifying valvular regurgitation, and calculating the chamber volume, particularly the left ventricular enddiastolic and endsystolic volumes, and the ejection fraction. Cardiac catheterization also permits cardiac pacing and electrophysiologic studies.

MEASUREMENT OF INTRAVASCULAR PRESSURES

Fluid-filled catheter systems are commonly used to record pressure curves from various cardiac chambers and great vessels. This system consists of an external strain-gauge type of pressure transducer that is connected to a fluid-filled catheter introduced into the vascular system. The disadvantages of such a system consist of catheter whip artifacts and an erratic frequency response. Careful technique, for example, elimination of air bubbles from the system, improves its frequency response and reliability. To overcome these difficulties even further, catheters have been devised that carry the pressure transducer at the tip. Their expense, however, precludes their widespread use.

Pressures are usually recorded from the right atrium, right ventricle, pulmonary artery and its main branches, pulmonary artery wedge position, left ventricle, and the aorta. Phasic and mean (electronically measured) pressures are recorded from the right atrium, pulmonary artery, pulmonary artery wedge and the aorta, whereas only phasic pressures are recorded from the ventricles.

Right atrial and pulmonary artery wedge pressure curves are characterized by two positive waves, a and v, and two negative waves, x and y. The a wave is due to atrial systole and the v wave is due to atrial filling during ventricular systole. Normally, the a wave is higher than the v wave in the right atrium. The x descent is due to atrial relaxation and is interrupted by a small positive c wave that is concomitant with tricuspid valve closure. The y descent is attributed to rapid inflow of blood from the right atrium into the right ventricle upon opening of the tricuspid valve. Pressure wave forms from the pulmonary artery wedge are similar to those of the right atrium, except that there is a delay in the wave form due to its travel time from the left atrium retrogradely to the pulmonary artery wedge position, the v wave is higher than the a wave, and the c wave is not usually seen.

Pressure curves from the pulmonary artery and aorta show a rapid rise to a peak systolic pressure, followed by a fall of pressure up to the dicrotic notch that is inscribed concomitant with closure of the semilunar valves. From the dicrotic notch, the pressure gradually declines further up to the enddiastolic point.

Pressure curves from the two ventricles show a rapid rise to the peak systolic pressure followed by an equally rapid decline. During diastole, a rapid filling wave, a slow filling wave, and an a wave due to atrial systole are recorded. The a wave is interrupted by the rapidly rising systolic pressure, and the enddiastolic pressure is measured at this distinct point.

Normally, the pulmonary artery diastolic, mean pulmonary artery wedge, mean left atrial, and the pre-a wave left ventricular diastolic pressures are similar. Thus, pulmonary artery diastolic or pulmonary artery wedge pressure are accurate reflections of the left ventricular filling pressure and can be readily monitored at the bedside by a Swan-Ganz catheter.

CARDIAC OUTPUT

Two methods are commonly used for measurement of cardiac output: the Fick method and the indicator dilution method.

Fick Method

This technique uses the principle of Adolph Fick (1870), which states that "total uptake or release of any substance by an organ is the product of blood flow to the organ and the arteriovenous concentration difference of the substance." Since the total oxygen consumption (ml/min) and concentration of oxygen in pulmonary arterial blood (ml/L of blood) and pulmonary venous blood (ml/L of blood, normally the same as in systemic arterial blood) can be readily measured and, since under normal circumstances pulmonary blood flow and systemic blood flow are identical, cardiac output (systemic blood flow) can be easily calculated as follows:

$$\text{Cardiac output (L/min)} = \frac{O_2 \text{ consumption (ml/min)}}{\begin{pmatrix} O_2 \text{ content of systemic} \\ \text{arterial blood (ml/L)} \end{pmatrix} - \begin{pmatrix} O_2 \text{ content of pulmonary} \\ \text{arterial blood (ml/L)} \end{pmatrix}}$$

Cardiac output is generally corrected for body surface area and is expressed as a cardiac index (L/min/m^2).

Indicator Dilution Method

This technique consists of injecting a bolus of a known amount of indocyanine green dye into the pulmonary artery and continuously recording its concentrations from the systemic side of circulation (left ventricle, aorta, or peripheral artery). Thus, a time-concentration curve is recorded that reveals a rapid rise to a peak followed by a gradual fall (in an exponential pattern), which is interrupted by a secondary peak representing a recirculation of the dye. The effect of recirculation is eliminated by extrapolating the initial linear portion of the curve to zero concentration; the cardiac output is then calculated as follows:

$$\text{Cardiac output (L/min)} = \frac{\text{Total amount of dye (mg)} \times 60}{\begin{pmatrix} \text{Average concentration} \\ \text{of dye (mg/L)} \end{pmatrix} \times \begin{pmatrix} \text{Total duration of} \\ \text{the curve (s)} \end{pmatrix}}$$

Thermodilution Method

In this method, temperature is used as an indicator for the measurement of cardiac output. A thermistor-tipped, multilumen catheter is placed in the right heart so that the proximal lumen opens into the right atrium and the catheter tip is in the main pulmonary artery. A bolus of cold saline, of known volume and temperature, is injected into the right atrium while the temperature is continuously sampled in the pulmonary artery. As the mixture of ice-cold saline and blood passes by the thermistor, its temperature rapidly falls. Subsequently, the thermistor registers a progressive rise of temperature over the next several seconds and a time-temperature curve is obtained. A computer is utilized to integrate the area under this curve and to compute the cardiac output by the Stewart-Hamilton method. The results correlate well with the Fick and indocyanine green dye methods. The advantages of the thermodilution method are that there is no need to draw blood, the effect of recirculation is negligible, the results are readily available and multiple measurements can be obtained after therapeutic interventions, and the equipment is relatively inexpensive.

Stroke volume (SV) is defined as the amount of blood ejected by the ventricle per beat. It is usually adjusted for the body surface area (stroke index) and is calculated as follows:

$$\text{Stroke index (ml/m}^2\text{)} = \frac{\text{Cardiac index (ml/m}^2\text{)}}{\text{Heart rate (beats/min)}}$$

Left ventricular (LV) performance can be expressed in terms of a stroke work index (SWI) that is a measure of external work performed by the left ventricle. Stroke work is determined on a per beat basis as gram-meters/meter^2 (g-meters/m^2) and is calculated as follows:

$$\text{LV SWI (g-meters/m}^2\text{)} = \frac{\left[\begin{pmatrix} \text{Mean LV} \\ \text{systolic} \\ \text{pressure} \end{pmatrix} - \begin{pmatrix} \text{Mean LV} \\ \text{enddiastolic} \\ \text{pressure} \end{pmatrix}\right] \times \text{Stroke volume} \times 0.0136}{\text{Body surface area}}$$

Mean arterial pressure can be substituted for mean LV systolic pressure, and mean pulmonary artery wedge pressure can be substituted for mean LV enddiastolic pressure. A constant of 0.0136 is used to convert mm Hg into the g-meters system.

MEASUREMENT OF VASCULAR RESISTANCES

Vascular resistance is calculated separately for systemic and pulmonary circulation as follows:

$$\text{Systemic vascular resistance (SVR) in Wood units} = \frac{\begin{pmatrix} \text{Mean aortic} \\ \text{pressure (mm Hg)} \end{pmatrix} - \begin{pmatrix} \text{Mean right atrial} \\ \text{pressure (mm Hg)} \end{pmatrix}}{\text{Systemic blood flow (L/min)}}$$

$$\text{Pulmonary vascular resistance (PVR) in Wood units} = \frac{\begin{pmatrix} \text{Mean pulmonary artery} \\ \text{pressure (mm Hg)} \end{pmatrix} - \begin{pmatrix} \text{Mean pulmonary} \\ \text{wedge pressure (mm Hg)} \end{pmatrix}}{\text{Pulmonary blood flow (L/min)}}$$

The vascular resistance is a useful index of the degree of vasoconstriction in a given vascular bed.

MEASUREMENT OF VALVE ORIFICE SIZE IN STENOTIC VALVES

The functional orifice area of the stenotic valves can be calculated by measuring the pressure gradient and blood flow across the stenotic valve. The pressure gradient and cardiac output should be determined simultaneously or in close sequence. The following equations are utilized:

$$\text{Aortic valve area (cm}^2\text{)} = \frac{\text{Flow (ml/s)} = \dfrac{\text{Cardiac output (ml/min)}}{\text{Systolic ejection period (s/min)}}}{44.5 \sqrt{\text{Mean systolic pressure gradient (mm Hg)}}}$$

$$\text{Mitral valve area (cm}^2\text{)} = \frac{\text{Flow (ml/s)} = \dfrac{\text{Cardiac output (ml/min)}}{\text{Diastolic flow period (s/min)}}}{38.0 \sqrt{\text{Mean diastolic pressure gradient (mm Hg)}}}$$

Flow patterns across the aortic and mitral valves account for the empirical constants 44.5 and 38.0 for the aortic and mitral valves, respectively.

Valve areas are fairly reliable when valvular regurgitation is absent. In the presence of coexistent valvular regurgitation, the blood flow across the stenotic valve as calculated from the cardiac output (the Fick method) is underestimated, resulting in an underestimation of the actual valve area.

MEASUREMENT OF VALVULAR REGURGITANT VOLUME

The Fick method measures only the forward stroke volume, that is, the blood being delivered downstream into the systemic circulation per beat. On the other hand, the stroke volume calculated by contrast left ventriculography (end-diastolic volume-end-systolic volume) indicates total amount of blood pumped by the ventricle per beat. Thus, angiographic stroke volume minus the Fick stroke volume indicates the amount of blood regurgitating across the incompetent valve. It is generally expressed as a percentage of angiographic stroke volume as shown below:

$$\text{Regurgitation fraction} = \frac{\begin{pmatrix}\text{Angiographic}\\ \text{stroke volume}\end{pmatrix} - \begin{pmatrix}\text{Fick stroke}\\ \text{volume}\end{pmatrix}}{\text{Angiographic stroke volume}} \times 100$$

DETECTION OF CARDIAC SHUNTS

Presence of abnormal communication between systemic and pulmonary circulation allows shunting of blood from one side to another without traversing the capillary bed. In intracardiac left-to-right shunt, oxygenated blood returning from the lungs passes through an abnormal opening to the right heart chamber, resulting in greater pulmonary blood flow than systemic blood flow. On the other hand, in intracardiac right-to-left shunt, systemic venous blood passes to the left heart chambers without traversing the lungs and lowers the oxygen saturation of the systemic arterial blood. This also causes sytemic circulation to be greater than pulmonary circulation. The magnitude of the shunts can be calculated by the following methods.

The oximetry method consists of collecting blood samples in rapid sequence from different cardiac chambers and great vessels and measuring their oxygen content. The amount of shunt can be determined by calculating separately systemic and pulmonary blood flows as follows:

$$\text{Systemic blood flow } (Q_S) \text{ in L/min} = \frac{O_2 \text{ consumption (ml/min)}}{\begin{pmatrix}O_2 \text{ content of}\\ \text{aortic blood}\\ \text{(ml/L)}\end{pmatrix} - \begin{pmatrix}O_2 \text{ content of}\\ \text{mixed venous blood*}\\ \text{(ml/L)}\end{pmatrix}}$$

*A sample of mixed venous blood is obtained from a right heart chamber upstream from the level of shunt.

$$\text{Total pulmonary blood flow } (Q_P) \text{ in L/min} = \frac{O_2 \text{ consumption (ml/min)}}{\begin{pmatrix}O_2 \text{ content of}\\ \text{pulmonary venous}\\ \text{blood (ml/L)}^{\dagger}\end{pmatrix} - \begin{pmatrix}O_2 \text{ content of}\\ \text{pulmonary arterial}\\ \text{blood (ml/L)}\end{pmatrix}}$$

$$\text{Left-to-right shunt} = Q_p - Q_s \text{ (L/min)}$$

$$\text{Right-to-left shunt} = Q_s - Q_p \text{ (L/min)}$$

Sometimes, communications between systemic and pulmonary circuits may allow bidirectional shunting of blood. Under these circumstances, the magnitude of left-to-right and right-to-left shunts can be calculated by determining Q_s and Q_p as mentioned above and additionally by calculating effective pulmonary blood flow (Q_{ep}).

Effective pulmonary blood flow (Q_{ep}) is the amount of mixed venous blood reaching the lungs. In other words, total pulmonary blood flow minus left-to-right shunt equals effective pulmonary blood flow and is calculated as follows:

$$Q_{ep} = \frac{O_2 \text{ consumption (ml/min)}}{\begin{pmatrix}O_2 \text{ content of}\\ \text{pulmonary}\\ \text{venous blood}\end{pmatrix} - \begin{pmatrix}O_2 \text{ content of}\\ \text{mixed venous}\\ \text{blood}\end{pmatrix}}$$

$$\text{Left-to-right shunt} = Q_p - Q_{ep}$$

$$\text{Right-to-left shunt} = Q_s - Q_{ep}$$

Indicator dilution technique: The shunting of blood between systemic and pulmonary circulations alters the configuration of the time-concentration curve obtained by injecting the indocyanine green dye in the pulmonary circulation and sampling from the systemic circulation. Left-to-right shunt causing continuous recirculation of a portion of the dye through the lungs will allow slow release of the dye into the systemic circulation. This results in a decrease of the peak concentration of the dye, prolonged disappearance time, and absence of a distinct recirculation peak. On the other hand, right-to-left shunt results in an early appearance time when the dye is injected in the right side of circulation upstream from the level of right-to-left shunt. Several formulas have been devised to quantify these shunts from the indicator dilution method.

Cineangiocardiography following selective injection of contrast material at various sites is helpful in localizing the shunt. This method provides only a qualitative indication about the magnitude of the shunt. However, the advantage of this method is that precise anatomic details are furnished.

INDICATIONS FOR CARDIAC CATHETERIZATION

Recent advances in noninvasive procedures, especially echocardiography and radionuclide imaging, have greatly influ-

†In the absence of a right-to-left shunt, oxygen content of pulmonary venous and aortic blood is identical.

enced the need and timing for cardiac catheterization. Under most circumstances, the history and physical examination along with various noninvasive tests are sufficient to exclude or confirm heart disease and to assess its severity. Only occasionally is it necessary to resort to cardiac catheterization to exclude heart disease, for example, catheterization may be needed in a young asymptomatic patient with a straight back, pectus excavatum, or idiopathic dilatation of the pulmonary artery to document the absence of an atrial septal defect to determine insurability or ability to participate in competitive sports. Similarly, cardiac catheterization is sometimes required to establish the presence of heart disease and to determine its severity when clinical findings are atypical and results of noninvasive tests are equivocal or are uninterpretable.

The primary role of cardiac catheterization at present is to furnish the surgeon with precise anatomic and physiologic details of the cardiac abnormality in patients in whom surgical intervention is being contemplated. Cardiac catheterization may also reveal additional abnormalities that were previously unsuspected or the severity of which was misjudged. This applies particularly to patients with multivalvular and congenital heart diseases.

Recent availability of the Swan-Ganz catheter has made bedside hemodynamic monitoring practical. Consequently, the role of cardiac catheterization has been extended to coronary and intensive care units. Thus, various therapeutic interventions may be applied in patients with severe heart failure and circulatory shock on a more rational basis. This technique is also helpful as a diagnostic tool, for example, in the differential diagnosis between acute mitral regurgitation and an acute ventricular septal defect in a patient with an acute myocardial infarction.

The indications for coronary arteriography are described later in this chapter in the Coronary Heart Disease section.

CONTRAINDICATIONS OF CARDIAC CATHETERIZATION

There are no absolute contraindications of cardiac catherization. Relative contraindications include febrile illnesses, digitalis toxicity, severe heart failure, serious ventricular arrhythmias, anemia, electrolyte imbalance, infective endocarditis, and pregnancy. If possible, some of these conditions should be controlled before cardiac catheterization, as it will not only reduce the risk of the procedure but also yield more accurate data.

COMPLICATIONS OF CARDIAC CATHETERIZATION

In general, the incidence of complications associated with cardiac catheterization is related to the underlying heart disease and experience of the operators. Right heart catheterization should be associated with minimal morbidity and zero mortality in adults. Most of the complications mentioned below occur as a result of left heart catheterization and coronary angiography. Acute myocardial infarction, impending myocardial infarction, severe heart failure, severe pulmonary hypertension, and severe cyanotic heart disease increase the risk of the procedure. High risk is also associated with coronary arteriography in patients with severe stenosis of the left main coronary artery. Major complications include death, myocardial infarction, serious ventricular arrhythmias, pulmonary edema, arterial thromboembolism, hypotension, cardiac rupture, and excessive blood loss that rarely, however, occur. In most cardiac catheterization laboratories and in the hands of experienced operators, the risk of death with coronary arteriography is 0.1 percent and the incidence of arterial complications is 2-3 percent. Minor complications include temporary arrhythmias, pyrogen reactions, vasovagal reactions, vessel spasm, reactions to contrast agents, and localized thrombophlebitis at the cutdown site.

Table 2 shows the normal values for various hemodynamic parameters.

CARDIAC ARRHYTHMIAS

The anatomy and physiology of the conduction system have already been described in the section under Electrocardiography.

MECHANISMS OF CARDIAC ARRHYTHMIAS

The mechanisms of cardiac arrhythmias can be broadly divided into abnormalities of impulse formation (automaticity) and/or impulse conduction.

Abnormalities of Automaticity

These abnormalities involve escape of subsidiary pacemakers, when the sinus node automaticity is depressed as in sick sinus syndrome. The rate of impulse formation from these subsidiary pacemakers is lower than the sinus rate. Also, increased automaticity of subsidiary pacemakers occurs in diseased hearts. For example, in digitalis toxicity or in acute myocardial infarction, the enhanced automaticity of the AV junction results in nonparoxysmal junctional tachycardia. Abnormal automaticity in atrial and ventricular working myocardial cells may occur in diseased hearts, resulting in premature beats. Atrial or ventricular parasystole may also be based on this mechanism. After potentials from previous beats have been shown to result in premature beats.

Abnormalities of Conduction

Reentry or circus movement has been proven to be responsible for some arrhythmias, for example, paroxysmal supraventricular tachycardia and premature ventricular beats. Reentry appears to be the predominant mechanism of arrhythmias. For its occurrence reentry requires two separate but contiguous pathways, one with unidirectional block and the other with slow conduction. As shown in Figure 8, impulse travelling

Table 2. Normal Values For Various Hemodynamic Parameters

Site	*Systolic Pressure (mm Hg)*	*Enddiastolic Pressure (mm Hg)*	*a Wave (mm Hg)*	*v Wave (mm Hg)*	*Mean Pressure (mm Hg)*
Right atrium	–	–	2.5-9	2-7	1-5
Right ventricle	15-30	0-8	–	–	–
Pulmonary artery	15-30	3-12	–	–	9-20
Pulmonary artery wedge	–	–	4-16	6-20	3-12
Left ventricle	90-140	4-14	–	–	–
Aorta	90-140	60-90	–	–	70-105
Cardiac index		2.5-4.2 L/min/m^2			
Stroke index		40-70 ml/m^2			
Stroke work index		40-80 g-meters/m^2			
Pulmonary vascular resistance		0.2-3 Wood units			
Systemic vascular resistance		10-20 Wood units			
Oxygen consumption		110-150 ml/min/m^2			
Arterio-venous oxygen difference		30-50 ml/L of blood			
Arterial saturation		94-100%			
Left ventricular					
End-diastolic volume		40-90 ml/m^2			
End-systolic volume		14-34 ml/m^2			
Ejection fraction		0.59-0.75			

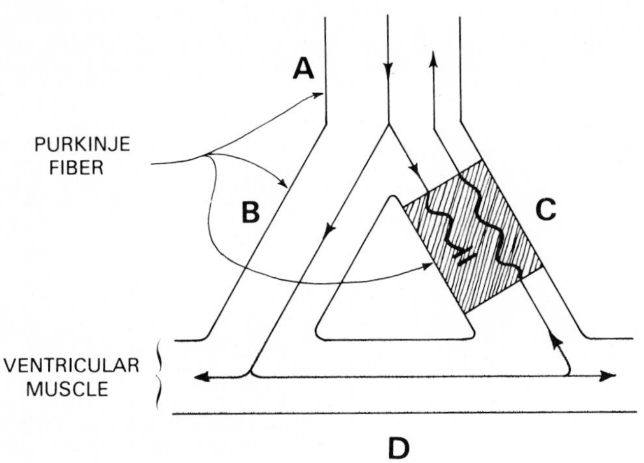

Figure 8. The reentry phenomenon. Impulse traveling antegrade in Purkinje fiber A is blocked in Purkinje fiber C (unidirectional block). However, the impulse can propagate through Purkinje fiber B and ventricular muscle D. The impulse travels retrograde through fiber C. By this time, fiber A has recovered and permits the impulse to reenter retrogradely.

antegrade in Purkinje fiber A is blocked in Purkinje fiber C (unidirectional block). However, the impulse can propagate through Purkinje fiber B and ventricular muscle D. The impulse travels retrograde through fiber C. By this time, fiber A has recovered and permits the impulse to reenter retrogradely. Conduction delay and block result in such arrthymias as sinoatrial (SA) block, AV block, and exit block from ectopic pacemakers.

HEMODYNAMIC CHANGES DURING ARRHYTHMIAS

Low cardiac output and hypotension may occur in various arrhythmias. Factors like ventricular rate, duration of arrhythmia, preservation of properly timed atrial contraction, and functional status of the myocardium contribute substantially toward the severity of hemodynamic changes. For example, occurrence of atrial fibrillation with a very rapid ventricular rate in a patient with acute myocardial infarction may have profound hemodynamic changes. On the other hand, atrial fibrillation with a slow ventricular rate in a relatively healthy heart may result in only minor or no hemodynamic changes. Furthermore, the status of blood vessels supplying various organs significantly affects the regional perfusion to these organs. An arrhythmia in a patient with atherosclerotic narrowing of the carotid arteries may produce symptoms of cerebrovascular ischemia, whereas the same arrhythmia in a patient with normal carotid arteries may be asymptomatic. Cerebral, coronary, renal, and mesenteric perfusion may be adversely affected by the cardiac arrhythmias, causing symptoms of ischemia in these organs.

DIAGNOSTIC APPROACH TO ARRHYTHMIAS

The following steps are suggested for making a correct diagnosis of a given arrhythmia.

1. ECG strips with three simultaneously recorded leads (e.g., I, II, III; aV_R, aV_L, aV_F; V_1, V_2, V_3; and V_4, V_5, V_6) are preferable for analysis of arrhythmias.
2. Determine the origin of P waves, that is, sinus, ectopic atrial, or junctional. Atrial activation from sinus node produces an upright P in leads I, II, III, aV_L, aV_F, and V_2-V_6. P waves are inverted in aV_R and diphasic in V_1. On the other hand, retrograde atrial activation from the AV junction gives rise to an inverted P in leads II, III, aV_F and upright P in leads I and aV_R. P waves arising from ectopic atrial focus appear distorted and bizarre.
3. Determine whether P-P and R-R intervals are regular or irregular.
4. Determine if the QRS complex is supraventricular or ventricular in origin. The supraventricular impulse, when conducted normally through the His-Purkinje system, produces a narrow QRS complex. However, an aberrantly conducted supraventricular impulse gives rise to a wide, bizarre QRS complex, and its differentiation from a QRS complex of ventricular origin presents considerable difficulty and sometimes may not be possible unless an invasive electrophysiologic study is performed. There are some clues on a surface ECG that may help in making this important differentiation. If the wide QRS complex in question occurs after a relatively long R-R interval, has a triphasic rSR pattern in lead V_1, is preceded by a P wave, has an initial portion resembling that of other normally conducted QRS complexes, it is likely to be an aberrantly conducted QRS complex. On the other hand, if the underlying heart rate is relatively slow, the broad QRS complex in question is followed by a pause, is not preceded by a P wave, and shows a monophasic or biphasic configuration in V_1, it is likely to be of ventricular origin.
5. Determine the relationship between P waves and QRS complexes. A normal P-R interval is 0.12-0.20 second and the P wave precedes the QRS complex. A P-R interval of <0.12 seconds indicates that the QRS is not causally related to the P wave with the only exceptions being the WPW syndrome and junctional beats. One should note whether the P-R interval of various beats is constant or widens progressively, as in Wenckebach's AV block, or shortens progressively, as in AV dissociation. In complete heart block, P waves and QRS complexes are totally independent of one another.
6. A beat that comes before its time may represent a premature atrial, junctional or ventricular beat, parasystolic beat, capture beat in the presence of AV dissociation, or a reciprocal (echo) beat.

   Premature atrial, junctional, or ventricular beats usually show a fixed coupling interval. Parasystolic beats, on the other hand, generally have a variable coupling interval. Demonstration of the longest interectopic interval, being a multiple of the shortest interectopic interval as well as presence of fusion complexes, further supports the diagnosis of parasystole. In the presence of AV dissociation a capture beat is recognized by its prematurity, presence of preceding P wave and normally or aberrantly conducted QRS complex. A reciprocal, or echo, beat may arise in the atrium, AV junction, or ventricles. A reciprocal ventricular beat may follow a premature ventricular beat (PVB), for example, a PVB may conduct retrogradely through the AV junction and may give rise to a retrograde P wave. The same impulse may turn around anterogradely through another portion of the AV junction and reactivate the ventricles, producing an echo, or reciprocal, beat.
7. Second-degree SA block, second-degree AV block, nonconducted premature atrial beats (PABs), and escape beats may be responsible for the occurrence of long pauses.

   Normal sinus rhythm arises from the sinus node that drives the heart at a rate of 60-100 beats/minute. P-QRS-T waves occur at regular intervals.

DISORDERS OF IMPULSE FORMATION

Supraventricular Arrhythmias

Sinus Tachycardia

Sinus rhythm with a heart rate of >100 beats/minute is defined as sinus tachycardia. P-QRS-T waves are normal and occur at regular intervals. The ST segment may show a J point depression. Sinus tachycardia may be physiologic, as during physical or emotional stress. Numerous disease states (e.g., heart failure, anemia, fever, thyrotoxicosis, hypoxia, hypotension, pulmonary embolism, as well as sympathomimetic drugs) produce sinus tachycardia. Sinus tachycardia usually represents a compensatory mechanism and is seldom harmful by itself. Therefore, it usually disappears with improvement of the primary disease state responsible for the tachycardia. It generally causes palpitation. The rate of tachycardia diminishes slightly and transiently during carotid sinus massage.

Sinus Bradycardia

Sinus rhythm, with a heart rate of <60 beats/minutes, is defined as sinus bradycardia. Physiologic sinus bradycardia occurs in elderly individuals and well-trained athletes in whom increased vagal tone results in a slow rate. Certain pharmacologic agents such as propranolol, digoxin, morphine, reserpine, as well as disease states like sick sinus syndrome, hypothyroidism, increased intracranial pressure, acute inferior myocardial infarction, and hypothermia result in sinus bradycardia. Generally, augmented stroke volume compensates for the slow rate and cardiac output remains normal. However, in the presence of myocardial damage as in acute myocardial infarction, as well as with extremely slow rates (<30 beats/minute), hypotension may result. Treatment depends on the primary disease; for example, in most patients with acute infarction, sinus bradycardia, and hypotension, 0.3-0.6 mg of atropine administered intravenously increases the heart rate as well as the blood pressure. In a symptomatic patient with sick sinus syndrome, a permanent pacemaker may be indicated.

Sinus Arrhythmia
Due to varying vagal tone, sinus rhythm in most people is slightly irregular. With accentuated vagal tone, the irregularity of sinus rhythm increases. When the difference between the longest and shortest P-P intervals exceeds 0.12 second, it is referred to as sinus arrhythmia. It should be noted that the change in P-P intervals is gradual. Sinus arrhythmia is said to be phasic when the rate is faster during inspiration and slower during expiration. When variation of the heart rate does not correspond with the phases of respiration, it is called non-phasic sinus arrhythmia. Phasic sinus arrhythmia is more common and is usually present in infants, young children, and elderly individuals. The only clinical consideration for sinus arrhythmia is that it should be differentiated from other types of rhythm disturbances.

Sinus Arrest
Sinus arrest is defined as a pause of variable duration resulting from failure of the sinus node to initiate an impulse. This pause is not an exact multiple of a normal P-P interval. Usually the pause is terminated by an escape beat from the AV junction or ventricles. In a symptomatic patient, a permanent pacemaker is the treatment of choice. Sinus arrest occurs in sick sinus syndrome, digitalis toxicity, ischemic injury to the sinus node, and in myocarditis.

Wandering Atrial Pacemaker
This self-explanatory term means that the pacemaker of the heart wanders back and forth from the sinus node to the AV junction. Electrocardiographically, it is recognized by a change in the configuration of P waves as well as variable P-R intervals in successive cardiac cycles. Usually there is a slight fluctuation of the P-P intervals as well. A wandering atrial pacemaker occurs because of periodic suppression of the sinus node due to enhanced vagal tone. This rhythm disturbance usually does not cause any hemodynamic changes.

Premature Atrial Beats (PABs)
The ECG diagnosis of a PAB is made by identifying a premature P wave with an abnormal contour. Depending on the degree of prematurity, the PAB may be blocked (no following QRS complex), abberrently conducted (wide QRS complex) or normally conducted (normal QRS complex). The P-R interval of a PAB is generally longer than that of a sinus beat. The pause after a PAB is usually less than compensatory. Strong tea, coffee, alcohol, smoking, emotional stress, or physical exhaustion may produce PABs in normal individuals. Certain disease states such as digitalis toxicity, atrial distension in heart failure, and myocardial infarction may be responsible for PABs. In these diseases, PABs may be the forerunner of paroxysmal atrial tachycardia, atrial flutter, or fibrillation. PABs may give rise to palpitations, a sensation of skipped beats, or may go unnoticed by the patient. The treatment of PABs depends on the underlying etiology. Removal of precipitating factors and mild tranquilizers may totally eliminate them. In unresponsive and symptomatic patients, drug therapy with digoxin and/or quinidine may be required. Treatment of heart failure in appropriate patients may control PABs.

Paroxysmal Supraventricular Tachycardia (PSVT)
Paroxysmal supraventricular tachycardias are characterized by an abrupt onset of rapid heart action that lasts for a variable period and terminates suddenly. In the majority of patients, the underlying mechanism of PSVT is considered to be a reentrant circuit involving the AV node. In others, reentry may occur in the sinus node, atrial tissue, or AV node and an accessory pathway. These tachycardias are generally initiated by a critically timed premature atrial, junctional, or ventricular beat. Some PSVTs are probably due to an increased automaticity of an ectopic atrial focus.

During an episode, the ECG shows normal QRS complexes occurring regularly at a rate of 150-250 beats/minute. Occasionally, the QRS complexes may become wide and bizarre due to aberrant conduction. It is difficult to determine the exact site of origin in these tachyarrhythmias from a surface ECG. However, certain features may be helpful in locating the origin of the PSVT. The occurrence of AV block during PSVT indicates that the tachycardia is either due to increased automaticity of an ectopic atrial focus or due to reentry at the sinus node or atrial muscle. R-R intervals may vary slightly in these types of tachycardias. On the other hand, PSVTs based on reeentry utilizing the AV node and accessory pathways manifest a fixed R-R interval and cannot, of necessity, block in the AV node without interruption of the tachycardia. Furthermore, in AV nodal reentrant tachycardia, P waves are hidden in QRS complexes and are not clearly identifiable, whereas in reentrant tachycardia utilizing accessory pathways, retrograde P waves may be seen following QRS complexes in the ST segment.

Frequently, PSVTs occur in patients with normal hearts. These individuals may be entirely asymptomatic or may experience anxiety and palpitations. However, patients with organic heart disease may experience angina, hypotension, dizziness, or dyspnea. During tachycardia, an abbreviated diastolic period results in decreased coronary blood flow and decreased ventricular filling causing reduced cardiac output. Myocardial oxygen supply demand imbalance may cause angina and hypotension. Attacks of PSVT are common in WPW syndrome. In some patients, strong coffee, tea, alcohol, smoking, and emotional or physical stress maybe the precipitating factors. The attacks last for several minutes to several hours.

Carotid sinus massage either terminates the attack or has no effect. Brief episodes of PSVT may be well tolerated and may not warrant treatment. Frequently, however, tranquilizers such as Valium are required to allay anxiety. Certain mechanical maneuvers, for example, Valsalva's, gagging, ingestion of cold water, and carotid sinus massage may terminate the attack by enhancing vagal tone and should be tried initially. If these maneuvers fail to terminate the attack, one of the following intravenous drugs should be tried: Tensilon, 10 mg

IV; phenylephrine, 0.5-1.5 mg IV (should be avoided in older hypertensive patients); Cedilanid, 0.8-1.2 mg IV; or propranolol, 0.5-1 mg IV (avoid in heart failure). Sometimes carotid sinus massage following the administration of Cedilanid or Tensilon is effective. Verapamil, a Ca^{++} channel blocker, 5 mg IV is the drug of choice for terminating an attack of PSVT. When drug treatment fails and adverse hemodynamic effects develop, electric countershock is the treatment of choice. Alternatively, a temporary pacemaker is inserted to deliver a critically timed premature atrial or ventricular stimulus to abolish the attack. Oral digoxin, quinidine, propranolol, and verapamil, either alone or in combination, are generally effective in preventing paroxysms of PSVTs.

Paroxysmal Atrial Tachycardia (PAT) with Block
Paroxysmal atrial tachycardia with block commonly occurs in patients with advanced digitalis toxicity, acute myocardial infarction, rheumatic mitral valvular disease, cor pulmonale, or following cardiac surgery. An ECG shows somewhat abnormal P waves occurring at a rate of 140 to 220 beats/minute (Fig. 9). P-P intervals may be regulr or somewhat irregular. P waves are upright in leads II, III, and aV_F. The ventricular rate depends on the degree of AV block. Usually there is a 2:1 AV block, and therefore the ventricular rate is 70-110 beats/minute. A fixed AV block will give rise to a constant R-R interval, whereas with variable AV block, R-R intervals will fluctuate. The mechanism of this tachyarrhythmia is probably based on an enhanced automaticity of an ectopic atrial focus. When the ventricular rate is near normal, adverse hemodynamic effects are not encountered. Carotid sinus massage may further slow the ventricular rate due to an increase in AV block. In contrast to PSVT, PAT with block indicates a much more serious prognosis. If a patient taking digitalis demonstrates PAT with block, digitalis toxicity should be suspected until proven otherwise. Digitalis must be discontinued and potassium supplements administered intravenously or orally, because most such patients have a deficit of cellular potassium. If the ventricular rate is unusually rapid (>120 beats/minute), intravenous dilantin or propranolol should be administered to slow the rate. On the other hand, when PAT with block is secondary to other cardiac disease, digitalis is the drug of choice to slow the ventricular response. Quinidine should be added later in an attempt to convert PAT with block into sinus rhythm.

Nonparoxysmal Supraventricular Tachycardia
Nonparoxysmal supraventricular tachycardia is characterized by a slow onset. The heart rate gradually increases and ranges from 60-150 beats/minute. This tachyarrhythmia is due to increased automaticity of the AV junction in most patients (nonparoxysmal junctional tachycardia, or NPJT) and ectopic atrial focus in other patients (nonparoxysmal atrial tachycardia, or NPAT). Localization of the origin of this arrhythmia is difficult on surface ECG. The most common causes are digitalis toxicity, acute inferior myocardial infarction, rheumatic myocarditis, and cardiac surgery. NPJT is commonly associated with AV dissociation such that the atria are under control of the sinus node and the ventricles are under control of the AV junction. When unrelated to digitalis, a rapid rate should be reduced with digitalis, quinidine, and/or propranolol. If it is digitalis-induced, the drug should be withheld and a potassium supplement administered.

Multifocal Atrial Tachycardia
Multifocal atrial tachycardia (MAT) is characterized by an atrial rate of >100 beats/minute, at least three different configurations of P waves in any one lead, variable P-P and R-R intervals, and fluctuating P-R intervals (Figure 10). Each QRS is preceded by a P wave. Chaotic atrial tachycardia and wandering atrial pacemaker with tachycardia are other names given to this arrhythmia. The mechanism of MAT is based on enhanced automaticity in the atria. It is usually a manifestation of myocardial hypoxia and occurs in elderly patients who have chronic obstructive pulmonary disease or coronary heart disease. Many patients also have diabetes mellitus. It usually indicates further deterioration of underlying cardiac disease and is associated with high mortality. Occasionally, MAT degenerates into atrial fibrillation. Carotid sinus massage has no effect. The usual antiarrhythmic medications are not effec-

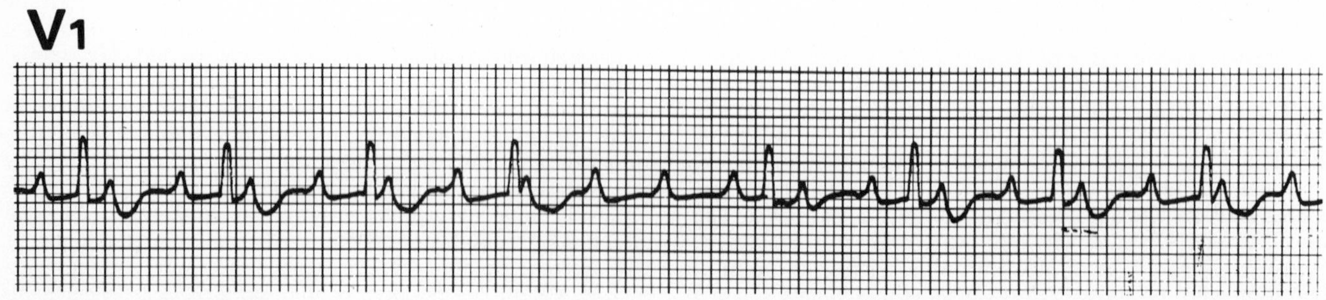

Figure 9. Paroxysmal tachycardia with variable block. Rapid atrial rate of 200 beats per min. Regular P-P intervals. Variable R-R intervals due to variable atrioventricular block.

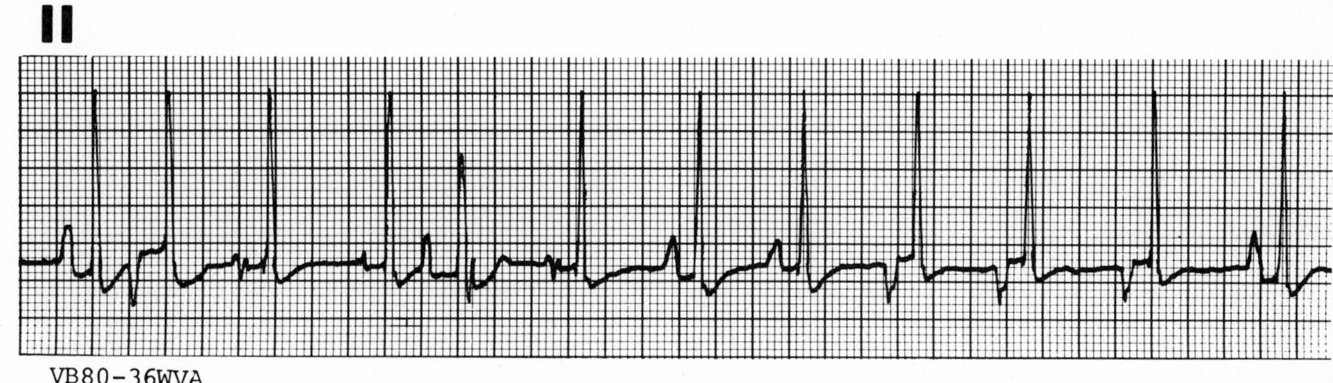

Figure 10. Multifocal atrial tachycardia. P waves show variable configuration.

tive in converting MAT to sinus rhythm. Improvement of the underlying cardiac and/or pulmonary disease is generally accompanied by conversion of MAT into sinus rhythm.

Atrial Flutter

Atrial flutter is a common arrhythmia that occurs either in a short-lived paroxysmal or sustained chronic form. Brief episodes of atrial flutter are frequently seen in acute pulmonary embolism, chronic lung disease, thyrotoxicosis, pericarditis, penumonia, after thoracotomy, alcohol intoxication, and sometimes in apparently healthy individuals. More sustained atrial flutter is usually seen in the sick sinus syndrome, rheumatic, hypertensive, or coronary heart disease, and chronic lung disease.

An ECG in atrial flutter shows flutter (F) waves occurring regularly at 250-350 beats/minute (Fig. 11). They appear in a saw-toothed pattern, are negative in leads II, III, and F, and do not have any isoelectric lines between them. The majority of patients reveal a 2:1 AV block resulting in a ventricular rate of 125-175/minute. A higher-grade AV block (that is, 3:1, 4:1, or variable) may occur. R-R intervals may be constant or variable. Carotid sinus massage increases the degree of AV block, slows the ventricular rate in a stepwise fashion, and brings out the otherwise obscure F waves in the surface ECG. Atrial flutter results from reentry circuit in the atrial tissue.

As a rule, patients complain of palpitations, dizziness, or syncope. A rapid ventricular rate may induce angina and worsen congestive heart failure.

The treatment of atrial flutter is directed at its conversion into sinus rhythm. If this attempt is unsuccessful, the next goal is to slow the ventricular rate. Treatment of the underlying disease, for example, pulmonary embolism or thyrotoxicosis, is usually accompanied by spontaneous emergence of sinus rhythm. When atrial flutter results in adverse hemodynamic effects such as deterioration of heart failure or hypotension and occurs in patients with organic heart disease (especially acute myocardial infarction), synchronous direct-current cardioversion is the treatment of choice. It is almost always successful and requires a small dose of 5- to 10-watt seconds. In less symptomatic patients, digoxin should be administered;

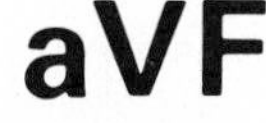

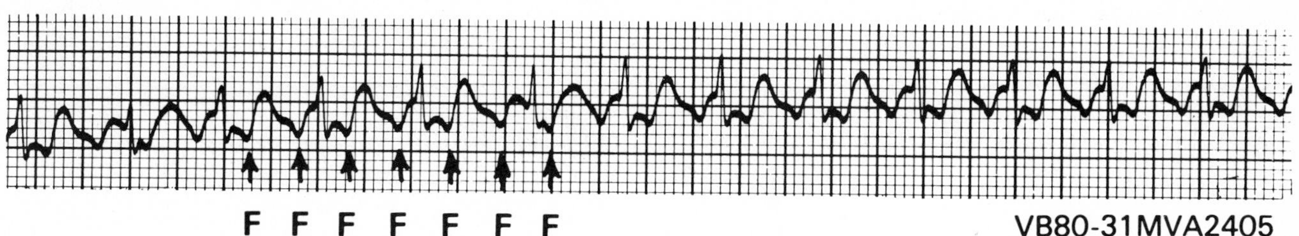

Figure 11. Atrial flutter with 2:1 block. The P waves are replaced by flutter waves (F waves) occurring at a rate of 300/min. They have a saw-toothed appearance. Ventricular rate is 150/min due to 2:1 atrioventricular block.

atrial flutter usually changes into atrial fibrillation and then sinus rhythm. If atrial flutter persists after full digitalization, quinidine should be added since it restores sinus rhythm in the majority of patients. Quinidine should never be used without starting digitalis first because, by slowing the atrial rate and augmenting AV conduction, 2:1 AV block may change into 1:1 conduction and cause an even more rapid ventricular rate. In intractable atrial flutter, propranolol may be used to slow the ventricular rate.

Atrial Fibrillation (AF)

Atrial fibrillation is a very common arrhythmia. It is characterized by total disorganization of atrial activity; the atria display only a writhing motion without any effective contraction.

On an ECG, P waves are absent and replaced by fibrillation (F) waves that are variable in size and occur irregularly at a rate greater than 350 beats/minute (Fig. 12). In certain diseases such as rheumatic mitral valve disease, the F waves are coarse, whereas in coronary heart disease either the F waves are very fine or totally absent. Since the AV node cannot transmit all the atrial impulses, second-degree AV block is always present and the ventricular rate is generally 100-160 beats/minute. R-R intervals are markedly irregular. When complete AV block or AV dissociation develops, the ventricles are controlled by the AV junction and the R-R intervals become regular. The mechanism of AF is believed to be based on reentry or circus movement in the atria.

Atrial fibrillation may be present in a paroxysmal form, with each paroxysm lasting for a few hours to a few days, or in a chronic established form. Paroxysmal AF may occur in apparently healthy individuals. More often, however, it occurs in thyrotoxicosis, early stages of rheumatic mitral valve disease, acute myocardial infarction, pulmonary embolism, lung infections, or with the onset of heart failure. Chronic AF occurs in advanced rheumatic mitral valve disease, hypertension, coronary heart disease, cardiomyopathy, constrictive pericarditis, an atrial septal defect, cardiac surgery, and sick sinus syndrome. Usually, AF indicates either pathologic involvement of the atrial muscle or atrial dilatation and hypertrophy due to atrial hypertension as in mitral valve disease or left heart failure.

Decreased diastolic filling time due to a rapid ventricular rate and loss of atrial contraction cause suboptimal ventricular filling, resulting in decreased cardiac output. A fast ventricular rate enhances myocardial oxygen demand, a deleterious effect in coronary heart disease. Moreover, thrombi form in the atria leading to systemic and pulmonary emboli. Systemic emboli are most common when the AF develops in mitral stenosis. Palpitations, increased heart failure, dizziness, and frequent angina occur in uncontrolled AF.

On physical examination, the peripheral pulse is irregular and each beat is of variable volume. Since during some beats very little stroke volume is ejected into the aorta, no pulsation is palpated peripherally. Therefore, the peripheral pulse rate is less than the apical heart rate (pulse deficit). The jugular venous pulse demonstrates total absence of a waves. The intensity of S_1 is variable.

The initiation or establishment of AF generally indicates progression of underlying cardiac disease. The main objectives of treating patients with AF are control of rapid ventricular rate, restoration of the sinus rhythm, and prevention of emboli. A rapid ventricular rate is best controlled by digitalis, administered orally or intravenously, depending on the clinical status. With adequate digitalization, the apical rate should be 60-80 beats/minute at rest and up to 110 beats/minute with slight exercise. If digitalis alone does not control the rapid ventricular rate, propranolol (40-80 mg) in divided daily doses should be added.

When AF is of the paroxysmal type or of recent origin, as seen in pulmonary embolism, acute myocardial infarction, thoracic operations, or recent heart failure, digitalis therapy restores sinus rhythm in many patients. If the sinus rhythm is not restored, quinidine should be started in doses of 300-400 mg q.i.d. Patients in whom a combination of digitalis and quinidine fails to convert AF into sinus rhythm, elective

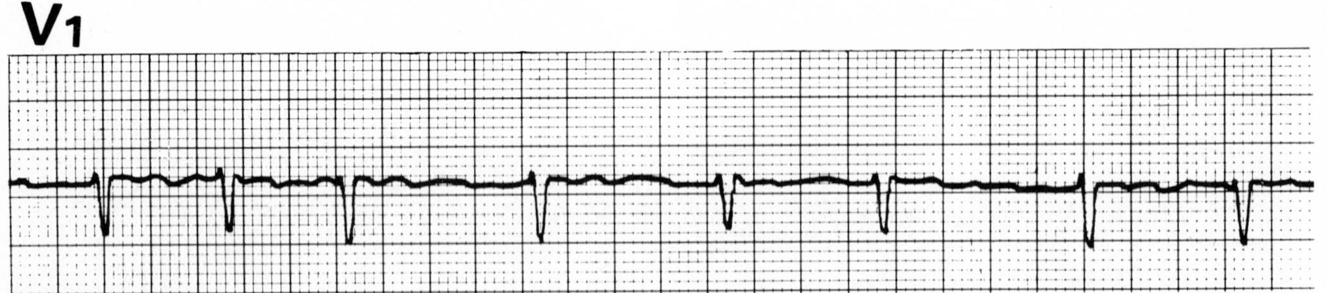

Figure 12. Atrial fibrillation. The P waves are replaced by fine, irregular, undulating fibrillatory waves (F waves). R-R intervals are irregular.

synchronized direct-current cardioversion should be attempted after withholding digitalis for 36-48 hours. The continuation of quinidine after successful cardioversion is helpful in preventing the recurrence of AF. When the onset of AF with rapid ventricular rate is associated with severe heart failure, low output state, or hypotension, synchronized direct-current cardioversion is the treatment of choice. If the AF has existed for more than 1 year, is associated with an enlarged left atrium (>5.5 cm), or recurs after repeat cardioversions, the primary objective should be to keep the ventricular rate under control with digitalis. Electric cardioversion should also be avoided in older patients who have AF with a slow ventricular rate. Long-term anticoagulant drug therapy should be strongly considered in patients with AF and mitral stenosis, gross congestive heart failure, and previous episodes of embolization.

Premature Junctional Beats (PJBs)

Premature junctional beats arise in the AV junctional tissue rather than the AV node, which lacks pacemaker cells. The impulse is transmitted anterogradely to the ventricles, producing a normal QRS complex. Occasionally, QRS becomes wide due to aberrancy. The impulse also conducts retrogradely to the atria, producing a retrograde P wave. Retrograde P waves may appear before, during, or after the QRS complex, depending on the relative velocity of the impulse conducting anterogradely and retrogradely. For example, if the retrograde impulse travels more slowly than the anterograde impulse, the P wave will appear following the QRS complex. When the P wave precedes the QRS, the P-R interval is usually <0.12 seconds. Ordinarily, the PJBs are followed by less than a compensatory pause because the sinus node is usually discharged by the retrograde impulse. They are less common than PABs and PVBs. When atrial activation precedes ventricular activation, a loud S_1 results. On the other hand, ventricular activation occurs simultaneously or following ventricular activation, S_1 is muffled and a cannon a wave is visualized in the jugular venous pulse. The clinical implication of, and therapy for, PJBs are similar to those of PABs.

Junctional Escape Beats (JEBs)

In the presence of sinus bradycardia, sinus arrest, or SA block, an impulse from the AV junction escapes, thereby activating the ventricles and usually the atria as well. The escape interval is greater than the basic P-P interval. The QRS complex is mostly normal but it may be abnormal occasionally due to aberrancy. The physical signs consist of an irregular pulse, variable S_1 intensity, and an occasional cannon a wave. Generally, no treatment is needed but if a patient is symptomatic because of an inadequate heart rate, a pacemaker or drug therapy may be required.

Junctional Rhythm

When there is prolonged sinus arrest or SA block, the AV junction escapes at a rate of 40-60 beats/minute, activating both the atria and the ventricles. The P waves are retrograde and may precede, follow, or be buried in the QRS complexes. On physical examination, the pulse is regular. The jugular venous pulse reveals regular giant a waves. When junctional rhythm is brief in duration and occurs during transient suppression of the sinus node due to increased vagal tone, no treatment is necessary. Furthermore, the reduction of heart rate is only modest and there are usually no adverse hemodynamic changes.

Atrioventricular Dissociation

Atrioventricular dissociation is defined as activation of the atria and ventricles by two different foci that are independent of each other. Usually, the atria are under the control of the sinus node, ectopic atrial focus, or a portion of the AV junction. Depending on the location of the atrial pacemaker, P waves are normal, ectopic, or retrograde. The ventricles are under control of the AV junction or the His-Purkinje system. Again, depending on the location of the ventricular pacemaker, the QRS complexes appear normal or somewhat bizarre.

Default of the sinus node as seen in marked sinus bradycardia, may permit the subsidiary pacemakers to escape and control the ventricles. Alternatively, enhanced automaticity of subsidiary pacemakers as in NPJT, may allow them to control the ventricles. The third mechanism may be failure of the sinus impulse to reach the ventricles, for example, AV block, again allowing the subsidiary pacemakers to escape and control the ventricles. It should be clear from these examples that AV dissociation is the result of underlying arrhythmias such as sinus bradycardia, NPJT, or AV block. AV dissociation is due to a physiologic block in the AV junction. Since the atrial and ventricular rates are nearly equal, atrial impulses cannot propagate to ventricles and vice versa (complete AV dissociation) because of refractoriness. Occasionally, the ventricles become responsive, thereby enabling an atrial impulse to capture them (ventricular capture). Similarly, atrial tissue occasionally becomes responsive, permitting the ventricular impulse to capture the atria retrogradely (atrial capture). In the presence of capture beats, the AV dissociation is described as incomplete.

Electrocardiographically, in AV dissociation atrial and ventricular rates are nearly similar (Fig. 13). There is no relationship between the P waves and QRS complexes. The P-P and R-R intervals are regular. The P waves can be seen marching through the QRS complexes. The patient may have atrial flutter or fibrillation. Occasional QRS complexes are premature, indicating ventricular capture beats. Premature retrograde P waves indicate atrial capture.

Physical examination reveals an S_1 of variable intensity and regular or occasional cannon a waves in the jugular venous impulse. AV dissociation is most commonly seen in digitalis toxicity and acute inferior myocardial infarction. It also may occur after heart surgery, acute rheumatic fever, and following electric cardioversion. The treatment depends on the etiology as well as the underlying arrhythmia responsible for the AV dissociation.

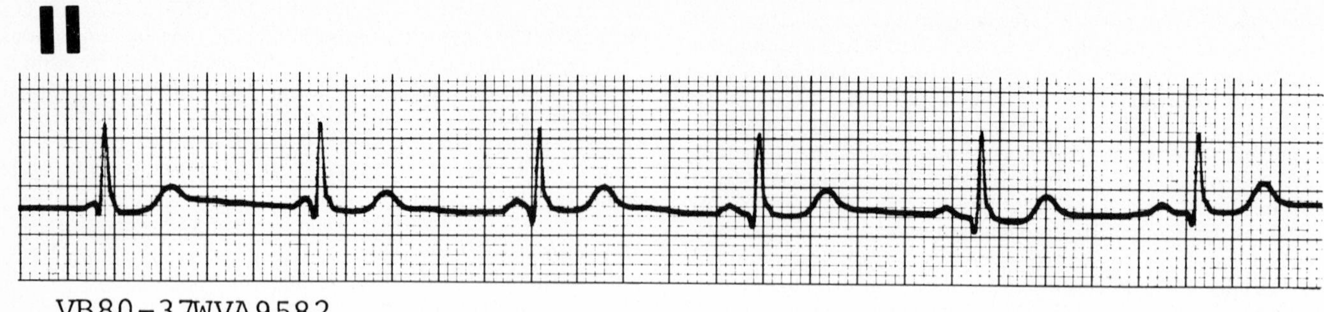

Figure 13. Atrioventricular dissociation. Regular atrial and ventricular rates of 65/min. Note lack of any relationship between P and R waves.

Ventricular Arrhythmias

Premature Ventricular Beats

Premature ventricular beats (PVBs) constitute the most commonly seen arrhythmia. The electrocardiographic characteristics of a PVB consist of a wide (⩾0.12) and an abnormal-looking QRS complex occurring before its time and without a preceding P wave, an ST-T wave pointing opposite to the main QRS complex, usually a complete postectopic compensatory pause (R-R interval containing PVBs is twice the basic R-R interval), and a fixed coupling interval. Sometimes the impulse transmits retrogradely to the atria and gives rise to a retrograde P wave. Moreover, the retrograde impulse may also discharge the sinus node and reset it; therefore, the postectopic pause is less than compensatory. Occasionally there is no compensatory pause so that the R-R interval containing PVB is identical to the basic R-R interval; this type of PVB is described as interpolated. A PVB arising from the septal region has a narrow QRS complex. When the origin of a PVB is from the right ventricle, the QRS resembles a pattern of left bundle-branch block. On the other hand, the left ventricular premature beat produces a right bundle-branch block pattern. PVBs with different configurations in the same lead are called multifocal or multiform. If a PVB alternates with a sinus beat for a period of time, it is described as bigeminal rhythm.

Most of the PVBs with a fixed coupling interval are believed to be on the basis of a reentry mechanism. The other possible mechanism for the origin of PVBs is an enhanced automaticity of an ectopic focus in the Purkinje system or ventricular myocardial tissue. This, however, is considered a more likely mechanism for ventricular parasystole.

Many patients are not aware of PVBs, others may feel a skipped heartbeat, or may be sensitive to forceful postectopic beats and experience palpitations. Frequent PVBs may cause dizziness or angina. Physical exertion reduces or eliminates PVBs in most patients. However, in some patients with coronary heart disease, exercise may increase their frequency. Physical examination reveals an irregular peripheral pulse, a more forceful pulse following the pause, irregular cannon a waves in the jugular venous pulse, and a widely split S_1 and S_2 corresponding to the PVB.

Healthy individuals, especially in their later years, may experience PVBs. Strong tea, coffee, alcohol, sympathomimetic amines, anxiety, hypoxia, occasionally exercise, anesthetic agents, and any type of heart disease may cause PVBs. They are most frequent in acute myocardial infarction, chronic coronary heart disease, digitalis toxicity, congestive heart failure, and mitral valve prolapse.

PVBs should be differentiated from ventricular parasystole and PABs or PJBs with aberrant conduction. Unlike PVBs, parasystolic beats have a variable coupling interval, fusion beats are present, and the longest interval between two consecutive parasystolic beats is a multiple of the shortest interval between two parasystolic beats. The differential features of a supraventricular beat with aberrancy have already been discussed.

The prognosis for patients with PVBs is largely determined by the underlying cause. In the absence of serious heart disease, PVBs do not seem to affect normal life expectancy. On the other hand, in both acute myocardial infarction and chronic coronary heart disease, PVBs increase mortality as well as the incidence of sudden death. The following features identify serious PVBs that may be forerunners of ventricular tachycardia (VT) and ventricular fibrillation (VF): multifocal PVBs, frequency of >6/min, in pairs, or occurring on T wave of previous beats. Recently, even late diastolic PVBs have been shown to cause VT and VF.

Asymptomatic patients without heart disease do not require treatment for PVBs. If palpitation is experienced, elimination of alcohol and strong coffee and the use of mild tranquilizers may be required. In acute myocardial infarction, PVBs must be vigorously treated. Since continuous monitoring has demonstrated PVBs in 80 to 90 percent of acute myocardial infarction patients, antiarrhythmic treatment may be employed routinely. Intravenous lidocaine is the drug of choice. After administering a 50-75 mg bolus, continuous infusion at a rate of 1-4 mg/minute is initiated. When lidocaine is ineffective, procainamide is used. Intravenous boluses of 100 mg should be administered at 5-minute intervals, carefully monitoring the blood pressure and ECG until the PVBs are suppressed or 1 gm of the drug has been given. A continuous infusion of 2-6 mg/minute can also be used. In a small number of patients, both lidocaine and procainamide may fail, and other drugs such as quinidine, propranolol, disopyramide (Norpace), and phenytoin may be tried. In refractory patients, overdrive suppression with a pacemaker may be required.

In patients with chronic coronary heart disease and frequent and multifocal PVBs, oral therapy with procainamide, quinidine, and disopyramide (singly or in combination) is usually effective. When QT interval is prolonged in the baseline ECG, these drugs are contraindicated; instead phenytoin and propranolol are advised. In exercise induced PVBs, propranolol is more effective. When multiple PVBs occur in a patient taking digitalis, it should be discontinued. On the other hand, when PVBs occur with congestive heart failure, digitalis should be started since the improvement of heart failure with digitalis may eliminate PVBs.

Ventricular Tachycardia

In ventricular tachycardia (VT), the ventricles beat rapidly at a rate of 100-250 beats/minute as a result of impulses arising within the ventricles (Fig. 14). The mechanism of VT is a reentry circuit or repetitive discharges from an ectopic ventricular focus; it is primarily an ECG diagnosis. The QRS complexes are broad (>0.12 s) and bizarre with ST and T pointing opposite to the QRS complexes. R-R intervals are fairly regular. Since atria are under control of the sinus node, AV disociation is usually present. Frequently, there is retrograde activation of the atria from the ventricles during each beat. The main differential diagnosis is supraventricular tachycardia (SVT) with wide QRS complexes due to preexisting bundle-branch block, Wolff-Parkinson-White syndrome, or aberrant conduction. Comparison of the QRS complexes with a previous ECG and examination of the ECG at the onset of arrhythmia are helpful. If the arrhythmia begins with a PAC, shows a right bundle branch-block pattern (rsR′), and is slowed or abolished by carotid sinus massage, it is most likely of supraventricular origin. On the other hand, if the arrhythmia begins with a PVB, is not affected by carotid sinus massage, resembles isolated PVBs on previous tracings, and is interrupted by fusion and ventricular capture complexes, it is most likely of ventricular origin. Wide QRS tachycardia showing a pattern of right bundle branch block with left anterior hemiblock is usually a VT. When ventricular rate is >250 beats/minute, it is called ventricular flutter.

By disturbing the sequence of ventricular contraction, VT generally has more profound hemodynamic effects than does SVT. However, the status of the underlying myocardium is a major determinant of hemodynamic deterioration. Symptoms of VT include palpitation, dyspnea, angina, and dizziness. Physical examination may reveal irregular cannon a waves in JVP; S_1 of variable intensity; rapid, regular, and feeble pulse, or hypotension and heart failure.

VT occurs in acute myocardial infarction, chronic coronary heart disease, digitalis toxicity, cardiac surgery, anesthesia, cardiac catheterization, and during administration of sympathomimetic amines, but rarely in healthy individuals. Acute myocardial infarction is the most common etiology of VT. VT may be as short as three consecutive beats or may be sustained for minutes to hours. The prognosis and therapy depends on the status of underlying cardiac disease.

When VT occurs in the presence of acute myocardial infarction or other severe heart disease, three intravenous lidocaine boluses (50-100 mg) at 2- to 3-minute intervals should be administered. If VT does not convert with lidocaine, procainamide should be injected intravenously (100 mg/min) under ECG control until termination of VT or a total of 1 g has been administered. If VT responds to lidocaine, continuous infusion of 1-4 mg/min should be started to prevent recurrence. If both drugs fail or the hemodynamic status deteriorates rapidly, electric cardioversion should be performed using 50- to 100-watt-seconds. To prevent recurrent bouts of VT, procainamide, quinidine, and disopyramide should be administered orally on a long-term basis. When QT interval is excessively prolonged in the baseline ECG, phenytoin and/or propranolol

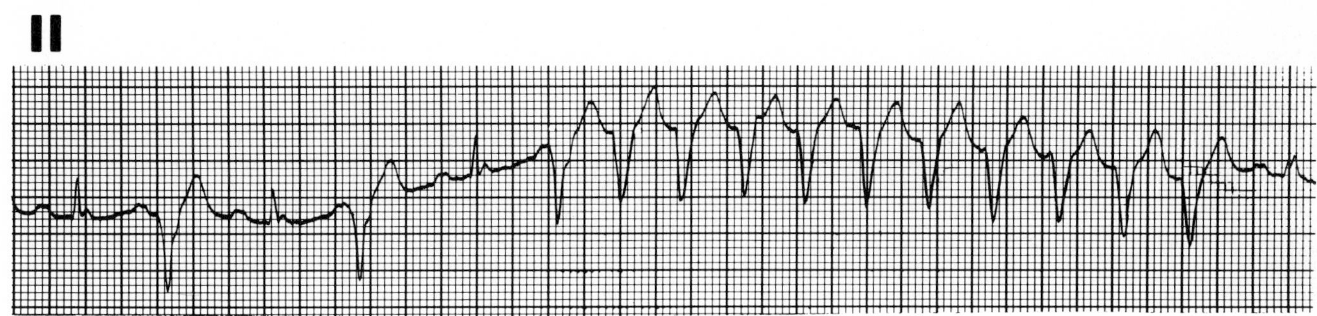

Figure 14. Paroxysmal ventricular tachycardia. Note wide QRS complexes occurring at a rate of 167/min. These QRS complexes are almost regular and identical to the premature ventricular beats occurring before the initiation of ventricular tachycardia (second and fourth QRS complexes).

should be started for further prevention. When VT is initiated by digitalis toxicity, digitalis should be discontinued. In addition, potassium chloride and lidocaine should be administered. In the presence of heart failure, VT is not a contraindication to digitalis therapy. Drug-resistant, recurrent VT can be controlled with overdrive suppression by a pace-maker. In patients with recurrent VT and ventricular aneurysm, aneurysmectomy has been successful in approximately 50 percent of the patients in controlling this arrhythmia.

Ventricular Escape Beats
When the supraventricular impulse defaults, as in sinus bradycardia, sinus arrest, SA, or AV block, the impulse arises from the ventricular Purkinje network and activates the ventricles. The resultant QRS complex is delayed and is described as a ventricular escape beat.

Idioventricular Rhythm
When the supraventricular pacemakers default for a prolonged period, the ventricular focus escapes and drives the heart at a rate of 20-60 beats/minute. The QRS complexes are bizarre and occur at regular intervals. Frequently, patients complain of dizziness or frank syncope during this rhythm. In symptomatic patients, a permanent pacemaker is indicated.

Accelerated Idioventricular Rhythm
The accelerated idioventricular rhythm (AIVR) is defined as three or more ventricular complexes occurring at a rate of 60-100 beats/minute, and it characteristically begins with a ventricular escape complex (Fig. 15). On the other hand, slow VT begins with a premature ventricular complex. Enhanced automoticity of ventricular tissue causes AIVR. Recently, it has been demonstrated that AIVR may lead to VT or VF. this rhythm disturbance. Since episodes of AIVR are brief and there is usually no hemodynamic disturbance, treatment is not needed. This rhythm disturbance may be abolished by accelerating the sinus rate by intravenous atropine and/or suppression of the AIVR with intravenous lidocaine.

Ventricular Fibrillation (VF) (Fig. 16)
Ventricular fibrillation is characterized electrocardiographically by base line undulations that have a variable amplitude and periodicity. There are no QRS complexes or T waves. Since there is no effective heart beat, ventricular fibrillation is a catastrophic event that is manifested by an absent pulse and blood pressure. The patient becomes unconscious, and death ensues within a few minutes of the inception of VF unless cardiopulmonary resuscitation is initiated within 3-4 minutes. The most common causes of VF include acute myocardial infarction, advanced coronary artery disease with severe left ventricular dysfunction, marked electrolyte disturbances (e.g., hypokalemia), drug intoxication (e.g., digoxin, quinidine), hypothermia, and electrocution. Ventricular fibrillation is the most common underlying cause of sudden death. Electrical defibrillation is required to abolish VF.

DISORDERS OF IMPULSE CONDUCTION

Sinoatrial Block
In sinoatrial (SA) block, an impulse arises in the SA node but fails to activate the atria. There is total absence of the P-QRS-ST-T for a variable period. In Mobitz Type-II SA block, the pause is an exact multiple of the basic P-P interval. In Wenckebach Type-I SA block, the pause is shorter than a multiple of the P-P interval. The clinical implications of SA block is similar to those of sinus arrest.

Atrioventricular Block
Block at the AV node is conventionally classified into three categories: first, second, and third degree block.

First-Degree AV Block
First-degree AV block is defined as delay of conduction from the sinus node to the ventricles. It is characterized by prolongation of the P-R interval ($\geq$0.21 s). The site of conduction delay is in the AV node. On physical examination, S_1 becomes

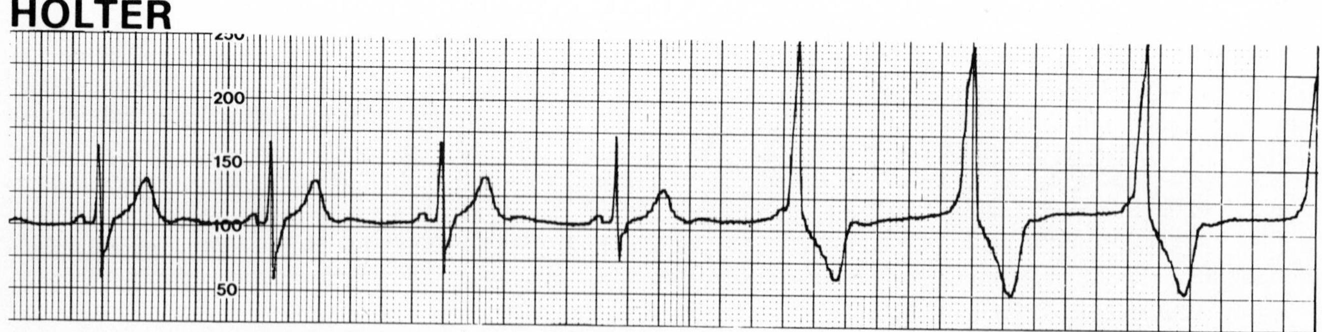

Figure 15. Accelerated idioventricular rhythm. Note wide bizarre QRS complexes occurring at a rate of 60/min following first 4 sinus beats. These QRS complexes are regular and there is concomitant atrioventricular dissociation.

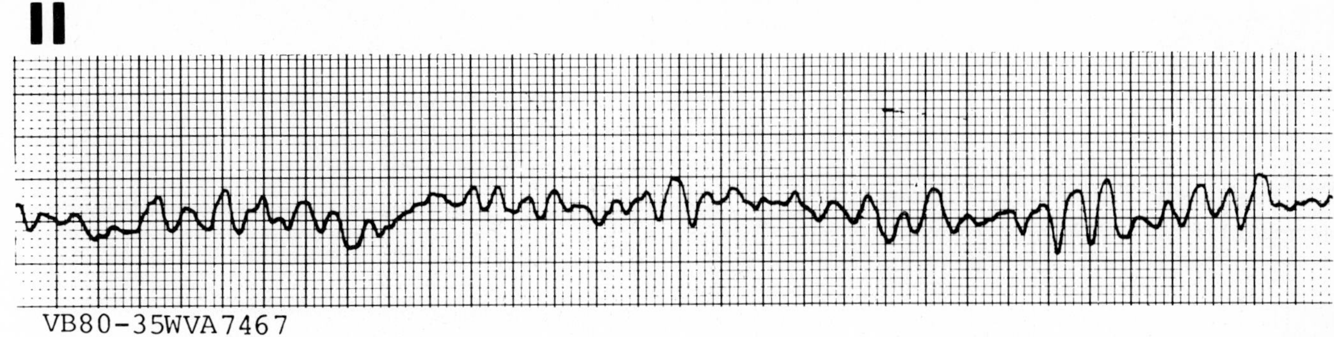

Figure 16. Ventricular fibrillation. Note broad bizarre complexes occurring rapidly and at irregular intervals. The configuration shows marked variability. There are no QRS complexes and T waves.

soft and S_4 becomes audible. Excessive digitalis, rheumatic myocarditis, and inferior wall infarction are common causes. When due to excessive digitalis, the dose should be slightly reduced. However, in a patient with heart failure and first degree AV block, digitalis can be administered cautiously. First-degree AV block does not usually progress to higher grades of block and does not require therapy.

Second-Degree AV Block

Second-degree AV block implies that some of the supraventricular impulses are blocked in the AV junction. It is further subdivided into the following categories: Wenckebach or Mobitz Type I, Mobitz Type II, 2:1 block, and high-grade block.

Wenckebach or Mobitz Type I is the most common variety of second degree AV block. It is characterized by progressive increase of the P-R interval from beat to beat followed by nonconduction of the P wave (Fig. 17). In addition, there is progressive shortening of the R-R intervals. The beat following the nonconducted P wave has the shortest P-R interval and the beat preceding the nonconducted P wave has the longest P-R interval. In an atypical Wenckebach type of AV block, which is more common than the classical variety, the increment of the P-R interval may be minimal from one beat to another or, after progressive increase, it may decrease before the blocked P wave. Therefore, it is important to compare the P-R intervals of the beat preceding and the beat following the blocked P wave because these beats should reveal the greatest difference.

In approximately 75 percent of patients, the AV node is the site of block. In such patients, the QRS complex is narrow and the prognosis is benign. This type of block is primarily due to decremental conduction in the AV node and occurs in digitalis toxicity, acute inferior myocardial infarction, and rheumatic myocarditis. Occasionally, the location of the Wenckebach block is in the His bundle and its branches. In these patients, the QRS may be broad. Sclerodegenerative disease of the conduction system is the usual origin. These patients may develop higher degrees of AV block manifested by syncope and thus require pacemaker therapy.

Mobitz Type-II AV block is characterized by sudden non-

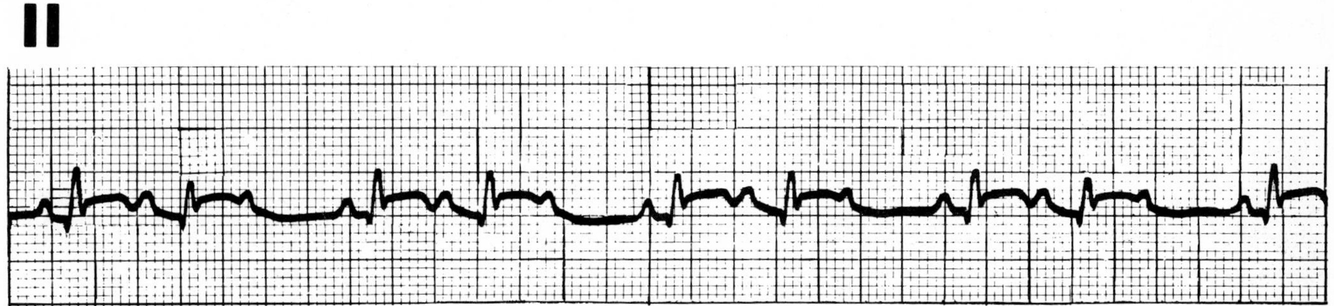

Figure 17. Wenckebach type of second-degree atrioventricular block. Note progressive prolongation of P-R interval until a P wave is blocked, following which the cycle restarts. 3:2 AV block (3 P waves to 2 QRS complexes).

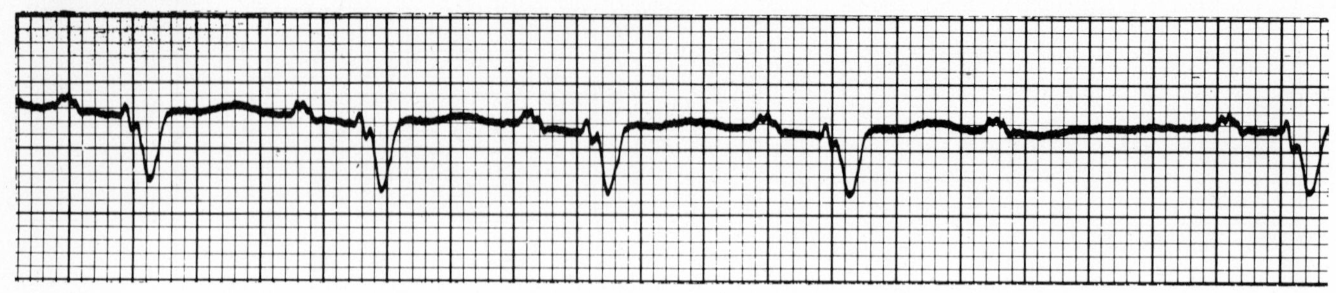

Figure 18. Mobitz type II, second-degree atrioventricular block. Note constant P-R intervals until suddenly a P wave is blocked.

conduction of the P wave. In contrast to the Wenckebach type of block, P-R intervals of beats preceding and following the nonconducted P wave are identical (Fig. 18). The location of the Mobitz type II block is almost always in the His bundle and its branches. The QRS complexes are generally broad and the majority of these patients have symptoms of dizziness and syncope. They are at risk of sudden death and a permanent pacemaker is usually indicated. Common causes of the Mobitz type II AV block include sclerodegenerative disease of the conduction system, anterior wall myocardial infarction, calcific aortic valve disease, hypertensive heart disease, and the cardiomyopathies.

A 2:1 AV block cannot be classified into either the Mobitz type II or the Wenckebach type I blocks because differentiation between them depends on the progressive behavior of the P-R intervals in several beats (Fig. 19). A careful review of long rhythm strips may sometimes show a 3:2 AV block that helps determine the correct classification.

High-grade AV block is recognized on ECG when several successive blocked P waves are followed by a conducted P wave. The ventricular rate is slow. Its clinical significance is similar to that of third-degree AV block.

Complete A V Block

Complete or third-degree block is characterized by total independence of the P waves and QRS complexes since propagation of atrial activity to the ventricles is totally blocked. The atria are generally controlled by the sinus node at a rate of 60-100 beats/minute and the P-P intervals are regular. The R-R intervals are also regular and QRS complexes may be narrow or wide, depending on the site of the block (Fig. 20). PVBs or VT on a reentry basis may occur because of inhomogeneous recovery rates of the ventricular muscle fibers due to the slow ventricular rate.

The site of block in the conduction system has great prognostic value. Block in the AV node is benign, whereas infranodal block (His bundle and its branches) is potentially hazardous and can cause sudden death due to ventricular asystole or fibrillation. Complete AV block can occur acutely as in acute myocardial infarction or in a more chronic form. Nodal block occurs in digitalis toxicity, acute inferior myocardial infarction, and myocarditis. In inferior myocardial infarction, complete AV block resolves spontaneously within 1 week and is usually asymptomatic. In congenital complete AV block, the site of block is in the AV node, the QRS complexes are

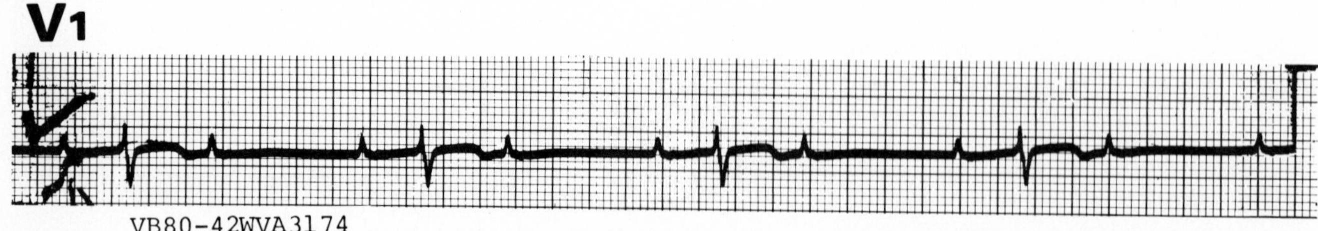

Figure 19. 2:1 Second-degree atrioventricular block. Since every alternate P wave is blocked, it cannot be further subclassified into Wenckebach or Mobitz Type II blocks.

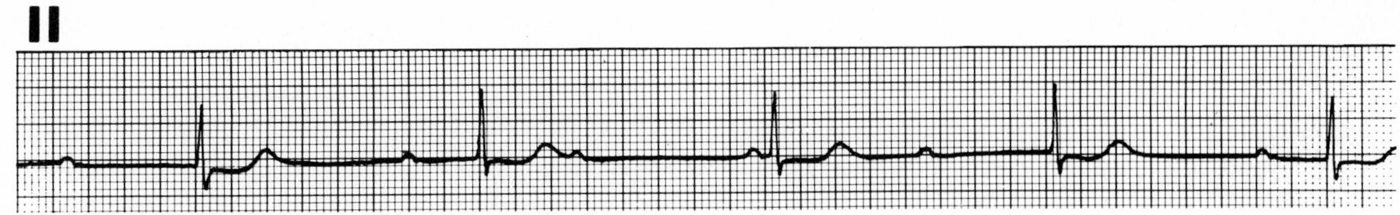

Figure 20. Third-degree or complete atrioventricular block. Note regularly occurring P waves at a rate of 64/min and regularly occurring QRS complexes at a rate of 44/min. There is no relationship between P waves and QRS complexes. Narrow QRS complexes suggest that the origin of ventricular impulse is located above the bifurcation of the His bundle.

narrow, and the patient is usually without symptoms as the ventricular rate is 40-60 beats/minute and increases with exercise. Infranodal block occurs in sclerodegenerative disease of the conduction tissue, calcific aortic stenosis, chronic coronary heart disease, surgical trauma, and cardiomyopathy. The QRS complexes are broad, and the ventricular rate is 20-40 beats/minute and does not increase with exercise. Infranodal block also occurs acutely in anterior myocardial infarction and has a high mortality of 70 percent. However, if the patient survives, the sinus rhythm is usually restored within 1 week.

Hemodynamic changes in complete AV block depend on the status of the myocardium and heart rate. A well-preserved myocardium may be able to compensate for the slow rate. However, a damaged myocardium does not provide this compensation and cardiac output is decreased. Filling pressures rise in both ventricles, as well as systemic vascular resistance. Blood flow to various organs is reduced. Bradycardia gives rise to increased systolic and pulse pressures.

Light-headedness, dizziness, or full-fledged Stokes-Adams attacks may occur in complete AV block. Stokes-Adams attacks are characterized by a total loss of consciousness for 10-30 seconds because of ventricular asystole, tachycardia, or fibrillation. Convulsions commonly accompany the attack. Consciousness rapidly returns on resumption of the heart beat. Patients are at high risk of sudden death during these attacks. Complete AV block may also initiate or worsen heart failure. Once Stokes-Adams attacks and/or heart failure begin, life expectancy is only a few months.

On physical examination, a slow bounding pulse, increased systolic and pulse pressures, cannon a waves in neck veins, and variable intensity of S_1 (loud S_1 is called cannon sound) are found. As increased stroke volume is ejected rapidly into the great vessels, systolic ejection murmurs over the cardiac base are common, and modest cardiomegaly is usually present. During Stokes-Adams attacks, the patient is pulseless, and the skin is cyanosed or pallid.

Bundle-Branch Blocks

Conduction of an impulse may be slowed or totally interrupted in the right bundle, main left bundle, or anterior and posterior fascicles of the left bundle.

Right Bundle-Branch Block (RBBB)

Delayed right ventricular activation gives rise to rsR′, broad bifid, or flat-topped R pattern in V_1 and V_2 leads, wide and slurred S in leads I, aV_L, V_5, and V_6. QRS duration is $\geq$0.12 s in complete RBBB. Mean QRS axis in the frontal plane remains normal. There are secondary ST-T changes. S_2 is widely split due to delayed closure of the pulmonic valve but maintains its respiratory variation. Incomplete RBBB (QRS duration 0.08-0.11 second) may indicate diastolic overloading of the right ventricle, as in an atrial septal defect. RBBB occurs in sclerodegenerative disease of conduction tissue, acute anterior myocardial infarction, acute pulmonary embolism, chronic coronary heart disease, and sometimes in individuals with no apparent cardiac disease. When R is $>$15 mm, it may indicate right ventricular hypertrophy. The clinical significance of RBBB lies in uncovering associated cardiac findings, if any exist. As an isolated finding, it is harmless. Progression of RBBB to complete AV block is rare.

Left Bundle-Branch Block (LBBB)

LBBB results because of slow conduction in the main left bundle or simultaneous slow conduction in its anterior and posterior fascicles. An ECG shows a normal mean frontal QRS axis; rsR′ or slurred R in I, aV_L, V_5, and V_6; deep S in V_1 and V_2; absence of Q in I, aV_L, V_5, and V_6; and secondary ST-T changes. LBBB is considered complete when the QRS width is $\geq$0.12 s and incomplete when it is $<$0.12 s. By affecting the initial portion of ventricular conduction, LBBB greatly interferes with the ECG diagnosis of myocardial infarction. Delayed closure of the aortic valve results in reversed or paradoxical splitting of S_2. LBBB occurs in sclerodegenerative disease of conduction tissue, cardiomyopathies, calcific aortic valve disease, and hypertensive or coronary heart disease. In most patients, incomplete LBBB is associated with left ventricular hypertrophy. LBBB is rarely seen in patients with no other demonstrable evidence of heart disease. Incidence of progression of LBBB to complete AV block is slight, and the prognosis depends on the associated cardiac disease.

Left Anterior Hemiblock (LAH)

This is the most common variety of conduction abnormality. Impaired conduction in the anterior fascicle causes some delay in activation of the anterosuperior portion of the left ventricle that produces the following ECG features: a left axis deviation $> -30^\circ$; qR pattern in I and aV_L; rS pattern in II, III, aV_F; and only negligible prolongation of QRS duration because of numerous interconnections between the two fascicles of the left bundle. LAH may also result in persistence of S waves in leads V_5 and V_6 and the absence of r in leads V_1 and V_2.

Left Posterior Hemiblock (LPH)
Impaired conduction in the posterior fascicle leads to some delay in activation of the posteroinferior portion of the left ventricle. ECG features of LPH consist of right axis deviation of $\geqslant +110^\circ$; presence of qR pattern in II, III, and aV_F; and presence of rS pattern in I and aV_L. Other conditions giving rise to right axis deviation, for example, lateral infarction, right ventricular hypertrophy, and vertical heart, must be ruled out. Since it is the broadest fascicle and has a dual coronary blood supply, isolated LPH is rare.

Bifascicular Blocks
Impairment of conduction can develop simultaneously in any two of the three fascicles; the impulse then propagates to ventricles through the remaining fascicle. RBBB, in combination with LAH, is the most common type (approximately 1 percent of all hospital ECGs) of bifascicular block. It is characterized by a mean QRS axis of $> -30^\circ$, rsR′ in V_1 and V_2, and slurred S in V_5 and V_6. Each year, approximately 5 percent of patients with RBBB plus LAH develop second or third degree AV block. RBBB and LPH is characterized by ECG changes of RBBB and right axis deviation of $> +110^\circ$. The incidence of progression to advanced AV block has been reported to vary from 5-10 percent annually. Simultaneous block in anterior and posterior fascicles manifests as LBBB.

Trifascicular Block
Simultaneous block in all three fascicles manifests as complete AV block. Incomplete trifascicular block indicates bifascicular block plus a prolonged P-R interval, indicating slow conduction in the third fascicle. It must be emphasized that in most patients a prolonged P-R interval results from a delayed impulse at the AV node rather than in the third fascicle. His-bundle electrocardiography is required to make this differentiation.

Patients with fascicular blocks can develop advanced AV block that may result in dizziness and syncope, at which time permanent pacemaker insertion is indicated. However, ambulatory ECG monitoring should be performed to document the fact that bradyarrhythmias are actually the cause of syncope. This documentation is required because syncope is sometimes due to tachycardia or is of unknown origin. Under the latter circumstances, pacemaker therapy is not beneficial.

PERMANENT PACEMAKERS

Indications for inserting a permanent pacemaker are as follows:

1. Complete AV block with accompanying dizziness, syncope, Stokes-Adams attacks, or heart failure.
2. Mobitz Type II AV block.
3. Bifascicular blocks accompanied by dizziness or syncope as a result of bradyarrhythmias.
4. Sick sinus syndrome in patients with symptoms.
5. Atrial fibrillation with slow (<40 beats/minute) heart rate and heart failure.
6. Bifascicular blocks and complete AV block persisting after acute myocardial infarction.
7. Overdrive suppression of drug-resistant ventricular tachycardia and multiple multifocal PVCs.

A permanent pacemaker consists of an electrode lead and a generator or battery. The electrode lead is inserted transvenously into the right ventricular apex or surgically implanted into the left ventricular wall (epicardium). The battery source is inserted into a subcutaneous pocket below the clavicle, in the axilla, or in the abdomen. The power source in the battery consists of mercury cells with a life expectancy of 3-5 years, lithium cells (8-10 years), rechargeable nickel-cadmium cells (8-12 years), or a nuclear power source with a life expectancy of 10-20 years. The choice of generator depends on the anticipated life expectancy and physical activity of the patient.

Several modes of pacing are available, namely, ventricular asynchronous (fixed-rate), ventricular synchronous (R-wave-inhibited on-demand, R-wave-triggered), atrial asynchronous, atrial synchronous, and AV sequential.

A ventricular asynchronous or fixed-rate pacemaker discharges at a constant, preselected rate. This type is ideally suited for patients with complete AV block who have extremely slow ventricular rates. However, it may interfere with the inherent ventricular complexes, for example, fusion complexes may result as the ventricles are depolarized by the pacemaker, as well as inherent ventricular focus. Moreover, the pacemaker spike may infringe on T waves and start ventricular fibrillation. To avoid these competitive rhythm problems, ventricular synchronous pacemakers were designed. An R-wave inhibited or a demand pacemaker is the most frequently used. The inherent R wave is sensed by the pacemaker, which is inhibited from discharging. However, when there is no R wave for a given interval, the pacemaker fires and captures the ventricles. R-wave-triggered is the other type of ventricular synchronous pacemaker that is used less frequently. It senses the inherent R-wave and discharges in its absolute refractory period. If the inherent R wave fails to arise, the pacemaker captures the ventricles. When appropriately timed atrial contractions are required to increase the cardiac output, an atrial pacemaker should be inserted. Permanent atrial pacemakers are usually implanted surgically. The atrial asynchronous type is like a fixed-rate pacemaker. An atrial synchronous pacemaker senses the P wave and stimulates the ventricles after a built-in delay. An AV sequential pacemaker stimulates the atria (P wave), followed by a built-in delay (P-R interval), and then stimulates the ventricles (R wave).

On an ECG, a pacemaker-induced complex shows a pacemaker spike (a vertical line), followed immediately by a broad QRS in a ventricular pacemaker, or a P wave in the presence of an atrial pacemaker. Since the electrode lead is placed in the right ventricular apex, the right ventricle is depolarized earlier than the left ventricle. The resulting QRS resembles an RBBB pattern. If the transvenously placed lead migrates into the coronary sinus, all the precordial leads record an R wave.

Complications of permanent pacing include infection and erosion at the site of battery implantation, or early failure to capture that is generally due to displacement or breakage of the electrode lead. The electrode lead may perforate the right ventricle and stimulate the diaphragm. Late failure to capture usually results from battery exhaustion. Failure to sense inherent R waves and, conversely, sensing of T waves are other complications of permanent pacemakers. Better shielding and inclusion of noise circuits in the newer pacemakers have decreased the incidence of pacemaker malfunction due to outside interference such as microwave ovens, electric shavers, and electrical cardioversion.

Patients with permanent pacemakers should be monitored periodically with ECGs to determine pacemaker function. Follow-up has been made convenient recently with the development of telephonic transmission of ECGs. Accurate measurement of heart rate is the most reliable criterion to assess pacemaker function. A decrease of even 2-3 beats per minute indicates imminent battery failure and should be an indication for battery change.

PREEXCITATION SYNDROMES

Preexcitation syndromes include the Wolff-Parkinson-White (WPW) syndrome and its variants. The ECG features of the WPW pattern consist of a short P-R interval (⩽0.12 s), prolonged QRS duration (⩾0.11 s) due to the addition of a delta wave to its initial portion, and secondary ST-T changes.

In these patients, existence of anomalous or accessory fibers bridging the AV groove has been demonstrated. The impulse from the sinus node conducts rapidly through the accessory pathway and activates a portion of the ventricles, resulting in a δ wave. The remainder of the sinus impulse travels normally through the AV node and depolarizes the remaining portion of the ventricles. Thus, the QRS complex in the WPW pattern represents a fusion complex due to near-simultaneous activation of the ventricles through two different pathways. The WPW pattern is customarily divided into types A and B. In Type A, the δ wave as well as the major portion of the QRS complex is upright in V_1. This is due to the posterior location of an accessory pathway (Kent's bundle) between the left atrium and the left ventricle. In Type B, the δ wave and major portion of the QRS complex is negative in V_1. This pattern is attributed to the anterior location of Kent's bundle bridging the right atrium and the right ventricle. In many other patients, the QRS complexes are of intermediate forms. In others, longitudinal dissociation is probably present in the AV node and His bundle, and the impulse propagates through these two portions of the AV node and His bundle at different speeds, resulting in a WPW pattern.

The prevalence of a WPW pattern in the general population is approximately 0.15 percent and ratio of males to females is 2:1. This anomaly is considered to be congenital in nature and is probably inherited. The WPW pattern may be associated with other cardiac anomalies, that is, Ebstein's anomaly, mitral valve prolapse, and idiopathic hypertrophic subaortic stenosis. Patients are at risk for tachyarrhythmias and may become symptomatic at any age. About two-thirds of the patients with a WPW pattern develop tachyarrhythmias. The most common variety of tachyarrhythmias is paroxysmal supraventricular tachycardia that occurs on a reentry basis. Usually the impulse transmits anterogradely through the AV node and His bundle and retrogradely through the accessory pathway, and this reentrant or reciprocating circuit perpetuates itself. During tachycardia, QRS complexes are generally normal or show functional bundle-branch block. The tachycardia starts and terminates with a premature atrial, junctional, or ventricular beat. In other patients, atrial fibrillation or atrial flutter occurs; QRS complexes are usually wide because the anterograde conduction is through the accessory pathway. Occasionally, a ventricular rate of >300 beats/minute may result due to 1:1 conduction through the accessory pathway. In general, rapid ventricular rates (>180 beats/minute) during supraventricular tachycardias are characteristic of a WPW syndrome. Many patients develop chest pain, heart failure, or syncope during these episodes of rapid tachycardia. The long-term prognosis is usually good, however, and the incidence of sudden death is extremely low.

Variants of WPW consist of a Lown-Ganong-Levine (LGL) pattern that is characterized by a short (⩽0.12 s) P-R interval and a normal QRS complex. This is probably due to the presence of an accessory pathway (James fibers) that bypasses the AV node. A minority of patients with this syndrome experience supraventricular tachycardias. Another variant form is characterized by a normal or prolonged P-R interval and a wide QRS complex due to a δ wave. This has been attributed to the presence of Mahaim fibers connecting the His bundle to the ventricular septum.

Treatment of the WPW syndrome comprises abolishing the acute attack of supraventricular tachycardia and then preventing further attacks. If the attack is accompanied by adverse hemodynamic effects, direct-current cardioversion should be performed; otherwise, intravenous procainamide or quinidine may be used. Pacemaker-induced PAC or PVC may also be utilized to terminate the tachycardia. When atrial flutter or fibrillation develops with a rapid ventricular rate, vagotonic maneuvers and acute digitalization should be avoided since the ventricular rate may increase even further due to a decrease of the refractory period of the accessory pathway. Direct-current cardioversion, intravenous procainamide, or quinidine should be tried. Most patients with preexcitation syndrome and recurrent tachyarrhythmias should have an electrophysiological study to evaluate an antiarrhythmic agent(s) best suited to prevent further episodes of arrhythmias. In patients with life-threatening or disabling tachyarrhythmias that are resistant to medical therapy, surgical interruption of the accessory pathway has recently proven useful in abolishing further attacks.

CONGESTIVE HEART FAILURE

Congestive heart failure (CHF) is clinically defined as a constellation of symptoms and signs denoting congestion of systemic and/or pulmonary venous beds and low cardiac output due to inability of the cardiac chambers to discharge their contents adequately. In this condition, despite adequate filling of the ventricles, cardiac output is relatively inadequate to meet the demands of the body. Several terms are used relative to CHF; for example, left heart failure indicates pulmonary venous congestion with low left ventricular output, right heart failure indicates systemic venous congestion, acute left heart failure is exemplified by acute pulmonary edema, chronic heart failure as in congestive cardiomyopathy secondary to alcohol abuse and low-output failure indicates higher than normal cardiac output that is still inadequate to meet the vastly increased demands of the body such as in thyrotoxic heart disease.

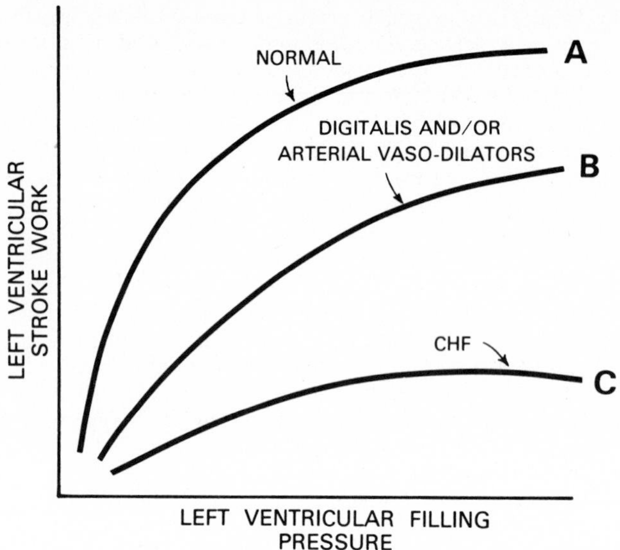

Figure 21. Ventricular function curves. (A) Normal ventricular function curve—a slight increase in left ventricular filling pressure (LVFP) should result in a large increase of left ventricular stroke work (LVSW). (B) Enhanced contractility due to digitalis and/or decreased impedance due to vasodilators in patients with CHF shift the ventricular function curve from C to B. Consequently, these agents augment LVSW at a given LVFP. (C) Markedly depressed ventricular function curve in congestive heart failure (CHF)—unlike normal curve, in CHF, a large increase in LVFP would result in a small increase of LVSW.

PATHOPHYSIOLOGY OF CONGESTIVE HEART FAILURE

Normal Circulation

The pump function of the heart is dependent on the contractile activity of the myocardium. Myocardial contraction is the summated result of shortening of each contractile element, namely, sarcomere, which is the anatomic and functional unit of myocardium. The amount of blood pumped by the heart per minute is described as cardiac output. Cardiac output is usually expressed as cardiac index, which is cardiac output per square meter of body surface area. Under basal conditions, normal cardiac index is 2.8-4.2 L/min/m^2 and outputs of the right and left ventricles are identical. Cardiac output is a product of heart rate and stroke volume, that is, the amount of blood ejected per beat (approximately 50 ml/m^2). Stroke volume is the difference between the end-diastolic volume (EDV) and the end-systolic volume (ESV). At rest the left ventricle normally discharges 60-70 percent of blood present at end-diastole. This represents the normal ejection fraction, which is EDV-ESV/EDV. Maintenance of adequate stroke volume is dependent on the factors described below.

Preload

Preload (presystolic or end-diastolic volume, end-diastolic pressure) greatly affects the amount of stroke volume. The relationship between preload and stroke volume is defined by Starling's law of the heart, that is the principal mechanism by which the output of the ventricle is adjusted to its venous input. This law states that, up to a certain limit, the stroke volume (or stroke work) is directly proportional to the presystolic or end-diastolic volume of the ventricle (Fig. 21). A curve defining this relationship is frequently referred to as Starling's, or the ventricular, function curve. Factors such as total intravascular volume, posture, and atrial function influence the end-diastolic volume. Normal left ventricular end-diastolic volume is attained at an end-diastolic pressure of up to 14 mm Hg. However, if the left ventricle becomes more rigid (less compliant) as in left ventricular hypertrophy, a higher end-diastolic pressure is required to distend the ventricle to a normal end-diastolic volume. Since measurement of left ventricular volume is difficult in vivo, left ventricular filling pressure (pulmonary artery wedge or left ventricular end-diastolic pressure) is utilized as a reflection of preload.

Afterload

Afterload (aortic impedance or resistance to left ventricular ejection) also influences the stroke volume. The most important factor that determines the impedance to left ventricular ejection is systemic vascular resistance (SVR). With a given preload and contractility, left ventricular stroke volume would be reduced in the presence of a high SVR and augmented when SVR is low. By an intrinsic homeometric adjustment, a normal ventricle can furnish a normal stroke volume when the impedance is altered. However, a diseased left ventricle loses this homeometric mechanism and its systolic performance becomes profoundly dependent on aortic impedance. With a given preload and contractility, reduced aortic impedance results in an upward and leftward shift of the ventricular function curve; conversely, an elevated aortic impedance will cause a downward and rightward shift of the ventricular function curve.

Myocardial Contractility

Myocardial contractility (inotropic state) indicates the intrinsic capacity of myocardial fibers to shorten independent of their preload and afterload. Maximum velocity of contraction (V_{max}) is an index of contractility. Sympathomimetic amines (epinephrine, isoproterenol, norepinephrine), digitalis, glucagon, and tachycardia enhance myocardial contractility, whereas β-adrenergic blocking agents such as propranolol reduce myocardial contractility. With a given preload and afterload, an upward and leftward shift of the ventricular function curve indicates increased contractility, whereas a downward and rightward shift indicates decreased contractility.

Synergy of Ventricular Contraction

Contraction of the ventricle in a normal sequence is important to maintain the normal stroke volume.

Systemic Circulation

Blood pressure (perfusion pressure for various organs) is the product of cardiac output and systemic vascular resistance. Depending on their needs, cardiac output is distributed to various organs. Autonomically mediated vasoconstriction or vasodilatation play a vital role in matching the perfusion of a particular organ to its demands.

At any time, the venous system contains approximately 75 percent of the blood in circulation. Thus, the veins function primarily as a reservoir for the circulation. The veins constrict in response to increased sympathetic activity, and generalized venoconstriction shifts the blood from the peripheral to the central circulation.

Circulatory Reserve

The cardiovascular system has the ability to provide increased amounts of oxygen to the body during physical exercise by augmenting cardiac output. In addition, peripheral tissues extract more oxygen from the arterial blood during exercise. During stressful situations, an increased sympathetic discharge augments myocardial contractility and increases heart rate, both of which increase the cardiac output. In athletes, or at more intense levels of exercise, left ventricular end-diastolic volume and cardiac output increase according to Starling's law. Moreover, through modification of vascular tone, more blood flow is diverted to regions with increased demands, for example, skeletal muscles during exercise.

Compensatory Mechanisms in Heart Failure

Impaired myocardial contractility leading to low cardiac output is the primary hemodynamic abnormality in heart failure. Several compensatory factors become operative in an attempt to restore cardiac output to normal. However, as these compensatory mechanisms are expended to maintain the output at rest, the ability of the cardiovascular system (cardiac reserve) to meet the demands under stressful situations becomes severely eroded. It should also be emphasized that there are several deleterious effects associated with each of these compensatory mechanisms.

Ventricular Hypertrophy and Dilatation

Since the contractility per unit mass of myocardium is impaired in heart failure, myocardial hypertrophy develops to compensate for impaired contractility. The hypertrophied ventricle can generate greater force to meet the increased afterload even though the contractility of the hypertrophied myocardium per unit mass is still subnormal. One of the reasons for subnormal contractility of hypertrophied muscle is that, beyond a certain limit, the blood supply cannot keep pace with the hypertrophy of the muscle fibers, resulting in diffuse and patchy fibrosis due to ischemic necrosis. In certain conditions, ventricular dilatation occurs to compensate for increased volume, for example, aortic regurgitation. An enlarged chamber can generate a greater stroke volume. However, as the ventricle enlarges wall tension also increases, raising the myocardial oxygen demand. Beyond a certain stage, the coronary arterial tree cannot meet these demands, again resulting in diffuse and patchy necrosis in the myocardium.

Starling's Law

The ventricular function curve becomes progressively depressed (rightward and downward shift) with increasing severity of heart failure; that is, large changes in preload (EDP or EDV) result in only small changes in stroke volume (Fig. 21). In heart failure, because of regional redistribution of an already low cardiac output renal blood flow is markedly reduced, which activates the renin-angiotensin-aldosterone system, causing retention of sodium and water and expansion of the intravascular volume. Systemic venous congestion also stimulates sodium and water retention by increasing pressure in the renal veins. Expanded central blood volume stretches the ventricles (increased preload) and activates the Starling mechanism in an attempt to increase the stroke volume. In contrast to ventricular hypertrophy, which takes time, this mechanism becomes operative immediately. However, the deleterious effects associated with this mechanism consist of increased myocardial oxygen demands and pulmonary and/or systemic venous congestion manifested by dyspnea, edema, and hepatomegaly.

Hyperadrenergic State

Increased sympathetic discharge is beneficial in maintaining the normal circulatory status in heart failure through several different mechanisms, for example, tachycardia, stimulation of contractility, arteriolar constriction, and venoconstriction. Tachycardia and enhanced myocardial contractility tend to increase cardiac output. Venoconstriction shifts blood from the periphery into the central circulation and is helpful for activation of the Starling mechanism. Arteriolar constriction tends to maintain normal blood pressure (perfusion pressure) in the face of falling cardiac output. Arteriolar constriction is predominantly mediated through the sympathetic nervous system. It is also caused by thickening of the arteriolar wall due to high sodium and water content. Sympathetic overactivity is also helpful in redistributing the blood flow. Thus, blood flow to vital organs, that is, the heart and brain, is maintained at the expense of less vital organs like the skin and kidneys. Even though the blood level of catecholamines is increased, the norepinephrine content of the failing myocardium is reduced. It is probably due to defects in its synthesis, uptake, and binding by cardiac sympathetic nerves. The primary disadvantage of this generalized arteriolar constriction is that it augments aortic impedance (afterload) with increased resistance to left ventricular ejection and a reduced stroke volume. This establishes a vicious circle of reduced cardiac output, increased sympathetic activity, increased arteriolar constriction, and further reduced cardiac output.

Increased Extraction of Oxygen by the Tissues

Normally, peripheral tissues extract 3.5-5.0 ml of O_2 from each 100 ml of arterial blood. Thus, the normal AV O_2 difference is 3.5-5.0 ml percent. In low-output states, tissues extract greater amounts of oxygen from slowly circulating arterial blood, giving much higher values of the AV O_2 difference. This represents one of the peripheral compensatory mechanisms to provide more oxygen to the tissues in heart failure.

Biochemical Basis of Heart Failure

Normally, as the myocardial cell is depolarized, sarcoplasmic reticulum releases Ca^{2+} in the vicinity of actin and myosin. In the presence of Ca^{2+} and Mg^{2+}, a linkage is established between actin and myosin. Myosin ATPase breaks this linkage, releasing energy that is utilized in the sliding of actin over myosin. The successive making and breaking of these linkages in rapid sequence causes repetitive shortening and relaxation of the sarcomeres and hence myocardium. Defective uptake and release of Ca^{2+} by the sarcoplasmic reticulum causes abnormality of excitation-contraction coupling. This is considered to be the basic mechanism of heart failure.

ETIOLOGY OF HEART FAILURE

Mechanical Abnormalities

Mechanical abnormalities cause heart failure by placing an abnormal load on the heart. Initially, contractility is normal. It becomes impaired secondarily after prolonged duration of abnormal loading conditions.

Pressure Overload

Pressure overload, such as in aortic stenosis, coarctation of the aorta, and systemic hypertension impose a pressure overload (increased afterload) on the left ventricle. Pulmonary stenosis and pulmonary hypertension place a pressure overload on the right ventricle. Hypertrophy of the ventricular wall occurs in response to a pressure overload in order to overcome the increased outflow resistance to ejection. A hypertrophied and thickened ventricular wall is more stiff (less compliant) to distend. Because of decreased compliance, end-diastolic pressure rises. Following several years of progressive ventricular hypertrophy, progressive contractile failure starts, resulting in ventricular dilatation.

Volume Overload

Volume overload, for example, aortic regurgitation, mitral regurgitation, patent ductus arteriosus, and ventricular septal defect place a volume overload on the left ventricle and tricuspid regurgitation; pulmonary regurgitation and atrial septal defect impose a volume overload on the right ventricle. To accommodate the increased volume, ventricular dilatation occurs relatively early, and over a span of several years ventricular hypertrophy also develops. The heart tolerates the volume overload better than the pressure overload.

Restriction to Ventricular Filling

Mitral stenosis and left atrial myxoma obstruct the mitral orifice and thus impede filling of the left ventricle. As left atrial emptying is hampered, left atrial and pulmonary venous hypertension arise. Similarly, systemic venous congestion develops in tricuspid stenosis, tricuspid atresia, and right atrial myxoma.

Pericardial effusion and constriction impair the filling of both right and left ventricles leading to increased filling pressures of both ventricles. Thus, symptoms and signs of both systemic and pulmonary venous hypertension develop.

A markedly hypertrophied left ventricle in idiopathic hypertrophic subaortic stenosis (IHSS) drastically decreases its compliance. It takes a powerful left atrial contraction to fill such a ventricle. This high left atrial pressure is transmitted into the pulmonary circulation and gives rise to dyspnea.

Myocardial Contractile Failure (Intrinsic Myocardial Failure)

Segmental myocardial damage occurs in myocardial infarction. In the presence of a small myocardial infarction, the remaining normal muscle can compensate and maintain a normal output. However, in the presence of a large myocardial infarction, the residual muscle and the compensatory mechanisms fail to sustain a normal output and heart failure and/or cardiogenic shock develop. In cardiomyopathies, myocardial contractility is reduced uniformly, resulting in global ventricular dysfunction and heart failure.

Precipitating Factors

Certain precipitating factors such as anemia, pulmonary emboli, infective endocarditis, infection in general, thyrotoxicosis, pregnancy, rheumatic myocarditis, tachyarrhythmia or bradyarrhythmia, and large intake of salt may either aggravate the previously existent heart failure or may result in clinical heart failure in a patient with a previously compensated cardiac abnormality.

CLINICAL FEATURES OF HEART FAILURE

The symptoms and signs of heart failure can be attributed to three main hemodynamic changes, that is, decreased cardiac output leading to inadequate perfusion of various organ systems, left atrial hypertension with pulmonary venous congestion, and right atrial hypertension with systemic venous congestion. Various clinical features are most conveniently discussed as belonging to left or right heart failure.

Left Heart Failure

Symptoms

Dyspnea is the cardinal symptom of left heart failure or mitral stenosis. Dyspnea implies a sensation of difficult breathing. Patients describe it as feeling breathless, short-winded, or not getting enough air. Dyspnea is generally attributed to decreased compliance of the lungs that occurs because of pulmonary venous hypertension (congestion) and exudation of fluid into the interstitial spaces. With mild heart failure, dyspnea occurs only on exertion. However, with progression of disease, the activity threshold further decreases.

Orthopnea indicates dyspnea during recumbency with relief on sitting up. Relief in an upright posture presumably occurs because of reduction of pulmonary venous congestion as the blood pools in the lower extremities. In addition, the diaphragm assumes a lower position, which increases the intrathoracic space.

Paroxysmal nocturnal dyspnea (PND) is a specific feature of left heart failure or mitral stenosis. Typically, the patient sleeps 1-2 hours and then awakes acutely short of breath with a feeling of suffocation. He sits upright at the edge of the bed gasping for breath, walks for a few minutes, or may open a window for fresh air. This may be accompanied by sweating, pallor, cyanosis, cold extremities, and cough. Approximately 10-30 minutes from the start of this episode the patient feels relief of dyspnea and sleeps comfortably the rest of the night. When the acute episode of breathlessness secondary to left heart failure is associated with wheezing, it is referred to as cardiac asthma.

Acute pulmonary edema indicates sudden and severe decompensation of the left ventricle or severe mitral stenosis. The episode starts with extreme shortness of breath and persistent cough productive of white or pink, frothy sputum. The accessory muscles of respiration are active. The extreme degree of anxiety and agony is obvious. The patient prefers the sitting posture and frequently leans forward. The skin is cold, pale, and grey with profuse sweating. The severity of pulmonary edema varies from mild to very severe. Usually the attack subsides spontaneously or with treatment after a few minutes to a few hours. However, severe pulmonary edema may result in death.

Persistent nocturnal cough is seen occasionally in patients with left heart failure or mitral stenosis. They may complain of a persistent, dry cough, restlessness, and insomnia.

Cheyne-Stokes breathing is defined as alternating periods of apnea and hyperpnea. It is generally observed in elderly patients with left heart failure who also have impairment of the central nervous system (CNS) and its vascular supply or who have been given sedatives. Cheyne-Stokes respirations are ascribed to a disturbance of feedback control of the respiratory center due to prolongation of circulation time.

Hemoptysis may occur in severe left heart failure or pulmonary edema. Red cells escape into the pulmonary alveoli resulting in rusty-colored or pink, frothy sputum.

Fatigue on mild exertion is a frequent symptom in patients with left heart failure and is probably due to low cardiac output and depletion of electrolytes, as seen in hypokalemia.

Many patients with heart failure report a history of dizziness, lightheadedness, weakness, and feeling unsteady on their legs. They may not experience total loss of consciousness. The majority of these episodes are brief and occur in an upright posture. Dizziness in cardiac disease is due to low cardiac output (heart failure and/or arrhythmia) resulting in poor perfusion to the brain.

Angina decubitus, or nocturnal angina, may be one of the manifestations of left heart failure.

Physical Signs

The physical signs in left heart failure are as follows:

Small volume pulse is due to low stroke volume.

Tachypnea is attributed to pulmonary venous congestion, which makes the lungs stiff and difficult to inflate and deflate.

Ventricular gallop (S_3). An audible ventricular gallop over the cardiac apex is commonly observed as an early sign of left heart failure. It indicates an enlarged and poorly contracting left ventricle with a high end-diastolic pressure. A soft S_3 that disappears with treatment indicates a relatively good prognosis. On the other hand, a persistent and loud S_3 despite therapy indicates a poor prognosis.

Pulmonary findings in left heart failure consist of bibasilar rales, diminished breath sounds over the bases, and occasionally bilateral rhonchi. These signs are secondary to exudation of fluid into the alveoli and to bronchiolar narrowing.

Functional mitral incompetence may develop in patients with persistent left heart failure. The left ventricular chamber enlarges markedly and the mitral valve leaflets do not coapt properly, resulting in functional mitral incompetence. As the left ventricle shrinks in response to therapy, mitral incompetence may disappear.

Pulsus alternans indicates an alternate strong and weak pulse even though the cardiac cycles are of equal duration. Pulsus alternans implies myocardial failure.

Tachycardia, pallor, cyanosis, and cold and clammy extremities indicate a hyperadrenergic state.

Laboratory Diagnoses

Chest x-ray is a valuable tool in first confirming and then following a patient with left heart failure. The transverse diameter of the heart may or may not be enlarged. The cardiac silhouette may show a configuration of left ventricular enlargement. Pulmonary venous markings in the upper lung fields become more prominent due to redistribution of blood. Vascular markings become hazy. Kerley's B lines appear near the costophrenic angles and are due to edematous interlobular septa. In fully developed pulmonary edema, confluent opacities appear in the central lung fields bilaterally near the hila. In persistent left heart failure, hydrothorax may develop either on the right side or bilaterally. Hydrothorax, however, is more common in biventricular failure.

Pulmonary function tests show a decreased vital capacity and decreased compliance of the lungs. However, at earlier stages of left heart failure, closing volume measurements show that peripheral airways tend to close prematurely at low lung volumes, causing maldistribution of intrapulmonary air.

Echocardiography demonstrates an enlarged and poorly contractile left ventricle.

Radionuclide ventriculogram reveals a decreased ejection fraction and a dilated left ventricle.

Cardiac catheterization shows high pulmonary artery wedge and left ventricular end-diastolic pressures, low cardiac output that remains unchanged or decreases with exercise, an abnormally wide arteriovenous oxygen difference, and subnormal ejection fraction.

A diagnosis of left heart failure is made on clinical grounds; the utility of echocardiography and cardiac catheterization lies in determining the etiology of left heart failure.

Right Heart Failure

The symptoms and signs of right heart failure are due to two primary factors, namely, systemic venous congestion and right ventricular dilatation. Systemic venous pressure rises as a result of an increased volume of blood in the systemic veins secondary to inadequate right ventricular emptying during systole, as well as generalized venoconstriction in response to sympathetic overactivity. In the vast majority of patients, left ventricular failure and mitral stenosis are the principal causes of right heart failure, that is, as the left heart fails and/or pulmonary venous hypertension occurs, pulmonary arterial hypertension develops passively in order to maintain the forward flow of blood. Once the pulmonary arterial pressure attains a certain level, pulmonary arterioles actively constrict by a reflex mechanism that makes the pulmonary hypertension even worse. This places a pressure overload on the right ventricle that subsequently fails as the compensatory mechanisms become ineffective in maintaining the forward output. The other factor that also probably has an important role is the continuity of myocardial layers enveloping the left and right ventricles. Failure of the contractile function starts in the myocardial layers of the left ventricle and eventually spreads to the right ventricular musculature. As the severity of right ventricular failure increases, the volume of blood ejected into the pulmonary circuit decreases. The signs and symptoms of pulmonary venous congestion (e.g., pulmonary vascular redistribution, dyspnea) become less marked. It is not uncommon for a patient with severe mitral stenosis to become comfortable in the supine position after right heart failure has developed. Although left heart failure is the major cause of right heart failure, pulmonary emboli, chronic obstructive pulmonary disease (COPD), and primary pulmonary hypertension result in isolated right heart failure.

Symptoms

Symptoms of right heart failure include fatigue, edema, right upper quadrant pain, and anorexia.

Dependent edema usually starts as swelling of the ankles and feet but may involve the legs and abdomen. It is bilateral and pitting in nature. In bedridden patients, edema is first detected over the sacrum. In the advanced stage, edema becomes widespread (anasarca) with hydrothorax, ascites, and edema of the external genital organs. Pleural effusion and ascites are probably due to inadequate lymphatic drainage into the high-pressure systemic veins. Another cause for pleural effusion may be a pulmonary infarction contiguous to the pleura.

Right upper quadrant pain in the abdomen occurs due to liver enlargement and the distention of its capsule.

Anorexia and nausea develop secondary to congestion of the gastrointestinal system. Absorption of nutrients is affected and, in persistent systemic venous congestion as seen in constrictive pericarditis, significant protein loss may result (protein-losing gastroenteropathy). All these factors cause gradual weight loss and ultimately cardiac cachexia.

Fatigue also occurs due to low cardiac output.

Nocturia and oliguria during the daytime are common.

Physical Signs

Signs indicating right heart failure include edema (see above), abnormal jugular venous pressure, right ventricular gallop, hepatomegaly, functional tricuspid incompetence, and cyanosis.

Jugular venous distention and jugular venous pressure (JVP) of greater than 3 cm above the sternal angle are indicative of right heart failure. Neck veins fill from below. A positive hepatojugular reflux, that is, persistent elevation of the JVP during sustained pressure in the right upper quadrant of the abdomen, is a sign of incipient right heart failure. On close examination of the venous pulse, one frequently finds a sharp y descent. As the right ventricule enlarges, tricuspid valve leaflets fail to coapt during systole, resulting in functional tricuspid incompetence. At this stage, the v wave of the venous pulse becomes very prominent.

Right ventricular gallop (S_3) is audible over the left lower sternal border and indicates enlarged right ventricular end-diastolic volume.

Hepatomegaly and occasionally splenomegaly occur in right heart failure. An enlarged liver is tender to light pressure. After prolonged or recurrent episodes of right heart failure, widespread necrosis followed by fibrosis develops in the liver due to ischemic injury of the liver cells (back pressure in hepatic veins and poor arterial perfusion). Ultimately, this leads to a shrunken liver, which is described as cardiac cirrhosis.

Functional tricuspid incompetence, as manifested by a pansystolic murmur over the left lower sternal border, prominent v waves in the neck veins, and a pulsatile liver, develops as the right ventricle dilates. Because the tricuspid valve no longer protects the systemic veins from right ventricular systolic pressure, systemic venous congestion becomes worse.

As the tissues extract more oxygen from a slowly circulating column of blood and the amount of deoxyhemoglobin exceeds 5 g/dl, peripheral cyanosis becomes evident.

Laboratory Diagnoses
Chest x-ray shows dilatation of the superior vena cava, inferior vena cava, right atrium, right ventricle, and main pulmonary trunks. Pleural effusion on the right side or on both sides is usually present.

Echocardiogram reveals dilatation of the right ventricle. It may also show evidence of volume overload of the right ventricle when functional tricuspid incompetence develops.

Liver function tests (e.g., SGOT) become elevated in advanced cases.

Urinalysis commonly shows slight proteinuria and high specific gravity. BUN may rise due to poor perfusion of the kidneys (prerenal failure).

Cardiac catheterization reveals high central venous, right atrial, and right ventricular end-diastolic pressures (>7 mm Hg mean). It may also demonstrate pulmonary arterial hypertension. When left heart disease or mitral stenosis have resulted in right ventricular failure, pulmonary artery wedge pressure is also elevated. On the other hand, when right ventricular failure is due to COPD or pulmonary emboli, pulmonary artery wedge pressure is normal.

These investigations help determine the specific etiology of right heart failure.

FUNCTIONAL CLASSIFICATION OF CONGESTIVE HEART FAILURE

It is useful to grade cardiac disability on the basis of symptoms. The classification developed by the New York Heart Association is widely used in practice. Dyspnea, angina, and fatigue are considered in classifying the patient.

Class I: No symptoms on ordinary activity.
Class II: Symptoms occur on ordinary activity.
Class III: Symptoms occur on less than ordinary activity.
Class IV: Symptoms are present even at rest.

PROGNOSIS

Long-term prognosis depends primarily on the underlying etiology of heart failure. Obviously milder degrees and initial episodes of heart failure, which are easily managed, have a better prognosis than severe and persistent heart failure. Correctable diseases, such as valve lesions, hypertension, and certain congenital lesions (when treated early) have a much better prognosis compared to untreatable diseases such as idiopathic congestive cardiomyopathy.

MANAGEMENT OF CONGESTIVE HEART FAILURE

The aim of management is to control heart failure and then treat the primary cardiac disease to prevent recurrence. As the surgical procedures on the heart are now performed at relatively lower risk, determination of the precise etiology of heart failure is extremely important. If the primary cardiac abnormality is amenable to surgical correction, control of heart failure by medical means prior to surgery reduces the surgical risk. Obviously, in patients with noncorrectable cardiac disease or in whom surgical risk is unacceptable, medical treatment is the only choice in the control and prevention of congestive heart failure. The following steps are recommended for treatment of heart failure.

General Measures

Depending on the severity of heart failure, complete bed rest or frequent rest periods should be advised in order to reduce the cardiac workload. Bed rest also promotes diuresis. However, one should be familiar with the hazards of bed rest such as phlebothrombosis and pulmonary emboli. The use of elastic stockings, passive exercises of the legs, and low-dose heparin therapy are some of the measures that can be undertaken to prevent these hazards. The head of the bed should be elevated to diminish ventricular preload by pooling the blood in the legs. If the patient is overweight, calories should also be restricted. In severe heart failure, oxygen should be administered.

Treatment of Precipitating Factors

Treatment of anemia, infection, pulmonary embolism, and infective endocarditis is extremely important in managing heart failure. Tachyarrhythmias and bradyarrhythmias should be controlled to maintain the optimal heart rate (60-90 beats/minute) to augment cardiac output.

Increasing Myocardial Contractility

Since depressed myocardial contractility is the basic feature of heart failure, its enhancement with pharmacologic agents is the cornerstone of medical treatment. Of the various pharmacologic agents available for this purpose such as sympathomimetic amines, glucagon, and digitalis glycosides, digitalis preparations are the ideal agents for long-term oral therapy. Digitalis glycosides enhance myocardial contractility by promoting the availability of Ca^{2+} to actin and myosin from Ca^{2+} stores in mitochondria and the sarcoplasmic reticulum. The direct effect of digitalis on systemic arteries and veins consists of vasoconstriction. However, as heart failure improves, sympathetic tone to systemic arteries and veins is withdrawn and the net result is vasodilatation. Enhanced contractility improves ventricular emptying (increased ejection fraction and stroke volume). As the systolic ventricular performance improves, there is reduced enddiastolic volume and end-diastolic pressure. In contrast to catecholamines, digitalis increases the myocardial contractility without concomitant tachycardia or systemic arterial constriction.

The most commonly used digitalis preparations are digoxin, digitoxin, and Cedilanid-D. Digoxin is prescribed orally as well as for intravenous use. Digitoxin is available only for oral use and Cedilanid-D only for intravenous use. Digoxin is available in 0.125-, 0.25-, and 0.5-mg tablets. Slightly more than three-fourths of the oral dose is absorbed. Effect starts within 1-2 hours and reaches a peak in 2-3 hours after ingestion. The half-life of digoxin is 1.6 days. It is excreted unchanged, predominantly through the kidneys. In mild heart failure, digoxin can be started at 0.25 mg/day and in approximately 5 days therapeutic digitalis levels are achieved. In moderate to severe heart failure, therapy is initiated with 0.75-1 mg of oral digoxin in divided doses during the first 24 hours and then continued at a maintenance dose of 0.125-0.25 mg daily. In acute pulmonary edema or atrial fibrillation with a very rapid ventricular rate associated with severe heart failure or hypotension, digoxin (0.5 mg) should be administered intravenously and 0.25 mg can be repeated 2 hours later; if needed, another 0.25 mg can be administered 8 hours later. This should be followed by oral digoxin in maintenance doses. In the presence of renal insufficiency, the digoxin dosage should be reduced to 0.125 mg daily or on alternate days, depending on the digitalis blood levels and clinical response. The therapeutic serum level of digoxin is usually 1-2 ng/ml. In patients with digitalis toxicity, the serum level of digoxin is generally >2 ng/ml. However, it must be emphasized that digitalis toxicity is a clinical and ECG diagnosis. Since there is a wide range of digitalis levels in toxic patients, blood level at best provides a supportive information. Blood levels of digoxin should be obtained when, in spite of an adequate dose, beneficial clinical effects are not apparent or the patient's compliance is questioned. Blood levels may also help in determining whether a given rhythm disturbance is due to digitalis toxicity or cardiac disease. Furthermore, in patients with renal insufficiency, blood levels are helpful in titrating the dose of digitalis. Digitoxin has a long half-life of approximately 7 days. It is used primarily for long-term maintenance in 0.1 mg daily doses. As digitoxin is predominantly metabolized in the liver, it is perhaps more useful as long-term therapy in patients with chronic renal insufficiency. Cedilanid-D is reserved for intravenous use only, the initial dose being 0.8-1.2 mg with 0.6 mg repeated in 2-4 hours.

Digitalis, in therapeutic doses, produces ST-segment depression and Q-T interval shortening. In higher amounts, it causes a variety of arrhythmias, such as multiple multifocal PVBs, bigeminy due to PVBs, atrial tachycardia with block, nonparoxysmal junctional tachycardia, atrioventricular dissociation, and first-, second-, or third-degree AV blocks. In addition, nausea, anorexia, vomiting, and yellow or green vision can also occur. Some of the precipitating factors for digitalis toxicity are hypokalemia, hypomagnesemia, hypoxia, and hypercalcemia. Patients with acute myocardial infarction, myocarditis, and cor pulmonale are perhaps somewhat more sensitive to digitalis. Treatment of digitalis toxicity consists of discontinuing the drug and administering a potassium supplement if serum K^+ is below or borderline normal. Occasionally, antiarrhythmic agents such as lidocaine, pronestyl, propranolol, or phenytoin are necessary to control the above-mentioned tachyarrhythmias. Rarely, a temporary pacemaker may be required when complete AV block with an extremely slow ventricular rate develops.

Other available inotropic agents are sympathomimetic amines (epinephrine, norepinephrine, isoproterenol, dopamine, dobutamine) and glucagon. These agents are available only for intravenous use. The chief disadvantages of epinephrine, norepinephrine, and isoproterenol are that they cause marked tachycardia, enhance myocardial oxygen demand, and provoke ventricular irritability. By contrast, dopamine and dobutamine produce no significant tachycardia and appear to be better suited for short-term use in refractory heart failure. Glucagon causes nausea and vomiting. These agents are occasionally used in advanced stages of heart failure as a temporizing measure. Amrinone is a new oral nonglycosidic inotropic agent that is presently undergoing clinical investigations.

Lowering of Ventricular Preload

Expanded intravascular volume due to abnormal salt and water retention by the kidneys in heart failure along with elevated ventricular filling pressure are responsible for pulmonary vascular congestion that results in dyspnea, orthopnea, and PND, and systemic vascular congestion causing edema, hepatomegaly, distended neck veins, and ascites. One way to reduce this expanded intravascular volume is to limit salt intake to 1-2 g/day (17-34 mEq Na^+). A sitting or semisitting posture reduces the ventricular preload by pooling blood in the periphery. However, the most effective way to reduce the preload is by the judicious use of diuretics that promote salt and water excretion. As the pulmonary congestion is relieved, oxygenation of blood and exercise tolerance improve. Since the ventricles are operating at the flat portion of Starling's curve, cardiac output is only slightly changed in spite of reduction of the preload (Fig. 21). However, it should be emphasized that overzealous use of diuretics causing excessive contraction of intravascular volume can reduce the cardiac output and also promote thromboembolic complications. The aim of diuretic therapy is to relieve symptoms of pulmonary and systemic venous congestion, yet not compromise the cardiac output. Obtaining dry weight in the patient is not the objective of diuretic therapy. The optimal dose of diuretics can be determined by serial clinical examinations, body weights, blood pressure in the supine and standing positions to detect postural hypotension, and BUN measurements. Thiazides, furosemide (Lasix), and ethacrynic acid (Edecrin) are the most commonly used diuretics. These agents interfere with reabsorption of sodium chloride in the renal tubules and thus promote natriuresis as well as diuresis.

Thiazide diuretics are effective orally. The daily dose of hydrochlorothiazide is 50-100 mg. The thiazides inhibit Na^+ reabsorption at the diluting site of the distal nephron. Thiazides also result in urinary loss of K^+ and Cl^-. Hypokalemia is common after intensive and prolonged therapy and can be prevented by increased intake of potassium-rich food (e.g., oranges, bananas). Supplementary potassium is required for correcting more than mild degrees of hypokalemia. Since Cl^- loss occurs also, causing hypochloremic alkalosis, potassium chloride is the agent of choice. Dilutional hyponatremia is another common side effect that should be treated by restriction of fluid intake. Other side effects of thiazides are hyperuricemia, hyperglycemia, hypercalcemia, nausea, vomiting, and skin rash. As the diuretic-induced volume contracts, and hyponatremia stimulates release of ADH and aldosterone which in turn promotes sodium and water retention, continuous diuretic therapy may result in total or partial refractoriness. Intermittent therapy is therefore encouraged.

Furosemide (Lasix) and ethacrynic acid (Edecrin) are the most powerful diuretic agents available. Diuresis occurs as a result of several different effects in the kidney such as increased renal blood flow due to reduction of renal arteriolar resistance, inhibition of sodium reabsorption at the ascending limb of Henle's loop, and loss of the ability to concentrate urine in the distal tubules. When given orally, action begins in 1 hour, reaches its peak in 2-3 hours, and lasts for 6-8 hours. The daily oral dose of furosemide is 20-600 mg, and ethacrynic acid is 50 to 200 mg. Following an intravenous dose, action begins in 10-15 minutes, reaches its peak in 30 minutes, and last for 2 hours. Usually the intravenous dose of furosemide is 40-80 mg and can be increased in refractory cases. Therapy should be initiated with smaller doses because larger doses causing profound volume loss may result in hypovolemic shock. These agents are also prone to cause hyperuricemia, hyperglycemia, hypercalcemia, hypochloremic alkalosis, dilutional hyponatremia, and hearing loss. The advantage of loop diuretics over thiazides lies in the rapid onset of action as well as their effectiveness in the presence of renal failure. They have proved extremely valuable in the treament of acute pulmonary edema.

Potassium-retaining diuretics such as spironolactone (Aldactone) and triamterene are weak diuretics that retain potassium. In combination with thiazides or furosemide, the diuretic effect is potentiated and potassium loss is reduced. In the presence of renal insufficiency, hyperkalemia can result. Their site of action is in the distal tubule. The daily dose of spironolactone is 100-400 mg. Side effects consist of nausea, vomiting, gynecomastia, and rarely agranulocytosis.

The second major class of pharmacologic agents used to decrease the ventricular preload are the venodilators such as nitrates. By pooling the blood in the periphery, they decrease the venous return, reducing the filling pressures of both ventricles. For the sake of convenience they are discussed in the next section.

Reduction of Left Ventricular Afterload (Outflow Impedance)

The recent introduction of vasodilators that lower the impedance to left ventricular ejection has provided useful adjunctive therapy in patients with severe or refractory heart failure. As described previously, in heart failure systemic vascular resistance, an important determinant of aortic impedance and ventricular afterload, is elevated. This represents one of the compensatory mechanisms to maintain a normal perfusion pressure in the face of reduced cardiac output. However, increased resistance to ejection further lowers the stroke volume and increases the myocardial oxygen demand. Vasodilating agents break this vicious cycle; lower systemic vascular resistance facilitates systolic emptying of the left ventricle; thus increasing cardiac output and decreasing myocardial oxygen demand. The vasodilators are particularly useful when acute mitral regurgitation is responsible for left heart failure since these drugs promote forward ejection into the aorta and reduce regurgitation into the left atrium. Vasodilator therapy is also useful in heart failure due to coronary heart disease, cardiomyopathy, aortic insufficiency, and ventricular septal defect.

Because of its potency and rapid onset of action, intravenous sodium nitroprusside is an ideal agent for short-term use in an intensive care environment. Pulmonary wedge pressure (left heart filling pressure), peripheral blood pressure, cardiac output, heart rate, and urine output must be monitored during sodium nitroprusside therapy. Besides dilating the arterioles, sodium nitroprusside dilates the veins. Therefore, in addition to afterload reduction, preload decreases as the blood is pooled in the peripheral veins. The dose of sodium nitroprusside is 1-5 μg/kg/min administered as a continuous drip. Side effects consist of hypotension and, after prolonged use, thiocyanate poisoning. Nitroglycerine, phentolamine (Regitine), and trimethaphan (Arfonad) are other agents that can be used intravenously. For long-term use, oral isosorbide dinitrate (20-60 mg every 6 hours) or nitroglycerine ointment (1-2 inches every 6 hours), both of which are predominantly venous dilators when administered in combination with hydralazine (50-100 mg every 6 hours), which is purely an arteriolar dilator, provide a potent form of vasodilator (unloading) therapy. Prazosin (Minipress) has an almost balanced effect on the arterial and venous beds and can be used effectively as a single agent. Captopril, a converting enzyme inhibitor, is also proving useful in the treatment of refractory heart failure.

Additional Measures

Persistent hydrothorax and ascites, by encroaching on the chest cavity, enhance dyspnea. If unresponsive to diuretic therapy, thoracentesis and paracentesis may be required.

CORONARY HEART DISEASE

In the industrialized countries of the world, coronary heart disease is a major cause of death. Over half a million deaths occur annually in the United States that are attributable to acute myocardial infarction, and most of these deaths occur suddenly. The clinical manifestations of coronary heart disease (CHD) consist of angina, myocardial infarction, sudden death, arrhythmias, and ischemic cardiomyopathy. Any of these clinical manifestations may be the prodrome of CHD. These manifestations are due to impairment of coronary blood flow that results from narrowing of the coronary arterial lumen by atheromatous plaques.

Atherosclerosis of the coronary arteries is a progressive disease; it is present for many years before the onset of clinical manifestations. The atheromatous plaques are usually present in the epicardial portions of the coronary arteries. The advanced atheromatous plaques consist of debris of degenerated cells, cholesterol, triglycerides, phospholipids, fibrous tissue composed of collagen and elastin fibers, and are generally calcified. Some plaques show hemorrhage. Aggregates of platelets may be deposited over atheromatous plaques. Platelets may also adhere to the irregular intimal surface of the artery, become organized, and result in arterial obstruction. The precise sequence of various pathologic processes such as intimal smooth muscle proliferation, lipid deposition, aggregation of platelets, and thrombosis in the final development of a complex atheromatous plaque is still controversial.

Several epidemiologic studies have stressed the role of various risk factors in the pathogenesis of coronary heart disease (CHD). Age and sex are important in the occurrence of this disease. The prevalence of myocardial infarction increases progressively with advancing age in both men and women. Prior to reaching the age of 50, the prevalence of CHD is much higher in men. However, after menopause, the prevalence of CHD in women approaches that in men. A high plasma cholesterol level, hypertension, cigarette smoking, heredity, obesity, diabetes mellitus, a sedentary life-style, and a Type A personality appear to be associated with accelerated atherogenesis. The risk of developing CHD is approximately 30 times greater in patients having all risk factors as compared to patients with no risk factors. It has been recently suggested that a high-density lipoprotein (HDL) level has a protective effect. For reasons that are not entirely clear, there has been a gradual downward trend in the prevalence of CHD since early 1970.

ANGINA

Stable Angina

Definition

Classic angina pectoris (Heberden's angina) is defined as a feeling of discomfort in the midanterior chest precipitated by exercise or emotion and relieved by rest. This episodic disorder is due to reversible myocardial ischemia that occurs secondary to an imbalance between myocardial oxygen supply and demand. Stable angina implies that the behavior of angina, that is, the activity threshold of developing angina, its intensity, duration, and relief with rest and/or nitroglycerine, is unchanged for months and years and is fairly predictable.

Etiology

Obstruction of one or more coronary arteries (⩾70% reduction in diameter) by atherosclerotic plaques is the major cause of angina pectoris in approximately 90 percent of the patients. In some patients, transient spasm of normal or atherosclerotic coronary arteries is being recognized as another cause of angina. Few patients with classical angina pectoris have entirely normal coronary arteries. Angina is commonly associated with aortic valve disease, especially with aortic stenosis, but also occasionally with aortic regurgitation. Systemic lupus erythematosus and polyarteritis nodosa, which affect small coronary vessels, are rare causes of angina. Marked right ventricular hypertrophy may occasionally result in angina.

Pathophysiology

Angina is generally attributed to an inadequate supply of oxygen (myocardial oxygen supply) relative to the needs of the myocardium (myocardial oxygen demand) at a given time (Figs. 22 and 23).

The supply of oxygen to the myocardium is directly related to the amount of coronary blood flow, provided the oxygen-carrying capacity of blood (hemoglobin level) and the ability of red cells to unload oxygen at the myocardial cellular level are normal. Even under basal conditions, the myocardium extracts nearly a maximal amount of oxygen from coronary arterial blood, resulting in a wide coronary arteriovenous difference. Therefore, the only mechanism of furnishing increased amounts of oxygen to the myocardium is by augmenting the coronary blood flow. Coronary blood flow in turn

MYOCARDIAL OXYGEN SUPPLY	=	MYOCARDIAL OXYGEN DEMAND
1. CORONARY BLOOD FLOW		1. HEART RATE
• AORTIC PRESSURE		2. CONTRACTILITY
• CORONARY RESISTANCE		3. WALL TENSION
2. ARTERIO-VENOUS OXYGEN DIFFERENCE		• VENTRICULAR VOLUME
		• VENTRICULAR PRESSURE

Figure 22. Factors determining myocardial oxygen supply and demand. Normally, under physiologic stress such as exercise, the myocardial oxygen supply can increase sufficiently to keep pace with the increase in myocardial oxygen demand. In obstructive coronary artery disease, myocardial oxygen supply is inadequate relative to the increased myocardial oxygen demand resulting in myocardial ischemia.

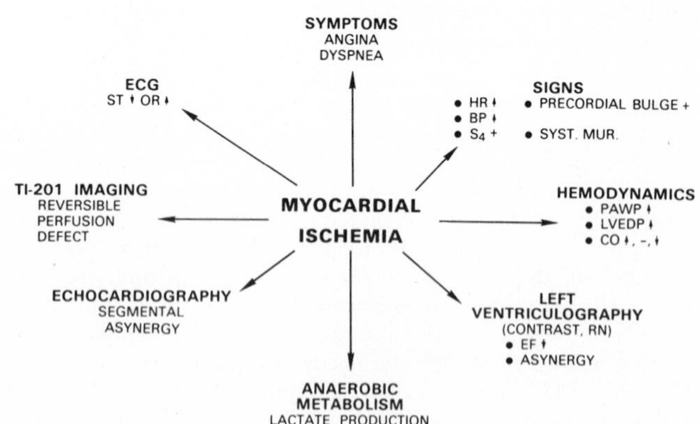

Figure 23. Various manifestations of myocardial ischemia. HR: Heart rate; BP: blood pressure; S_4: fourth heart sound; Syst. Mur.: systolic murmur; PAWP: pulmonary artery wedge pressure; LVEDP: left ventricular end-diastolic pressure; CO: cardiac output; RN: radionuclide; EF: ejection fraction; Tl-201: thallium-201; ↑: increase; ↓: decrease; –: no change.

is dependent on coronary vascular resistance and arterial pressure (perfusion pressure). Under normal conditions, coronary vasodilatation (decreased coronary vascular resistance) is the primary mechanism to enhance coronary blood flow. However, in obstructive coronary artery disease (CAD), atherosclerotic plaques impose fixed high resistance in the coronary arteries and impede coronary blood flow. To compensate for this hampered blood flow, coronary arterioles distal to the obstructing athersclerotic plaques dilate and tend to maintain normal blood flow. In the presence of mild to moderately severe (50-90%) coronary stenosis, this mechanism is successful in maintaining normal coronary blood flow at rest. Since the compensatory mechanism of arteriolar dilatation is expended in an attempt to maintain adequate coronary blood flow at rest, it is no longer available to further augment coronary blood flow during exercise. Thus, in the presence of mild and moderate stenosis, coronary blood flow is unable to increase adequately during exercise. On the other hand, in severe (⩾90%) coronary stenosis, even maximal vasodilatation distal to the obstructive lesions cannot sustain normal coronary blood flow, even at rest. As the coronary arterioles distal to the obstructing lesion are already maximally dilated and are unable to further augment coronary blood flow, an optimal arterial pressure becomes critically important in maintaining normal coronary blood flow in the presence of coronary artery disease. Thus, hypotension in the presence of severe (⩾90%) coronary stenosis will drastically reduce the coronary blood flow. Enlargement of preexistent but dormant collateral vessels represents another compensatory mechanism to maintain coronary blood flow. Several studies have demonstrated that blood flow provided by collateral vessels is inadequate to meet the myocardial metabolic demands, particularly during stress. However, blood flow via the rapidly enlarging collateral vessels may prevent or limit the occurrence of a large myocardial infarct in the distribution of a slowly occluding coronary artery.

Myocardial oxygen demands are determined by three major factors: heart rate, contractility, and left ventricular wall tension. In turn, wall tension is dependent on the diameter of the left ventricle and left ventricular systolic pressure. Thus, increased heart rate, contractility, left ventricular chamber size, and/or systolic blood pressure augment the myocardial needs for oxygen. When the myocardial demand for oxygen exceeds the capability of coronary blood flow to supply oxygen, myocardial ischemia results. If myocardial ischemia is brief, it is manifested subjectively as angina. By contrast, if ischemia is prolonged, irreversible myocardial damage may occur, manifesting as a myocardial infarction. Certain factors that adversely affect the oxygen-carrying capacity of blood include anemia, polycythemia, hypoxia due to lung disease, and states that enhance myocardial oxygen demand such as tachycardia, hypertension, thyrotoxicosis, and fever.

As to the mechanism of angina, it has been generally believed that increased myocardial oxygen demand in face of limited oxygen supply is responsible for angina. Recently it has become obvious that in a significant number of patients, myocardial oxygen demand may not be altered, however a reduction of oxygen supply by coronary-vasospasm plays an important role in the production of myocardial ischemia. The precise mechanism underlying coronary vasospasm is not clear. It has been suggested that minor coronary atherosclerotic plaque inhibits the production of prostacyclin thereby permitting the release of thromboxane A_2 which stimulates platelet clumping and is also a potent vasoconstrictor and results in coronary spasm. Autonomic imbalances and abnormal activation of serotonin receptors in coronary arteries have also been implicated as responsible for spasm.

Symptoms

Angina pectoris is episodic chest discomfort induced by exercise and/or emotion and relieved by rest. It has a deep achelike character of a visceral pain and is usually described as tightness, heaviness, or a burning or choking sensation in the chest. Occasionally it is described as indigestion that may be somewhat relieved by belching. The chest discomfort may be accompanied by acute anxiety, nausea, sweating, and dyspnea, and is most commonly experienced in the substernal region or across the anterior chest and occasionally in the precordial area. Pain in the region of the cardiac apex is not typical of angina. The pain may radiate to one or more of the following regions: inner aspect of the left arm, right arm, shoulders, neck, throat, jaw, cheeks, teeth, upper abdomen, and interscapular area. Less commonly, the pain may be limited to any of these areas. Angina is precipitated by physical activity, especially if it is performed in a hasty manner to which the patient is not accustomed. Sexual intercourse, walking uphill, exposure to cold wind, consumption of a heavy meal, arm work, hurrying to answer a telephone, and emotional buildup (anger, fright, excitement) represent some of the common situations precipitating angina. Episodes of angina are generally more common during the morning hours. The intensity of pain is variable. Frequently, the discomfort builds up quickly with activity, forcing the patient to rest. Occasionally, it builds up to a tolerable intensity, continuing until activity is discontinued. Occasionally, there is spontaneous relief of angina during continued activity and the patient can exercise at an even greater level without interruption. This has been called walk-through or second-wind angina. Most episodes of angina last 3-5 minutes, aborting after sublingual nitroglycerine and/or rest; however, a severe attack may last as long as 30 minutes.

Physical Signs

Cardiovascular examination is generally normal between attacks of angina. Physical examination during an episode of angina may reveal tachycardia, hypertension, abnormal precordial pulsation, and an atrial gallop or mitral insufficiency murmur secondary to papillary muscle dysfunction.

Laboratory Tests

Electrocardiography. In one-half to two-thirds of the patients with stable angina, a standard 12-lead electrocardiogram (ECG) is normal. In the remaining patients, an ECG may show evidence of old myocardial infarction or repolarization changes (ST-T abnormalities). During a spontaneous attack of angina, most patients demonstrate an abnormal ST-segment depression, indicating subendocardial ischemia. A horizontal or down-sloping ST-segment depression of ⩾0.1 mV is generally considered diagnostic of subendocardial ischemia.

Exercise stress test. Since the majority of patients with stable angina have normal ECGs at rest, exercise stress tests have been devised to evaluate patients with suspected CHD. There are two types of stress tests: symptom limited (maximal) and submaximal. In the former, the subject exerts to maximal capacity or is limited by symptoms, whereas in the latter, exercise is terminated at a predetermined level of activity or target heart rate. The Master's two-step test is a submaximal type that is performed on stairs with the work load predetermined. Recently, this has been largely replaced by submaximal graded exercise tests whereby the subject exercises at progressively greater loads until 85-90 percent of the maximal age-predicted heart rate is achieved. Either a treadmill or an upright bicycle is used to perform the exercise. Continuous ECG monitoring and frequent measurements of blood pressure are made during the test. Usually a single bipolar ECG lead from the CM5 position is used for monitoring. However, use of 12-lead ECG monitoring increases sensitivity of the exercise stress test by approximately 10 percent.

A subject should be in a fasting state for approximately 4-6 hours before testing. Drugs such as digitalis and diuretics interfere with interpretation of the test and should preferably be withheld for several days. Propranolol prevents the attainment of a maximal heart rate and, if feasible, should be slowly withdrawn and discontinued for at least two days before the test. A completed clinical examination and control 12-lead ECG before the test are absolutely essential to rule out recent myocardial infarction or unstable angina, which are contraindications of the stress test. Other contraindications include uncontrolled congestive heart failure, uncontrolled hypertension (⩾200/100), accelerating peripheral vascular insufficiency, any acute illness, disabilities of the musculoskeletal or neurologic systems, and dangerous arrhythmias such as complex ventricular arrhythmias and heart blocks. When the test is performed, a physician should be present. The endpoints to terminate the exercise are significant angina, ⩾3 mm ST-segment depression of ischemic type, ventricular tachycardia, frequent and/or multiform premature ventricular complexes, staggering gait, mental confusion, fall of systolic blood pressure (>20 mm Hg systolic), physical exhaustion, drop in heart rate, and left bundle-branch block. The generally accepted electrocardiographic criterion of a positive stress test is horizontal or downsloping ST depression of ⩾1 mm for more than 80 milliseconds. The P-R segment is used as the reference for determining the degree of ST depression. ST depression indicates subendocardial ischemia that occurs because augmented myocardial oxygen demand during stress surpasses the limited oxygen supply available through the obstructed coronary arteries. An ST elevation occurs more frequently in patients with left ventricular aneurysms. The following parameters are observed during the stress test: degree of ST-segment depression or elevation, level of activity at which the ST change begins, duration of the ST change after cessation of stress, any arrhythmias, blood pressure, amplitude of the R wave, atrial gallop, ventricular gallop, and apical systolic murmur. Abnormalities of T wave, conduction defects, and arrhythmias are not specific signs of myocardial ischemia. A significant fall of systolic blood pressure (⩾20 mm Hg) indicates left ventricular dysfunction. The indications for an exercise stress test are as follows:

1. Confirmation of suspected CHD is one of the primary indications for an exercise stress test. The symptom-limited stress tests have shown an overall sensitivity of 70 percent for detection of CHD. The incidence of false-positive tests is approximately 10 percent; however, this is much higher in women.
2. Assessment of severity of CHD is interrelated to the first indication. Marked ST depression at lower exercise level (< 5METS*) or a heart rate of <120 beats/minute, persistence of the ST depression for >5 minutes postexercise, and a sustained fall of systolic blood pressure during exercise correlate with severe and extensive CHD. This is very beneficial in selecting patients for coronary angiography as well as estimating the cardiovascular risks of anesthesia and noncardiac surgery. For example, in an asymptomatic or mildly symptomatic patient with prior myocardial infarction, exercise stress testing is not performed for diagnosis of CHD since this has already been established by virtue of myocardial infarction; however, it is performed to determine the extent and severity of CHD. In such a patient, attaining a near maximal heart rate with no ST depression or minimal ST depression only at a higher exercise level indicates mild CHD. This patient can be followed with medical therapy, and cardiovascular risk for noncardiac surgery should be minimal. On the other hand, if exercise stress testing indicates severe CHD, coronary angiography should be recommended.
3. Exercise stress testing is valuable in establishing the efficacy of medical or surgical therapy in CHD patients. It can also be beneficial in follow-up of these patients. Conversion of a negative test to a positive test may indicate increasing obstruction in the coronary arteries and/or occlusion of bypass grafts.
4. As a screening procedure for predicting CHD in asymptomatic patients, exercise stress testing is an excellent means of predicting future coronary events in asymptomatic subjects. One study revealed a 20-fold increase of coronary events in subjects with a positive stress test. In asymptomatic subjects, this test is indicated in the following categories: patients with major risk factors, subjects >40 years of age who wish to join strenuous exercise programs, subjects in certain occupations (e.g., airplane pilots) that place the public at potential risk, and for insurance purposes.

*METS indicates multiples of basal total body oxygen consumption, for example, in the basal state, total body oxygen consumption is 3.5 ml/kg/min; 2 METS would be 7 ml/kg/min.

5. As a prerequisite for entry into physical training programs for CHD patients and normal subjects >40 years of age to determine the exercise prescription.
6. For evaluation of functional status of heart disease patients.
7. For evaluation of cardiac arrhythmias and to determine the efficacy of antiarrhythmic medications.

Nuclear Imaging. Recent developments of new radionuclides, high-resolution scintillation cameras, and computers have made nuclear cardiology one of the most rapidly growing fields in cardiovascular diagnosis. The ability of these techniques to measure various physiologic parameters of cardiac function in a nontraumatic manner makes them particularly attractive to the practicing physician. The current clinical applications of ^{201}Tl imaging and radionuclide ventriculography are summarized below.

1. Detection of CHD in patients with
   (a) Chest pain and negative exercise ECG
   (b) Chest pain and uninterpretable exercise ECG (LBBB, WPW pattern, digitalis, LVH, inadequate heart rate during exercise)
   (c) Atypical angina
   (d) Nonspecific chest pain
2. Asymptomatic patients with positive exercise ECG
3. In patients with known CHD
   (a) To evaluate the functional significance of specific coronary artery lesions
   (b) To evaluate the site and extent of myocardial infarction
4. Radionuclide ventriculography is extremely helpful in following left ventricular function on a long-term basis in these patients.
5. Evaluation of patients following coronary artery bypass surgery

Hemodynamics. Cardiac output and intracardiac pressures at rest are generally normal if a patient has not had a prior myocardial infarction. If angina occurs spontaneously or is provoked by stress (exercise, atrial pacing) during a cardiac catheterization study, left ventricular end-diastolic and pulmonary artery wedge pressure become abnormally elevated. This hemodynamic response, indicating left ventricular dysfunction, is probably due to a transient decrease of left ventricular compliance caused by ischemia. Transient left ventricular failure may also explain the elevated left ventricular end-diastolic pressure. In addition, tachycardia, hypertension, and low cardiac output may be present. Increased serum lactate in coronary sinus blood indicates anaerobic metabolism in myocardium during angina.

Coronary Arteriography. Selective coronary arteriography enables the visualization of major coronary arteries and their subbranches down to vessels with a diameter of 100 μm. One can estimate the size of the vessel, the degree of narrowing, status of the coronary artery distal to the lesion, presence or absence of collateral channels to the obstructed artery, and the number of diseased coronary arteries. It should be remembered that coronary arteriography delineates the anatomic characteristics of the coronary arteries and yields little information regarding coronary blood flow. Coronary arteriography is performed either by the brachial approach (Sones' technique) or by the percutaneous femoral approach using preformed catheters (Judkin's technique). The technique consists of selective catheterization of each coronary artery, injection of contrast material (Renografin-76), and simultaneous imaging in cine mode with x-rays in multiple views. There is an 0.1 percent mortality associated with this procedure. Occasionally myocardial infarction, coronary artery dissection, stroke, hypotension, arrhythmias, thromboembolic complications, and local trauma to the artery can occur. The incidence of these complications is extremely low in most laboratories. Patients with disease of the left main trunk and/or severe left ventricular dysfunction are at the greatest risk for serious complications. Coronary angiography is indicated under the following circumstances:

1. Patients with disabling angina pectoris despite adequate medical therapy, the objective being to define the coronary anatomy for possible coronary artery bypass surgery
2. As a diagnostic measure in patients with chest pain of unclear origin
3. Patients > 40 years of age who are undergoing cardiac catheterization for evaluation of valve disease
4. For evaluation of graft patency or progression of disease in the native coronary circulation in postcoronary artery bypass patients who have redeveloped disabling angina
5. Patients with angina and a strongly positive exercise stress test at a low level of stress (<5 METS, or heart rate <120 beats/min)
6. Patients suspected of having coronary artery anomalies or other congenital heart disease

Some cardiologists recommend coronary angiography in patients with significant angina even if the angina is well controlled by medical therapy. Another controversial indication is in postinfarction asymptomatic patients. Other factors such as age, presence of disability from a previous cerebrovascular accident, and other life limiting conditions such as cancer should be carefully considered before advising coronary angiography. Acute myocardial infarction and acute infections are relative contraindications of coronary angiography.

Natural History of Stable Angina

Patients with stable angina have a variable risk for future cardiac events such as myocardial infarction and/or sudden death. The number of obstructed coronary arteries and left ventricular function are the most reliable long-term prognostic indicators. The annual mortalities from single-, double-, and triple-vessel disease are 2 percent, 6 percent, and 10 percent, respectively. Stenosis of the left anterior descending coronary artery has an annual mortality of 4 percent. Stenosis of the left main coronary artery indicates the most ominous prognosis. Fifty percent of these patients die by the fifth year, and 80 percent by the tenth year. The presence of global or multiple segmental contraction abnormalities greatly worsen the prognosis. Thus, severe left ventricular dysfunction with CHD carries a 1-year mortality of 50 percent and a 5-year mortality of 85 percent. The symptom-limited stress test is also helpful in identifying patients with a poor long-term prognosis. The following indicate a poor prognosis: the occurrence of marked ST depression (≥2 mm) of down-sloping type at low levels of stress (stage 1 of Bruce's protocol or heart rate < 120 beats/min); persistence of ST depression for several minutes after termination of exercise; fall of systolic blood pressure during exertion; and ventricular ectopy in association with ST depression. In addition, congestive heart failure, systemic hypertension, electrocardiographic abnormalities in a resting ECG, as well as the occurrence of angina at rest or with minimal effort, constitute poor prognostic signs. In general, the severity of angina is a poor guide to prognosis.

Patients with stable angina may follow any of the following patterns: continuation of stable angina without any change; occurrence of unstable angina that may be followed by myocardial infarction; sudden death; multiple myocardial infarctions complicated by a picture of ischemic cardiomyopathy; and, rarely, disappearance of angina, presumably due to infarction in the ischemic region or development of adequate collateral vessels.

Patients with angina and normal coronary arteries have an excellent long-term prognosis.

Differential Diagnosis

Pericarditis, myocardial infarction, reflux esophagitis, peptic ulcer, cholecystitis and cholelithiasis, musculoskeletal pains from the chest wall and neck, and neurocirculatory asthenia may have to be considered in the differential diagnosis of angina. The diagnosis of angina pectoris is based on history. Until proven otherwise, discomfort in the midanterior chest on exertion and/or emotion relieved with rest and/or nitroglycerine should be considered as angina. Pericardial pain is sharper, more often precordial in location, and is aggravated by recumbency, deep breathing, and coughing. Pain of myocardial infarction is prolonged, more intense, usually not relieved by rest and/or nitroglycerin, and is generally accompanied by sweating, nausea, and vomiting. Serial ECGs and enzymes show characteristic changes. Reflux esophagitis is associated with low substernal pain of burning quality that may radiate to the neck, is accompanied by belching and precipitated by recumbency or stooping, and relieved with antacids. An acid perfusion test, esophagoscopy, and upper gastrointestinal series are diagnostic. Pain of peptic ulcer is epigastric in location and related to food intake rather than exertion. It is relieved by antacids and is accompanied by epigastric tenderness. Localized tenderness is the main clinical feature of rib fracture, costochondritis, and other nonspecific musculoskeletal pains. The pain is aggravated by rotation of the trunk, pulling, bending, and lifting. Cervical radiculopathy causes pain in the neck, and upper chest, radiating into the arms.

Management

The objectives of treating a patient with angina pectoris are: relief of angina and prevention of further episodes of angina; and, if possible, prevention of the progression of underlying coronary artery disease so that future catastrophic events such as myocardial infarction and sudden death can be prevented.

Medical Treatment. As stated previously, angina occurs when myocardial oxygen demand and supply imbalance occurs. Pharmacologic agents that improve this imbalance are useful in the treatment of angina.

Glyceryl trinitrate (nitroglycerin) is the drug of choice for immediate relief of angina. It causes dilatation of venous and arteriolar beds, thus reducing both the preload and afterload on the ventricle. The vasodilatation is more marked in the venous bed. Consequently, the left ventricular chamber becomes smaller and the myocardial oxygen demand is curtailed. Nitroglycerin causes mild hypotension that reflexly produces slight tachycardia, which in turns tends to increase myocardial oxygen demand. However, the net effect is the reduction of myocardial oxygen demand. Nitroglycerin, by reducing the left ventricular end-diastolic pressure, facilitates the blood supply to the subendocardial region. In addition, some studies suggest that nitroglycerin dilates the coronary collateral vessels, resulting in enhanced perfusion to the ischemic zone of the myocardium. Recently it has been shown that nitrites also dilate the stenotic segments of coronary arteries thereby enhancing blood flow. Thus, nitroglycerin, through its multifaceted effects, reverses the myocardial ischemia and relieves angina. It is available as tablets (0.3, 0.4, or 0.6 mg) for sublingual use. It becomes effective in 2 minutes, and the hemodynamic effects last 15-30 minutes. Occasionally, nitroglycerin can cause significant hypotension and syncope; therefore, minimal effective doses should be prescribed. A throbbing headache is the other main side effect. The potency of nitroglycerin deteriorates over time; therefore, tablets 3-6 months old should be discarded. The patient should be encouraged to carry nitroglycerin tablets at all times, to be used at the first sign of angina. Moreover, nitroglycerin should be used prophylactically before certain activities that are anticipated to give rise to angina. Nitroglycerin has recently become available for intravenous use. In the coronary care unit, it can be administered as a continuous infusion at a rate of 50-200 μg/minute for the control of refractory myocardial ischemia.

Long-acting nitrates are indicated for the prevention of angina. Isosorbide dinitrate is effective for $1\frac{1}{2}$-2 hours following sublingual administration. The sublingual dose is 2.5-10 mg every 2 hours. Following oral administration, the absorption is somewhat erratic, but the hemodynamic effect generally lasts up to 4 hours. The recommended oral dose is 10-20 mg every 4-6 hours. Recently, the use of nitroglycerin ointment has become increasingly popular. After local application of 1-2 inches of 2 percent nitroglycerin ointment, sustained blood levels and hemodynamic effects are achieved for 6-8 hours. Nitroglycerin ointment is ideally suited for use at bedtime as it permits the angina patient to have restful sleep.

The introduction of beta-adrenergic blocking agents has been a major advance in the treatment of angina pectoris. By blocking the beta receptors in the heart, these agents reduce heart rate, contractility, and blood pressure; all three effects lead to a decrease of myocardial oxygen demand. Propranolol is particularly effective in preventing an exercise-induced increase in heart rate, blood pressure, and contractility. Depression of contractility tends to cause left ventricular enlargement, thereby increasing oxygen demand. However, this effect is more than counterbalanced, and reduced oxygen demand is the net effect. Propranolol is an example of a nonselective beta-blocking agent. In addition to blocking β_1 receptors in the heart, it also blocks β_2 receptors in the bronchial tree and the peripheral circulation. Metoprolol (Lopressor), however, is a cardioselective beta-blocking agent that selectively blocks β_1 receptors in the heart, having little effect on those in the lungs. The usual starting dose of propranolol is 10 mg four times daily. At intervals of 2-4 days, the dose is increased to a maximum of 100 mg four times daily. In most patients, the effective dose is 40-60 mg four times daily. The end points for determining the maximal dose are abolition of angina, resting heart rate of approximately 50 beats/minute, or serious side effects such as hypotension, heart failure, and/or bronchoconstriction. Fatigue, depression, skin rash, impotence, cold limbs, and worsening of claudication may also occur. Gross congestive heart failure, asthma, 2 or 3 degree AV block, allergic rhinitis, and hypoglycemia are contraindications to the use of propranolol. Mild heart failure, left ventricular dysfunction, or cardiomegaly are not contraindications to propranolol use, especially when accompanied by frequent angina. By ameliorating myocardial ischemia, propranolol may actually improve left ventricular function in such patients. The combined use of digitalis and propranolol in these patients is very helpful since digitalis prevents the negative inotropic effect of propranolol at rest; propranolol prevents exercise-induced angina by limiting heart rate, blood pressure, and contractility responses during exercise. The combination of propranolol and nitrates is beneficial in preventing angina. Propranolol avoids nitrate-induced tachycardia and increased contractility, and nitrates prevent propranolol-induced left ventricular enlargement. Propranolol therapy should not be abruptly discontinued as it may result in severe angina or myocardial infarction.

If angina is not well controlled by a combination of nitrites and beta blocking agents, Ca^{2+} channel blocking agents (nifedipine, verapamil, diltiazem) may be added to the medical regimen. These agents are potent vasodilators and exert a negative ionotropic action. Of the three Ca^{2+} channel blockers available at present, verapamil has the most potent negative ionotropic effect and nifedipine is the most potent vasodilator. In addition, verapamil has the most profound effect on the pacemaker and conduction systems of the heart whereas nifedipine is minimally effect in this regard. Because of marked negative ionotropic effects of both verapamil and beta blocking agents, this combination should be avoided in patients with left ventricular dysfunction as it may precipitate frank congestive heart failure. Instead, nifedipine and beta blocking agents should be combined for such patients.

Other therapeutic measures, such as good control of hypertension, treatment of tachyarrhythmias and bradyarrhythmias, correction of anemia, polycythemia, hypoxia, thyrotoxicosis, and congestive heart failure are extremely valuable for adequate control of angina. The patient should be encouraged to achieve an ideal body weight, discontinue smoking, eat low-cholesterol food, and use alcohol in moderation. The judicious use of tranquilizers is beneficial. Supervised physical training provides adequate cardiovascular training and permits a patient to accomplish a greater work load without developing angina or any objective evidence of myocardial ischemia. In the management of stable angina, the use of antiplatelet agents remains controversial.

Coronary Artery Bypass Surgery. The technique of direct myocardial revascularization consists of performing aortocoronary bypass using short segments of the saphenous vein or internal mammary artery. These conduits are anastomosed to the coronary artery(ies) distal to the obstruction(s). Presently, the mortality from this operation is 1-2 percent, and the incidence of perioperative myocardial infarction is 3-4 percent in patients with adequate left ventricular function. The efficacy of such bypasses in supplying an increased amount of blood to the ischemic myocardium has been proven by several methods. Approximately 89 percent of the bypasses stay open and functional 1 year after the operation. The incidence of graft occlusion after 1 year has been very low. Approximately 50 percent of the patients undergoing surgery become totally asymptomatic and, in an additional 20 percent of patients, angina is markedly relieved. Moreover, serial exercise stress tests and ^{201}Tl imaging postoperatively have furnished objective data showing a decrease or abolition of myocardial ischemia. Surgical therapy is more effective than medical therapy in preventing episodes of unstable angina. Left ventricular function is improved, especially during exercise. Most of the studies have shown that surgery improves the long-term survival in a subset of patients with left main coronary artery stenosis. Other studies have also indicated that survival is probably prolonged in patients with multivessel CAD. In addition to the extent and severity of CAD, left ventricular function, severity of angina, response of angina to medical therapy, and results of the exercise stress test, other factors like age, occupation, and general condition of the patient deserve strong consideration before surgical intervention. In patients with double- or triple-vessel coronary artery disease and disabling angina, coronary artery bypass surgery is generally recommended. In most medical centers, surgical procedures are performed in patients who have left main CAD, even when angina is mild or absent. In single-vessel disease, medical therapy is usually advisable. However, if disabling angina persists despite maximal medical therapy, or if there is a severe obstruction of the proximal left anterior descending artery with strongly positive exercise stress test at low level, surgery should be performed.

Percutaneous Transluminal Coronary Angioplasty (PTCA): Approximately 5-10% of patients with CHD who undergo coronary artery bypass surgery have discrete single vessel disease in the proximal portion of the coronary vessel. These patients are amenable to PTCA which consists of passing a balloon catheter selectively into the coronary artery, positioning the balloon in the stenotic segment and inflating the balloon under high pressure (up to 14 atmospheric pressure) in order to compress the lesion and opening up the coronary artery. This technique has proven successful in a high percentage of properly selected patients.

Unstable Angina

There are a group of patients whose description of ischemic cardiac pain falls between exercise-induced brief anginal episodes and the intense and prolonged chest pain of myocardial infarction. Several descriptive terms have been used for these clinical situations, for example, preinfarction angina, acute coronary insufficiency, status anginosus, and unstable angina. Such patients are presumably at higher risk for myocardial infarction or of sudden death than are patients with stable angina. This group represents a heterogeneous mixture of patients with different prognoses and, as such, they should be subdivided into the following three groups:

1. Angina of recent onset within the previous three months represents the group with the most benign prognosis.
2. Changing pattern of angina comprises the majority of patients with unstable angina. These patients with previously stable angina start having angina at rest, at night, or at a decreased level of exertion than previously. More intense angina, prolonged episodes, greater frequency, and only partial or no response to the usual dose of nitroglycerin are also characteristic of this group. When factors like anemia, tachyarrhythmia, and increased emotional or physical activity are excluded, change in the pattern of angina suggests increased severity of underlying CAD.
3. *Intermediate syndrome.* In these patients, the pain lasts >30 minutes, is poorly controlled with nitroglycerin, and is accompanied by ST-T changes. Serial cardiac enzymes (CPK, SGOT, LDH) may show only a minimal rise (less than twofold). This group represents patients at the highest risk for developing myocardial infarction or of sudden death.

Diagnosis

Physical examination is generally unremarkable in these patients. An atrial gallop and apical systolic murmur may be audible during an episode of acute myocardial ischemia.

An electrocardiogram may show depression or elevation of the ST segments and flattening or inversion of T waves. Generally, these ST-T changes accompany the episodes of chest pain and may revert to normal with relief of pain.

Radionuclide studies. Thallium-201 myocardial perfusion images may demonstrate regional hypoperfusion at rest, indicating intense regional myocardial ischemia. In some patients with unstable angina, ^{99m}Tc-stannous pyrophosphate (PYP) scintigraph may also be positive. Even though other laboratory tests do not indicate the occurrence of clinical myocardial infarction, necrosis of a small amount of myocardium cannot be ruled out in these patients.

Coronary angiography generally reveals multivessel coronary artery disease. The incidence of left main coronary artery stenosis is approximately 10 percent in patients presenting with unstable angina. Approximately 5-20 percent of all patients have entirely normal coronary arteries. Coronary vasospasm has been demonstrated to be responsible for unstable angina in a significant number of patients. The risk of performing coronary arteriography is essentially similar in stable and unstable angina.

The ejection fraction and segmental wall motion may be entirely normal if there is no active myocardial ischemia present at the time of left ventriculography. If, however, critical stenoses are present that are compromising nutrient blood flow at rest, segmental wall motion abnormalities may be demonstrated. On repeat ventriculogram following nitroglycerin administration, segmental wall motion may become normal in such cases.

Natural History

Natural history depends on a multitude of factors in a given patient. The presence of hypertension, heart failure, cardiomegaly, previous myocardial infarction, recurrent prolonged anginal episodes at rest that respond poorly to nitroglycerin and are accompanied by ST-T changes, critical multivessel or left main CAD, abnormal left ventricular end-diastolic pressure, low cardiac output, and a low ejection fraction increase the risk for myocardial infarction or of sudden death. Unstable angina patients without the above-mentioned factors obviously carry a better prognosis. The overall incidence of myocardial infarction is 5-15% and hospital mortality is 1-2%.

Treatment

Patients with unstable angina must be admitted to the coronary care unit and placed on full bed rest. Tranquilizers may be needed to treat apprehension. A combination of beta-adrenergic blocking agents and nitrates are the mainstay of medical treatment. Propranolol should be initiated at a dose of 10 mg every 6 hours, and rapidly increased up to 100 mg every 6 hours. The end point for adjusting the dose of propranolol is control of the angina or the development of side effects, that is, hypotension, heart failure, or marked bradycardia (<50 beats/minute). Isosorbide dinitrate is started at a dose of 2.5-10 mg sublingually every 4 hours. For relief of nocturnal angina, nitroglycerin ointment (1 inch) can be applied at bedtime. Sublingual nitroglycerin is prescribed for each episode of angina. Intravenous nitroglycerin may have to be used for relief of acute intractable ischemia. If the patient is hypertensive, blood pressure should be rapidly controlled. If there is coexistent heart failure, digitalis should be added. If these measures are not effective Ca^{2+} blockers may be added to the regimen. With this aggressive medical regimen, episodes of angina are controlled in a majority of patients. Serial enzymes, ECGs, and PYP scan should be performed to rule out myocardial infarction. Cardiac rhythm is monitored continuously. If arrhythmias occur, they should be controlled and an optimum heart rate achieved. If the unstable angina is well controlled and myocardial infarction has been ruled out, the patient can leave the coronary care unit and supervised progressive ambulation can be initiated. Coronary angiography is performed during the second week to determine the extent and severity of CAD. If critical multivessel or left main CAD is demonstrated, coronary artery bypass surgery should be recommended. Patients whose anginal episodes fail to respond to vigorous medical therapy should undergo coronary angiography during the second or third day. If the coronary anatomy is suitable for coronary artery bypass surgery, it should be performed without further delay. Several studies have demonstrated that coronary artery bypass surgery is extremely effective in relieving angina and preventing further bouts of unstable angina. Its role in preventing myocardial infarction and prolonging life remains to be fully established. Some patients with unstable angina do not respond to medical therapy and develop pump failure. In these patients, it is wise to support the circulation with intra-aortic balloon counterpulsation, then perform coronary angiography and myocardial revascularization if feasible.

Prinzmetal's (Variant) Angina

In some patients, episodes of angina occur at rest without any obvious precipitating factor, and are accompanied by ST-segment elevation and ventricular ectopy. Angina and electrocardiographic changes totally disappear following sublingual nitroglycerine. The attacks are common at night and frequently occur at similar times. Elevation of the ST segment indicates transmural rather than subendocardial ischemia. Coronary angiography demonstrates severe (>90%) fixed atherosclerotic lesions in the proximal region of one or more major coronary arteries in the majority of patients with Prinzmetal's angina. In the remaining patients, the coronary arteries are either entirely normal (approximately 10-15%) or demonstrate mild CAD. In the latter group, coronary angiography shows spasm of the major coronary artery either during a spontaneous attack of variant angina or in response to a provocative test consisting of intravenous administration of ergonovine maleate (0.05-0.2 mg). Patients with variant angina and coronary artery spasm have a more benign course than those with variant angina and severe coronary atherosclerosis. A small number of patients develop myocardial infarction and sudden death. Since the mode of treatment is different in these two angiographically different groups of angina patients, it is obvious that coronary angiography should be the first step in planning the management of these patients. Patients with severe fixed stenosis should be treated with beta-adrenergic blocking agents and Ca^{2+} blockers and/or nitrates. Also, in view of the critical coronary arterial lesions and severe recurrent angina, coronary artery bypass surgery should be performed in most of these patients. Surgery is generally very effective in the relief of angina in this category of patients. By contrast, coronary artery bypass surgery is contraindicated in patients with no or mild CAD and coronary artery spasm. Moreover, beta-adrenergic blocking agents may induce attacks of variant angina in these patients. The mainstay of treatment in this group consists of calcium antagonists such as nifedipine, diltiazem and verapamil as well as nitrates.

Atypical Angina Pectoris

Some patients experience episodic chest pain that has some characteristics of typical angina pectoris except that it has no definite relationship with exertion or emotion. It may occur after the cessation of exertion rather than during exertion. It may not have the characteristic radiation, quality, or location of classic angina. Many patients with atypical angina have mitral valve prolapse, hypertrophic subaortic stenosis, or other types of cardiomyopathies. In some patients who do not have readily available evidence of cardiomyopathy, cardiac catheterization shows left ventricular dysfunction at rest or during exercise. Electrocardiography reveals repolarization changes in approximately 50 percent of the patients. A significant proportion of patients also have positive exercise stress tests. Coronary angiography demonstrates minimal or no CAD. The long-term prognosis of these patients is generally excellent. The underlying cardiac disease, for example, mitral valve prolapse or idiopathic subaortic stenosis, rather than chest pain influences the prognosis. Most of the patients experience relief of chest pain with propranolol and/or nitroglycerin.

ACUTE MYOCARDIAL INFARCTION

The term myocardial infarction indicates necrosis of the myocardium due to compromised coronary blood flow. It is characterized by severe and prolonged anterior chest pain, evolutionary electrocardiographic changes, and transient cardiac enzyme rise in the blood.

Etiology

Myocardial infarction usually occurs due to a sudden and severe occlusion of a major coronary artery. Thrombosis over a preexistent atheromatous plaque or subintimal hemorrhage into the plaque may be responsible for sudden coronary occlusion. If coronary artery obstruction occurs slowly with a relatively rapid development of collateral channels, infarction may not occur or may be small. Generally, occlusion of the left anterior descending coronary artery can be demonstrated in an anterior wall infarction. Occlusion of the right or circumflex coronary artery occurs in an inferior or inferolateral infarction. Rare cases of documented infarction and normal coronary arteries have been reported. Coronary embolism or spasm has been incriminated in such patients. Whereas most patients who die suddenly following myocardial infarction demonstrate CAD at autopsy, only a few show fresh thrombotic occlusion of the coronary artery(ies). The immediate cause of myocardial infarction in such patients is unclear. On the other hand, survivors of myocardial infarction usually have total occlusion of the coronary artery(ies).

Pathology

The earliest histologically recognizable changes begin to occur 6-12 hours after the initiation of an infarction. These changes consist of an eosinophilic appearance of myocardial fibers, and cross striations of these myocardial fibers appear indistinct and fuzzy. Polymorphonuclear infiltration begins in 18-24 hours. Forty-eight hours later, the infarcted zone appears pale with interspersed hemorrhagic areas. The border zone between the necrotic and healthy zones consists of a mixture of injured and viable islets of myocardium. Fibrosis starts after the third week, and scar formation is completed in 6-8 weeks.

Symptoms

The most common presenting symptom is the substernal pain that is usually more intense than the pain of angina, radiates along one or both arms and the neck, lasts from 30 minutes to several hours (usually $<$24 hours), and is generally accompanied by nausea, vomiting, sweating, marked weakness, anxiety, and fear of impending death. It does not respond to nitroglycerin or rest and, as a rule, is not precipitated by effort. The majority of patients experience either new onset angina or a change in the pattern of angina prior to the occurrence of myocardial infarction. Elderly and some diabetic patients may not experience any pain during acute infarction. In them, acute myocardial infarction may manifest as arrhythmia, exacerbation or onset of heart failure, or a cerebrovascular accident. In some patients, myocardial infarction is totally asymptomatic and is detected on a routine ECG.

Physical Signs

During the initial few hours of acute myocardial infarction, the patient is in pain, acutely anxious, and the skin is pale, cold, and clammy. Bradycardia and hypotension, which are signs of parasympathetic overactivity, are frequently seen, especially in an inferior wall infarction. Conversely, tachycardia and hypertension, which are signs of sympathetic overactivity, may be observed. When pain has been relieved, the blood pressure usually settles down to the preinfarction level. An abnormal systolic bulge, representing the dyskinetic anteroapical segment, may be visualized and palpated in the precordial region in patients with anteroapical infarction. S_1 is frequently soft due to decreased myocardial contractility. S_2 may be paradoxically split; however, this is an uncommon finding. An atrial gallop (S_4) is usually audible over the apex. A pericardial friction rub may develop on the second or third day and disappear within 1-2 days. Slight fever may also occur early during the first week. Physical findings of heart failure and other complications are described later. Killip has suggested the following clinical classification of acute myocardial infarction: Class I, uncomplicated; Class II, mild left ventricular failure (ventricular gallop, pulmonary rales); Class III, acute pulmonary edema; and Class IV, cardiogenic shock.

Laboratory Diagnosis

Electrocardiography

The earliest ECG change during the evolution of a transmural myocardial infarction is in the T wave. In the leads facing the infarcting region the T wave becomes tall and spiked (hyperacute T wave), which is probably due to ischemia in the subendocardial layer of the myocardium. This change is very early and short-lived and is therefore overlooked in most patients. Elevation of the ST segment in leads facing the infarcting region follows the hyperacute T wave change. Reciprocal depression of the ST segment is recorded in the opposite leads. ST segment elevation is due to injury current in the subepicardial layers of the myocardium. The potential gradient between injured cells and the adjoining healthy cells is responsible for the injury current. At this stage, the T wave is usually obscured by the elevated ST segment. ST-segment elevations last from a few hours to a week or so, and become isoelectric by 2 weeks at the most.

A few hours to a few days after the onset of ST-segment elevation, a pathologic Q wave appears in the leads facing the infarcted zone. Since the infarcted muscle is electrically inert, the initial QRS vector is directed away from it and is recorded as a negative (Q) wave. The Q wave persists for months, years, or indefinitely and serves as an ECG sign of an old scar.

As the ST-segment regresses towards the isoelectric line, a symmetrically inverted T wave becomes more clear. T-wave inversion reflects transmural ischemia. This change persists for several months to years. Thus, ST-segment elevation is the only ECG sign of acute myocardial injury and, when accompanied with the development of a new Q wave, indicates acute transmural myocardial infarction. An ECG may not show any changes during the very early stages of myocardial infarction and should be repeated daily for at least 3 days to determine if evolutionary changes described above develop in patients suspected of having a myocardial infarction.

The standard 12-lead ECG permits an approximate localization of myocardial infarction: Q waves in leads V_1 and V_2, anteroseptal; in V_3 and V_4, midanterior; in I, aV_L, V_5, and V_6, anterolateral; in I, aV_L, and V_1-V_6, extensive anterior; in II, III, and aV_F, inferior or diaphragmatic. In cases of true posterior myocardial infarction, leads V_1 and V_2 register a tall, broad R wave and an upright T wave since these leads are separated from the infarcted region by the healthy anterior wall. If one obtains leads V_7-V_9, they might show Q waves. A subendocardial infarction produces ST-segment depression and T-wave inversion.

The ECG has several limitations when used in the diagnosis of myocardial infarction. In the presence of conduction defects such as LBBB and WPW patterns, changes of myocardial infarction are not apparent. In patients with multiple prior infarcts, electrical forces may counterbalance one another and a new infarct may not produce any ECG changes. Infarction involving the left ventricular apex or high lateral wall, as well as a small infarction anywhere in the myocardium, may not result in any ECG changes.

Chest X-Ray

Serial chest x-rays in acute myocardial infarction are helpful for the diagnosis and follow-up of left heart failure. Since the chest x-rays are usually portable (obtained in the CCU), they are not reliable for the assessment of cardiac size.

Blood Tests (Serum Enzymes)
Slight leukocytosis with a shift to the left usually occurs on the second or third day. The erythrocyte sedimentation rate (ESR) also becomes elevated during the second or third day.

Myocardial cell necrosis results in leakage of certain enzymes, notably creatine phosphokinase (CPK), serum aspartate transaminase (SGOT), and lactate dehydrogenase (LDH) into the blood. Determination of the level of these enzymes has been used as a diagnostic and prognostic aid in acute myocardial infarction. Serum CPK rises within 6 hours of the onset of acute myocardial infarction, reaches a peak level in 24 hours, and becomes normal within 4 days. The SGOT level rises within 6-12 hours, peaks in 24-48 hours, and returns to normal within 4 days. The serum LDH activity starts rising in 12-24 hours, peaks in 48-72 hours, and returns to normal within 14 days. However, these enzymes are present in other organs as well and, consequently, their elevations are not specific for myocardial infarction. For example, CPK is present in brain and skeletal muscle and its level becomes elevated in diseases of skeletal muscle, intramuscular injections, convulsions, and central nervous system diseases; SGOT is present in the liver and its activity rises in inflammatory disease of the liver, ischemic necrosis of the liver due to heart failure or shock as well as pericarditis, electric cardioversion, and rapid tachycardia; LDH is present in the liver, red cells, kidney, and lung and its acitivity rises in hemolytic anemia, leukemia, neoplastic diseases, pulmonary or renal infarction, and liver diseases. To improve the specificity, isoenzymes of CPK and LDH are measured. Elevation of MB isoenzyme of CPK is the most specific indicator of myocardial injury and is a useful laboratory diagnostic aid if the patient is seen within the first 48 hours of onset of chest pain. Elevation of fast-moving fraction of LDH (LDH-1) occurs in acute myocardial infarction as well as hemolytic anemia, gastric carcinoma, and renal infarction. Myoglobin is also released into the blood after acute myocardial infarction; its presence in urine is indicative of acute myocardial infarction. In patients with prolonged chest pain and in patients who have nondiagnostic ECG changes, serial measurements of serum enzymes are useful in the diagnosis of acute myocardial infarction.

Myocardial Imaging
Myocardial imaging with ^{99m}Tc-PYP is a useful diagnostic tool in acute myocardial infarction. This isotope concentrates in the acutely necrotic myocardium and appears as a hot spot. The precise mechanism of binding to the acutely damaged myocardium is not clear. An abnormally increased binding of calcium with mitochondria of the acutely injured myocardial cells is considered the likely mechanism. This test is positive from 24 hours up to 6 days after onset of infarction. The sensitivity and specificity are excellent for transmural infarction, but the technique is less reliable for subendocardial infarction. Positive images may also be obtained in patients with ventricular aneurysm in patients following electrical defibrillation, myocardial contusion, and calcified cardiac valves. The chief clinical utility of PYP imaging is to confirm and localize myocardial infarction in patients with equivocal ECG and serum enzyme changes. Serial imaging may be valuable in monitoring the size of the myocardial infarction.

On thallium-201 myocardial perfusion imaging, the infarcted region appears as a cold spot because the isotope is not accumulated by the infarcted zone. Its chief advantage is that, unlike PYP imaging, it becomes positive immediately after onset of infarction; however, its disadvantage is that it does not distinguish between an old or an acute infarction, or between an infarction and severe ischemia.

Radionuclide angiography can reliably estimate the ejection fraction of the left ventricle (global function) as well as segmental wall motion abnormalities (regional function). Akinetic or dyskinetic segments determined by this method correspond to the old or acute infarcts, and the ejection fraction is helpful in determining the prognosis in myocardial infarction.

Echocardiography
Cross-sectional echocardiography is useful in evaluating the segmental wall motion in an acute myocardial infarction. Segmental wall motion abnormalities appear almost instantaneously following infarction and can be reliably detected and localized using cross-sectional echocardiography. Ventricular aneurysms and intraventricular mural blood clots may also be visualized. M-mode echocardiography is helpful in identifying the development of pericardial effusion in acute infarction. Occasionally, abnormal mitral valve motion can be visualized in acute mitral regurgitation due to a ruptured papillary muscle. Echocardiography is also helpful in detecting and localizing a ventricular septal rupture and can provide an accurate estimate of the anatomic size of the defect.

Holter Monitoring
Holter monitoring is useful in documenting cardiac arrhythmias after the patient has been discharged from the cardiac care unit of the hospital. It is a useful technique in assessing the effectiveness of various antiarrhythmic medications.

Hemodynamic Monitoring
The introduction of a balloon-tipped, flow-directed catheter by Swan and Ganz has made possible the monitoring of hemodynamics at the patient's bedside. It has greatly advanced the understanding of cardiac performance as a pump during the acute phase of infarction and has permitted the management of heart failure and cardiogenic shock on a much more rational basis. The triple-lumen thermodilution catheter allows measurement of pulmonary artery and right atrial pressures as well as cardiac output. The central venous or right atrial pressure does not reliably reflect the status of the left ventricle, for example, it may be low or normal in the presence of acute pulmonary edema. By contrast, in a patient with an inferior wall myocardial infarction with coexistent right ventricular ischemia or infarction, the central venous or right atrial pressure may be very high, even though the left ventricular filling pressure is low. Pulmonary artery wedge pressure accutely reflects the mean left atrial pressure or left ventricular filling pressure. It also reflects the pre-a wave left ventricular diastolic pressure. Serial measurements of left ventricular filling pres-

sure, cardiac output, systemic vascular resistance, and peripheral blood pressure are extremely helpful in introducing various therapeutic interventions for heart failure and cardiogenic shock. The necessity of hemodynamic monitoring has become more obvious with the realization that physical signs do not reliably reflect the underlying hemodynamic changes. Moreover, there is a great degree of lag between physical signs, x-ray signs of heart failure, and changes of intracardiac pressures. It is also possible to measure the oxygen content of blood samples from various right heart chambers, further enabling one to differentiate between a rupture of the ventricular septum and acute mitral regurgitation secondary to a ruptured papillary muscle. Routine measurements of the left ventricular stroke work index (LVSWI) and left ventricular filling pressure (LVFP) have shown that acute myocardial infarction patients fall into five categories: Patients with normal LVSWI and LVFP have generally no complications; patients with high LVSWI and normal or low LVFP represent a hyperadrenergic state and would probably benefit from beta-adrenergic blocking agents; patients with modest reduction of LVSWI (20-40 g-meters/m^2) and high LVFP ($\geq$15 mm Hg) have heart failure; patients with markedly reduced LVSWI ($<$20 g-meters/m^2) and elevated LVFP have cardiogenic shock and have a mortality in excess of 80 percent; and patients with low LVSWI and low LVFP have hypotension on the basis of hypovolemia and respond readily to volume therapy. It should be remembered that invasive hemodynamic monitoring is not required in uncomplicated myocardial infarction.

Coronary and Left Ventricular Angiography

These procedures generally are not indicated during the acute phase of a myocardial infarction and actually have a slightly higher mortality and morbidity. However, it becomes essential to perform these procedures if a patient develops severe heart failure due to a mechanical complication, for example, a papillary muscle rupture, a ventricular septal rupture, and a ventricular aneurysm or pseudoaneurysm, and when surgical correction is contemplated. Continuation of intractable angina that is totally unresponsive to aggressive medical therapy, is another indication for coronary arteriography.

Differential Diagnosis

The initial presenting features of acute myocardial infarction can be confused with several acute clinical problems such as acute pulmonary embolism, dissection of the aorta, acute pericarditis, acute pancreatitis, biliary colic, and rupture of a peptic ulcer. It is extremely important to hospitalize a patient suspected of having an acute myocardial infarction without delay and then confirm or exclude this diagnosis. When the serial ECGs show characteristic evolutionary changes consisting of ST-segment elevation, T-wave inversion, Q waves, and serum enzymes rising in a typical fashion, the diagnosis of an acute myocardial infarction is obvious. However, in patients with prolonged chest pain, only ST-T changes in the ECGs, and borderline rise of serum enzyme levels, it becomes extremely difficult to differentiate between an infarction and unstable angina. In some patients, the demonstration of a well-localized hot spot on PYP imaging may confirm the diagnosis of a myocardial infarction.

Natural History and Prognosis

More than 50 percent of the deaths due to acute myocardial infarction occur suddenly and before the patient reaches a hospital. The vast majority of these deaths are presumably due to ventricular fibrillation. Of the patients admitted to the coronary care unit, the inhospital mortality is approximately 15-20 percent, with most of these deaths occurring during the first or second day; mortality then declines progressively. The most important determinants of inhospital mortality are age, total amount of damaged myocardium during the current and any previous episodes of infarction, and the presence of hypertension and/or diabetes mellitus. Mortality is high in elderly patients with infarction. The following are indicative of a large infarct and, hence, an increased risk of mortality: development of heart failure (tachycardia, ventricular gallop, rales), cardiogenic shock, cardiomegaly, magnitude of enzyme elevation, the number of leads in a standard ECG showing ST-segment elevation and Q waves, depressed left ventricular ejection fraction, low LVSWI, high LVFP, intractable ventricular arrhythmias, complete heart block, bundle-branch blocks, and/or persistent pain. The in-hospital mortality of uncomplicated myocardial infarction is approximately 5 percent. The long-term mortality of patients discharged from the hospital depends on the status of the left ventricle and the severity and extent of the coronary artery disease.

Treatment

The course of an acute myocardial infarction can be divided into four distinct phases, prehospital phase, coronary care unit (CCU) phase, post-CCU hospital phase, and posthospital discharge phase. Treatment of myocardial infarction is discussed according to these phases. Treatment during the prehospital phase is discussed under the section on sudden death.

The objective of the treatment is to relieve symptoms, decrease myocardial oxygen requirements in order to limit infarct size, and to recognize and manage complications. Patients with suspected acute myocardial infarction should be admitted to the coronary care unit (CCU). The primary goal of the CCU is to provide continuous monitoring of cardiac rhythm and have the specialized personnel quickly recognize and then treat the arrhythmias. Since the availability of CCUs, deaths from arrhythmias have been markedly reduced. Pump failure due to destruction of a large mass of myocardium continues to be the major cause of death in acute myocardial infarction.

General Measures

Patients with an acute myocardial infarction require complete physical and mental rest. Rest lowers the myocardial oxygen demand by decreasing the heart rate and blood pressure. This decreased cardiac work load helps in the healing process. Ideally, patients should be in private rooms where they are not disturbed by noisy respirators, lights constantly being turned on and off, and other patients in the CCU. Patients should be confined to bed for the first 24 hours. Following this period, if it is an uncomplicated infarction, the patient can be assisted to a chair or sit on the bedside. Cardiac work is somewhat less in a sitting as compared to a supine posture. In addition, sitting reduces the hazards of prolonged bed rest such as pulmonary embolism, deconditioning of the body, shoulder-hand syndrome, hypostatic pneumonia, and difficulty in voiding. While in bed, passive exercises of the leg muscles are advisable. Most patients require tranquilizers to relieve mental tension. In the majority of patients, diazepam (Valium), 2.5-10 mg q.i.d., is effective. Flurazepam (Dalmane), 15-30 mg, may be used when retiring to ensure a restful night's sleep. All visitors, except the immediate family, and all telephone calls should be prohibited.

A liquid diet (1,000 calories) should be prescribed for the first 24-48 hours, after which time it can be changed to a soft, easily digestible diet. Most patients will tolerate a regular diet after 5 days. The amount of salt in the daily diet should not exceed 4 g. Patient education about heart disease should begin in the CCU, including instruction in a low-cholesterol diet. If the patient is overweight, calories must be restricted. The use of cigarettes and alcohol should not be permitted while the patient is in the hospital.

A stool softener is prescribed to avoid straining during bowel movements. Dioctyl calcium sulfosuccinate (Surfak, 240 mg tablet), bisacodyl (Dulcolax), milk of magnesia, or mineral oil are usually effective in achieving gentle bowel action. Catheterization of the urinary bladder should be avoided unless there is severe difficulty in voiding.

Patients with acute myocardial infarction must have an intravenous line inserted; 1,000 ml of 5 percent dextrose with half-normal saline should be dripped continuously to keep the line open. Relief of pain can be achieved with intravenous administration of 2 mg of morphine sulfate or 25 mg of demerol. Morphine sulfate can be repeated in 2 mg doses at 5-minute intervals until the pain is fully relieved or until 20 mg of morphine sulfate have been administered. Subsequent to control of the initial pain, only 2 mg of morphine for intravenous use should be prescribed to relieve recurrent pain. Morphine has a sympatholytic effect and in excessive doses may cause hypotension, bradycardia, respiratory depression, nausea, and/or vomiting. Some patients experience angina after the first 24 hours; sublingual nitroglycerin (0.3-0.4 mg) may be prescribed for relief of this pain.

Although most patients have mild arterial hypoxia, oxygen therapy is not necessary in patients with uncomplicated disease who do not demonstrate arterial hypoxia. However, patients who develop heart failure, cardiogenic shock, or pulmonary embolism benefit greatly from the administration of oxygen (2-4 L) through a nasal cannula.

Use of Anticoagulants

Anticoagulants are useful in preventing venous thrombi and probably avoid the occurrence of mural thrombus, but their role in preventing arterial thrombi is questionable. The routine use of anticoagulants has become less important recently because early ambulation is encouraged in patients with uncomplicated infarctions. However, anticoagulants may be used in the following circumstances: large infarct, heart failure, cardiomegaly, cardiogenic shock, persistent atrial fibrillation, previous episodes of venous thrombi and pulmonary emboli, or when prolonged bed rest is anticipated.

Limitation of Infarct Size

It has now become clear that the prognosis of an infarction patient depends on the size of the infarcted myocardium. It has also been shown that there is a significant amount of ischemic heart muscle that constitutes the border zone between the irreversibly necrotic myocardium and the healthy myocardium. The ultimate fate of this ischemic border zone as to whether it will eventually become necrotic or recover depends on the balance between oxygen supply and demand. Several pharmacologic agents such as sodium nitroprusside, nitroglycerin, steroids, glucose-insulin-potassium infusion, and propranolol have been evaluated in an attempt to save the jeopardized border zone and thus limit the size of the myocardial infarction. However, their role in the routine care of acute myocardial infarction has not been established. Moreover, there is no ideal method to accurately measure the size of a myocardial infarction. Of the various available methods, that is, ST-segment mapping, CPK isoenzymes, and radionuclide techniques, the CPK isoenzymes appear to be the most reliable method to date, but has its limitations. In a patient with acute infarction and hypertension, the consensus is that blood pressure should be controlled; heart failure in association with infarction should be treated with unloading agents such as nitroglycerin or sodium nitroprusside; and continuing ischemia and sinus tachycardia should be treated with propranolol provided there are no contraindications to its use. Recently intracoronary streptokinase infusion has been shown to be successful in lysing the clot and in establishing perfusion to the jeopardized myocardium in acute myocardial infarction patients. Furthermore, this procedure has been shown to salvage the jeopardized myocardium and favorably influence the eventual size of myocardial infarction. The exact indications of this technique are not well defined at present.

The time a patient remains in the CCU depends on whether there are any complications. Patients with uncomplicated infarctions are usually transferred to a step down unit after 3-4 days where monitoring of cardiac rhythm is continued for a few more days.

Complications of Myocardial Infarction

Angina and Extension of Infarction

Some patients continue to have rest angina after relief of the initial pain of infarction, especially following subendocardial infarction. Nitroglycerin should be administered sublingually for the relief of angina. If the anginal episodes are recurrent, long-acting nitrates or nitroglycerine ointment, Ca^{++} blockers, and progressively increasing doses of propranolol should be initiated. If the angina is intractable, coronary arteriography may be necessary, followed by urgent coronary artery bypass surgery. It should be emphasized that the hazards of coronary artery bypass surgery in a patient with recent infarction are greater than in a patient with unstable angina without an infarct.

Extension of an infarction indicates occurrence of another infarction within 3 weeks of a previous episode of infarction. Generally, electrocardiographic changes occur in the same leads as during the previous infarction and should be treated as a new episode of myocardial infarction.

Cardiac Arrhythmias

Atrial arrhythmias result from ischemia of the sinus node that is supplied by the right coronary artery in 55 percent of the patients and the left cirumflex artery in the remaining 45 percent. Sudden left atrial hypertension secondary to left ventricular failure and hyperactive vagal tone that has a profound effect on the sinus node can also lead to atrial arrhythmias. Sinus bradycardia commonly occurs in the early phase of acute myocardial infarction. When associated with hypotension, PVBs, and/or accelerated junctional or idioventricular rhythm, it should be treated with 0.4-0.6 mg of intravenous atropine, repeated in 2 hours if necessary. If sinus bradycardia persists, a temporary pacemaker should be inserted. Sinus tachycardia frequently indicates heart failure or pulmonary embolism. Atrial tachycardia, atrial flutter, and atrial fibrillation occur due to left atrial hypertension or ischemia of the atrial tissue. When associated with very rapid ventricular rates resulting in hemodynamic impairment, these rhythms should be terminated with electric countershock. Digoxin should be administered to control ventricular rate.

Premature ventricular beats (PVBs) and other ventricular arrhythmias are observed in approximately 90 percent of the patients admitted with acute myocardial infarction. Ventricular arrhythmias arise as a result of ischemic myocardial damage. The rationale of aggressively suppressing PVBs in the acute phase of myocardial infarction is that, if uncontrolled, they are likely to provoke ventricular tachycardia (VT) and ventricular fibrillation (VF). The likelihood of developing VT and VF is much higher during the first few hours of myocardial infarction. Therefore, if a patient is admitted within the first 4-6 hours after onset of myocardial infarction, routine prophylactic antiarrhythmic drug therapy is indicated. When admission to the hospital is late (after 6 hours), treatment of PVBs is warranted only if they are multifocal, occur in salvos, show an R-on-T phenomenon, or their frequency is more than 5 PVBs/minute. Intravenous lidocaine is the drug of choice for prophylaxis as well as treatment of PVBs. If lidocaine fails, procainamide, quinidine, disopyramide (Norpace), phenytoin, bretylium tosylate, or aprindine may be administered. If these drugs are ineffective, overdrive suppression by a temporary pacemaker may be employed. Drug treatment of VT is similar to that of PVBs and should be attempted initially when the hemodynamic status is stable. If drug therapy fails or severe hemodynamic impairment accompanies VT, electric countershock (100 watt-seconds) should be employed. Treatment of VF is discussed in the section on sudden death.

Nodal and infranodal atrioventricular blocks also occur during acute myocardial infarction. The atrioventricular (AV) node and His bundle are supplied by the right coronary artery in 90 percent of the patients and the left circumflex artery in the remaining 10 percent. Since the right coronary artery supplies the inferior wall of the left ventricle, AV node, and His bundle, ischemia of these structures commonly occurs in acute inferior infarction, resulting in first-, second- (Wenckebach Type I), or third-degree AV block. When complete, or third-degree, AV block occurs, escape rhythm arises from the His bundle and is stable at 50 to 60 beats/minute. In an acute inferior infarction, these conduction blocks are generally transient and spontaneously resolve in 2-3 days. If the escape rate is unusually slow and is associated with hypotension or ventricular instability, atropine or a temporary pacemaker is advisable. The right bundle and left anterior fascicle of the left bundle are perfused by the left anterior descending coronary artery, occlusion of which may result in an anterior myocardial infarction. The posterior fascicle of the left bundle is supplied by the left circumflex and right coronary arteries. Since the conduction fascicles are involved in the ischemic process, the occurrence of bundle-branch blocks (usually bifascicular block, left axis plus right bundle-branch block) may occur in anterior myocardial infarction. This may progress to second-degree (Mobitz Type II), and third-degree or complete heart block. When complete heart block develops in an acute anterior infarction, the escape rhythm arises from the distal bundle branches or Purkinje fibers. Not only is the escape rate slow, it is also unstable and the possibility of developing VF is very high. In addition, the amount of damaged muscle mass is much greater in an anterior myocardial infarction. Thus, development of a complete heart block in acute anterior infarction carries a high mortality of approximately 70 percent. Insertion of a temporary pacemaker is advocated when right bundle-branch block, RBBB with left anterior or left posterior hemiblock, or complete heart block develops during the first few days after an anterior myocardial infarction. Pacemaker insertion does not appear to greatly influence the high mortality in acute anterior infarction that is related to destruction of large muscle mass; however, it probably tilts the balance favorably in a few patients. In survivors of acute myocardial infarction, complete heart block usually resolves by the end of the second week; however, bundle-branch blocks may persist. Long-term follow-up of these patients has revealed a higher incidence of complete heart block and sudden death during the first year after infarction. Some physicians recommend permanent pacemakers in such patients.

Heart Failure

Acute myocardial infarction is usually accompanied by hemodynamic changes, indicating left ventricular dysfunction such as a high left ventricular filling pressure. Clinical manifestations of heart failure, however, are less frequent. Sinus tachycardia, tachypnea, pulmonary venous congestion and left ventricular gallop are early signs of heart failure. Oral or intravenous administration of furosemide is generally sufficient to control mild heart failure. If severe heart failure or pulmonary edema develops, hemodynamic monitoring with a Swan-Ganz balloon-tipped catheter is helpful in managing the patient. In addition to hemodynamic monitoring, cardiac rhythm, blood pressure, urine flow, electrolytes, and BUN should be monitored and serial chest x-rays obtained. A potent and rapidly-acting diuretic (furosemide or ethacrynic acid) is administered. Digoxin should be started, especially if cardiomegaly is present. By improving contractility, digoxin shrinks the left ventricular chamber size and reduces the myocardial oxygen demand. If the blood pressure is normal, a continuous infusion of sodium nitroprusside or nitroglycerine should be initiated to unload the heart and maintain the left heart filling pressure in a 10-15 mm Hg range. It is common for severe heart failure and cardiogenic shock to coexist, in which case inotropic support with dopamine or dobutamine may be required. In the presence of severe heart failure, the use of a Swan-Ganz catheter is invaluable in detecting mechanical complications (rupture of ventricular septum or papillary muscle) as the cause of heart failure. If these complications are identified, drastic measures such as intraaortic balloon counterpulsation are generally required to stabilize the circulatory status prior to surgical intervention to correct the mechanical complications.

Acquired Ventricular Septal Defect (Rupture of the Ventricular Septum)

Rupture of the ventricular septum occurs in approximately 1 percent of the patients with an anterior or inferior myocardial infarction. This catastrophic event suddenly causes severe congestive heart failure and/or cardiogenic shock and usually occurs in the first week after infarction. It is recognized by the sudden appearance of a loud pansystolic murmur and a systolic thrill over the left lower parasternal area. It is extremely difficult to differentiate this condition from acute mitral regurgitation resulting from rupture of the papillary muscle. In an acquired ventricular septal defect, right heart catheterization shows a step-up of oxygen saturation in the right ventricle. On the other hand, in mitral regurgitation, the pulmonary artery wedge pressure curve shows a prominent v wave. If the patient's condition can be stabilized, it is preferable to wait a few weeks before undertaking surgical repair of the septal defect. However, in the majority of patients, circulatory impairment is too severe to wait. In such patients, the circulatory status should be stabilized with medical means and intraaortic balloon counterpulsation, emergency left ventriculography and coronary arteriography should be performed and, if feasible, followed by urgent surgical repair of the ventricular septal defect by plication or patch graft. In many cases, coronary bypass surgery is also required.

Papillary Muscle Rupture (Acute Mitral Regurgitation)

Complete rupture of the belly of the papillary muscle causes acutely severe mitral regurgitation that results in severe heart failure, cardiogenic shock, and is rapidly fatal. However, rupture of the tip of one of the heads of the papillary muscle also leads to acute mitral regurgitation that initiates heart failure and/or cardiogenic shock; the patient may survive only for several days to several weeks. Acute mitral regurgitation is clinically detected by the development of a new apical systolic murmur. Intensity of the systolic murmur is influenced by the state of the left ventricle. If there is marked left ventricular failure, the murmur is soft. The pulmonary artery wedge pressure tracing records a prominent v wave. Treatment consists of stabilization of the circulatory status by a medical regimen, intraaortic balloon counterpulsation, followed by surgical replacement of the mitral valve and bypasses to the coronary arteries.

Cardiac Rupture

Rupture of the free wall of the left ventricle occurs in approximately 3 percent of patients with an acute infarction and accounts for 10 to 15 percent of all deaths in acute myocardial infarction. Rupture is common in elderly hypertensive patients and is more frequent in women. In some patients, this event is preceded by strenuous coughing or straining during bowel movements. The majority of patients die suddenly and others, with perhaps a slow oozing of blood, may survive for a few hours or days. Most patients complain of continuing or recurrent chest pain that is due to myocardial ischemia or pericarditis. A pericardial friction rub may be detected. The peripheral pulses may be barely palpable, and neck veins may be grossly distended due to cardiac tamponade. Electromechanical dissociation is common, as shown by the absence of palpable blood pressure, while the ECG demonstrates a regular rhythm. Hemopericardium causes intense vagotonia resulting in sinus bradycardia and AV junctional rhythm. As mentioned earlier, most patients die before medical assistance can be delivered. However, if the condition is suspected, immediate pericardiocentesis and the institution of a saline and isoproterenol infusion, followed by emergency repair of the rupture, could be life saving. A few successful outcomes have been reported.

Cardiogenic Shock

In myocardial infarction, cardiogenic shock represents the extreme stage of pump failure and is defined as a reduction of the systolic blood pressure below 90 mm Hg with clinical evidence of decreased perfusion to various organ systems. In a hypertensive patient, fall of systolic blood pressure ($\geqslant$80 mm Hg) from the usual systolic pressure is considered significant. The clinical diagnosis of cardiogenic shock is based on hypotension, weak and thready peripheral pulsations, cool and clammy skin, disturbed mentation (agitation, restlessness, confusion, somnolence), and urine flow ($<$20 ml/h) with Na^+ concentration ($<$20 mEq/L). Symptoms include weakness, dizziness, and prostration. On physical examination, the patient is lethargic and signs of heart failure may be present. Persistent shock results in metabolic acidosis due to anaerobic metabolism. Cardiogenic shock occurs in approximately 10-15 percent of all patients and carries a mortality of 80 percent; it is more common in association with an anterior myocardial infarction.

Shock occurs when more than 40 percent of the total myocardial mass is damaged by infarction (old and new). Hemodynamic abnormalities consist of a low cardiac index ($<$2 L/min), high systemic vascular resistance ($>$20 units), low arterial pressure, elevated left ventricular filling pressure, arterial hypoxemia, and moderate pulmonary hypertension. Right atrial or central venous pressure may be normal or elevated. An inferior wall infarction, when accompanied by right ventricular infarction, can give rise to a distinctive hemodynamic picture characterized by a high right ventricular filling (central venous) pressure and a low or normal left ventricular filling pressure.

Since all the essential information cannot be obtained by clinical examination, monitoring of cardiac rhythm, urine output by a bladder catheter, urine Na^+ concentration, blood gases, arterial pressure by an intraarterial line, left heart filling pressure, and cardiac output by a Swan-Ganz catheter are essential for a rational approach to management of cardiogenic shock.

The objective of treatment is to improve the cardiac output and perfusion of various organ systems including the heart; this is accomplished by manipulating the preload, afterload, contractility, and heart rate. To maintain optimum perfusion to various organs, a mean arterial pressure of >80 mm Hg should be maintained. Due to inadequate fluid intake, diaphoresis, and vomiting, hypovolemia is usually present. Its presence is suggested by a low left heart filling (pulmonary artery wedge) pressure and low cardiac output. To maintain a left heart filling pressure in the vicinity of 18-20 mm Hg, dextran, albumin, or saline should be administered intravenously. If volume infusion does not improve the circulatory status, inotropic agents are indicated. Previously popular drugs (epinephrine, norepinephrine, and isoproterenol) have, for the most part, been abandoned since they cause marked tachycardia, which in turn increases the myocardial oxygen demand and tends to extend the size of the myocardial infarction. These agents have a very pronounced effect on the peripheral vascular system and are markedly arrhythmogenic. Currently, dopamine and dobutamine are the most commonly used inotropic agents since they produce little tachycardia, have a less prominent effect on the peripheral vascular system, have a more pronounced inotropic effect, and produce less ventricular irritability. Use of afterload-reducing agents should be combined with inotropic agents when low cardiac output coexists with a high left ventricular filling pressure. Bradyarrhythmias and tachyarrhythmias, if present, should be corrected to optimize the heart rate at 60-100 beats/minute. Parasympathetic overactivity manifested by bradycardia and hypotension occasionally dominates the clinical picture, especially during the first 12 hours after an inferior myocardial infarction. It responds readily to intravenous atropine (0.6-0.8 mg).

Intraaortic balloon counterpulsation may be attempted in patients who fail to respond to conventional management. This technique has a beneficial effect on the circulation; it decreases the preload and afterload, augments cardiac output, and improves the coronary blood flow. It is an excellent temporizing method to enable performance of angiographic studies, followed by surgical intervention. If the patient does not have a surgically correctable complication and cardiogenic shock is due simply to a massive loss of myocardium, the likelihood of recovery—even with counterpulsation—is extremely low. Presently, the use of a polarizing solution (glucose plus insulin plus potassium) and corticosteroids is controversial.

Electromechanical Dissociation

This term is defined as severe impairment of the force of ventricular contraction in the presence of regular electrical activity. Electromechanical dissociation is encountered in massive hemopericardium secondary to rupture of the left ventricular free wall, acute mitral regurgitation due to transection of the belly of the papillary muscle, massive pulmonary embolism, following prolonged cardiopulmonary bypass, and in advanced triple-vessel CHD. This complication is usually fatal.

Pericarditis

Pericarditis is a frequent complication of myocardial infarction. It occurs on the second to fourth day of acute infarction and becomes manifest by a pleuritic type of chest pain that is aggravated by deep inspiration and relieved by sitting up. Sinus tachycardia and other atrial tachyarrhythmias, pericardial friction rub, low-grade fever, dyspnea, and diffuse ST-segment elevation complete the clinical picture. The pericardial friction rub is evanescent. Salicylates, indomethacin, or a short course of corticosteroids resolve various manifestations of pericarditis within a few days.

Thromboembolic Complications

A mural thrombus may form at the site of endocardial injury due to infarction. Systemic emboli from this thrombus may occur a few days to a few weeks after a myocardial infarction. Heparin therapy, followed by coumadin therapy, is sufficient. Thrombi also develop quite rapidly in the deep leg and pelvic veins and may embolize to the lungs.

Post-Coronary Care Unit Hospital Period

In acute infarction, almost one-third of inhospital deaths occur after transfer from the CCU to a general medical ward during the second or third week. Consequently, some hospitals have developed a step-down or intermediate coronary care unit where cardiac rhythm is monitored by telemetry or frequent ECG rhythm strips. A patient with an uncomplicated infarction should be started on progressively increasing ambulation, beginning with walking under supervision on the sixth day. The goal during this period is to achieve an activity level sufficient for self-care by the time of hospital discharge. In complicated patients, an ambulatory program is initiated after controlling the complication, and the degree of physical activity is allowed to progress at a slower pace. Patients with an uncomplicated infarction are discharged from the hospital after 2-3 weeks of total hospital stay. The value of psychologic support cannot be overemphasized. Patients generally progress through stages of denial, fear of death, and depression. Prior to discharge, a low-level exercise stress test (to a maximum heart rate of 120 beats/minute) should be performed. Besides identifying patients at high risk, it serves to boost the patient's morale and self-confidence. During this phase, the patient and the family should be educated regarding the nature of the disease and given advice about avoiding various risk factors, medications, resumption of various activities, and future plans. Several recent studies have shown that routine administration of beta blocking agents in post-myocardial infarction patients starting 5-21 days after the onset of infarction significantly reduces the incidence of recurrent infarction and sudden death.

The following complications can develop during this or the subsequent phases of myocardial infarction.

Angina

As the activity level increases, the patient may start experiencing angina. Recurrent angina should be treated medically and, if it is severe and difficult to control, direct myocardial revascularization deserves consideration.

Dressler's Syndrome (Postmyocardial Infarction Syndrome)

This syndrome most commonly occurs 2 weeks to several months after an acute myocardial infarction. It occurs in approximately 3 percent of all patients and is characterized by fever, pericardial type of chest pain, pericardial friction rub, serosanguineous pericardial and/or pleural fluid, and leukocytosis. This postmyocardial infarction syndrome has been attributed to an immunologic reaction to necrotic myocardium. The attacks may be recurrent; however, the development of constriction is unlikely. An acute attack is treated with aspirin, indomethacin, or steroids.

Left Ventricular Aneurysm and False Aneurysm

A left ventricular aneurysm following trasmural infarction usually involves the anterolateral or apical segments and, when large, can give rise to congestive heart failure, systemic emboli from a mural thrombus, and/or ventricular arrhythmias. Large aneurysms produce abnormal pulsations in, or somewhat medial to, the apical area. On a posteroanterior chest x-ray, an aneurysm may cause a bulge on the left heart border. Occasionally a calcium deposit is observed in the mural thrombus or in the wall of the aneurysm. An ECG may reveal persistent elevation of the ST segment in leads showing Q waves. Left ventricular aneurysms have an unfavorable influence on a long-term prognosis. A neurysmectomy is indicated under the following circumstances: intractable heart failure despite medical therapy, recurrent systemic emboli despite anticoagulants, and drug-resistant ventricular tachycardia. It should be emphasized that an aneurysmectomy can be undertaken only when the remaining portion of the left ventricle has a normal wall motion.

Shoulder-Hand Syndrome

Presently, this syndrome occurs less frequently becuase of early ambulation in managing patients with infarction. The clinical features of this late complication consist of pain and stiffness, usually of the left shoulder and left hand. The hand may also show significant swelling. In difficult patients, treatment consists of physiotherapy and the use of steroids.

Posthospitalization Period

The objective is to prepare the patient physically and mentally to be able to return to work at the end of 8-12 weeks. The patient is permitted to perform minor chores. Isometric exercise should be avoided. The patient should be instructed to maintain the level of activity achieved, such as walking, during the latter period of hospitalization and slowly increase the pace and duration of exercise. The occurrence of angina, shortness of breath, and excessive fatigue are general indications that the exercise level should be reduced. A greater number of hospitals are providing supervised training programs that are beneficial for rehabilitation. The patient should be seen about 1 month after discharge and again 1-2 months later before returning to work in order to assess the progress made during these periods. In order to better advise the patient regarding return to work, a symptom-limited exercise stress test should be an integral part of the second visit to establish safe limits of activity. This test is also utilized to prescribe the level of exercise for conditioning programs. In order to achieve cardiovascular training, 30 minutes of dynamic exercise (preferably involving both arms and legs, including warm-up and cool-down periods) three times weekly on alternate days performed at a level to achieve 70 percent of a safely attained maximal heart rate during a symptom-limited stress test, should be prescribed. Long-term training programs enable the patient to perform extended work with a lesser increment of heart rate and blood pressure. These programs are extremely beneficial for the psychologic well-being of the patient.

It should be kept in mind that uncontrolled hypertension, heart failure, arrhythmias, and disabling angina are contraindications of exercise training. These complications should be controlled before embarking on a high-intensity training program.

SUDDEN DEATH

Sudden death is defined as unexpected death occurring instantaneously or within 1 hour after the onset of symptoms; it is more common in males. Athersclerotic CHD is the most frequent cause of sudden death. Approximately 50-60 percent of all deaths due to CHD are sudden in nature. The risk factors for sudden death are heavy cigarette smoking, hypertension, electrocardiographic evidence of left ventricular hypertrophy, complex ventricular arrhythmias, cardiomegaly, and excessive obesity. Approximately one-fourth of sudden death patients experience angina, undue fatigue, or dyspnea on the day of death. Other cardiovascular causes of sudden death include aortic stenosis, cardiomyopathy, Wolff-Parkinson-White syndrome, prolonged Q-T syndrome, acute massive pulmonary embolism, primary pulmonary hypertension, idiopathic hypertrophic subaortic stenosis, myocarditis, and cardiac tamponade secondary to rupture of an infarcted left ventricular wall. In the majority of patients, the immediate mechanism of death consists of ventricular fibrillation. In the remainder, asystole, complete heart block, or ventricular tachycardia is responsible for sudden death. Approximately one-third of the survivors reveal an acute myocardial infarction. Pathologic examination of the coronary arteries shows severe multivessel disease in the majority of patients and fresh thrombosis over old plaques in about one-third of the patients. Recent experience has demonstrated that, if cardiopulmonary resuscitative measures can be instituted within 3-4 minutes of the onset of ventricular fibrillation, some patients can be saved. In many cities, paramedical personnel trained in cardiopulmonary resuscitation and mobile coronary care units have become available. Large segments of the general population are being encouraged to become acquainted with cardiopulmonary resuscitative measures. Subsequent to resuscitation, patients should be admitted to a CCU for further observation since the recurrence of ventricular arrhythmia is very high. Coronary angiography is also recommended, especially in younger patients; in patients with critical lesions, coronary artery bypass surgery should be considered. More importantly, certain preventive measures such as discontinuation of smoking, control of complex ventricular arrhythmias, and the use of beta-adrenergic blocking agents especially in postinfarction patients, should be undertaken. Recent studies have demonstrated that routine use of sulfinpyrazone (Anturane) following myocardial infarction decreases the prevalence of sudden death. Some studies have suggested that coronary artery bypass surgery should be performed in patients with severe multivessel disease; however, there does not appear to be any definitive evidence that it prevents sudden death.

One should also keep in mind the noncardiac causes of sudden death such as cerebral hemorrhage, chronic obstructive lung disease, drug poisoning, and so forth.

ISCHEMIC CARDIOMYOPATHY

Some patients with atherosclerotic CHD develop multiple patchy infarcts over the left ventricle along with diffuse left ventricular fibrosis, and ultimately present with a clinical picture of congestive cardiomyopathy. Angina or myocardial infarction may not be prominent in their clinical course. Coronary arteriography is required to differentiate this condition from the usual types of congestive cardiomyopathy. The prognosis is poor, and treatment consists of supportive measures to control heart failure.

VALVULAR HEART DISEASE

Recent improvements in diagnostic techniques and cardiovascular surgical procedures have emphasized the importance of recognizing and properly managing patients who have valvular heart disease. Although the incidence of acute rheumatic fever is declining in the United States, rheumatic heart disease continues to be a common form of valvular heart disease. In addition, valvular malfunction due to degenerative, ischemic, or congenital lesions, and acute valvular incompetence due to infective endocarditis are being recognized more frequently and treated more vigorously. An understanding of the functional anatomy of valvular heart disease will allow the clinician to predict clinical findings and the natural history in these patients. A thorough evaluation is essential in order to properly make a decision concerning the need and timing of valve replacement.

ACUTE RHEUMATIC FEVER

Rheumatic fever is an inflammatory disease that may involve the joints, muscles, brain, and heart. Rheumatic fever is initiated by an infection with group A beta-hemolytic streptococci, appearing 1-4 weeks after an episode of tonsillitis, nasopharyngitis, or otitis media. The streptococcal antigen-antibody response causes a perivascular granulomatous reaction and vasculitis (Aschoff's bodies) in the endocardium, myocardium, pericardium, and in other organs, including the joints, peritoneum, lungs, and pleura.

Clinical Manifestations

Rheumatic fever primarily affects children between the ages of 5 and 15 years, but may also occur in adults. Epidemics of streptococcal infection and subsequent rheumatic fever are seen in conditions of poverty, malnutrition, and overcrowding. Children usually have a more fulminant form of illness than adults, making the diagnosis more obvious. Rheumatic fever may present as a mild illness, particularly in young adults, and the diagnosis is often difficult to make.

The disease usually presents as fever and arthritis in a patient who has recently recovered from a beta-hemolytic streptococcal infection. The fever may be low grade and intermittent or may be severe, protracted, and associated with general malaise, anorexia, and weight loss. The arthritis of rheumatic fever is characteristically a migrating polyarthritis that involves the large joints in a sequential fashion.

The symptoms of carditis may be quite minor and easily overlooked. Congestive heart failure can occur in severe cases. Pericardial and pleural inflammation may produce characteristic pain syndromes. Sydenham's chorea appears with brain involvement. Chorea is manifest as purposeless jerking movements of the limbs, trunk, and face that are worsened by anxiety and disappear during sleep.

Physical findings include the general appearance of chronic debility and acute discomfort. Arthritis is manifest as hot, red, swollen, tender joints with palpable effusion. Severe myocardial involvement may be reflected by signs of gross heart failure, including cardiac enlargement and pulmonary congestion. Tachycardia may be the only feature if rheumatic carditis is mild. A pansystolic murmur of mitral regurgitation may appear during the course of rheumatic fever. Occasionally a short diastolic rumble (Carey-Coombs' murmur) can be heard, but usually disappears as recovery occurs. Mild aortic regurgitation appears in about one-third of patients and may persist after recovery.

Small, firm, painless, subcutaneous nodules are frequently

found in children with rheumatic fever. Erythema marginatum rheumaticum may also appear. These skin lesions are characterized by enlarging, raised macules shaped as crescents or rings with clear centers.

Laboratory Findings

General features of an inflammatory illness, such as leukocytosis and elevation of the erythrocyte sedimentation rate, are present. Slight anemia and proteinuria are common. A high or increasing antistreptolysin O (ASO) titer indicates recent streptococcal infection, but does not mean that rheumatic fever is present. Throat cultures are positive for beta-hemolytic streptococci in about one-half of patients.

The electrocardiogram usually shows P-R prolongation and, occasionally, second-degree antrioventricular block. Nonspecific T-wave changes may also be present. The chest x-ray may show cardiac enlargement in the presence of severe myocarditis or pericardial effusion. Echocardiography is helpful in detecting pericardial fluid and in measuring chamber size.

Differential Diagnosis

Rheumatic fever is easily confused with a wide variety of inflammatory and infectious diseases that share the features of fever, skin lesions, and polyserositis. In addition, a definite diagnosis of rheumatic fever can be exceedingly difficult because the clinical manifestations vary widely and the antecedent streptococcal infection may have been asymptomatic. A helpful schema for making a diagnosis of rheumatic fever is the Jones criteria, devised by T. Duckett Jones in 1944, and since updated by the American Heart Association. The criteria are divided into major and minor categories; the presence of two major criteria or one major plus two minor criteria strongly suggests a diagnosis of rheumatic fever (Table 3).

Table 3. Modified Jones Criteria for the Diagnosis of Acute Rheumatic Fever

Major Criteria	*Minor Criteria*
Carditis	Fever
Polyarthritis	Arthralgia
Chorea	Elevated erythrocyte sedimentation rate or leukocytosis
Subcutaneous nodules	Elevated ASO titer
Erythema marginatum	Prolonged P-R interval
	History of rheumatic fever or rheumatic heart disease

Treatment

Patients with rheumatic fever should be placed on bed rest as long as signs of active inflammation persist. Salicylates markedly reduce fever, pain, and swelling and should be employed liberally. Severe or persistent inflammation responds dramatically to corticosteroid administration.

Penicillin should be administered to eradicate streptococcal infection. Recurrent episodes of rheumatic fever should be prevented with prophylactic antibiotic therapy, either parenteral benzathine penicillin G, 1.2 million units intramuscularly once per month; oral penicillin V, 250 mg/day; or sulfadiazine, 1 g orally per day. Prophylaxis should be continued for at least 5 years in adults or until age 30 when initiated during childhood.

Prognosis

Initial episodes of rheumatic fever usually persist a few weeks or even months. Persistent inflammation indicates a poor prognosis. Severe myocarditis occasionally results in death, but the overall prognosis is good. Approximately one-third of children with rheumatic fever have evidence of valvular damage immediately after the attack. An additional one-third will eventually develop evidence of rheumatic valvular disease. Residual cardiac damage is less frequent in adults.

MITRAL STENOSIS

Although mitral stenosis can be congenitally acquired and obstruction to left ventricular inflow is occasionally caused by degenerative calcification of the valve, acute rheumatic fever continues to be by far the most common cause of mitral stenosis. Clinically manifest mitral stenosis generally occurs 10-20 years after an episode of acute rheumatic fever. A history of rheumatic fever may be difficult to elicit.

The pathologic changes of rheumatic mitral stenosis are chordal fusion, valve leaflet thickening and calcification, and commissural fusion. The consequence of these changes is obstruction to the flow of blood from the left atrium to the left ventricle. In general, significant obstruction and the resultant symptoms do not occur until the normal valve area is reduced by one-half. At this point, resistance to flow across the valve produces a pressure gradient with elevation of left atrial pressure and subsequent pulmonary venous hypertension. The left atrium hypertrophies and dilates and eventually loses the ability to maintain sinus rhythm. Loss of atrial systole leads to a decrease in cardiac output, and atrial fibrillation with rapid ventricular response decreases atrial emptying time and increases left atrial pressure. Sluggish blood flow in the distended, fibrillating atrium predisposes to thrombus formation and subsequent systemic embolization.

As a result of left atrial hypertension, pulmonary venous pressure is also elevated. Pulmonary congestion and pulmonary edema produce symptoms of dyspnea. Pulmonary arterial hypertension may ultimately result from pulmonary venous hypertension, initially by passive transmission of pressure, and worsened by reflex arteriolar vasoconstriction. Severe pulmonary hypertension in turn may cause right ventricular hypertrophy and failure, functional tricuspid regurgitation, systemic venous hypertension, and the attendant symptoms of right heart failure. Paradoxically, severe pulmonary hypertension may prevent pulmonary congestion and mask the symptoms of pulmonary venous hypertension.

Clinical Manifestation

Mitral stenosis is usually a slowly progressive disease. Symptoms appear gradually, and patients often unconsciously modify their life-style, masking the true limitations imposed by significant mitral stenosis. The first symptom is usually dyspnea, which is commonly precipitated by the onset of atrial fibrillation. If pulmonary hypertension and right ventricular failure predominate, left atrial pressure and cardiac output may fall, resulting in the relief of dyspnea but substituting symptoms of easy fatigability.

Pulmonary venous congestion commonly causes dry cough and paroxysmal nocturnal dyspnea. Frank hemoptysis occurs when pulmonary hypertension is severe. Angina pectoris without coronary obstruction occurs in a few patients with mitral stenosis and appears to be related to severe pulmonary hypertension and right ventricular strain.

Systemic emboli occur in up to 25 percent of patients with mitral stenosis. Emboli commonly lodge in the brain but may also occlude vessels to the viscera, heart, or limbs. The occurrence of systemic emboli is not directly related to the severity of stenosis and may occasionally be the first presenting symptom. The diagnosis of mitral stenosis should be considered in any patient presenting with systemic emboli.

The classic physical findings of mitral stenosis are an opening snap and a diastolic rumble. The first heart sound is usually quite loud and may provide the first clue to diagnosis; however, the first heart sound may be muffled if the valve is heavily calcified. The interval between aortic valve closure and the opening snap is usually shorter in more severe stenosis. In mild mitral stenosis, the diastolic rumble is confined to mid-diastole and may exhibit presystolic accentuation when sinus rhythm is present. Prolongation of the diastolic rumble encompassing all of the diastole is a feature of severe stenosis.

Pulmonary hypertension may produce accentuation of the pulmonary component of the second heart sound as well as a right ventricular lift. The left ventricle is not notably enlarged and no left ventricular impulse should be palpable in pure mitral stenosis.

Laboratory Diagnosis

The electrocardiogram is an insensitive index of the presence and severity of mitral stenosis, although it may show several abnormalities. If sinus rhythm is present, the P wave may exhibit a broad-notched left axis deviation in lead II and enlargement of a terminal negative component in lead V1, indicating left atrial enlargement. In atrial fibrillation, the fibrillatory pattern appears to be more coarse in rheumatic mitral stenosis than in other diseases. A prominent R wave in lead V1 or an rsr′ pattern may be present, indicating right ventricular hypertrophy.

The chest x-ray is helpful in estimating chamber size and in detecting pulmonary venous congestion. Left atrial enlargement is recognized by straightening of the left heart border together with the presence of a double density over the heart and posterior displacement of the esophagus. The left main stem bronchus may be elevated. Right ventricular enlargement may be appreciated by a filling in of the retrosternal space on the lateral chest x-ray. The left ventricular shadow should not be enlarged in pure mitral stenosis. Pulmonary venous hypertension produces a reversal in the distribution of blood, with increased prominence of the upper lobe veins. Interstitial edema may be recognized as Kerley's B lines and diffuse haziness of the lung fields. The pulmonary trunk appears prominent when pulmonary arterial hypertension is present. Valvular calcification can be observed during fluoroscopy.

Echocardiography is helpful in establishing both the presence and severity of mitral stenosis. The classic M-mode echocardiographic features of mitral stenosis include: thickening of the valve leaflets, decreased leaflet excursion, decreased E-F slope, and anterior diastolic motion of the posterior valve leaflet. Left atrial size can be accurately determined, and pulmonary hypertension may be diagnosed by alteration in the motion of the pulmonary valve. Although M-mode echocardiography provides a sensitive and specific means of diagnosing mitral stenosis, quantification of the severity of stenosis is better accomplished with two-dimensional echocardiography. With this technique, the mitral valve orifice is directly visualized on the short axis and the actual limiting valve area planimetered from stop-action photographs of the valve. These measurements of valve area correlate well with similar measurements made at the time of surgery and with valve area calculated from cardiac catheterization data.

The cardinal feature of mitral stenosis at cardiac catheterization is the presence of a diastolic pressure gradient between the left atrium and left ventricle. The pressure gradient varies directly with cardiac output and the amount of blood flow through the mitral valve orifice. Actual valve area can be calculated by measuring the diastolic gradient and the diastolic blood flow using Gorlin's formula. Left ventricular cineangiography is also performed to establish the presence and severity of any associated mitral regurgitation.

Management

The medical management of mitral stenosis consists of administering digitalis to control the ventricular response to atrial fibrillation and the use of diuretics to control symptoms of pulmonary congestion and right ventricular failure. If no significant contraindications exist, warfarin (Coumadin) should be administered to patients with atrial fibrillation and enlarged atria to prevent thrombus formation. Antibiotic prophylaxis should be administered before dental and surgical procedures to prevent subacute bacterial endocarditis. Continuous antibiotics should be administered to prevent recurrent episodes of rheumatic fever in patients under 30 years of age or in patients exposed to children.

Surgical management consists of either mitral valvotomy or valve replacement. Valvotomy can be performed when the valve retains reasonably pliability and is not heavily calcified. If technically feasible, valvotomy is the surgical procedure of choice since it affords good relief of mitral obstruction and is not associated with the long-term complications inherent in a prosthetic valve. Mitral valve replacement is necessary when the valve is heavily calcified and fibrotic or if significant mitral regurgitation is also present. Since mitral valvotomy is effective and is associated with low morbidity and mortality (approximately 1%), it is indicated for patients who have symptoms with ordinary levels of exertion. Mitral valve replacement is generally reserved for patients who are either symptomatic at rest or symptomatic with minimal exertion. The objective determination of mitral valve area is also useful in determining the need for surgery. Patients with valve areas of 1 sq cm or less are considered operative candidates.

MITRAL REGURGITATION

Although some degree of mitral regurgitation commonly accompanies rheumatic mitral stenosis, rheumatic heart disease is probably no longer the most common cause of mitral regurgitation. Mitral regurgitation may be seen due to papillary muscle dysfunction caused by ischemic heart disease, degeneration of components of the mitral valve apparatus, and as a consequence of the mitral valve prolapse syndrome. Important forms of acute mitral regurgitation include bacterial endocarditis and rupture of chordae tendineae or the papillary muscle.

The common result of these various forms of mitral valve disease is systolic regurgitation of blood from the left ventricle into the left atrium. When significant chronic mitral regurgitation is present, both the left atrium and left ventricle dilate to accommodate the regurgitant volume. The left ventricular stroke volume may be dramatically augmented in order to maintain adequate forward cardiac output. Pulmonary venous and pulmonary arterial pressures are variably elevated. The left atrium may be massively dilated and serve as a damper, muting the transmission of pressure back to the pulmonary bed. In acute mitral regurgitation, the left atrium may be small and noncompliant, directly transmitting the ventricular pressure back to the pulmonary veins, giving rise to pulmonary venous and pulmonary arterial hypertension.

Clinical Manifestations

Dyspnea and fatigue are the major symptoms of mitral regurgitation. If cardiac output is maintained at relatively normal levels and if left atrial dilatation is not marked, pulmonary congestion is the primary manifestation. More commonly, the left atrium dilates severely, the cardiac output falls, and fatigue rather than dyspnea predominates. Right ventricular failure occurs relatively late in the course of mitral regurgitation and is usually progressive and intractable. Acute mitral regurgitation may present as pulmonary edema and cardiovascular collapse.

An apical systolic murmur is the outstanding feature of mitral regurgitation. The murmur usually starts immediately after the first heart sound and occupies all of systole, extending beyond the second heart sound. The murmur is plateaulike in quality and usually radiates from the apex into the axilla. Unlike the murmur of tricuspid regurgitation, the murmur of mitral regurgitation becomes softer with inspiration. A systolic thrill may be palpated in the presence of a very loud murmur. A third heart sound followed by a middiastolic flow rumble is usually present when mitral regurgitation is of hemodynamic significance. The apical impulse is displaced toward the midclavicular line and a hyperdynamic left ventricular impulse can usually be appreciated. Atrial fibrillation is often present also. In acute mitral regurgitation, sinus rhythm is maintained, heart size may be normal, and the murmur may not be pansystolic.

Laboratory Diagnosis

In chronic mitral regurgitation, the chest x-ray shows left ventricular and left atrial enlargement. The left atrium in mitral regurgitation is usually larger than the left atrium in pure mitral stenosis and can reach gigantic proportions. When left ventricular failure ensues, pulmonary markings are increased and pulmonary edema may be seen. A calcified mitral annulus may be seen during fluoroscopic examination.

The electrocardiogram may show evidence of left ventricular hypertrophy. Left atrial enlargement is suggested by presence of the left axis of the P wave and enlargement of the terminal negative component in lead V1.

Echocardiography can be used to evaluate the diameter of the left atrium and left ventricle in patients with mitral regurgitation. Serial examinations are helpful in assessing progression of the disease. Direct visualization of the mitral valve may reveal evidence of rheumatic heart disease and associated mitral stenosis. Left ventricular wall motion can be evaluated by two-dimensional echocardiography; in particular, the motion of the papillary muscles can be assessed. Mitral valve prolapse, flailing or fenestration of the valve leaflets, and bacterial vegetations can be recognized. The echocardiogram is also useful in detecting mitral annular and valvular calcification. Radioisotopic left ventriculography is helpful in monitoring left ventricular function in patients with chronic mitral regurgitation. Gated radionuclide ventriculograms can be performed during supine bicycle exercise and hold promise of identifying early left ventricular dysfunction.

At cardiac catheterization, left atrial pressure is elevated. Evidence may also be seen of pulmonary venous and pulmonary arterial hypertension as well as right ventricular failure. The pressure tracing taken in the left atrium or in the pulmonary artery wedge position shows a tall, peaked v wave that is caused by regurgitation of blood from the left ventricle to the left atrium. If the left atrium is small and noncompliant, the height of the v wave may be quite large. In the presence of left atrial dilatation, the v wave may be damped. Left ventricular cineangiography is helpful in defining left ventricular wall motion and function. The degree of mitral regurgitation can be assessed by observing the amount of contrast material that passes from the left ventricle to the left atrium during systole.

Treatment

Significant degrees of mitral regurgitation may be well tolerated for many years. The left ventricle compensates for the backward leak by dilating, becoming hypertrophied, and increasing its stroke volume. However, some patients progress to left ventricular failure, which may become irreversible despite valve replacement. Therefore, the object of following patients with mitral regurgitation is to intervene with mitral valve replacement at a point in time when serious symptoms have occurred and left ventricular failure is in its early stages before irreversible damage occurs. In general, progressive enlargement of the heart on either chest x-ray or echocardiography, or a decline in the exercise ejection fraction as determined by radionuclide ventriculography, is a sign that the patient may be approaching the stage of irreversible left ventricular failure. Valve replacement is generally recommended for these patients. Prolonged medical therapy with digitalis and diuretics should not be undertaken in patients with significant left ventricular failure due to mitral regurgitation.

Acute mitral regurgitation presents a different management problem since these patients are often critically ill. Bedside Swan-Ganz catheterization may be undertaken to detect the regurgitant v wave and to differentiate acute mitral regurgitation from acute ventricular septal rupture. If the left ventricular reserve is exhausted, these patients deteriorate quite rapidly and require emergency valve replacement. Patients may be supported with the use of digitalis, diuretics, afterload reduction, and even intraaortic balloon counterpulsation to prepare them for valve replacement.

AORTIC STENOSIS

The etiology of aortic stenosis has been the subject of controversy for many years. Rheumatic heart disease was previously considered to be a frequent cause of aortic stenosis, but it now appears that isolated aortic stenosis is rarely the result of rheumatic fever. It is quite likely that patients in the 40-50 year age group who present with isolated aortic stenosis probably have congenital bicuspid valves that, over a period of years, have undergone fibrosis and calcification. Even older patients presenting with isolated aortic stenosis may have had a previously normal valve that has calcified with age. Aortic stenosis accompanying mitral and tricuspid valvular lesions is usually of rheumatic origin.

Clinical Findings

Obstruction to outflow of blood from the left ventricle is responsible for the clinical manifestations of aortic stenosis. The aortic orifice must be reduced to approximately one-quarter of its normal size in order to produce significant hemodynamic change. Obstruction to outflow results in left ventricular pressure overload and consequent left ventricular hypertrophy. Myocardial hypertrophy reduces left ventricular compliance, increasing left ventricular pressure for any given increment of diastolic filling. Myocardial contractility is also impaired.

The cardinal symptoms of aortic stenosis are dyspnea, angina pectoris, and syncope. Dyspnea and congestive heart failure due to the left ventricular hypertrophy of aortic stenosis carries an ominous prognosis. Few patients with aortic stenosis live five years after the onset of heart failure. Left ventricular hypertrophy also causes an increase in myocardial oxygen demand and decreased subendocardial myocardial perfusion. Typical angina pectoris is present in about 15 percent of patients with aortic stenosis even in the absence of coronary arterial obstruction.

Syncope in aortic stenosis usually follows physical effort and is probably related to an inappropriate decrease in total peripheral resistance. Patients with aortic stenosis are also at increased risk of sudden death. The pathogenesis of sudden death is unknown, but may be related to ventricular dysrhythmia.

A careful physical examination usually permits reasonable assessment of the severity of aortic stenosis. However, physical findings may be misleading, particularly in older patients. A sustained left ventricular lift can usually be palpated in younger patients, but this finding is often absent in patients who have rigid barrel-shaped chests. The carotid pulse is of small amplitude, rises slowly, and falls away slowly (pulsus parvus et tardus). A palpable thrill may be felt. The carotid pulse tracings often show a prominent anacrotic notch or shoulder on the ascending limb. In older patients, atherosclerosis of the peripheral arteries may obscure this change in the carotid upstroke.

Auscultation reveals a rough, high-pitched, ejection-type murmur over the aortic area. The murmur usually radiates toward the neck, peaks in midsystole, and is completed just prior to the second heart sound. A systolic thrill may also be palpated at the base of the heart. In older patients, the murmur of aortic stenosis may be less intense and may not radiate clearly to the neck. An early systolic ejection click may precede the systolic ejection murmur. The aortic component of the second heart sound is characteristically faint or absent when aortic valve motion is severely restricted. A palpable and audible fourth heart sound reflects the decrease in left ventricular compliance due to significant aortic stenosis.

Laboratory Evaluation

The chest x-ray and electrocardiogram are not particularly sensitive indices of the severity of aortic stenosis. Left ventricular hypertrophy may not be manifest by enlargement of the cardiac silhouette on the chest x-ray. Poststenotic dilatation of the aorta may be seen. Calcification of the aortic valve may be recognized on cardiac fluoroscopy. Significant aortic stenosis is rarely seen in the adult patient in the absence of calcification, and the extent of calcification correlates roughly with the severity of obstruction. The electrocardiogram typically shows left ventricular hypertrophy but may be entirely normal in younger patients. The ECG is helpful in following patients with aortic stenosis. Development of signs of left ventricular hypertrophy and strain on serial ECGs should alert the clinician to the possible need for further investigation.

Echocardiography is useful for measuring left ventricular wall thickness and chamber dimensions in patients with aortic stenosis and is more accurate than either the chest x-ray or the electrocardiogram. In younger patients who do not have a history of hypertension or ischemic heart disease, the wall thickness can be used to predict the severity of stenosis. Thickening and calcification of the aortic valve can be observed with M-mode echocardiography, but it is difficult to predict the severity of stenosis from these findings. Two-dimensional echocardiography can be used to directly visualize the opening of stenotic valve leaflets. Hemodynamically significant stenosis can generally be excluded if the diameter of the valve opening is more than 15 mm. Lesser degrees of opening suggest significant aortic stenosis, and further evaluation may be warranted.

The definitive diagnostic procedure for assessing the severity of aortic stenosis is measurement of the systolic pressure gradient between the left ventricle and the aorta together with the systolic blood flow across the valve. In general, gradients of over 50 mm Hg indicate severe stenosis if the cardiac output and aortic blood flow are maintained in the normal range. At lower cardiac outputs, it is particularly important to calculate the actual aortic valve area using Gorlin's formula. Valve areas of less than 0.7 sq cm indicate severe obstruction. In the presence of significant aortic regurgitation, the valve area cannot be accurately calculated and more reliance must be placed on the gradient across the valve.

Differential Diagnosis and Treatment

The diagnosis of aortic stenosis should be considered in all patients who present with left ventricular failure, particularly if a systolic murmur is heard and there is a history of syncope or dizziness. In older patients and in patients presenting with heart failure, it is particularly important to consider a diagnosis of aortic stenosis, realizing that the physical findings may be obscured and that the murmur may be very soft. Aortic stenosis can usually be differentiated from mitral regurgitation and a ventricular septal defect by physical examination, although very loud murmurs are often confusing. Idiopathic hypertrophic subaortic stenosis may occasionally be confused with valvular aortic stenosis, but the true diagnosis can be made by physical examination and echocardiography.

The appearance of significant symptoms and demonstration of significant obstruction of aortic outflow at catheterization are indications for valve replacement. Drug therapy with digitalis and diuretics is effective in treating left ventricular failure due to aortic stenosis but should be considered only as a temporizing measure while preparing for surgery. The prognosis of patients with aortic stenosis after the development of signs and symptoms of heart failure is poor. Aortic valve replacement is usually effective, even after the onset of heart failure, and can usually be carried out with acceptable morbidity and mortality, even in very old patients.

AORTIC REGURGITATION

The most common cause of chronic aortic regurgitation is rheumatic heart disease. Syphilis, Marfan's syndrome, ankylosing spondylitis, hypertension, ascending aortic aneurysms, and congenital lesions are less commonly associated with chronic aortic regurgitation. Acute aortic regurgitation is largely a result of infective endocarditis or aortic dissection. Acute and chronic aortic regurgitation are quite distinct entities. Chronic aortic regurgitation may be well tolerated for many years before the onset of symptoms. Acute aortic regurgitation usually presents as a medical emergency.

Clinical Features

Hemodynamically significant aortic regurgitation creates an increase in the volume work of the left ventricle. Blood flows back across the aortic valve during diastole and must be ejected during systole. Chronic aortic regurgitation results in marked peripheral vasodilatation. This, in combination with an increased stroke volume of the left ventricle, may allow maintenance of a normal forward cardiac output. The peak systolic arterial pressure tends to be increased, and the aortic diastolic pressure is lower because of a rapid runoff of blood into the peripheral arterial bed and back into the left ventricle. With dynamic exercise, the cardiac output increases and further peripheral vasodilatation occurs in the arteries and capillary bed of the muscles. The proportion of the left ventricular stroke volume that returns to the left ventricle during diastole falls, and the hemodynamic status of the patient may actually improve. By contrast, isometric exercise, sympathetic stimulation, and cardiac failure all tend to raise the systemic vascular resistance, thus increasing the volume of blood returning to the ventricle during diastole. The diastolic blood pressure rises and the forward cardiac output decreases. Chronic aortic regurgitation leads to left ventricular dilatation and hypertrophy. In time, this long-standing hypertrophy almost inevitably leads to myocardial fibrosis that may be irreversible even with valve replacement. Frank sympatoms of congestive heart failure occur late in the course of chronic aortic regurgitation and may occur after irreversible fibrosis has taken place.

Acute aortic regurgitation produces distinct hemodynamic alterations because incompetence develops either instantaneously or over a few days or weeks. The left ventricle is incapable of undergoing dilatation or hypertrophy over such a short period and is unable to maintain a normal forward cardiac output. The hemodynamic load falls largely to the lungs with the rapid appearance of pulmonary edema progressing to peripheral cardiovascular collapse.

The characteristic physical sign of both acute and chronic aortic regurgitation is a high-pitched, blowing diastolic murmur that begins immediately after the second heart sound. The murmur may be most intense over the aortic area, the lower left sternal border, or even the cardiac apex. Faint murmurs may be accentuated by having the patient lean forward in a sitting position while holding the breath in expiration. A functional systolic ejection murmur may also be present due to the increase in left ventricular stroke volume. In chronic aortic regurgitation, a widened pulse pressure is usually present with high systolic and low diastolic pressures. The carotid pulsations are prominent and may even result in up and down bobbing of the head. Capillary pulsations can be seen in the fingertips. Systolic and diastolic murmurs can be heard over the femoral arteries. The left ventricular impulse is hyperdynamic. The apex is displaced downward and to the left. When aortic regurgitation is severe, an apical diastolic (Austin Flint) murmur may be present in middiastole or presystole. This murmur, which resembles the diastolic rumble of mitral stenosis, is thought to be due to fluttering of the mitral cusp that is caught in the two streams of blood flowing into the ventricle from both the left atrium and the aorta.

Signs of rapid runoff of the blood from the aorta during diastole may be absent in acute aortic regurgitation. The signs of acute pulmonary congestion, peripheral vasoconstriction, and low cardiac output predominate.

Laboratory Findings

The cardiac silhouette on x-ray in chronic aortic reguritation shows evidence of left ventricular enlargement. The aortic root is commonly dilated, and calcification of the aortic annulus and aortic arch may be seen. In acute aortic regurgitation, left ventricular enlargement may be absent. Evidence of pulmonary congestion on chest x-ray is common in acute aortic regurgitation and may appear in the late phases of chronic aortic regurgitation.

The electrocardiogram usually shows evidence of left ventricular hypertrophy in chronic aortic regurgitation, but may be normal in acute lesions. Left bundle-branch block is common. Atrial fibrillation is rarely seen in pure aortic regurgitation.

Echocardiography is useful for monitoring the dilatation and hypertrophy caused by chronic aortic regurgitation. Diastolic fluttering of the anterior mitral valve leaflets is usually noted. Vegetations may be seen in patients who have infectious endocarditis. Premature closure of the mitral valve is a bad prognostic sign in patients with acute severe aortic regurgitation.

Cardiac catheterization and cineangiography are useful in demonstrating the degree of aortic regurgitation and in assessing left ventricular hemodynamic responses. Determination of the left ventricular ejection fraction during exercise using gated radionuclide left-ventricular angiography has recently been introduced as a means of detecting earlier forms of left ventricular failure.

Treatment

Aortic valve replacement is the obvious treatment for aortic regurgitation, but the timing of aortic valve replacement remains one of the most problematic areas of cardiology. The left ventricle may be able to withstand severe aortic regurgitation for many years before decompensating. Nonetheless, the onset of symptoms due to chronic aortic regurgitation may be associated with irreversible fibrosis of the left ventricle. Symptoms may not regress following valve replacement. The onset of symptoms of congestive heart failure is an undeniable indication for aortic valve replacement. Ideally, valve replacement should be undertaken shortly before the onset of symptoms in order to avoid the problem of irreversible myocardial fibrosis. Progressive dilatation of the left ventricle on either echocardiography or chest x-ray is an indication for consideration of surgery; more recently, failure of the radionuclide ejection fraction to increase with exercise has been used to select patients for consideration of valve replacement.

Valve replacement is almost always necessary in patients with acute severe aortic regurgitation. These patients generally deteriorate rapidly, and valve replacement must be undertaken as an emergency procedure.

TRICUSPID VALVE DISEASE

Organic lesions of the tricuspid valve are generally uncommon. Tricuspid stenosis usually is seen in the setting of rheumatic mitral stenosis. Tricuspid stenosis should be suspected when severe right-sided venous congestion is found in the absence of marked pulmonary hypertension. On physical examination, the jugular a wave is quite prominent if sinus rhythm is present. The diastolic rumble of tricuspid stenosis can be augmented by inspiration to differentiate it from mitral stenosis.

Tricuspid regurgitation is most commonly a functional lesion caused by severe right-sided heart failure. Rheumatic tricuspid regurgitation may be seen as part of multivalvular disease. Severe tricuspid regurgitation causes large jugular v waves and systolic pulsation of the liver. A pansystolic murmur that is intensified by inspiration can be heard at the lower left sternal border.

Other causes of tricuspid valve disease include infective endocarditis and trauma, and congenital malformations such as Ebstein's anomaly. The murmur of functional tricuspid regurgitation due to pulmonary hypertension is usually pansystolic, whereas the murmur of organic tricuspid regurgitation with normal pulmonary pressure commonly ends earlier in systole or may be absent.

MITRAL VALVE PROLAPSE

The mitral valve prolapse syndrome is an entity that is pehraps best defined by its classic physical findings: a midsystolic click and late systolic murmur. Although midsystolic clicks and late systolic murmurs were long thought to be extracardiac in origin, it has become apparent in recent years that these sounds emanate from the mitral valve apparatus. Such patients are found to have pathologic abnormalities of the mitral valve apparatus that include a scalloped or hooded appearance, redundant valve leaflet tissue, annular dilatation, and microscopic evidence of myxomatous degeneration. The use of echocardiography to detect abnormal valve motion indicative of mitral prolapse has resulted in the increasingly frequent recognition of this entity.

Clinical Manifestations

Mitral valve prolapse is found in all age groups but seems particularly prevalent in young women. It is commonly associated with a general appearance of asthenia and skeletal abnormalities including pectus excavatum, scoliosis, kyphosis, and a high arched palate. Most patients with mitral valve prolapse are asymptomatic and have an excellent prognosis. Fatigue, dyspnea, and atypical chest pain are seen in some patients. Palpitations are quite common.

The classic auscultatory features of mitral valve prolapse include the midsystolic click and the late systolic murmur. The systolic clicks may be multiple, and the late systolic murmur is variable in length. Both the click and the murmur appear earlier in systole after standing or administration of amyl nitrate. In some cases, the murmur is pansystolic, assuming the usual features of mitral regurgitation. Mitral prolapse may also be seen in the absence of any abnormal auscultatory findings.

Laboratory Diagnosis

The classic echocardiographic feature of mitral valve prolapse is a late systolic posterior bowing of the mitral valve leaflets. Holosystolic posterior motion is a less specific feature since it may be highly dependent on the orientation of the ultrasound transducer. Two-dimensional echocardiography is helpful in detecting the abnormal scalloping of the mitral valve and systolic displacement of valve tissue into the left atrium.

Electrocardiographic abnormalities are present in as many as two-thirds of patients with mitral valve prolapse. The most common abnormality is T-wave flattening or inversion in leads II, III, and aV_F. ST-segment depression is common during exercise. Arrhythmias, particular PVCs, are quite common.

Left ventricular cineangiography may show systolic scalloping of the mitral valve leaflets and segmental differences in left ventricular contraction. Hemodynamic measurements are normal unless significant mitral regurgitation is present.

Natural History and Treatment

Mitral prolapse is a recently recognized syndrome that is being diagnosed with increasing frequency. The natural history of this entity is largely unknown, but the disease appears benign in most patients. Three major complications can occur: infective endocarditis, sudden death, and hemodynamically significant mitral regurgitation. Patients who have systolic murmurs should receive antibiotic prophylaxis for endocarditis. Although much feared, sudden death rarely occurs. Ventricular arrhythmias presumably underlie this event. Thus, complex ventricular arrhythmias should be treated. Propranolol is frequently employed to control ventricular ectopy and may ameliorate chest pain as well. Mitral regurgitation of hemodynamic significance may appear gradually or follow chordal rupture as an acute event.

DISEASES OF THE PERICARDIUM

The pericardium is a thin, double-walled sac that surrounds the heart and is attached to the roots of the great vessels. An inner or visceral layer of the pericardium adheres to the heart, while an outer parietal layer lies free, leaving a potential space between the two layers. The pericardium can be affected by a wide variety of diseases that may be either isolated in the pericardium or secondary manifestations of disease occurring elsewhere. Important clinical types of pericardial disease include acute inflammatory pericarditis, pericardial effusion, and chronic constrictive pericarditis.

ACUTE PERICARDITIS

Acute inflammation of the pericardium can be caused by an extremely wide variety of conditions. The most common clinical entities are idiopathic or viral pericarditis, pericarditis associated with acute myocardial infarction, pericarditis due to metastatic carcinoma, and uremic pericarditis. Less commonly seen are pericarditis due to connective tissue disorders, rheumatic fever, bacterial infection, and dissecting aortic aneurysm.

Clinical Features

Most patients with acute pericarditis experience acute onset of sharp central chest pain that is worsened by inspiration. Unlike angina pectoris, the pain of acute pericarditis is persistent, not particularly affected by exertion, and frequently radiates to the shoulder or back. Relief may be obtained by sitting or leaning forward. True dyspnea is absent, but splinting of the chest may occur because of the adverse effect of respiration on pain. A low-grade fever usually accompanies acute pericarditis. Malaise, anorexia, and myalgia are common. When pericarditis accompanies another disorder, features of the underlying illness may dominate the clinical presentation.

The pathognomonic sign of acute pericarditis is a percardial friction rub. Friction between the inflamed layers of the pericardium produces a rough, scratchy sound. The rub characteristically has three major components that occur during the three abrupt phases of cardiac motion—systole, early diastole, and atrial systole. Pericardial friction rubs are notoriously evanescent, and only one or two components may be audible. Most rubs are best heard at the left lower sternal border and apex. The coarse, superficial sound of a rub usually radiates widely, but can be localized to a very small area. Rubs can usually be easily distinguished from murmurs by their characteristic monotonal nonmusical quality and their relationship to the heart sounds. Pleural friction rubs can be distinguished from pericardial rubs by having the patient hold his breath.

Laboratory Findings

The electrocardiogram is extremely helpful in the diagnosis of acute pericarditis. The visceral layer of the pericardium is closely adherent to the epicardium. Consequently, inflammation of the pericardium usually causes some inflammation of the myocardium. Myocarditis is rarely apparent clinically but does cause characteristic electrocardiographic findings. Initial ECG changes consist of ST-segment elevation in all left ventricular leads. Unlike acute myocardial infarction, the ST segments are upwardly concave, and reciprocal ST depression in opposing leads is absent except in lead aV_R. Q waves do not appear. As the pericarditis evolves, the ST segment returns to baseline. Later, the T wave flattens and inverts in most or all leads. The electrocardiogram eventually returns toward normal.

The chest x-ray in acute pericarditis may be entirely normal. Cardiac enlargement suggests the presence of significant pericardial effusion, which should be investigated with echocardiography. Lymphocytosis is usually present in viral pericarditis. The sedimentation rate is commonly elevated, and cardiac enzymes may rise if a significant degree of myocarditis occurs. Other abnormalities, such as the elevation of creatinine or serologic abnormalities, depend on the underlying etiology of disease.

Differential Diagnosis and Treatment

It is particularly important to distinguish acute pericarditis from myocardial infarction. Acute viral pericarditis can usually be recognized by the abrupt onset of pain worsened by inspiration, fever, and general malaise. ECG changes, particularly on serial tracings, confirm the diagnosis. Pericarditis can also occur during the course of a myocardial friction rub or can be present during the first few days following a transmural myocardial infarction, but rarely causes pain. The postpericardiotomy syndrome, which occurs about 3-6 weeks following acute myocardial infarction or cardiac surgery, causes both pericardial and pleural inflammation and is treated much differently than recurrent myocardial ischemia or infarction.

Treatment of acute pericarditis is symptomatic unless the primary cause can be identified and corrected. Pain and fever are usually relieved by aspirin. Indomethacin is particularly effective and should be employed for persistent pain. Agents such as phenylbutazone and corticosteroids should be reserved for persistent severe cases. Rarely, pericardiectomy is employed as a last resort for intractable pain, but with limited success.

The prognosis of acute viral pericarditis is generally excellent if associated myocarditis is minimal. In other cases, the prognosis is largely dependent on the course of the underlying disease. In a few instances, pericardial inflammation may, over a period of months or years, cause chronic fibrosis. Pericardial calcification or chronic constrictive pericarditis may appear.

PERICARDIAL EFFUSION

Fluid may accumulate between the visceral and parietal pericardium as a result of inflammation, bleeding into the pericardial sac, or as part of a generalized process of fluid accumulation, such as congestive heart failure. The fluid may cause no problem, or it can compress the heart, impeding diastolic filling. The determinants of the effects of pericardial effusion are the rate of fluid accumulation and the distensibility of the pericardial sac. If pericardial fluid accumulates slowly, the pericardium may stretch, accommodating large quantities of fluid without compressing the heart. If the effusion accumulates rapidly, or if the pericardium cannot stretch due to fibrosis, pressure within the pericardial cavity may rise rapidly, impairing diastolic relaxation of the heart and causing cardiac tamponade.

Clinical Features

Pericardial effusion may be accompanied by no symptoms or be associated with findings of percardial inflammation. Cardiac tamponade causes symptoms ranging from anxiety, dizziness, and dyspnea to frank cardiovascular collapse and shock.

If the effusion is large, the heart sounds may be muffled, but this finding is neither specific nor sensitive. The hallmark of pericardial tamponade is pulsus paradoxus, an exaggerated fall in systolic blood pressure during inspiration. This sign is elicited by inflating the blood pressure cuff above systolic pressure and then slowly lowering the pressure until the first Korotkoff's sounds are heard. These sounds disappear during normal quiet inspiration and return during expiration. Pressure is then slowly lowered until the sounds are present continuously during both inspiration and expiration. Normally, the difference between the pressure at which the first sounds are heard and the pressure at which all sounds are heard is 10 mm Hg. A greater than 10 mm Hg inspiratory fall in blood pressure suggests tamponade, but pulsus paradoxus may also be seen in severe asthma or right heart failure. Other signs of cardiac tamponade include tachycardia, hypotension, and jugular venous distension that increases rather than decreases with inspiration (Kussmaul's sign). These are not specific signs of tamponade. Pericardial tamponade should be suspected in any patient exhibiting the combination of a rising pulse rate, rising jugular venous pressure, and falling arterial pressure (Beck's triad).

Laboratory Findings

The electrocardiogram shows no specific changes in pericardial effusion or tamponade, but the T waves are commonly abnormal. QRS voltage may be reduced, and features of acute pericarditis may be seen. Electrical alternans, a phasic change in the amplitude of the QRS, is occasionally present.

The chest x-ray in cardiac tamponade may be entirely normal if a small amount of pericardial fluid has accumulated rapidly. Large pericardial effusions, with or without tamponade, cause enlargement of the cardiac silhouette but no signs of specific chamber enlargement.

Echocardiography is extremely helpful in the diagnosis of pericardial effusion. Very small amounts of fluid are recognized by the presence of an echo-free space lying posterior to the heart. Two-dimensional echocardiography may be useful in quantifying the degree of effusion and in detecting loculated fluid. Echocardiographic features of cardiac tamponade are, however, nonspecific.

Cardiac catheterization may be employed to measure intracardiac pressures in patients suspected of having pericardial tamponade. Pericardial effusion can be detected by measuring the distance between the right atrial endocardium and the epicardial surface (normally less than 1 cm), but this method is less specific than echocardiography. Similarly, pericardial effusion can also be recognized as a radiation-free halo around the heart on radionuclide angiography.

Treatment

Pericardial effusion may present as an inconsequential manifestation of another disease such as heart failure. Small pericardial effusions are common in acute pericarditis and should cause no particular concern. On the other hand, percardial effusion resulting in cardiac tamponade is a medical emergency. Immediate therapy with intravenous volume infusion is indicated. Relief of intrapericardial pressure by pericardiocentesis (percutaneous needle drainage) can be life saving. Open surgical pericardiectomy is usually the definitive procedure in pericardial effusion of hemodynamic significance. This procedure is also commonly required in bacterial pericarditis and in malignant pericardial effusion.

CHRONIC CONSTRICTIVE PERICARDITIS

Constrictive pericarditis is an uncommon disease of insidious onset that mimics right heart failure and may be confused with cirrhosis because ascites is a common feature. In the past, tuberculosis was the primary cause of pericardial constriction. At present, constrictive pericarditis is more commonly a late sequela of acute inflammatory pericarditis. In many patients, the cause of pericardial constriction cannot be determined.

Clinical Features

The earliest symptoms of constrictive pericarditis are peripheral edema and ascites. Dyspnea, while usually present, is not severe. Chest pain and pericardial effusion are generally absent, although an intermediate syndrome—effusoconstrictive pericarditis—is occasionally seen, combining manifestations of inflammatory pericarditis and chronic constrictive pericarditis.

Pulsus paradoxus can be present in constrictive pericarditis but is infrequent. The key to diagnosis on physical examination is the presence of marked jugular venous distention with a rapid y descent and an early diastolic filling sound (pericardial knock). The jugular venous pressure may be quite elevated, with filling above the angle of the jaw even in the upright position. Recognition of elevated jugular pressure is a key to differentiating constrictive pericarditis from other causes of ascites and edema, such as cirrhosis. The pericardial knock is an early diastolic sound that is related to the abrupt cessation of rapid early diastolic filling of the indistensible ventricle. The pericardial knock usually occurs slightly earlier than the third heart sound. Edema, ascites, pleural effusion, and hepatic enlargement are all common results of the elevated venous pressure caused by pericardial constriction. Jaundice may be seen in severe cases.

Laboratory Findings

The electrocardiogram in constrictive pericarditis shows no specific features. A finding of left or right ventricular hypertrophy is evidence against the diagnosis of constrictive pericarditis. On x-ray, the heart in constrictive pericarditis is not enlarged, although mild pulmonary congestion may be present. Calcification of the pericardium is occasionally seen.

Echocardiography is helpful in evaluating other conditions that might be confused with constrictive pericarditis. The abrupt cessation of ventricular filling and thickening of the pericardium can also be observed on the echocardiogram, but these findings may not be specific for constrictive pericarditis.

Pericardial effusion is not present in most cases of chronic constrictive pericarditis. An intermediate syndrome, effusoconstrictive pericarditis, combines features of acute pericarditis and constrictive pericarditis. Pericardial effusion and active inflammation are present in this entity.

Cardiac catheterization is usually performed to confirm the diagnosis of constrictive pericarditis. Characteristic findings include elevated right heart pressures with equalization of diastolic pressure in the four chambers of the heart and in the pulmonary artery. The characteristic diastolic wave form in the right and left ventricles resembles the square-root sign, a rapid early diastolic dip, followed by a high diastolic plateau.

Differential Diagnosis and Treatment

Constrictive pericarditis is usually easy to differentiate from other causes of edema and ascites such as cirrhosis, superior vena cava syndrome, cor pulmonale, and tricuspid stenosis. Restrictive cardiomyopathy, however, may present with quite similar symptoms and hemodynamic abnormalities. The distinction of these two entities may require surgical exploration.

Medical treatment of constrictive pericarditis, other than treatment of underlying illnesses such as tuberculosis, is ineffective. Surgical resection of the pericardium is nearly always recommended for symptomatic patients. If the myocardium has not been damaged, pericardial resection results in relief of symptoms and a good long-term prognosis.

INFECTIVE ENDOCARDITIS

The widespread availability of antibiotics and prosthetic heart valves, the use of immunosuppressive drugs, and the increased prevalence of intravenous drug abuse have markedly influenced the current status of endocarditis. *Streptococcus viridans* still causes this infection in patients with rheumatic heart disease, but new forms of endocarditis are appearing with increasing frequency. Acute fulminant endocarditis due to *Staphylococcus aureus* may destroy a previously normal valve. Emergency valve replacement can be life saving. Endocarditis involving a prosthetic heart valve may also necessitate operative intervention. Infections caused by fungi, Gram-negative, and other rare organisms have also changed the spectrum of endocarditis. This section deals with the clinical presentation and hemodynamic aspects of endocarditis. Specific etiologic agents and antibiotic therapy are discussed in the chapter on infectious diseases.

Pathogenesis

The development of infectious endocarditis is dependent on the entrance of microorganisms into the bloodstream. Transient bacteremia is quite common, particularly following dental extraction and urologic procedures, but may appear with no discernible cause. When these microorganisms are implanted on the endocardial surface of the heart, they characteristically form vegetations. Vegetations are broad-based protrusions from the valve surface consisting of degenerating valve tissue, platelet thrombi, fibrin, and the offending microorganisms.

Parts of the vegetations may dislodge, causing peripheral embolization. In addition, the destructive effects of vegetative lesions may lead to perforation of a valve leaflet, rupture of chordae tendineae, or formation of mycotic aneurysms, particularly in the aortic root and myocardium, resulting in severe valvular incompetence.

Predisposing Factors and Prevention

Endocarditis frequently affects previously abnormal or damaged valves. Of particular importance is the incidence of endocarditis in patients with congenitally bicuspid aortic valves. The bicuspid aortic valve is a common congenital anomaly that often has no symptoms and may remain undetected well into adulthood. Although hemodynamically insignificant, this frequent abnormality of the aortic valve does predispose to endocarditis.

Rheumatic heart disease, particularly in the presence of mitral and aortic regurgitation, predisposes to endocarditis. A ventricular septal defect, pulmonary stenosis, mitral valve prolapse, the presence of a prosthetic heart valve, or any cardiac lesion causing high pressure turbulent blood flow results in increased susceptibility to the development of endocarditis following transient bacteremia.

Intravenous drug users frequently develop endocarditis in previously normal heart valves. The tricuspid valve is most commonly affected. Similarly, hospitalized patients with long-term indwelling venous catheters are susceptible to the development of endocarditis, particularly if they are receiving immunosuppressive drugs. Fungal endocarditis is common in these patients.

Patients with cardiac abnormalities prone to the development of endocarditis should receive antibiotic prophylaxis prior to any anticipated transient bacteremia, such as that occurring during dental manipulation or operative procedures. Recommended prophylaxis for dental work is penicillin V, 250 mg orally 1 hour before the procedure and every 6 hours thereafter until 2 days following the procedure. For genitourinary and gastrointestinal procedures, prophylaxis may be achieved with ampicillin 25-50 mg/kg orally 1 hour before the procedure, and 25 mg/kg every 6 hours until 2 days following the procedure, plus streptomycin 1-2 g intramuscularly 1 hour before, and daily for 2 days following the procedure.

Clinical Features

The onset of endocarditis may be chronic and insidious or abrupt and fulminant. The diagnosis of subacute endocarditis may be missed for weeks or months. Presenting symptoms are usually nonspecific and include fever, arthralgia, malaise, and muscle pain. Fever is found in virtually all patients with endocarditis but may be masked in the elderly, in uremia, and in patients taking corticosteroids.

Acute systemic embolization may be responsible for the first presenting symptoms of endocarditis. The emboli, which represent pieces of vegetation that have become dislodged, are generally small and multiple. Major emboli frequently lodge in the brain. Other arterial systems may also be occluded. Septic pulmonary emboli are seen in the presence of tricuspid endocarditis. Pulmonary infiltrates in a drug addict should alert the clinician to the possibility of endocarditis.

Petechiae are frequently present in both acute and subacute endocarditis. The petechiae are believed to result from deposition of immune complexes. Petechiae may be best seen in the conjunctiva, on mucous membranes, the skin or ocular fundi. White-centered retinal hemorrhages, called Roth's spots, may also be present. Vertical hemorrhage streaks in the skin under the nails—splinter hemorrhages—are also a characteristic finding of endocarditis.

Janeway lesions are characteristic but infrequent findings in endocarditis. These small erythematous or hemorrhagic lesions usually occur on the palms or hands. They are sometimes raised and nodular, but not painful. Osler's nodes are small painful nodules that appear in the pads of the fingers and toes. These lesions, which are the result of embolization, strongly suggest the presence of endocarditis, but are rarely seen. Splenomegaly is present in most patients with endocarditis, but may be absent in the more acute forms of endocarditis.

The cardiac manifestations of endocarditis are essentially those of the underlying cardiac lesion. Changes in the character and site of the murmur may occur, or new murmurs may appear during the period of observation. Heart murmurs are absent in a significant number of patients, particularly when endocarditis is confined to the tricuspid valve. An ominous prognostic finding is the development of signs of congestive heart failure, including the presence of a third heart sound and pulmonary congestion.

Laboratory Findings

The most important feature of endocarditis is bacteremia or fungemia. Blood cultures are necessary to establish an etiologic diagnosis and to determine the antibiotic sensitivity of the organism. Five or six aerobic and anaerobic blood cultures should be performed before instituting antibiotic therapy if the patient's clinical condition permits. Blood cultures are positive in approximately 90 percent of patients with endocarditis. Negative blood cultures may be due to improper technique, to the paucity of microorganisms in the blood at the moment of sampling, or due to previous antibiotic therapy.

Anemia is usually present. Leukocytosis is also characteristic, but less commonly found. The erythrocyte sedimentation rate is frequently elevated. The urinalysis often reveals red blood cell casts, indicating low-grade glomerulonephritis from immune complex deposition in the glomerular capillaries.

The chest x-ray is helpful for identifying cardiomegaly and pulmonary congestion in patients with mitral and aortic endocarditis. Septic pulmonary emboli may be seen in patients with tricuspid endocarditis. Echocardiography can be used for the direct noninvasive visualization of valvular vegetations in some patients with endocarditis. The echocardiographic diagnosis of a vegetation is based on the presence of a masslike lesion attached to the valve. Other causes of masslike lesions such as myxomatous degeneration cannot be distinguished from vegetations. In addition, vegetations are generally seen only when the endocarditis is fairly advanced and the vegetations sizable. Echocardiography thus cannot exclude the presence of endocarditis, but is helpful in identifying the location of vegetations in patients who are more likely to have a complicated course. Echocardiography can also identify the hemodynamic consequences of endocarditis, such as chamber enlargement and early mitral valve closure in acute severe aortic regurgitation.

Cardiac catheterization is commonly employed if valve replacement is being contemplated for patients with endocarditis. Vegetations are rarely visualized with angiography, but valvular regurgitation can be identified. Particularly important is the identification of occult mitral regurgitation in patients with aortic valve endocarditis, indicating extension of the disease to involve two valves. It is also important to visualize the aortic root when planning surgical replacement of the aortic valve.

Differential Diagnosis and Therapy

The firm diagnosis of endocarditis requires a murmur caused by an organic valvular lesion or congenital heart defect, fever, positive blood cultures, and embolic phenomena. However, a significant number of cases, particularly early in their course, present without one or more of these features. The devastating and destructive effects of endocarditis require early diagnosis and therapy. Thus, a diagnosis of endocarditis may be based on lesser criteria. The diagnosis of endocarditis should be assumed probable whenever a patient with an organic heart murmur experiences fever of 1 week's duration with no other apparent cause. It may be necessary to initiate therapy based on a presumptive diagnosis after sufficient numbers of blood cultures have been taken.

Numerous diseases that cause prolonged fever may be confused with endocarditis. Rarely, diseases such as lupus erythematosus and acute rheumatic fever are mistaken for endocarditis. More commonly, a secondary manifestation of endocarditis, such as stroke or heart failure, may alert the clinician to the possibility of endocarditis.

Primary therapy for endocarditis is obviously the administration of an antibiotic to which the causative microorganism is sensitive. These considerations are discussed in the chapter on infectious diseases. However, endocarditis may result in hemodynamic deterioration and death despite prompt administration of appropriate antibiotics, particularly in acute endocarditis. Emergency valve replacement, even prior to completion of a course of antibiotics, may be life saving in some patients. The primary indications for early valve replacement are intractable heart failure and resistance of the offending microorganism to antibiotics. Valve replacement is occasionally necessary in patients with repeated bouts of major embolization. Careful attention must be given to detecting early signs of hemodynamic deterioration when treating patients with infectious endocarditis.

PRIMARY MYOCARDIAL DISEASES

Primary myocardial disease is a term used to describe a group of diseases that share the common feature of cardiomyopathy or myocardial dysfunction in the absence of any of the common causes of heart disease—ischemia, valvular disease, congenital malformation, and systemic hypertension. The etiology of many of the primary myocardial diseases remains unknown. A variety of connective tissue, metabolic, and neurologic diseases may affect the myocardium. These relatively rare causes of cardiomyopathy are listed in Table 4.

Table 4. Systemic Diseases Associated With Myocardiopathy

Amyloidosis	Myotonia dystrophica
Sarcoidosis	Muscular dystrophy
Scleroderma	Hemochromatosis
Lupus erythematosus	Glycogen storage disease
Polyarteritis nodosa	Hurler's syndrome
Friedrich's ataxia	

Primary myocardial disease can be classified on the basis of anatomic and physiologic manifestations. Major groups include hypertrophic, congestive, obliterative, and restrictive cardiomyopathies.

HYPERTROPHIC CARDIOMYOPATHY

The central feature of hypertrophic cardiomyopathy is massive left ventricular hypertrophy that principally affects the interventricular septum, but may extend to involve the entire left ventricle and even the right ventricle. This disease has a genetic basis in most cases, although overt evidence of familial involvement may be clinically inapparent.

When myocardial hypertrophy is largely restricted to the interventricular septum, the disease is termed asymmetric septal hypertrophy (ASH). This entity appears to be genetically transmitted as a nonsex-linked autosomal dominant trait. Pathologic examination of the septum in ASH reveals a distinct pattern of bizarre cellular hypertrophy with a disordered pattern of cell arrangement and variable degrees of interstitial fibrosis. The anatomic, hemodynamic, and clinical features of hypertrophic cardiomyopathy vary considerably. Asymmetric septal hypertrophy may present only as an echocardiographic abnormality without any clinical symptoms or manifest hemodynamic abnormalities. In general, the abnormal hypertrophied myocardium is stiff and inelastic. If the amount of myocardium involved in this process is sufficient, diastolic filling of the heart is impaired. Systolic function of the heart may also be abnormal. At the other end of the spectrum of hypertrophic cardiomyopathy is the syndrome of idiopathic hypertrophic subaortic stenosis (IHSS). This disease is characterized by marked septal hypertrophy. During systole, the anterior leaflet of the mitral valve abuts the septum, narrowing the outflow tract and obstructing left ventricular ejection.

Symptoms

The most frequent symptoms of hypertrophic cardiomyopathy are exertional dyspnea and angina pectoris. Dizziness and syncope are common, but do not carry the same ominous prognosis as does valvular aortic stenosis. Frank congestive heart failure with pulmonary congestion and peripheral edema may also occur. Sudden death occurs with increased frequency in IHSS, particularly in younger patients. This event is presumably related to arrhythmia and is not closely correlated with other symptoms or hemodynamic abnormalities.

Physical Examination

A left ventricular lift and a protodiastolic gallop are commonly observed in patients with hypertrophic cardiomyopathy. In the presence of outflow obstruction, a systolic murmur is heard. Usually the murmur is loudest at the left sternal border and apex and does not radiate well to the neck. Provocative maneuvers are quite useful in differentiating the murmur of IHSS from those of aortic stenosis and mitral regurgitation. Valsalva's maneuver decreases left ventricular volume and thus increases the degree of obstruction, causing the murmur to become louder. Similarly, inhalation of amyl nitrate causes the murmur of IHSS to increase in intensity, while it has no effect on the murmur of aortic stenosis and causes the murmur of mitral regurgitation to become softer.

Laboratory Diagnosis

The carotid pulse tracing in IHSS rises sharply and then falls in midsystole, with a secondary rise or plateau during late systole. This peculiar spike and dome configuration is difficult to appreciate on physical examination, but can be readily appreciated on carotid pulse tracings.

The electrocardiogram is almost always abnormal in IHSS. In most instances, there is evidence of left ventricular hypertrophy. Abnormal Q waves simulating infarction are seen in about one-fourth of patients with IHSS. The Q waves may be seen in leads II, III, aV_F, or over the left precordium and are the result of hypertrophy of the septum, not infarction.

Echocardiography has emerged as the most useful noninvasive technique for the evaluation of patients with hypertrophic cardiomyopathy. The location and degree of left ventricular hypertrophy can be readily assessed. Asymmetric septal hypertrophy is defined as the presence of septal thickness more than 1.3 times the thickness of the posterior wall. This finding may be used as a genetic marker to screen asymptomatic relatives of patients presenting with hypertrophic cardiomyopathy. The hallmark of IHSS on echocardiography is systolic anterior motion of the mitral valve, which produces outflow obstruction. In addition, the aortic valve may be seen to close in midsystole if severe obstruction is present.

Cardiac catheterization in IHSS reveals a subaortic pressure gradient. The severity of obstruction is quite variable and labile. It may be necessary to use drugs or other maneuvers, such as isoproterenol, amyl nitrate and Valsalva's maneuver, which precipitate or increase the degree of obstruction, to elicit a gradient. Analysis of pressure tracings after an extrasystole is also helpful. Normally, the left ventricle contracts more forcefully and the peripheral pulse is increased after an extrasystole as the compensatory pause allows for more diastolic filling. In IHSS, the vigorous contraction increases the degree of obstruction, raises the subaortic gradient, and results in a fall in peripheral pulse pressure.

Angiography characteristically shows marked left ventricular hypertrophy and a small left ventricular cavity; hypertrophy of the septum may be recognized by its inward bulging. Simultaneous biventricular angiograms may be used to better outline the septum. Mitral regurgitation, usually mild, is present in about one-half of patients with IHSS, and may be significant in a small number of patients.

Treatment

No treatment is necessary for asymptomatic patients with asymmetric septal hypertrophy. Patients with outflow obstruction should be advised to avoid strenuous activities, particularly exercise with a large isometric component. Digitalis, isoproterenol, nitroglycerin, and vigorous diuresis are best avoided as they may worsen outflow obstruction. Atrial fibrillation and congestive heart failure may, however, require digitalis therapy. Propranolol is used to decrease sympathetic stimulation of the heart and reduce myocardial oxygen demand. A daily dose of 160-320 mg of propranolol diminishes the frequency of angina, tends to reduce outflow obstruction, and may prevent arrhythmia. Verapamil, a calcium antagonist, has recently been used for similar reasons with apparent success.

Patients with severe outflow obstruction who remain disabled despite medical therapy may be considered for surgical treatment. The operation consists of incising or removing part of the hypertrophied septum. Patients with significant mitral regurgitation may also need mitral valve replacement. Results are variable, but some patients experience substantial clinical improvement following operation.

CONGESTIVE CARDIOMYOPATHY

Congestive cardiomyopathy is a syndrome consisting of isolated cardiomegaly, striking dilatation of the left and right ventricles, and heart failure. The coronary arteries and valves are normal. Heart weight is increased, but the thickness of the walls may not be increased due to thinning associated with chamber dilatation. Microscopic examination of the myocardium shows fibrosis, cellular infiltrates, and mitochondrial abnormalities, but fails to demonstrate the actual etiology of the disease in most cases.

The causes of congestive cardiomyopathy are poorly understood and probably multiple. In many cases, cardiomyopathy is probably the late result of prior viral myocarditis that may or may not have been clinically apparent. Toxins including alcohol and antineoplastic drugs such as doxorubicin (Adriamycin) and daunorubicin (Daunomycin) are recognized causes of cardiomyopathy. Immunologic disorders may be implicated in some cases. The term peripartum cardiomyopathy is used to describe the syndrome of heart failure occurring in a mother during late pregnancy or the puerperium without obvious cause.

Clinical Features

The symptoms of congestive cardiomyopathy are those of heart failure. Exertional and nocturnal dyspnea are frequent. Fatigue occurs due to reduced cardiac output. Left-sided heart failure may be followed by right-sided heart failure, with peripheral edema, ascites, and hepatic congestion.

The physical signs of congestive failure include a diastolic gallop, pulmonary rales, and jugular venous distention. The left ventricular impulse is displaced outside the midclavicular line and is of poor quality. Massive ventricular dilatation may cause functional incompetence of the mitral and tricuspid valves, with resultant pansystolic murmurs.

Laboratory Diagnosis

The electrocardiogram usually shows nonspecific flattening of the T wave. Left atrial enlargement or left ventricular hypertrophy patterns may be seen. Q waves simulating myocardial infarction are present in 15-20 percent of patients. Intraventricular contraction disturbances occur frequently.

The chest x-ray shows cardiomegaly due to biventricular enlargement. The atria may also be enlarged. Evidence of pulmonary congestion and pleural effusion may also be seen.

Echocardiography shows dilatation of both the left and right ventricles with reduced systolic wall motion and diminished wall thickening throughout. Valvular motion may be altered by increased diastolic pressure and reduced cardiac output. Left ventricular thrombi and pericardial effusion can also be detected.

Cardiac catheterization findings are those of pump failure. The stroke volume and ejection fraction are reduced. The systolic and diastolic left ventricular volumes are increased, and wall motion is diffusely depressed. Diastolic ventricular pressures are elevated and pulmonary hypertension may be present.

Treatment

The treatment of congestive cardiomyopathy is symptomatic and supportive. The course of the disease is usually steadily downhill, and the prognosis for recovery is poor. Digitalis, diuretics, afterload reduction, and prolonged bed rest improve symptoms of congestive failure. Anticoagulation should be considered to prevent both pulmonary and systemic thromboembolism. Antiarrhythmic therapy is often necessary. Surgical treatment is limited to cardiac transplantation, which is currently performed only at a few medical centers as an experimental procedure.

OBLITERATIVE CARDIOMYOPATHY

This rare condition is characterized by obliteration of the ventricular cavities, decreased myocardial contractility, and valvular distortion. Endomyocardial fibrosis, the most common type of obliterative cardiomyopathy, is usually restricted to tropical countries. Löffler's endocarditis is a rare disease in which peripheral eosinophilia is associated with plaquelike deposits in the heart. These diseases may predominantly affect either the right or left ventricle, with subsequent symptoms of heart failure. The etiology is unknown and treatment is supportive.

RESTRICTIVE CARDIOMYOPATHY

This rare condition mimics the hemodynamic abnormalities of constrictive pericarditis. Diastolic filling of the ventricles is impaired by primary myocardial disease, although systolic function can remain normal. Symptoms and physical findings are quite similar to those of pericardial constriction, and exploratory surgery may be required to differentiate the two. Amyloidosis and hemochromatosis are known causes of restrictive cardiomyopathy but the etiology is unknown, and no specific treatment is available.

CONGENITAL HEART DISEASES

New techniques for cardiopulmonary bypass and open heart surgery were first introduced in the 1950s. These procedures were initially applied to patients with congenital anomalies, virtually revolutionizing the therapeutic approach to congenital heart disease. These procedures have been continually perfected, and today even very young children with complex congenital lesions can frequently undergo corrective surgery. The prompt recognition and accurate diagnosis of patients with congenital cardiac anomalies have thus achieved great importance for the practitioner. In addition, these improved surgical procedures have allowed many children, who would otherwise have died, to reach adulthood. Patients who have previously undergone surgical correction of congenital cardiac anomalies are being seen with increasing frequency by general practitioners. A working knowledge of congenital heart disease is essential for physicians caring for these patients.

Incidence

Congenital heart disease occurs in 0.5-1.0 percent of all live births. Overall, congenital heart diseases are more common in males.

Etiology

Congenital heart disease occurs as a result of abnormal embryonic development of the heart. Certain environmental factors, for example, maternal viral illnesses such as rubella and the ingestion of drugs like thalidomide during early pregnancy, are known to be associated with congenital heart disease in offspring. In addition, certain chromosomal abnormalities and the mutation of single genes are associated with congenital heart diseases. These diseases are generally not inherited in a predictable manner according to mendelian laws. However, there is a twofold to fourfold increase in the prevalence of congenital disease in children of affected parents.

Immunization of children with rubella vaccine is expected to eliminate maternal rubella. All drugs with teratogenic potential and unnecessary radiation from x-rays should be strictly avoided in pregnant women.

Classification

Congenital heart diseases have been classified in a variety of ways, with the following being the most convenient:

1. Abnormal communications between the pulmonic and systemic circulation with
   (a) Left-to-right shunt (acyanotic) (e.g., atrial septic defect, ventricular septal defect, patent ductus arteriosus).
   (b) Right-to-left shunt (cyanotic) with
      (1) Decreased pulmonary vascularity (e.g., cyanotic type of tetralogy of Fallot, complete transposition of great vessels with severe pulmonic stenosis)
      (2) Increased pulmonary vascularity (e.g., complete transposition of great vessels, truncus arteriosus).
2. Without shunts (e.g., coarctation of the aorta, aortic stenosis, mitral incompetence, pulmonary stenosis, cor triatriatum, Ebstein's anomaly).
3. Cardiac malpositions (e.g., dextrocardia).

ATRIAL SEPTAL DEFECT

Atrial septal defects (ASD) are classified according to their location in the atrial septum.

1. Sinus venosus defect is an upper defect in which the superior vena cava opens into both the right and left atria.
2. Ostium secundum defect is located in the middle portion (region of fossa ovalis) of the atrial septum.
3. Endocardial cushion defect is a low defect involving the mitral and/or tricuspid valves and/or upper portion of the ventricular system. This is further classified as
   (a) Incomplete–ostium primum defect with cleft mitral or tricuspid valves;
   (b) Complete–persistent atrioventricular canal.

Ostium Secundum Defect

This is the most common type of congenital heart disease in adolescents and adults. It is two to three times more common in women and may have a familial pattern. The defect varies in size from 1-3 cm and occupies the middle portion of the atrial septum.

Pathophysiology

During prenatal life, the right ventricle is thicker and less compliant in comparison to the left ventricle. This is responsible for normal right-to-left shunt through the foramen ovale before birth. Soon after birth, there is a rapid involution of the pulmonary arterioles and the right ventricle becomes relatively thin and more compliant in comparison to the left ventricle, which becomes relatively thick and less compliant. This change in relative compliance and hence inflow resistances of the two ventricles results in higher left-sided filling (left atrial) pressure and lower right-sided filling (right atrial) pressure, causing functional closure of the foramen ovale. However, in the presence of an abnormal communication between the two atria, gradually decreasing inflow resistance of the right ventricle in relation to that of the left ventricle initiates a left-to-right shunt. In addition to the difference in inflow resistance of the ventricles, the magnitude of left-to-right shunt also depends on the size of the interatrial communication. In the presence of a large nonrestrictive defect, pressures in the two atria become equal. Later in life the pulmonary vascular resistance may rise, resulting in pulmonary hypertension and right ventricular hypertrophy. In this situation, high right ventricular inflow resistance causes right-to-left shunt through the ASD (Eisenmenger's syndrome).

Clinical Features

The majority of adolescents and young adults with ASD are asymptomatic. Patients with unusually large left-to-right shunts may develop effort intolerance due to fatigue and dyspnea. In later life (after age 40), patients commonly develop atrial arrhythmias (atrial fibrillation, flutter, tachycardia) and heart failure. The development of pulmonary hypertension and high pulmonary vascular resistance (Eisenmenger's syndrome) is uncommon. However, most patients are symptomatic after age 60.

Adolescents may have a thin and fragile body build. Arterial pulse may have normal or low volume. The jugular venous pulse shows a and v waves of equal size. The precordium reveals a hyperdynamic left parasternal region, indicating right ventricular volume overload. The first heart sound is frequently normal. A fixed wide split of S_2 is the hallmark of an ASD. Increased stroke volume of the right ventricle necessitates a longer right ventricular ejection period, resulting in delayed pulmonic valve closure. At the same time, smaller left ventricular stroke volume requires a shorter ejection period, causing early aortic valve closure. The early A_2 and delayed P_2 result in a wide splitting of S_2. Since venous return to the atria during various phases of respiration is equalized across the septal defect, a widely split second sound shows little variation with inspiration or expiration (fixed split). Increased diastolic flow across the tricuspid valve results in an S_3 and a middiastolic flow rumble at the left lower parasternal area. Clinically, this finding indicates a greater than 2:1 left-to-right shunt. Increased systolic flow across the pulmonic valve causes a grade 2 to 3 midsystolic ejection-type murmur over the left upper parasternal area.

Laboratory Diagnosis

Electrocardiogram

The rhythm is usually sinus in young patients, but atrial fibrillation is very common in the elderly. The axis is commonly in the normal range or rightward. Right precordial leads reveal an rSR′ or RSR′ pattern that is referred to as an incomplete right bundle-branch block and indicates right ventricular volume overload.

Chest X-ray

The heart size may be normal or modestly increased. The right atrium and right ventricle are enlarged. The main pulmonary arteries are markedly enlarged and may become aneurysmatic. The peripheral pulmonary arteries and veins are also prominent, reflecting a left-to-right shunt. The aortic knuckle is small.

Echocardiogram

The echocardiogram displays an enlarged right ventricle and paradoxical motion of the ventricular septum. This pattern is indicative of right ventricular volume overload that may occur in tricuspid insufficiency, pulmonary incompetence, and anomalous pulmonary venous drainage, in addition to an ASD. Some ASD patients demonstrate mitral valve prolapse.

Cardiac Catheterization

The primary reasons for performing cardiac catheterization are to exclude any associated cardiac anomalies, to identify the location of ASD, and to quantify the left-to-right shunt. Passage of the catheter across the defect confirms the diagnosis and suggests the location of the ASD. The magnitude of the left-to-right shunt is estimated by the amount of step-up of oxygen saturation in the right atrium. In the majority of young patients, pulmonary artery pressure and pulmonary vascular resistance are normal. Passage of the catheter into pulmonary veins directly from the right atrium and high oxygen saturation in the superior vena cava indicate a sinus venosus type of ASD or partial anomalous venous drainage. Contrast cineangiocardiography and selective indicator-dilution curves from right and left pulmonary arteries can demonstrate the location and number of anomalous pulmonary veins.

Natural History

Although a few patients present with large left-to-right shunts in their infancy, in the vast majority of patients, clinical manifestations of isolated ASD rarely appear before 4-6 years of age. Most patients have normal pulmonary artery pressure and vascular resistance in their childhood and early adult life. With advancing age, the incidence of pulmonary hypertension and Eisenmenger's syndrome increases; after age 40, there is approximately a 20 percent incidence of Eisenmenger's syndrome. The life span is shortened in patients who develop high pulmonary vascular resistance. Death is usually due to heart failure. The annual mortality rate is 0.6 percent during the first decade, 4.5 percent during the fourth decade, and 7.5 percent during the sixth decade of life. Since the left-to-right shunt through an ASD is a low-velocity shunt (because of low pressures in the right and left atria) there are no jet lesions, which explains an extremely low (<0.15 annually) incidence of infective endocarditis in ASD.

Differential Diagnosis

Rheumatic heart disease with mitral stenosis or regurgitation, ventricular septal defect, mild pulmonary valve stenosis, straight-back syndrome, and idiopathic dilatation of the pulmonary arteries frequently enter into the differential diagnosis.

Management

An ASD that allows 1.5:1.0 or greater left-to-right shunt should be considered for surgical closure. The risk of mortality is extremely low (<1%), and results are excellent after surgery. The ideal age for corrective surgery is after infancy and before 5 years of age. However, even in adolescents and adults, surgical closure is advisable if the shunt is predominantly left to right. Development of severe pulmonary vascular disease with reversal of shunt (Eisenmenger's syndrome) is a contraindication to surgery.

If heart failure develops in an ASD patient, the usual medical measures, that is, digitalis, diuretics, low salt diet, and bed rest, should be employed.

Endocardial Cushion (Atrioventricular Canal) Defects

Pathology

Endocardial cushion defects exist in incomplete and complete forms. The incomplete variety (ostium primum defect) is characterized by a low defect in the atrial septum. The upper margin of the defect has a crescent shape, and the lower margin consists of mitral and tricuspid valve tissue. In the majority of these patients, the anterior mitral valve leaflet shows a cleft and has abnormal chordal attachments. In some individuals, the septal leaflet of the tricuspid valve is hypoplastic. A complete atrioventricular canal defect exhibits a high ventricular septal defect (VSD) in addition to a low atrial septal defect and cleft mitral and tricuspid valves.

Pathophysiology

The shunting of blood in endocardial cushion defects occurs via atrial and ventricular septal defects. The direction of shunt is determined by relative resistances in the pulmonary and systemic circuits. Initially, the shunt is left to right, from left atrium to right atrium, and from left ventricle to right ventricle. The cleft mitral and tricuspid valves may be incompetent. Both left and right ventricles face an increased volume work that eventually results in biventricular failure. Patients with endocardial cushion defects present with a wide variety of pathophysiologic disturbances, left-to-right shunt through the ostium primum defect, left-to-right shunt via ventricular septal defect, left-to-right shunt from left ventricle to right atrium, mitral incompetence, tricuspid incompetence, or combinations of these disturbances.

Clinical Features

The ostium primum defect is two to three times more common in women, whereas a complete atrioventricular canal is equally common in both sexes. Heart failure, poor growth and development, and respiratory infections generally begin in late childhood or adolescence. In many cases, atrial fibrillation or flutter mark the beginning of heart failure and occur at an earlier age than in ostium secundum defects. Patients with an ostium primum defect are at a considerably higher risk for infective endocarditis because of coexistent mitral regurgitation than patients with an ostium secundum defect.

Due to more severe circulatory disturbances, patients with complete forms of atrioventricular canal defects become symptomatic during infancy.

Almost 50 percent of the patients with endocardial cushion defects have Down's syndrome. Slight cyanosis, particularly on effort, and physical underdevelopment are frequent. The arterial pulse may be normal, of small volume in patients with predominant left-to-right shunt via an ostium primum defect, or may display a brisk upstroke in patients with predominant mitral valve incompetence. Jugular venous pressure is normal until the development of right heart failure when it becomes elevated. A large a wave indicates decreased right ventricular compliance that occurs as the right ventricle develops hypertrophy in response to pulmonary hypertension. A prominent v wave indicates coexistent mitral or tricuspid valve incompetence or both. Bulging precordium and Harrison's groove (horizontal depression along the lower border of the chest) are frequently present. The left parasternal region is hyperdynamic due to right ventricular volume overload. In patients with dominant mitral valve incompetence or ventricular septal defect, the apical impulse is also hyperdynamic because of left ventricular volume overload. A systolic thrill over the apex and left lower parasternal area may be palpated. The auscultatory signs of an ostium primum defect closely mimic those of an ostium secundum defect with the addition of a pansystolic murmur of mitral valve incompetence. The murmur of mitral valve incompetence in endocardial cushion defects differs from that of rheumatic mitral insufficiency in that it selectively radiates toward the sternum. Ejection of left ventricular blood directly into the right atrium via the cleft mitral valve is the underlying basis for this radiation. In complete forms of endocardial cushion defects, pansystolic murmurs of a ventricular septal defect and mitral valve incompetence are superimposed. Physical signs of pulmonary hypertension become evident relatively early.

Laboratory Diagnosis

Electrocardiogram

Depending on the predominant hemodynamic abnormality, right atrial, left atrial, or a combination of both are commonly observed. Some patients show first-degree atrioventricular block. Atrial arrhythmias and atrioventricular blocks are seen with advancing age. In right precordial leads, the QRS complex shows an rSR′ pattern. A vast majority of patients with endocardial cushion defects show left axis deviation. Left ventricular hypertrophy occurs secondary to significant mitral incompetence, and right ventricular hypertrophy develops with the occurrence of pulmonary hypertension.

Chest X-ray

The x-ray appearance is greatly influenced by the underlying pathology. In ostium primum defects, the x-ray appearance is indistinguishable from that of a secundum type of ASD. If mitral regurgitation is the dominant component, left atrial and left ventricular enlargement are predominant. In the case of a complete endocardial cushion defect, cardiomegaly is invariably present. The right atrium, right ventricle, and left atrium are enlarged. Pulmonary plethora is obvious, and the pulmonary artery and its branches are enlarged.

Echocardiogram

Echocardiography shows the right ventricular volume overload. In addition, the anterior mitral valve leaflet lies in close proximity to the ventricular septum, both during systole and diastole, and the tricuspid valve echo traverses the ventricular septal echoes.

Cardiac Catheterization

Cardiac catheterization shows a step-up of oxygen at the right atrial level. Passage of a catheter across the atrial septal defect in an unusually low position is suggestive of a primum defect. On left ventriculography, a gooseneck deformity of the left ventricular outflow tract is pathognomonic of a primum defect. Left ventriculography also shows mitral regurgitation and a shunt from the left ventricle to the right atrium.

Natural History

The long-term prognosis of patients with a primum-type defect and mild mitral incompetence is similar to that of those with an ostium secundum defect. Patients with more prominent mitral incompetence may develop heart failure early. Patients with complete types of endocardial cushion defects usually have heart failure during infancy and die at an early age.

Management

Medical management consists of prophylaxis for infective endocarditis and treatment of heart failure and frequent respiratory infections. In primum defects, surgical correction is advisable between the ages of 5-6 or earlier. In patients with marked mitral incompetence, valve replacement is generally required and the operation is therefore deferred to a later age. To prevent the development of Eisenmenger's syndrome, patients with a complete AV canal should undergo total correction before 2 years of age.

VENTRICULAR SEPTAL DEFECT

In adults, ventricular septal defects (VSD) constitute approximately 10 percent of all congenital heart diseases, being equally as frequent in men as in women. When viewed from the right ventricle, 80 percent of the defects are present in the outflow region of the ventricular septum, that is, between the pulmonary valve above and septal leaflet of the tricuspid valve below. The majority of these are located in the membranous portion and are infracristal in location; an occasional defect is supracristal in location. The remaining 20 percent occur in the inflow region or muscular portion of the ventricular septum.

Pathophysiology

The size of the defect greatly influences the pathophysiology. VSDs are generally described as large, medium-sized, or small.

The large VSD has a cross-sectional area greater than or equal to the cross-sectional area of the aortic valve and offers little resistance to blood flow from the left to the right ventricle. Because of this unrestrictive communication between left and right ventricles throughout the cardiac cycle, the systolic pressures in the left ventricle, aorta, right ventricle, and pulmonary artery are equal. Thus, a patient with a large VSD has severe pulmonary hypertension. The left-to-right shunt depends on the relative resistance of systemic and pulmonary circuits. If the pulmonary vascular resistance falls progressively and is considerably lower than the systemic vascular resistance, a large left-to-right shunt develops. Volume overload on the left ventricle distends it and may result in left ventricular failure. In the medium-sized VSD, the left-to-right shunt is dependent on the resistance offered by the defect, as well as the relative resistances of pulmonary and systemic vascular beds. Because of the restrictive nature of medium-sized VSD, the systolic pressure in the right ventricle and pulmonary artery is only moderately elevated. In the case of a small VSD, the defect imposes much more resistance to blood flow from the left to the right ventricle. Consequently, the systolic pressure in the right ventricle and pulmonary artery is nearly normal. In patients with large left-to-right shunts and pulmonary hypertension, pulmonary vascular disease develops over the course of years, increasing the pulmonary vascular resistance. This results in a decrease of left-to-right shunt and ultimately causes right-to-left shunt (Eisenmenger's syndrome).

Clinical Features

Infants with moderate and large VSDs develop symptoms of heart failure, that is, dyspnea, fatigue, effort intolerance, and respiratory infections, usually during the second month. With the spontaneous reduction in the size of VSD, symptoms slowly disappear. Weight gain and growth are slow. Patients with small VSDs are usually asymptomatic.

Arterial pulse is normal in patients with a small left-to-right shunt, and somewhat brisk in patients with a large left-to-right shunt. Jugular venous pulse is essentially normal. Chest deformity in the precordial region and Harrison's groove may be present. In patients with significant left-to-right shunts, the apical impulse is hyperdynamic. A systolic thrill is frequently palpable in the left parasternal region. The first heart sound is usually covered by the holosystolic murmur, and the second heart sound may be widely split. In the presence of greater than or equal to 2:1 left-to-right shunt, the third heart sound and a brief middiastolic murmur are generally audible over the apical region. A holosystolic murmur over the left parasternal region is the most prominent auscultatory sign. The murmur is commonly uniform or plateau shaped throughout systole and may show a slight midsystolic accentuation. The murmur decreases in response to vasodilators (amyl nitrite inhalation) and accentuates in response to vasopressors (phenylephrine). In a very small VSD, left-to-right shunt is interrupted during midsystole as contraction of the ventricular septum closes the opening. Consequently, in such patients the systolic murmur is confined to early systole.

Laboratory Diagnosis

Electrocardiogram

Left ventricular hypertrophy is present in large left-to-right shunts without pulmonary hypertension. Large R waves, deep narrow Q waves and tall T waves are usually seen in left precordial leads. This QRS pattern reflects volume overload of the left ventricle. In patients with large left-to-right shunts and pulmonary hypertension, large equiphasic R and S waves (Katz-Wachtel phenomenon) indicating biventricular hypertrophy, are encountered in midprecordial leads. Left atrial hypertrophy is frequently seen in patients with large left-to-right shunts.

Chest X-ray

Chest x-ray frequently shows moderate cardiomegaly with enlargement of the left ventricle, right ventricle, and left atrium, with a normal or small ascending aorta. In an occasional patient, the aortic arch is right sided. The main pulmonary artery and its branches are enlarged. The peripheral pulmonary arterial branches are also enlarged, giving an appearance of pulmonary plethora in predominant left-to-right shunts.

Echocardiogram

In most patients, M-mode echocardiography is not reliable in predicting VSD. In a few patients with very large VSDs, echocardiography may demonstrate a discontinuity of the ventricular septal echoes.

Cardiac Catheterization and Angiography

The objectives of cardiac catheterization are to determine the magnitude of the left-to-right shunt, to locate the site of the VSD, and to detect any additional malformations. Serial blood samples from right heart chambers show a step-up of oxygen saturation in the right ventricle. The pulmonary artery pressure is normal or variably elevated, depending on the size of the VSD. A left ventricular angiogram reveals the location and size of a VSD.

Natural History

Progressive decrease in size of the defect is very common and, in a significant number of children, it eventually disappears completely. The majority of children remain asymptomatic as the majority of VSDs are restrictive. Children with larger defects develop CHF early in life, with most being managed medically. Occasionally a child needs pulmonary artery banding as a palliative measure. Eisenmenger's syndrome rarely develops in childhood, occuring most frequently in young adults. Some patients develop aortic incompetence that adversely influences their prognosis, while others may develop pulmonary infundibular stenosis and present with a picture of tetralogy of Fallot. Patients with VSD are at risk for infective endocarditis.

Differential Diagnosis

A septum primum defect, infundibular pulmonary stenosis,

and mitral regurgitation should be considered in the differential diagnosis.

Management

Medical management consists of prophylaxis against infective endocarditis, treatment of CHF (common during the first year of life), and advising surgical closure. In infants with large VSD and unmanageable CHF, surgical palliation or repair is indicated. In medium-sized VSDs with left-to-right shunt ($\geqslant$1.5:1), surgical closure is recommended before entering school.

PATENT DUCTUS ARTERIOSUS

Patent ductus arteriosus (PDA) is the second or third most common congenital heart disease in adults and is two to three times more common in women. The occurrence of German measles during pregnancy makes the offspring prone to develop PDA, particularly in combination with pulmonic stenosis. The pulmonary orifice of the ductus is located immediately distal to the bifurcation of the main pulmonary trunk, and the aortic orifice of the ductus lies distal to the origin of the left subclavian artery. Coarctation of the aorta and VSD can occur with PDA.

Pathophysiology

During fetal life, oxygenated maternal blood bypasses the lungs and reaches the aorta via the ductus arteriosus. Normally, the ductus closes functionally within several hours to 1 week, and anatomically within a few days to several weeks, after birth. However, if the ductus remains patent after birth, it shunts blood from the aorta into the pulmonary artery, both during systole and diastole. This left-to-right shunt causes volume overloading of the left ventricle. In addition, the left atrium and pulmonary vasculature are exposed to increased blood volume. The size of left-to-right shunt is determined by the caliber of the ductus and level of pulmonary vascular resistance. A small ductus allows a small left-to-right shunt and pulmonary artery pressure remains normal. By contrast, a ductus with a large lumen is nonrestrictive and permits direct transmission of the aortic pressure into the pulmonary artery, causing pulmonary hypertension. In such patients, the size of left-to-right shunt is determined by the relative pulmonary and systemic resistances. When the pulmonary resistance is considerably lower than the systemic resistance, there is a large left-to-right shunt resulting in volume overload of the left ventricle and pressure overload of the right ventricle. When the pulmonary resistance is similar to systemic resistance or only slightly lower, the left-to-right shunt is small, which imposes less volume overload on the left ventricle; however, pulmonary hypertension places considerable pressure overload on the right ventricle. When the pulmonary resistance is higher than the systemic resistance, there is a right-to-left shunt and the right ventricle faces a high-pressure work load.

Clinical Features

Heart failure can occur during infancy in patients with large left-to-right shunts through a PDA. During adult life, CHF is more common during the third and fourth decades in patients with large left-to-right shunts. Patients with small left-to-right shunts remain asymptomatic. All patients are prone to develop infective arteritis.

Children with large shunts and CHF may be underdeveloped and may also show Harrison's groove, pigeon chest, and precordial asymmetry. In patients with large shunts, a bounding pulse (wide pulse pressure) is present; this is attributed to rapid runoff of blood from the aorta into a low-resistance pulmonary vascular bed. In such patients, the left ventricular impulse is hyperdynamic. A continuous thrill with systolic accentuation may be palpable in the first and second left intercostal spaces. On auscultation, a continuous murmur (continuous from systole to diastole without interruption or change of character) over the left upper sternal border is a typical feature of PDA. The murmur peaks around the second heart sound and is rough in character. An S_3 and middiastolic flow rumble over the apex are audible and are due to an augmented diastolic blood flow across the mitral valve. These findings suggest at least 2:1 left-to-right shunt.

Laboratory Diagnosis

Electrocardiogram

In patients with medium-sized and large PDA, the electrocardiogram shows left ventricular hypertrophy. Left ventricular hypertrophy is usually of the volume-overloading type.

Chest X-ray

In patients with medium-sized and large PDA, the chest x-ray reveals cardiomegaly. More specifically, the left ventricle, left atrium, ascending aorta, and aortic arch are enlarged. The pulmonary artery and its branches are also enlarged. Pulmonary vascular markings are prominent (pulmonary plethora) up to the periphery secondary to enlargement of both the pulmonary arteries and veins. In older persons, a chest x-ray may reveal a calcified ductus.

Echocardiography

Echocardiography does not permit direct visualization of the ductus. However, it is a good technique to demonstrate enlargement of the left atrium and left ventricle and is useful in following patients with PDA.

Cardiac Catheterization

The objective of cardiac catheterization is to confirm the clinical diagnosis and to identify any other coexistent congenital heart abnormality. Sequential blood sampling from right heart chambers shows a significant oxygen step-up in the main pulmonary artery over that of the right ventricle. Pulmonary artery pressure is either normal or elevated, depending on the size of the PDA. Pulmonary vascular resistance is normal or slightly elevated initially. Manipulation of the catheter from the pulmonary artery into the descending aorta via the PDA provides the most direct diagnosis. Aortography furnishes information regarding the size and precise location of the ductus.

Differential Diagnosis

Other conditions with a continuous murmur over the precordium should be considered in the differential diagnosis of PDA; these include aorticopulmonary septal defect, ruptured aneurysm of the sinus of Valsalva into the right heart chamber, combination of VSD and AR, coronary arteriovenous fistula, branch stenosis of the pulmonary artery, pulmonary arteriovenous fistula, and cervical venous hum.

Natural History

As mentioned earlier, the natural history of the ductus is greatly influenced by its size, which in turn determines the degree of left-to-right shunting. A small ductus has no adverse effect on the cardiovascular system and does not shorten life expectancy. The only clinical implication is that it is a potential site for infective arteritis. Most patients with a medium-sized ductus tolerate the volume overload of the left ventricle well and are asymptomatic. Aneurysm of the ductus rarely develops. These patients, as well as patients with a large ductus, are at risk for infective endarteritis. Patients with a large ductus may develop CHF during infancy or early childhood. Some suffer from frequent respiratory infections and their growth is retarded. A few patients gradually develop high pulmonary vascular resistance and reversal of a left-to-right shunt (Eisenmenger's syndrome).

Treatment

All patients with a ductus should be instructed in antibiotic prophylaxis against infective endarteritis. The role of medical therapy is to control heart failure in inoperable patients. The definitive treatment consists of surgical division of the ductus as soon as the diagnosis is established, regardless of the presence, absence, or severity of symptoms. The mortality of surgery is essentially zero. The development of Eisenmenger's syndrome is the only contraindication to surgical division. Surgery may not be advisable in middle-aged and elderly patients who have a small ductus and are asymptomatic since, in this age group, the risk of surgery exceeds the risk for infective endarteritis.

EISENMENGER'S SYNDROME

Eisenmenger's syndrome is defined as the development of pulmonary hypertension at a systemic level due to a high pulmonary vascular resistance, resulting in a reversed or bidirectional shunt through communication between the systemic and pulmonic circuits of circulation such as VSD, ASD, and PDA, which originally allow a large left-to-right shunt.

In some patients with large left-to-right shunts, pulmonary vascular resistance gradually rises relative to the systemic resistance and results in a gradual decrease of the left-to-right shunt. When resistance in the pulmonary and systemic vascular beds becomes equal, the shunt disappears or becomes bidirectional. In some, the pulmonary vascular resistance surpasses the systemic vascular resistance and a right-to-left shunt is established. The pulmonary artery pressure approaches the systemic level and imposes a pressure overload on the right ventricle. The pulmonary blood flow decreases and is lower than the systemic flow, which remains at a normal level.

Clinical Features

Eisenmenger's syndrome occurs more frequently in large VSD and PDA than in large ASD. In most patients with VSD and PDA, the onset of Eisenmenger's syndrome starts during infancy or childhood; in most patients with ASD, it starts during adult life. Dyspnea on exertion is frequent. In addition to dyspnea, angina pectoris (presumably due to right ventricular hypertrophy), syncope, hemoptysis, and heart failure occur in Eisenmenger's syndrome. Squatting is uncommon in these patients. When this syndrome occurs with PDA, it is tolerated better than in other conditions since the head and neck still receive arterial blood and only the lower body receives desaturated blood.

Physical signs are due to a right-to-left shunt and pulmonary hypertension. Central cyanosis is present in most patients. Patients with PDA and reversal of the left-to-right shunt demonstrate differential cyanosis; that is, cyanosis is observed in the toenails, whereas the fingernails are pink. Clubbing and polycythemia are also present. The pulse is generally of low volume or normal. The jugular venous pulse reveals a prominent a wave. When functional tricuspid incompetence develops, the v wave also becomes prominent. On palpation, a heaving right ventricle is commonly found. Right-sided S_4, a pulmonary ejection click, and an ejection systolic murmur at the upper left parasternal area are frequent. Some patients develop functional pulmonary incompetence due to severe pulmonary hypertension. This is recognized by a high-frequency early diastolic (Graham-Steell's) murmur along the upper left parasternal area. The pulmonic component of S_2 is loud. The splitting of S_2 becomes narrow; in many cases, the S_2 is single. However, patients with ASD retain a fixed splitting of S_2, even after development of Eisenmenger's syndrome. Eventually, signs of right heart failure become manifest and many patients develop functional tricuspid incompetence.

Laboratory Diagnosis

Electrocardiogram

In most patients, the ECG shows right ventricular hypertrophy with strain and right atrial hypertrophy.

Chest X-ray

The characteristic features consist of marked enlargement of the main pulmonary artery and its major branches. The distal pulmonary arteries in the peripheral regions are markedly attenuated, giving a truncated tree appearance. The greatest enlargement of central pulmonary arteries occurs in patients with ASD when Eisenmenger's syndrome develops. The right ventricle and right atrium become enlarged.

Cardiac Catheterization

The pulmonary artery and right ventricular systolic pressures are at a systemic level. The right atrial pressure may be elevated with a prominent a wave. The pulmonary artery wedge pressure is usually normal. The pulmonary blood flow is decreased and systemic blood flow is normal. Pulmonary vascular resistance is markedly increased (>10 Wood units). The arterial blood shows moderate to marked desaturation. Shunts may be right to left, bidirectional, or absent. In most patients, the catheter may be manipulated across the defect. Dye dilution curves, obtained after injecting indocyanine green dye upstream (right heart chambers) and sampling downstream (left heart chambers or aorta), demonstrate a right-to-left shunt. Selective angiocardiography also helps locate the site of the shunt.

Differential Diagnosis

Chronic cor pulmonale, primary pulmonary hypertension, persistent truncus arteriosus, and transposition of the great vessels with VSD should be considered in the differential diagnosis of Eisenmenger's syndrome. In patients with Eisenmenger's syndrome, it is extremely difficult to locate precisely the site of the shunt on a clinical basis.

Natural History

The average age of demise in these patients is the middle thirties. The most common causes of death are hemoptysis, cardiovascular collapse, and heart failure. Occasionally, cerebral thrombosis, cerebral abscess, and infective endocarditis occur. Pregnancy carries a very high risk of mortality.

Treatment

Treatment is strictly medical and consists of management of heart failure and long-term anticoagulant therapy for thromboembolic complications. Surgical closure of the defect is contraindicated.

VENTRICULAR SEPTAL DEFECT WITH PULMONARY STENOSIS (TETRALOGY OF FALLOT)

The combination of a large nonrestrictive VSD and pulmonary stenosis has a wide physiologic and clinical spectrum. At one extreme, pulmonary stenosis is mild to moderate, permitting a left-to-right shunt through the VSD. This is called the acyanotic type of tetralogy of Fallot. At the other extreme, there is pulmonary atresia resulting in right-to-left shunt, and the pulmonary circuit is supplied via bronchial collateral vessels. This is the most extreme type of cyanotic variety of tetralogy of Fallot. Most cases, however, consist of severe pulmonary stenosis, which allows a right-to-left shunt, and are described as a cyanotic type of tetralogy of Fallot. In addition to VSD and pulmonary stenosis, right ventricular hypertrophy and a variable degree of overriding of the aorta complete the tetrad described by Fallot. Pulmonary stenosis is frequently of the infundibular type, and occasionally of the valvular type. It should be remembered that pulmonary obstruction is progressive and, therefore, a previously acyanotic type of tetralogy of Fallot can progress to a cyanotic type. A right-sided aortic arch, persistent left superior vena cava, hypoplastic pulmonary artery, incomplete pulmonary valve, and an abnormal origin of the left anterior descending coronary artery from the right coronary artery can occur with tetralogy of Fallot.

Pathophysiology

The degrees of pulmonary obstruction and systemic vascular resistance determine the hemodynamics. As the right ventricle communicates with the aorta via its overriding origin as well as a large VSD, its systolic pressure is always at a systemic level. When the pulmonary resistance (due to pulmonary stenosis) is modest relative to systemic vascular resistance, the shunt is predominantly left to right. As resistance to ejection into the pulmonary artery increases, the left-to-right shunt decreases; when the pulmonary resistance is greater than the systemic resistance, the shunt is entirely right to left.

Clinical Features

Cyanosis becomes evident during the first few days after birth. Many patients complain of dyspnea, and squat or assume a knee/chest position to relieve it. Patients with severe tetralogy of Fallot may become unconscious due to anoxia. In adults, tetralogy of Fallot is the most common type of cyanotic congenital heart disease, with most patients being underdeveloped.

Fingers and toes are clubbed, and arterial and jugular venous pulses are normal. Right ventricular heave is generally not conspicuous. S_1 is normal, P_2 is soft and delayed or totally absent, and A_2 is loud. An aortic ejection click is frequently audible; this is due to a dilated aorta as it receives the stroke volume of both the left and right ventricles. The systolic ejection murmur, audible over the mid-left sternal border, arises from the pulmonary infundibular stenosis. The intensity of the murmur has an indirect relationship to the severity of tetralogy of Fallot. A loud and long murmur indicates milder pulmonary stenosis and, hence, significant pulmonary blood flow. In cases of extreme tetralogy of Fallot and pulmonary atresia, continuous murmurs over the chest wall can be heard that are due to bronchial collaterals.

Laboratory Diagnosis

Electrocardiogram

Right atrial hypertrophy is only occasionally present. Typically, an ECG shows moderate right axis deviation and moderate right ventricular hypertrophy with a tall monophasic R in V_1 and rS pattern in V_2-V_6. This is in contrast to severe pulmonary stenosis with intact ventricular septum, in which tall R waves persist from V_1-V_3 and deep S waves are seen from V_4-V_6. In the acyanotic type of tetralogy of Fallot, there is biventricular hypertrophy.

Chest X-ray

The pulmonary artery segment is absent and the aorta is enlarged. A right-sided aortic arch is present in 25 percent of the patients. Heart size is frequently normal or slightly increased, with the cardiac silhouette being described as boot shaped. This appearance is due to concentric hypertrophy of the right ventricle and an underfilled left ventricle that lifts the cardiac apex. The lung fields show oligemia in the cyanotic type of tetralogy. In the acyanotic type, pulmonary vascular markings may be normal or even increased.

Echocardiography
Echocardiogram shows the biventricular origin of the aorta. Continuity between the posterior aortic wall and the anterior leaflet of the mitral valve is preserved.

Cardiac Catheterization
Cardiac catheterization is required to estimate the site and size of VSD, degree of pulmonary obstruction, and to detect the presence of other congenital heart abnormalities. Selective angiocardiography is extremely important in delineating the anatomy of the right ventricular outflow tract.

Differential Diagnosis

Pulmonary stenosis with patent foramen ovale, Eisenmenger's syndrome, Ebstein's anomaly, tricuspid atresia, and transposition of the great vessels should be considered in the differential diagnosis.

Natural History

The life history of this abnormality is related to the magnitude of the right-to-left shunt. Many patients can survive into adulthood, and survival into the sixties is not rare. Infective endocarditis of the pulmonary valve, paradoxical embolism, cerebral abscess, and cerebral thrombosis can punctuate the course of this disease.

Treatment

Medical treatment consists of antibiotic prophylaxis against infective endocarditis and control of hemoglobin levels by treating both anemia and excessive polycythemia. Propranolol has been found useful in the prevention of anoxic spells.

Treatment is primarily surgical, and the type of surgery is dependent on the weight of the patient at the time of diagnosis and the anatomy of the right ventricular outflow tract. If the body weight is less than 10 kg and the right ventricular outflow tract and pulmonary artery are well developed, total correction (closure of VSD and relief of pulmonary obstruction) should be carried out. Otherwise, palliative surgery consisting of a Blalock-Taussig operation (shunt between the pulmonary artery and subclavian artery) or a Waterston operation (shunt between the ascending aorta and pulmonary artery) should be performed. This shunting procedure permits increased pulmonary blood flow and results in improved oxygenation of blood. As these children improve and gain weight, total correction can follow. Complete right bundle-branch block and left axis deviation usually develop after total correction of the disease.

TRANSPOSITION OF THE GREAT ARTERIES

In this condition, the septum dividing the aorta from the pulmonary artery develops abnormally and results in the aorta arising from the right ventricle and the pulmonary artery arising from the left ventricle. The aorta lies anterior and parallel to the pulmonary artery that is located posteriorly.

Pathophysiology

The transposition described above in its pure form is incompatible with life; a mixing of blood between right and left side of the circulation through ASD, VSD, or PDA is required for survival. Most patients have an ASD, approximately two-thirds have a PDA, and one-third have VSD. As the pulmonary and systemic circulations are operating in parallel rather than in series, the shunt has to be bidirectional.

Clinical Features

This condition is more common in males and in offspring of diabetic mothers. The most common manifestations are dyspnea, cyanosis, heart failure, and growth retardation.

The aortic second sound is very loud due to the anterior location of the aorta. The type of murmur depends on associated abnormalities such as VSD, PDA, or pulmonic stenosis.

Laboratory Diagnosis

Electrocardiogram
Generally, the ECG shows right atrial enlargement, right axis deviation, and right ventricular hypertrophy. In patients with pulmonary stenosis, left ventricular hypertrophy is present.

Chest X-ray
Cardiomegaly is very common. The narrow mediastinum with cardiomegaly gives rise to an egg-shaped heart. The lung fields show pulmonary plethora.

Echocardiography
M-mode echocardiography, by demonstrating the anterior location of the aorta, is a useful diagnostic tool. Two-dimensional echocardiography is helpful in delineating the anatomic relationships of the great vessels.

Cardiac Catheterization
Cardiac catheterization reveals that oxygen saturation is much lower in the aorta than in the pulmonary artery. Sequential sampling is helpful in locating the level of the shunt. Pullback pressures show pulmonic stenosis. Angiocardiography is of primary importance in establishing a diagnosis and in defining the precise anatomy.

Natural History

Approximately 75 percent of untreated patients die by 6 months of age, and the remainder rarely survive to adulthood. Patients with large ASD or VSD and significant pulmonary stenosis have a good possibility of surviving infancy.

Treatment

Medical treatment consists of digitalis, diuretics, and oxygen for treatment of heart failure. In many infants, palliative procedures, for example, atrial septostomy, pulmonary artery banding, or systemic-pulmonary anastomosis may be required. Recently, Mustard's operation (rearranging the venous inflow) and Rastelli's operation (correcting the ventricular outflow) have been successful.

CORRECTED TRANSPOSITION OF THE GREAT ARTERIES

Inversion of the ventricles along with transposition of the great arteries results in physiologic correction of circulation. Venous blood from the systemic veins flows into the right atrium, across the mitral valve (bicuspid), into a ventricle having the anatomic characteristics of the left ventricle (fine trabeculation and no infundibulum), and is ejected into the pulmonary artery. Oxygenated blood from pulmonary veins flows into the left atrium, across the tricuspid valve into a ventricle that has characteristics of the right ventricle (coarse trabeculation and the presence of an infundibulum) and is ejected into the aorta; this arrangement is well tolerated. However, these patients are prone to other associated abnormalities such as incompetence of the tricuspid (left-sided) valve, VSD, pulmonary stenosis, and complete heart block causing circulatory difficulties. A_2 is very loud because of the anterior location of the aortic valve. An ECG shows absence of septal forces (q waves) in the left precordial leads and the presence of q waves in the right precordial leads. Chest x-ray demonstrates concavity in the region of the pulmonary segment and a smooth convexity of the high left border of the heart produced by a displaced ascending aorta. Diagnosis is established by angiocardiography. Treatment consists of surgical correction of associated abnormalities.

COARCTATION OF THE AORTA

Coarctation of the aorta occurs in one of every 2,000 people in the general population and is more common in men. Anatomically, there is a curtainlike infolding of the media at or just distal to the origin of the left subclavian artery and ligamentum anteriosum that causes obstruction to blood flow. This is called an adult-type coarctation. The infantile type of coarctation involves the segment of aorta proximal to the origin of the patent ductus arteriosus and has other associated abnormalities. The bicuspid aortic valve, VSD, mitral incompetence, endocardial fibroelastosis, and cerebral aneurysms may be associated with coarctation. Twenty percent of patients with Turner's syndrome exhibit coarctation.

Pathophysiology

The mechanism of hypertension in coarctation is still unclear. The major factor seems to be renal hypertension due to lack of pulsatile flow to the kidneys. Increased resistance at the site of coarctation also tends to increase the blood pressure.

Clinical Features

Many patients are asymptomatic while others complain of headaches, nosebleeds, cold feet, chest pain, and pain in the calves on walking. On physical examination, there is modest hypertension in the arms with absent, weak, or delayed pulses in the legs. A systolic pressure gradient of greater than 30 mm Hg between the right arm and legs is present. To establish a diagnosis of coarctation, simultaneous palpation of the radial and femoral pulses is extremely important. Many patients have only systolic hypertension, and hypertensive retinopathy is unusual. Thrills are palpable over the scapular areas and ribs, and continuous murmurs are audible because of marked enlargement of the collateral channels. The precordium reveals a left ventricular heave and S_4 due to left ventricular hypertrophy. S_1 is normal and A_2 is loud. An aortic ejection click may be present, indicating dilatation of the ascending aorta. A systolic ejection murmur over the right upper sternal border is usually present. It may be due to turbulence in the ascending aorta or to an associated bicuspid aortic valve. An early diastolic murmur due to aortic incompetence may be present. In the left interscapular area, a continuous murmur arising from the coarcted segment may be audible.

Laboratory Diagnosis

Electrocardiogram
The ECG shows left ventricular hypertrophy with systolic overload (pressure overwork).

Chest X-ray
The heart size is normal or moderately increased. The ascending aorta is also enlarged. Enlargement of the aortic knuckle and left subclavian artery, concavity of the coarcted region, and poststenotic dilatation give rise to a 3 sign (a figure-three configuration of the left margin of the aorta at the point of coarctation) on an anteroposterior chest x-ray. On esophagogram, there is a reversed 3 sign. The lower margin of the ribs reveal notching due to enlarged intercostal vessels.

Cardiac Catheterization and Angiocardiography
Cardiac catheterization is required to measure the pressure gradient across the coarcted segment and to detect associated conditions such as aortic valve disease due to a bicuspid aortic valve. Aortography is extremely important to define the degree and extent of coarctation.

Differential Diagnosis

Pseudocoarctation of the aorta (kinking and tortuosity without obstruction) and saddle embolism in the descending aorta should be considered in the differential diagnosis.

Natural History

Twenty-five percent of the patients survive into adulthood; the remaining 75 percent die from infective endocarditis, aortic rupture, heart failure, stroke, or coronary artery disease. Only 10 percent live beyond 50 years of age. Stroke can occur due to rupture of an associated cerebral aneurysm. Myelopathy may be caused by thrombosing anterior spinal arteries. A mycotic aneurysm may occur in the region of the poststenotic dilatation. Dissection of the aorta may occur. These patients are prone to develop infective endarteritis at the coarcted segment and endocarditis of the bicuspid aortic valve.

Treatment

The treatment is primarily surgical, the ideal age for surgical correction being 8-16 years. Surgical mortality is less than 5 percent. Due to the small size of the aorta during infancy, surgical correction may result in relative aortic stenosis and may require repeat surgery. In most patients, the blood pressure returns to normal within several weeks after surgery. Surgery is relatively contraindicated in elderly patients with coarctation who are asymptomatic and have a severely calcified aorta. Medical management consists of antibiotic prophylaxis against infective endocarditis and treatment of heart failure and hypertension.

PULMONARY STENOSIS

A valvular type of pulmonary stenosis is the most common type of obstructive disease in the right ventricular outflow tract. Obstruction of the supravalvular and subvalvular levels is less common. Right ventricular hypertrophy develops in response to an increased pressure overload on the right ventricle. Patients with mild (systolic gradient across the pulmonic valve, <50 mm Hg) and moderate (systolic gradient, 50-100 mm Hg) may be asymptomatic. Patients with severe obstruction (gradient >100 mm Hg) suffer from fatigue, dyspnea, and syncope. The jugular venous pulse shows a prominent a wave. A right ventricular heave is palpable. S_1 is normal, P_2 is soft and delayed or may be absent. A pulmonic ejection click may be audible. S_4 of right ventricular origin may also be present. The length of murmur and its peak correlate with the severity of stenosis. A longer murmur with a late peak indicates severe stenosis. With the development of right heart failure, functional tricuspid incompetence and right-to-left shunt through the foramen ovale may become manifest. The ECG shows right atrial enlargement, and right axis and right ventricular hypertrophy with strain. The height of R in lead V_1 correlates well with the degree of pulmonic stenosis. Chest x-ray shows prominent poststenotic dilatation and pulmonary oligemia in severe stenosis. In addition, the right atrium and right ventricle are enlarged. The objective of cardiac catheterization and angiocardiography is to localize the obstruction, estimate its severity, and rule out additional abnormalities. In patients with severe or moderately severe pulmonic stenosis, the treatment is primarily surgical.

EBSTEIN'S ANOMALY

The tricuspid valve tissue is redundant, and the septal and posterior valve leaflets are attached lower than normal so that the upper right ventricle becomes a portion of the right atrium. The tricuspid valve is frequently incompetent, the right ventricle is hypoplastic, and the foramen ovale is patent with a right-to-left shunt. Patients have features of tricuspid incompetence (tall v waves, pulsatile liver, systolic murmur with inspiratory accentuation), cyanosis, and atrial arrhythmias. S_1 and S_2 are widely split; S_3 and S_4 are frequently present. The ECG shows P pulmonale, right bundle-branch block, and a prolonged P-R interval. Chest x-ray reveals marked enlargement of the right atrium, a small right ventricle, and normal or oligemic lung fields. Echocardiography shows that tricuspid valve closure follows mitral valve closure. Careful pullback of the electrode catheter from the right ventricular apex demonstrates a chamber (between the right atrium above and right ventricle below) in which the pressure curve is characteristic of the right atrium and electrogram is characteristic of the right ventricle. Many patients survive only to the third or fourth decade. Treatment is the same as for heart failure. In a few patients, surgical replacement of the tricuspid valve is beneficial.

MALPOSITIONS OF THE HEART

When the cardiac apex lies on the right side of the midline, it is called dextrocardia; when it is located in the midline, it is described as mesocardia. Normally, the cardiac apex is located on the left side of the midline and is described as levocardia. Generally, no serious abnormality of the heart exists when dextrocardia is a part of situs inversus, that is, mirror image reversal of all body organs. On the other hand, serious congenital heart malformation occurs in patients with isolated dextrocardia or in levocardia with situs inversus.

QUESTIONS

(One or more answers for each question may be correct.)

1. The major technical limitations in obtaining an adequate echocardiographic examination are encountered in
   A. Obese patients
   B. Children
   C. Patients with obstructive lung disease
   D. Patients with myocardial infarction
2. A patient known to have Wolff-Parkinson-White syndrome is admitted to the emergency room with palpitations and a blood pressure of 80/40 mm Hg. An electrocardiogram shows grossly irregular wide QRS complexes occurring at a rate of 260/min. Which of the following statements concerning this condition are true?
   A. The patient has ventricular tachycardia that should be converted with electrical shock.
   B. The patient has atrial fibrillation but digitalis is contraindicated since it may result in ventricular fibrillation.
   C. The patient has atrial fibrillation; electrical cardioversion should be performed without delay.
   D. Propranolol should be used to reduce the ventricular rate.
   E. Quinidine or procainamide may be used on a long-

term basis to prevent recurrences of this tachyarrhythmia.

3. Atrial flutter with 2:1 atrioventricular block may be caused by
   A. Digitalis intoxication
   B. Pulmonary embolism
   C. Wolff-Parkinson-White syndrome
   D. Thyrotoxicosis
4. Atrioventricular dissociation due to nonparoxysmal junctional tachycardia is consistent with
   A. Myocardial infarction
   B. Digitalis toxicity
   C. Post open heart surgery
   D. Myocarditis
5. Which of the following statements regarding accelerated idioventricular rhythm are correct?
   A. It may cause atrioventricular dissociation.
   B. It usually occurs in patients with myocardial infarction.
   C. It usually does not cause hemodynamic deterioration and therefore needs no specific treatment.
   D. It causes marked hemodynamic deterioration and therefore requires immediate treatment.
   E. It commonly indicates disease of the His-Purkinje system.
6. Which of the following statements regarding ventricular tachycardia are correct?
   A. It is a benign rhythm and requires only observation.
   B. It is a serious cardiac arrhythmia and requires immediate attention.
   C. It usually does not cause any hemodynamic impairment.
   D. It may be associated with clinical and ECG manifestations of atrioventricular dissociation.
   E. It usually occurs in patients with no underlying heart disease.
7. Which of the following ECG features are helpful in differentiating between aberrantly conducted supraventricular beats and ventricular beats?
   A. Aberrantly conducted supraventricular beats show a triphasic rSR′ pattern in V_1.
   B. Aberrantly conducted supraventricular beats are likely to be followed by full compensatory pauses.
   C. Ventricular beats may be preceded by P waves.
   D. Beats showing different durations of QRS complexes depending on the coupling interval are more likely to be aberrantly conducted supraventricular beats.
   E. In a sustained wide QRS complex tachycardia, presence of ventricular capture and fusion beats favor ventricular tachycardia.
8. Which of the following statements concerning different types of second-degree atrioventricular block are correct?
   A. Mobitz Type II block is characterized by constant P-R intervals preceding a nonconducted P wave.
   B. Mobitz Type I (Wenckebach) block is characterized by variable P-R intervals preceding a nonconducted P wave.
   C. Location of second-degree atrioventricular block does not influence the prognosis.
   D. Mobitz type II block commonly occurs in acute inferior wall myocardial infarction.
   E. Mobitz type II block is frequently an indication for placement of a permanent pacemaker.
9. Which of the following features may be associated with an acquired complete atrioventricular block?
   A. Irregular cannon a waves and loud first heart sound
   B. Wide pulse pressure, reduced cardiac output, and systolic murmur at the base and apex
   C. Narrow pulse pressure and increased cardiac output
   D. Wide QRS complexes
   E. Ventricular rate usually faster than atrial rate
10. Which of the following hemodynamic findings are likely to be present in chronic congestive heart failure?
   A. Low cardiac output
   B. High left ventricular filling pressure
   C. Wide arteriovenous oxygen difference
   D. Increase of left ventricular filling pressure, arteriovenous oxygen difference, and decrease or no change in cardiac output during mild exercise
11. Which of the following physical signs are compatible with isolated left heart failure?
   A. Jugular venous distention
   B. Apical ventricular gallop
   C. Pulsus alternans
   D. Apical atrial gallop
   E. Pulmonary rales
12. Which of the following signs suggest excessive depletion of intravascular volume in a patient with heart failure who has been taking diuretics?
   A. Rising blood urea nitrogen
   B. Postural hypotension
   C. Excessive fatigue
   D. Loud ventricular gallop
13. Which of the following statements regarding the use of digitalis in heart failure are correct?
   A. Although digitalis causes vasoconstriction by a direct action, as heart failure improves there is withdrawal of excessive sympathetic tone; the net effect is decrease of systemic vascular resistance.
   B. Rapid administration of digitalis by an intravenous route may be potentially dangerous, since by causing

direct vasoconstriction it may increase the afterload excessively.

C. In a patient with chronic congestive heart failure and frequent premature ventricular beats (>6/min), digitalis is contraindicated.

D. Digitalis is very useful in a patient with tight mitral valve stenosis and sinus rhythm who suddenly develops pulmonary edema.

E. Digitalis is of little benefit in a patient who develops heart failure with the onset of atrial fibrillation with a rapid ventricular rate.

14. Which of the following conditions are compatible with rapid development of high jugular venous pressure?

A. Large acute pulmonary embolism
B. Rupture of the ventricular septum
C. Right ventricular infarction
D. Pericardial tamponade

15. Which of the following statements regarding the use of vasodilators for the treatment of marked heart failure are true?

A. Vasodilators decrease the systemic vascular resistance, cardiac output, and blood pressure.
B. Vasodilators increase the systemic vascular resistance, cardiac output, and blood pressure.
C. Vasodilators decrease the systemic vascular resistance, increase the cardiac output, and may have little influence on the blood pressure.
D. Vasodilators increase the preload by increasing the venous return.
E. Vasodilators reduce the preload.

16. Which of the following statements regarding acute pulmonary edema are correct?

A. It is almost always accompanied by jugular venous distention.
B. It is usually associated with hypoxia.
C. It is rarely associated with hypercarbia.
D. The patient should be encouraged to lie flat in this condition.
E. IV administration of morphine and rapidly acting diuretics, oxygen, and vasodilators constitute important steps in its treatment.

17. A 50-year-old man complains of epigastric discomfort along with dyspnea during exercise and relief after several minutes of rest. Which of the following conditions is this chest discomfort characteristic of:

A. Hiatus hernia
B. Angina pectoris
C. Aneurysm of the descending thoracic aorta
D. Gastric ulcer
E. Intestinal ischemic attacks due to mesenteric artery stenosis

18. A 45-year-old woman is hospitalized with episodes of anterior chest pain, palpitations, and dyspnea occurring almost daily at 4-5 AM for the last 3 months. Cardiac physical examination, routine ECG, and chest x-ray are entirely normal. Which of the following laboratory tests should be ordered first to detect the likely cause of her chest pain?

A. Repeat ECG
B. Echocardiogram
C. Exercise ECG
D. Upper gastrointestinal series
E. ECG during chest pain
F. Coronary angiography

19. Which of the following factors enhance the myocardial oxygen demand?

A. Enlarged left ventricular chamber
B. Slow heart rate
C. Increased contractility
D. Hypertension

20. A 60-year-old man enters the Coronary Care Unit with an acute inferior myocardial infarction. Physical examination reveals low amplitude pulse of 107 beats per minute, blood pressure 78/60 mm Hg, grossly distended neck veins, no apical S_3, and no pulmonary rales. Chest x-ray reveals normal lung fields. Which of the following therapies is indicated?

A. Patient has right heart failure and digitalis and diuretics are indicated.
B. Patient has cardiogenic shock and intravenous infusion of dopamine is indicated.
C. Intravenous digitalis is indicated to slow down the heart rate.
D. Swan-Ganz catheter should be inserted; pulmonary artery wedge pressure is likely to be low or normal, and low molecular weight dextran is indicated.
E. Patient is in cardiogenic shock and insertion of intra-aortic balloon for counterpulsation is indicated.

21. A patient with known history of hypertension is admitted to the Coronary Care Unit with an acute anterior myocardial infarction. Physical examination reveals that the patient is diaphoretic and tachypneic. Pulse is 156 beats per minute, and blood pressure is 98/50 mm Hg. ECG reveals atrial flutter with 2:1 AV block. Which of the following steps should be first in this patient's management?

A. Patient is in cardiogenic shock, intravenous dopamine is indicated.
B. Rapid ventricular rate is probably a major contributory factor for cardiogenic shock, immediate electrical cardioversion should be performed.
C. Intravenous propranolol should be administered to slow down the rapid ventricular rate.

D. Patient should be started on oral doses of digitalis to improve contractility and to slow down the ventricular rate.

E. Intravenous sodium nitroprusside and dobutamine are indicated to treat cardiogenic shock.

22a. A 45-year-old man is admitted to the CCU with acute inferior myocardial infarction. Physical examination reveals blood pressure of 80/50 mm Hg and ECG rhythm strip shows sinus bradycardia (heart rate 40/min). Which of the following should be the first step to treat hypotension and bradycardia?

A. Fluid challenge
B. Intravenous isoproterenol
C. Intravenous dopamine
D. Intravenous atropine
E. Temporary pacemaker

22b. The clinical status improved markedly after appropriate treatment. On the second hospital day the blood pressure is 110/70 mm Hg and ECG rhythm strip shows 5:4 Wenckebach type of second degree atrioventricular block. Which of the following steps should be taken for treating this arrhythmia?

A. Temporary pacemaker
B. Intravenous isoproterenol
C. Intravenous atropine
D. Oral ephedrine
E. Observation

22c. Sinus rhythm resumes on the fourth hospital day. In the afternoon of fourth hospital day, patient suddenly develops diaphoresis, shortness of breath, rales on lung bases, and blood pressure drops to 70/40 mm Hg. Careful physical examination reveals a grade 2/6 systolic murmur over the left lower sternal border. Which of the following conditions should be considered in the differential diagnosis?

A. Rupture of chordae tendineae
B. Rupture of ventricular septum
C. Rupture of left ventricular free wall
D. Partial rupture of papillary muscle

22d. Which of the following steps may be required to confirm the diagnosis and for further management?

A. Swan-Ganz catheterization
B. Left ventricular and coronary cineangiograms
C. Administration of vasodilators and Dopamine
D. intraaortic balloon counterpulsation
E. Surgical repair

23. Which of the following constitute(s) the most significant indicator of increased cardiovascular risk in a patient undergoing noncardiac surgery?

A. Right bundle-branch block
B. Transmural myocardial infarction 5 years ago
C. Atrial gallop (S_4)
D. Left anterior hemiblock
E. Ten multifocal premature ventricular beats per minute

24. Match the drugs in the column on the left to one of the statements on the right.

A. isosorbide dinitrate
B. hydralazine
C. prazosin
D. sodium nitroprusside

1. oral agent which blocks the alpha-adrenergic receptor and has a balanced vasodilatory effect in the systemic arterial and venous beds
2. direct-acting vasodilator agent, has a predominant effect in the systemic venous bed
3. vasodilator agent having a predominant effect in reducing severe pulmonary hypertension
4. rapidly acting vasodilator, administered as an intravenous infusion, balanced effect on the systemic arterial and venous beds
5. direct-acting vasodilator having a predominant effect on the arterial bed

25. Match the drugs in the column on the left to one of the statements on the right.

A. nitroglycerin
B. propranolol
C. verapamil

1. influences myocardial oxygen supply and demand balance favorably by reducing myocardial contractility and heart rate.
2. Influences myocardial oxygen supply and demand favorably by increasing coronary blood flow due to increased myocardial contractility and cardiac output.
3. Influences myocardial oxygen supply and demand balance favorably by decreasing preload and probably by increasing blood flow to the ischemic regions in the myocardium.
4. Causes vasodilatation by blocking Ca^{2+} channels

and is useful in variant angina.

26. A 50-year-old man with a history of exertional anterior chest discomfort for the last 2 years, complains of increased frequency and decreased exercise threshold of chest discomfort for the last 2 months. During these 2 months, he has experienced chest pain at rest and at night several times. Some of the chest pain episodes were prolonged, over 20 minutes, and were only partly relieved with sublingual nitroglycerin. Which one of the following steps should be taken for further management?
    A. Exercise stress test to further define the etiology of chest pain.
    B. Exercise thallium-201 scintigraphy to further clarify the etiology of chest pain.
    C. Refer the patient for emergency coronary angiography and coronary artery bypass surgery.
    D. Continue with sublingual nitroglycerin and start oral propranolol and isosorbide dinitrate as an outpatient.
    E. Admit the patient to the hospital and start propranolol and isosorbide dinitrate in progressively increasing doses. Following control of chest pain, consider performing coronary angiography and if critical narrowings are visualized, consider the patient for coronary artery bypass surgery.
27. Rheumatic fever most commonly affects:
    A. Indigent men
    B. Women in their 50's
    C. Children
    D. Newborn babies
28. Treatment of acute rheumatic fever may require use of which of the following drugs:
    A. Aspirin
    B. Penicillin
    C. Corticosteroids
    D. Isoproterenol
29. Significant obstruction to flow through the mitral valve does not occur until the normal valve area is reduced by:
    A. 10%
    B. 50%
    C. 90%
    D. 95%
30. The first presenting symptom of mitral stenosis may be:
    A. Dyspnea or easy fatigability
    B. Stroke
    C. Cough or hemoptysis
    D. Chest pain
31. The best way to assess the severity of mitral stenosis is:
    A. Cineangiography
    B. Electrocardiography
    C. Two-dimensional echocardiography
    D. M-mode echocardiography
32. A 29-year-old mother of two preschool age children presents for routine examination. She is noted to have sinus rhythm, a loud first heart sound, and a diastolic rumble with presystolic accentuation. Chest x-ray shows clear lung fields. Echocardiography shows mild mitral stenosis with a valve area of 2.2 square cm and a slightly dilated left atrium. Treatment should include:
    A. Digitalis
    B. Benzathine penicillin 1.2 million units intramuscularly each month
    C. Full dose antibiotic administration prior to dental procedures to prevent bacterial endocarditis
33. Which of the following is the most common complication of atrial fibrillation in patients who have mitral stenosis?
    A. Stroke
    B. Pulmonary embolism
    C. Heart failure
    D. Angina pectoris
34. Which of the following is least likely to be present in a patient with severe rheumatic mitral regurgitation?
    A. Atrial fibrillation
    B. Loud third heart sound
    C. Left ventricular enlargement
    D. Mitral opening snap
    E. Reversed splitting of the second heart sound
35. Which of the following is least likely to be seen in a patient with isolated severe aortic stenosis?
    A. Atrial fibrillation
    B. Syncope
    C. Peripheral edema
    D. Pulmonary congestion
    E. Left ventricular hypertrophy
36. Which of the following is least likely to be seen in a patient with isolated severe aortic regurgitation?
    A. Dyspnea on exertion
    B. Syncope
    C. Systolic murmur radiating to the neck
    D. Angina pectoris
    E. Paroxysmal nocturnal dyspnea

37a. A 50-year-old woman with severe isolated aortic regurgitation presents for her yearly examination; she is asymptomatic. Which of the following diagnositic procedure is unnecessary?
    A. Echocardiography
    B. Exercise radionuclide ventriculography
    C. Cineangiography

D. Electrocardiography

E. Chest roentgenography

37b. Which of the following modes of therapy is inappropriate?

A. Bacterial endocarditis prophylaxis

B. Digitalis

C. Diuretics

D. Rheumatic fever prophylaxis

38. The diagnostic procedure of choice for pericardial effusion is:

A. Chest x-ray

B. Echocardiogram

C. CO_2 infusion

D. Cardiac catheterization

39. Symptoms of acute pericarditis include all of the following *except*:

A. Chest pain

B. Fever

C. Dyspnea on exertion

D. Malaise and anorexia

40. All of the following statements concerning pericardial effusion and cardiac tamponade are true except:

A. Large quantities of fluid may cause no hemodynamic decompensation if the fluid accumulates slowly.

B. Tamponade should be suspected in any patient with a rising pulse rate, rising jugular pressure, and falling blood pressure.

C. Pulsus paradoxicus is recognized as a fall in blood pressure during deep inspiration.

D. Needle pericardiocentesis should be performed in patients with cardiac tamponade if open surgical pericardiectomy cannot be performed before severe hemodynamic deterioration occurs.

41. All of the following are common symptoms of constrictive pericarditis *except*:

A. Ascites

B. Dyspnea

C. Hepatic congestion

D. Edema

E. Chest pain which increases with inspiration

42. The best indication for urgent valve replacement in patients with acute endocarditis is:

A. Severe heart failure

B. Endocarditis of the aortic valve

C. Recurrent pulmonary emboli

D. Signs of systemic embolization such as petechiae and Roth's spots

43. Which of the following valves is most commonly affected by endocarditis in heroin addicts?

A. Aortic

B. Mitral

C. Pulmonary

D. Tricuspid

E. Eustachian

44. Which of the following statements about hypertrophic cardiomyopathy is/are true?

A. IHSS is a frequent cause of death in young patients.

B. The most frequent symptoms of IHSS are angina and dyspnea.

C. Valsalva's maneuver causes the systolic murmur of IHSS to become softer.

D. The electrocardiogram is almost always abnormal in patients with significant IHSS.

E. Characteristic echocardiographic findings of IHSS include asymmetric septal hypertrophy and systolic anterior motion of the mitral valve.

45. Which of the following physical signs indicate the presence of a large intracardiac left-to-right shunt?

A. Loud S3

B. Loud S4

C. Middiastolic rumble across atrioventricular valves

D. Hyperkinetic precordium

E. Cyanosis

46. Which of the following physical signs and laboratory tests indicate the development of pulmonary vascular disease and pulmonary hypertension in a patient previously known to have left-to-right shunt?

A. Prominent a waves in the jugular venous pulse

B. Loud pulmonary component of S2

C. High frequency early diastolic murmur along left upper sternal border

D. Progressively diminishing intensity and duration of previously loud systolic murmur

E. Progressive prominence of central pulmonary vessels and diminution of peripheral pulmonary vessels

F. Right axis deviation

G. Development of functional tricuspid incompetence

47. Which of the following statements concerning an atrial septal defect of the secundum variety are correct?

A. Second heart sound is widely split and varies little with phases of respiration.

B. Second heart sound is widely split and shows considerable variation with phases of respiration.

C. Precordial systolic murmur is usually produced by left-to-right shunt occurring at the atrial level.

D. Precordial systolic murmur is usually produced by augmented pulmonary blood flow across the pulmonary valve.

E. In young adults, large left-to-right shunt causes high pulmonary artery pressure but the pulmonary vascular resistance is usually normal.

F. Middiastolic rumble at left lower sternal border showing an inspiratory increase in intensity usually indicates >2:1 left-to-right shunt.

48. A 19-year-old boy is referred for evaluation of a heart murmur. On physical examination the blood pressure is 110/60 mm Hg, jugular venous pulse is normal, and pulse is regular. The apical impulse is displaced downward and leftward. There is a systolic thrill over the left midsternal area. A grade 4/6 pansystolic murmur is audible over the left midsternal area. S1 is covered by the murmur. S2 is widely split with considerable respiratory variation. An S3 followed by a middiastolic rumble is heard over the apex. ECG shows biventricular hypertrophy and chest x-ray shows increased pulmonary vascularity. Which of the following conditions are compatible with the above mentioned findings?
   A. Atrial septal defect
   B. Ventricular septal defect
   C. Patent ductus arteriosus
   D. Aortopulmonary septal defect (window)
   E. Transposition of great vessels

49. Which of the following conditions can develop in the natural history of a ventricular septal defect?
   A. Aortic regurgitation
   B. Congestive heart failure
   C. Infective endocarditis
   D. Progressive decrease in the size of the defect
   E. Eisenmenger syndrome
   F. Infundibular stenosis

50. A 14-year-old girl is diagnosed as having a moderate left-to-right shunt through a patent ductus arteriosus (PDA). She is quite active in several sports and is entirely asymptomatic. What would you recommend?
   A. Antibiotic prophylaxis against infective endarteritis until surgical division of PDA
   B. Long-term rheumatic prophylaxis
   C. Curtailment of intense physical activity
   D. Surgical division of PDA on an elective basis
   E. Regular observation until the development of cardiac symptoms and then recommend surgical treatment

ANSWERS

1. C
2. B, C, E
3. A, B, C, D
4. A, B, C, D
5. A, B, C
6. B, D
7. A, C, D, E
8. A, B, E
9. A, B, D
10. A, B, C, D
11. B, C, E
12. A, B, C
13. A, B
14. A, B, C, D
15. C, E
16. B, C, E
17. B
18. E
19. A, C, D
20. D
21. B

22a. D
22b. E
22c. B, D
22d. A, B, C, D, E

23. E
24. A, 2; B, 5; C, 1; D, 4
25. A, 3; B, 1; C, 4
26. E
27. C
28. A, B, C
29. B
30. A, B, C
31. C
32. B, C
33. A
34. E
35. A
36. B

37a. C
37b. D

38. B
39. C
40. C
41. E
42. A
43. D
44. A, B, D, E
45. A, C, D
46. All correct
47. A, D, E, F
48. B
49. All correct
50. A, D

BIBLIOGRAPHY

TEXTBOOKS AND MONOGRAPHS

General Textbooks

Bonchek LI, Brooks HL (eds): Office Management of Medical and Surgical Heart Disease: A Concise Guide for Physicians. Boston: Little, Brown & CO, 1981.

Braunwald E (ed): Heart Disease. Philadelphia: W B Saunders Co, 1980.

Fowler NO: Cardiac Diagnosis and Treatment, ed. 3. Hagerstown: Harper & Row, Publishers Inc, 1980.

Hurst JW, Logue RB (eds): The Heart, Arteries and Veins, ed. 4. New York: McGraw-Hill, 1978.

Phillips RE: Cardiovascular Therapy: A Systematic Approach. Volume 1, Circulation. Philadelphia: W B Saunders Co, 1979.

Selzer A: Principles of Clinical Cardiology: An Analytical Approach. Philadelphia: W B Saunders Co, 1975.

History and Physical Examination

Gazes PC: Clinical Cardiology: A Bedside Approach. Chicago: Year Book Medical Publishers Inc, 1975.

Leatham A: Auscultation of the Heart and Phonocardiography, ed. 2. New York: Churchill Livingstone Inc, 1975.

Tavel ME: Clinical Phonocardiography and External Pulse Recording, ed. 3. Chicago: Year Book Medical Publishers Inc, 1978.

Electrocardiography

Fisch C (ed): Complex Electrocardiography. Cardiovascular Clinics, Volume 5, No. 3. Philadelphia: F A Davis Co, 1973.

Fisch C (ed): Complex Electrocardiography. Cardiovascular Clinics, Volume 6, No. 1. Philadelphia: F A Davis Co, 1974.

Lipman BS, Kleiger RE, Massie E: Clinical Scalar Electrocardiography. 6th Edition. Chicago: Year Book Medical Publishers Inc, 1972.

Schlant RC, Hurst JW (eds): Advances in Electrocardiography. Volume 2. New York: Grune & Stratton Inc, 1976.

Noninvasive Techniques of Cardiac Diagnosis

Ellestad MH: Stress Testing: Principles and Practices, ed. 2. Philadelphia: F A Davis Co, 1980.

Feigenbaum H: Echocardiography, ed. 3. Philadelphia: Lea & Febiger, 1981.

Soin JS, Brooks HL (eds): Nuclear Cardiology for Clinicians. Mount Kisco, New York: Futura Publishing Co Inc, 1980.

Congestive Heart Failure

Braunwald E, Ross J, Sonnenblick EH: Mechanisms of Contraction of the Normal and Failing Heart, ed. 2. Boston: Little, Brown & Co, 1976.

Mason DT: Congestive Heart Failure: Mechanisms, Evaluation and Treatment. New York: Yorke Medical Books, 1976.

Coronary Heart Disease

Cohn PF (ed): Diagnosis and Therapy of Coronary Artery Disease. Boston: Little, Brown & Co, 1979.

Karliner JS, Gregoratos G: Coronary Care. New York: Churchill Livingstone Inc, 1981.

Rackley CE, Russell RO Jr: Coronary Artery Disease: Recognition and Management. Mount Kisco, New York: Futura Publishing Co Inc, 1979.

Primary Myocardial Disease

Fowler NO: Myocardial Diseases. New York: Grune & Stratton Inc, 1973.

Congenital Heart Disease

Perloff JK: The Clinical Recognition of Congenital Heart Disease, ed. 2. Philadelphia: W B Saunders Co, 1978.

Roberts WC (ed): Congenital Heart Disease in Adults. Philadelphia: F A Davis Co, 1979.

ARTICLES

Electrocardiography

Kennedy HL, Caralis DG: Ambulatory electrocardiography: A clinical perspective. *Ann Intern Med* 87:729-739, 1977.

Rosen KM: Cardiac electrophysiology symposium. *Arch Intern Med* 135:387-479, 1975.

Noninvasive Techniques of Cardiac Diagnosis

Morganroth J, Pohost GM: Symposium: Two-dimensional echocardiography versus cardiac nuclear imaging techniques. *Am J Cardiol* 47: 1093-1288, 1980.

Cardiac Arrhythmias

Wit AL, Rosen MR, Hoffman BF: Electrophysiology and pharmacology of cardiac arrhythmias. *Am Heart J* 88: 380-385, 515-524, 664-670, 798-806, 1974. 89: 115-122, 253-257, 391-399, 526-536, 665-673, 804-808, 1975. 90: 117-122, 265-272, 397-404, 521-533, 665-675, 795-803, 1975.

Congestive Heart Failure

Braunwald E: Regulation of the circulation. *N Engl J Med* 290: 1124-1129, 1420-1425, 1974.

Chatterjee K, Parmley WW: The role of vasodilator therapy in heart failure. *Prog Cardiovasc Dis* 19:301-325, 1977.

Cohn JN, Franciosa JA: Vasodilator therapy of heart failure. *N Engl J Med* 297:27-31, 254-258, 1977.

Goldberg LI, Hsieh YY, Resnekov L: Newer catecholamines for treatment of heart failure and shock: An update on dopamine and a first look at dobutamine. *Prog Cardiovasc Dis* 19:327-340, 1977.

Mason DT: Symposium on vasodilator and inotropic therapy of heart failure. *Am J Med* 65:101-216, 1978.

Coronary Heart Disease

Braunwald E: Control of myocardial oxygen consumption: Physiologic and clinical considerations. *Am J Cardiol* 27:416-432, 1971.

Braunwald E: Protection of the ischemic myocardium. *Circulation* 53 (3 Suppl 1):I1-228, 1976.

Corday E, Dodge HT: Symposium on identification and management of the candidate for sudden cardiac death. *Am J Cardiol* 39:813-937, 1977.

Forrester JS, Diamond G, Chatterjee K, Swan HJC: Medical therapy of acute myocardial infarction by application of hemodynamic subsets. *N Engl J Med* 295:1356-1362, 1404-1413, 1976.

Hillis LD, Braunwald E: Coronary-artery spasm. *N Engl J Med* 299: 695-702, 1978.

McIntosh HD, Garcia JA: The first decade of aortocoronary bypass grafting, 1967-1977. A review. *Circulation* 57:405-431, 1978.

Proudfit WL, Bruschke AVG, Sones FM Jr: Natural history of obstructive coronary artery disease: Ten-year study of 601 nonsurgical cases. *Prog Cardiovasc Dis* 21:53-78, 1978.

Ross RS: Ischemic heart disease: An overview. Am J Cardiol 36:496-505, 1975.

Schwartz A (ed): Symposium on Cardiovascular Disease and Calcium Antagonists. *Am J Cardiol* 49:497-636, 1982.

Sheldon WC, Rincon G, Pichard AD, Razavi M, Cheanvechai C, Loop FD: Surgical treatment of coronary artery disease: Pure graft operations, with a study of 741 patients followed 3-7 years. *Prog Cardiovasc Dis* 18:237-253, 1975.

Valvular Heart Disease

Devereux RB, Perloff JK, Reichek N, Josephson ME: Mitral valve prolapse. *Circulation* 54:3-14, 1976.

Perloff JK: Clinical recognition of aortic stenosis: The physical signs and differential diagnosis of the various forms of obstruction to left ventricular outflow. *Prog Cardiovasc Dis* 10:323-352, 1968.

Perloff JK, Roberts WC: The mitral apparatus: Functional anatomy of mitral regurgitation. *Circulation* 46:227-239, 1972.

Rahimtoola SH: Outcome of aortic valve surgery: Key references. *Circulation* 60:1191-95, 1979.

Reichek N, Shelburne JC, Perloff JK: Clinical aspects of rheumatic valvular disease. *Prog Cardiovasc Dis* 15:491-537, 1973.

Selzer A, Cohn KE: Natural history of mitral stenosis: A review. *Circulation* 45:878-890, 1972.

Diseases of the Pericardium

Spodick DH: Acute pericardial disease: Pericarditis, effusion and tamponade. *J Contin Educ Cardiol* 14:9-27, 1979.

Wood P: Chronic constrictive pericarditis. *Am J Cardiol* 7:48-61, 1961.

Infective Endocarditis

Weinstein L, Schlesinger JJ: Pathoanatomic, pathophysiologic and clinical correlations in endocarditis. *N Engl J Med* 291:832-837, 1122-1126, 1974.

Primary Myocardial Disease

Maron BJ, Epstein SE: Hypertrophic cardiomyopathy: Recent observations regarding the specificity of three hallmarks of the disease: asymmetric septal hypertrophy, septal disorganization and systolic anterior motion of the anterior mitral leaflet. *Am J Cardiol* 45:141-154, 1980.

Congenital Heart Diseases

Dave KS, Pakrashi BC, Wooler GH, Ionescu MI: Atrial septal defect in adults: Clinical and hemodynamic results of surgery. *Am J Cardiol* 31:7-13, 1973.

Hallidie-Smith KA, Goodwin JF: The Eisenmenger syndrome. *In* Progress in Cardiology, Vol. 3, PN Yu and JF Goodwin (eds.). Philadelphia: Lea & Febiger, pp. 211-25, 1974.

Higgins CB, Mulder DG: Tetralogy of Fallot in the adult. *Am J Cardiol* 29:837-846, 1972.

Weidman WH, Blount SG Jr, DuShane JW, Gersony WM, Hayes CJ, Nadas AS: Clinical course in ventricular septal defect. *Circulation* 56 (Suppl I): I 56-69, 1977.

ACKNOWLEDGMENTS

The following sections have been contributed by Virinderjit S. Bamrah: History, Physical Examination, Electrocardiography, Other Noninvasive Techniques of Cardiac Diagnosis, Cardiac Catheterization, Cardiac Arrhythmias, Congestive Heart Failure, Coronary Heart Disease, and Congenital Heart Diseases.

The following sections have been contributed by L. Samuel Wann: Valvular Heart Disease, Diseases of the Pericardium, Injective Endocarditis, and Primary Myocardial Diseases.

CHAPTER 4
DISEASES OF THE SKIN AND APPENDAGES

Charles Zugerman

The overall scope of cutaneous disease is difficult to assess, considering the overwhelming differences between populations and subpopulations. The region of the world must be precisely defined, as well as whether the research is dealing with normal individuals, hospitalized patients, or outpatients visiting a variety of primary care or specialty medical facilities. Age, race, and socioeconomic factors must also be considered in detail.

Between 1971 and 1974, the United States Department of Health, Education, and Welfare performed the "Health and Nutritional Examination Survey" on 20,749 individuals between the ages of 1 and 74. Their findings suggest that 31.2% of these Americans had some significant dermatologic pathology, while roughly 6.4% had two diseases, and 3.1% had three diseases. The incidence increased until the age of 24 (as a result of acne), at which time it began to decline. The most common groups of diseases included sebaceous gland pathology (acne), a dermatophytosis (tinea, ringworm), benign and malignant tumors, and seborrheic dermatitis (dandruff).

Besides considering the volume of dermatologic disease, the overall impact cutaneous disease can have on these patients should be discussed. It has been estimated that skin disease costs Americans in excess of 1.5 billion dollars annually in disability. A worker whose hands do not function cannot perform adequately and must either be laid off or moved to a different job. A person who cannot stand or move about because of foot dermatitis cannot function adequately. Second, dermatologic disease is a source of severe discomfort. Patients may present to the dermatologist earlier with severe pruritus or burning than with jaundice or malaise. The inability to sleep because of intense nocturnal pruritus is an extremely convincing stimulus. Third, cutaneous disease can lead to severe cosmetic disfigurement resulting in job loss, loss of self-esteem, psychiatric decompensation, and alienation from friends and family. The patient with facial lesions such as acne vulgaris may develop a distorted image that may be difficult, if not impossible, to correct. Changes in the skin also may be important clues to serious internal disease. A cutaneous eruption may lead an observant physician to the correct diagnosis of an internal malignant tumor, connective tissue disease, or endocrine disease.

The chapter is divided into three major sections. The first deals with initial evaluation and basic therapy of skin diseases. The second is a more specific discussion of commonly encountered skin disorders. The last section deals with dermatologic clues that may suggest the presence of serious internal disease.

EVALUATION AND BASIC THERAPY OF DERMATOLOGIC DISEASES

EVALUATION OF THE PATIENT

The history allows the physician to characterize correctly both the patient and the disease, while the physical examination records the nature of the disease at the time the patient is seen by the physician.

History

There are three important aspects of the disease that need to be determined by a complete history: the characteristics of the disease, the relationship of the patient to the disease, and the role of medications in the disease.

The Illness

In the course of elucidating the patient's chief complaint, it is important to know its temporal sequence of involvement including when the patient first noted a problem, whether the problem has waxed and waned, when the problem became worse, and over what period the different lesions developed. Pityriasis rosea is a good example of the importance of this sequence. Classically, a herald patch develops several days to a few weeks prior to the onset of the entire eruption.

A second important characteristic of the disease is the pattern of involvement of the skin. On what area of the skin did the problem begin and what additional areas became involved as the problem progressed? The initial area of involvement is important in determining the cause of the patient's contact dermatitis. The next question is: How ill does the disease make the patient feel? Certain diseases are accompanied by high fever, malaise, weakness, and loss of appetite. In taking a history it is important to elicit from the patient such systemic symptoms since frequently these symptoms are caused by serious sytemic disease. Finally, has the patient's lesion itched, bled, ulcerated, or spread beyond its original borders? Some of these features may be signs of a malignant tumor.

The Patient

The patient's age is particularly important. There are diseases that are age specific such as acne vulgaris, atopic dermatitis, tinea infections, tumors, and seborrheic dermatitis. Acne occurs in the teens and early twenties. Atopic dermatitis is primarily a disease of children and some tinea infections disappear as the patient reaches puberty. Seborrheic dermatitis begins in infancy, subsides during childhood, returns in puberty, and increases in severity until old age.

The physician must also be aware of the patient's occupational background, including previous jobs, materials handled on the job, environment, hobbies, and materials handled at home. A worker in a manufacturing plant has a much higher incidence of chrome sensitivity and the dermatitis may easily represent a contact allergy to chrome. A worker in the petrochemical industry may be at significantly higher risk for developing mycosis fungoides. A patient who continually washes his hands with industrial solvents (such as turpentine) may develop an irritant contact dermatitis.

Racial considerations are important since certain diseases affect one race more than others and certain dermatologic diseases are manifest differently in different groups. For instance, black patients have a significantly higher incidence of sarcoidosis, but because of their deep pigmentation are less likely to have basal cell carcinoma. An eczematous eruption on a black patient is more likely to cause lichenification than it is on a white person. On the other hand, white patients with Kaposi's sarcoma have a more benign course than a black African with the same disease.

Family history is important in several respects. Diseases such as ichthyosis, psoriasis, acne, and baldness frequently appear in families. In addition, an individual with an eczema who has a strong family history of asthma, hay fever, urticaria, or other allergies may be more likely to have atopic eczema. Finally, it is beneficial to become aware of genetic malformations that appear in the patient's family.

The patient's birthplace and areas of the world visited are important considerations in the dermatologic history. It has already been pointed out that the prognosis of Kaposi's sarcoma in a black African differs markedly from that of a white American. Moreover, a patient presenting with a warty tumor on his face, who recently visited the San Joaquin Valley, may be suspected of having coccidioidomycosis, which is a deep fungal infection of the skin. Likewise, yaws is primarily a tropical disease, while blastomycosis is frequently discovered in the midwestern United States.

Finally, the patient's past medical history is important. Has the patient had the disease in the past? For instance, if the patient has pityriasis rosea and develops a similar eruption two or three times, the diagnosis should be seriously questioned. Has the patient been or is she now pregnant? Not only does pregnancy dictate which drugs may not be used but, in addition, there are diseases and physiologic processes that are more common in pregnant women.

The Medications

The patient's medication list is extremely important in determining both the etiology and future treatment of the disease process. If the patient has urticaria and is taking penicillin, the drug may be causing the urticaria. In evaluating the patient's medications, it is important to determine the length of time on the drug, the reason for taking it, and whether its administration preceded the patient's current problem.

Physical Examination

On physical examination specific note is made of features of the skin, condition of the hair, nails, and mucous membranes, and the type, grouping, and distribution of lesions.

Features of the Skin

The skin of the entire body should be examined, even if only one area is involved, since lesions can be discovered in places impossible for the patient to visualize. For example, lesions in the intergluteal cleft suggest psoriasis, whereas lacy-white mouth lesions may imply lichen planus. The texture, moisture, and color of the skin should also be inspected. In dermatologic examinations, it is important to feel the skin; it may feel smooth and soft, rough and scaly, or hard. Change in texture may lead to the diagnosis of pituitary abnormalities, scleroderma, myxedema, or amyloidosis. It may also imply that metabolic substances are being deposited in the skin or that the growth patterns of the skin are abnormal. Excessive moisture of the skin may imply thyrotoxicosis or fever. Abnormal dryness may be observed with diseases such as atopic dermatitis, ichthyosis, chronic nephritis, or myxedema. In addition, dryness can be caused by large doses of drugs such as atropine. Finally, color of skin can change based on changes in its vascularity, deposition of melanin exogenous pigments, or hyperkeratosis. Cyanosis of the skin may be caused by a reduced blood hemoglobin, while erythema may be observed as a result of excessive blood flow to the area. Carotene, a derivative of certain plants, may give the body an overall yellow hue, whereas normal pigmentation such as melanin is brown.

Condition of the Hair, Nails, and Mucous Membranes

Examination of the hair, nails, and mucous membranes constitutes an important part of the dermatologic evaluation; even if they are not directly involved by disease, there can be changes in these areas that may direct a physician toward the correct diagnosis.

During the lifetime of an individual, hair follows a certain pattern of evolution. In the neonate, hair rapidly changes from the anagen to telogen phase and is usually lost between the ages of 6-12 weeks. Prior to puberty, as the sex hormones begin secreting, hair grows in the axillary and pubic areas. Baldness begins with aging, can occur in both men and women, and follows a pattern of predominant loss at occipital and frontal areas and recession of the hairline. Hair patterns closely follow the development of an individual as a whole. The physician should determine if there is excessive (hypertrichosis) or too little (hypotrichosis) hair, and the distribution of the abnormality should be noted. Bitemporal hair loss suggests a male pattern baldness, while generalized hair loss is more suggestive of a drug reaction or a systemic disease. Examination of the hair implies examination of the scalp and, in this regard, the presence or absence of scarring and inflammation is important. In addition, the hair shaft should be examinated under a microscope in order to determine whether hair loss is secondary to breakage or to narrowing of the hair shaft. Finally, the relative number of anagen versus telogen hair should be noted. Anagen hair may be recognized by its size, as well as by the presence of a normal sheath or covering, and normal pigmentation near the root. Telogen hairs are smaller, have a white bulb, and lack a normal sheath. Anagen hairs represent growing hairs, while telogen are resting hairs. A large percentage of telogen hairs may also indicate disease.

Fingernails and toenails serve to protect the digits and are important diagnostic aids for the physician. There is a long list of skin diseases that present with nail manifestations. In several instances, it may be almost impossible to make a correct diagnosis of the skin disorder without examining the nails. For instance, psoriasis can present with pitting of the nails, with hyperkeratosis, or discoloration of the nails. Lichen planus, on the other hand, can also present with pitting but more commonly the nails become dystrophic. In severe cases of alopecia areata, the nails show pitting suggestive of psoriasis. Nails can be involved in severe cases of Norwegian scabies. Connective tissue disease, such as lupus erythematosus and dermatomyositis, may present with telangiectasis surrounding the nail bed. Nails can also be involved in systemic disease, including connective tissue diseases, and infectious diseases, such as subacute bacterial endocarditis (splinter hemorrhage). Clubbing of the nails may be an important sign of systemic disease. Half-and-half nails, which appear white proximally and normal distally, have been seen in cases of renal failure, and white parallel bands on the nail are observed in some albuminemic patients. Typical nail changes may be noted in iron deficiency anemia, thyroid disease, and argyria. Nail involvement with typical brown pigmentation may be a sign of malignant melanoma arising in the nail bed. Finally, drugs such as arsenic or silver may cause typical silver discoloration of the nail plate and lunula.

Examination of mucous membranes of the mouth, nose, eyes, and vagina is important in the diagnosis of certain illnesses such as Addison's disease and Peutz-Jeghers syndrome because of distinctive pigmentary patterns. In addition, typical changes of lichen planus (lacy-white infiltrates) can be seen in the mouth (Plate 1). Certain blistering diseases such as bullous pemphigoid, pemphigoid, pemphigus vulgaris, and erythema multiforme are sometimes diagnosed because they present with mouth lesions. Finally, *Candida* infection of the mucous membranes may at times suggest severe systemic illness.

Type of Lesions

Skin lesions may be either primary or secondary. Primary lesions are those that appear on the skin as a result of the disease. Secondary lesions are created by the patient as he responds to the disease. Secondary lesions therefore are of little help in determining the type of disease affecting the skin. An example of a primary lesion is a blister of herpes simplex. An example of a secondary lesion is an excoriation created by the patient as a result of intense pruritus. The following is a list of the primary skin lesions and their definitions:

1. *Macule.* A macule is a nonpalpable circumscribed area that differs from surrounding skin because of changes in vascularity or pigmentation. An example is the macular depigmentation of vitiligo.
2. *Papule.* A papule is an elevated lesion usually less than 5 mm in diameter. Examples are lichen planus, psoriasis, and warts.
3. *Nodule.* A nodule is usually deeper than a papule and ranges in size from 5-50 mm. An example is a common nevus.
4. *Tumor.* A tumor is an extremely large palpable lesion usually greater than 5 cm in diameter. Tumors frequently represent serious cutaneous disease. Examples are squamous cell carcinoma and deep fungal infection.
5. *Plaque.* A plaque is a lesion that has a large surface area compared to its depth. Usually plaques are larger than 2 cm in diameter and may form as a result of coalescence of papules. Examples are psoriasis, parapsoriasis, and mycosis fungoides.
6. *Vesicles and bullae.* Vesicles and bullae can be included in the same classification. A vesicle is a lesion that is elevated and contains clear fluid; it is usually less than 5 mm in

diameter. A bulla is basically the same lesion but is greater than 5 mm. An example of a vesicle is herpes simplex; examples of bullae are burn blisters and bullous pemphigoid.

7. *Pustule.* A pustule is an elevated lesion containing purulent material rather than clear fluid. Examples include acne, impetigo, and pustular psoriasis.
8. *Wheal.* A wheal is a palpable lesion that is formed secondary to edema in the upper dermis. Wheals are generally transient and rapidly change in size and shape. An example is urticaria.
9. *Cyst.* A cyst is a lesion that has an epithelial lining and contains liquid or semisolid material. Examples are acne and epidermal cysts.
10. *Scale.* A scale is a lesion that forms secondary to the accumulation of squamous debris. Examples include psoriasis, and pityriasis rosea.

The following is a list of lesions that are usually secondarily produced by the patient:

1. *Crust.* A crust is an accumulation of serum, bacteria, and cells on top of damaged epidermis. An example of this is impetigo.
2. *Lichenification.* Lichenification is an accentuation of skin markings resulting from severe itching and scratching. Lichenification is typical of diseases such as neurodermatitis and atopic dermatitis.
3. *Fissure.* A fissure is a crack in the epidermis frequently seen with chronic contact dermatitis.
4. *Erosion.* An erosion usually occurs after a blister has broken and results from a loss of the epidermis. Erosions are usually not as deep as ulcerations and rarely result in scarring. An example of an erosion is herpes simplex.
5. *Ulcers.* Ulcers are much deeper than erosions and frequently extend into the dermis or even subcutaneous spaces. Marked scarring usually occurs. Ulcers can either be primary or secondary, depending upon the disease in question. Examples are diabetic and stasis ulcerations.
6. *Excoriations.* Excoriations are linear erosions of the skin that are self-induced by the patient's scratching. Excoriations can be observed in cases of chronic pruritus or scabies.
7. *Scars.* Scars represent normal physiologic healing of the skin after deeper injury. Scars are usually secondary to other disease processes and are seen in acne and after infections or deep lacerations of the skin.
8. *Atrophy.* Atrophy implies thinning of the skin. Either the epidermis or the dermis can be thinned, and in each case different diseases should be considered. In many instances, atrophy is a secondary phenomenon such as when corticosteroids are injected into the skin causing it to atrophy. However, there are a few diseases of the skin in which atrophy is of primary importance such as lichen sclerosus et atrophicus.

Grouping of Lesions

Grouping implies the relationship of one lesion to its neighbor. The following is a list of the common groupings seen in dermatology.

1. *Linear.* Lesions are present in a straight line. For instance, in plant dermatitis the patient casually brushes against an allergenic plant such as poison ivy and the antigen is applied to the skin in a linear fashion. Linear lesions can also be seen with diseases that disseminate along lymphatic channels such as sporotrichosis.
2. *Arcuate.* This implies an arc-shaped lesion and is commonly seen with urticaria.
3. *Serpiginous.* This lesion is snakelike and is typical of urticaria.
4. *Herpetiform or zosteriform.* These lesions exist in small groups and frequently have a dermatomal distribution. As the name implies, zosteriform lesions are present in herpes zoster, while herpes simplex is herpetiform.
5. *Reticulated.* These are netlike lesions present in livedo reticularis.
6. *Iris.* Iris or target lesions consist of a dark inner circle with a surrounding light circle and a second dark outer circle. Iris lesions are typical of erythema multiforme.
7. *Guttate.* Guttate lesions are droplike in appearance and are present in individuals with psoriasis or parapsoriasis.
8. *Round Lesions.* There are various kinds of round lesions, including nummular, or coin-shaped; discoid, or disc-shaped; annular, or ring-shaped; and circinate, or circle-shaped. Nummular lesions are commonly seen in nummular eczema, while discoid lesions are observed in discoid lupus erythematosus, and annular lesions are seen in common tinea.

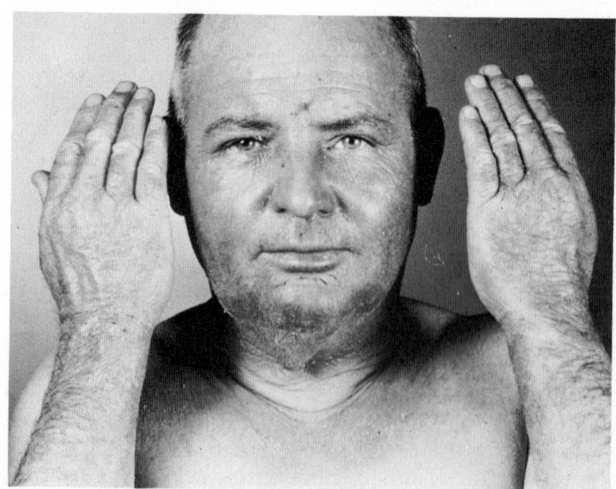

Figure 1. The classic distribution of photodermatitis includes the V of the neck, the face, and the hands.

Distribution of Lesions

In certain instances, knowing the distribution of lesions on the body is essential to make the correct diagnosis. Contact dermatitis, for instance, occurs over the area of distribution of the antigen. In shoe dermatitis, the area of contact is the dorsum of the feet, whereas in nickel dermatitis, eczema is frequently seen at the site where jewelry is worn. On the other hand, if the patient is allergic to sunlight, one might notice distribution of the eczema over the areas normally exposed to the sun. Therefore, one would expect to see an erythematous eruption on the face, chin, the V-area of the neck, and perhaps the hands and arms, with notable sparing of the submental areas and the skin beneath the nose (Fig. 1). If the patient has Koebner's phenomenon (develops lesions in areas exposed to trauma), psoriasis or lichen planus should be seriously suspected since this is a common finding. If the lesions occur in the antecubital space and posterior popliteal surfaces of the skin, atopic dermatitis should be seriously considered. A symmetric, bilateral eruption is most likely a drug eruption and not contact dermatitis.

Procedures and Techniques

Biopsy of the Skin

The cutaneous biopsy is an important adjunct to the diagnosis of skin diseases and is more useful when both the type of lesion and the site of biopsy are carefully selected. Skin biopsy is beneficial in the diagnosis of vasculitis, bullous eruptions, malignant tumors, lichen planus, granuloma annulare, and adnexal tumors. On the other hand, it is rarely helpful in determining the origin of eczematous eruptions.

The biopsy should be performed on an unaltered, fresh primary lesion. A new or fully developed lesion is considerably more useful than one that is old and healing. When a blister is biopsied, it is important to include a rim of normal tissue with the biopsy specimen. Once a correct site is selected, the area should be cleansed and locally anesthetized with either xylocaine or procaine. Dermatologists employ a number of techniques in performing a biopsy including cutaneous punch, excision, curettage, shave biopsy, or incisional biopsy. A few of these methods will be described briefly in the following paragraphs.

In a cutaneous punch, the instrument is driven through the skin with a rotary motion to a depth of 4 mm (Fig. 2). The physician must insert the punch deep enough to include areas of pathology. If the pathologic process is deep, a superficial punch biopsy may be inadequate. When performing a punch biopsy, tension is provided on the skin perpendicular to the normal skin lines. In this manner, when the tension is released, the skin biopsy site forms an oval in the direction of the skin lines, giving the patient a more suitable cosmetic effect. A disposable punch is now readily available, and punch biopsy sets can be obtained in all sizes (2-10 mm). At completion of the biopsy procedure, the skin can be closed with a suture that is removed in 5-10 days, or the wound can remain open to heal spontaneously.

Excisional biopsies are useful for larger lesions that may not be easily removed with a punch. This procedure is generally somewhat more difficult and requires a more extensive area of anesthesia. It is useful to outline the biopsy site with a dye such as gentian violet to localize it before the anesthesia obscures normal markings. The excision is made along skin lines with a No. 15 scalpel blade to provide the most cosmetically acceptable results. At the completion of the biopsy procedure, the skin is again closed with sutures.

Curettage can also be used as a biopsy technique, but it is usually reserved for tumors whose structure is unimportant. Because curettage fragments the lesions, this technique is performed only on lesions such as basal cell carcinomas and seborrheic keratoses. The area to be curetted is anesthetized and a small ring-shaped curette is applied to the lesion. A scraping or digging motion is used to remove a clump of tissue.

Shave biopsies are usually performed on superficial lesions such as seborrheic keratoses. The lesion is anesthetized and is raised by pressure between the thumb and first finger. A single-edge razor or a No. 11 blade can be used to shave the lesion, while hemostasis is obtained by using either a hot-tipped cautery or trichloroacetic acid.

Finally, dermatologists occasionally employ an incisional biopsy technique. Incisional biopsy is reserved for keratoacanthomas that may be too large to excise. An elliptic incision is made into the lesion, including normal tissue on both sides.

After the biopsy is performed, the specimen must be handled correctly. It should not be squeezed with forceps. It should be carefully removed from the normal skin and placed in a bottle containing 10% formaldehyde. The bottle should be labeled as to type of lesion, patient's name, and area of the body from which the lesion was obtained.

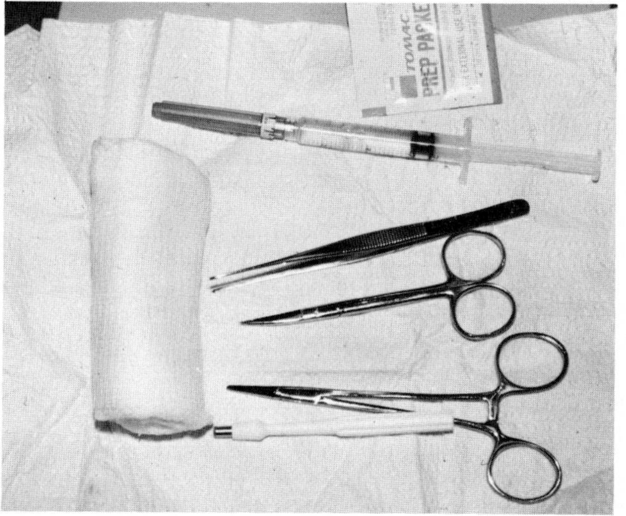

Figure 2. A punch biopsy setup including a cutaneous punch, forceps, iris scissors, and the anesthetic.

Potassium Hydroxide (KOH) Mount

The potassium hydroxide (KOH) mount is useful for identification of hyphae and spores. Consequently, KOH preparations are vital in the diagnosis of candidiasis, tinea, and, in some cases, deep fungal disease such as blastomycosis. In addition, KOH preparations are useful in the diagnosis of scabies and pediculosis pubis.

Dry scaly lesions are usually scraped with a No. 15 blade or the edge of a microscope slide. Vesicular lesions are examined by first removing the roof of the vesicle with a No. 11 blade and then placing the overlying skin on a microscope slide. It is of little benefit to examine the vesicular fluid in such infections. In cases of scabies, potassium hydroxide or mineral oil can be placed on the skin over a burrough or vesicle and the entire lesion can then be scraped.

The tissue is placed on a microscope slide and covered with one or two drops of 10 or 20% potassium hydroxide. A coverslip is placed over the specimen and the slide gently heated for a few seconds to dissolve the keratin. It is important not to boil the tissue since this can destroy hyphae, making diagnosis impossible. The specimen is then examined at high magnification under a dry microscope objective looking for fungal hyphae, spores, or mites.

Diascopy

Diascopy is a technique that is useful in delineating purpura from erythema secondary to vascular dilatation. The diascope is a clear piece of glass, and frequently a microscope slide is used for this purpose. The slide is placed against the lesion and slight pressure is applied. Blanching indicates that the vessels are intact, while lack of blanching suggests purpura.

Wood's Lamp Examination

A Wood's lamp is a source of ultraviolet light containing a filter that transmits light at a wavelength of 365 nm. The patient is placed in a darkened room and the lesion in question is examined under Wood's light. This technique may be used in the detection of a number of diseases including ringworm, tinea versicolor, erythrasma, vitiligo, and porphyria. Ringworm caused by the microorganisms *Microsporum canis* and *Microsporum audouini* fluoresces blue-green, whereas tinea versicolor fluoresces a golden color. Erythrasma, a disease caused by a bacterium, *Corynebacterium minutissimum*, fluoresces red because of porphyrins produced by the bacterium. Vitiligo, which is a depigmenting disease, is revealed by Wood's light because the lack of pigment causes light to be reflected. Wood's light is also useful in detecting the presence of certain drugs in the skin. It is occasionally necessary to determine whether a patient prescribed tetracycline for acne is actually taking the drug. If yellow fluorescence of tetracycline, especially in the mouth and around the hair follicles, is evident under Wood's light, the patient may be taking the medication as prescribed.

Patch Testing

The cutanous patch test is a technique useful in detecting allergic contact dermatitis (Fig. 3). Rather than being injected under the skin, the material in question is placed in a specific form under a gauze patch that is then taped to the patient's back (Fig. 4). The patch is removed in 48 hours and the skin examined for erythema or vesiculation. The skin is again examined in 96 hours and a positive reaction suggests the presence of allergic contact dermatitis (Plate 2). A group of chemicals in standard form is available from the American Academy of Dermatology (P.O. Box 552, Evanston, Illinois, 60201). In addition, the chemicals, patches, and tape are available from Hollister-Stier Laboratories (P.O. Box 14957, Dept. F74, Atlanta, Georgia 30325) and Tro-Lab (6 B.A.N., Hansen Alle, Denmark). Because of the differences between irritation and allergy, chemicals must be placed in the correct concentration so irritation to the skin is minimized. In addition, the chemicals may cause irritation if they remain on the skin for more than 48 hours. Therefore, the test must be performed correctly with the proper materials in order to obtain useful information.

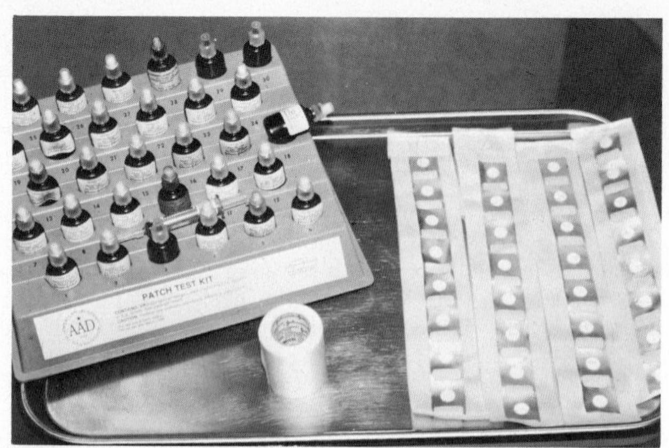

Figure 3. A patch test kit including Al-test aluminum strips and Dermacel tape.

Cytologic Smears

The cytologic smear is used in the diagnosis of viral and some other blistering processes. It is important to obtain an early, nontraumatized lesion. The blister is opened and the floor of the lesion scraped with a No. 15 blade or a curette. After the specimen is placed on a slide, it is air-dried and stained with either Wright's stain or Giemsa stain. The stained material is then observed under a low or high dry objective. Bizarre, virally altered giant epidermal cells or inclusion bodies indicate the presence of viral vesicles.

PRINCIPLES OF TOPICAL TREATMENT

The goals of treating a patient with topical medications may include the relief of a cutaneous symptom such as pruritus or pain, protection of an area of skin, treatment of inflammation, for peeling off scales, and removing or killing microorganisms or parasites. To accomplish these objectives, different forms of

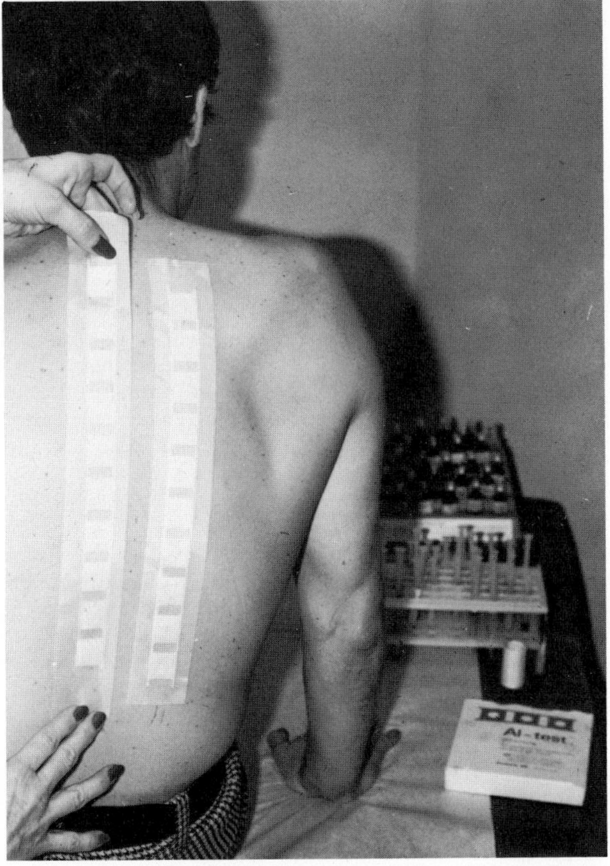

Figure 4. Al-test strips being placed on a patient's back.

external therapy are used. For instance, wet dressings alter the flow of blood. When the skin is dry, emollients are useful, while lotions containing menthol, phenol, or tar control itching. The following is a discussion on treatment modalities most frequently used by dermatologists.

Dressings and Baths

Dressings are applied as moist compresses, whereas a bath implies that the patient is submerged in liquid. Both forms of therapy are employed in the treatment of acute weeping dermatoses in order to dry the lesions, prevent bacterial superinfection, and allow regulation of skin temperature. In addition, wet dressings are very soothing to pruritic skin. In order to apply the dressing, soft cloths such as handkerchiefs, bed linen, or gauze fluffs can be used. Dressings are frequently left in place for 1 hour at a time and should be changed at least three times daily to avoid drying out. If the dressing becomes dry, the patient may frequently complain of increasing pain or itching.

Aluminum acetate or aluminum subacetate is a commonly used chemical for wet dressings and soaks. Aluminum acetate is available as Burrow's (USP) stock solution. It is used in strengths of 1:16, 1:30, or 1:40 dilutions and functions as an astringent. Aluminum subacetate is available in the form of either Domeboro tablets or powder. A packet of Domeboro powder contains 2.5 g of chemical. It is then placed in 1 pint of water in order to make a 1:20 dilution.

Silver nitrate may be prepared in a dilute solution of 1 part silver nitrate to 750 or 1,000 parts water; it is not only an astringent and mild antipruritic, but also has an antibacterial effect. Silver nitrate may stain both clothing and skin, but the stains can be removed with 2% iodine and water or with 10% potassium iodide. Stronger solutions of silver nitrate should be avoided over larger areas of skin, since both systemic absorption and coagulation of protein may occur. A normal saline solution, obtained by adding 1 level teaspoon of sodium chloride to 1 pint of water, is an excellent drying agent. Indeed, plain water can be used to dry an area and provide some relief from pruritus.

Finally, magnesium sulfate (Epsom salts) is an age-old and highly effective treatment for acute dermatitis. Wet dressings can be made in a dilution of 1 part magnesium sulfate to 65 parts water by dissolving a tablespoon of the chemical in a quart of water.

In cases where the cutaneous involvement is over such a large area of the body that wet dressings are impractical, medicated baths are employed. Many of the same materials mentioned above can be used in the bath and serve to draw out eczematous lesions. In a patient who is suffering from pruritus secondary to dryness of the skin, frequent bathing may only aggravate the problem. Oatmeal is frequently used in the bathtub to provide an additional therapeutic effect. Currently, Aveeno can be used to provide debridement of lesions and relief from pruritus. If Aveeno is not available, corn starch can be used. Two cups of corn starch are mixed with 4 cups of tap water to form a paste. The paste is then added to a tub of warm water, stirring constantly. Starch is antipruritic and helps soothe the skin. Finally, a patient with psoriasis frequently gains a great deal of relief by adding tar to the bathtub and soaking for up to 20 minutes daily in a tar bath. Tar preparations including Balnetar, Zetar emulsion, juniper tar bath, and liquor carbonis detergent (LCD) can be used successfully in the bathtub for this purpose.

Lotions

In treating acute or subacute dermatitis and pruritus, lotions represent suspensions of powder in water and are applied topically. In preparing a lotion, powder can be added to either water or alcohol, in which case the cooling effect is increased. Some lotions represent emulsions of an oil-in-water that are stabilized by surface-acting agents. All lotions separate when standing and should be shaken prior to administration. Various kinds of lotions exist in dermatology. Most of the major corticosteroids exist in a lotion form and are useful in the treatment of acute dermatitis.

The following is a very brief list of a few of the more representative nonsteroidal types of lotions:

BASIC SHAKE LOTION (USEFUL AS A VEHICLE)*

Zinc oxide	30%
Talc	30%
Glycerin	10%
Distilled water (to make)	100%

BASIC SHAKE LOTION WITH MENTHOL AND TAR (USED IN TREATING PRURITUS)*

Menthol	0.3 grams
LCD	6.0 ml
Basic shake lotion (to make)	120.0 ml

CALAMINE LOTION

LOTIO ALBA (USP)

Zinc sulfate	40 g
Sulfurated potash	40 g
Purified water (to make)	1,000 ml

Ointments and Creams

Ointments and creams represent the foundation of dermatologic therapy. There are specific indications for each type of vehicle.

The choice of a particular base depends on the nature of the medication that is incorporated into the base, the type of action desired, the area of the body on which the material is to be placed, and the shelf life of the finished product.

When the term ointment is used in its purest sense, it represents a semisolid preparation intended for external application. When used in this sense, there are four different ointment bases:

1. Hydrocarbon bases are insoluble and incapable of absorbing water. Consequently, this type of preparation is used primarily to protect and moisturize the skin. Inasmuch as they do not wash off easily, hydrocarbon bases such as white petroleum jelly, are somewhat unacceptable cosmetically.
2. The absorbent ointment base differs from hydrocarbon bases in that it absorbs water and as such is more acceptable cosmetically. These bases are extremely useful as vehicles for certain medications. Examples of absorbent ointments include Aquaphor and hydrophilic petrolatum.
3. Emulsion bases consist of two types: oil-in-water (O/W) emulsions such as Unibase or Neobase, and water-in-oil (W/O) types. An O/W emulsion contains small droplets of oil suspended in a water vehicle. This type of emulsion is commonly called a cream and, besides being an effective vehicle, is readily accepted by most patients. A W/O type of emulsion contains droplets of water in an oil vehicle and is commonly called an ointment. W/O emulsions are more greasy and as such are less readily acceptable. Both creams and ointments have their own uses. Creams are useful in situations where cosmetic appearance is important and high potency is neither needed nor desired. On the other hand, ointments allow for much greater potency and absorption of the medication, but are less cosmetically acceptable and can occasionally lead to maceration, yeast infection, striae, or cutaneous atrophy if they are used incorrectly or too often.
4. The last type of therapeutic ointment is the water-soluble base, such as polyethylene glycol, which is both water-soluble and water-absorbent. Water-soluble bases are the least occlusive of all ointments and are therefore the most cosmetically acceptable. Because the vehicle penetrates the skin easily, medications placed in this base are highly potent.

*Both of the above can be prepared with alcohol instead of water.

Pastes

Pastes are made by incorporating powder into an ointment. Powders usually constitute between 20 and 50% of the paste. This type of vehicle is rarely used in dermatology except in protection of the skin. The most common paste currently used is called Lassar's paste and consists primarily of zinc oxide, corn starch, and white petrolatum.

COMMON DISORDERS OF THE SKIN

The common disorders of the skin can be classified as shown in Table 1.

THE PAPULOSQUAMOUS DISORDERS

The papulosquamous disorders consist of a group of inflammatory diseases that are characterized by both papules and scaling. This important class of diseases includes psoriasis, lichen planus, parapsoriasis, pityriasis rosea, syphilis, and dermatophytosis. In general, the correct diagnosis can be made by carefully observing the distribution and morphologic appearance of individual lesions, presence or absence of nail or mouth involvement, and the typical histologic features. The following is a discussion of the more common noninfectious papulosquamous diseases.

Psoriasis (Fig. 5, Plate 3, Fig. 6)

Clinical Characteristics

The classic lesion of psoriasis is a large red plaque with an overlying silvery white scale. The border is sharp and the surrounding skin appears normal. The brightness of plaque color depends primarily on pigmentation of the patient. In white patients, the plaque appears as a much brighter red than it does in black patients. The scales are normally somewhat loosely adherent and, when removed, tiny bleeding points

Table 1. Classification of Skin Disorders

I.	Papulosquamous disorders
	A. Psoriasis
	B. Pityriasis rosea
	C. Lichen planus
II.	Vesiculobullous disorders
	A. Pemphigus
	B. Bullous pemphigoid
	C. Dermatitis herpetiformis
	D. Porphyria cutanea tarda
III.	Vascular disorders
	A. Urticaria
	B. Erythema multiforme
IV.	Dermatitis
	A. Contact dermatitis
	B. Atopic dermatitis
	C. Stasis dermatitis
	D. Seborrheic dermatitis
V.	Benign tumors of the skin
	A. Seborrheic keratosis
	B. Actinic keratosis
	C. Benign melanocytic nevi
	D. Acrochordon
	E. Keloids
VI.	Malignant tumors of the skin
	A. Basal cell epithelioma
	B. Squamous cell carcinoma
	C. Malignant melanoma
VII.	Acne
	A. Acne vulgaris
	B. Acne rosacea
VIII.	Fungal infections of the skin
	A. Dermatophytes
	B. Tinea versicolor
	C. Candidiasis
IX.	Bacterial diseases
	A. Impetigo
	B. Folliculitis, furuncles, and carbuncles
X.	Syphilis
XI.	Viral infections
	A. Verruca vulgaris
	B. Molluscum contageosum
	C. Herpes simplex
	D. Herpes zoster
XII.	Infestations
	A. Scabies
	B. Pediculosis
XIII.	Disordered Pigmentation
	A. Vitiligo

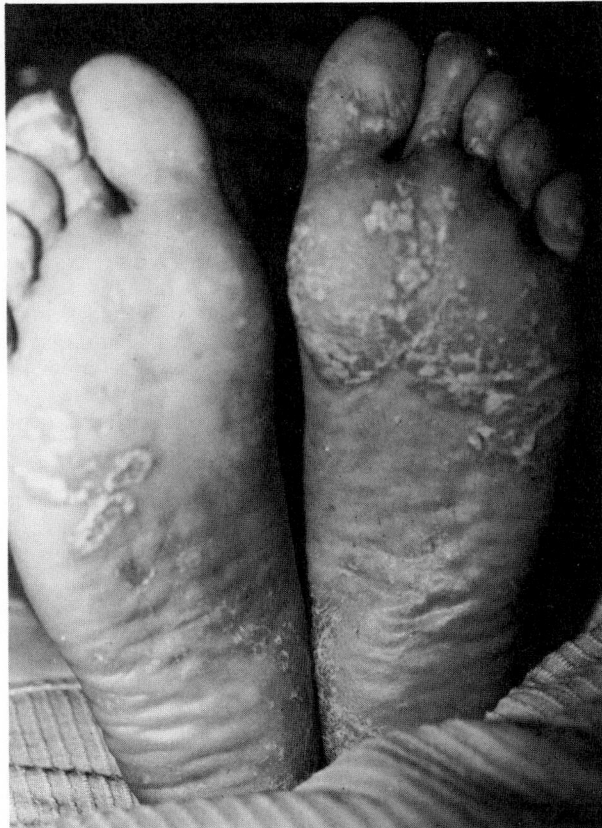

Figure 5. Typical psoriatic lesions on the feet.

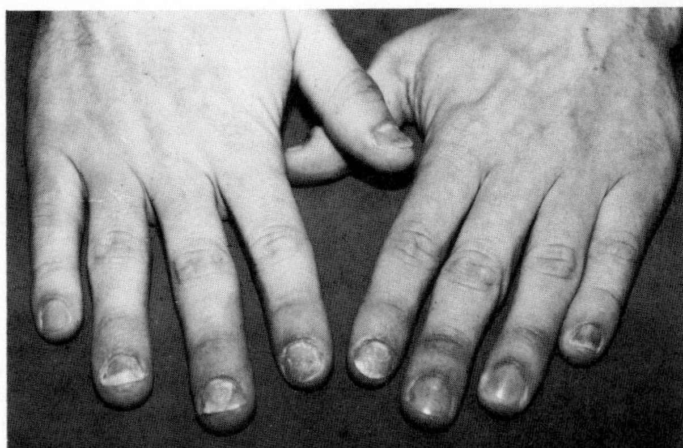

Figure 6. Psoriatic nail changes consist of subungual keratosis and multiple small pits.

remain on the plaque. Psoriasis may present with several clinical variations including pustular, exfoliative, and guttate psoriasis. The elbows, knees, scalp, and lumbosacral area are the sites most commonly involved because of the tendency of psoriasis to occur in areas that are traumatized (Koebner's phenomenon). Mucous membranes are rarely involved with psoriasis. In addition to the skin, the nails and joints may also be affected with the resultant deformity extremely disabling.

Etiology and Pathogenesis

The true cause of psoriasis is still unknown. Basically, three major areas are of interest to researchers at the present time. The first of these involves structure and possibly biochemical alterations of the skin. Various techniques have demonstrated that the turnover time of cutaneous epidermis is shortened in a psoriatic from the normal 28 days to approximately 3-4 days. This rapid turnover may be the result of a markedly shortened basal cell cycle. Due to this tremendous state of hypermetabolism, the skin is thickened, and abnormal maturation gives rise to the typical silvery white scale. In addition, the massive proliferation of blood vessels necessary to support a hypermetabolic cutis probably results in the development of the petechial bleeding points mentioned previously. Although the biochemistry has been well established, the basic reason for these alterations is still unclear. A second area of interest involves the genetics of psoriasis. It is well known that psoriasis appears in families, but the disease does not conform to a specific mode of inheritance. An increased frequency of antigens HLA-B13 and HLA-BW17 has been detected. Unfortunately, its relationship to the etiology of this disease is not clear.

Finally, it is well known that certain precipitating factors induce psoriasis. This is called Koebner's or the isomorphic, phenomenon. The precipitating factors may be trauma or may involve abnormal endocrine factors, emotion, stress, or change in climate. For instance, a patient sitting in the sun to treat psoriasis who develops a sunburn may exacerbate the psoriasis as a result of Koebner's phenomenon.

Differential Diagnosis

Psoriasis must be differentiated from other papulosquamous diseases including lichen planus, which is violaceous in color and frequently demonstrates mouth lesions, parapsoriasis, and pityriasis rosea occurring on the chest and back in the distribution of Langer's lines. In addition, one must consider lichen simplex chronicus, contact dermatitis, which occurs only in the area of contact, and tinea infection, which should demonstrate a positive potassium hydroxide mount.

Therapy

The average psoriatic patient does quite well without the intervention of either a pharmacist or physician. For patients who do not respond to very simple measures, additional treatment with either powerful topical drugs or systemic medications may be indicated. The following is a brief discussion of some of the treatments available to the psoriatic.

The general measures include relaxation to relieve emotional stress, sunlight, and awareness on the part of the patient that Koebner's phenomenon may be precipitating new lesions. It is an important adjunct to psoriatic therapy to keep the patient's bedroom warm and humid in the winter months. Some over-the-counter medications may also be helpful, including emollients and ointments to moisturize the psoriatic skin, medications containing sulfur, and those containing salicylic acid. When the psoriatic no longer responds to these very simple measures, prescription medications may be necessary.

There is no cure for psoriasis and therefore most therapy is palliative. The foundation of prescription topical therapy is the topical corticosteroid. It is best to begin with a mild steroid, using more potent ones only if it becomes necessary. Steroid ointments are preferred in situations where an emollient effect is needed. In addition, the steroid ointment is more potent because percutaneous absorption is enhanced. In mild cases and in patients who cannot tolerate ointments, steroid creams are recommended. In situations where enhanced penetration is required, it may be possible to occlude the area of skin involved with either polyethylene plastic or with polyvinyl. With psoriasis of the hands or feet, a plastic bag or glove is useful in achieving this effect.

Various tars have been employed in the treatment of psoriasis. Medicinal tar may be incorporated into baths, dressings, or shampoos, as well as ointments and creams. Medicinal tar and ultraviolet light are individually effective in treating psoriasis. Some years ago it was discovered that tar and ultraviolet light have an additive effect, which led to the development of the Goeckerman treatment involving a combination of tar and ultraviolet light. Various types of tar can be used including crude coal tar in a 1-5% solution, liquor carbonis detergents (LCD) in a 5-10% solution, and a tar-salicylic acid combination. Recently, several highly effective tar gels have been introduced on the market. Finally, in certain instances where psoriasis is localized in small areas, low concentrations of corticosteroids may be injected directly into the plaques.

When topical therapy fails, several forms of systemic therapy may be considered. Included in this group of modalities is methotrexate, immunosuppressive agents, and a combination of psoralen and long-wave ultraviolet light (PUVA) therapy. PUVA is the oral or topical administration of methoxypsoralen 2 hours prior to total body or local irradiation with long-wave ultraviolet light in the A range (320-400 nm). Its efficacy in the treatment of psoriasis is impressive, but because its safety is questionable it is not currently approved for general use by the Food and Drug Administration. Oral corticosteroids are probably never indicated for the treatment of psoriasis. It is well known that an individual treated with systemic corticosteroids may develop a rebound or pustular flare when the therapy is discontinued.

Pityriasis Rosea (Fig. 7)

Clinical Characteristics

In a classic case of pityriasis rosea, a mild prodromal period is followed by the onset of an asymptomatic herald patch. This

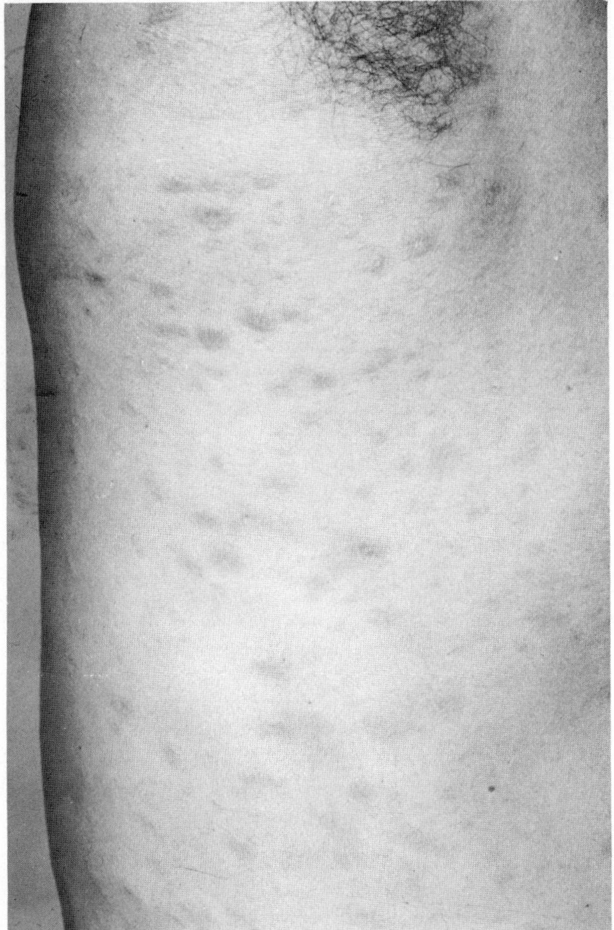

Figure 7. Pityriasis rosea–Notice how the lesions follow Langer's lines.

is a solid, oval to circular lesion approximately 4 cm in diameter. The herald patch most commonly occurs on the trunk. Three to 14 days after the herald patch is noticed, the secondary eruption occurs. This eruption is characterized by small fawn-colored plaques that have the same characteristics as the herald patch but are numerous and form in Langer's lines. The lesions usually have fine scales that peel off peripherally and produce the so-called collarette. During the first several weeks of eruption new lesions occur, but most lesions disappear within 6-8 weeks without scarring.

Differential Diagnosis

The most serious disease with which pityriasis rosea may be confused is secondary syphilis. Consequently, it is important to obtain a serologic test for syphilis in these patients. Other diseases that may be confused with pityriasis rosea include seborrheic dermatitis, psoriasis, parapsoriasis, and drug eruption.

Therapy

Unless there is severe pruritus, no treatment except reassurance is necessary. If pruritus is a problem, the patient can be treated with an antipruritic lotion containing 2% LCD (tar) and ¼% menthol or, alternatively, the patient may be treated with topical corticosteroids. Occasionally, ultraviolet light treatment or systemic corticosteroids are beneficial. If pityriasis rosea does not clear within 3 months, a reevaluation is necessary.

Lichen Planus (Plates 1 and 4)

Clinical Characteristics

The classic lesions of lichen planus are polygonal, violaceous, flat-topped papules that coalesce into plaques. White radiating lines, called Wickham's striae, may overlie the papule. Lichen planus can involve any area of the body but the most common is the lumbar region, anterior lower legs, wrists, ankles, and genitalia. Mucous membrane involvement is common and usually manifests itself as lacy-white infiltrates (Plate 1).

The nails, which are commonly involved with lichen planus, may show thinning, longitudinal striations, and splitting. In addition, a wing-shaped scar extending from the nail matrix called a pterygium is commonly observed in lichen planus. If the scalp is involved, scarring alopecia may be noted.

Variation in the morphology of this disease is a common occurrence, including follicular lichen planus, annular lichen planus, and hypertrophic lichen planus.

Etiology and Pathogenesis

The etiology of this disease remains obscure, but it is apparent that stress and drugs play a significant role.

Differential Diagnosis

The differential diagnosis of cutaneous lichen planus includes psoriasis, lichen simplex chronicus, and lichenoid drug eruptions. Oral lesions of lichen planus must be differentiated from leukoplakia, oral candidiasis, and trauma to the mucous membranes from rubbing or cheek biting.

Therapy

Treatment of lichen planus is frustrating for both the physician and the patient. Occasionally therapy will be effective but, in many cases, the patient may have to tolerate his disease for long periods of time. It is important for the physician to reassure the patient repeatedly that the disease will eventually resolve. In addition to reassurance, local treatment with corticosteroid creams, as well as with systemic antipruritic agents such as antihistamines, may be indicated. Occasionally, a severely disabled patient may be given a short (10-14 days) course of oral corticosteroids.

Course and Prognosis

Uncomplicated cases of lichen planus resolve in 6-18 months, however, the more involved forms (e.g., the hypertrophic form of lichen planus) may take more than 10 years. The only serious complication of lichen planus is an occasional squamous cell carcinoma that may develop in the hypertrophic variety.

VESICULOBULLOUS DISORDERS

Blistering of the skin occurs when fluid accumulates either between or within the cells of the epidermis or dermis. Vesicles represent accumulations of fluid that are less than 0.5 cm in diameter, while blisters (or bullae) have a diameter greater than 0.5 cm. Both vesicles and bullae are considered equivalent, hence the term vesiculobullous. Some blisters occur as a result of deposition of immune globulins in the skin; this group includes pemphigus vulgaris, pemphigoid, and dermatitis herpetiformis. In addition, infectious agents may cause blistering as seen in impetigo, tinea, and herpes simplex. Finally, blisters can occur with severe inflammatory diseases of the skin such as acute contact dermatitis.

In addition to knowing the etiology of a blister, the physician should also be aware of the depth of skin involvement. Accumulations of fluid in the skin occur either within or just beneath the epidermis. In each case, there are numerous diseases that are characterized by blistering in particular areas; therefore, to diagnose vesiculobullous disease reliably, the physician must biopsy an early lesion.

A few of the typical vesiculobullous disorders are described below.

Pemphigus

Two varieties of pemphigus exist (pemphigus vulgaris and pemphigus foliaceus), each having a clinical variant. Pemphigus vulgaris has a variant called pemphigus vegetans, while pemphigus foliaceus has a variant called pemphigus erythematosus. Both types have blisters that form in the epidermis and are characterized by acantholytic, or noncohesive, cells. Pemphigus vulgaris is probably the most common form of pemphigus.

Pemphigus Vulgaris

Clinical Features

The disease frequently begins as a localized eruption in the mouth or on the scalp, and within 1 year extends to other areas. The characteristic blister of pemphigus vulgaris is flaccid, and pressure on the blister causes it to spread to adjacent normal skin (Nikolsky's sign). Pemphigus vulgaris occurs on the scalp, midface, nostrils, mouth, sternum, back, umbilicus, and groin. Inasmuch as the blisters are flaccid, large areas of skin become denuded. Consequently, patients with pemphigus vulgaris are more susceptible to bacterial and candidal infections, perhaps exacerbated by treating these people with systemic corticosteroids and immunosuppressive agents.

Etiology and Pathogenesis

There is increasing evidence that pemphigus vulgaris represents an autoimmune disease. It is quite possible that antibodies are formed against the intercellular cement of the epidermal cells. Immune globulins have been found to be deposited in the intercellular spaces and, in addition, there have been reports of circulating immunoglobulins that are active against the intercellular spaces of the epidermis.

Differential Diagnosis

The differential diagnosis of pemphigus vulgaris includes several of the diseases discussed below; these include bullous pemphigoid, bullous erythema multiforme, and dermatitis herpetiformis.

Diagnostic Procedures

The diagnosis of pemphigus is made by both clinical and histopathologic examination of the skin. Skin biopsy reveals an intraepidermal blister. Direct immunofluorescence demonstrates immunoglobulins that have been deposited in the intercellular spaces. Finally, diagnosis can be made by detecting pemphigus antibodies to intercellular cement.

Therapy

Treatment of pemphigus vulgaris should be undertaken only by a physician who is familiar with both the disease and the drugs employed. Two forms of therapy are commonly utilized. Corticosteroids such as prednisone (80-300 mg/day) have been used to control the disease. As might be expected with such doses, side effects are substantial including osteoporosis, gastric ulcers, diabetes mellitus, suppression of the pituitary-adrenal axis, and hypertension.

In addition, immunosuppressive therapy may be used to treat the disease, as well as allowing the physician to decrease steroid dosage. Among the immunosuppressive agents employed are methotrexate, azathioprine, and cyclophosphamide.

Bullous Pemphigoid (Plate 5)

Clinical Characteristics

Bullous pemphigoid is a chronic blistering eruption occurring most frequently in the elderly. It is characterized by large, tense, irregular blisters that do not break easily and rarely become superinfected. Blisters usually involve the groin, inner aspects of the thigh, abdomen, and flexor aspects of the forearms. Mucous membrane involvement occurs in 10-20% of the cases. The notable absence of Nikolsky's sign and the presence of bullae, both on normal and on erythematous skin, are points of differential diagnosis.

Etiology and Pathogenesis

Like pemphigus vulgaris, pemphigoid represents a disease of autoimmunity. IgG and the third component of complement (C3) have been found to be deposited along the basement membrane of the epidermis.

Disease Associations

In the past, it has been stated that bullous pemphigoid is strongly associated with internal malignancy. Because bullous pemphigoid and internal malignancy are both common in elderly patients, they are more likely to occur simultaneously in the same patient. In addition, bullous pemphigoid is an autoimmune disease and may be associated with other autoimmune disorders such as systemic lupus erythematosus, rheumatoid arthritis, and pernicious anemia.

Differential Diagnosis
Bullous pemphigoid should be considered in the differential diagnosis of other blistering eruptions including pemphigus vulgaris, erythema multiforme, benign mucosal pemphigoid, dermatitis herpetiformis, and acute contact dermatitis.

Diagnosis
The diagnosis of bullous pemphigus may be suggested by clinical presentation alone. Numerous tense, centrally distributed bullae, occurring both on normal and erythematous skin, strongly suggest bullous pemphigoid, especially if Nikolsky's sign is negative. In addition, several laboratory tests are beneficial in establishing this diagnosis, including skin biopsy and biopsy for direct immunofluorescence.

Histopathologic examination reveals a subepidermal blister with detachment of the epidermis from the dermis. There is very little inflammatory change within the dermis. The direct immunofluorescence shows deposition of IgG and C3 throughout the basement membrane of the epidermis. Occasionally, antibasement membrane antibodies are detected in the serum.

Therapy
Bullous pemphigoid may remit spontaneously. Nevertheless, because it commonly occurs in the elderly and because patients with this disease are prone to infection, it is important that the disease be brought under control. Two forms of therapy have been employed in the treatment of this disease. Systemic corticosteroids, in moderate to high doses, are an effective treatment. Immunosuppressive agents such as methotrexate and azathioprine also have been used in combination with corticosteroids.

Dermatitis Herpetiformis

Clinical Characteristics
Dermatitis herpetiformis is a severely pruritic eruption occurring on extensor surfaces such as the scapula, as well as the buttocks and scalp. The eruptiosn consist of small symetrically grouped vesicles with marked surrounding erythema. The disease is persistent and, although it may occur at any age, it is most common between the ages of 30 and 60. Alternatively, it may present with no vesicles but simply severe itching and multiple excoriations. Therefore, it is common for a patient to have an extremely pruritic eruption without vesicles and frequently have excoriated lesions in a herpetiform distribution.

Etiology and Pathogenesis
Since IgA has been found in the dermal papillae on direct immunofluorescence, this probably represents an autoimmune phenomenon.

Associated Conditions
Dermatitis herpetiformis is most commonly associated with small bowel abnormalities that may vary in severity and include villous atrophy. Occasionally, cases of dermatitis herpetiformis have improved with a gluten-free diet, implying that dermatitis herpetiformis may be linked to gluten sensitivity. Although an association with internal malignancy has been suggested in the past, there is little evidence that it is real.

Differential Diagnosis
Dermatitis herpetiformis must be differentiated from other diseases such as scabies, neurotic excoriations, pityriasis lichenoides et varioliformis acuta, contact dermatitis, tinea infections, bullous pemphigoid, and bullous lichen planus.

Diagnosis
The diagnosis of dermatitis herpetiformis may at times be exceedingly difficult and as such a careful history and physical examination are essential. If typical vesicles are not found, a KOH preparation to determine the presence of scabies is indicated. In addition, a biopsy of a vesicular lesion is of benefit. Finally, direct immunofluorescence of the paralesional or normal skin may reveal IgA in the dermal papillae.

Treatment
There are several forms of therapy that are highly effective in the treatment of dermatitis herpetiformis, with the treatment of choice being diaminodiphenylsulfone (DDS or Dapsone). In other cases, the use of sulfapyridine has been very successful. Although a gluten-free diet may be helpful, poor patient compliance may be an overwhelming problem. Finally, in cases not responding to the above treatment, a trial of systemic corticosteroids may be indicated.

Porphyria Cutanea Tarda (Plate 6)

Clinical Characteristics
This disease most commonly occurs in middle-aged patients and is characterized by vesicles and scarring, primarily on sun-exposed areas. The presence of these vesicles is associated with a tearing or burning sensation. Occasionally, these areas become hardened and take on a sclerodermoid appearance. In addition, they may show marked fragility with erosion and subsequent scarring. Along with vesiculation there is hypertrichosis, primarily confined to the face.

Etiology and Pathogenesis
This disease represents an abnormality in porphyrin metabolism caused by decreased levels of uroporphyrin III cosynthetase (uroporphyrinogen decarboxylase). The relative presence of this enzyme may be genetically controlled and the disease may be triggered by various other processes such as ingestion of birth control pills, iron overload, barbiturates, estrogens, tolbutamide, and hexachlorobenzene.

Associated Conditions
Porphyria cutanea tarda may be associated with diabetes mellitus, lupus erythematosus, hemolytic anemias, and hepatoma.

Diagnosis
Diagnosis of porphyria cutanea tarda can be established by

finding significant amounts of uroporphyrin in the urine. Elevated fecal coproporphyrin and protoporphyrin, although present, are of less diagnostic importance. Biopsy of a lesion may reveal a subepidermal bulla.

Differential Diagnosis
Porphyria cutaneous tarda must be differentiated from other eruptions including polymorphous light eruption, neurotic excoriations, and pellagra. Histologically, the disease may resemble bullous pemphigoid, bullous erythema multiforme, and dermatitis herpetiformis.

Therapy
Before considering any specific form of therapy in this disease, the patient must completely avoid alcohol, estrogens, barbiturates, and any other offending drugs. In addition, it may be helpful for the patient to avoid direct sunlight by wearing a chemical sunscreen. Once this has been accomplished, there are several specific therapies that may be successful.

Phlebotomy, which has been advocated in the treatment of the disease, may be effective by removing excessive iron from the blood. Relatively small amounts of blood (5-10 pt) are removed from the patient over a period of several months. A second form of therapy involves small doses of antimalarial agents such as chloroquine and hydroxychloroquine. To prevent severe hepatic damage, the dosage of antimalarial agent must be minimal. Finally, alkalinization of the urine has been tried in an attempt to increase porphyrin excretion.

VASCULAR DISORDERS

This common but important group of diseases occurs because of abnormalities in the blood vessels. Three processes may give rise to vascular disorders. Vasodilatation occurs when the blood vessels enlarge and blood flow to the involved skin increases. The skin appears erythematous and, if enough blood flows into an area, edema or swelling occurs. The next level of damage to the vessel involves a mild perivascular inflammatory reaction, causing extravasation of red cells and induration of involved skin. Because there is hemorrhage under the skin, it does not blanch on pressure. The third and least common type of vascular disorder involves actual damage to, and necrosis of, the vessel wall. This process, called vasculitis, results in hemorrhage of red blood cells through the vessel wall with induration of the involved area. If the vessel wall is completely destroyed, infarction, necrosis, and ulceration of the skin may occur. Vasculitis is a complex disease process that cannot be dealt with adequately in this brief discussion. However, two of the more common vascular diseases will be reviewed below.

Urticaria (Hives)

Clinical Characteristics (Plate 7)
The basic lesion of urticaria is the wheal, which is very pruritic and ranges in size from several millimeters to several centimeters. Multiple configurations such as arcuate, serpiginous, circular, and geographic may be present. At times, the configuration may be exceedingly bizarre and change rapidly, often with a complete resolution within several hours. Occasionally, however, individual wheals may persist for as long as 24 hours. Wheals occurring on the palms of the hands and soles of the feet may cause a prickly stinging sensation as well as pruritus. Angioedema, a deep edematous process without superficial erythema, may occur at times. Mucous membranes may be involved with massive swelling, which can compromise the upper respiratory tract. Dermographism, an urticarial lesion that can be induced by external pressure, is a different manifestation of urticaria. Patients with dermographism may demonstrate linear wheals in scratched areas.

Etiology and Pathogenesis
The many causes of urticaria are listed in Table 2. Frequently the physician is unable to determine the reason for urticaria. Ingested or injected drugs are an important etiology in cases for which a cause can be found. Foods are an occasional source of urticaria, with the responsible agents being proteins, preservatives, colors, dyes, salicylates, citric acid, penicillin, yeast, and breakdown food products. The most common nutritive causes of urticaria are nuts, fish, eggs, strawberries, egg whites, tomatoes, and lobster.

In the past, infections were regarded as a common etiology of urticaria. Presently, infectious origins are quite rare but should still be considered. Classic infections causing urticaria include bacterial infections of the teeth, sinuses, chest, gastrointestinal tract, and the genitourinary tract. Other infectious causes include candidiasis, dermatophytosis, viral hepatitis, mononucleosis, and Coxsackie virus infections. Insect and arthropod bites are an occasional cause of urticaria and angioedema.

Table 2. Etiology of Urticaria

Drugs
Foods
Food protein
Food colors, dyes
Food preservatives
Penicillin
Yeasts
Breakdown products
Inhaled allergens
Infections
Insect bites
Contactants
Medications
Cosmetics
Plants
Internal diseases
Connective tissue diseases
Carcinomas
Lymphomas
Physical agents
Pressure
Cholinergic
Cold, heat, sunlight

Recently, it has been found that certain contact agents may cause urticaria. Numerous medications, when applied to the skin, will result in localized, or sometimes generalized, urticaria. Occasionally, urticaria may be caused by physical agents such as dermographism, pressure, cold, heat, sunlight, and cholinergic drugs. Finally, internal diseases as possible causes for urticaria should be mentioned. Although extremely rare, they should not be overlooked in cases of chronic unresponsive urticaria. Considered in this group are connective tissue disease, carcinoma, lymphoma, hyperthyroidism, hepatitis, and rheumatoid arthritis.

Recently, much has been discovered about the pathogenesis of this disease. It is well known that two kinds of urticaria occur, one of which is immunologically mediated and involves either the classic or alternate pathways of the complement chain or the IgE-mast cell system. Alternatively, the urticaria may occur because of nonimmunologic reactions with direct release of histamine from mast cells. The major mediators of urticaria are histamine, kinens, slow-reacting substance of anaphylaxis and, possibly, prostaglandin E_2, serotonin, however, probably has no role in urticaria. Each of these factors is released from the mast cell by the etiologic agents already discussed.

Evaluation of a Patient with Urticaria

A complete history and physical examination must be obtained from a patient with urticaria. Frequently this is the only evaluation necessary; however, if the urticaria persists or if the history and physical examination provide an indication, various laboratory tests may be helpful in determining the etiology of the disease.

Laboratory tests that may be indicated in some patients with urticaria include the erythrocyte sedimentation rate (ESR), antinuclear antibodies, complement levels, Venereal Disease Research Laboratories test (VDRL), cryoglobulins, and cryofibrinogens. If infection is a possibility, examination of stools for ova and parasites, vaginal smears for *Candida*, and x-rays of the sinuses, chest, and teeth are indicated. In cases of inhaled allergens, serum IgE levels and scratch testing of the skin may be useful. If physical urticaria is suspected, it is sometimes beneficial to scratch the skin lightly in search of dermographism. In addition, an ice cube when placed on the skin might detect cold urticaria, while light testing may be helpful in detecting solar urticaria. Finally, in a few cases, skin biopsy or elimination diets are indicated in the evaluation of this disease.

Treatment

To treat urticaria effectively, it is best to remove exacerbating factors, but sometimes this cannot be done and urticaria must be treated empirically. In cases of severe acute urticaria, epinephrine 1:1000 (0.1-0.3 cc) subcutaneously is effective. In less severe cases, the treatment of choice is antihistamines. Hydroxyzine (Atarax, Vistaril) is a particularly effective antihistamine and is frequently used as the initial drug of choice. There are several groups of antihistamine that can be administered, and it is useful in refractory cases to use antihistamines from two groups simultaneously. Table 3 lists some of the commonly used antihistamines.

Systemic corticosteroids occasionally may be useful in the treatment of urticaria. More often, however, they are ineffective and should not be utilized as initial therapy.

Finally, emollients or lubricants may make the patient feel more comfortable and thus be marginally useful in treating this disease.

Erythema Multiforme (Plate 8, Fig. 8)

Clinical Characteristics

Although erythema multiforme is most common between the ages of 20 and 40, it may occur at any age. It is characterized by a symmetric eruption consisting of macules, papules, vesicles, and occasionally bullae. The characteristic lesions is an iris or target lesion that has concentric rings with occasional central necrosis or vesiculation. Occasionally, ocular or oral lesions may occur with this form of the disease.

A more severe form of erythema multiforme is Stevens-Johnson syndrome. This occurs more commonly in men, and is most common in young adults or children. The rash related to Stevens-Johnson syndrome may look similar to that of erythema multiforme. Significantly, however, the patient is more toxic and has significant mucous membrane involvement with multiple bullae and considerable crusting. If the eyes are involved, scarring and blindness may result, and this syndrome also has significant mortality.

Etiology and Pathogenesis

At least 50% of cases of erythema multiforme or Stevens-Johnson syndrome are idiopathic. Otherwise, the most

Table 3. Commonly Used Antihistamines

Class	*Generic Name*	*Trade Name*	*Tablet or Capsule Strength (mg)*	*Single Adult Dose (mg)*
Ethanolamines	Diphenhydramine	Benadryl	25, 50	50
Ethylenediamines	Triplenamine	Pyribenzamine	25, 50; long acting: 50, 100	50
Alkylamines	Chlorpheniramine		4; long acting: 8, 12	2-4
	Chlor-trimeton	Teldrin, Histaspar		
Phenothiazines	Trimeprazine	Temaril	2.5; long acting: 5	2.5
Miscellaneous	Hydroxyzine	Atarzx, Vistaril	10, 25, 50, 100	25-100

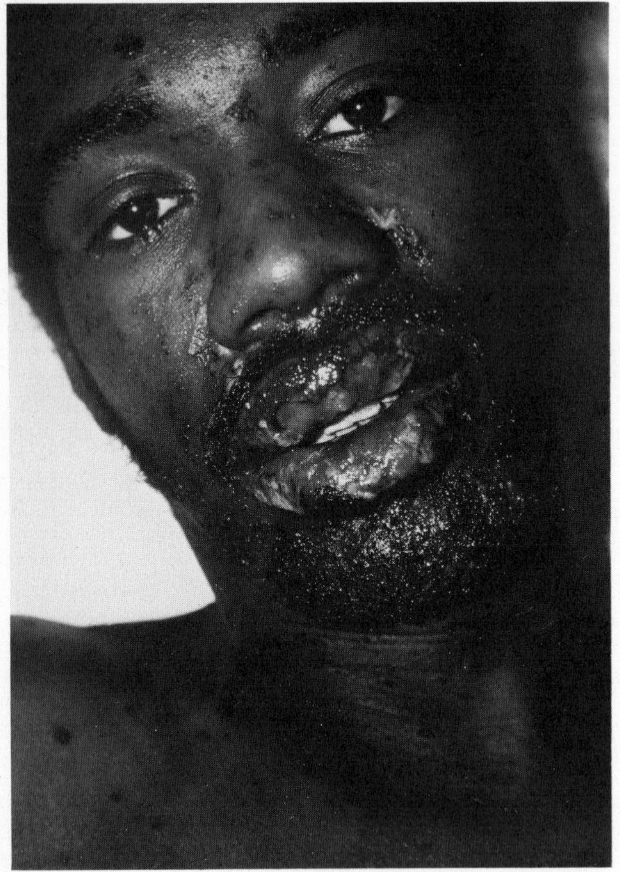

Figure 8. Marked mucous membrane involvement in a patient with the Stevens-Johnson form of erythema multiforme.

common causes of erythema multiforme include drugs, infection, ingested material, connective tissue disease, immunizations, and occasionally malignancy. Pathogenetically, this probably represents a hypersensitivity phenomenon.

Differential Diagnosis

The differential diagnosis includes urticaria, toxic erythemas, blood-borne infections, syphilis, bullous diseases such as bullous pemphigoid, and connective tissue diseases.

Diagnosis

An accurate diagnosis of this disease is aided by a thorough history and physical examination. In addition, biopsy for light microscopy and direct immunofluorescence should be performed to help rule out other blistering processes.

Treatment

The importance of good supportive care should not be underestimated. If the patient has eye lesions, a consultation with an ophthalmologist is helpful, while symptomatic care of mouth and skin lesions is also of importance. In most cases of mild erythema multiforme, the disease will clear in 2-3 weeks. In more severe cases, systemic corticosteroids (prednisone, 60-120 mg/day) are often administered but proof of their effectiveness is lacking. Fluid replacement and good topical and medical care are important additional considerations.

DERMATITIS

Dermatitis means inflammation of the skin and, as such, there are many entities that may be within the scope of this definition. Because the skin lacks expressiveness, a variety of processes result in the same reaction pattern. Dermatitis is classified into at least two groups: acute and chronic. Acute dermatitis appears rapidly, is markedly pruritic, and vesicular or bullous. Marked weeping, oozing, and crusting, as well as secondary infection, may occur (Plate 9). On the other hand, chronic dermatitis is a scaly, poorly marginated lesion that is occasionally lichenified and usually itches. It appears over a relatively long period and demonstrates marked thickening of the skin (Fig. 9).

The following paragraphs describe the more common forms of dermatitis.

Contact Dermatitis

Clinical Characteristics (Plates 10, 11)

Contact dermatitis is an inflammatory disease caused by external contact of the skin with an irritating or allergenic material. This process may be either acute or chronic, and is confined to the area of contact. The shape and localization of this disease is important in determining its etiology. For example, a patient who develops contact dermatitis by brushing against the leaves of poison ivy will demonstrate linear lesions in the area of exposure.

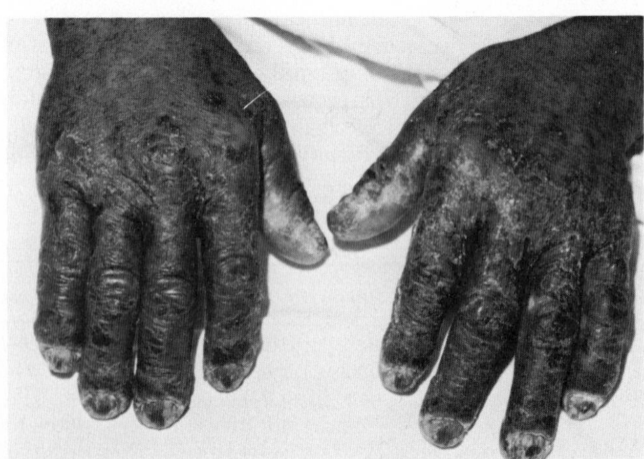

Figure 9. Chrome dermatitis in a patient chronically exposed to solvents.

Pathogenesis
Contact dermatitis is classified as two distinct entities: allergic and irritant. An irritating substance is one that can cause a reaction in most persons if it is applied for a period of time in a significant concentration. Percutaneous penetration of the material occurs and a nonimmunologically mediated inflammatory reaction takes place. Irritation may occur through several mechanisms including denaturation of epidermal proteins, which alters the capacity of the stratum corneum to hold water. Because this reaction is not immunologically mediated, the concentration of an irritant must exceed its threshold before a reaction takes place; this threshold may be high, and varies according to the irritancy of the compound. An irritant contact dermatitis will occur immediately after contact with the compound and requires no induction period. Strong acids, for example, will cause an irritant contact dermatitis in most individuals.

Allergic contact dermatitis, on the other hand, is mediated by the T-lymphocyte system and is therefore a delayed hypersensitivity phenomenon. As such, a period of 7-14 days is required before the rash appears. If the antigen is reapplied, the intensity of the eruption reaches a peak in 24-48 hours. Although only a small number of individuals have the capacity to react to any particular antigenic material, the threshold for eliciting an allergic contact dermatitis is very low in these individuals.

Etiology
Virtually any material in a patient's environment is capable of causing either an irritant or an allergic dermatitis. Irritant compounds include materials that are mechanically abrasive such as fiberglass; chemical irritants such as soap, water, and detergents; and biologic irritants, which include infectious agents. Allergic contact dermatitis may be caused by a number of compounds commonly present both at home and at work. For instance, foot dermatitis may be an allergic contact dermatitis to compounds present in shoes including rubber accelerators, glue, dyes, and dichromates. Furthermore, dermatitis may even develop if a material is used by the patient for long periods of time. Thus, it is possible to develop allergic contact dermatitis to cosmetics, hair sprays, nickel-plated utensils, medications, toothpaste, perfumes, elastics in clothing, and to airborne contactants. Patients who work in industrial environments are exposed to multiple biologic, physical, mechanical, and chemical causes of both irritant and allergic contact dermatitis. Chrome, mercury, nickel, and cobalt are common allergic sensitizers found in industry. Those who work with plants or plant products may develop an allergic contact dermatitis, or even a photoallergy, to the materials with which they are in contact. Individuals employed in the rubber industry may develop allergies to rubber accelerators, antioxidants, or even to synthetic rubber, while those working in the plastic industry are occasionally sensitized to either monomers or to hardening agents.

Diagnosis and Evaluation
With this multitutde of potential sensitizers, proving the cause for allergic dermatitis is quite difficult. A thorough history and physical examination are two of the most useful diagnostic aids. The points of historical interest will vary from patient to patient but, in general, it is important to determine onset of the eruption, whether it is intermittent or constant, whether it clears when the patient leaves home or work, and its relationship to the patient's exposure to perfumes, cosmetics, metals, or rubber products. Determining the origin requires a great deal of persistence.

A patch test is the major laboratory test used to diagnose contact dermatitis, and is useful only in instances of allergic contact dermatitis. When the material to be tested is a strong irritant, it is of no benefit. The procedures used in patch testing have already been described.

Therapy
In order to treat allergic or irritant contact dermatitis successfully, the correct diagnosis must be established. In cases of acute dermatitis, the provoking agent must be discontinued and the patient treated with lotions, baths, or soaks. In more chronic cases, a topical corticosteroid in either a cream or ointment base is the treatment of choice. Oral antihistamines are useful as antipruritic agents.

Atopic Dermatitis (Fig. 10)

Clinical Characteristics
Atopic dermatitis is a disease that commonly begins between the ages of 2 months and 2 years. Early in its evolution it is characterized by a weeping, oozing dermatosis present on the buttocks, face, scalp, and/or neck. Occasionally, the eruption may involve the entire body. As the disease progresses it develops into a lichenified pruritic eruption involving the flexor surfaces, particularly the anticubital and posterior popliteal fossae. These individuals also have markedly xerotic skin and frequently, on questioning, have a strong family history of allergic disease.

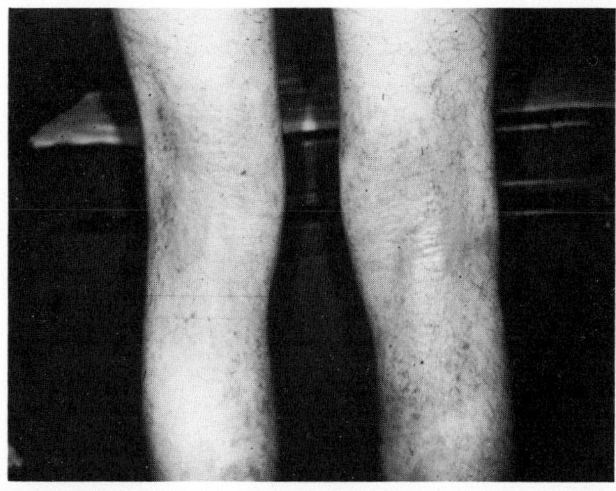

Figure 10. Atopic dermatitis localized to the posterior popliteal space.

Whereas most atopic disease improves by adolescence, a few individuals have persistent eruptions into adulthood. These eruptions are more localized and frequently involve single areas such as the hands or feet.

Etiology and Pathogenesis
The cause of this disease is unknown; however, many factors seem to be involved in its etiology. These factors include allergy, abnormal cell-mediated immunity, high serum IgE levels, infections, dry skin, a genetic tendency to develop the disease, and abnormal response of cutaneous vessels to injury.

Associated Condition
Patients with atopic dermatitis are predisposed to widespread cutaneous dissemination of certain viruses, including herpes simplex and vaccinia. Patients with active disease should not be vaccinated with a living virus and should be protected from siblings who may have herpes simplex. In addition, patients with atopic dermatitis have a higher incidence of cataracts, and may be more prone to develop a penicillin allergy.

Treatment
Excessive dryness of the skin should be avoided. Frequent bathing with strong soaps in hot water is contraindicated in patients with this disease. When bathing, it is important for the patient to use a good lubricant to preserve moisture in the skin. In addition, materials that irritate the skin (harsh detergents, wool, and strong chemicals) should be avoided.

Beyond these basic instructions, the major therapeutic modalities include topical corticosteroids and oral antihistamines. Topical corticosteroids should be used in the lowest available concentration that is effective, and should be applied daily as often as possible. Oral antihistamines are most useful in preventing itching, which may be particularly annoying at night.

Stasis Dermatitis (Fig. 11)

Clinical Characteristics
This disease occurs in either older patients or in those who have damaged the vasculature of their legs as a result of varicosities, phlebitis, prolonged severe edema, or trauma. The earliest form of this disease is characterized by edema and stasis with pigmentary changes secondary to deposition of hemosiderin in the skin. As the disease progresses, erythema and pruritus occur with the development of small areas of petechial bleeding. The dermatitis increases in severity, becomes scaly, and eventually appears as a hyperpigmented, dry, scaly dermatosis present bilaterally over the lower legs, especially around the ankles. Finally, as the disease reaches its peak ulceration and/or secondary infection may occur.

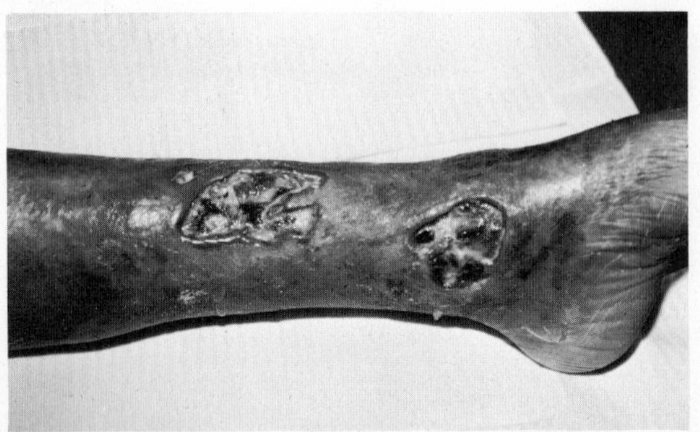

Figure 11. Stasis dermatitis with ulceration.

Treatment
Standing or sitting positions for prolonged periods should be avoided. The patient should maintain a supine position whenever possible, with the legs elevated at least 15 degrees above the horizontal. The obese patient should lose weight. Support hose or gelatin boots may be necessary to prevent stasis of blood. Chronic stasis dermatitis responds to corticosteroid creams or ointments. Acute or subacute lesions may require Burrow's or tap water soaks. If superinfection intervenes, oral or topical antibiotics may be necessary.

If ulceration occurs, there is no single treatment that is effective in all cases. Bed rest is mandatory. In addition, soaking with Burrow's solution or tap water and applying an antibiotic cream or ointment is important in preventing superinfection and providing debridement. Neomycin applied to the ulcer may cause allergic contact dermatitis and should not be used. In large ulcerations, pinch grafting or surgical intervention may be necessary. In smaller lesions, applying small plastic beads (Debrisan) is an excellent means of decreasing exudation and removing bacteria from wounds.

Seborrheic Dermatitis (Plates 12, 13)

Clinical Characteristics
Seborrheic dermatitis initially occurs in infants as cradle cap. This is a greasy yellow inflammatory plaque confined to the scalp. Eventually the disease disappears only to recur at puberty when it involves the scalp, ear canals, chest, back, axillae, eyebrows, nasolabial fold, and eyelids. Frequently, the lesions affect only one area of the body. The typical lesion of seborrheic dermatitis is a greasy yellow plaque with mild erythema and scaling, which generally increases in severity with age. This disease may be associated with severe acne, parkinsonism, and phenytoin ingestion.

Differential Diagnosis
The differential diagnosis of seborrheic dermatitis includes contact dermatitis, psoriasis, tinea, and lupus erythematosus.

Treatment
It is important that the patient be made aware that the disease is chronic and may recur if the treatment is discontinued. Severe forms of seborrheic dermatitis may be treated with topically applied corticosteroids. If the disease occurs over the eyelashes or on the eyelids, application of corticosteroids can increase intraocular pressure. Milder cases of the disease may

be treated with shampoos containing salicylic acid, sulfur, or tar. These shampoos can be used on a routine basis and are available without a prescription. In order to suppress the eruption, it is important to shampoo frequently.

BENIGN TUMORS OF THE SKIN

Seborrheic Keratosis (Fig. 12)

Seborrheic keratosis is a benign epithelial tumor of the skin, usually occurring after age 30, and commonly in older patients. Clinically, it is a verrucous, or warty brown to black lesion that appears on the face, chest, or back. The lesion has a stuck-on appearance and looks as though it can be flicked off with a fingernail. It is sharply marginated and grows slowly, darkening in color.

There is no malignant potential for this lesion and it is treated only for cosmetic reasons. The treatment of choice is surgical removal, either by shaving and dessicating or by curettage. Alternatively, cryotherapy with liquid nitrogen is a reasonable treatment in patients who do not want surgery. It is seldom necessary to excise seborrheic keratosis and, indeed, excision usually gives a less than adequate cosmetic effect.

Actinic Keratosis (Fig. 13)

The actinic keratosis is a rough hyperkeratotic patch present on an erythematous base that occurs on sun-damaged skin and is associated with multiple telangiectasias and marked actinic damage. Inasmuch as the tumor is not sharply marginated, it is frequently easier to detect its presence by feeling the skin rather than by looking at it. The surface of the actinic keratosis has a sandpaperlike quality. Skin biopsy is indicated in the diagnosis of this disease. Histologic findings include dermal actinic degeneration, nuclear dysplasia, and columns of parakeratotic cells in the stratum corneum.

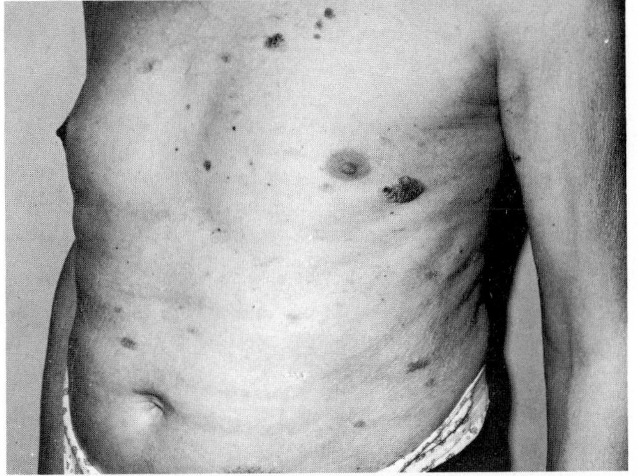

Figure 12. Multiple seborrheic keratoses of the chest.

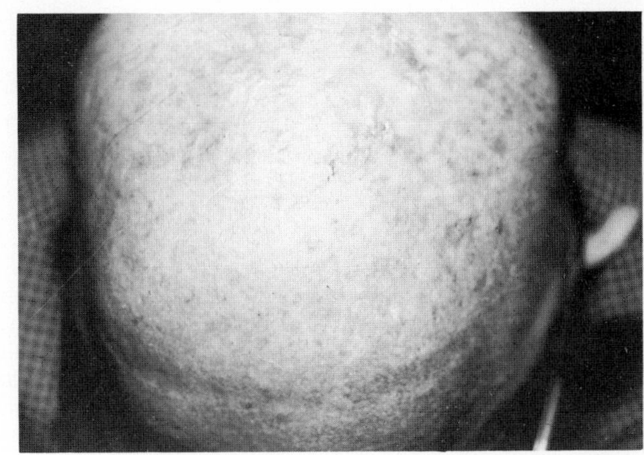

Figure 13. Actinic keratoses of the scalp.

Because there is significant malignant potential, actinic keratosis should definitely be treated. Topical 5-fluorouracil cream or lotion in a 1-5% concentration is the treatment of choice. It is applied twice daily to the entire involved area for a period of 3 weeks. Following a 3-week application, areas of potential malignancy become bright red. At this point, the topical 5-fluorouracil is discontinued and a topical corticosteroid cream is started. Alternatively, if the number of actinic keratoses is relatively small, each one can be frozen with liquid nitrogen. Finally, individual lesions may be curetted, or shaved and dessicated. In any case, the patient must be carefully observed for recurrence of the problem.

Benign Melanocytic Nevi (Plates 14, 15)

Melanocytic nevi arise from pigmented nevus cells and usually appear shortly after birth, eventually numbering 40 per individual. There are three varieties of melanocytic nevi including the junction nevus, compound nevus, and intradermal nevus. The junction nevus is a flat, tan, well-defined macule of uniform color that has most of the nevus cells confined to the basal cell layer of the epidermis. Junction nevi are replaced by compound nevi as the patient ages. The compound nevus has nevus cells in both the junctional area and in the dermis. These are elevated, regularly-pigmented lesions that may be dome-shaped, verrucoid, or papillomatous. Finally, as the patient becomes older, a larger number of intradermal nevi appear. These are elevated, soft nonpigmented tumors that also may be dome-shaped, polypoid, or papillomatous. The nevi may be widely distributed over the entire body including the palms of the hands, soles of the feet, and the genitalia.

Melanocytic nevi are usually removed for one of the following reasons: the patient wants it removed for cosmetic reasons; the patient is concerned that the lesion may be malignant; and the physician is concerned that the lesion may be malignant. Any pigmented lesion should be removed if it ulcerates, bleeds, enlarges, undergoes pigmentary change, develops satellite lesions, itches, becomes inflamed, is painful, or develops a rough, scaly, or irregular surface. All pigmented, surgically removed lesions should be subjected to histopathologic confirmation. In all cases, malingnat melanoma must be thoroughly ruled out.

Complete, simple excision is the treatment of choice for melanocytic nevi. Shave biopsy or curettage may not be adequate since the resultant histologic specimen may be incomplete or disrupted.

Acrochordon (Skin Tags) (Fig. 14)

A skin tag is a papillomatous polypoid lesion commonly appearing in middle age. The usual location for an acrochordon is the upper trunk, the neck, or the axillae. Occasionally, acrochordons may become inflamed secondary to trauma and may be symptomatic. The differential diagnosis of this lesion includes intradermal nevi and neurofibromatoses. The treatment of choice is excision of the lesion, or shave and dessication.

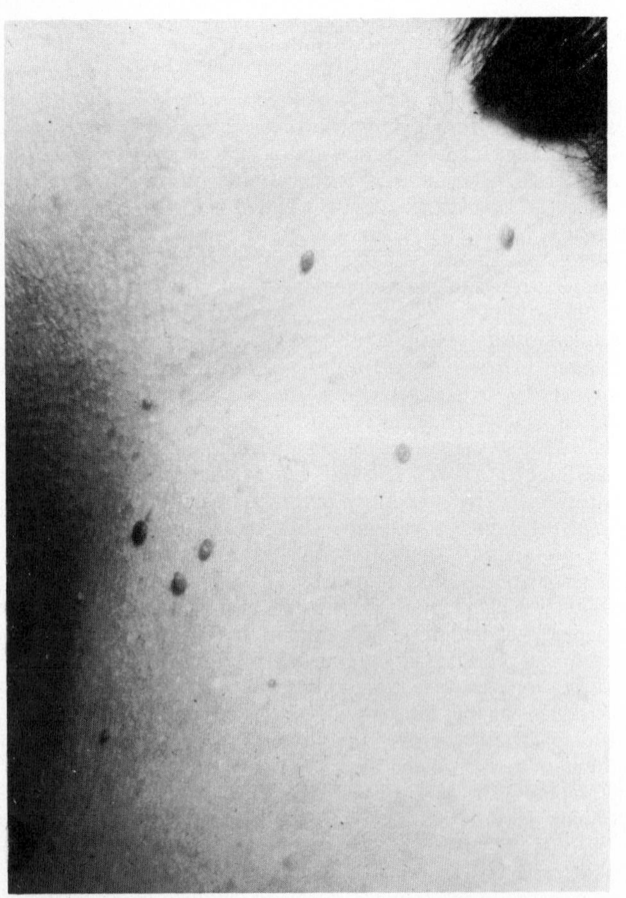

Figure 14. Multiple acrochordons.

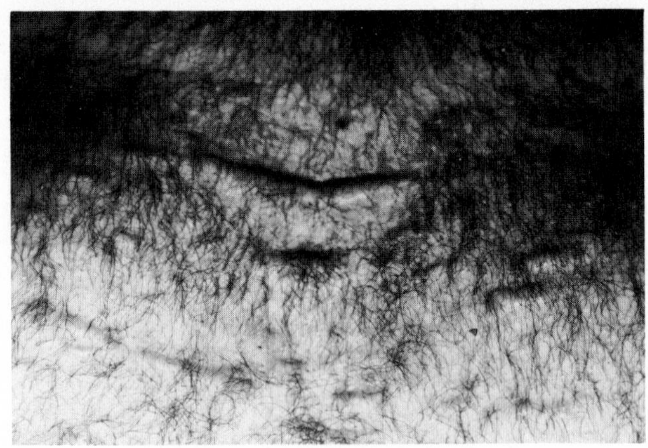

Figure 15. Linear keloids of the chest.

Keloids (Fig. 15)

The keloid represents an exaggeration of the normal fibroblastic response to injury and presents as thickened, painful scar tissue. Keloids occur more commonly in blacks and are most prevalent over the sternum, ears, back, legs, and neck. Although they are benign, they may be most disturbing to the patient—both symptomatically and cosmetically. Keloids may be treated in several ways. First, it is best to avoid elective surgery on regions of the body that are prone to develop keloids in high risk patients. When a keloid has formed, intermediate doses of potent corticosteroids may be injected into the lesion at 2-4-week intervals in order to cause atrophy of the keloid. Occasionally, when this type of therapy fails, it is possible to excise the original keloid and, after a period of several weeks, begin injecting the excision line with corticosteroids.

MALIGNANT TUMORS OF THE SKIN

Basal Cell Epithelioma (Plates 16, 17)

Basal cell epithelioma is the most common malignant tumor affecting males. It is more prevalent in light-skinned individuals who have had extensive sun exposure. It also occurs commonly in patients who have ingested arsenic for medicinal purposes, and in those who have received radiation therapy. In addition, the basal cell carcinoma may occur along with congenital syndromes such as xeroderma pigmentosa or basal cell nevus syndrome. The basal cell epithelioma is probably related to benign adnexal tumors that have proliferated in an undifferentiated manner. It may arise from basal cells of the surface epidermis or from the external root sheath of hair follicles. Basal cell epitheliomas do not possess the ability to undergo differentiation when they are removed from the epidermis or the dermis and, as such, they rarely metastasize. Most of the damage is done by their direct extension from the skin to underlying tissue.

There are several clinical varieties of basal cell carcinoma, the most common being the noduloulcerative form. This type of basal cell carcinoma appears as nodules or papules that are pearly in color and surrounded by telangiectasias. As the lesion grows, ulceration of the center occurs and the typical ulcerated translucent papule with surrounding telangiectasias results. There are several other types of basal cell carcinomas including the superficial, pigmented, and sclerosing. The superficial basal cell carcinoma presents as a lightly pigmented, sharply defined plaque with a scaly surface. The plaque has a pearly telangiectatic border and spreads outward as it grows. Pigmented basal cell carcinomas appear as brown to black and may easily be misdiagnosed as malignant melanomas. The most dangerous type of basal cell carcinoma is the sclerosing (morphea) variety, which is characteristically yellow, waxy, white, and indurated (like morphea). These lesions are more dangerous because they are more difficult to cure. The basal cells insinuate themselves between collagen bundles and cannot easily be removed.

The diagnosis of basal cell carcinoma is made clinically and on histologic examination. The typical basal cell carcinoma is composed of irregular masses of basaloid cells lying either under the epidermis or within the dermis. The periphery of the cell masses forms a palisade pattern, resembling the basal layer of the epidermis. There is a marked fibrous proliferation surrounding the masses of basaloid cells.

The initial treatment of uncomplicated basal cell carcinomas yields a 95% cure with most surgical techniques. Curettage and electrodessication is most commonly employed, although surgical excision has been successfully performed in selected cases. A method of microscopically controlled chemosurgery has also been recommended. The tissue is fixed in vivo and is sectioned. Each section is carefully examined histologically, and additional cuts are made in areas where tumor cells remain. Radiation therapy may also be useful in treating selected basal cell carcinomas, especially in elderly or debilitated patients. Also, cryotherapy may occasionally be indicated. It is important to advise the patient with basal cell carcinoma to prevent further sun damage by using appropriate sun screening agents. To monitor recurrence, the patient should be seen two or three times annually.

Squamous Cell Carcinoma (Fig. 16)

The squamous cell carcinoma is a truly malignant epithelial cancer that arises from keratinizing epidermal cells. This tumor occurs more frequently in elderly individuals and, like basal cell carcinoma, is associated with exposure to sunlight, ionizing radiation, and arsenic. In addition, squamous cell carcinomas can occur in actinic keratoses, burns, and scars.

Clinically, squamous cell carcinoma is found more commonly on the upper face, lower lips, hands, ears, and chest. It is frequently associated with marked actinic degeneration of the skin. This type of carcinoma is usually a solitary lesion that slowly enlarges and develops an indurated base. The surface of the nodule becomes crusted and eventually ulcerates. Occasionally, the lesions appear verrucous or form plaques.

Histologically, the squamous cell carcinoma consists of irregular masses of epithelial cells that, depending on their degree of differentiation, may be able to form keratin. Well-differentiated tumors form keratin masses called horn pearls, while highly malignant, poorly differentiated squamous cell carcinomas may possess a large number of mitotic figures, marked dysplasia, and an inability to make keratin.

Squamous cell carcinoma must be differentiated from basal cell epitheliomas, other malignant tumors, infectious granulomas, syphilis, and keratoacanthomas.

Treatment for squamous cell carcinoma is similar to that of basal cell carcinoma. The skin must be protected from carcinogenic hazards such as sunlight. Possible therapeutic modalities include surgical excision, curettage and electrodessication, microscopic chemosurgery, and radiation therapy. Finally, because squamous cell carcinomas metastasize via the lymphatic channels in approximately 2% of cases, a workup for systemic involvement may be indicated, especially with squamous cell carcinomas that metastasize early such as those on the glans penis, vulva, perianal area, lip, and ear. If regional lymphadenopathy exists, a lymph node biopsy should be performed however, prophylactic lymph node dissection is usually not indicated.

The prognosis of this type of cancer depends on the clinical appearance, the histology, and the depth to which the lesion extends into the skin. Squamous cell carcinomas that arise in actinic keratosis have a better prognosis, whereas those that arise on mucosal surfaces (in burn scars or secondary to radiation) have a poor prognosis. Also, squamous cell carcinomas that form keratin are probably less malignant.

Malignant Melanoma (Plate 18)

The malignant melanoma is a dangerous pigmented tumor that is often conveniently classified into three varieties: nodular, superficial, and lentigo maligna. The nodular melanoma is an elevated brown to black lesion that appears in any age group

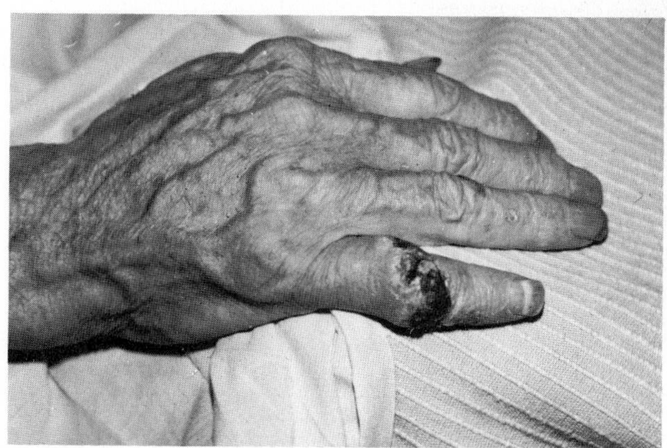

Figure 16. A squamous cell carcinoma on a patient who had received medicinal arsenic years before.

on any area of the body. Because it metastasizes early, it is by far the most dangerous type of melanoma. Superficial spreading malignant melanomas are large, relatively flat, irregularly pigmented lesions with irregular borders and crusted or ulcerated surfaces. This variety is more common and has a higher incidence in younger individuals. Finally, the lentigo maligna melanoma is a nodular lesion that occurs in a flat, mottled, pigmented lesion called a lentigo maligna. These are most commonly seen on the face of elderly patients and have the best prognosis of any melanoma.

In distinguishing a benign, pigmented nevus from a malignant melanoma, the features described in Table 4 are considered: however, none of the features mentioned are diagnostic of malignant melanoma. If present, they serve as a warning that a biopsy is indicated.

The prognosis of melanoma depends on several factors including sex (women have a slightly lower incidence than men), size, location on the body, depth of penetration, thickness of tumor, presence of satellite lesions, presence of nodal or systemic metastases, and the relative number of mitoses present on histologic examination. As previously mentioned, patients with lentigo maligna melanoma do better than those with nodular melanomas. Thus, a nodular melanoma on the back of a young male patient would be more aggressive than a lentigo maligna melanoma on the face of an elderly woman. This would, of course, dictate how the lesion would be treated.

If the physician suspects a malignant melanoma, it should be completely excised if possible and sent to a pathologist. Current therapies for malignant melanoma include primary wide excision of the lesion with a graft and nodal dissection, chemotherapy with single or multiple agents (Dacarbozinc nitrosoureas), chemosurgery, immunotherapy, and radiotherapy.

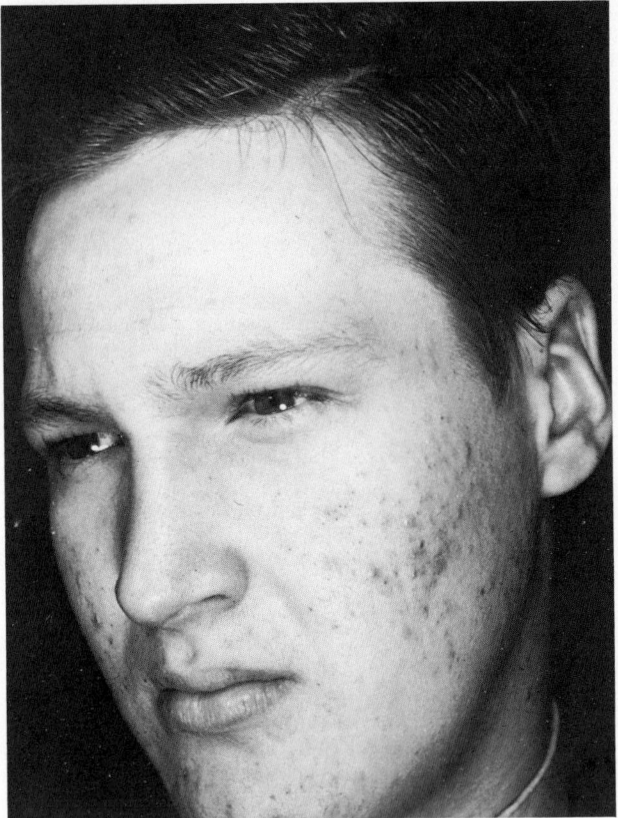

Figure 17. Inflammatory acne of the face.

ACNE

Acne Vulgaris (Figs. 17-19)

Clinical Characteristics

Acne vulgaris is a chronic inflammatory disorder, common in young individuals, that involves the pilosebaceous units. The disease occurs primarily on the face, neck. upper arms, back, and/or chest, and is frequently accompanied by an oily complexion. Acne lesions are usually divided into two major groups, that is, inflammatory and noninflammatory. Closed and open comedones constitute the major noninflammatory lesions of acne. An open comedo (blackhead) contains keratin in which melanin has been deposited, making the lesion appear black. In most instances, open comedones do not lead to the development of inflammatory acne. On the other hand, a closed comedo (whitehead) contains cheesy, white keratin along with some sebum and hair. These lesions may obstruct pilosebaceous openings and therefore lead to the development of inflammatory acne lesions. Inflammatory acne is probably the most devastating variety; this consists of papules, pustules, nodules, and cysts that may occur on the cheeks, forehead, chin, chest, and back Inflammatory acne is disfiguring and may result in extensive scarring of involved areas. Scars that form may be small, pitlike depressions or may cut deep, jagged furrows through the skin. Keloids or hypertrophic scars may be the unwelcome sequelae of this type of acne.

Table 4. Differentiation Between Nevus and Melanoma

Feature	*Nevus*	*Melanoma*
Color	Regularly distributed, usually brown	Irregularly distributed, red, blue, white, or black
Border	Regular	Irregular with pseudopods
Surface	Regular, possesses normal skin lines	Skin lines gone; crusting, bleeding, or ulceration
Satellite lesions	Absent	Present
Symptoms	None	Itching, burning, or pain
Growth	Grows in proportion to patient	Rapidly growing

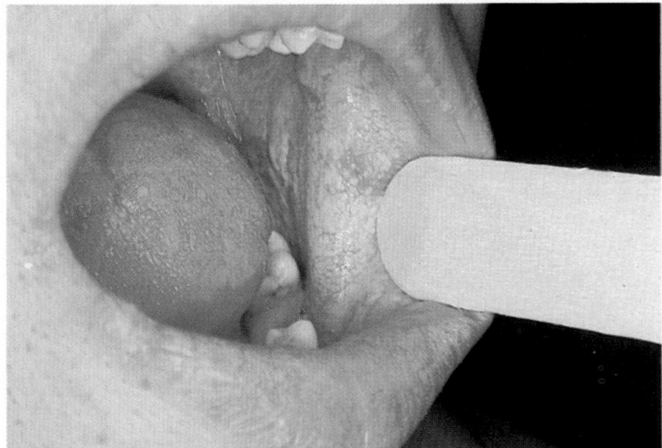

Plate 1. Lacy white infiltrates of lichen planus are present on the buccal mucosa.

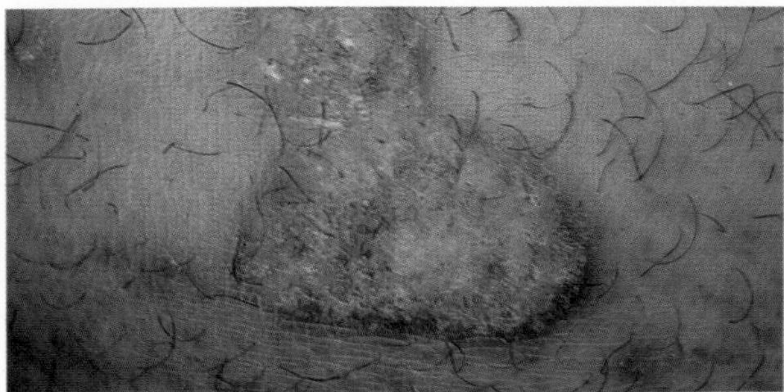

Plate 4. Large violaceous plaques of lichen planus.

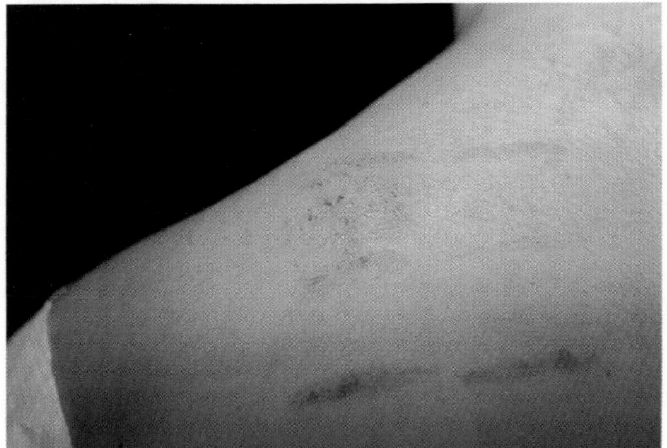

Plate 2. A positive patch test in a patient allergic to nickel.

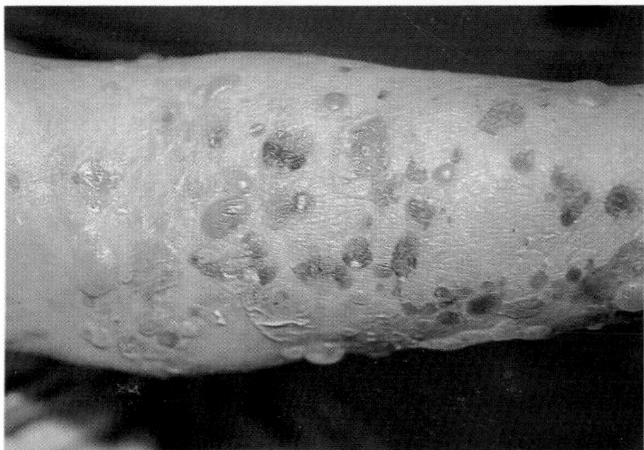

Plate 5. A patient with bullous pemphigoid showing multiple tense vesicles.

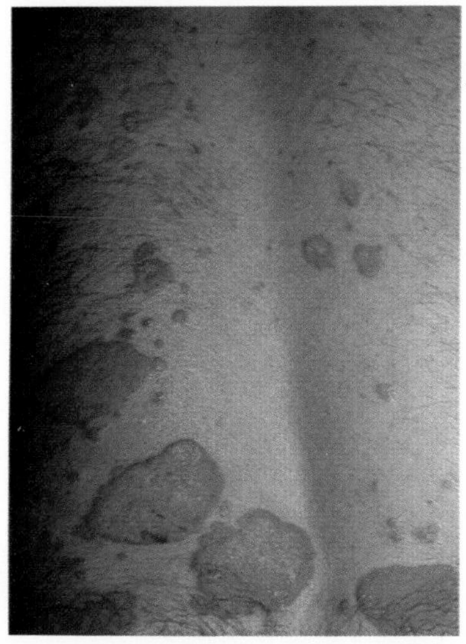

Plate 3. Large red plaques with silvery-white scales are typical of psoriasis.

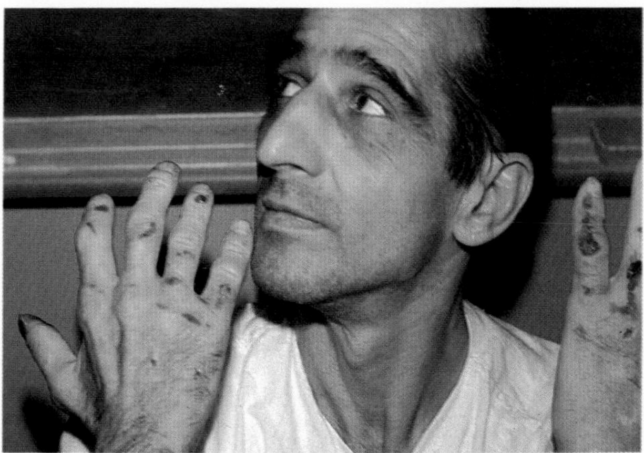

Plate 6. A patient with porphyria cutanea tarda who demonstrates hypertrichosis and excoriated vesicles in a photo distribution.

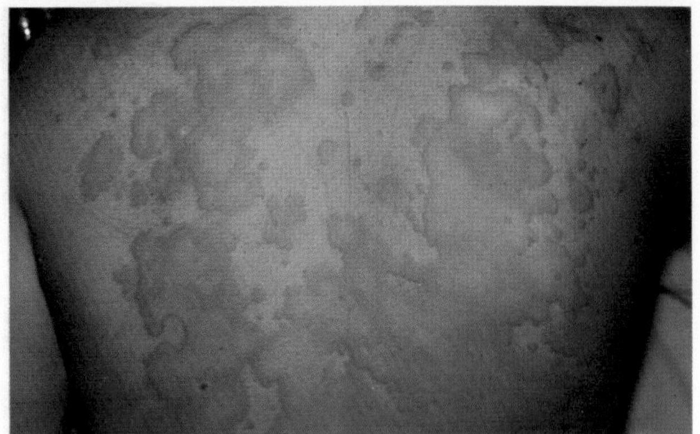

Plate 7. Urticaria.

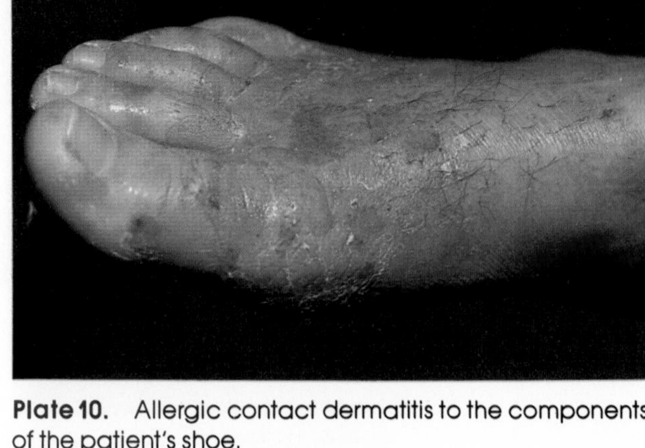

Plate 10. Allergic contact dermatitis to the components of the patient's shoe.

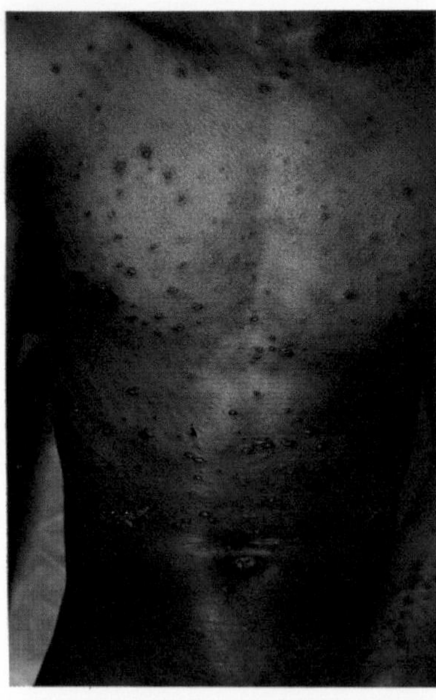

Plate 8.
Erythema multiforme of the chest.

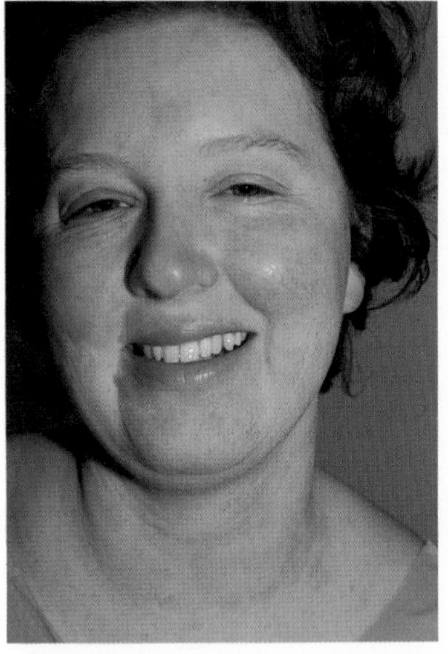

Plate 11.
Allergic contact dermatitis to the patient's cosmetics.

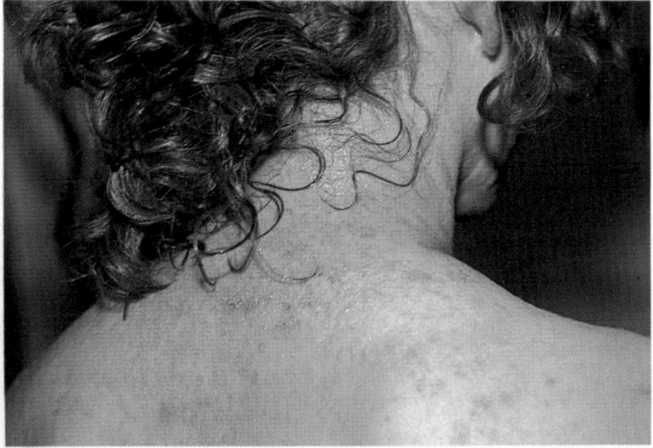

Plate 9. Acute contact dermatitis in a patient with hair dye allergy.

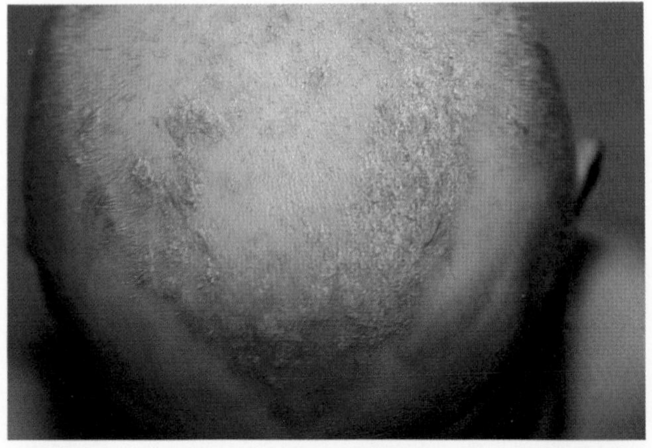

Plate 12. The greasy, yellow scales of seborrheic dermatitis.

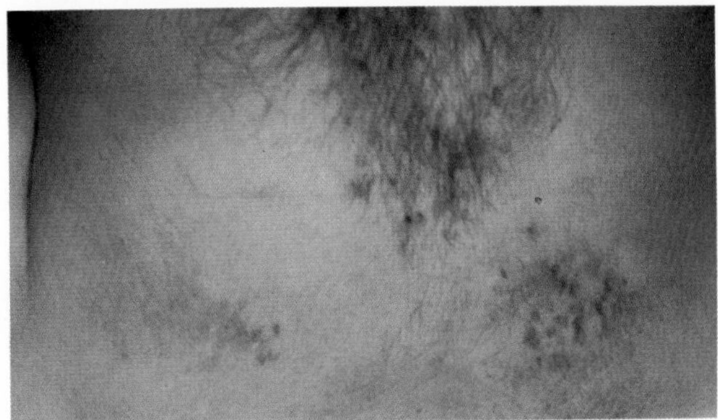

Plate 13. Seborrheic dermatitis of the chest.

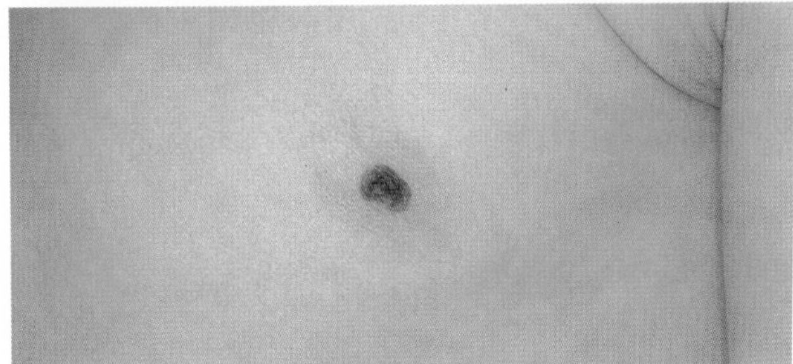

Plate 14. Intradermal nevus.

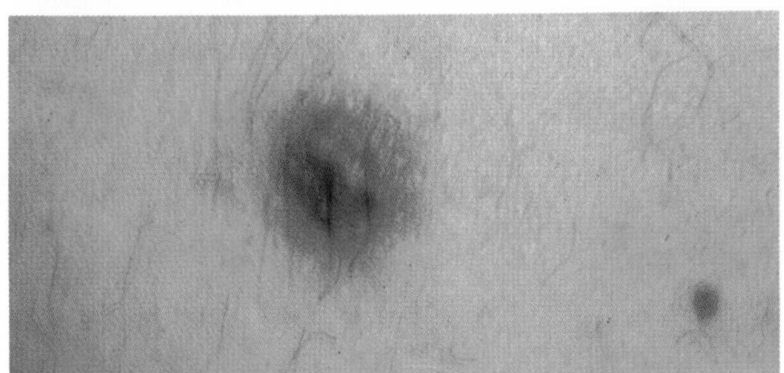

Plate 15. Compound nevus.

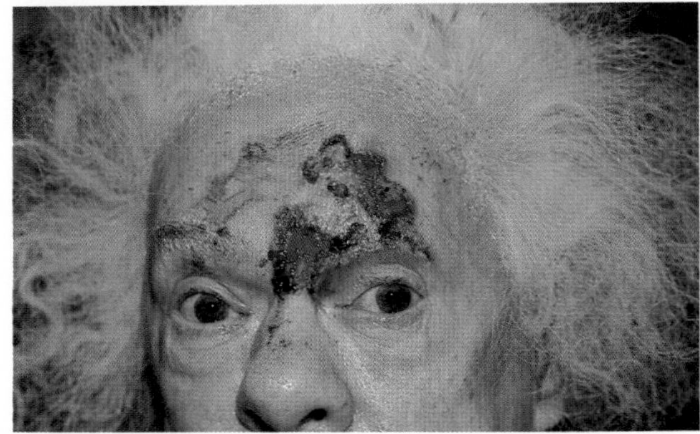

Plate 16. A large, destructive basal cell carcinoma is present on this patient's forehead.

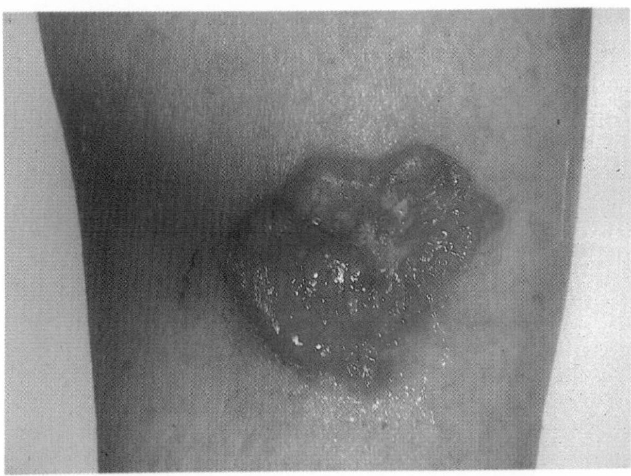

Plate 17. A basal cell carcinoma with the typical waxy, or pearly, appearance.

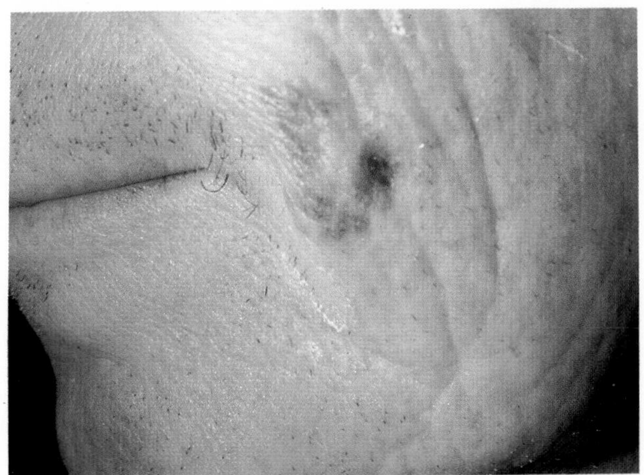

Plate 18. Lentigo maligna melanoma.

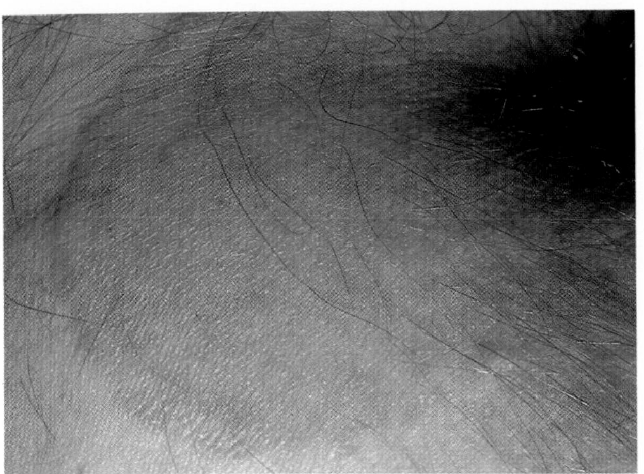

Plate 19. A plaque of tinea corporis showing an indurated border and scaly center.

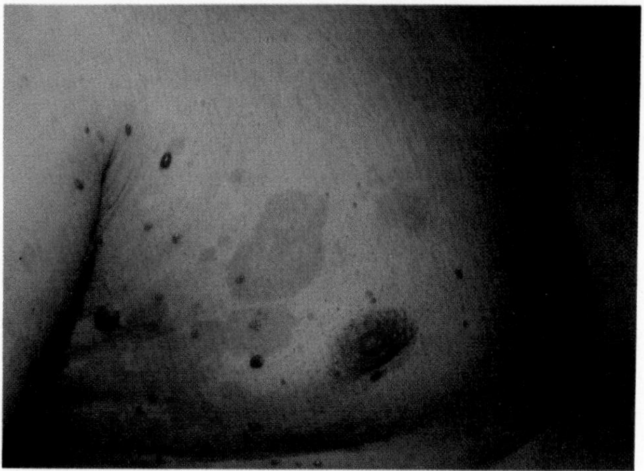

Plate 20. Tinea versicolor in a patient with multiple acrochordons.

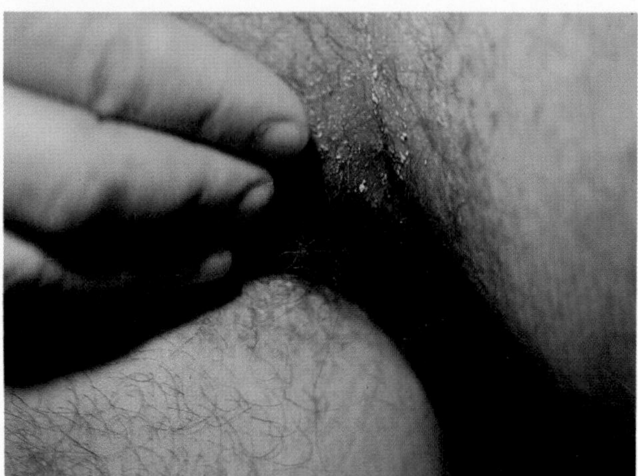

Plate 21. Intertriginous candidiasis. Notice the presence of satellite lesions surrounding the main plaque.

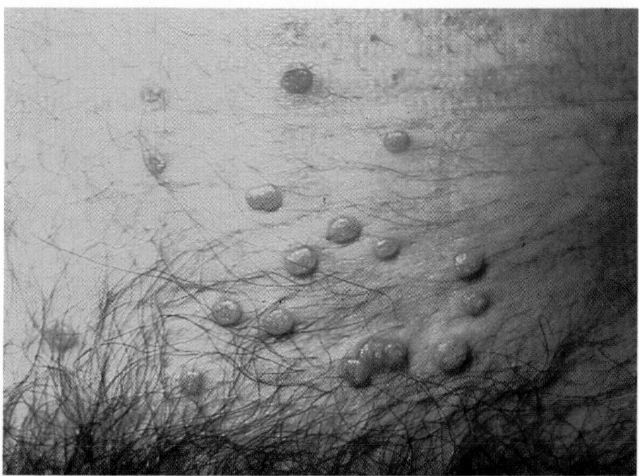

Plate 22. Molluscum contagiosum.

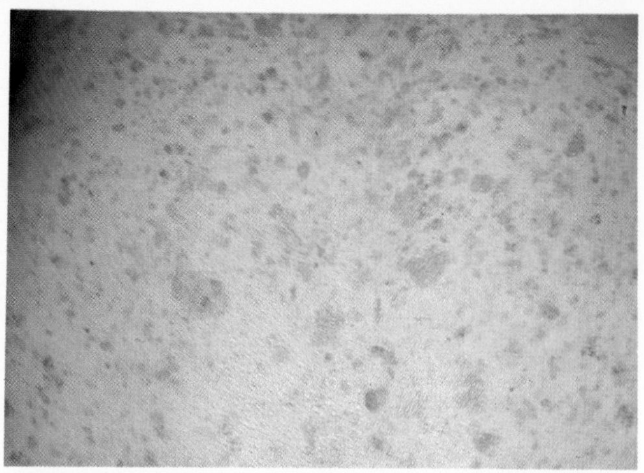

Plate 23. Arsenical keratoses commonly present in patients with internal malignancy.

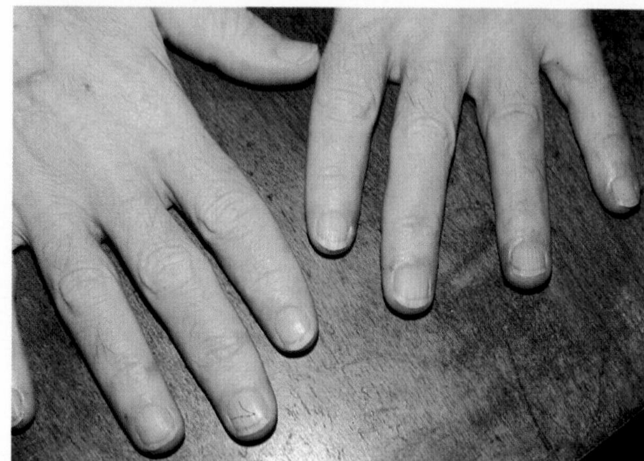

Plate 24. Dermatomyositis in a cancer patient — periungual telangiectasias.

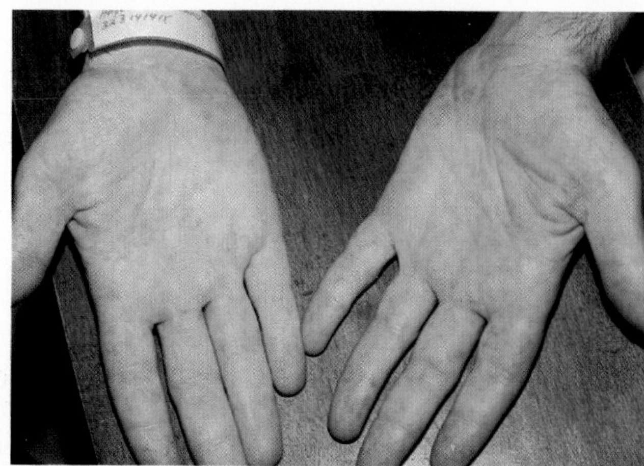

Plate 25. Dermatomyositis in a cancer patient — palmar erythema.

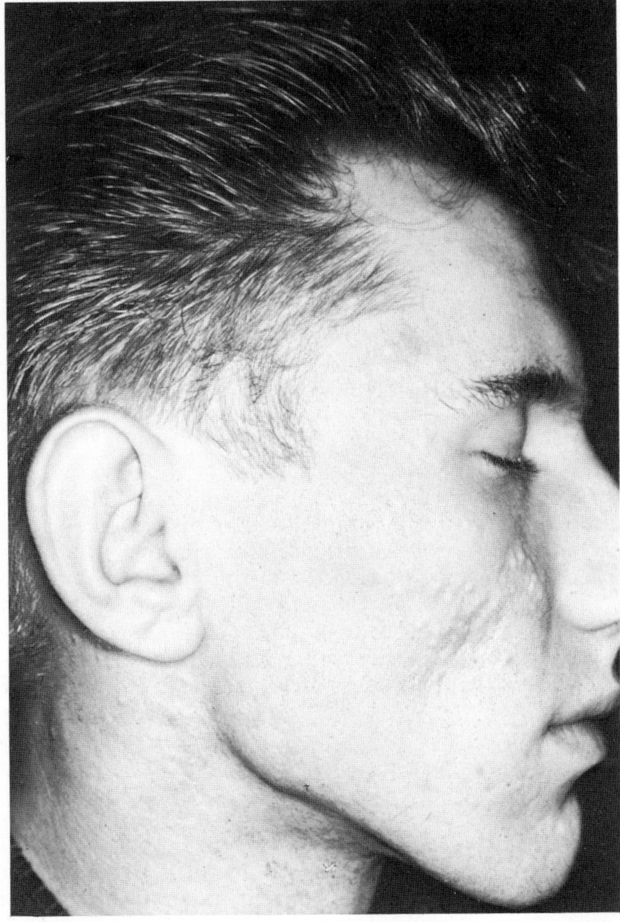

Figure 18. Noninflammatory closed comedo type acne.

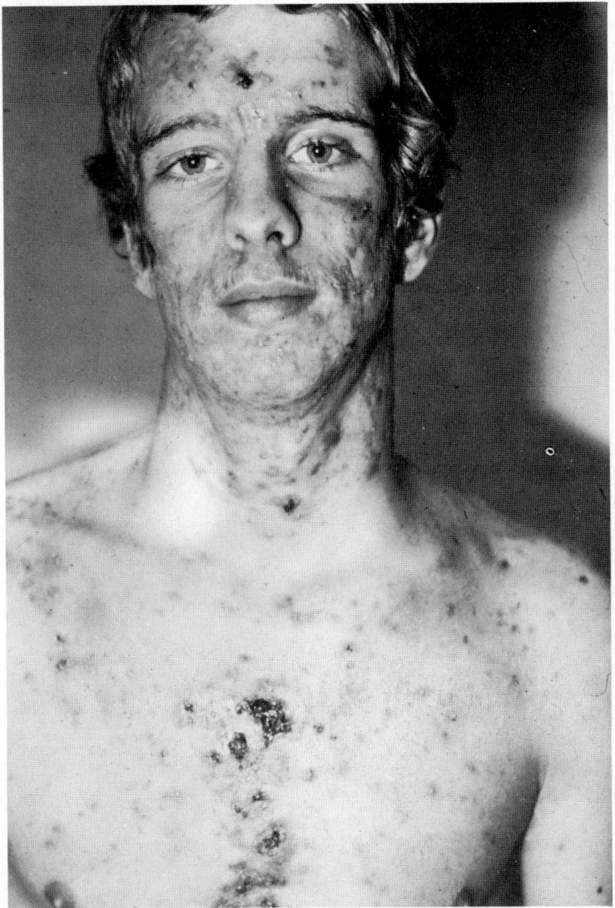

Figure 19. Severe scarring acne conglobata.

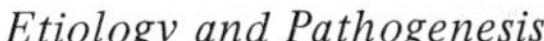

Etiology and Pathogenesis

The cause of acne vulgaris is unknown; however, there are many factors that may exacerbate a patient's acne. It is well known that emotions play an important role in the development of acne. Individuals who are distressed or who have undergone traumatic experiences frequently develop severe flares of acne vulgaris. In addition, the ingestion of drugs such as corticosteroids, phenytoin, bromide, and iodides may result in acne vulgaris. Chemicals, both domestic and industrial, may be important factors in causing acne; these include various cosmetics, moisturizing creams, petrochemicals, tar, and halogens. Interestingly enough, oral contraceptives may either induce or suppress acne; many women frequently experience a flare of acne just prior to the onset of menstruation.

Differential Diagnosis

Included in the differential diagnosis of acne vulgaris are the following diseases: folliculitis, pseudofolliculitis, acne rosacea, perioral dermatitis, and acneiform drug eruptions.

Treatment

Acne vulgaris can be an emotionally disabling disease. Many patients need a good deal of support from the physician, and frequent office visits may be helpful. In many instances, the elimination of environmental factors that can be identified to exacerbate the condition is beneficial. If possible, discontinuing the drugs that may be exacerbating the acne is often helpful. Dietary restriction for the control of acne is rarely useful. Nonprescription medications include benzoyl peroxide lotion, sulfur, and salicylic acid. Ultraviolet light or sunlight may be helpful in some cases of acne. When the above treatment has failed, there are several prescription medications available. Closed comedo acne may be treated with vitamin A acid (Retin A) as long as the patient does not receive significant concomitant sun exposure. This medication, however, is very irritating to the skin and may make the acne appear initially worse before it begins to improve. The patient should be mentally and physically prepared to use vitamin A acid. Benzoyl peroxide gel (5 or 10%) is considerably more effective than benzoyl peroxide lotion in the treatment of both inflammatory and noninflammatory acne. Oral and topical antibiotics constitute an important treatment for acne vulgaris. Tetracycline and erythromycin, 250-1500 mg/day in divided doses, are the two most commonly used oral antibiotics. Topically applied clindamycin has been shown to be safe and almost as effective as oral tetracycline.

Surgery is a useful adjunct in the treatment of the disease. Liquid nitrogen or carbon dioxide slush applied to acne lesions has a noticeable drying effect. In addition, opening closed comedones, and opening and removal of large cysts by incision and drainage are sometimes helpful. Finally, long-acting corticosteroids such as triamcinolone (Kenalog), 5 mg/ml, may be injected directly into pustular, nodular, or cystic lesions. Other rarely used therapeutic modalities include oral vitamin A, zinc, x-ray therapy, and dapsone. Each of these may be effective and indeed indicated in some cases of acne, but are potentially dangerous and should be employed only by physicians experienced in their use.

Acne Rosacea (Fig. 20)

Clinical Characteristics

Clinical characteristics of acne rosacea include erythema of the face, with telangiectasias located mainly over the nose, chin, and malar areas. Along with the telangiectasias, there may be multiple pustules and papules located over the central portion of the face. The lesions of acne rosacea frequently occur in individuals over 30 years of age, a large percentage being women. In the most severe form, hypertrophy of sebaceous glands of the nose leads to the development of rhinophyma.

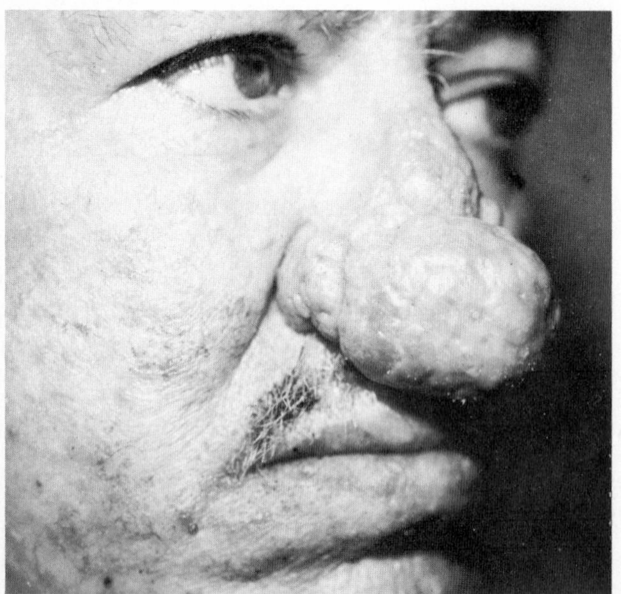

Figure 20. Severe long-standing acne rosacea with sebaceous hyperplasia of the nose (rhinophyma).

Etiology and Pathogenesis

The etiology of the condition is unknown. It is more common in those who blush easily. The consumption of large quantities of coffee, tea, alcohol, tobacco, and hot or spicy food predispose to acne rosacea. In addition, those who work in hot environments may develop this disease.

Differential Diagnosis

This disease must be differentiated from acne vulgaris, seborrheic dermatitis, lupus erythematosus, and photosensitivity.

Therapy

The treatment of acne rosacea begins with the elimination of exacerbating factors. Nonfluorinated corticosteroids such as hydrocortisone are frequently helpful. However, fluorinated corticosteroids may be associated with the development of acneiform eruptions. Precipitated sulfur cream or ointment (2-10%) is useful in treating many cases of acne rosacea. Finally, oral tetracycline (250-1,000 mg/day) is highly effective, but the use of this drug must be avoided during pregnancy.

FUNGAL INFECTIONS OF THE SKIN

Dermatophytes (Fig. 21, Plate 19, Fig. 22)

Clinical Characteristics

Dermatophytic infections are caused by true fungi that inhabit the stratum corneum of hair, skin, and nails, and are single-cell microorganisms lacking chlorophyll that form septate hyphae. These organisms are unable to exist in deeper layers of the skin and rarely cause systemic disease. They are transmitted either from man to man, or from infected animals to man. The major groups of dermatophytes that cause infections in human beings are *Microsporum*, *Epidermophyton*, and *Trichophyton*. Clinically, fungal disease is named for the region of the body involved including tinea capitis (ringworm of the scalp), tinea barbae (ringworm of the beard), tinea pedis (athlete's foot), tinea manus (ringworm of the hand), tinea cruris (ringworm of the groin) (Fig. 21), tinea corporis (infection of nonhair areas of the body) (Plate 19), and onychomycosis (infection of the nails). In addition to infection in these areas, the body can react in uninfected areas with a dermatophytid reaction. This is an immunologic response of the body to dermatophyte infection. The clinical characteristics of each of the different fungal infections are briefly described in the following paragraphs.

There are three clinical variations of tinea capitis: the papulosquamous variety, black dot ringowrm, and kerion, each caused by a different organism. The papulosquamous variety appears as round to oval patches of alopecia with hairs being

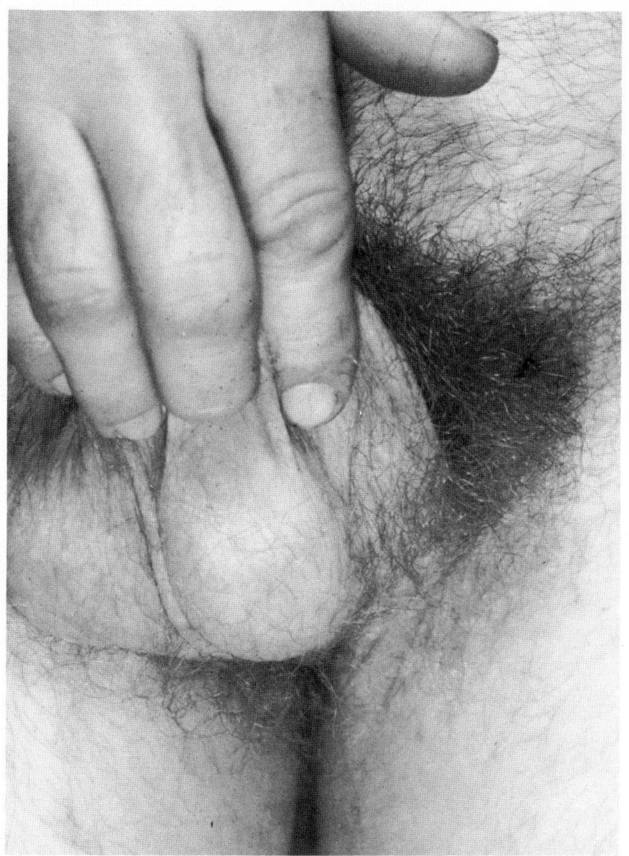

Figure 21. The well-defined scaly plaque of tinea cruris on the inner aspect of thigh.

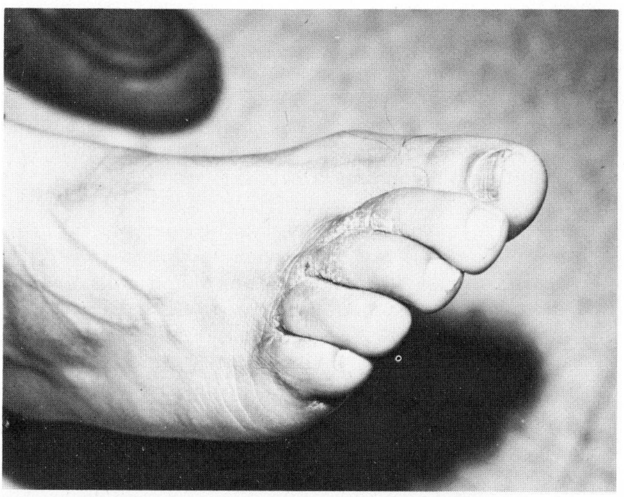

Figure 22. The intertriginous type of tinea pedis.

broken off close to the surface of the skin. The scalp shows marked scaling and various degrees of erythema and inflammation. This type of tinea capitis is unusual in adults. The black dot ringworm is smooth with sharp borders and no scales. Hair is broken off close to the level of the scalp and, as such, small black dots are seen on the scalp. The *kerion* type is extremely inflammatory and is characterized by crusting erythematous pustular nodules that lead to scarring.

A second type of cutaneous dermatophyte infection is tinea barbae or ringworm of the beard. This occurs in individuals such as butchers and farmers who handle animals. The lesions may be inflammatory with crusting and erythema, or they may be noninflammatory with plaque formation and peripheral scaling.

Tinea pedis, or athlete's foot, is a very common problem in individuals living in warm climates who wear occlusive shoes. Tinea pedis may be intertriginous with maceration and scaling between the toes, inflammation with blisters and vesicles mostly around the instep of the foot, or bullae with generalized scaling and mild erythema covering the entire foot.

Tinea manus or tines of the hands, is one of the least common types of dermatophyte infections. Usually the infection is unilateral and consists of asymptomatic, dry, scaly hyperkeratosis of the palm. Frequently, tinea pedis occurs in the same individual.

Tinea cruris is a mildly erythematous, scaling eruption that occurs in the inguinal fold, and may involve the scrotum and the upper thigh. No satellite lesions of pustules occur in this type of lesion, but frequently there is a slightly indurated active border. Tinea cruris occurs in individuals who have tinea infections elsewhere and who have experienced significant sweating and maceration in the groin.

Finally, tinea infections of the nail, onychomycosis, may involve any number of nails and generally begins at the distal edge of the nail and extends proximally. The typical lesion is brittle, yellow, and the nail plate appears discolored and opaque. Toenails are more commonly involved in this process than are fingernails.

Diagnosis

The diagnosis of dermtophyte infection of the skin is made through careful clinical examination of the patient. Potassium hydroxide (KOH) mounts have already been described in detail earlier in this chapter. They allow the rapid diagnosis of most types of tinea infections. Frequently, it is necessary to obtain several specimens for diagnosis. The active border of an expanding lesion is probably best for obtaining a KOH specimen. In addition, Wood's light examination may be helpful in the diagnosis of tinea capitus caused by *M. canis* or *M. audouinii*. Finally, the causative organism may be cultured on Sabouraud's agar. Several specimens should be obtained from each involved region of the body. Culture results usually take about 15 days.

Differential Diagnosis

The differential diagnosis of various dermatophyte infections includes the following:

DISEASE	DIFFERENTIAL DIAGNOSIS
Tinea capitis	Alopecia areata
	Psoriasis
	Folliculitis
	Irritant or allergic contact dermatitis
	Seborrheic dermatitis
	Lupus erythematosus
Tinea pedis	Candidiasis
	Psoriasis
Tinea cruris	Candidiasis
	Erythrasma
	Psoriasis
	Seborrheic dermatitis
Tinea corporis	Pityriasis rosea
	Psoriasis
	Seborrheic dermatitis
	Nummular eczema
Onychomycosis	Psoriasis
	Lichen planus
	Candidiasis
	Paronychia

Treatment of Fungal Diseases

Griseofulvin is the systemic treatment of choice for dermatophyte infection. The average adult dose for this drug is 1 g/day but as much as 2 g/day may be necessary. In the treatment of most dermatophyte infections, griseofulvin should be continued for 4 weeks to 3 months. However, in treating infections of the nail, a 1-year trial of the drug may be necessary. The side effects of griseofulvin include phototoxicity, allergic reactions, headaches, and exacerbations of porphyria. Griseofulvin is the only effective drug in the treatment of tinea capitis or onychomycosis. These diseases are usually not successfully treated with topical agents. In other infections such as tinea corporis or tinea pedis, systemic agents are probably unnecessary and may even be less effective than topical agents.

Some topical agents useful for the treatment of fungal infections include miconazole (Monistat), clotrimazole (Lotrimin, Mycelex), and haloprogin (Halotex). These are available in cream and liquid formulations and are effective against a wide range of dermatophytes and yeasts. Tolnaftate (Tinactin), available as a cream, powder, or solution, is ineffective against yeast infections. Whitfield's ointment (salicylic acid, and benzoic acid in zinc oxide ointment) is successful in treating indolent chronic infections. In some instances, carbol-fuchsin dye (Castellani's paint) may be used in treating chronic tinea of the feet, or as an adjunct to other types of therapy. For the most part, topically applied antifungal agents should be used two or three times daily for up to 1 month.

Tinea Versicolor (Plate 20)

Clinical Characteristics

Tinea versicolor is an asymptomatic or slightly pruritic eruption occurring over the chest, back, and upper arms of young adults. It consists of well-defined, slightly pigmented plaques that are covered by a fine white scale. Because these areas do not pigment, they appear lighter in color than normal skin in the summer, and darker in the winter.

Etiology

The etiologic agent for this disease is a filamentous yeast, *Malassezia furfur*, which on KOH preparation looks like spaghetti and meatballs because there are multiple short filaments with groups of spores. Culture of *M. furfur* is difficult and is usually unnecessary.

Therapy

Many agents are useful in the treatment of tinea versicolor. The disease must be treated over a prolonged period and, apparently, uninvolved areas must also be treated. Selenium sulfide (Selsun), 2.5%, may be applied three times a week to the entire area between the neck and the groin. The material is left on overnight or for at least 12 hours. The applications are continued twice a week for 6 weeks, once a week for 6 weeks, and then every other week until a 6-month period of treatment has been completed. Skin color does not immediately return to normal. There is usually rapid improvement in itching, scaling, and redness if they are present.

Other topical agents used in treatment of this disease include sodium hyposulfite, miconazole, salicylic acid, sulfur preparations, clotrimazole, and haloprogin. Sodium hyposulfite and selenium sulfide are the least expensive of these agents.

Candidiasis (Plate 21)

Clinical Characteristics

Candida albicans infection involves intertriginous areas of the groin, breasts, and fingers. Lesions in these areas are moist, erythematous, macerated, and well demarcated. Frequently, little pustules form within the area of maceration. There are numerous small satellite papules or pustules surrounding the main mass of erythema. The involved areas often become denuded, leaving a raw, painful mass. *C. albicans* sometimes involves the mouth, causing a disease called thrush. Oral candidiasis, occurring more commonly in newborn infants, may be contracted from the mother's vaginal canal. The lesions are present on the pharynx, tongue, gingiva, and oral mucosa, and consist of creamy white plaques that later become painful erythematous erosions.

Candidiasis can involve the corners of the mouth, in which case it is called angular cheilitis. This commonly occurs in edentulous patients, or in those having an overbite with overlapping of the corners of the mouth. The warm, moist environment allows for the growth of *Candida* as well as bacteria. The lesions are red, fissured, and frequently painful. *C. albicans* can cause a chronic paronychia. This is an inflammatory, painful, and somewhat edematous lesion that occurs around the base of the fingernails and gives rise to nail dystrophy.

Etiology

The infections described above are caused by *C. albicans*. This organism grows in the keratin layer of the skin, and colonizes all types of damaged and inflamed skin. The predisposing factors include drugs such as corticosteroids, birth control pills, and systemic antibiotics; local factors such as irritation, moisture, heat, or obesity; and immunosuppressed states such as diabetes mellitus, leukemias, lymphomas, and carcinomas.

Treatment
The removal of underlying predisposing causes of infections are of paramount importance in the effective treatment of *C. albicans*. Therefore, an obese individual must lose weight. All patients with recurrent *Candida* infections should be examined for the possibility of the systemic diseases listed above.

The specific treatment of choice for *C. albicans* infections is nystatin (Mycostatin), which is available as a cream or vaginal inserts Alternatively, amphotericin B lotion (Fungizone) may be used. The newer antifungals such as miconazole and haloprogin are also useful in the treatment of candidiasis. Older modalities such as gentian violet are especially valuable in treating chronic cases of intertriginous candidiasis.

BACTERIAL DISEASES

Impetigo

Clinical Characteristics
Impetigo is a superficial bacterial infection of the skin that occurs on the face, hands, scalp, and genitalia. It is an extremely pruritic vesicular eruption that gives rise to exudative pustules that form a typical golden crust. The lesions, which expand in an annular fashion, are contagious to other individuals. It is common for satellite lesions to form.

Etiology
This disease is caused by coagulase-positive staphylococci or by β-hemolytic streptococci. Acute glomerulonephritis may occur in 2-5% of patients with this disorder.

Therapy
In an uncomplicated case of impetigo, the disease responds rapidly to topical antiseptics such as betadine or topical antibiotics. It is often beneficial to remove the crust and wash with an antibacterial soap. Direct contact with family members should be avoided. If the lesions are moist and exudative, soaks with Burrow's solution may be helpful. In rare instances when the disease is unresponsive to topical therapy, or when it is recurrent or an epidemic is possible, a culture should be obtained and treatment initiated with systemic antibiotics such as penicillin, erythromycin, or dicloxacillin.

Folliculitis, Furuncles, and Carbuncles (Fig. 23)

Clinical Characteristics
Folliculitis is a superficial eruption consisting of small pustules that are very pruritic, and frequently occur in moist intertriginous areas. Furuncles, on the other hand, represent small perifollicular abscesses that destroy the hair and hair follicles, and lead to deep inflammation and subsequent scarring. When several furuncles coalesce, a carbuncle results. Carbuncles occur on the back, neck, and intertriginous areas, and may lead to scarring.

Etiology
Staphylococcus aureus is the usual causative organism.

Therapy
In treating folliculitis, all exacerbating factors must be removed. The patient is instructed about good hygiene, and an antibiotic soap is prescribed. Topical antibiotics such as neomycin and topical antiseptics such as povidone-iodine (Betadine) are also useful in treating folliculitis. Because of their antibacterial and drying effects, acne lotions may also be administered. In treating furuncles and carbuncles it is vital to incise and drain the lesions, followed by packing with antiseptic gauze. These lesions should be cultured and, if the clinical appearance of the patient warrants, systemic antibiotics may be started. If carbuncles or furuncles recur on a regular basis, underlying illness should be suspected and tests made for diabetes, leukemia, or lymphoma.

SYPHILIS (Fig. 24)

Clinical Characteristics
Ten to 90 days after exposure, during sexual contact, to *Treponema pallidum*, the primary lesion of syphilis occurs. This lesion is called a chancre and is typically a solitary, painless, ulcerated, indurated plaque. Most syphilitic chancres occur on the genitalia, but they may be present in any area of sexual contact. They resolve spontaneously in 7-14 days. Usually, when the chancre appears, serologic tests for syphilis are negative; the diagnosis must be made with a dark-field examination. A serologic test for syphilis typically becomes positive 4-6 weeks after initial contact. Occasionally, if lesions of syphilis are superinfected with bacteria, they may be painful. On occasion there are multiple lesions.

Syphilis is known as the great imitator because the clinical appearance of the lesions of secondary syphilis is extremely varied. Practically any type of lesion may be seen in secondary

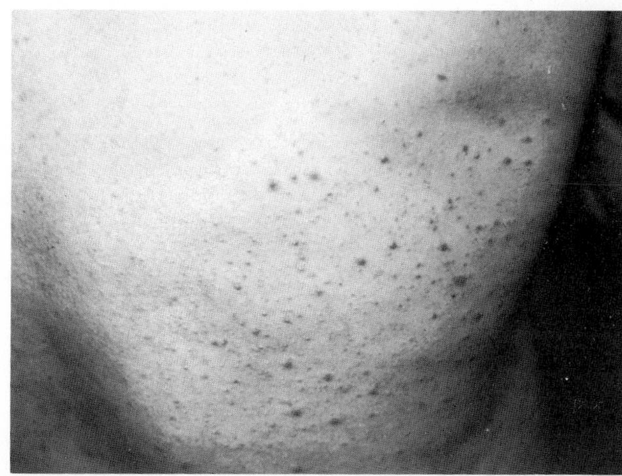

Figure 23. Folliculitis.

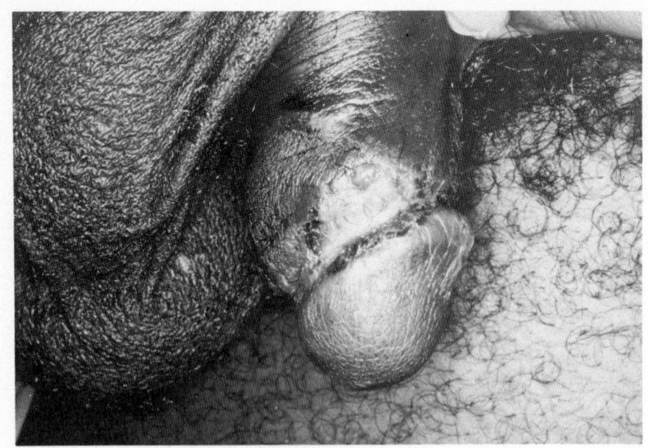

Figure 24. A chancre of primary syphilis.

syphilis, with the exception of blisters, which do not occur in adults. Lesions of secondary syphilis may be macular, papular, pustular, or scaly. They occur 2-6 months after initial exposure and resolve spontaneously in 4-12 weeks. White patches may be present on the buccal mucosa. In addition, highly contagious, moist patches called condylomata lata occur in the anogenital areas. Palmar lesions of secondary syphilis are small, scaly, asymptomatic plaques. Alopecia, with a moth-eaten appearance, occurs accompanied by lymphadenopathy. A diagnosis of secondary syphilis can be established with a dark-field examination of a lesion or by typical serologic changes in the VDRL or fluorescent treponemal antibody (FTA).

The lesions of late syphilis involve the central nervous system, cardiovascular system, skin, or bones. The typical lesions on the skin are called gummas and are painless granulomatous nodules with central ulceration. FTA and VDRL tests are positive in active tertiary syphilis.

Diagnosis

Syphilis may be diagnosed by dark-field examination or by serologic testing. This examination is most useful in primary syphilis, and in moist lesions of secondary syphilis. The VDRL test is an example of a routine, nonspecific serologic test for syphilis and is useful in screening for this disease. It usually becomes positive 4-6 weeks after initial contact with the organism. In adequately treated individuals, the VDRL and other nonspecific serologic tests will become negative 1 year after treatment has been initiated. If, however, the patient is treated later in the course of the disease, he may become serofast and low-titer positive VDRLs may persist. Treponemal tests such as the FTA test are not used for general screening. They are highly specific for the diagnosis of syphilis and may become positive slightly before the VDRL. Once they are positive, they remain so for the lifetime of the individual and are not useful for following the course of treatment of the disease.

Therapy

In early syphilis, which includes primary, secondary, or latent syphilis of less than a 1-year duration, the treatment of choice is benzathine penicillin G (2.4 million units) by intramuscular (IM) injection administered 1.2 million units in each buttock, or aqueous procaine penicillin G (4.8 million units) by IM injection (600,000 units daily for 8 days). In patients allergic to penicillin, tetracycline hydrochloride (500 mg) four times daily by mouth for 15 days, or erythromycin (500 mg) four times daily by mouth for 15 days may be substituted.

If syphilis has existed for more than 1 year or onset of the disease is unknown, treatment is as follows: benzathine penicillin G, 7.2 million units (2.4 million units IM weekly for 3 weeks), or aqueous procaine penicillin G, 9 million units (600,000 units by IM injection for 15 days). In this case, a cerebrospinal fluid examination is mandatory. Patients who are allergic to penicillin and who have had syphilis for more than 1 year may be treated with tetracycline (500 mg) four times a day for 30 days, or with erythromycin (500 mg) four times a day for 30 days.

All patients with early syphilis should be followed with VDRL tests at 3, 6, and 12 months. Patients who have syphilis for more than 1 year should have a repeat test at 24 months. If clinical signs and symptoms of the disease persist, or if there is a sustained fourfold elevation in the titer of anontreponemal serologic test, retreatment should be considered. Also, retreatment should be given if an initially high titer fails to fall at the rate of a fourfold decrease within 1 year.

VIRAL INFECTIONS

Verruca Vulgaris

Clinical Characteristics

The common wart, or verruca vulgaris, is a brown, elevated tumor with rough-pointed projections and a warty surface. It may occur singularly or in large numbers, and involves the

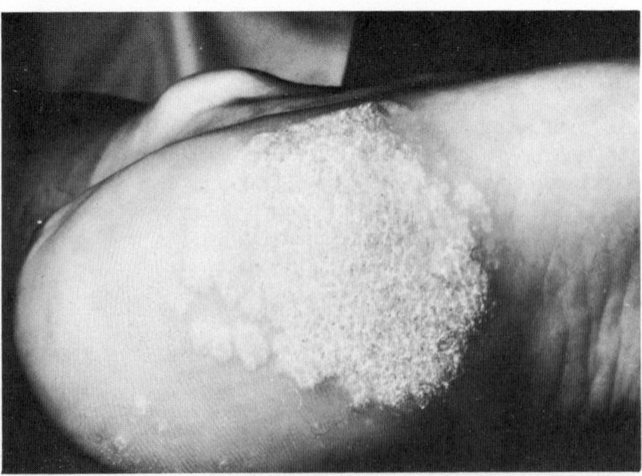

Figure 25. Plantar warts.

dorsum and palmar surfaces of the hands, fingers, legs, arms, and trunk. Warts occurring on the soles of the feet are called plantar warts (Fig. 25); they differ from common warts in that the pressure on the sole of the foot forces the wart into the skin rather than outward. Therefore, these warts are flat, sharply circumscribed lesions with a tender, overlying callus. When these are trimmed with a razor blade, multiple black dots that bleed easily are seen on the surface of the wart. In addition, the fact that normal skin lines are lost over the wart may be important in establishing a diagnosis. The flat wart, or verruca plana, occurs most commonly on the face but can also appear on the hands or legs. As the name implies, it is a flat, skin-colored to slightly brown lesion that may be sliightly raised and is frequently asymptomatic. Finally, the genital wart or condyloma acuminatum (Fig. 26) occurs in moist regions such as the perianal, groin, and vulvar areas. The lesions frequently appear red, soft, and papillomatous with a cauliflowerlike appearance. These lesions are highly contagious, and additional warts often can be found in the anus.

Etiology

Warts caused by a papovavirus (a DNA virus) are contagious and can be inoculated to other areas of the body. The course of this disease is completely unpredictable, although two-thirds of all untreated warts disappear within 2 years without scarring. Therefore, treatment of warts should not be vigorous.

Treatment

Verruca vulgaris and flat warts may be treated surgically with curettage and desiccation. Multiple flat warts of the face may be treated with salicylic acid, lactic acid, or vitamin A acid. Warts on the hands respond well to liquid nitrogen or to carbon dioxide slush. Occasionally, warts may be witched away; in children, treating one wart (the mother wart) and telling the child that the little warts will eventually disappear sometimes succeeds. In addition, warts can be circled with gentian violet and the child told that, when the gentian violet fadės, the warts will disappear. Plantar warts must be treated differently. If the wart is thickly calloused, a salicylic acid preparation in the form of a plaster or liquid may be useful in softening the callous so that it can be trimmed. In addition, trichloroacetic acid (50 or 80% solution) may be directly applied to the wart once following trimming. Formaldehyde and cantharone have also been used in treating plantar warts. In any case, it is important to minimize the use of surgery in treating plantar warts, since scarring on the sole of the foot may be very disabling.

Finally, genital warts may be a therapeutic problem. Podophyllin (20-25%), in tincture of benzoin or alcohol, is used to treat these lesions. The patient is instructed to remove the podophyllin within 4 hours by soaking in a tub of warm water. Podophyllin application is repeated in 3 to 4 weeks. Genital warts can also be removed by liquid nitrogen, or by curettage and desiccation. It should be emphasized that the natural course of this disease is one of eventual resolution without scarring. Therefore, in choosing the treatment the physician should minimize the use of modalities that cause scarring, especially on the soles of the feet and overlying joints.

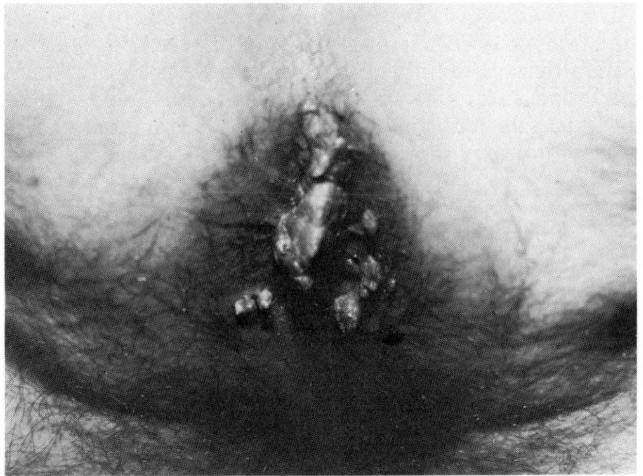

Figure 26. Condyloma acummata.

Molluscum Contagiosum (Plate 22)

Molluscum contagiosum is a common disease affecting children, and is caused by a large DNA virus. As such, it is a contagious disease and autoinoculation can occur. The patient usually presents with multiple, slightly pink, smooth, round, dome-shaped, somewhat translucent lesions with central umbilication. Unless they become inflamed, the lesions may heal spontaneously and are usually minimally symptomatic.

This common lesion can easily be treated by puncturing the center of the molluscum and expressing it with a comedo expressor. In addition, catharidin in flexible collodion may be applied to the lesions, or they may be curetted and lightly desiccated, or frozen with liquid nitrogen.

Herpes Simplex (Fever Blister, Cold Sore) (Fig. 27)

Herpes simplex is a common infection caused by a DNA virus that classically presents as a painful group of small vesicles overlying an erythematous base. Frequently, the lesion is preceded by mild pruritus and is somewhat painful when it develops. The blisters eventually break, emitting serous fluid that crusts and heals within 14 days. Adenopathy and low-grade fever may accompany the primary lesions of herpes simplex. Primary infections with herpes simplex are often very severe, with marked erythema and swelling of the involved tissue. Secondary or recurrent infections may be less severe and may be triggered by a number of events such as fever, trauma, sunlight, menstruation, and systemic illness.

Multiple areas of the body can be involved by herpes simplex. One can have gingivostomatitis, whitlow (infection of the finger), vulvovaginitis, and, in more severe cases, systemic dissemination with meningoencephalitis or pneumonia. The

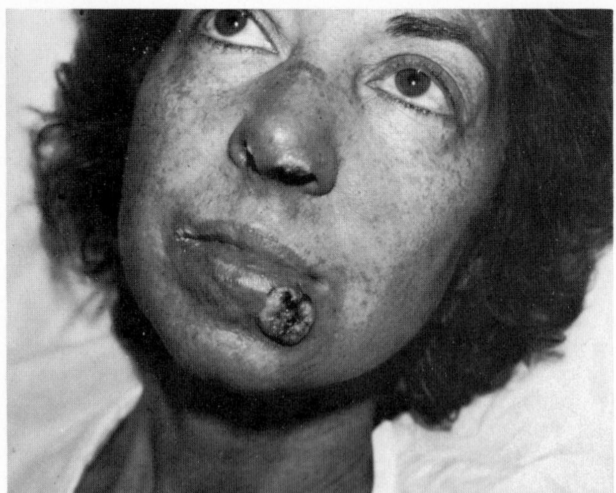

Figure 27. Herpes simplex in a leukemia patient.

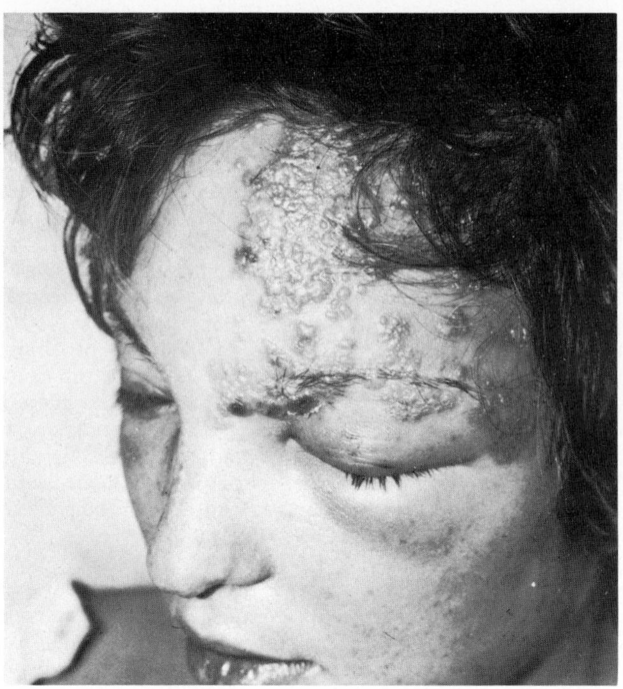

Figure 28. Trigeminal herpes zoster.

differential diagnosis of herpes simplex includes impetigo, herpes zoster, and aphthous stomatitis.

Diagnosis
A diagnosis of herpes simplex is based on an accurate history of recurrent lesions that, on physical examination, appear to be grouped vesicles on an erythematous base. A Tzanck smear that examines tissue from the floor of a lesion is useful in determining whether multinucleated giant cells are present. Serologic tests such as fluorescent treponemal antibody or complement fixation may be used to verify the diagnosis. Finally, the lesions may be cultured to distinguish the infection from herpes zoster.

Treatment
Inasmuch as no therapeutic regimens have been proven effective in controlled studies, treatment of herpes simplex is symptomatic. Patients have been treated with topical agents such as menthol, flexible collodion, and low-potency topical corticosteroids. The smallpox vaccination used in the past is rarely employed today because of the severe side effects. Dye inactivation, using a photoactive dye plus light, is no longer employed since there is no proof that the treatment is successful and since this treatment also may be carcinogenic. Although effective in cases of herpes conjunctivitis, idoxuridine does not have adequate percutaneous penetration to successfully treat skin disease. Topical acyclovir ointment (Zovirax) may be indicated for primary genital herpes and for herpes in immune suppressed hosts.

Herpes Zoster (Fig. 28)

Clinical Characteristics
The primary infection of the varicella virus is chickenpox, which has an incubation period of 2-3 weeks, is spread via the respiratory tract, and appears primarily in children. It is associated with malaise, weakness, and low-grade fever. Small vesicles that later become pustular rupture with crust formation, and may result in significant scarring.

The secondary form of this infection, herpes zoster, occurs in older patients who have had chickenpox in the past. Classically, the pain precedes the appearance of typical grouped vesicles on an erythematous base. The primary lesions are usually unilateral, and frequently present in a dermatomal distribution. Unlike herpes simplex, herpes zoster is not recurrent. Occasional lesions may occur outside the involved dermatome. Significant dissemination of vesicles should serve as a warning of the presence of an internal malignant tumor. In addition, older patients may develop postherpetic neuralgia, or severe pain persisting in the involved dermatome beyond the period of resolution of the primary skin lesions.

Therapy
The treatment is primarily symptomatic. When the lesions are in a vesicular stage, warm soaks with tap water or Burrow's solution may be useful. In order to prevent superinfection with bacteria, topical antibiotics may be required. In patients over 50 years of age, intermediate doses of oral corticosteroids given early in the course of the disease may prevent the development of postherpetic neuralgia. In individuals with marked dissemination of zoster or with central nervous system involvement, zoster immune globulin may be administered. Systemic administration of adenosine arabinoside is reserved for life-threatening cases.

INFESTATIONS

Scabies (Figs. 29, 30)

Clinical Characteristics

Symptoms and clinical findings of scabies occur as a result of a hypersensitivity reaction to the causative organism and, as such, the patient remains asymptomatic for the first 3 to 4 weeks. When the overt signs of disease appear, the typical lesion of scabies is a pruritic, crusted, excoriated papule or vesicle that occurs between the fingers, flexor surface of the wrist, anterior axillary folds, nipples, penis, and groin (Fig. 29). These lesions rarely appear on the face. In addition to typical vesicles, burrows that appear as fine elevated lines on the skin may occur.

Etiology

Scabies is caused by a mite called *Sarcoptes scabiei*. The organism causes epidemics that occur every 15 to 25 years. The disease is passed from one person to the next by direct contact, and it is rare to be infected by soiled bedclothes or towels. The usual number of mites on an average patient is very small, numbering less than 50 per case. Excoriation and bacterial superinfection actually limit the progress of scabies and, as such, individuals who do not excoriate themselves possess a much larger number of mites and are much more infectious.

Diagnosis

Scabies is frequently diagnosed by observing the mites on a KOH preparation of a burrow, an unexcoriated papule, or vesicle (Fig. 30). Occasionally, if excoriated lesions are not found, material from beneath the patient's nails may be used. In addition, a very fine needle may be passed through a burrow and the removed tissue examined by KOH. Scabies must be differentiated from contact dermatitis, dermatitis herpetiformis, and neurodermatitis.

Treatment

The most common treatment for scabies is gamma benzene hexachloride (Kwell). It is important to stress to the patient that this medication should be used with caution since it tends to be irritating to the skin of adults. After bathing, this medication is applied simultaneously by the patient and all involved members of the family. It is washed off 24 hours later and reapplied, if necessary, after 5 days. The bedsheets and linens simply need washing in hot water.

Other satisfactory treatments for this disease include benzyl benzoate (20-25%), which is used in the same manner as Kwell, and crotamiton (Eurax), with two applications at 24-hour intervals. In addition to being a scabicide, crotamiton is successful in relieving pruritus. The above medications may not be safe in infants for whom a 10% sulfur ointment is recommended, applied twice daily for 7 days.

Part of the therapy of scabies involves prevention. Therefore, the patient should be told not to associate closely with other people until they are treated. Antipruritic agents such as topical corticosteroids, and occasionally systemic steroids, may be useful in helping relieve symptoms of scabies, which can persist well beyond the period of infection.

Pediculosis

Clinical Characteristics

Pediculosis is caused by lice that commonly affect the scalp, body, or pubis. Pediculosis capitis usually occurs in adults and children with poor hygiene, and may result in epidemics. This extremely pruritic disease demonstrates nits or egglike concretions and lice in the scalp. Pediculosis pubis is caused by the crab louse, *Phthirus pubis*, and is localized to the groin, axilla, or chest in hairy individuals. The nits and lice may also be present, and frequently there are small nodules or excoriations in the involved area. Interestingly enough, the organism causing pediculosis capitis rarely causes pediculosis pubis.

The third member of the triad is pediculosis corporis that, as the name implies, is an infestation of the body caused by *Pedi-*

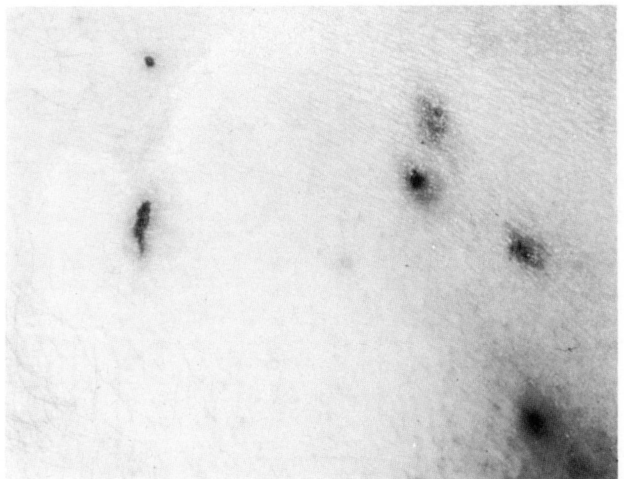

Figure 29. Typical excoriations in a patient with scabies.

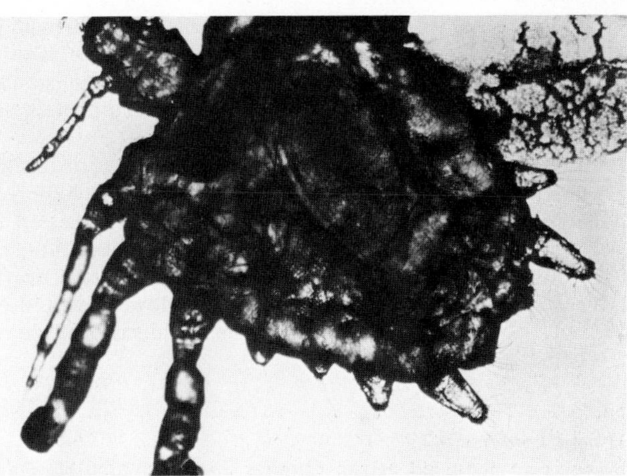

Figure 30. *Sarcoptes scabiei*

culus humanus corporis. Because the organism generally does not live on the body but in the seams of clothing, it occurs primarily in vagabonds and individuals with poor hygiene. The characteristic lesion is an excoriation; primary lesions are rarely seen in this disease.

Diagnosis
A diagnosis of pediculosis capitis or pubis is established by observing nits or lice on the hair, and of pediculosis corporis by finding the causative organism or its eggs in the seams of clothing worn nearest the body.

Therapy
Pediculosis capitis and pediculosis pubis may be treated with gamma benzene hexachloride (Kwell). Pediculosis corporis may also be treated in the same manner, but it is only necessary to thoroughly clean clothing and wash the patient. Concomitant pruritus may be treated with low-potency topical corticosteroids.

PIGMENTARY DISORDERS

Although not the only pigment in human skin, melanin is certainly the most important. Melanin, which may be brown to black (eumelanin) or yellow to red (pheomelanin) is produced in melanocytes that transfer the pigment through dendrites to 36 surrounding keratinocytes. Melanin is held in packages called melanosomes, and the number, type, size, and distribution of these melanosomes determines the depth and extent of cutaneous pigmentation. This pigmentation is under genetic control that regulates the activity of melanocytes, the production of melanosomes, and their degree of melanization. In addition, hormones such as melanocyte-stimulating hormone (MSH) and ACTH produced by the intermediate lobe of the pituitary gland lead to darkening of the skin by causing dispersal of melanosomes within melanocytes.

Tyrosinase, an aerobic oxidase found in melanocytes, converts the amino acid tyrosine to dihydroxyphenylalanine (levodopa), thus beginning the process of melanogenesis. Immediate tanning is produced by ultraviolet light through its effect on melanosomes already formed. Delayed tanning occurs in 2-3 days through stimulation of new melanin production. In any case, melanin pigmentation serves to protect the skin against damage by ultraviolet light.

Disorders of pigmentation are generally categorized into those causing hypopigmentation, depigmentation, or hyperpigmentation. These pigmentary aberrations can result from increasing or decreasing the rates of melanosome formation, the number of melanocytes, the degree of melanization, or the degree of degradation of melanin. The following is a short discussion of a common but cosmetically disastrous depigmenting disease—vitiligo.

Vitiligo

Clinical Characteristics
Vitiligo is an acquired, often familial disease characterized by chalk-white macules several millimeters to several centimeters in diameter that are oval with fairly distinct margins. The extent of the disease is variable, with one to hundreds of lesions being present in a bilaterally symmetric distribution. Occasionally, total or near total amelanosis is present. Extensor bony surfaces, particularly digits, knees, and elbows, are most frequently involved but periorificial, pretibial, axillae, and low back areas may be involved, possibly as a result of Koebner's (the isomorphic) phenomenon. The hair, palms, and soles may also show vitiliginous changes.

There may be considerable variation in the appearance of individual lesions of vitiligo with intermediate tan colors being present (trichrome vitiligo). In addition, hyperpigmented margins have been described and, rarely, a vitiliginous macule may show a raised, erythematous, pruritic, inflammatory border. Finally, multiple pinpoint macules may be present.

Etiology and Pathogenesis
The cause of vitiligo is unknown. Current theories include an immune hypothesis suggesting aberration of immune surveillance resulting in melanocyte destruction or dysfunction; a neural hypothesis suggesting that a neurochemical mediator inhibits melanogenesis; and a self-destruct hypothesis, which suggests that a metabolite of melanogenesis causes melanocyte dysfunction.

Diagnosis
Vitiligo is a disease that is often easily diagnosed clinically. Occasionally, light or electron microscopy can aid the clinician in its diagnosis.

Treatment
The most effective treatment for vitiligo is psoralen and ultraviolet light administered twice to three times weekly by a physician experienced in its use. Slow improvement is usually evident after many months of therapy. 8-methoxypsoralen, 40-50 milligrams, is administered 2 hours before measured sun exposure. The patient must use sunglasses for 6-8 hours after

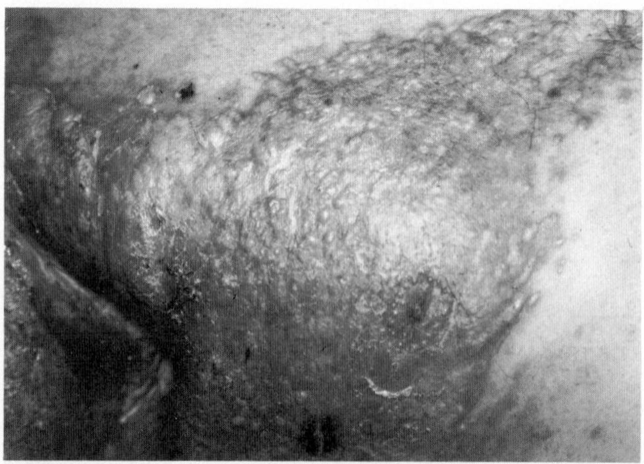

Figure 31. Metastatic malignant melanoma infiltrating the axilla.

taking psoralen to prevent the development of cataracts, and sunscreens should be used after the therapeutic dose of light is administered in order to prevent burning. The patient should be exposed to sunlight only on reasonably clear days and only between 10 AM and 3 PM. At each subsequent exposure, the amount of light may be slowly increased as long as burning has not previously occurred. With the invention of artificial light sources for the production of ultraviolet light in the A range, this treatment, in the hands of physicians experienced in its use, promises to be highly effective.

Alternative forms of therapy for this disease are far less satisfactory. Oral and topical glucocorticoids have been used with minimal success in inflammatory vitiligo. Hydroquinone has been used in extensive vitiligo in order to depigment normal skin. Finally, a waterproof cosmetic agent may be used to cover up involved areas.

CUTANEOUS MANIFESTATIONS OF SYSTEMIC DISEASES

CUTANEOUS SIGNS OF INTERNAL MALIGNANCIES (Figs. 27, 31, 32, Plates 23, 24, 25)

It has been estimated that one in every five patients seen in an internist's or family practitioner's office has a cutaneous eruption. A wide variety of these disorders are associated with significant internal disease, including malignancy. It is therefore vital that the primary care physician be capable of recognizing cutaneous eruptions associated with potentially serious systemic disease. This association may be made in several ways. First, the cutaneous disease begins or ends at the same time as the internal malignancy. For example, a cancer is removed surgically and an otherwise intractable cutaneous eruption resolves. Second, the tumor produces a metabolic product that is known to affect the skin. For instance, the patient has a virilizing syndrome or a tumor that produces melanocyte-stimulating hormone, causing typical cutaneous signs. Third, the rarity of a cutaneous eruption makes its association with a tumor statistically significant. Finally, the tumor is associated with a genetic syndrome (such as tuberous sclerosis) that also has cutaneous manifestations.

Complete classification of these eruptions and tumors is complex, and is beyond the scope of this textbook. Table 5 is a partial list of cutaneous lesions that serve as clues to internal disease, some of which are discussed in more detail elsewhere in this chapter.

Some of the cutaneous disorders frequently associated with internal malignancies are briefly discussed here.

Adult Onset Dermatomyositis (Plates 24, 25)

Dermatomyositis occurs in patients over the age of 50 and is associated with malignant tumors in 7-25% of the cases, depending on the criteria for diagnosis and for the patient population. Malignancies of the stomach and large bowel are the most common lesions. The most common cutaneous manifestation of dermatomyositis is a butterfly erythema over the malar area that, unlike lupus, extends to the upper eyelids giving rise to a purple periorbital eruption known as a heliotrope erythema. Erythema may also be present over the knuckles (Gottron's sign) or overlying other joints. Unlike lupus, the skin between the joints of the fingers is spared. Finally, like lupus, dermatomyositis causes erythema and telangiectasia of the proximal nail folds (Plate 24).

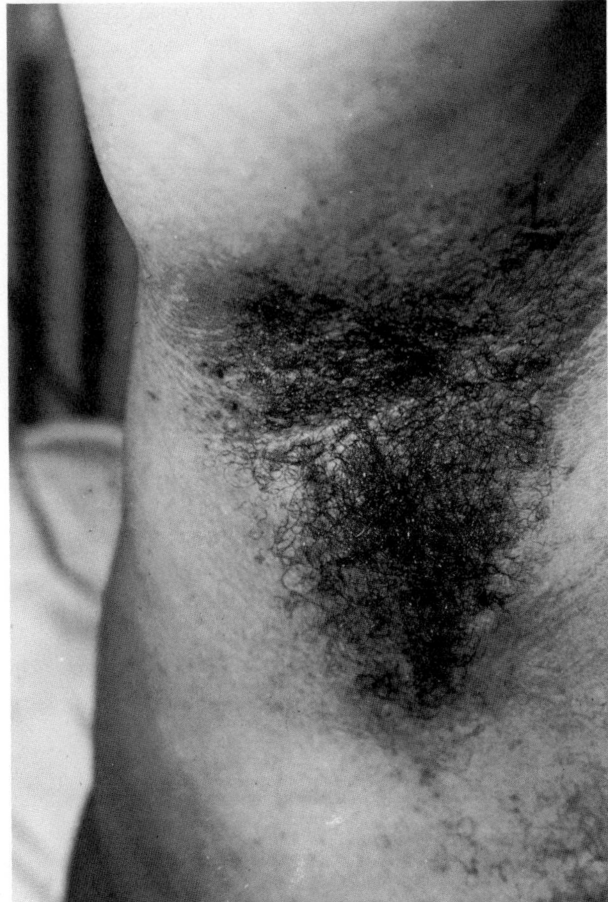

Figure 32. Acanthosis nigricans of the axilla.

Acanthosis Nigricans (Fig. 32)

Acanthosis nigricans may occur as a benign idiopathic entity present at birth or developing in childhood. Alternatively, it occurs secondary to endocrine diseases such as acromegaly, or as a result of ingestion of drugs such as nicotinic acid or corticosteroids. It is an important aspect of genetic diseases such as Bloom's syndrome. Nevertheless, this disease has gained notoriety as a strong indicator for the existence of internal malignancy. Malignant acanthosis nigricans occurs in

Table 5. Classification of Cutaneous Signs of Internal Malignancies (Partial List)

I. *Nonspecific changes*
- Color — Erythema, pallor, pigmentation, jaundice
- Pruritus
- Vascular — Purpura, vasculitis, thrombosis with gangrene
- Gynecomastia
- Infections — Herpes simplex, herpes zoster, opportunistic fungi, recurrent pyodermas, disseminated candidiasis

II. *Carcinogens causing both internal and cutaneous malignancy*
- Arsenic exposure: cutaneous basal cell carcinomas, squamous cell carcinomas, and arsenical keratotis

III. *Metastatic or multicentric internal malignancy that may involve the skin through infiltration*
- Metastatic carcinoma
- Lymphomas and leukemias
- Paget's disease of breast

IV. *Specific cutaneous diseases associated with internal malignancy*
- Frequently associated
  - Adult onset dermatomyositis
  - Acanthosis nigricans
  - Acquired ichthyosis
  - Erythema gyratum repens
  - Hypertrichosis lanugosa
- Occasionally associated
  - Bullous pemphigoid: association in doubt
  - Dermatitis herpetiformis
  - Urticaria
  - Erythroderma
  - Erythema multiforme
  - Poikiloderma vasculare atrophicans (association with mycosis fungoides)

V. *Syndromes that produce humoral substances affecting the skin*
- Carcinoid syndrome
- Urticaria pigmentosum
- Virulizing syndrome

VI. *Genetic associations*
- Autosomal dominant
  - Neurofibromatosis: malignant neurolemmoma pheochromocytoma
  - Gardner's syndrome: colonic adenocarcinoma
  - Plantar-palmar hyperkeratosis: esophageal carcinoma
- Autosomal recessive
  - Ataxia, telangiectasia, lymphomas and leukemia
  - Bloom's syndrome: leukemia
  - Chediak-Higashi: lymphoma
- X-linked recessive
  - Dyskeratosis congenita: carcinomas

both men and women, localizing to body folds such as the groin and axillae, although it may occur in other locations as well. It is characterized by large velvety, hyperkeratotic, asymptomatic, hyperpigmented plaques on body folds, and around the nipples and umbilicus. Malignant acanthosis nigricans is associated with internal malignancy in almost all cases. Most commonly, the patient has a localized adenocarcinoma with the gastrointestinal tract, stomach, pancreas, liver, and colon being the most common locations.

Acquired Ichthyosis

This disease is characterized by dryness, cracking, and hyperkeratosis in which the involved area (usually large portions of the body) are covered with rhomboid scales. Individuals who acquire ichthyosis later in life have an unusually high incidence of malignancies such as Hodgkin's disease, mycosis fungoides, and breast and lung carcinoma.

Erythema Gyratum Repens

This is a group of diseases characterized by transitory erythematous macules and plaques in a gyrate, annular, or serpiginous grouping. Erythema gyratum repens is distinctive, however, in its resemblance to knotty pine or the cross section of a tree trunk. It is strongly associated with the development of breast or lung carcinoma or adenocarcinoma.

Hypertrichosis Lanuginosa

In an adult, the excessive and sudden growth of fine lanugolike hair over most of the body suggests the possibility of internal malignancy. Tumors associated with this process include gastrointestinal carcinomas, as well as lung and uterine malignancy.

CUTANEOUS SIGNS OF NONMALIGNANT SYSTEMIC DISEASES

Many internal diseases are characterized by pathognomonic skin lesions. Table 6 summarizes some of the cutaneous signs observed in systemic diseases.

Essential Generalized Pruritus

Pruritus is a prominent feature in many of the diseases described previously in this chapter. Pruritus with no apparent primary skin eruption, however, may present the physician with a diagnostic as well as therapeutic dilemma. After unsuccessfully treating the patient for environmental causes of pruritus, particularly sweat retention or xerosis, the astute physician must begin to consider systemic causes for the condition.

Pruritus is a well-recognized result of obstructive biliary diseases such as drug-induced cholestasis, extrahepatic obstruction from a tumor, or hepatitis. In addition, severe pruritus following bathing is a well-recognized symptom of polycythema vera. Although rare, thyrotoxicosis may be associated with pruritus, and hypothyroidism with concomitant xerosis may also present with itching. Finally, end-stage renal failure can induce chronic unremitting pruritus.

Pruritus may be a vitally important symptom when it serves to alert the physician to the possibility of internal malignancy. Generalized pruritus may be the presenting symptom in Hodgkin's disease, mycosis fungoides, leukemia, lymphoma, and with various visceral carcinomas.

Treatment of pruritus must be directed at breaking the relentless itch-scratch-itch cycle. To accomplish this, antihistamines, topical antipruritics such as menthol and tar, topical steroids, various emollients, and ultraviolet light may be used.

Table 6. Cutaneous Manifestations of Systemic Disorders

Organ	*Disease*	*Cutaneous Signs*
GI tract	Gardner's syndrome	Multiple cysts
	Peutz-Jeghers syndrome	Pigmented macules around lips
	Osler-Rendu-Weber syndrome	Telangiectasis on lips, face, and hands
	Pseudoxanthoma elasticum	Ivory-colored plaques in intertriginous spaces
	Pyoderma gangrenosum	Painful ulcers on extremities
Endocrine	Hyperthyroidism	Acne Sparce hair Warm, moist skin
	Hypothyroidism	Myxedema Dry, cold skin Alopecia
	Addison's disease	Diffuse hyperpigmentation
	Diabetes	Cutaneous infection Necrobiosis lipoidica Dermopathy Granuloma annulare Pruritus Bullae Xanthomas
	Pheochromocytoma	Neurofibromas Cafe-au-lait spot
Neuron system	Tuberous sclerosis	Adenoma Periungual fibromas Ash leaf spots
	Neurofibromatosis	Neurofibromas Cafe-au-lait spots Axillary freckling
Connective tissues	Systemic lupus erythematosus	Butterfly rash on nose & malar area Photosensitivity Periungual telangiectasias Palmar erythema at fingertips Erythema between knuckles
	Dermatomyositis	Discussed in text
	Scleroderma	Hyperpigmentation & depigmentation Periungual telangiectasias Bound-down skin

A patient whose itching does not respond to routine therapeutic modalities, however, should undergo a workup for systemic disease.

QUESTIONS

1. Match each nail problem with its corresponding disease.
   - A. splinter hemorrhage
   - B. silver nails
   - C. periungual telangiectasia
   - D. half-and-half nails
   - E. nail pitting

   1. lupus erythematosus
   2. bacterial endocarditis
   3. alopecia areata
   4. renal failure
   5. arsenic poisoning

2. Each of the following will show fluorescence when viewed with a Wood's light, except
   - A. tetracycline
   - B. involved skin in vitiligo patients
   - C. involved skin in *Microsporum rubrum* infection
   - D. involved skin in *Microsporum audouini* infection
   - E. porphyrins in the bones, blood, or urine
3. Which of the following is true about psoriasis?
   - A. Mucous membranes are frequently involved in this disease.
   - B. The elbows and knees are frequently involved, probably because of Koebner's phenomenon.
   - C. The turnover time in epidermis actively affected by psoriasis is 28 days.

D. Potassium hydroxide mounts are typically positive in patients with psoriasis.
E. Systemic corticosteroids are both safe and effective in this disease, and are frequently used.

4. Match each of the following:

A. bullous pemphigoid	1. Wickham's striae
B. pityriasis rosea	2. IgG and C_3 along the basement membrane
C. pemphigus vulgaris	3. collarette scales
D. lichen planus	4. small, symmetrically grouped vesicles with severe pruritus
E. dermatitis herpetiformis	5. large, flacid, intradermal blisters

5. Which one of the following is NOT true about erythema multiforme.
A. It may occur at any age.
B. The characteristic lesion is an iris or target lesion.
C. Many cases are idiopathic.
D. It may involve the mucous membrane.
E. Systemic corticosteroids, when administered to patients with severe erythema multiforme, have been shown to decrease the mortality rate.

6. Allergic contact dermatitis (only one answer is correct):
A. is mediated by the B-lymphocyte system.
B. may be caused by virtually any material in the patient's environment.
C. may occur immediately after initial exposure to a chemical.
D. may be associated with a reaction in most people if they are exposed for a long enough period to high concentrations of a chemical.
E. may occur immediately after reexposure to a chemical.

7. Atopic dermatitis is associated with each of the following except:
A. a predisposition to the development of malignancy
B. high serum IgE
C. cataracts
D. disseminated herpes simplex or vaccinea
E. abnormal cell-mediated immunity

8. Each of the following factors predisposes a patient to the development of basal cell carcinoma except:
A. sunlight
B. ingestion of arsenic
C. x-radiation
D. systemic corticosteroids
E. lack of pigmentation

9. Which of the following rarely plays an exacerbating role in the pathogenesis of acne?
A. diet
B. cosmetics
C. ingestion of corticosteroids, bromides, or iodides
D. menstruation

10. Match the following:

A. *Microsporium canis*	1. impetigo
B. *Candida albicans*	2. pityriasis rosea
C. *Malassezia furfur*	3. thrush
D. *Staphylococcus aureus*	4. Wood's light positive
E. *β-hemolytic streptococci*	5. folliculitis

11. Each of the following is true about syphyilis except:
A. there are never multiple chancres.
B. the incubation period is 10-90 days.
C. the lesions of secondary syphilis occur 2-6 months after initial exposure.
D. the VDRL usually becomes positive 4-6 weeks after initial exposure.
E. the VDRL routinely becomes negative 1 year after treatment

12. The average number of mites infesting a human host with scabies at the height of the disease is closest to:
A. 5
B. 10
C. 50
D. 100
E. 500

13. Match the following:

A. acquired ichthyosis	1. Poikiloderma vasculare atrophicans
B. gardner's syndrome	2. Heliotrope rash
C. erythema gyratum	3. Breast adenocarcinoma
D. mycosis fungoides	4. Hodgkin's disease
E. dermatomyositis	5. Colonic adenocarcinoma

14. Match the following:

A. cafe-au-lait spot	1. gastrointestinal tract
B. necrobiosis lipoidica	2. systemic lupus erythematosus
C. ash leaf spots	3. neurofibromatosis
D. pyoderma gangranosum	4. diabetes mellitus
E. periungual telangiectasia	5. tuberous sclerosis

ANSWERS

1. A, 2; B, 5; C, 1; D, 4; E, 3
2. C
3. B
4. A, 2, B, 3, C, 5, D, 1, E, 4
5. E
6. B
7. A
8. D
9. A
10. A, 4, B, 3, C, 2, D, 5, E, 1
11. A
12. C
13. A, 4, B, 5, C, 3, D, 1, E, 3
14. A, 3, B, 4, C, 5, D, 1, E, 2

BIBLIOGRAPHY

TEXTBOOKS

Short Textbooks

Sauer GC: *Manual of Skin Diseases*, ed 4. Philadelphia: JB Lippincott, 1980.

Stewart WD, Danto JL, Maddin WS: *Dermatology*, ed 4. St. Louis: CV Mosby, 1978.

Sutton RL, Waisman M: *The Practitioners' Dermatology*. New York: Yorke Medical Books, 1975.

Comprehensive Textbooks

Demis DJ, Dobson RL, McGuire J (eds): *Clinical Dermatology* (4-volume looseleaf). Hagerstown: Harper & Row, 1972.

Fitzpatrick TB (ed): *Dermatology in General Medicine*, ed 2. New York: McGraw-Hill Book Co, 1979.

Moschella SL, Pillsbury DM, Hurley HJ Jr (eds): *Dermatology*. Philadelphia: WB Saunders Co, 1975 (2 volumes).

Took AJ, Wilkinson DS, Ebling FJG (eds): *Textbook of Dermatology*, ed 3. Oxford: Blackwell Scientific Publications, 1979 (2 volumes).

Therapeutics

Arndt KA: *Manual of Dermatologic Therapeutics: With Essentials of Diagnosis*, ed 2. Boston: Little, Brown & Co, 1978.

Dermatopathology

Lever WF, Schaumburg-Lever G: *Histopathology of the Skin*, ed 5. Philadelphia: JB Lippincott Co, 1975.

REVIEW ARTICLES AND MONOGRAPHS

Papulosquamous Disorders

Baker H: Psoriasis: A review. Part I and II. *Dermatologica* 150:16-25, 136-53, 1975.

Black MM: The pathogenesis of lichen planus. *Br J Dermatol* 86:302-5, 1972.

Farber EM, Pearlman D, Abel EA: An appraisal of current systemic chemotherapy for psoriasis. *Arch Dermatol* 112:1679-88, 1976.

Vesiculobullous Disorders

Lever WF: Pemphigus and pemphigoid: A review of the advances made since 1964. *J Am Acad Dermatol* 1:2-31, 1979.

Vascular Disorders

Monroe EW, Jones HE: Urticaria: An updated review. *Arch Dermatol* 113:80-90, 1977.

Tonnesen MG, Soter NA: Erythema multiforme. *J Am Acad Dermatol* 1:357-64, 1979.

Dermatitis

Fisher AA: *Contact Dermatitis*, ed 2. Philadelphia: Lea & Febiger, 1973.

Malignant Tumors

Sober AJ, Fitzpatrick TB, Mihm MC Jr: Primary melanoma of the skin: Recognition and management. *J Am Acad Dermatol* 2:179-97, 1980.

Acne

Kligman AM: An overview of acne. *J Invest Dermatol* 62:268-87, 1974.

Syphilis

Musher DM, Schell RF, Knox JM: The immunology of syphilis. *Int J Dermatol* 15:566-76, 1976.

Skin Infections and Infestations

Clayton YM: Therapy of fungal infections: Comment. *Br J Dermatol* 89:423-5, 1973.

Ive FA: Diseases of the skin: Treatment of skin infections and infestations. *Br Med J* 4(5890):475-8, 1973.

Marples MJ: The Ecology of the Human Skin. Springfield, Illinois:, Charles C Thomas, 1965.

Orkin M, Maibach HI: Scabies and Pediculosis. Philadelphia: JB Lippincott Co, 1977.

Sanders BB, Stretcher GS Jr: Warts: Diagnosis and treatment. *JAMA* 235:2859-61, 1976.

Cutaneous Manifestation of Systemic Diseases

Newbold PCH: Skin markers of malignancy. *Arch Dermatol* 102:680-92, 1970.

Miscellaneous References

Norton LA: Nail disorders: A review. *J Am Acad Dermatol* 2:451-67, 1980.

Storrs FJ: Use and abuse of systemic corticosteroid therapy. *J Am Acad Dermatol* 1:95-106, 1979.

CHAPTER 5
ENDOCRINOLOGY AND METABOLISM

Ved V. Gossain

Steven R. Gambert

PITUITARY AND HYPOTHALAMUS

The hypophysis or pituitary gland is about 10 × 13 mm in size, 0.5 g in weight, and is located in the sella turcica. In most mammals, the gland is composed of anterior, posterior, and intermediate lobes. In man, only the anterior (adenohypophysis) and posterior (neurohypophysis) lobes are present. In the anterior pituitary, eosinophilic, basophilic, and chromophobe cells can be identified on light microscopy. By electron microscopy and specific stains, special secretory cells can be demonstrated for each of the anterior pituitary hormones. The secretions of both lobes of pituitary are under the control of the hypothalamus. The hypothalamus exerts a direct control on the posterior pituitary secretion via neuronal connections but influences anterior pituitary hormones humorally.

HYPOTHALAMIC HORMONES

The releasing hormones, previously called releasing factors before their structures were recognized, are now more generally referred to as hypophysiotrophic hormones. Recent neuropharmacologic studies have shown that the secretion of the hypophysiotropic hormones is under the influence of biogenic aminergic neurons. The catecholamines that serve as neurotransmitters thus exert a significant influence on endocrine secretion. For example, injection of norepinephrine and dopamine in the third ventricle leads to growth hormone release and inhibition of prolactin release, respectively. Thyrotropin releasing hormone (TRH), a tripeptide, when given intravenously or orally causes release of thyrotropin (TSH) and prolactin. Similarly, administration of gonadotropin releasing hormone (GnRH), structurally a linear decapeptide, results in release of leutinizing hormone (LH) and follicle-stimulating hormone (FSH).

Somatostatin (growth hormone release-inhibiting factor) has been found not only in brain but in the gastrointestinal (GI) tract and pancreas. It is a 14-amino acid polypeptide that is capable of inhibiting growth hormone secretion in every test system in which it has been evaluated. In addition, somatostatin can inhibit secretion of insulin, glucagon, gastrin, and TRH-stimulated TSH release. The existence of growth hormone releasing factor (GHRF), prolactin inhibiting factor

(PIF) and prolactin releasing factor (PRF) has been suggested by experiments with crude hypothalamic extracts but their structures have not been identified. The identification of the structure of corticotropin releasing factor (CRF) and its synthesis was accomplished in 1982.

Prolactin inhibiting factor (PIF) exerts a tonic inhibitory influence on prolactin secretion. Dopamine has a potent inhibitory effect on prolactin release, but its significance as PIF is still uncertain. Although TRH has prolactin-releasing activity, a separate PRF has been postulated.

Multiple actions of hypothalamic hormones indicate that these hormones are not as specific as their names suggest. Hypothalamic hormones are also found in significant concentrations in other areas of the brain. In addition, the presence of pituitary and gastrointestinal hormones has been demonstrated in the brain, but their roles in the central nervous system have not been fully elucidated.

ANTERIOR PITUITARY HORMONES

Adrenocorticotropic Hormone (ACTH)

This single peptide chain of 39 amino acids regulates growth and secretion of the adrenal cortex. It stimulates the synthesis and release of glucocorticoids and sex steroids from the adrenal cortex. It also causes a modest increase in secretion of aldosterone, but the effect is not sustained. Extra-adrenal actions of ACTH include the stimulation of lipolysis and uptake of amino acids and glucose by muscle. The secretion of ACTH is regulated by the hypothalamic CRF and the circulating cortisol levels. CRF increases the secretion of ACTH, while cortisol levels exert a negative feedback effect on the adenohypophysis. Glucocorticoids may also act on the brain to inhibit CRF secretion. There is normally a diurnal pattern of secretion of ACTH. The levels are highest in the early morning hours, gradually fall in the afternoon, and are lowest late in the evening. In addition, many stressful situations such as injury or illness stimulate CRF, resulting in an increase in ACTH levels that may override the diurnal rhythm (Fig. 1).

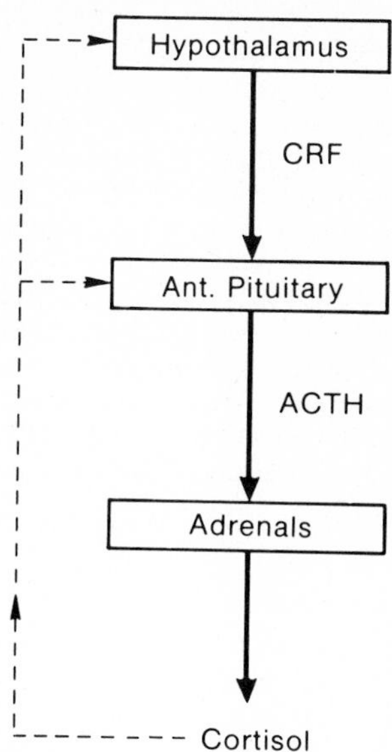

Figure 1. The hypothalamic-hypophyseal-adrenal (cortisol) axis. The solid arrows indicate a positive (stimulatory), and the arrows with broken lines indicate a negative (inhibitory), effect. Corticotropin releasing factor (CRF) is stimulated by a decrease in plasma cortisol level, hypoglycemia, and other stressful stimuli, and inhibited by an increase in cortisol level.

β-Melanocyte-Stimulating Hormone (β-MSH) and β-Lipotrophin (β-LPH)

Until recently, β-MSH was considered to be the main pigmentary hormone in man. In various situations studied (e.g., in Addison's disease, Nelson's syndrome, and in response to various stresses) the alterations in plasma β-MSH were parallel with ACTH. β-MSH was thus a constant companion of endogenous ACTH. It now appears that the adult human pituitary synthesizes and stores only two ACTH-like peptides, β-LPH and ACTH, which are both derived from a common precursor. β-LPH is a larger molecule that contains the entire amino acid sequence of β-MSH within itself. In animals with an intermediate lobe, these larger peptides are cleaved into smaller peptides: β-LPH to β-MSH, with γ-LPH as a molecular intermediate and ACTH into a corticotropin-like intermediate lobe peptide (CLIP) and α-MSH. Recent studies have demonstrated that in man β-MSH does not exist in vivo but is merely an extraction artifact formed by enzymatic degradation of β-LPH and that the β-MSH immunoreactivity is actually due to β-LPH. The role played by β-LPH or by its natural degradation products in the physiologic control of human pigmentation remains to be defined (Fig. 2)

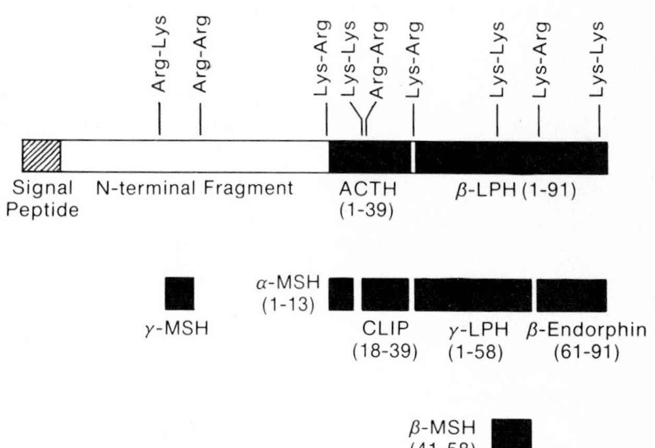

Figure 2. Schematic representation of the precursor molecule for ACTH and β-LPH (bovine) as proposed by Nakanishi et al (*Nature* 278:423-427, 1979). Structure of related peptides is also represented.

Thyroid Stimulating Hormone (TSH)

This glycoprotein increases the uptake of iodide by the thyroid gland and facilitates most of the steps required in the synthesis and release of thyroid hormones. The secretion of TSH is regulated by an interaction of TRH and thyroid hormones. TRH exerts a stimulatory influence, whereas thyroid hormones (thyroxine and triiodothyronine) exert negative feedback on TSH secretion at the pituitary level. Their effects on TRH secretion are not well established. Both a stimulatory and an inhibitory effect of thyroid hormones on TRH secretion have been described. The levels of the thyroid hormones seem to determine the response of TSH to TRH administration in that only a slight elevation of these levels inhibits the TSH response to TRH (Fig. 3).

Gonadotropins

Follicle stimulating hormone (FSH) and luteinizing hormone (LH) are required for the normal growth and maturation of the ovarian follicle in women and for spermatogenesis in men. LH, also known as interstitial cell stimulating hormone in men, promotes the secretion of testosterone by the Leydig cells of the testes. The gonadotropin levels are low in infants, increase to detectable levels well before puberty, remain in the adult normal range during the reproductive phase, and are markedly increased following menopause. In both sexes, the gonadotropins are released in an episodic, pulsatile manner. In men the level of gonadotropins is sustained, but in women it is characterized by midcycle surges of LH and FSH. The secretion of gonadotropins is increased by GnRH in both sexes. In men, testosterone in sufficient doses suppresses both LH and FSH. FSH is also selectively inhibited by a nonsteroidal substance secreted by seminiferous tubules called inhibin. The existence of a similar substance in the follicular fluid has been suggested but not yet established for women. In women, estrogens like the androgens exert a negative feedback, but there is also an element of positive feedback control. Shortly before the middle of the menstrual cycle there occurs a sharp increase in the concentration of estradiol that triggers the release of LH and, to a lesser extent, of FSH resulting in ovulation (Fig. 4).

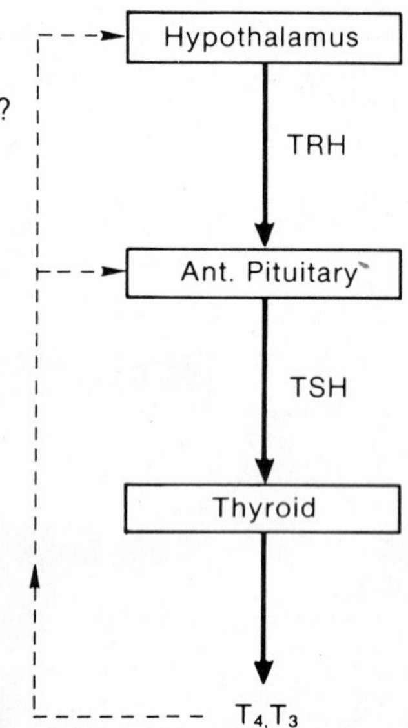

Figure 3. The hypothalamic hypophyseal thyroid axis. Solid arrows indicate a positive (stimulatory) effect, and the broken line arrows a negative (inhibitory) effect. The effect of T_4 and T_3 on hypothalamus is not definitely known, and is indicated by (?). T_4 = thyroxine-T_3 = triiodothyronine.

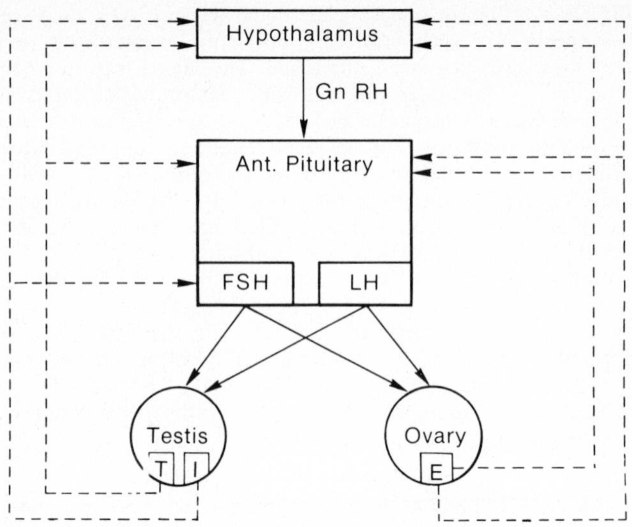

Figure 4. The hypothalamic-hypophyseal-gonadal axis. Solid arrows indicate a positive (stimulatory) effect, and the broken line arrows indicate a negative (inhibitory) effect. Testosterone in sufficient doses inhibits both LH and FSH. Estradiol has a negative and positive feedback effect. Inhibin selectively inhibits FSH secretion. T = testosterone-I = inhibin-E = estradiol.

Growth Hormone

Human growth hormone consists of 191 amino acids with a molecular weight of approximately 20,500. The major effect of this hormone is on somatic growth beginning in early infancy. Hypophysectomy leads to narrowing of the epiphyseal cartilage, which is restored by the administration of growth hormone. Growth hormone exerts its effects on cartilage by stimulating the release of a second hormonal mediator called somatomedin. The latter then acts directly on target tissues. Growth hormone also promotes growth of muscle, connective tissue, and viscera. Metabolic effects of growth hormone include increased protein synthesis, increased serum glucose, and lipolysis. When administered to hypophysectomized patients, growth hormone leads to retention of sodium, potassium, magnesium, calcium, and phosphorus. Growth hormone secretion is controlled by two hypothalamic hormones. GHRF, although not yet identified, is believed to stimulate, and somatostatin (GHRIF) inhibits growth hormone release. Basal plasma levels of growth hormone are low but are increased by estrogens, stress, hypoglycemia, exercise, sleep, glucagon, and α-adrenergic stimuli, whereas β-adrenergic stimulation and hyperglycemia have an inhibitory effect. Somatomedin may also exert negative feedback on growth hormone secretion.

Prolactin

The only established function of prolactin is initiation and maintenance of lactation in women; its function in men remains unknown. Prolactin secretion is under the tonic inhibitory control of prolactin inhibitory factor (PIF). A PRF has also been postulated. Afferent impulses from the breasts and nipples reach the hypothalamus and increase the secretion of prolactin. A number of drugs that affect dopaminergic mechanisms influence secretion of prolactin. Most of the psychotropic drugs increase, whereas levodopa (L-Dopa) and bromocriptine decrease, the secretion of prolactin.

EVALUATION OF PITUITARY FUNCTIONS

With the availability of radioimmunoassays, minute quantities of hormones can be measured in blood. Measurements of these hormones have become the most direct method to evaluate pituitary and other endocrine functions. ACTH can be measured directly, but it is difficult to distinguish low from normal levels. Consequently, ACTH function has to be evaluated indirectly by evaluating adrenal function. For this purpose, metyrapone, insulin-induced hypoglycemia, lysine vasopressin, and pyrogen tests have been utilized. However, only metyrapone and insulin-induced hypoglycemia are the ones most often employed. Administration of metyrapone results in inhibition of the enzyme 11β-hydroxylase that is required for the synthesis of cortisol. The block in synthesis of cortisol causes an increase in ACTH secretion, resulting in a twofold increase in the 24-hour excretion of urinary 17-hydroxysteroids. A subnormal response indicates hypofunction of the pituitary-adrenal axis. Adequacy of normal adrenal function can be determined by administration of exogenous ACTH. In primary adrenal failure, there is no increase in plasma or urinary hydroxycorticoids. In pituitary deficiency with secondary adrenal failure, subnormal response is present; however, continued administration of ACTH over several days leads to a stepwise increase in 17β-hydroxysteroid excretion.

For the insulin test, hypoglycemia is induced by administration of insulin in the dose of 0.1 unit/kg (higher doses may be required for obese and diabetic patients), and plasma cortisol is measured at frequent intervals. The test has the advantage that growth hormone and prolactin function can also be evaluated at the same time. Since it can result in the development of severe hypoglycemia, especially in those with pituitary or adrenal insufficiency, the patient should therefore be under constant monitoring during the test. Performed with care, this test has been found to be safe, sensitive, and reliable with fewer side effects than the lysine vasopressin or pyrogen test.

Radioimmunoassay of TSH is often employed to evaluate pituitary-thyroid axis function. The test is most useful in primary hypothyroidism where TSH levels are markedly elevated. TSH levels are undetectable in hyperthyroidism, but this finding is of limited diagnostic value since many normal people also have undetectable TSH. Although some newer TSH assays can differentiate between the normal levels and low levels found in hyperthyroidism, these assays are not generally available. A low or normal level of TSH in the presence of hypothyroidism is suggestive of either pituitary or hypothalamic insufficiency. A TRH stimulation test can be used to differentiate between these two possibilities. A delayed but significant increase in the TSH level after administration of TRH indicates normal pituitary function, and localizes the lesion in the hypothalamus.

A deficiency of growth hormone can be confirmed by failure of growth hormone levels to increase in response to hypoglycemia, arginine infusion, L-Dopa, or exercise. If growth hormone fails to increase with one stimulus, a second stimulus should be used before diagnosing growth hormone deficiency. Patients with acromegaly have high growth hormone levels that are not suppressed with administration of glucose. Occasionally, acromegalic patients may have a paradoxical increase of growth hormone with glucose administration

By radioimmunoassay, levels of plasma FSH and LH found in normal adults are relatively low. The assay is therefore more useful when gonadotropin levels are elevated, for example, after menopause. Low levels of gonadotropin in postmenopausal women are suggestive of pituitary hypofunction. Similarly, a markedly elevated level of gonadotropins in young hypogonadal patients indicates primary gonadal failure, whereas a normal or low level in hypogonadism is suggestive of hypothalamic or pituitary insufficiency. Pituitary gonadotropic function can be further evaluated by administration of clomiphene and gonadotropin-releasing hormone but the latter is not widely available.

DISEASES OF THE ANTERIOR PITUITARY

TUMORS OF THE ANTERIOR PITUITARY

About 10% of the intracranial tumors arise in the anterior pituitary. Nearly 80% of these tumors are chromophobe adenomas by light microscopy; the remainder arise from eosinophilic or basophilic cells. Almost all such tumors are benign. The manifestations of these tumors include pressure symptoms, as well as the characteristic syndromes resulting from excess production of individual hormones. Hypofunction of the anterior pituitary may result from compression by the tumor. The majority of these patients seek medical attention due to headaches or visual disturbances. The headache does not have any characteristic pattern. Enlarging pituitary tumors compress the optic chiasm producing various types of visual field defects, the most characteristic of which is bitemporal hemianopsia. Involvement of cranial nerves (III, IV, and VI) may occur, resulting in paralysis of extraocular muscles and diplopia. The extension of the tumor into the hypothalamus may result in disturbances of sleep or appetite, but diabetes insipidus rarely occurs. Diagnostic evaluation of these tumors should include skull x-ray, which may reveal enlargement of the sella turcica, erosion of anterior or posterior clinoid processes, or a "double floor" of the sella. If the plain x-ray film of the skull is normal, a polytomography of the sella turcica or a computerized axial tomography (CAT scan) is performed. Pneumoencephalography may be necessary to delineate the size of the tumor and exclude empty sella syndrome.

The treatment of pituitary tumors is determined by the size and extent of the tumor, its hormonal effects, and the facilities available locally. Tumors with large suprasellar extension and visual field defects are best handled by a transfrontal hypophysectomy. Functioning adenomas without suprasellar extensions may be managed by transsphenoidal hypophysectomy. Proton beam irradiation has been used. It appears to offer good results for these patients, but it is available only at a few centers. In some cases hypersecreting adenomas may be treated with conventional x-ray therapy alone, but there may be a delay of several months before a significant therapeutic effect is achieved. Conventional x-ray therapy is most frequently employed for treatment of patients with nonfunctioning adenomas limited to the confines of sella turcica, although transsphenoidal hypophysectomy or proton beam irradiation appear to be equally effective. Local implantation of yttrium and gold radioisotopes is now seldom employed because of the increased incidence of associated complications.

ACROMEGALY AND GIGANTISM

The term *acromegaly* is derived from *akron* (extremities) and *mega* (large). The disease is a result of chronic overproduction of growth hormone by a pituitary tumor, usually an eosinophilic or a chromophobe adenoma The onset of the disease in childhood, before the closure of epiphyses of the long bones, results in gigantism and in adults, after the epiphyses have closed, in acromegaly. Excessive growth hormone affects the skeletal tissues and viscera. In acromegaly increase in subcutaneous connective tissue results in thick and fleshy hands and feet. Patients may report an increase in glove, shoe, or hat size. The skin also thickens, resulting in exaggerated skin folds. Enlargement of the tongue and lips is also encountered. Hypertrophy of cartilage causes arthralgias and arthritis. Increased periosteal bone formation results in thickening of bones. There is overgrowth of the supraorbital ridges and enlargement of the frontal and maxillary sinuses. The ramus of the mandible grows longer, producing prognathism. Overgrowth of the mandible and maxilla results in the widening of the spaces between the teeth. The anteroposterior diameter of the vertebral bodies is increased. The long bones may become massive and bowing deformities may occur. Bone resorption is also increased and osteoporosis frequently results. Enlargement of liver, spleen, kidneys, and heart is common, and many patients develop congestive heart failure. About 25% of the patients have goiters. Enlargement of the adrenal cortex and parathyroids is also encountered. Growth hormone is diabetogenic and is responsible for the frequently impaired carbohydrate intolerance among acromegalics.

The disease most frequently occurs between the ages of 30 and 50 years. The onset is usually so slow that several years may elapse before the diagnosis is suspected. Comparison with previous photographs frequently helps in detecting subtle changes. Patients usually complain of headaches, and visual field defects are frequently encountered Although the classical visual field defect is bitemporal hemianopsia, quadrantic and irregular field defects are not uncommon. Women may complain of amenorrhea or infertility, though loss of libido is common in both sexes. Thick skin, coarse facial features, and large hands and feet make the diagnosis fairly easy in advanced cases.

Diagnostic work-up should include x-rays of the skull, which frequently reveal enlargement of the sella turcica. Elevated basal levels of growth hormone or, if the basal levels are not elevated, inadequate suppression following administration of glucose provide confirmation of the diagnosis. Paradoxical increases in the growth hormone levels are occasionally seen in patients with acromegaly. Administration of TRH may cause an increase in growth hormone levels in 80-90% of acromegalics, whereas no increase occurs in normal subjects.

The treatment of pituitary tumors as discussed above also applies to the management of tumors associated with acromegaly. Medical treatment with chlorpromazine and medroxyprogesterone has been suggested but is usually not successful. Treatment with bromocriptine has been reported to result in clinical improvement and some lowering of growth hormone levels, but much more clinical experience needs to be accumulated before it can be recommended for routine use.

GALACTORRHEA-AMENORRHEA SYNDROME

Galactorrhea implies inappropriate lactation in nonpuerperal women and men. It is one of the most common hypothalamic-pituitary disorders seen in clinical practice and is discussed here because many patients with this syndrome harbor prolactin secreting pituitary tumors. It has been observed that the incidence of galactorrhea in men and women with hyperprolactinemia is about 30%. The presence of galactorrhea is not always associated with an increase in circulating prolactin levels. The patient may complain of galactorrhea, or the disorder may be observed during physical examination. Gonadal dysfunction is frequently associated with hyperprolactinemia, and it may manifest as impotence in the male and amenorrhea in the female. Reduction of elevated prolactin levels is associated with the return of normal menstrual cycles in the majority of the cases. The mechanism of hypogonadism associated with hyperprolactinemia is not entirely clear. Prolactin may partially block the action of gonadotropins on the gonads with resultant decrease in gonadal steroid production. It has also been suggested that a common pathophysiologic basis for the development of hyperprolactinemia and associated acyclic gonadotropin secretion may be a dysfunction of hypothalamic dopamine.

Although there are many other causes of galactorrhea, as many as 30-70% of the patients with galactorrhea-amenorrhea have been found to have pituitary tumors. Prolactin secreting adenomas, that secrete only prolactin, account for about 50% of chromophobe pituitary adenomas. About 25% of acromegalics also have hyperprolactinemia. Diagnosis of prolactin producing adenomas is made by the combination of radiologic studies and prolactin assay. Some of these tumors produce enlargement of the sella. which may be readily visible on plain x-ray films of the skull, whereas others may produce only subtle changes. However, many such lesions are missed by routine x-ray, and polytomograms of the sella turcica are required for their detection. The presence of radiologic abnormalities, however, does not prove the presence of a tumor, since this syndrome has also occurred in association with "empty sella." Markedly elevated prolactin levels in patients who are not taking a prolactin secretagogue are considered to be presumptive evidence of the microadenoma of the pituitary, even if the pituitary fossa is normal radiologically. A large number of conditions besides pituitary tumor may produce hyperprolactinemia; the common ones are primary hypothyroidism, chronic renal failure, psychotropic drugs, estrogens, antihypertensive drugs (reserpine and methyldopa), antiemetics (metoclopramide), and opiates (morphine, methadone). Ectopic production of prolactin by malignant tumors has also been reported. In spite of intensive investigations, the etiology of galactorrhea may remain undetermined in as many as one-third of the patients.

Treatment of the galactorrhea-amenorrhea syndrome depends on the cause. Correction of hypothyroidism and successful renal transplant (but not hemodialysis) will normalize prolactin levels. The mainstays of treatment of idiopathic galactorrhea with hyperprolactinemia, however, are dopamine agonists. L-Dopa was first used to treat hyperprolactinemia; but, due to its short duration of action, it was found to be of little clinical value. Bromocriptine has been found to be very effective in the medical management of these patients. It restores serum prolactin levels to normal and abolishes galactorrhea in 80-90% of the patients. Although the drug is frequently used in patients with galactorrhea-amenorrhea syndrome associated with infertility to induce ovulation and subsequent pregnancies, the drug is not approved by the FDA for this purpose. Large tumors with supra-sellar extension generally require surgery Transphenoidal hypophysectomy is also increasingly being performed for microadenomas with excellent results and very low morbidity. After removal of a microadenoma, about ¾ of the patients resume normal menses and conceive spontaneously. Although bromocriptine has been used in Europe for patients with microadenomas, it has not been approved by the FDA for such use in this country.

EMPTY SELLA SYNDROME

The term *empty sella* was first introduced by Busch in 1951 to describe an anatomical variation observed at autopsy in individuals without known pituitary disease. It is now a well characterized entity in which the sella turcica forms an extension of the subarachnoid space through a partially defective diaphragma sella. The pituitary fossa is partially or completely filled with cerebrospinal fluid and the pituitary gland is flattened and often compressed against the posterior wall of the pituitary fossa. The development of an empty sella due to the anatomic defect in the diaphragma sella is called primary (or idiopathic). It may also develop following surgery or radiation therapy and is then referred to as secondary.

The primary empty sella syndrome is most commonly found in middle-aged, hypertensive, obese women. The most common presenting complaint is headache and the sellar abnormality may be noticed on routine skull films. Most patients with this syndrome have normal endocrine functions, although occasionally hypopituitarism, amenorrhea-galactorrhea syndrome and increased growth hormone secretion with acromegaly have been described. The clinical importance of this syndrome is to differentiate this entity from pituitary tumor. Enlarged sella, with visual field defects and pituitary dysfunction are signs suggestive of a pituitary tumor; whereas visual field defects as a rule are absent and the sella turcica is often enlarged symmetrically giving a ballooned appearance in patients with empty sella syndrome. Pneumoencephalography or computerized axial tomography should therefore be done whenever empty sella syndrome is suspected to avoid unnecessary surgical or radiation therapy. On pneumoencephalography it should be demonstrated that the sellar space is occupied by air.

HYPOPITUITARISM

Insufficiency of the anterior pituitary may result from destruction of the gland by surgical removal, radiation treatment, inflammation, infarction and various tumors. The latter may include adenomas of the anterior pituitary, craniopharyngiomas, and less often gliomas. Other causes include tuberculosis, syphillis, scarcoidosis, Hand-Schuller-Christian disease, basal meningitis and head injuries. Development of spontaneous pituitary failure following excessive postpartum hemorrhage and shock first described by Sheehan is now well recognized. Any of the above processes may result in loss of one or more hormonal functions of the anterior pituitary. Insufficiency of all pituitary hormones (panhypopituitarism) is also called Simmond's disease.

Clinical features of hypopituitarism depend on the age of onset and associated failure of the other target endocrine glands. In prepubertal children, panhypopituitarism, usually due to supracellar cyst or craniopharyngiomas, is characterized by dwarfism and lack of secondary sexual characteristics. However, the mental development is normal.

In patients with Sheehan's syndrome, lack of lactation and atrophy of the breasts are the first manifestations appearing after a prolonged labor and postpartum hemorrhage. These are followed by symptoms of chronic debility, lethargy, loss of libido, and loss of axillary and pubic hair. Diabetes insipidus does not commonly develop since the neurohypophysis is less dependent on portal vessels and escapes destruction. It should be noted that there may be a latent period of several years between the postpartum hemorrhage and onset of the symptoms of hypopituitarism. Whatever the cause of panhypopituitarism, the secondary effects on other endocrine glands are the same. Patients with pituitary tumors usually lose growth hormone and gonadal function first, followed by loss of TSH and lastly ACTH function; however, exceptions to this sequence are frequent and isolated deficiencies also occur.

Physical findings of hypopituitarism consist of bradycardia, hypotension, and loss of axillary and pubic hair. The skin is pale, fine and atrophic. There is a general loss of secondary sex characteristics. The development of secondary adrenal failure is characterized by nausea, vomiting and hypotension; but hyperpigmentation is not seen. The low Na^+/high K^+ characteristic of primary adrenal failure is also absent since aldosterone secretion is generally unimpaired. Hyponatremia, when present, is due to excessive water retention from cortisol deficiency rather than sodium loss. Correction of hyponatremia in these patients by administration of cortisol contrasts with the syndrome of inappropriate antidiuretic hormone (SIADH). Symptoms of hypothyroidism include lethargy, constipation, and cold intolerance but myxedema is unusual. Coarse thick skin, goiter and elevated cholesterol levels seen in patients with primary myxedema are absent.

The diagnosis of hypopituitarism must be confirmed by the laboratory procedures outlined below before a lifelong treatment is undertaken. A skull x-ray should always be performed to rule out the presence of pituitary tumor. Craniopharyngioma usually can be identified by the presence of calcification in the suprasella region. If the sella is enlarged, pneumoencephalogram or CAT scan should be performed to exclude the "empty sella syndrome." Adrenal function can be evaluated by measurement of plasma cortisol and urinary 17-hydroxysteroids and 17-ketosteroids, all of which may be low. Further evaluation of pituitary-adrenal function can be carried out by use of metyrapone and ACTH infusion test as previously outlined. If ACTH assay is available, ACTH insufficiency may also be diagnosed by low or "normal" level of ACTH when simultaneously obtained plasma cortisol is also low.

Growth hormone secretion is evaluated by direct radioimmunoassay under basal conditions, followed by conditions which normally stimulate its secretion such as exercise and administration of L-DOPA. Insulin-induced hypoglycemia as previously described, may be utilized to evaluate growth hormone and ACTH function simultaneously. Failure of growth hormone and cortisol to increase following induction of hypoglycemia (glucose level should decrease to 50% of the baseline value) confirms the deficiency of these hormones.

Radioimmunoassay of TSH provides direct evidence to distinguish primary from secondary hypothyroidism. If TSH level is not elevated in the presence of hypothyroidism, it indicates hypothalamic or pituitary dysfunction.

Direct assay of gonadotropin is most useful when LH and FSH are elevated. This test thus excludes failure of the pituitary to secrete gonadotropins. If the levels are "normal" in association with hypogonadism, it is suggestive of pituitary insufficiency. Secretory capacity of the pituitary for gonadotropins can be evaluated by administration of clomiphene (Clomid) or when available by gonadotropin releasing hormone, both of which normally increase gonadotropin secretion.

The aim of treatment in hypopituitarism is to provide the hormones that are deficient so as to restore the hormonal milieu of the patient to normal. Although pituitary hormones are available, their use is not practical as they must be given parentrally. They are derived from nonhuman sources and may result in antibody formation and lowering of their biologic effects. Hormonal preparations are, therefore, given to replace the secretions of the thyroid, gonads, and adrenals. Hydrocortisone or cortisone should be given orally in doses of 30 mg or 37.5 mg daily, respectively divided into two doses with about $\frac{2}{3}$ administered in the morning and $\frac{1}{3}$ in the afternoon. Additional doses are required at times of stress or other intercurrent illnesses. Mineralocorticoids are not required by many patients, but may be given as a 9-α fluorohydrocortisone when needed. Thyroid hormone can be replaced as USP thyroid or preferably as L-thyroxine. The latter is a more reliable synthetic preparation and its dose is more easily monitored by measurement of circulating thyroxine levels compared to USP thyroid. The starting dose of L-thyroxine is 0.025 mg daily with gradual increase to full replacement of 0.15 to 0.2 mg daily. It is important that in panhypopituitarism cortisol administration is started before or at least simultaneously with administration of thyroid to avoid precipitation of adrenal crisis. Replacement therapy with androgens is usually given in the form of testosterone esters (testosterone enanthate and testosterone cypionate are the preferred preparations). Usual dosage is 100-250 mg intramuscularly every two to three weeks. The dosage should be adjusted for each individual. Testosterone maintains secondary sex characteristics, the degree of return of sexual potency and libido is variable; and it does not restore spermatogenesis. The adverse side effects are usually minimal, but priapism, water retention and edema may occur. In children there is risk of premature closure of epiphysis and eventual short stature, whereas in older men, prostatic hypertrophy may occur. The risk of jaundice is small with these preparations compared to 17 α alkyl-substituted androgens (e.g., methyl testosterone). In females administration of estrogens helps restore vaginal mucosa to normal and may be combined with progesterone to produce cyclic withdrawal bleeding. It is also possible to restore fertility in the female by administration of gonadotropins but the restoration of male fertility is more difficult.

NEUROHYPOPHYSIS (POSTERIOR PITUITARY)

The posterior lobe of the pituitary, although anatomically a part of the pituitary gland, functionally is a part of neurosecretory system concerned with the secretion of antidiuretic hormone (ADH) and oxytocin. These hormones are formed in the nerve cell bodies of supraoptic and paraventricular nuclei, from where they travel along the axons of the neurohypophysial tract to be stored in the neurohypophysis. Both hormones appear to be bound reversibly to a large protein molecule called neurophysin which serves as a "carrier protein" for the intraneuronal transport of these hormones. Once released from the posterior pituitary by appropriate stimuli, both hormones are rapidly cleared from the circulation, with a half-life of approximately five minutes. Structurally they are similar and consist of 9 amino acids, arranged in a hexapeptide ring bridged by a disulfide bond and a tripeptide "tail" (Fig. 5).

Antidiuretic Hormone (Vasopressin, ADH)

ADH secretion is controlled by three major stimuli. These are changes in the osmolality of blood, alterations in the blood volume, and psychogenic stimuli such as pain, fear, and emotional stress. The osmoreceptors that control the secretion of ADH are located in the hypothalamus. The volume receptors are located in the left atrium and also in other parts of the cardiovascular system, particularly in the aortic arch baroreceptors and the carotid sinus. The concentration of extracellular fluid is maintained in a relatively narrow range. An increase in the tonicity of the extracellular fluid by as little as 1% leads to an increased secretion of ADH but a much larger decrease in the effective plasma volume is required for ADH release. Thus under normal circumstances the osmolar mechanism serves as the more dominant regulator of ADH secretion. In addition, many pharmacological agents affect the secretion of ADH. Alcohol inhibits while acetylcholine, nicotine, morphine, and barbiturates stimulate release of ADH.

The major physiological role of antidiuretic hormone is to control the reabsorption of water in the distal convoluted tubules and the collecting ducts of the kidney. In the presence of ADH, the water permeability of these portions of the nephron is increased allowing the hypotonic fluid in the distal tubule to equilibrate with the hypertonic fluid in the interstitial space of the medulla. Increased ADH secretion thus leads to increased water absorption and urine of higher concentration. In the absence of antidiuretic hormone, water reabsorption does not occur, thus, resulting in dilute urine.

In addition to its effects on water metabolism, antidiuretic hormone has a mild pressor effect. Large doses of hormone also produce smooth muscle contraction. The effect on splanchnic vascular bed has been employed in the treatment of bleeding esophageal varices. Large doses of vasopressin also cause a release of ACTH from the anterior pituitary.

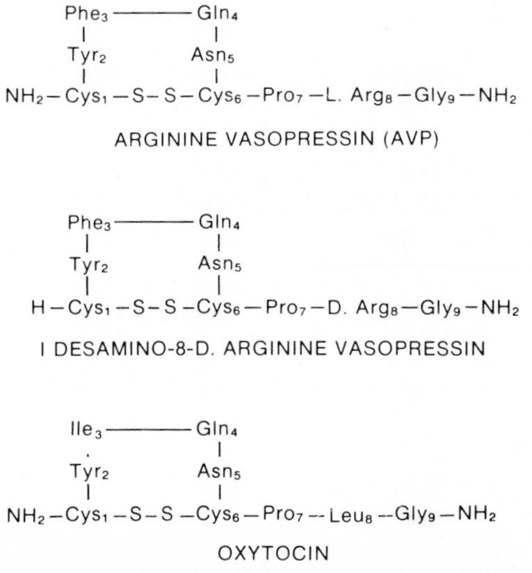

Phe_3 — Gln_4
Tyr_2 — Asn_5
$NH_2-Cys_1-S-S-Cys_6-Pro_7-L.\ Arg_8-Gly_9-NH_2$

ARGININE VASOPRESSIN (AVP)

Phe_3 — Gln_4
Tyr_2 — Asn_5
$H-Cys_1-S-S-Cys_6-Pro_7-D.\ Arg_8-Gly_9-NH_2$

I DESAMINO-8-D. ARGININE VASOPRESSIN

Ile_3 — Gln_4
Tyr_2 — Asn_5
$NH_2-Cys_1-S-S-Cys_6-Pro_7-Leu_8-Gly_9-NH_2$

OXYTOCIN

Figure 5. Structural formulae of oxytocin, and antidiuretic hormones.

DIABETES INSIPIDUS

Etiology

Diabetes insipidus is a clinical condition characterized by inadequate action of antidiuretic hormone. This may result from a deficiency of ADH secretion (central diabetes insipidus) or inability of renal tubules to respond to the antidiuretic hormone (nephrogenic diabetes insipidus).

Central diabetes insipidus has been classified into a primary and a secondary group. About 50% of cases of diabetes insipidus have no apparent cause and are classified as idiopathic. Familial diabetes insipidus is a very rare condition and accounts for less than 1% of the cases of diabetes insipidus. Even more rarely, diabetes mellitus and diabetes insipidus may coexist in some families. The major causes of secondary diabetes insipidus are trauma (head injury and neurosurgery) and tumors (primary pituitary or other intracranial and metastatic tumors most commonly from carcinoma of breast). Rarely diabetes insipidus may also result from involvement of the hypothalamic area by histocytosis X, tuberculosis, sarcoidosis, syphilis, and following encephalitis.

Nephrogenic diabetes insipidus may also be primary or secondary. Primary nephrogenic diabetes insipidus is a sex-linked recessive disorder that presents during the first few weeks of life. The common causes of secondary nephrogenic diabetes insipidus include hypercalcemia and hypokalemia. In addition, nephrogenic diabetes may develop in a variety of chronic renal diseases such as pyelonephritis, analgesic nephropathy, obstructive uropathy and after lithium therapy.

Clinical Features

Polyuria and polydipsia are the characteristic features of diabetes insipidus. The symptoms are usually of sudden onset. The urine specific gravity is low with the urine osmolality being almost always lower than serum osmolality. Only with severe dehydration, the urine osmolality may approach or even exceed the plasma osmolality. As long as the patient's thirst mechanism is normal and there is free access to water, no serious consequences occur, but serious or fatal dehydration may occur if the patient is unable to obtain water as may happen during periods of unconsciousness or persistant vomiting.

Diagnosis

The differential diagnosis of polyuria with a urine of low specific gravity generally includes central and nephrogenic diabetes insipidus and psychogenic polydipsia. Diabetes mellitus, a much more common cause of polyuria, and polydipsia, is associated with urine that contains glucose and is of high specific gravity. Patients with psychogenic polydipsia have an unsatiable desire to drink large quantities of water and often have accompanying other mental symptoms, but have normal ADH secretory capacity. In the absence of availability of a reliable assay of antidiuretic hormone, the following indirect tests are utilized to differentiate between these conditions.

In the water deprivation test the patient is deprived of water, and changes in the urine and serum osmolality are serially observed. Careful observation should be maintained to insure that the patients with psychogenic polydipsia do not have access to water and those with diabetes insipidus do not get severely dehydrated. The test should be discontinued if body weight is reduced by three to five percent. After about eight hours of dehydration, most normal subjects will produce a urine with an osmolality of at least 800 mOsm/kg while the plasma osmolality remains unchanged. Patients with true central diabetes insipidus are unable to raise the urine osmolality above 200-300 mOsm/kg but the plasma osmolality rises significantly. At the end of the dehydration period, when the urine osmolality has stabilized, administration of ADH results in an increase in the urine osmolality of more than 15% in diabetes insipidus, and less than 5% in normals and those with psychogenic polydipsia. An increase between 5 and 15% in the urine osmolality upon ADH administration suggest partial diabetes insipidus. The accompanying figure (Fig. 6) shows the results of water deprivation test in three patients. Patient A and B have diabetes insipidus while the response of patient C is normal. Patients with nephrogenic DI are unable to concentrate their urine on water deprivation and also do not respond to vasopressin administration.

Administration of hypertonic saline infusion is another means of differentiating between various types of polyuria. The principle of this test is that administration of hypertonic saline leads to an increase in serum osmolality. In normal subjects and in psychogenic polydipsia, this results in increased release of ADH which causes a decrease in the urine volume, while in diabetes insipidus no significant change in the urine volume occurs.

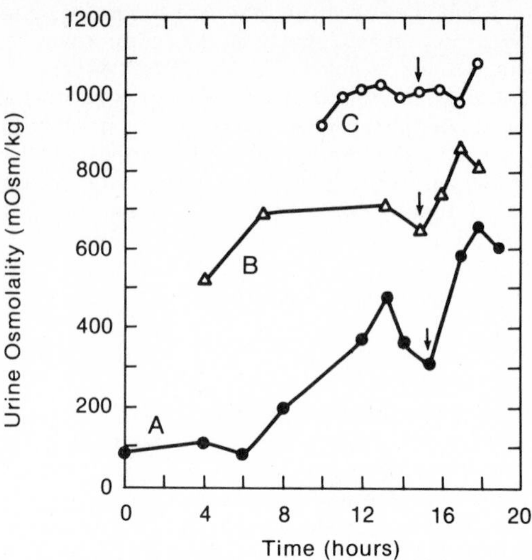

Figure 6. Results of fluid deprivation in 3 brothers with diabetes mellitus. In patient A, on dehydration plasma osmolality increased from 282-315 mOsm/kg. Maximum urine osmolality was 475 mOsm, but declined to 316 mOsm on continued dehydration. Two hours after vasopressin, urine osmolality increased to 666 mOsm/kg. Patient B was able to concentrate his urine to 720 mOsm/kg, but urine osmolality increased to 868 mOsm/kg (a 20% increase over fluid deprivation alone). Patient C was able to concentrate his urine normally, and no further increase occured after administration of vasopressin. Thus, patients A and B have diabetes insipidus also, whereas the response of patient C is normal. ↓ indicates the time when vasopressin was given (Reproduced from *J. Clin Endo & Metab* 41:1020, 1975, with permission).

Treatment

Lysine vasopressin may be administered as a nasal spray with one to two applications per nostril every three to four hours. It has been largely replaced by a long acting vasopressin analog DDAVP (1-desamino-8-D-arginine vasopressin) which produces a prolonged antidiuresis after a single intranasal application. To those patients who find nasal application of drugs unacceptable, pitressin tannate in oil can be administered intramuscularly. It is a long acting preparation and administration of five units may produce relief of symptoms for periods varying from 24 to 72 hours.

Chlorpropamide, a hypoglycemic agent, also exerts an antidiuretic effect by potentiating the action of endogenous ADH. It may decrease the urine output to half or one third and may be useful in patients with partial ADH deficiency. Diuretics remain the only satisfactory treatment for nephrogenic diabetes insipidus, and may also decrease the urine volume in central diabetes insipidus by decreasing glomerular filteration rate.

SYNDROME OF INAPPROPRIATE SECRETION OF ANTIDIURETIC HORMONE (SIADH)

This syndrome is defined as consisting of the signs and symptoms resulting from excess ADH secretion which continues despite hypotonicity of the plasma. A large number of conditions can produce this syndrome. Some of the more common ones include ectopic production of ADH by bronchogenic and other carcinomas; central nervous system lesions; and lung infections. Many drugs have also been associated with this syndrome and include clofibrate, vincristine, chlorpropamide, and carbamazepine. The clinical features of this syndrome relate to a low serum sodium level which may result in disorientation, mental confusion and in cases of severe and prolonged hyponatremia, convulsions and coma. The diagnosis should be suspected in any patient with hyponatremia and hypoosmolality of plasma who secretes urine that is not maximally dilute with urinary sodium being inappropriately increased.

The treatment of the syndrome of inappropriate ADH secretion is water restriction. Only very rarely is the infusion of hypertonic saline required. In those patients where prolonged water restriction is not possible, demeclocycline or lithium may be used. These drugs limit the reabsorption of water in the distal nephron resulting in excretion of dilute urine. Demeclocycline in doses of 600-1200 mg has been found to be effective with few side effects. However, nephrotoxicity has been reported and patients with cirrhosis are particularly prone to develop renal damage.

Oxytocin

Besides ADH, neurohypophysis contains another hormone, oxytocin. It is structurally similar to ADH and has a very mild antidiuretic effect. The major actions of oxytocin are contraction of uterine musculature, myoepithelial cells surrounding the alveoli and small ducts in the breast resulting in milk ejection. A spurt release of oxytocin occurs during labor and suckling suggesting that this hormone may play a role in the initiation of labor and lactation. Like prolactin, it serves no known function in the male.

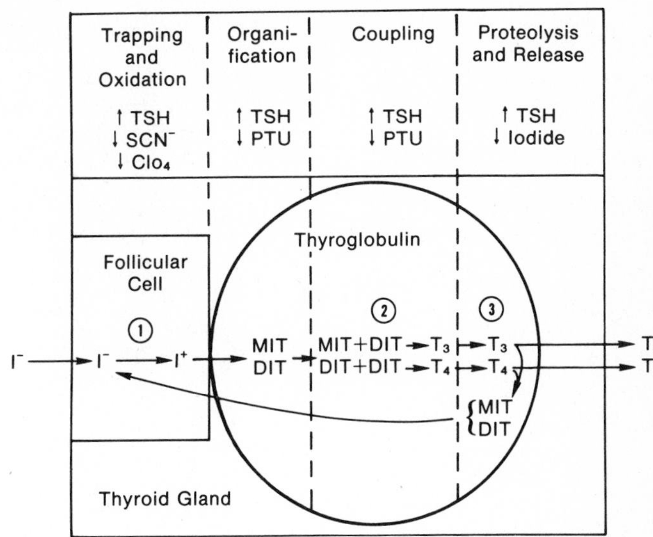

Figure 7. Intrathyroidal, biosynthesis of thyroid hormones. The numbers in the circle indicate enzymes that facilitate the reactions indicated. 1-Peroxidase 2-Coupling enzyme 3-Protease agents that enhance (↑) or inhibit (↓) the reactions are indicated on the top portion of the figure.

THE THYROID GLAND

Anatomically, the thyroid gland consists of a right and left lobe connected by an isthmus. The gland is located in the anterior aspect of the neck, and in the healthy adult, weighs approximately 15 to 25 grams. Microscopically, the gland consists of follicles which are filled with clear, proteinaceous material called colloid. The wall of the follicle is normally lined by a single layer of cuboidal cells. The gland receives its blood supply from superior and inferior thyroidal arteries and is supplied by both the adrenergic and cholinergic nerves.

Synthesis of Thyroid Hormones

The steps for synthesis of thyroid hormones are summarized in Figure 7. The substrate for the synthesis of thyroid hormones is provided by circulating iodides. The thyroid gland by virtue of an active, energy requiring mechanism, is able to trap iodide from the blood stream. As a result of this process, the concentration of iodides within the thyroid gland is much greater than what could be achieved by a simple diffusion process. This mechanism can be blocked by agents like perchlorate and thiocyanate. The trapped iodide is oxidized by the enzyme peroxidase. The next step in the synthesis of tetraiodothyronine (thyroxine, T_4) and triiodothyronine (T_3) is the iodination of tyrosine to moniodotyrosine (MIT) and diiodotyrosine (DIT). Coupling of two molecules of DIT and condensation of one molecule of MIT and one molecule of DIT result in the production of T_4 and T_3 respectively. T_3 may also be derived from intrathyroidial deiodination of T_4. Some of the MIT and DIT formed is diodinated and the released iodide becomes available for reaccumulation by the thyroid gland. The formed T_4 and T_3 are stored in the thyroid gland in combination with thyroglobulin. The latter is a large glycoprotein molecule (molecular weight 65,000) and contains about 10% carbohydrates by weight. T_4 and T_3 are cleaved from thyroglobulin by proteolysis and enter the blood stream. Both hormones circulate in the blood stream predominantly bound to an inter-alpha globulin, thyroxine binding globulin (TBG), and to a lesser extent to albumin. T_4 is also bound to prealbumin, but T_3 is not. Only about 0.05% of T_4 and 0.5% of T_3 is free. Only the free component of these hormones is considered to be metabolically active. About 20% of the total circulating T_3 is secreted by the thyroid gland; the remainder is derived from peripheral monodeiodination of T_4. Some of the T_4 is deiodinated to reverse T_3 (rT_3) which is believed to be metabolically inactive. (Fig. 8) It appears that there are separate enzymes which deiodinate T_4 to T_3 on one hand, and rT_3 on the other. It has also been demonstrated that T_3 is about four times more potent than T_4. This has led to the speculation that T_4 by itself is inactive and must be converted to T_3 in order to act. The evidence, although indirect, indicates that T_4 does possess some intrinsic biological activity. There is no doubt, however, that the biologic activity of T_4 is increased by conversion to T_3.

Regulation of Thyroid Function

The secretion of the thyroid hormones T_3 and T_4 is under the control of thyroid-stimulating hormone (TSH). The latter is responsible for the growth and maintenance of the thyroid gland, as well as for stimulating the synthesis and secretion of thyroid hormones. Both T_4 and T_3, in turn, exert a negative feedback effect on the secretion of TSH. As mentioned earlier,

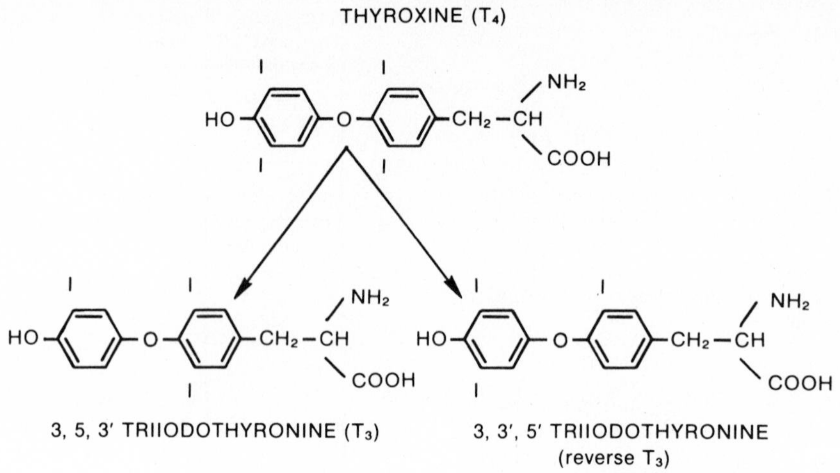

THYROXINE (T_4)

3, 5, 3′ TRIIODOTHYRONINE (T_3)

3, 3′, 5′ TRIIODOTHYRONINE (reverse T_3)

Figure 8. Structural formulas of thyroid hormones.

the secretion of TSH is under the influence of hypothalamic TRH. In addition to regulation by the anterior pituitary, the thyroid gland is unique in that it regulates its own secretion. Autoregulation is provided by modifying the mechanism for trapping iodide. In iodine deficiency, a greater proportion of administered ^{131}I is taken up by the gland, whereas the ^{131}I uptake is decreased when there is excessive ingestion of iodides. In addition, a variety of intrathyroidal processes are influenced by iodides. Small amounts of iodides abruptly increase the rate of synthesis of thyroid hormones, at least for a time. Larger doses of iodides acutely decrease the formation of total organic iodide within the thyroid gland to a level below the normal range, and synthesis of T_4 and T_3 is markedly suppressed. This acute inhibitory effect on the synthesis of the thyroid hormones is called the Wolff-Chaikoff effect. If the administration of iodides is continued, however, an escape from this continued inhibition occurs and synthesis of T_4 and T_3 resumes normally. Failure to escape from the Wolff-Chaikoff effect may result in enlargement of the thyroid and hypothyroidism. This has been referred to as iodide myxedema, which is encountered in some patients with chronic obstructive pulmonary disease who have received iodides for long periods, in many patients with Hashimoto's thyroiditis, and in some patients with Graves' disease previously treated with radioactive iodine. In addition, iodides inhibit release of T_4 and T_3 from the thyroid gland. This effect of iodides provides an immediate therapeutic benefit in the treatment of severe thyrotoxicosis. Iodides may, under certain circumstances, induce hyperthyroidism. This phenomenon (Jod-Basedow) is described later.

THYROID FUNCTION TESTS

A large number of thyroid function tests are available. Each test provides only a limited amount of information. Therefore, for efficient use of these tests, an understanding of the physiology of thyroid hormones and some understanding of the techniques involved are required. A brief classification of the frequently employed thyroid function tests is presented below:

1. Tests dependent upon levels of thyroid hormones
   (a) Determinations of PBI, T_4, T_3, and rT_3
2. Tests dependent on alterations of thyroxine-binding proteins
   (a) T_3 resin uptake
   (b) Radioimmunoassay of TBG
3. Dynamic tests of thyroid function
   (a) Radioisotope uptake and scan
   (b) TSH stimulation test
   (c) T_3 suppression test
4. Test of functional integrity of hypothalamic pituitary axis
5. Tests to establish the etiology of thyroid dysfunction

Tests Dependent Upon Levels of Thyroid Hormones

Protein-bound iodine was used for many years as a measure of thyroid function but, because of frequent contamination with exogenous iodides and due to the availability of tests that directly measure levels of T_4 and T_3, it has been largely abandoned.

The measurement of T_4 by radioimmunoassay or competitive protein-binding assay is the most frequently employed test of thyroid function. Both these techniques measure the total (bound and unbound) concentration of T_4. Hyperthyroidism is associated with increased levels and hypothyroidism with low levels of T_4. In clinical situations associated with alterations of thyroxine-binding globulin, the levels of T_4 parallel the levels of thyroxine-binding globulin, but since the free concentration of thyroid hormones is not changed, the metabolic status of the patient remains normal (euthyroid).

Total serum T_3 is also measured by radioimmunoassay. Alterations of TBG affect the measurement of T_3 in the same way as they affect the T_4 levels. In hyperthyroidism, levels of T_4 and T_3 are increased but the elevation of serum T_3 concentration is usually greater. Therefore serum T_3 measurement may be of help in establishing the diagnosis of hyperthyroidism when T_4 (and free T_4 index) are only minimally elevated. In some patients, only levels of T_3 are increased without a concomitant increase in T_4 concentrations, a condition known as T_3 toxicosis. A modest reduction of T_3 levels has been encountered in healthy elderly persons. T_3 levels are low in patients with hypothyroidism, but they are also frequently decreased in patients with nonthyroidal systemic disease due to a defect in the peripheral monodeiodination of T_4 to T_3. This observation makes T_3 a less useful test for the diagnosis of hypothyroidism.

Recently, immunoassay of rT_3 has also become available. The rT_3 levels are increased in hyperthyroidism, but they are of no diagnostic value since they are also increased in many euthyroid patients with nonthyroidal systemic illnesses who have decreased peripheral conversions of T_4 to T_3. Elevated rT_3 with low T_3 levels have been described in a variety of systemic illnesses, including (but not limited to) cirrhosis, renal failure, myocardial infarction, trauma, burns, advanced malignancy, and malnutrition.

Tests Dependent on Alterations of Thyroxine-Binding Globulin

To determine whether an alteration in the levels of T_4 and T_3 is related to the functional status of the thyroid gland or is due to an abnormality in thyroxine-binding globulin, direct measurement of free hormones can be employed, but these are not generally available. Consequently, indirect tests that measure the residual binding capacity of thyroxine-binding globulin have been employed. The most common of these tests is the T_3 resin uptake. In this test, the patient's plasma is incubated with an excess of T_3 labeled with ^{125}I. The labeled T_3 occupies the free binding sites on the patient's thyroxine-binding globulin and the surplus remains free in solution. The labeled T_3 is subsequently removed by either a resin sponge, red blood cells, or Sephadex particles. The radioactivity bound to the binding agent is counted and expressed as a ratio relative to a standard reference serum. The T_3 resin uptake, therefore, represents the number of unoccupied binding sites on the TBG. The T_3 resin uptake is increased in hyperthyroidism and decreased in hypothyroidism. Increased T_3 resin uptake is also observed in patients with decreased TBG. In patients with an increase in TBG the T_3 resin uptake is low. The table below describes conditions associated with an increase and a decrease in TBG.

INCREASE IN TBG	DECREASE IN TBG
Pregnancy	Nephrotic syndrome
Oral contraceptives	Severe liver failure
Estrogen preparations	Androgen therapy
	Familial decrease of TBG

Drugs like Dilantin compete with thyroxine for binding sites on TBG and also result in a low T_4 and an increased T_3 resin uptake. A change in the level of TBG may be confirmed by a direct measurement, but is usually not required for clinical purposes.

By multiplying the obtained T_4 and T_3 resin uptake values, a free thyroxine index can be calculated. This calculation takes into account the alterations of the binding proteins and provides a better discrimination of hyperthyroid, euthyroid, and hypothyroid patients than can be obtained by T_4 values alone. In most circumstances, the free T_4 index correlates well with the levels of free hormone.

Dynamic Tests of Thyroid Functions

In the radioactive iodine uptake (RAI) test, a small dose of radiolabeled iodine is administered and the amount of the administered dose trapped by the thyroid is calculated. In general, radioactive iodine uptake is increased in hyperthyroidism and decreased in hypothyroidism. However, the uptake is substantially affected by alteration of the total body iodine pool and also by drugs that interfere with the trapping mechanism. Consequently, radioactive iodine uptake is a poor test to determine hyperthyroidism or hypothyroidism. In general, for 24-hour uptake, usually ^{131}I is most convenient, but ^{123}I may be preferable due to its shorter half-life, weaker γ-radiation, and absence of β-radiation. It is becoming widely available and may become the isotope of choice in the future.

^{131}I or technetium (^{99m}Tc) radioisotope scans may be obtained to get an estimate of the functional anatomy of the thyroid. ^{99m}Tc is preferred because it gives the best results with the least radiation. However, the scan provides only a measure of the relative ability of different areas of the thyroid to trap the isotope and is not a test of the functional status of the gland. The scan is a useful procedure in the evaluation of certain single nodules in the thyroid gland.

The T_3 suppression test and TSH stimulation test determine the functional integrity of the thyroid by measuring radioactive iodine uptake in response to exogenous administration of T_3 or TSH, but have limited clinical use. The T_3 suppression test detects autonomy of the thyroid function and is therefore used to evaluate equivocal hyperthyroidism and/or functioning thyroid nodules. The TSH stimulation test was used to determine the capacity of the thyroid gland to respond to pharmacologic doses of exogenously administered TSH to differentiate between primary and secondary hypothyroidism. Measurement of serum TSH, however, provides the same information more reliably and easily, and has replaced the TSH stimulation test for this purpose.

Tests of Hypothalamic Pituitary Function

The utility of serum TSH and the TRH stimulation test is described in the section on the pituitary and hypothalamus.

Tests to Establish the Cause of Thyroid Dysfunction

Antibodies to various components of the thyroid gland are found in some patients with primary hypothyroidism, and in Hasimoto's and Graves' diseases. These antibodies appear to have a pathogenetic role in inducing thyroid lesions, and the presence of these antibodies in the serum of patients is used as evidence to designate these diseases as autoimmune. The most commonly employed tests are estimation of antithyroglobulin antibodies and thyroid microsomal antibodies. The thyroglobulin antibodies may be of any class but are usually of the IgG class. They are not complement fixing and, for the most part, are species specific. The thyroid microsomal antibodies are IgG and complement fixing. These antibodies can be detected by tanned red cell agglutination, immunofluoresence, or by complement fixation. Another group of immunoglobulins called thyroid-stimulating antibodies are found only in the sera of patients with Graves' disease. These antibodies are unique in that they stimulate thyroid hormone production. It has been shown that these antibodies bind to a TSH receptor site (or a closely contiguous site) on the thyroid cell surface. These antibodies are known by various names, depending on the method employed for their assay. LATS (long-acting thyroid stimulator) was first demonstrated to be present by mouse bioassay. Subsequently LATS-protector (LATS-P), human thyroid stimulator (HTS), and human thyroid adenyl cyclase stimulator (H-TACS) have been demonstrated by utilizing human thyroid tissue. Thyroid stimulating antibodies are considered a diagnostic marker of Graves' disease. Also, the continued presence of these antibodies indicates a greater chance of relapse, whereas their disappearance signifies a greater probability of a prolonged remission in patients undergoing treatment.

Metabolic Effects of Thyroid Hormones

Both T_4 and T_3 act directly on tissues to increase cellular metabolism. In thyroidectomized animals, administration of thyroid hormones increases protein synthesis, but large doses inhibit protein synthesis and increase the concentration of free amino acids in the plasma. Thyroid hormones influence carbohydrate metabolism in many ways. Epinephrine-induced glycogenolysis is increased, possibly by increasing the sensitivity of the cyclic AMP system. The rate of absorption of glucose from the gastrointestinal tract is increased. Glucose uptake by muscle and fat is also increased. Increased degradation of insulin has also been described. Synthesis and degradation of lipids are also increased by thyroid hormones, but the lipolysis exceeds synthesis resulting in decreased stored and plasma levels of triglycerides, cholesterol, and phospholipids. The interactions with catecholamines are complex, but increased amounts of thyroid hormones appear to induce a state of increased adrenergic activity.

HYPERTHYROIDISM

Hyperthyroidism implies increased circulating levels of thyroid hormones. It may result from many causes as indicated below. Causes 1-4 account for over 90% of patients.

1. Graves' disease
2. Toxic multinodular goiter
3. Toxic adenoma
4. Thyroiditis (subacute, silent or Hashimoto's type)
5. Excess TSH secretion (pituitary adenoma or "inappropriate secretion").
6. Iodide induced
7. Trophoblastic malignancy
8. Struma ovarii
9. Factitious (self-administration of thyroid hormones)
10. Thyroid carcinoma

Graves' Disease

Etiology and Pathogenesis

Graves' disease is the most common cause of hyperthyroidism. It is a systemic illness of undetermined etiology, but autoimmune processes appear to have an important role in its pathogenesis. A hereditary factor in the etiology of Graves' disease has been suggested by several descriptions of families in which several instances of Graves' disease occurred. Abnormalities of thyroid function among the relatives of patients with Graves' disease, and a higher rate of concordance of Graves' disease among monozygotic twins as compared to dizygotic twins, have also been described. Recent studies of histocompatibility (HLA) antigens have demonstrated that HLA B8 and DW3 antigens are associated with an increased risk of Graves' disease. These same antigens are also found with increased frequency in other autoimmune disorders, namely, chronic autoimmune hepatitis, celiac disease, diabetes mellitus, and others. It appears that the hereditary factor may be a tendency toward autoimmunity. This line of thought is supported by the fact that other diseases of autoimmunity, such as pernicious anemia and perhaps systemic lupus erythematosus, are also inordinately common in these families.

For a long time, the pituitary hypersecretion of TSH was considered a pathogenetic mechanism for hyperthyroidism. However, the recent demonstration by radioimmunoassay that TSH levels are actually decreased in patients with hyperthyroidism has made this hypothesis untenable.

LATS, an immunoglobulin IgG present in many patients with Graves' disease, was postulated several years ago to be the cause of this disorder. This view is also currently in disfavor because LATS is not invariably present in patients with Graves' disease, the concentration of LATS does not correlate with the severity of the disease, and it is occasionally found in euthyroid subjects. As mentioned previously, thyroid-stimulating immunoglobulins have been described in patients with Graves' disease and are regarded to be of pathogenic importance in this disorder. Abnormalities of cell-mediated immunity are also frequently demonstrated in patients with Graves' disease and Hashimoto's thyroiditis. The primary cells involved in immune response are lymphocytes. T lymphocytes are derived from a bone marrow precursor cell that differentiates in the thymus (thymus dependent). They participate in the cell-mediated reactions and also interact with B lymphocytes to regulate antibody production. B lymphocytes (bursa-equivalent lymphocytes) are precursor cells that proliferate and differentiate into plasma cells. The latter are responsible for production of humoral antibodies. Based on the altered cell-mediated immunity and presence of humoral antibodies, Volpe has suggested that Graves' disease and Hashimoto's thyroiditis are defects of immune surveillance which permits a specific randomly mutating self-reactive "forbidden" clone of "helper" T lymphocytes to survive, interact with its complimentary antigen and induce a cell mediated immune response. In addition, T cells also direct and cooperate with the B cells that produce the humoral component of the disease. However, the mechanisms by which cell mediated immunity or antibodies alter the function of the thyroid have not been completely clarified.

The pathogenesis of ophthalmopathy is even less well understood, but the favored hypothesis is that it is also an autoimmune phenomenon. Lymphatic connections between the thyroid and orbit have been demonstrated. Lymphocytic infiltration in the extraocular tissues provides support for this hypothesis.

Many anecdotal observations suggest that emotional stress may precipitate Graves' disease, but a cause and effect relationship has not been established. It has been speculated that if such a mechanism were to operate, it may act by stimulating the CRF-ACTH cortisol axis. Increased cortisol, in turn, may suppress T lymphocytes and immune surveillance.

Table 1. Clinical Manifestation of Graves' Disease

Symptoms	*Frequency (percent)*	*Signs*	*Frequency (percent)*
Nervousness	99	Tachycardia	100
Increased sweating	91	Goiter	100
Hypersensitivity to heat	89	Skin changes	97
Palpitation	89	Tremor	97
Fatigue	88	Bruit over thyroid	77
Weight loss	85	Eye signs	71
Tachycardia	82	Atrial fibrillation	10
Dyspnea	75	Splenomegaly	10
Weakness	70	Gynecomastia	10
Increased appetite	65	Liver palms	8
Eye complaints	54		
Swelling of legs	35		
Hyperdefecation (without diarrhea)	33		
Diarrhea	23		
Anorexia	9		
Constipation	4		
Weight gain	3		

(Adapted from Williams RH: *J Clin Endocrinol* 6:1, 1946.)

Clinical Features

The disease is about five times more common in women than men. In a large Mayo Clinic series, it was estimated that the incidence of this disease was 36.8 women and 8.3 men per 100,000 population. In its full-blown form, the disease is characterized by a diffuse goiter with hyperthyroidism, infiltrative ophthalmopathy, and dermopathy. The components of the disease may occur singly or in combination. Some patients may even present as euthyroid Graves' disease. The clinical manifestations and their frequency are summarized in Table 1.

The spectrum of ophthalmopathy is represented by a continuum that varies from minimal exophthalmos, chemosis of the conjunctiva, and weakness of extraocular muscles to a complete loss of vision due to corneal ulcerations or optic nerve involvement. Ophthalmopathy, when accompanied by hyperthyroidism, usually improves when the latter is treated but may progressively worsen or remain unchanged.

Dermopathy of Graves' disease consists of pretibial myxedema and thyroid acropachy. Pretibial myxedema is characterized by thickening of the skin, erythema, and accentuation of hair follicles. It is usually accompanied by itching and sometimes pain. It is not always pretibial in location, and trauma may determine the site of these lesions. Acropachy includes soft tissue swellings in the digits of the hands and feet with underlying bony abnormalities. Like the ophthalmopathy, infiltrative dermopathy may not be associated with hyperthyroidism.

The clinical picture is variable in that patients may present with many of the signs and symptoms presented in the table above or may have practically none of them. Nervousness, which is probably the most common symptom, may manifest as anxiety, apprehension, inability to concentrate, and emotional lability. In some patients, muscular weakness is a prominent symptom. This thyrotoxic myopathy generally improves when hyperthyroidism is controlled. Increased metabolic rate is responsible for loss of weight in spite of an increased appetite.

The thyrotoxic patient manifests increased sympathetic nervous system activity leading to tachycardia, arrhythmias, and even congestive heart failure. It is debated that if thyrotoxicosis alone can cause congestive heart failure, its development may signify underlying heart disease. There is also increased frequency of bowel movements. Oligomenorrhea is a common finding in women, and amenorrhea may sometimes occur. These abnormalities improve after treatment. In men, there may be some decrease in libido, and gynecomastia is frequently reported.

Glucose intolerance is a frequent accompaniment of hyperthyroidism. In patients with diabetes mellitus, insulin requirements usually increase.

The characteristic physical signs are exophthalmos and a diffusely enlarged thyroid gland. A slight lid lag is often present due to increased sympathetic activity without other signs of ophthalmopathy. In addition, patients may appear fidgety and manifest fine tremors in extended hands. The skin is soft, velvety, warm, and moist. The precordium is hyperactive, the heart rate is generally increased, and a systolic murmur may be audible. A bruit may be heard over the thyroid gland due to increased vascularity. Reflexes are brisk in all the extremities, especially the return phase of the reflex. The nails are thin and the distal part of the nail separates easily (Plummer's nails).

Diagnosis

The diagnosis of hyperthyroidism is readily confirmed by obtaining a serum T_4 and T_3 resin uptake. The serum T_4 is almost always elevated. T_3 resin uptake is obtained to differentiate those cases in which T_4 elevation is due to an elevation of TBG. Elevation of serum T_3 is observed in nearly all cases of hyperthyroidism. In a small number of patients only T_3 is elevated, but T_4 is within the normal range (T_3 toxicosis). The clinical picture of T_3 toxicosis is indistinguishable from the usual variety of hyperthyroidism.

Although radioiodine uptake as a single test does not confirm the diagnosis of hyperthyroidism, it is useful in distinguishing Graves' disease from a silent variety of subacute thyroiditis. The radioiodine uptake is extremely low in silent thyroiditis, whereas it is generally elevated in patients with Graves' disease. RAI uptake also gives a low result in hyperthyroidism due to exogenous hormone (factitious or iatrogenic hyperthyroidism), struma ovarii, and iodine-induced hyperthyroidism.

A T_3-suppression test or a TRH stimulation test are occasionally employed when the diagnosis is not obvious. A T_3-suppression test simply indicates whether the thyroid gland is functioning autonomously. This has largely been replaced by the TRH-stimulation test. Patients with endogenous or exogenous excess of thyroid hormones do not respond to TRH with TSH elevation.

Treatment

There are three different modes of therapy available for hyperthyroidism. The treatment should be selected jointly by the physician and the patient after the latter has been fully informed about the relative risks and benefits of each one of them.

Antithyroid Drugs. The most useful drugs for the treatment of thyrotoxicosis are the thionamide class of drugs. The drugs most commonly employed are propylthiouracil and methimazole (Tapazole). These drugs exert their antithyroid action by inhibiting the oxidation of iodide, iodination of tyrosines, and the coupling of tyrosines to form T_4 and T_3. More recently it has been shown that propylthiouracil, but not methimazole, inhibits the extrathyroidal conversion of T_4 to T_3. This give prophylthiouracil a slight advantage over methimazole. The drugs are otherwise quite similar in their effectiveness and associated side effects. Due to their short half-life, the drugs are given at 6- to 8-hour intervals, although some studies have suggested that a single large dose or two equivalent doses often may be sufficient.

Propylthiouracil is usually administered in a dose of 100-200 mg every 8 hours (the equivalent dose of methimazole is 10-20 mg every 8 hours). The daily dosage may have to be increased to as much as 900-1000 mg of propylthiouracil in severe cases. Patients generally note improvement in their status in about 2 weeks, and a normal metabolic state can be established in about 4-6 weeks in most patients. The dosage of the drugs can then be reduced and maintained at a lower level. It has been customary to give these drugs for as long as 12-18 months. However, some recent studies have suggested that the relapse rate may not be higher even if the drugs are discontinued after a shorter period; however, not all physicians agree with this point of view. After discontinuation of the drugs, about 30-40 percent of the patients may be in permanent remission, while others relapse. In recent years, there has been a decrease in the remission rate achieved by antithyroid drugs. The reasons for this change are not apparent but may be related to increased ingestion of iodides. Most common adverse reactions to these drugs are pruritus and skin rashes. They can be managed successfully with antihistamines without discontinuing the antithyroid drugs. Agranulocytosis is the most serious complication but is encountered in only about 0.2 percent of drug-treated patients. Its onset may be indicated by a fever and sore throat. All patients taking antithyroid drugs should therefore be advised to discontinue the drug and contact their physician immediately if any of these symptoms appear. This precaution is more important than the frequent measurement of leukocyte counts, since agranulocytosis can appear suddenly over 1 or 2 days. If agranulocytosis occurs, the drug should be withdrawn and appropriate treatment instituted. Thereafter the offending drug should never be readministered. Other less common side effects include myalgia, arthralgia, neuritis, hepatitis, cholestasis, and a lupuslike syndrome.

Sympatholytic drugs such as reserpine and guanethidine have been used for symptomatic relief in patients with hyperthyroidism. More recently, they have been replaced by β-adrenergic blocking agents, such as propranolol. Propranolol is initiated in doses of 10-20 mg four times a day and increased as necessary. By its β-blocker effect, propranolol relieves almost all the symptoms of hyperthyroidism but has no effect on the underlying disease. Recent studies have also shown that propranolol decreases extrathyroidal conversion of T_4 to T_3; this may contribute to its beneficial effects.

Iodides. The ability of iodides to inhibit the release of thyroid hormone, especially from a hyperfunctioning gland, makes these agents a useful adjunct in the medical management of patients with hyperthyroidism. Addition of 1 mg iodide daily to propylthiouracil therapy results in more rapid fall of serum hormone levels during the early phase of therapy as compared to drug therapy alone. They also decrease the vascularity of the gland and are used for this purpose in patients being prepared for thyroid surgery. Toxic reactions to iodides may occur and include skin rash, salivary gland swelling, and gynecomastia.

Radioactive Iodine. The treatment of choice for hyperthyroidism in nonpregnant adults is radioactive iodine (^{131}I). It is safe and simple to administer, is generally free of major side effects, and does not require hospitalization. It is somewhat controversial if ^{131}I should be the treatment of choice for children and young adults with hyperthyroidism. This is mainly due to the possibility of future development of tumors or the effects of radioactive iodine on the gonads of patients being treated. Experience from a large number of adult patients treated with radioactive iodine suggests that the incidence of leukemias or cancers of the thyroid is not increased in these patients as compared to those treated with other modalities. In some clinics, children with hyperthyroidism have been treated with radioactive iodine. The experience is somewhat limited but suggests that there is no increased incidence of cancer, leukemias, or birth defects in the children born to patients treated with radioactive iodine. The major side effect of radioactive iodine appears to be the development of hypothyroidism. Efforts to decrease the incidence of hypothyroidism by treating patients with smaller doses of radioactive iodine have not been successful over the long term. The incidence of hypothyroidism following radioactive iodine treatment appears to be cumulative at the rate of 2-3% per year. Therefore, patients treated with radioactive iodine should be monitored indefinitely to detect hypothyroidism so that it can be treated early.

Surgery. The third modality of treatment available for hyperthyroidism is surgery. It should be emphasized that patients cannot be operated on while they are still hyperthyroid. Therefore, initial treatment consists of antithyroid drug therapy until the patient is rendered euthyroid. The surgical procedure consists of removing a major portion of the thyroid gland, and the majority of patients are rendered euthyroid after the surgical procedure. A smaller percentage of patients will relapse even after surgery, and some become hypothyroid. The incidence of hypothyroidism following surgery, although somewhat smaller as compared to radioactive iodine treatment, is not insignificant. An incidence of 25-40% has been reported. The major disadvantages of surgery are the required hospitalization and the associated small increase in morbidity and mortality. In addition, vocal cord paralysis and permanent hypoparathyroidism can occur. The incidence of all these complications, however, is quite low in the hands of an experienced surgeon.

Treatment of Infiltrative Ophthalmopathy and Dermopathy. The treatment of ophthalmopathy is unsatisfactory. Mild forms of ophthalmopathy do not require any treatment. Various modalities of treatment of hyperthyroidism do not seem to influence the course of ophthalmopathy, except that hypothyroidism appears to make it worse and should be avoided. Large doses of glucocorticoids have been recommended for progressive, severe infiltrative manifestations such as chemosis, marked proptosis, and corneal exposure. One hundred to 120 mg of prednisone may be administered as the initial daily dose; as improvement occurs, the dose is gradually reduced. If glucocorticoids do not improve the ophthalmopathy, surgical procedures like tarsorrhaphy in an attempt to obtain closure of the lids may be performed. Finally, if vision is threatened due to corneal ulceration or changes in the retina or optic nerve, an orbital decompression should be performed. Dermopathy often does not require specific therapy. If the lesions are bothersome, local applications of corticosteroids are usually helpful.

Multinodular Goiter

Multinodular goiter refers to an enlargement of the thyroid gland in which several nodules can be clinically palpated or demonstrated by scan. These goiters are usually of long-standing duration. The etiology and pathogenesis of multinodular goiter are unknown. Mild deficiency of thyroid hormone production, either as a result of iodine deficiency or as a result of an inherited partial defect in thyroid hormone synthesis, have been suggested as possible etiologies. Deficiency of thyroid hormones results in continued stimulation of the thyroid gland, perhaps by increased TSH secretion. Periods of alternating stimulation and regression result in multinodular goiter. Histologically, the gland shows a variable appearance and the nodules may consist of colloid cysts or adenomas. There may be considerable fibrosis or hemorrhage into the nodules, and lymphocytic infiltration may also be present.

The most common complication of a multinodular goiter is the development of hyperthyroidism (Plummer's disease) due to uncontrolled hyperfunction in one or more of the nodules in the goiter. This is common in patients over 50 years of age. The manifestations of hyperthyroidism in general are the same as those of Graves' disease; however, the cardiovascular manifestations tend to be more prominent, probably because of the older age of the patients. Muscular weakness is usually prominent but the nervousness demonstrated by younger patients is uncommon. The diagnosis is readily confirmed by an elevation of T_4 and T_3 resin uptake. The scan may demonstrate usually more than one hyperfunctioning area within the thyroid gland.

Treatment of multinodular goiter depends upon its size and associated dysfunction. A nontoxic, small multinodular goiter does not require any treatment. When hyperthyroidism develops, these patients can be managed by administration of radioactive iodine. The usual dose required for management of a nodular goiter is generally greater than those required for patients with Graves' disease. If the goiter is very large or is producing obstructive symptoms, surgical treatment is indicated.

Toxic Adenoma

Toxic adenomas are true follicular adenomas and are a rare cause of hyperthyroidism. These occur generally in the younger age group. The clinical manifestations of toxic adenomas are generally milder than those of Graves' disease. Ophthalmopathy is uniformly absent. Toxic adenomas appear on the ^{131}I scans as hot nodules. The ^{131}I uptake may also be elevated. The treatment of toxic adenomas is indicated only if local symptoms are present or hyperthyroidism develops. Hyperthyroidism associated with toxic adenomas can be managed by radioactive iodine or surgery. Antithyroid drugs have little to offer for long-term management. Since the radioactive iodine is primarily concentrated by the hot nodule, hypothyroidism rarely, if ever, develops.

Hyperthyroidism associated with thyroiditis (including the silent variety) is discussed in the section on thyroiditis.

Rare Causes of Hyperthyroidism

Excess TSH Secretion (pituitary adenoma or "inappropriate" secretion)

TSH-producing adenomas are an extremely rare cause of hyperthyroidism. Contrary to the usual cases of hyperthyroidism, TSH levels are absolutely or inappropriately elevated.

Many of these patients have pituitary tumors associated with acromegaly or hyperprolactinemia. Treatment with radiation or surgery directed toward the pituitary tumors is curative for associated hyperthyroidism. The nontumor patient can be treated with radioactive iodine or subtotal thyroidectomy, but the disease may be unusually resistant requiring multiple doses of radioactive iodine or several operations for control of thyrotoxicosis.

Iodide-Induced Hyperthyroidism

That iodides may induce hyperthyroidism has been known for a long time; this phenomenon is known as the Jod-Basedow effect. Typically, this type of hyperthyroidism develops in patients living in iodine-deficient areas when supplemental iodides are provided, but a similar phenomenon has been described in patients who were not iodine deficient. Most of these patients have had multinodular goiter and typically the resulting hyperthyroidism is mild requiring only symptomatic treatment. If hyperthyroidism is severe, antithyroid drugs are the treatment of choice.

Hyperthyroidism Associated With Trophoblastic Malignancy. The association between molar pregnancy and hyperthyroidism has been known since 1955. The mechanism, however, was not clarified until recently. It has been shown that human chorionic gonadotropin has some TSH-like biologic activity.

In patients with hydatidiform mole, serum HCG concentration greatly exceeds those found in normal pregnancy. These data indicate that the intrinsic thyroid-stimulating activity of HCG is responsible for hyperthyroidism associated with hydatidiform mole and choriocarcinoma. The clinical features of hyperthyroidism are usually mild despite elevated T_4 and T_3 levels. The diagnosis is made by the clinical features of the molar pregnancy (e.g., abnormal uterine bleeding, large-for-date uterus, or molar tissue passed per vagina). Treatment is directed toward the mole. Hyperthyroidism subsides rapidly after removal of the tumor.

Struma Ovarii

Struma ovarii are ovarian teratomas containing thyroid tissue. They are an extremely rare cause of hyperthyroidism. The diagnosis should be considered in women who are hyperthyroid and have a low radioactive iodine uptake in the thyroid. The ovarian lesions are usually palpable and a high ^{131}I uptake may be present in the pelvis.

Factitious Hyperthyroidism

Factitious hyperthyroidism results from self-administration of exogenous thyroid hormones. These patient have a variety of personality disorders characterized by hysterical, perfectionist, or immature behavior. The diagnosis can be suspected in a patient with such personality disorders an hyperthyroidism with very low ^{131}I uptake and the absence of a goiter.

Thyroid Carcinoma
Associated with Hyperthyroidism

Although follicular carcinoma has the ability to concentrate iodide, it produces hyperthyroidism very rarely. In the majority of the instances it is the metastases that, even though they function suboptimally, result in thyrotoxicosis because of their large mass. Even more rare are a few case reports in which the cervical thyroid carcinoma contributed significantly to the development of thyrotoxicosis.

Thyrotoxic Crisis (Thyroid Storm)

Thyroid crisis is defined as life-threatening hyperthyroidism. It is a rare disorder and accounts for about 2% of all hospital admissions for hyperthyroidism. In the majority of cases, the thyroid crises is brought about by a precipitating event in previously untreated severely hyperthyroid patients. The precipitating events include infections, cardiovascular diseases, gastrointestinal disorders, emotional upset, toxemia of pregnancy, onset of labor and delivery, surgical procedures, and trauma.

The clinical features of thyrotoxic crisis are those of severe hyperthyroidism. Fever is almost universally present and may be high. Patients are generally restless, confused, and frank psychosis may be present. Cardiac arrhythmias are frequently present. Congestive heart failure may be precipitated in patients with even mild underlying cardiovascular disease.

The diagnosis must be made on clinical grounds and treatment must be instituted pending confirmation by definitive tests. A high 2-hour radioiodine uptake is a useful confirmatory procedure. Blood for serum T_4 measurement must be obtained prior to institution of treatment. Specific treatment for the disorder includes the administration of antithyroid drugs in large doses. Propylthiouracil (800-1,200 mg) or methimazole 80-120 mg per day may be given by mouth or by nasogastric tube. Ten to 20 drops of Lugol's iodine by mouth or 1-2 g sodium iodide are administered by slow intravenous drip. Iodides inhibit the release of the preformed hormone and therefore are immediately useful. However, it is important that iodide be administered after propylthiouracil has been given since iodide also acts as a substrate for thyroid hormone synthesis. The use of sympathetic inhibitors in patients with thyrotoxic storm can be lifesaving. Propranolol has a rapid onset of action and a short half-life. The usual dose is 1-5 mg intravenously or 20-80 mg orally every 4 hours. Glucocorticoids (hydrocortisone 200-300 mg a day or equivalent doses of dexamethasone) are administered to prevent the development of relative adrenal insufficiency. Both propranolol and dexamethasone decrease peripheral monodeiodination of T_4 to T_3, and dexamethasone also acutely inhibits the release of thyroid hormone in patients with Graves' disease. These effects provide additional basis for their therapeutic benefit in thyroid storm. A careful search for the precipitating event should be made and, if detected, appropriately treated. In addition, the general supportive measures should be applied as necessary. Recently, plasmapheresis and peritoneal dialysis have been used in patients with thyroid storm with some success. However, these procedures still remain experimental.

THYROTOXICOSIS AND PREGNANCY

Hyperthyroidism complicates pregnancy in approximately 0.1% of patients. The diagnosis of hyperthyroidism is difficult during pregnancy since many of the signs and symptoms of hyperthyroidism and pregnancy are similar. These include tachycardia, goiter, tremors in extended extremities, and presence of palmar erythema. However, ophthalmopathy, dermopathy, muscle wasting, and oncholysis are present only in thyrotoxicosis and if present are helpful in the differential diagnosis. In addition, during pregnancy many of the laboratory test results are altered in the direction of hyperthyroidism. This is because of an increase in the thyroxine-binding globulin that results in an increased T_4 and T_3 measurement. However, the T_3 resin uptake is a useful test to distinguish between pregnancy and hyperthyroidism. The T_3 resin uptake is decreased in pregnancy, whereas it is increased in hyperthyroidism. Elevated free thyroxine, if available, is also a useful test to establish the diagnosis of hyperthyroidism during pregnancy.

The therapy for hyperthyroidism during pregnancy includes antithyroid drugs and surgery, since treatment with radioactive iodine during pregnancy is contraindicated. The preferred therapy for hyperthyroidism during pregnancy is antithyroid drugs. It should be remembered that propylthiouracil and methimazole cross the placenta and influence the fetal thyroid. Drugs, therefore, are employed in minimal effective doses. Once euthyroidism has been achieved, the dosage of the drug is further decreased especially in the latter part of the pregnancy. Hypothyroidism should be carefully avoided since it seems to have a detrimental effect on the fetus. Iodides should be avoided during pregnancy since their use has been associated with the development of large goiters in the fetus. Similarly, large doses of propylthiouracil and/or methimazole have also been associated with the development of goiters in the fetus. Most patients can be adequately controlled with drugs alone until the end of the pregnancy. β-Adrenergic drugs have been used to a very limited extent for management of hyperthyroidism during pregnancy, but they may compromise placental blood flow and produce bradycardia, neonatal respiratory depression, and hypoglycemia in the fetus. In some institutions, subtotal thyroidectomy is performed after euthyroidism has been achieved. If surgery is to be performed, the optimal time is the second trimester, since there is an increased risk of abortion during the first and premature labor during the third trimester. If antithyroid drugs are continued postpartum, the mother should not breast-feed since propylthiouracil, and to a lesser extent, propranolol is excreted in the milk.

THYROIDITIS

Hashimoto's Thyroiditis (Chronic Lymphocytic Thyroiditis)

Hashimoto's thyroiditis is an autoimmune disease most frequently encountered in women in the age group of 30-50 years. About 95% of the patients with Hashimoto's thyroiditis have antibodies to thyroglobulin, antimicrosomal antibodies, and antibodies reacting with a second colloid antigen that is distinct from thyroglobulin. In practice, only thyroglobulin and microsomal antibodies are measured in most situations.

Patients with autoimmune thyroiditis generally present with an enlargement of the thyroid. They are usually euthyroid; however, some patients present with hyperthyroidism (Hashitoxicosis) or hypothyroidism. The natural history of the disease appears to be that of slow destruction of the thyroid gland; the majority of patients eventually develop hypothyroidism. On physical examination, characteristically the gland is three to five times normal size, and the surface is granular but distinct nodules are usually not palpable. Sometimes when the process is rapid, the patient may complain of pain, and tenderness may be elicited on palpation.

Presence of antithyroglobulin antibodies in high titers or a strongly positive test for antimicrosomal antibodies nearly confirms the diagnosis. In case of doubt, a needle biopsy can be obtained. Microscopic examination of the tissue reveals that the normal thyroid structure is replaced by a dense infiltrate of lymphocytes. In many cases, firbosis is a prominent feature. Serum thyroxine determination reflects the metabolic status of the patient and may be increased, normal, or decreased.

The treatment is by replacement of thyroid hormone in patients who have developed hypothyroidism. Where only a simple goiter is evident, replacement of thyroid hormone may lead to a decrease in the size of the goiter, especially if it is of recent origin. If the patient is euthyroid and the goiter is small, not causing disfiguration, it may simply be followed.

Subacute Thyroiditis Medicine

Subacute thyroiditis (de Quervain's or granulomatous thyroiditis) is an inflammatory condition of the thyroid, probably of viral origin. The illness is usually preceded by an upper respiratory tract infection. A few days later, the patient notices gradual onset of pain in the thyroid area, usually radiating across the lateral aspects of the neck to the jaw and the ear. There may be systemic symptoms of fever, malaise, and muscle aches. On examination, the gland is only slightly or moderately enlarged and there is mild to severe tenderness that may be present in one lobe or in the entire thyroid area. Cervical lymph nodes are generally not enlarged. Signs of mild hyperthyroidism may be present in the early phase. Diagnosis is made by typical history of upper respiratory tract infection followed by pain in the thyroid area accompanied by enlargement of the thyroid and diffuse tenderness. Leukocytosis is usually not present but ESR is elevated. The serum thyroxine and PBI are frequently elevated in the early phase of the disease because of release of thyroid hormones during the acute inflammatory phase. Radioiodine uptake, on the other hand, is markedly suppressed and is often zero. Treatment in mild cases consists of administration of anti-inflammatory agents. Salicylates and propoxyphene have frequently been used with success; in severe cases, adrenal steroids may be used with beneficial effects. In the event of repeated exacerbations, administration of thyroid hormones is of considerable benefit and appears to prevent further recurrences. Obviously, thyroid hormones should not be given if the patient is clinically or chemically hyperthyroid. Almost all cases of subacute thyroiditis eventually recover completely. Rarely, some patients may develop permanent hypothyroidism.

Silent Thyroiditis

Silent (or painless) thyroiditis is considered to be a variant of subacute thyroiditis. It is characterized by thyroiditis and is accompanied by spontaneously resolving hyperthyroidism. It has been known for several years that many patients with subacute thyroiditis did not complain of neck pain and had no tenderness in the thyroid. In recent years, this has received a lot of attention because an increasing number of case reports of this entity have appeared in the literature. It has been suggested that this disorder may represent 15% of all hyperthyroid patients in North America. The other clinical features of this variant are similar to classic subacute thyroiditis, that is, there is an early phase of hyperthyroidism accompanied by elevated T_4 and T_3, a low radioiodine uptake, and eventual recovery in a few months, sometimes preceded by a period of transient hypothyroidism. Clinically, the only difference is the lack of pain. There are some differences in the laboratory values, however. ESR is markedly elevated in the painful variety, but may be normal or minimally elevated in the painless variety. A higher frequency of antithyroid antibodies in high titers has been reported in the silent variety. Biopsy studies in the painless disorder have shown predominant lymphocytic infiltration, and even formation of lymphoid follicles has been reported, but features consistent with granulomatous (subacute) thyroiditis have not been demonstrated. This has led to the conclusion by some investigators that this disorder is a variant of chronic lymphocytic thyroiditis. It has, in fact, been suggested that it may represent a heterogeneous disorder. The importance of this variety of hyperthyroidism is to make the correct diagnosis and to avoid inappropriate treatment. Because of its frequent occurrence, it has been suggested that a radioiodine uptake test should be reinstituted in the routine work-up of patients with hyperthyroidism. A low radioiodine uptake easily distinguishes this disorder from Graves' disease but not from other causes of hyperthyroidism with low ^{131}I uptake, for which additional studies may be needed. The treatment of choice is propranolol for symptomatic control.

Ablative (surgery and ^{131}I) treatment is contraindicated, and drugs are unlikely to be effective.

HYPOTHYROIDISM (MYXEDEMA)

Etiology

Hypothyroidism or functional inactivity of the thyroid gland may result from a primary defect in the gland or secondarily due to a deficiency of TSH. Many cases of primary hypothyroidism that appear to be idiopathic are due to the end stages of Hashimoto's or autoimmune thyroiditis. This is supported by the fact that many cases of idiopathic hypothyroidism have antithyroid antibodies in high titers in their plasma. Perhaps the most common cause of primary hypothyroidism is the administration of radioactive iodine for hyperthyroidism. Less commonly, hypothyroidism may result from surgery, congenital defects of thyroid hormone biosynthesis, administration of antithyroid drugs, or administration of iodides in large doses. Secondary hypothyroidism may result from an isolated deficiency of TSH or may occur as part of the total picture of panhypopituitarism. A deficiency of TRH has also been reported to result in hypothyroidism (tertiary or hypothalamic hypothyroidism).

Clinical Features

Patients with primary hypothyroidism usually present with fatigue, unusual sluggishness, weight gain, or sleepiness. A majority of the patients also complain of increased sensitivity to cold. The skin becomes dry, thickened, and puffy due to its infiltration with mucopolysaccharide material. There is a generalized thickening and puffiness of the face and extremities. This edema, however, is nonpitting and is characteristic of hypothyroidism. The hair also becomes coarse; loss of hair may occur from the scalp and the lateral third of the eyebrows. Patients may complain of generalized aches, and pains in muscles rather than the joints. Irregular menstruation and menorrhagia are frequent in young women although hypomenorrhea is also encountered. On physical examination, the thyroid may not be palpable or may be enlarged depending upon the etiology. The skin feels cool and a faint yellow coloration of the skin may be present due to carotenemia. Speech is characteristically slow in addition to being hoarse. The precordium is unusually quiet and the heart sounds are muffled. The heart may be enlarged and there may be evidence of pleural or pericardial effusions. These effusions are of the exudative variety. The relaxation phase of the deep tendon reflexes is delayed although the contraction phase may remain brisk. This is best elicited in the Achilles tendon although it is present in other reflexes as well. Many of these patients appear inappropriately humorous and frank psychosis may develop in some of them (myxedema madness).

Secondary (or tertiary) hypothyroidism, while usually milder, may present in a manner similar to primary hypothyroidism. There may be symptoms and signs of other associated endocrine gland dysfunction. Clinical features suggesting a pituitary origin are a thin pale skin, and loss of axillary and pubic hair in combination with other features of hypothyroidism.

Diagnosis

In fairly advanced cases, the diagnosis may be clinically obvious and is readily confirmed by a low T_4. A serum T_3 measurement is also generally low but is not as helpful as T_4 because it is frequently found to be low in other nonthyroidal systemic illnesses. Electrocardiogram shows bradycardia and low voltage. X-ray of the chest may show cardiomegaly (small heart in secondary hypothyroidism). Serum enzymes, SGOT, LDH, and CPK are frequently elevated. Serum sodium is frequently depressed because of inability to excrete free water. Serum cholesterol is frequently elevated in primary hypothyroidism but is not necessarily of diagnostic value. Serum TSH measurement is the most useful test to distinguish between primary and secondary hypothyroidism. If pituitary hypothyroidism is suspected, other end-organ functions should be evaluated. Serum level of cortisol is generally normal in patients with primary hypothyroidism but urinary 17-hydroxysteroid excretion is decreased due to a decrease in cortisol metabolism. Growth hormone response to insulin hypoglycemia and the results of metapyrone administration may be abnormal in the presence of hypothyroidism. These tests, however, return to normal after hypothyroidism is corrected if anterior pituitary function is basically normal. Treatment of choice is administration of synthetic levothyroxine. It is safe, effective, and results in normal T_4 and T_3 levels in plasma; desiccated thyroid is therefore no longer indicated.

Treatment

The treatment is initiated with small doses of 0.025-0.05 mg of levothyroxine. Replacement therapy should be given together with glucocorticoids in patients with hypopituitarism. Replacement with thyroxine alone may precipitate adrenal crisis in these patients. Dosage is gradually increased every 7-14 days until a full replacement dose is achieved. The usual full replacement dose varies from 0.15-0.2 mg of thyroxine. The optimal thyroid replacement dose should be judged by the clinical response, although TSH level can be used as a guideline. The treatment of permanent hypothyroidism is lifelong and patients should be carefully informed of this fact so that they continue the medication once they feel better.

Myxedema Coma

Myxedema coma is the end stage of untreated hypothyroidism. It usually occurs in long-standing severe cases and, like thyroid storm, is often precipitated by intercurrent illnesses; fortunately, it is rare. The majority of patients with myxedema coma have primary hypothyroidism. These patients present with severe manifestations of hypothyroidism, including dry skin, puffy face, loss of scalp and eyebrow hair, and delayed relaxation of the reflexes. Often the patients are severely obtunded rather than comatose. Hypothermia is a common accompaniment; temperature may be as low as 24°C (75°F). Hypoventilation is also commonly present.

Sinus bradycardia is present on electrocardiogram together with low voltage, diffuse T-wave depression, and prolonged QT and P-R intervals. Carbon dioxide retention, hypoxia, and hyponatremia are frequently found, as is hypoglycemia. The diagnosis can be confirmed by finding a low serum level of T_4, but treatment should begin without waiting for results. The major principle of treatment of myxedema is to administer immediately a relatively large dose of thyroid hormone. This can be administered as 300-500 μg of T_4 intravenously followed by 100-200 μg daily thereafter. Some experts prefer triiodothyronine because of its rapid absorption. The latter can be used in equivalent doses (75-125 μg) via a nasogastric tube. Although most patients have normal adrenal function, 200-300 mg of hydrocortisone should be administered during the first 24 hours to prevent adrenal crisis. These doses can be rapidly tapered. In addition to the specific treatment, attention should be paid to general supportive measures. Respiratory insufficiency may require intubation or tracheostomy. The hyponatremia and hypoglycemia should receive appropriate treatment. If the treatment is successful, most patients with myxedema coma show a significant improvement in 24 hours and a marked improvement within 1 week.

THYROID CARCINOMA

Thyroid carcinoma is a rare disease. The average annual incidence per 100,000 population has been reported to be between 1 and 5. In one survey, thyroid carcinoma accounted for 0.5% of all cancer deaths in women and only 0.2% of all cancer deaths in men. Like other malignant tumors, the etiology of thyroid carcinoma is not well known, but prior exposure of the thyroid to external radiation in childhood is associated with an increased incidence. Thyroid carcinoma may be subdivided into the following types.

Papillary Carcinoma

This is the most benign of thyroid cancers and accounts for approximately 50% of all thyroid carcinomas. Peak incidence of this type occurs during the third and fourth decades of life and is more frequent in women. The disease tends to remain localized in the thyroid gland and is especially benign in children and young adults. The metastases occur to local lymph nodes, although distant metastases may also arise. On histologic examination, it is composed of columnar epithelium that is thrown into folds forming papillary projections.

Follicular Carcinoma

This accounts for about 25% of thyroid cancers. The peak incidence occurs in the fifth decade of life. It may be divided into two subgroups: encapsulated, which shows little capsular or vascular invasion and is associated with a favorable prognosis, and invasive, which shows evidence of rapid growth and marked vascular invasion. Metastases to lymph nodes, and distant metastases to bone and lung, occur in most patients. Most carcinomas have histologic features of both papillary and follicular types.

Clinically, many papillary or follicular carcinomas present with a single nodule in the neck. The decision to be made then is which of these nodules harbors the malignancy. In general, single nodules in young patients (less than 40 years of age), especially in men, have a greater chance of being malignant. The other characteristics of the nodule, namely, hardness, fixation to the surrounding tissues, and presence of enlarged lymph nodes, are highly suggestive of malignancy. The ^{131}I or ^{99m}Tc scans are helpful in that cold nodules are more likely to be malignant and hot nodules are almost never malignant. If the nodule is cold, ultrasound study may be helpful in differentiating cystic from solid lesions. Purely cystic lesions are unlikely to be malignant. If malignancy is not very likely, the patient may be given suppressive doses of thyroid hormones and the growth of the nodule observed. Although carcinomatous lesions have been known to increase in size even while the patient has been taking thyroid, lack of growth or a decrease in size of the nodule favors the diagnosis of a benign lesion. By the considerations outlined above, one can considerably reduce the number of patients who require surgery to exclude the presence of malignancy. Fine needle biopsy and aspiration cytology are being increasingly utilized with reasonable degrees of success to achieve this goal.

Anaplastic Carcinoma

Anaplastic carcinoma accounts for about 10% of all thyroid carcinomas. It is a highly malignant lesion, rapidly invades the surrounding structures, and metastasizes extensively throughout the body. The patients are usually older than 50 years of age and present with a hard, fixed mass in the neck. Evidence of invasion or compression of recurrent laryngeal nerve, trachea, and esophagus may be present at the time of the diagnosis.

Medullary Carcinoma of the Thyroid

This carcinoma arises from the parafollicular (C cells) of the thyroid gland and accounts for 5% to 10% of thyroid carcinomas. Like the other types, it is also slightly more common in women. The disease may occur sporadically, although frequently it is familial and apparently inherited as an autosomal dominant trait. It may also occur as part of the multiple endocrine adenomatosis type II. The other associated features of the syndrome are pheochromocytomas, which are often bilateral, and hyperparathyroidism. The characteristic feature of this tumor is the production of calcitonin, and plasma calcitonin levels are frequently elevated. The cells may also secrete serotonin, prostaglandins, ACTH, and histaminase with resulting clinical syndromes. In relatives of patients with this disease, elevated plasma calcitonin levels are considered a forerunner of the clinically evident disease. It is recommended that plasma calcitonin levels, either with or without pentagastrin stimulation, be measured in close relatives of patients with medullary carcinoma of the thyroid. A high basal level of calcitonin or hyper-response after stimulation with pentagastrin suggests an occult carcinoma.

Treatment of Thyroid Carcinoma

Papillary and follicular carcinomas are malignancies of low grade associated with prolonged survival. The treatment of these lesions is, therefore, somewhat controversial. Small lesions can be treated with lobectomy or total thyroidectomy, leaving the posterior capsule behind. Radical neck dissections are generally not indicated. If lymph nodes are involved, the dissection of lymph nodes is performed. All patients should be given adequate doses of thyroid hormones to suppress the TSH level since the growth and function of these tumors appear to be TSH dependent. Following thyroidectomy, radioactive iodine administration has been suggested to ablate the remainder of the thyroid tissue, but the advantages of ^{131}I are difficult to prove. If subsequent metastases occur, they can sometimes be treated with radioactive iodine administration. The treatment of medullary carcinoma of the thyroid is also total thyroidectomy. The therapy of anaplastic carcinoma is generally unsatisfactory. Surgical removal, external radiation, and chemotherapy, singly or in combination, have been tried; but rapidly progressing tumors often show no response.

PARATHYROID AND CALCIUM METABOLISM

Calcium is a major component of the human skeleton and has a major role in numerous physiologic processes, including blood coagulation, neuromuscular function, hormonal secretion, and the maintenance of cell membranes and enzyme function. Ninety-nine percent of body calcium is present in bone, 1% of which is freely exchangeable with the extracellular fluid. The rest of body calcium is distributed in other body tissues with 0.3% in muscle. Although the normal range for serum calcium is 8.5-10.5 mg/dl, or 4.7-5.2 mEq/L, less than 50% of the circulating calcium is in the free, or unbound, form. Calcium is largely bound to serum proteins; however, a small amount circulates as complexes with citrate and phosphate. Alkaline pH increases calcium binding, as does a significant increase in plasma protein concentration. For every gram change in serum albumin concentration, serum calcium changes approximately 0.8 mg/dl in the same direction.

Since only the ionized, or unbound, fraction has physiologic activity, changes only in total calcium content do not alter body function unless there is a concomitant alteration in the unbound portion.

CALCIUM HOMEOSTASIS

Under usual conditions, there exists a balance between calcium intake and excretion. Although less than 1% of the enormous skeletal reservoir is available for ion exchange, the body can, in times of calcium need, increase bone resorption and gut absorption with a concomitant decrease in calcium excretion.

Normal dietary calcium intake varies from 0.5-1.0 g, of which 25-75% is absorbed depending on the need. Calcium absorption can also be influenced by age and vitamin D. Vitamin D has a major role in the active transport of calcium against an electrochemical gradient through calcium-dependent ATPase. In addition, vitamin D is essential for gut absorption of inorganic phosphorus and for normal mineralization of bone matrix. Although calcium is secreted into the gastrointestinal tract in digestive juices, variations in fecal calcium appear to have little influence on overall calcium balance. The body can also lose calcium during sweating; usually insigificant, this loss can approach 100-200 mg/day in times of severe loss. The kidney is the major route of calcium excretion, with a normal 24-hour daily output of 150-400 mg. Approximately two-thirds of calcium resorption, like that of sodium, takes place in the proximal tubule, perhaps through a common pathway. Conditions favoring sodium excretion, such as saline infusions, also favor calcium excretion. Growth hormone leads to hypercalciuria by direct action of the kidney; phosphate also has a direct effect on the kidney and reduces renal calcium excretion. In states of extreme phosphate depletion, however, an increase in urinary calcium is noted. Glucocorticoid administration causes an increased urinary calcium excretion by altering skeletal calcium homeostasis. Parathyroid hormone reduces urinary calcium excretion directly, exerting most of its effect on the distal renal tubules despite most of the calcium resorption occurring in the proximal tubules. When calcium deprivation results in a slight lowering of ionized calcium, parathyroid hormone is secreted, resulting in reduced urinary calcium excretion to maintain normal serum calcium levels. An increased serum calcium, on the other hand, leads to reduction in parathyroid hormone secretion and increases in urinary calcium clearance. Although glucocorticoids and growth hormone are capable of modifying serum calcium, they are not secreted in response to changes in blood calcium and are thus not part of the homeostatic process.

Role of Vitamin D

Vitamin D is a key factor in calcium homeostasis. One major site of production is the skin, utilizing 7-dehydrocholesterol as a precursor to produce cholecalciferol (vitamin D_3). Vitamin D can also be obtained from plant sterols called ergocalciferol (vitamin D_2). Both of these sources of vitamin D yield a relatively metabolically inert form that must undergo conversion into active metabolites. Vitamin D_3 is first converted into 25-hydroxyvitamin D_3 (25-hydroxycholecalciferol) in the liver, which then is converted by the kidney to 1,25-dihydroxyvitamin D_3 (1,25-dihydroxycholecalciferol, the physiologically active form) and 24,25-dihydroxyvitamin D_3. Calcium, phosphate, parathyroid hormone, and calcitonin have been reported to affect hydroxylation. The production of 1,25-dihydroxyvitamin D_3 is stimulated by parathyroid hormone and by a reduction in intracellular phosphate. A high calcium or phosphorous suppresses 1,25-dihydroxyvitamin D_3 synthesis in the kidney. In the absence of stimuli, vitamin D metabolism preferentially produces relatively inert products such as 24,25- and 25,26-dihydroxyvitamin D_3.

Vitamin D regulates the efficiency of calcium absorption by the gut, probably by stimulating the transcription of messenger RNA that directs the synthesis of protein components acting as a transport system in both bone and intestine. Vitamin D probably also acts directly to influence bone calcium turnover. Patients with vitamin D deficiency appear to be resistant to the actions of parathyroid hormone.

Parathyroid Hormone (Parathormone, PTH)

Ionized blood calcium concentration regulates the secretion of parathyroid hormone from four parathyroid glands located on the posterior aspect of the thyroid. Parathyroid hormone is a polypeptide consisting of 84 amino acids and acts in the kidney, gut, and bone to stimulate the renal excretion of phosphorous, sodium, and potassium, and to raise urinary cyclic AMP levels while reducing the excretion of calcium and magnesium. Parathyroid hormone also decreases fecal calcium excretion and promotes an increased rate of calcium release from the skeleton by increasing osteoclastic activity. After secretion, the polypeptide chain is broken into two major fragments, N- and C-terminal portions. The N-terminal fragment is thought to be the active component; however, due to its shorter half-life, in many assays a better correlation exists between the C-terminal fragment and presence of hyperparathyroidism. Because of dependency on renal clearance, it is important to remember that the C-terminal fragment may be elevated in renal failure, regardless of the calcium state. In addition, levels must be interpreted in association with the level of calcium. An increased parathyroid hormone level does not necessarily indicate hyperparathyroidism; a normal level, on the other hand, in association with a high serum calcium may indicate hyperparathyroidism.

Calcitonin (Thyrocalcitonin)

Calcitonin is a polypeptide hormone synthesized and secreted by the parafollicular cells of the thyroid gland. The hormone is continually secreted at physiologic concentrations unless challenged by hypercalcemia, with resultant hormone elevations. Calcitonin is thought to oppose parathyroid hormone action and appears to work by stimulating cyclic AMP in specific bone and kidney cells. Although this hormone is considered part of the calcium homeostatic mechanism, it appears to have a minor role in regulating serum calcium and phosphorus.

PHOSPHORUS HOMEOSTASIS

Phosphorus is found largely in the skeleton in association with calcium; however, approximately 15% is present outside bone, widely distributed in the body as organic compounds such as nucleic acids, phospholipids, phosphoproteins, and high-energy phosphate compounds. Dietary deficiency of phosphorus and disorders in homeostasis are rare and usually encountered only in severe malnutriton, renal disease, or hormonal imbalance. Because of abrupt shifts between extracellular and intracellular compartments, phosphorus concentrations vary considerably; glucose, insulin, epinephrine, and glucagon lead to a decrease in serum phosphorus through the formation of intracellular organic phosphorus compounds involved in carbohydrate metabolism.

Intracellular phosphorus concentrations can influence the renal transport of calcium; increased dietary phosphorus increases the renal clearance of calcium. Although the concentration of phosphorus in the kidney affects vitamin D metabolism, there is no direct effect of serum phosphorus on parathyroid hormone. A phosphorus deficiency increases renal hydroxylation of 25-hydroxy vitamin D_3, and a high phosphorus has a negative effect in this regard. Severe deficiency results in proximal muscle weakness and a decrease in erythrocyte 2,3-diphosphoglycerate with alterations in the oxyhemoglobin dissociation curve. Excessive levels of phosphorus may result in ectopic calcifications and deposition of calcium phosphate crystals in body tissues.

Phosphorus is rapidly absorbed in the jejunum, apparently by active transport; however, the absorption efficiency is dependent on phosphorus intake. Average intake is 800-900 mg a day with the major sources being dairy products, cereal, and meat. Absorption is also affected by aluminum hydroxide-containing antacids that bind phosphates and retard absorption. The kidneys are the principal site for regulation of blood phosphorus. Phosphorus excretion is increased by parathyroid hormone and estrogens, and reduced by glucocorticoids, vitamin D, and growth hormone. Urinary excretion of phosphorus involves glomerular filtration and tubular reabsorption; 85-95% of filtered phosphorus is normally reabsorbed. Urinary excretion equals dietary intake under normal conditions. The upper limit of tubular phosphate reabsorption is approximately 2-6 mg per minute with maximal excretion occurring at night. Alterations in homeostasis can also result from changes in blood phosphorus levels and glomerular filtration rate. Rarely, loss of phosphorus can occur as a result of an inherited tubular defect or secondary to renal tubular damage. Severe renal phosphorus wasting may also occur as a result of hyperparathyroidism.

HYPERCALCEMIA

Hypercalcemia is a common clinical problem with multiple etiologies, the two leading causes being malignancy and hyperparathyroidism. In recent years, routine automated laboratory screening has increased the frequency of diagnosis. The differential diagnosis of an elevated serum calcium includes numerous possibilities, for example, vitamin D intoxication, milk alkali syndrome, malignancy, sarcoidosis, thiazide usage, immobilization, hyperthyroidism, Addison's disease, and parathyroid hormone excess. Hypercalcemia complicating malignancy can result from osteolytic metastases, ectopic production of parathyroid hormone, or the production of similar humoral substances chemically distinct from parathyroid hormone, but with similar biologic actions.

Hypercalcemia may present in a variety of ways; however, the earliest manifestations are usually polyuria and nocturia, thought to be secondary to an impaired concentrating ability in the kidney. Clinical clues suggesting hypercalcemia include the following:

Renal: Nephrolithiasis, nephrocalcinosis, renal tubular defects, and renal failure

Gastrointestinal: Peptic ulcers, pancreatitis, constipation, anorexia, and nausea

Psychiatric: Apathy, depression, or psychosis

Neuromuscular: Muscle weakness, hyporeflexia, and coma

Skin: Pruritus, band keratopathy, and palpebral calcification

Cardiovascular: Shortened QT interval on ECG and increased digoxin sensitivity

Skeletal: Mild, generalized osteoporosis with mild, generalized radiolucency seen on radiographs (osteitis fibrosa generalisata) and cystic lesions in the long bones and skull (osteitis fibrosa cystica)

Treatment

The treatment of hypercalcemia should be aimed at reducing calcium levels while searching for an underlying etiology.

Although the cutoff for urgent treatment remains controversial, a calcium greater than 12.5% must be reduced immediately. If renal function is adequate, volume repletion with normal saline, often up to 10 liters per day, helps increase urinary calcium excretion. The use of furosemide in doses of 40-100 mg intravenously every 2-4 hours enhances calcium excretion and lowers serum calcium levels. Large electrolyte losses may occur under this regimen and must be replaced.

Phosphate salts given orally are useful adjunctive therapy. Intravenous usage increases the risk of ectopic calcifications and should be avoided. It is felt that phosphorus decreases serum calcium by making the bones refractory to parathyroid hormone (PTH) as well as causing calcium deposition in body tissues. Caution must also be used to prevent hypocalcemia, as the effects may linger for several days after use.

Mithramycin, a cytotoxic agent used to treat certain neoplasms, is also capable of lowering plasma calcium by direct action on bone. The hypocalcemic effect from mithramycin is usually not seen for 24 hours and may last for several days. Repeat administration should not be considered until serum calcium begins to rise again. Recommended dosage is 15-25 μg/kg IV at 24-48-hour intervals as needed. There is the potential for hepatic, renal, or hematologic toxicity, and a maximal dose of 150 μg/kg per week should not be exceeded. Administration of calcitonin (2 units/kg subcutaneously) has been successful in lowering calcium.

Nonurgent treatment for hypercalcemia involves hydration and oral phosphate supplementation such as Neutra-Phos, 1 g three times a day. Surgical exploration is recommended for suspected hyperparathyroidism in patients thought to be good surgical risks. Treatment of hypercalcemia from causes other than hyperparathyroidism should be aimed at correcting the underlying disorder. Steroids can be used to decrease the absorption of calcium from the gut in cases of vitamin D intoxication and sarcoidosis; they are also useful in lowering elevated calcium levels associated with malignancies. Chemotherapy on occasion may also help reduce hypercalcemia due to malignancy. Prostaglandin inhibitors, such as indomethacin, have been used successfully to treat hypercalcemia resulting from certain tumors.

Primary Hyperparathyroidism

Primary hyperparathyroidism is most commonly seen in women aged 40-49. A single parathyroid adenoma is by far the most common cause, with four-gland hyperplasia occurring in approximately 15% of cases. Adenomas occur in the lower parathyroid glands three times more commonly than in the upper glands. Mediastinal lesions are found in 5-20% of the reported series.

Although the hallmark of diagnosis is an elevation of serum calcium and depression of serum phosphorus, often repeated calcium determinations are necessary to confirm the suspicion due to the potential for episodic excess parathyroid hormone secretion. Diagnosis is made by documenting an elevated parathyroid hormone level by radioimmunoassay in relation to the serum calcium level. Because parathyroid hormone causes retention of the hydrogen ion, serum chloride usually is greater than 102 mEq/L. A chloride to phosphorus ratio greater than 35 is often detected, and serum alkaline phosphatase may be elevated. Elevations in urinary calcium are generally present. Rarely, a selective parathyroid venous catheterization is required to aid further in diagnosis, especially after unsuccessful surgical attempts to cure the illness. This procedure helps localize elevations in hormone secretion to a specific region, such as the neck, chest, or other areas.

Definitive treatment is the surgical removal of the abnormal gland(s). In cases of single adenomas, the diseased gland is removed. In cases of four-gland hyperplasia, usually three of the glands are removed, leaving the fourth in place.

Postoperatively, there is a prompt fall in phosphorus and calcium returns to normal within a day, the phosphorus often remaining low for up to 1 week. Magnesium deficiency may also be seen, as well as transient hypocalcemia due to either edema of the remaining parathyroid tissue or the hungry bone syndrome; rarely, surgery results in permanent hypocalcemia if excess tissue is removed. A calcium elevated for more than 1 week after surgery, or recurrent hypercalcemia within a few weeks, implies surgical failure.

Treatment of asymptomatic hypercalcemia due to primary hyperparathyroidism has not been clearly defined. Patients may be treated surgically to prevent the future development of complications, particularly renal function impairment. Alternatively, careful follow-up of serum calcium and renal function may be embarked upon if the patient understands the importance and is fully cooperating. Familial hypocalciuric hypercalcemia is being increasingly recognized; surgery does not appear to help these patients.

Secondary Hyperparathyroidism

Secondary hyperparathyroidism results from excessive production of parathyroid hormone as a result of constant stimulation from hypocalcemia. Serum calcium remains low because compensation by increased PTH is not complete, but other effects may occur in bone disease. Secondary hyperparathyroidism occurs in patients suffering from chronic renal disease, osteomalacia, and pseudohypoparathyroidism.

HYPOCALCEMIA AND HYPOPARATHYROIDISM

Hypocalcemia is encountered not only in hypoparathyroidism but also in malabsorption, osteomalacia, vitamin D deficiency or resistance, renal failure, pancreatitis, and acute nutritional deficiency. The most common cause of hypoparathyroidism is surgical removal or damage interference with the vascular supply to the parathyroid glands on the neck. Transient hypoparathyroidism may occur immediately following thyroid surgery, although it is not yet clear whether this results from edema of the parathyroid glands or release of calcitonin. Parathyroid glandular failure may, in some cases, be partial rather than absolute. Idiopathic hypoparathyroidism, a rare entity, can occur as an isolated condition, in association with agenesis of the thymus or as an autoimmune familial disorder in which there may be an associated deficiency of the thyroid, adrenal and ovarian function, pernicious anemia, and other defects.

Pseudohypoparathyroidism, due to deficient end-organ (kidneys, bone) response to PTH, is characterized by decreased calcium and increased phosphorus, parathyroid hyperplasia, clinical features of hypoparathyroidism, and distinctive skeletal and developmental defects that frequently include short fourth and fifth metacarpal bones.

Signs and symptoms of hypoparathyroidism involve primarily neuromuscular irritability from decreased concentration of ionized calcium. Contraction of the facial muscles on tapping the facial nerve (Chvostek's sign) and carpopedal spasm of the fingers on application of pressure around the arm (Trousseau's sign) are often present. Carpopedal spasm, tetany, and even frank convulsions may occur. Soft tissue calcification, involving the lens and basal ganglia, is noted in as many as 50 percent of the patients.

Laboratory abnormalities of hypoparathyroidism include hypocalcemia and hyperphosphatemia in the presence of normal renal function. Radioimmunoassayable parathyroid hormone level is low or absent in idiopathic or postsurgical hypoparathyroidism, but may be normal or elevated in pseudohypoparathyroidism. Measurement of urinary cyclic adenosine 3′,5′-monophosphate (AMP) excretion following parathyroid hormone injection may help differentiate true from pseudohypoparathyroidism. In the former, cyclic AMP excretion rises ten to twentyfold.

Treatment usually consists of supplementary dietary calcium and vitamin D. Hypercalcemia and hypercalciuria should be avoided by frequent monitoring of blood and urinary calcium. It may take several weeks of therapy before serum calcium level reaches the desired range of 8.5-9 mg/dl.

OSTEOPENIA AND OSTEOPOROSIS

The skeleton is composed of minerals, cells, and a matrix. Although cells comprise less than 5% of bone volume, they are of major importance in bone architecture. Osteoblasts form bone; and osteoclasts, located in hollow spaces within layers of bone, resorb small amounts of local bone. Bone is composed of 50% matrix, of which most is fibrous tissue, mucopolysaccharides, and collagen. The remaining volume of bone is composed of minerals, primarily hydroxyapatite. When abnormalities in this carefully orchestrated balance occur, bone disease results.

Osteoporosis is a skeletal disorder characterized by a reduction in the entire bone tissue leading to increased porosity. This entity is most commonly found in postmenopausal women and elderly men. Symptoms range from no pain to some pain, severe statural shortening, kyphosis, and compression fractures. There are numerous causes of premature osteoporosis including increased parathyroid hormone, hyperthyroidism, growth hormone excess, glucocorticoid administration, and immobility. Osteoporosis is rare among blacks, probably due to increased bone mass throughout early life.

Treatment is aimed at preventing further bone loss and replacement of lost bone. One gram of elemental Ca^{2+} per day is recommended. Calcitonin and phosphate therapy are of little benefit. Estrogen in low doses to postmenopausal women generally slows the progression of bone loss and, if otherwise not contraindicated, should be tried. Some investigators advocate fluoride supplementation to stimulate new bone formation, although the new bone formed is often poorly mineralized and secondary hyperparathyroidism and osteomalacia may also occur. The use of vitamin D is presently controversial; recent evidence suggests further mineral loss with its usage to treat osteoporosis.

Osteomalacia and rickets are characterized by decreased mineralized bone and increased osteoid or bone matrix. Rickets occurs in children, due to vitamin D deficiency prior to epiphyseal closure. Osteomalacia is the adult form and results from vitamin D deficiency; hypophosphatemia, either from vitamin D-resistance rickets, renal tubular defects, or phosphate depletion; defective vitamin D metabolism; fluoride intoxication; hypophosphatasia; chronic renal failure; prolonged phenytoin, phenobarbital, and glutethimide therapy; and postgastrectomy. Symptoms include bone pain or fracture from minor trauma, weakness, hypocalcemia, hypophosphatemia, increased alkaline phosphatase, and pseudofractures (so-called milkman's fractures) on x-ray. The treatment consists of vitamin administration.

PAGET'S DISEASE OF THE BONE

Paget's disease of the bone (osteitis deformans) is usually focal in nature, although it may be widespread. It is characterized by excessive resorption of bone with replacement of normal marrow by vascular, fibrous connective tissue. The resorbed bone is replaced by coarse, dense trabecular bone organized in a haphazard fashion, with multiple irregular cement lines giving the bone a mosaic pattern. Although usually asymptomatic, it can cause devastating effects. Only rarely reported before middle age, estimates suggest it to affect 3% of the population over age 40. Its etiology is unknown. Although increased bone resorption is balanced by increased bone formation, an imbalance may occur. When resorption predominates, the bones become osteopenic with a negative calcium balance. A decreased resorption leads to hard, dense bone and a positive calcium balance. The rate of urinary hydroxyproline excretion and plasma alkaline phosphatase correlates well with bone turnover rate and disease activity. Radiologic findings also reflect the disease state. Changes in cortical density, deformity of the long bones, and cyst formation can be seen. The pelvic bones are most commonly involved. The skull, femur, lumbosacral spine, clavicles, ribs, and tibia are also commonly affected.

The disease may remain asymptomatic or present as a swelling or deformity of a long bone with resultant gait alteration. A change in hat size may indicate enlargement of the skull. In some, bone pain may be the first symptom. Hearing loss due to temporal bone involvement is seen, as well as other neurologic findings due to basal skull compression from pagetic bone growth. Fractures of the long bones and spinal column can result from abnormal bone formation. When the disease is widespread, the increased blood flow through the skeleton may result in high cardiac output and heart failure. Serum calcium and phosphorus are usually normal; however, alkaline phosphatase is increased in relation to disease activity. Hypercalciuria may lead to urinary stone formation. The most serious complication is sarcoma transformation seen in 1-2% of patients. Rarely, hypercalcemia results from immobilization.

Although there is no specific cure for Paget's disease, aspirin therapy can provide analgesia as well as suppress disease activity. Corticosteroids are not usually indicated since only high doses have a beneficial effect, although relief of high output cardiac failure within days has been reported. The best treatment to date is salmon calcitonin, 50-100 MRC units daily given subcutaneously, although this should be reserved for disease exhibiting a rapid course with widespread destruction and potential neurologic compromise. Other potentially useful drugs include cytotoxic agents such as mithramycin and actinomycin D, administered intramuscularly, and disodium etidronate, a diphosphonate compound given orally. Serum alkaline phosphatase and urinary hydroxyproline are indicators of disease activity and should be monitored during therapy.

ADRENAL CORTEX

The two adrenal glands are located in the vicinity of the upper poles of the kidney. The glands consist of an outer portion (the cortex) and an inner portion (the medulla). Histologically, the adrenal cortex is divided into three zones. From outside to inside, these are zona glomerulosa, zona fasciculata, and zona reticularis. The zona glomerulosa produces aldosterone and the fasciculata and reticularis secrete glucocorticoids and adrenal androgens.

PHYSIOLOGY OF THE ADRENAL CORTICOSTEROIDS

The adrenal cortex produces three groups of hormones.

Glucocorticoids

Hydrocortisone (cortisol) is the representative steroid of the glucocorticoid group. Its major actions include suppression of ACTH, protein catabolism, gluconeogenesis, impairment of glucose utilization, and potent anti-inflammatory actions. It also has a weak sodium-retaining activity. The secretion of cortisol is predominantly controlled by ACTH; cortisol, in turn, exerts a negative feedback influence on CRF and ACTH secretion. The pattern of secretion of cortisol closely follows the diurnal rhythm of ACTH, resulting in higher levels in the morning and lower in the evening. Stress, a well-known stimulus for an increase in the secretion of ACTH, also results in higher cortisol levels. The stimulus of stress is strong and may override the basic diurnal pattern.

Mineralocorticoids

The most potent mineralocorticoid secreted by the human adrenal cortex is aldosterone, and its predominant effects include sodium retention and potassium excretion. 11-Deoxycorticosterone (DOC) is normally secreted at about the same rate as aldosterone, but its mineralocorticoid effects are far less than that of aldosterone. The secretion of aldosterone is predominantly under control of the renin-angiotensin system. Renin is an enzyme secreted by the juxtaglomerular apparatus of the kidney. Juxtaglomerular cells in the wall of the afferent arterioles function as baroreceptors. A fall in the plasma volume or renal arterial pressure stimulates renin secretion by decreasing the stretch on these receptors. In addition, net concentration of Na^+ at the macula densa and renal sympathetic nerves regulates renin secretion. β-Adrenergic receptors appear to be involved in this regulation since β-adrenergic blocking agents decrease renin secretion but α-adrenergic blockers do not. Hypokalemia and prostaglandins also increase renin release. Hyperkalemia inhibits, and the concentration of angiotensin II may also exert a negative feedback effect on the secretion of renin. Renin acts on the renin substrate in the α_2-globulin fraction of blood, also called angiotesinogen, and leads to the formation of a decapeptide, angiotensin I, which is further converted to an octapeptide, angiotensin II. Besides being a potent vasoconstrictor, angiotensin II is a powerful stimulator of aldosterone secretion. An increase in the secretion of aldosterone leads to sodium retention and restoration of the effective plasma volume, thus completing the feedback circuit for secretion of aldosterone. In addition, the secretion of aldosterone is increased by increased concentration of potassium and ACTH; the effects of ACTH are, however, only transient (see Fig. 9).

Adrenal Androgens

The third group of hormones secreted by the adrenal cortex are adrenal androgens. These have only weak androgenic activity. Their secretion is significantly increased by administration of ACTH, but they do not have a significant negative feedback effect on the secretion of ACTH.

Synthesis and Metabolism of Adrenal Steroids

The substrate for steroid synthesis is cholesterol. The common biosynthetic pathway from cholesterol is via pregnenolone. Pregnenolone represents the precursor for all the three major groups of adrenal steroids. The subsequent synthesis of cortisol, aldosterone, and the androgens occurs in a stepwise, systematic fashion. Each step is facilitated by the action of a specific enzyme. The enzymes involved are shown in Figure 10.

Cortisol is reversibly bound to an α_2-globulin in circulation. It is metabolized by the liver and reduced to tetrahydrocortisol via dihydrocortisol, and finally excreted as tetrahydrocortisol glucuronide by the kidney. The metabolic products of cortisol are measured in the urine as 17-hydroxycorticosteroids by the Porter-Silber reaction. The latter is a color reaction developed by addition of phenylhydrazine in sulfuric acid with steroids having 17,21-dihydroxy 20-keto side chain. The metabolic products of the adrenal androgens are excreted as 17-ketosteroids. They contribute about two-thirds to the urinary 17-ketosteroids in men as measured by Zimmermann's reaction. The other one-third is contributed by the testes in

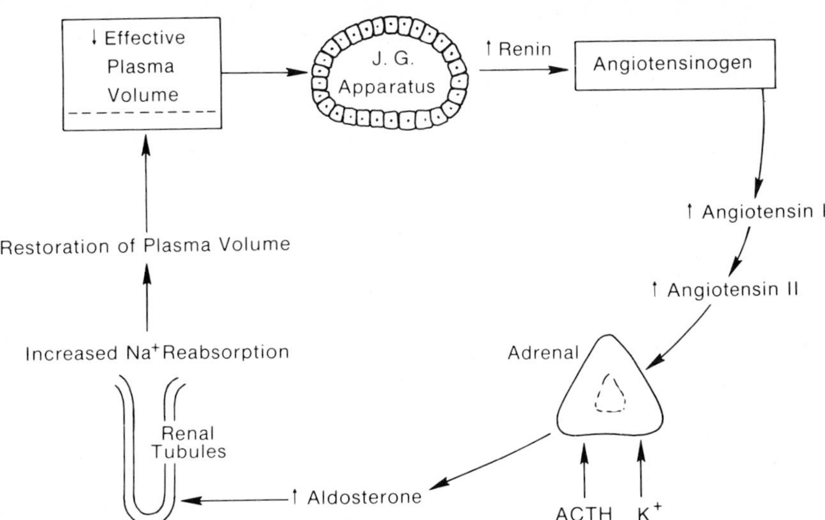

Figure 9. Renin Angiotensin-Aldosterone System. A decrease in effective plasma volume leads to increased renin secretion, resulting in increased production of angiotensin II, and in turn, aldosterone. ACTH and K^+ directly stimulate aldosterone secretion. Increased Na^+ absorption, as a result of increased aldosterone levels, restores the plasma volume.

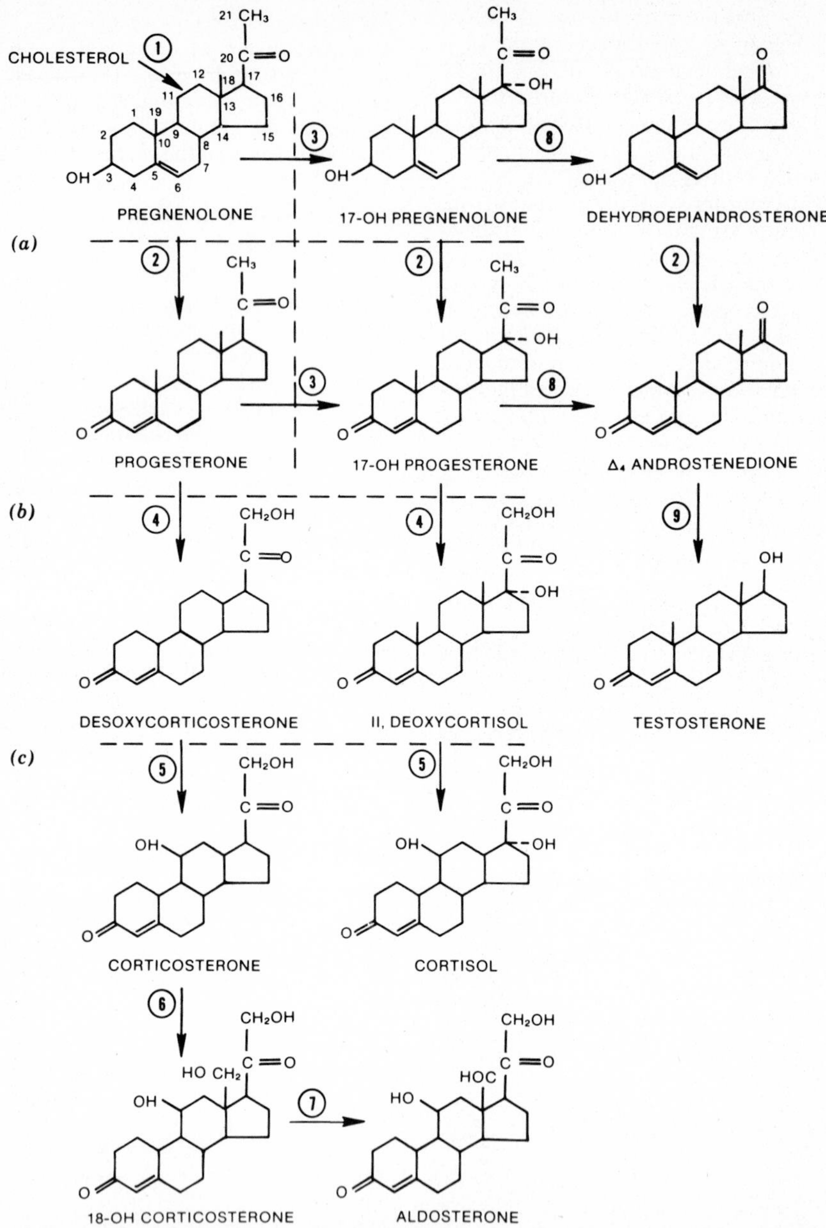

Figure 10. Biosynthesis of adrenal steroids. (1) Desmolase; (2) 3-β-0H dehydrogenase: Δ^5-Δ^4 Isomerase; (3) 17-hydroxylase; (4) 21-hydroxylase; (5) 11-hydroxylase; (6) 18-hydroxylase; (7) 18 0H-dehydrogenase; (8) 17, 20, Lyase; and (9) 17-keto reductase. A, B, and C indicate the site of block in 17-hydroxylase, 21-hydroxylase, and 11-hydroxylase deficiency, respectively. The numbers shown on the pregnenolone structure indicate the conventional way of numbering the carbons in the steroid molecule.

men. 17-Ketosteroids excretion is about one-third lower in women as compared to men.

EVALUATION OF ADRENAL FUNCTIONS

The basal adrenal glucocorticoid function can be evaluated by measurement of plasma cortisol and 24-hour urinary 17-hydroxycorticoid excretion. Plasma cortisol can be conveniently measured by radioimmunoassay. This method has essentially replaced the older fluorimetric method for measurement of plasma cortisol. Normally, the plasma cortisol levels are higher in the morning than in the evening. Twenty-four hour urinary excretion of 17-hydroxysteroids varies from 4-12 mg per 24 hours.

ACTH Stimulation Test

When hypofunction of the adrenal cortex is suspected, adrenal reserve can be measured by either a short or long ACTH stimulation test. The short stimulation test is performed by drawing blood for cortisol before and 30-60 minutes after injection of 0.25 mg (about 25 units) of cosyntropin (Cortrosyn). Cortrosyn is a synthetic product that contains the first 24 amino acids of ACTH. Usually the plasma cortisol increases by at least 8 μg, or to an absolute level of 20 μg/dl. The test is simple to perform, can be carried out in the office, and is useful as a screening procedure for evaluation of adrenal function since a normal response rules out Addison's disease. If a suboptimal response is obtained, 25 units of ACTH is administered as an infusion over 8 hours. Plasma cortisol and 24-hour urinary hydroxysteroids are measured before and after the infusion. An increase in the plasma cortisol level of 10-25 μg/dl in the first hour and 15-40 μg/dl by 8 hours of the ACTH infusion indicates a normal response. The urinary 17-hydroxysteroids excretion should increase to 12-25 mg/24 hours after an 8-hour infusion of ACTH.

Metyrapone (Metapyrone) Test

This drug is widely used in testing the pituitary-adrenal axis. It inhibits the enzyme 11-β hydroxylase that blocks the secretion of cortisol, which in turn stimulates ACTH secretion. Since cortisol cannot be produced, the latter leads to an increase in the secretion of 11-deoxycortisol. Increased plasma levels of 11-deoxycortisol can be measured, but urinary measurement of 17-hydroxysteroids is simpler and more satisfactory. The test is performed by oral administration of metyrapone. The usual adult dose is 750 mg every 4 hours for six doses. Urine is collected prior to the day of administration of metyrapone (control urine), on the day of, and the day after administration of the drug. In normal individuals, the urinary 17-hydroxysteroids increase slightly during the day of administration and rise further on the following day. A twofold or greater increase of urinary 17-hydroxysteroids constitutes a normal response.

Dexamethasone Suppression Test

When hyperfunction of the adrenal cortex is suspected, its suppressibility is often evaluated by administration of dexamethasone. Normal individuals decrease their secretion of 24-hour urinary 17-hydroxysteroids to less than 3 mg after administration of dexamethasone given in doses of 0.5 mg every 6 hours for 2 days. Failure of 17-hydroxysteroids to decrease below 3 mg per 24 hours suggests hypercortisolism. An overnight dexamethasone suppression test is useful in screening patients suspected of hyperfunction of the adrenals. A 1 mg dose of dexamethasone is given at 11:00 PM. A suppression of AM cortisol to less than 5 μg/dl is considered a normal response.

PHARMACOLOGIC USES OF STEROIDS

The physiologic use of steroids is in the management of adrenal insufficiency. In addition, glucocorticoids have been widely used in a variety of illnesses because of their many useful pharmacologic effects. The most beneficial among these are the anti-inflammatory effects. The glucocorticoids decrease the vascular permeability and inhibit the migration of inflammatory cells from capillaries. They may also suppress the release or action of histamine on surrounding tissues. These effects reduce inflammatory swelling by decreasing edema fluid formation. They also produce suppression of lymphoid tissue activity. The latter effect has been used to suppress immune responses in disease states related to hyperimmunity. This has lead to the widespread use of steroids in autoimmune disorders and in organ transplantation.

Whenever glucocorticoids are administered in greater than physiologic doses, side effects begin to appear. In general, these include the catabolic effects of glucocorticoids, namely, muscle weakness, thinning of the skin, easy bruisability, and osteoporosis. The anti-insulin effects of glucocorticoids may lead to glucose intolerance. In children, linear growth may be inhibited. Many patients experience euphoria after the initial dose of steroids; only a few may develop psychosis and depression. Since cortisol also has inherent mineralocorticoid activity, mineralocorticoid side effects may also occur with administration of hydrocortisone. These include sodium and water retention, potassium loss, and hypertension. These effects are not usually seen with synthetic steroids that primarily have glucocorticoid effects. Pharmacologic use of steroids also results in inhibition of the hypothalamic-pituitary axis. Continued suppression of ACTH results in suppression of adrenal function. When steroids are abruptly withdrawn, or if the patient is exposed to stress, this may result in adrenal crisis. Use of steroids on alternate days minimizes the suppression of the hypothalamic-hypophysial-adrenal axis.

HYPERFUNCTION OF THE ADRENAL CORTEX

Cushing's Syndrome

Cushing's syndrome results from the effects of large amounts of glucocorticoids over a prolonged period of time. Cushing's syndrome may result from excess production of glucocorticoids by the adrenal cortex either as a result of an adrenal adenoma or carcinoma. It may also result from excess production of ACTH either by the pituitary (referred to as Cushing's disease) or by ectopic production of ACTH. In addition, a frequent cause of Cushing's syndrome is exogenous administration of glucocorticoids or ACTH in pharmacologic doses.

Pathogenesis and Clinical Features

Large doses of glucocorticoids lead to the redistribution of fat resulting in rounding of the face (moon facies), fat deposit in the lower part of the neck on the back (buffalo hump), and central obesity. The catabolic effects of glucocorticoids lead to a reduction in muscle mass and connective tissue causing weakness, proximal myopathy, osteoporosis, easy bruisability, and purple striae. The glucogenic effects of glucocorticoids are responsible for elevation of blood sugar and glycosuria frequently encountered in these patients. The weak but unopposed mineralocorticoid effects of cortisol are reflected in sodium retention, potassium loss, and hypertension. Overproduction of adrenal androgens results in hirsutism, acne, and menstrual disturbances in women. An excess of glucocorticoids may also result in depression and even frank psychosis may occasionally develop in these patients.

Diagnosis

The diagnosis is made by characteristic clinical features. It should be noted that several years may elapse before typical features of Cushing's syndrome develop. Therefore, it is often helpful to compare the patient's appearance with previous pictures if available. Differentiation between Cushing's syndrome of pituitary or adrenal origin is made by biochemical procedures. Patients with ectopic ACTH production often do not have the cushingoid appearance, presumably because the underlying malignancy and shortened survival of the patients do not allow enough time for these clinical features to develop. Simple obesity and hirsutism often enter into the differential diagnosis of patients with Cushing's syndrome but the dexamethasone suppression test is helpful in differentiating these from true Cushing's syndrome. The diagnosis is confirmed by demonstrating abnormalities of cortisol secretion. Patients with Cushing's disease have loss of diurnal variation; this can be demonstrated by elevated plasma cortisol (and, when available, ACTH) in the evening, relatively early in the course of the disease. Subsequently, plasma cortisol levels are found to be elevated in the morning and evening.

Administration of 1 mg dexamethasone at 11:00 PM and measurement of plasma cortisol the next morning at 8:00 AM constitutes a useful screening test. In most normal patients, plasma cortisol levels suppress to a level below 5 μg/dl. Those patients who do not suppress to this level are evaluated by a more definitive dexamethasone suppression test as outlined in Table 2. Thus, the dexamethasone suppression test not only helps in confirming the diagnosis but also helps localize the site of the lesion.

The metyrapone test (performed as described previously) may also be helpful in the differential diagnosis. Patients with Cushing's disease have a hyperactive response, wheras patients with adrenal or ectopic tumors do not respond.

In the pituitary form of the disease, skull x-ray should be obtained to rule out a large pituitary tumor, but such tumors are rare. Microadenomas, on the other hand, are common and may be detected by polytomograms of the sella. Because many microadenomas are too small to deform the sella turcica, a normal tomogram does not exclude the diagnosis of a functional adenoma.

Adrenal tumors may be detected by physical examination if large, or by radiologic techniques including arteriography, performance of ^{131}I-C19 cholesterol and NP-59 (6β-iodomethyl-19-norcholesterol) scanning. Ultrasonic studies and CAT scan are also increasingly being performed for the diagnosis of adrenal tumors. Adrenal hyperplasia may also be visualized by these techniques.

Detection of ectopic tumors producing ACTH requires a careful physical examination, and may require additional radiologic and endoscopic procedures. Lung cancer remains the most frequent cause and chest x-ray may be diagnostic in over half of the cases.

Treatment

The treatment of Cushing's syndrome depends upon the cause. In cases of ectopic ACTH production, removal of the offending neoplasm may be corrective. The adrenal tumors are also best treated surgically. It should be emphasized that after unilateral adrenalectomy it may take up to a year before the remaining adrenal gland recovers its function. In patients with adrenal carcinoma, if total removal is not possible, mitotane (*o,p′*-DDD) has been used to destroy the adrenal cortical cells and to block the metabolism of corticosteroid; complete cures are rare. Metyrapone and aminoglutethimide have also been

Table 2. Interpretation of Glucose Tolerance Test[a]

Adults (nonpregnant)			*Children*		
Fasting	*($\frac{1}{2}$ to $1\frac{1}{2}$ h)*[b]	*2h*	*Fasting*	*($\frac{1}{2}$ to $1\frac{1}{2}$ h)*[b]	*2h*
Normal <115	<200	<140	<130	–	<140
Diabetic <140	⩾200	⩾200	⩾140	⩾200	⩾200
Impaired <140	⩾200	140-200	<140	–	>140

[a]All values are for venous plasma

[b]Indicates anytime between $\frac{1}{2}$ hour to $1\frac{1}{2}$ hour

tried but are less effective. The management of Cushing's disease of pituitary origin is somewhat controversial. External radiation to the pituitary is often successful, especially in children but less so in adults. Total bilateral adrenalectomy provides another means of complete biochemical cure. On the day of surgery, these patients should receive 200-300 mg of hydrocortisone that is gradually tapered over the next several days until physiologic doses are achieved. Postoperatively, about 10-15% of these patients develop pituitary tumors associated with enlargement of the sella turcica, excess production of ACTH, and β-LPH and hyperpigmentation (Nelson's syndrome). Some of these tumors may become large, produce pressure symptoms, and may require hypophysectomy. In addition, they also appear to have an increased tendency to develop pituitary infarction. As mentioned previously, many patients with Cushing's disease are found to have pituitary microadenomas. Selective removal of these tumors by transsphenoidal microdissection has frequently led to total remission with preservation of pituitary function. A number of pharmacologic agents also have been found to be useful adjuncts in the management of patients with Cushing's disease. Cyproheptadine (a serotonin antagonist) suppresses ACTH release by acting on the hypothalamus. Although not effective uniformly, it has been reported to produce cures in some patients. Bromocriptine suppresses ACTH, as well as growth hormone and prolactin production by pituitary tumors, and has been successful in reducing cortisol secretion in some patients. None of these agents, however, can be recommended for long-term treatment at this time because of limited experience.

Aldosteronism

Overproduction of aldosterone may result from a lesion within the adrenal gland (primary aldosteronism), or it may result from overactivity of the renin-angiotensin system (secondary aldosteronism).

Primary Aldosteronism

Primary aldosteronism was first described by J.W. Conn in 1955. It may result from a single adenoma (Conn's syndrome), or may be due to bilateral adrenal hyperplasia. The clinical features are direct results of excess production of aldosterone and consist of hypertension, hypokalemia, and metabolic alkalosis. The level of blood pressure is variable but, characteristically, vascular changes are moderate. It can be differentiated from essential hypertension only by laboratory studies. Although estimates vary, it is estimated that primary aldosteronism is responsible for about 1% of the cases of hypertension. The plasma volume is slightly expanded but edema is rare. Potassium depletion leads to muscular weakness, polyuria, and polydipsia. The metabolic alkalosis accompanied by hypokalemia can result in development of tetany-like symptoms. Carbohydrate intolerance is frequently present. The diagnosis is confirmed by elevated secretion or excretion of aldosterone. The elevated levels are not suppressed by fluid overloading or sodium administration. In addiion, one must demonstrate that the plasma renin activity is low, and not stimulated by low sodium intake or diuretics. This can be done by measuring plasma renin activity when the patient is on a low-sodium diet (<20 mEq) and in upright posture for 2 hours, or by administration of furosemide. These stimuli lead to an increase in plasma renin activity in normal subjects but fail to do so in patients with primary aldosteronism.

The differential diagnosis includes patients with essential hypertension and low renin activity. The aldosterone secretion of these patients, however, is normal. Excessive ingestion of licorice also results in a syndrome similar to primary aldosteronism. The active principle of licorice (glycyrrhizic acid) has actions similar to aldosterone. The aldosterone level, however, is low and the treatment is discontinuation of licorice. Once the diagnosis of primary aldosteronism has been confirmed, differentiation between adenoma and bilateral hyperplasia should be made. This is important because surgical removal of adenoma results in cure of hypertension, but patients with hyperplasia are usually not cured by adrenalectomy. Various techniques have been utilized for this purpose. In some cases, adrenal arteriography or venography may demonstrate the adenoma, but their small size makes them difficult to visualize. CAT scan and ^{131}I-19-iodocholesterol scans have also been used with success. Biochemical measures are also helpful in that patients with adrenal hyperplasia show a normal increase of aldosterone production with upright posture, but patients with adenoma may show an anomalous decrease. Measurement of aldosterone in the adrenal veins by selective catheterization shows a high level of aldosterone on the side of the adenoma and a suppressed level on the other side, whereas in hyperplasia both sides have high levels.

The aims of treatment are to lower the blood pressure and to correct biochemical abnormalities. This can be best achieved by removal of the adenoma when found. In patients with bilateral hyperplasia, administration of spironolactone results in lowering of the blood pressure and correction of electrolyte abnormalities. Side effects of high-dose spironolactone include the development of gynecomastia and impotence in men, and menstrual irregularities in women.

Secondary Aldosteronism

Many edematous states are associated with increased plasma renin activity and, as a result, increased aldosterone levels. Such conditions include cirrhosis of the liver with ascites, nephrotic syndrome, and severe congestive heart failure. Secondary aldosteronism may develop in association with renal artery stenosis. These patients have hypertension, and plasma renin activity is increased due to renal ischemia. Patients taking oral contraceptive agents develop an increase in renin substrate and in plasma renin activity, but only a few develop hypertension. A few patients with hyperplasia or adenomas of the juxtaglomerular apparatus have been described. They are characterized by severe hypertension, hypokalemia, marked increase in plasma renin activity, and secondary hyperaldosteronism. Hyperplasia of the juxtaglomerular apparatus, with hyperreninemia and hyperaldosteronsim but without hypertension is known as Bartter's syndrome.

ADRENOCORTICAL INSUFFICIENCY

Insufficient secretion of adrenocortical hormones may occur as a result of primary disease of the adrenal cortex, or secondary to a deficiency of ACTH secretion.

Addison's Disease

Etiology and Pathogenesis

Primary adrenal insufficiency, or Addison's disease, is a rare disorder affecting one in 100,000 of the population. The most common cause of the disorder is a bilateral adrenal atrophy of unknown etiology, most likely of autoimmune origin. Other causes include hemorrhage, tuberculosis, fungus infections, lymphomas and leukemic infiltrations, and bilateral adrenal infiltration with metastases. Although carcinoma of the lung metastasizes frequently to the adrenal glands, it rarely produces clinical adrenal insufficiency, presumably because more than three-fourths of both adrenal glands have to be destroyed before clinical evidence of insufficiency develops. Antiadrenal antibodies are frequently present in the plasma of patients with Addison's disease; adrenal insufficiency is often associated with other autoimmune diseases such as Hashimoto's thyroiditis and pernicious anemia.

Clinical Manifestations

The signs and symptoms of adrenal insufficiency can be directly explained by the lack of glucocorticoid and mineralocorticoid activity. The glucocorticoid deficiency leads to weakness, fatigue, weight loss, and hypoglycemia. In the absence of cortisol's negative feedback, the anterior pituitary ACTH and β-LPH secretion is markedly increased, and is accompanied by increased pigmentation of the skin. Pigmentation may be particularly evident in the palmar creases, along the edges of recent scars, and on the lips and gums. Minerocorticoid deficiency leads to dehydration, hypovolemia, hypotension, and shock. Gastrointestinal symptoms like nausea and vomiting are frequently present. Some patients have unexplained calcification of the external ear. Laboratory abnormalities typically include hyponatremia and hyperkalemia. Increased BUN concentration and eosinophilia also may be present. Adrenal glands may be calcified in patients in whom adrenal insufficiency is a result of granulomatous disease.

Diagnosis

The diagnosis of adrenal insufficiency is confirmed by a low plasma cortisol, a low 24-hour urinary 17-hydroxysteroid excretion, and an elevated ACTH. If ACTH measurement is not readily available, an attempt should be made to demonstrate the inability of the adrenal glands to respond to ACTH infusion. This can be done conveniently in the office or outpatient department by intramuscular administration of synthetic ACTH. A normal response to this test excludes primary adrenal insufficiency. If a subnormal response is obtained, a prolonged ACTH infusion test should be carried out as previously described in the section on the hypothalamus and pituitary.

Secondary adrenal insufficiency may occur due to a selective loss of ACTH secretion or as part of panhypopituitarism. Characteristically, patients with secondary adrenal insufficiency are not hyperpigmented. The electrolyte abnormalities of primary adrenal insufficiency are generally not observed because aldosterone secretion is maintained via the renin-angiotensin system. Direct evidence of ACTH insufficiency may be obtained by insulin hypoglycemia or by a metyrapone test. Associated deficiencies of other pituitary hormones may also be present and should be sought.

Treatment

Treatment of adrenal insufficiency consists of replacement of glucocorticoids and mineralocorticoids. Most patients can be managed conveniently by the daily administration of 25-37.5 mg of cortisone (or an equivalent) given orally. It is usually administered in divided doses, with two-thirds of the dose being administered in the morning and one-third in the evening. Many of these patients can be managed without any additional mineralocorticoid if their dietary intake of sodium is liberalized. Mineralocorticoid activity can be provided by administration of 9-α-fludrocortisone (Florinef) in doses of 0.05-0.1 mg a day when required. All patients receiving chronic steroid replacement should increase their dosage at times of increased stress like minor intercurrent illnesses, especially if fever is present. If serious illness is suspected, patients should be hospitalized and an increased dose of steroid administered. Every patient should wear a bracelet indicating the diagnosis of adrenal insufficiency. They should also have a supply of injectable steroids at home for use in adrenal crisis.

Acute Adrenal Insufficiency or Addisonian Crisis

This is a life-threatening medical emergency. It usually occurs in patients receiving maintenance glucocorticoid therapy for adrenal insufficiency or steroid therapy for other disease processes. Various stressful situations like surgery, severe infections, and trauma may precipitate this event if the steroid dosage is not increased. Rarely, it may occur in children in association with meningococcal septicemia due to bilateral adrenal hemorrhage. It is characterized by weakness, hypoglycemia, and rapidly progressive hypotension leading to vascular collapse, shock, and death. If the diagnosis is suspected, treatment should be instituted immediately without waiting for confirmation by the laboratory results. Prior to administration of treatment, blood samples for plasma cortisol and measurement of ACTH are drawn. Immediately thereafter, 100 mg of hydrocortisone is administered intravenously. This should be followed by 5% glucose in normal saline to correct hypoglycemia and hyponatremia. About 200-300 mg of hydrocortisone is generally required in the first 24 hours. Thereafter, the dosage of hydrocortisone is gradually reduced until the maintenance dose is achieved, usually within 4 or 5 days.

Syndrome of Selective Hypoaldosteronism

Isolated hypoaldosteronism is a rare disorder that is characterized by selective deficiency of aldosterone production, but normal cortisol function. The patients usually present with asymptomatic hyperkalemia and, in a few cases, cardiac arrhythmias due to hyperkalemia may also occur. Salt wasting and dehydration occur occasionally in adults. When dietary sodium is restricted, dehydration and hypotension may occur. The pathogenetic basis of deficiency of aldosterone secretion may be a defect in the aldosterone biosynthesis, or a deficiency of stimuli for aldosterone production (renin-angiotensin system). An acquired defect in 18-hydroxylase and 18-dehydrogenase in adults, and a congenital defect in children responsible for hypoaldosteronism, have been described but are very rare. In recent years, a deficiency of renin synthesis or secretion as a cause of hypoaldosteronism (hyporeninemic hypoaldosteronism) has been described with increased frequency as a cause of unexplained hyperkalemia. The majority of these patients have mild to moderate renal failure and/or diabetes mellitus. The syndrome is diagnosed by a low aldosterone secretion when the dietary intake of sodium and potassium is normal, and by an inability of aldosterone secretion to increase appropriately with sodium restriction. In patients with hyporeninemic hypoaldosteronism, plasma renin activity under the same conditions is also low, and is considered to be the basis of low aldosterone secretion. In patients in whom a biosynthetic defect in the aldosterone secretion exists, plasma renin activity has been normal or high. Normal glucocorticoid function should be demonstrated in these patients by use of ACTH stimulation to rule out Addison's disease. Administration of mineralocorticoids leads to correction of hyperkalemia, and the tendencies to hypotension and sodium loss.

Congenital Adrenal Hyperplasia

The biosynthesis of cortisol is an orderly process involving a series of enzymatic steps. A number of enzymatic blocks occur as congenital defects. The consequences of an enzymatic block are insufficient secretion of cortisol that results in excessive secretion of ACTH, leading to adrenal hyperplasia. Due to a block in cortisol synthesis and increased ACTH secretion, the steroid precursors are diverted to the synthesis of adrenal androgens. The resulting increased synthesis of adrenal androgens and accompanying virilization constitute the typical features of most of these defects.

21-Hydroxylase deficiency is the most common defect inherited as an autosomal recessive trait. The result of 21-hydroxylase block is to inhibit the synthesis of both glucocorticoids and mineralocorticoids. The excess androgen production results in virilization of the female infant varying from a mild clitoral hypertrophy to an almost normal-appearing male phallus with hypospadias; of course, no testes are palpable. No genital abnormalities are obvious in the male infant. However, in subsequent years this may lead to precocious puberty. Approximately one-third of patients with this enzymatic defect are found to have overt aldosterone deficiency with salt wasting. Such infants develop apathy, vomiting, dehydration, and vascular collapse; death may occur during infancy. The patients also have all the signs of adrenal insufficiency including hyperkalemia, hyponatremia, and low cortisol levels. It is confirmed by low plasma cortisol, and excessive excretion of urinary 17-ketosteroids and pregnanetriol. Plasma levels of dehydroepiandrosterone, androstenedione, and testosterone are also elevated. The treatment consists of replacement with glucocorticoids to suppress the excessive secretion of ACTH. Those with salt wasting may also need additional mineralocorticoids.

11-Hydroxylase deficiency leads to a syndrome similar to that of 21-hydroxylase defect, except that these patients also secrete desoxycorticosterone and deoxycortisol. The presence of virilization in women, accompanied by hypertension and hypokalemia (due to elevated desoxycorticosterone), should suggest this diagnosis. The urinary 17-ketosteroids are elevated, but, because there is no defect in 21-hydroxylation, plasma 17-hydroxyprogesterone and urinary pregnanediol are not increased. The treatment is by replacement doses of glucocorticoids to suppress the ACTH levels to normal.

Other enzymatic defects are rare and are not accompanied by virilization. A defect in the conversion of cholesterol to pregnenolone is lethal because no steroids can be produced. A defect in 3 β-hydroxy-dehydrogenase is also fatal if complete. A defect in the 17-hydroxylase is associated with an inability to synthesize estrogens and androgens. All of the patients are therefore phenotypically female, but do not develop secondary sexual characteristics and have primary amenorrhea. Corticosterone and desoxycorticosterone are produced in increased quantities and are responsible for hypertension and electrolyte abnormalities seen in these patients. The treatment consists of replacement doses of cortisol and administration of estrogens to induce development of female secondary sexual characteristics.

ADRENAL MEDULLA

PHYSIOLOGY OF THE ADRENAL MEDULLA

The adrenal medulla, although close in proximity to the adrenal cortex, is functionally a part of the sympathetic nervous system. The hormones of the sympathetic nervous system are dopamine, epinephrine, and norepinephrine. As a group, these hormones are referred to as catecholamines. Chemically, these hormones are dihydroxylated phenolic amines. Besides the adrenal medulla, the synthesis of catecholamines occurs in the brain, sympathetic nerve endings, and other sites of chromaffin tissues, including the organs of Zuckerkandl and other ectopic remains of neural crest tissues. The substrate for catecholamine synthesis is the dietary amino acid tyrosine, which is hydroxylated by the enzyme tyrosine hydroxylase to dihydroxyphenylalanine (Dopa). Dopa is then converted by the enzyme decarboxylase to dopamine. β-Hydroxylation of dopamine results in the synthesis of norepinephrine. In the adrenal medulla, norepinephrine is further methylated to epinephrine.

Circulating catecholamines are metabolized to vanillylmandelic acid (VMA) by the actions of the enzymes catecholamine *O*-methyltransferase (COMT) and monamine oxidase (MAO).

While epinephrine and norepinephrine exert major peripheral effects, the effects of dopamine are mainly limited to the central nervous system. Important quantitative differences exist between the actions of epinephrine and norepinephrine when these hormones are infused in small physiologic doses. However, the effects are obliterated when these hormones are released in large quantities, for example, in patients with pheochromocytoma. Epinephrine produces an increase in heart rate, cardiac output, and systolic pressure; diastolic pressure either remains unchanged or may fall slightly. Norepinephrine causes an increase of both systolic and diastolic pressures by generalized vasoconstriction. The rise in blood pressure may reflexively slow the heart rate and decrease cardiac output. The metabolic effects of these catecholamines include increased lipolysis and hyperglycemia. The latter is a result of increased glycogenolysis, as well as inhibition of insulin release from the islets of Langerhans.

PHEOCHROMOCYTOMA

Pheochromocytoma is a benign (10% are malignant) tumor of the sympathetic nervous system most commonly located in the adrenal medulla but that may also arise from other chromaffin tissues. Although rare (less than 1% of the hypertensive population), these tumors are clinically important because they represent a curable cause of hypertension. The majority of these tumors occur sporadically, but in 10-20% of the cases pheochromocytomas are inherited. About 1-5% of familial pheochromocytomas occur in association with Von Recklinghausen's disease. In addition, pheochromocytomas may be inherited as part of multiple endocrine adenomatosis type II (Sipple's syndrome). The pattern of inheritance appears to be autosomal dominant with variable penetrance. The other components of multiple endocrine adenomatosis type II include medullary carcinoma of the thyroid and parathyroid adenomas. In some instances, medullary carcinoma of the thyroid and pheochromocytomas are associated with multiple mucosal neuromas. This constellation has been referred to as multiple endocrine adenomatosis type III.

Clinical Manifestations

The clinical features include a constellation of distinctive and dramatic signs that represent the effects of an excessive release of catecholamines. Hypertension is the most common clinical finding. Although episodic hypertension is a characteristic feature of pheochromocytoma, nearly one-half of these patients may present with sustained hypertension. The episodes of hypertension may be associated with attacks that consist of sudden development of tachycardia, palpitation, or cardiac arrythmia. They may be accompanied by the development of severe headache, excessive sweating, and pallor or flushing. A feeling of anxiety or impending doom may occur frequently. Physical examination during the attack will reveal significant hypertension, tachycardia, cardiac arrhythmia, and excessive perspiration. Weight loss is common and patients are rarely obese. The basal metabolic rate is frequently increased. Glucose intolerance is frequently present but severe hyperglycemia rarely occurs. Congestive heart failure may result because of hypertension, or due to the development of catecholamine cardiomyopathy.

Diagnosis

Because of its varied clinical expression, the diagnosis of pheochromocytoma is frequently delayed for several years. Clinical entities like essential hypertension with or without lability, thyrotoxicosis, functional bowel complaints, and various psychiatric disorders are often considered in the differential diagnosis. The diagnosis is established by biochemical investigations. These include increased levels of free catecholamines, total metanephrines, or VMA in a 24-hour urine. In some patients in whom these measurements are normal, a timed collection of urine for these measurements during an acute attack reveals elevated values. Because of the availability of sensitive and specific tests for these chemical determinations, the pharmacologic tests used in the past for diagnosis of pheochromocytoma are rarely employed. For localization of the tumor, radiologic techniques are employed. Intravenous pyelogram with laminography may show a suprarenal mass. Pheochromocytomas are vascular tumors and adrenal arteriography may demonstrate the tumor, but may induce hypertensive crisis and should not be done without adequate preparation of the patient or facilities with the expertise to manage the crisis. CAT scan appears promising for localizing the adrenal lesions, but experience with pheochromocytomas is limited.

Treatment

The treatment of pheochromocytoma is surgical removal. Preoperatively, the patients should be prepared by adequate α-adrenergic blockade. This can be achieved by administration of phenoxybenzamine. Phenoxybenzamine has a long duration of action and is effective orally. Another α-adrenergic blocking agent, phentolamine is used primarily for acute intravenous administration to lower the blood pressure rapidly. The β-adrenergic blocking drugs like propranolol are particularly useful in the treatment of troublesome tachyarrhythmias that may occur in some patients during therapy and especially during surgery. However, β-adrenergic blocking drugs should not be used alone since exaggeration of pressor effects of catecholamines may occur due to the unopposed effects of their α-adrenergic actions. Patients who cannot be operated on, or in whom complete removal of the tumor is not possible, can be managed by phenoxybenzamine and propranolol, which block the effects of catecholamines. α-Methyltyrosine reduces biosynthesis of catecholamines by inhibiting the enzyme tyrosine hydroxylase. It has been used both for preoperative preparation and for chronic therapy of pheochromocytomas, but at present the drug is investigational.

THE OVARY

At birth, the ovaries contain several hundred thousand primordial germ cells from which all ova subsequently develop;

approximately 400 reach maturity during a woman's lifetime. During childhood, the ovary secretes small amounts of estrogen. Although this amount is insufficient to stimulate genital growth, the production of estrogens early in life is thought to influence the more rapid maturation of the skeleton and earlier onset of puberty in girls.

Luteinizing hormone-releasing hormone (LHRH) is secreted by the hypothalamus, and stimulates the secretion of follicle-stimulating hormone (FSH) and luteinizing hormone (LH) in preparation for gonadal development, reproduction, and the onset of puberty. Between the ages of 8 and 12, FSH secretion results in the maturation of ovarian follicles that are now producing higher levels of estrogen. Although FSH levels are not high enough during early puberty to evoke ovulation, pubertal changes occur in the following order: broadening of the pelvis, budding of the nipples and breasts, development of the vaginal mucosa, growth of the internal and external genitalia, nipple pigmentation, breast enlargement, and menarche. Estrogens are also important in the maturation of the bony skeleton and in the deposition of subcutaneous fat. Between the ages of 12 and 15, most women experience their first menstrual flow. During the childbearing years, hormonal balance is aimed at providing an optimal milieu for conception. FSH and LH stimulate the ovaries to secrete estrogen and progesterone, respectively, with a negative feedback system serving to further regulate hormonal balance.

MENSTRUAL CYCLE

The first half of the menstrual cycle is characterized by proliferation of the uterine endometrium by ovarian estrogens in preparation for the implantation of a fertilized ovum. Although FSH secretion results in the maturation of several ovarian (or graafian) follicles, only one follicle reaches maturity; the others atrophy. At midcycle, an LH surge causes the mature graafian follicle to rupture and an ovum is released. The high estrogen content of the follicular fluid increases the circulating estrogen to levels that begin to inhibit the pituitary secretion of FSH.

The ruptured follicle becomes a corpus luteum, now under the control of persistent LH secretion, and secretes both estrogen and progesterone. During the second half of the menstrual cycle, the proliferated endometrium is ready to accept a fertilized ovum. The corpus luteum remains functional for 12-14 days, unless a fertilized ovum is implanted. The high levels of estrogen and progesterone cause feedback on the pituitary with the resultant inhibition of LH. Unless implanatation occurs, the corpus luteum dissolves with a resultant decline in estrogen levels and the disappearance of progesterone. With the decline in estrogen and progesterone levels, there is a shedding of the endometrium to its basal layers, resulting in menstruation.

As a woman ages, changes in ovarian function result in the climacteric (menopause). There is a depletion of primordial follicles, and their ability to mature declines. Ovulation stops, and the cyclic production of progesterone ceases. Estrogen levels fall below the minimum necessary to maintain the endometrial lining; menstruation becomes less frequent and eventually stops. The onset of menopause is frequently associated with emotional disturbances and hot flashes. The pituitary now secretes high amounts of FSH and LH in the absence of negative feedback.

AMENORRHEA

Primary Amenorrhea

It is imperative that the clinician distinguish delayed menarche accompanied by normal sexual development from complete lack of sexual maturation. Isolated primary amenorrhea rarely has endocrinologic implications and usually resolves spontaneously. Congenital disorders such as uterine agenesis must be considered, as must imperforate hymen. Less common causes include testicular feminization syndrome and an end-organ unresponsiveness to FSH. Turner's syndrome, characterized by short stature, shield chest, webbed neck, and an XO karyotype, must also be considered.

Primary amenorrhea without sexual development usually implies a serious endocrine disorder, and a thorough work-up for causes of delayed puberty is warranted. Although debilitating illness and gonadal dysgenesis are common causes, abnormalities should be sought in pituitary, hypothalamic, or ovarian function. Chromosomal and hormonal analyses, and radiograms of the sella turcica are helpful. A low estradiol level with elevated LH and FSH in a woman who is not menopausal suggests primary ovarian disease.

Secondary Amenorrhea

Failure of menstruation to occur for more than 6 consecutive months after normal menstrual function has been established is called secondary amenorrhea. Although the majority of cases are due to functional causes, an evaluation as outlined previously is warranted. One must exclude pathology in the hypothalamus, pituitary, and ovary, and excessive androgenic activity must be ruled out. Pituitary disease is suggested by low levels of FSH and LH in the setting of a low or normal estradiol level.

THE TESTIS

Testes serve two major functions; spermatogenesis, and the synthesis and secretion of testosterone. Testosterone is made in Leydig's cells that are regulated by LH, also known in men as the interstitial cell-stimulating hormone. FSH regulates spermatogenesis in the seminiferous tubules that comprise three-fourths of testicular volume.

Although Leydig's cells and limited spermatogenesis are present at birth, these regress rapidly; FSH and LH are barely detectable in the serum of prepubertal males. As puberty approaches, there is widening of the seminiferous tubule lumen and an increase in germinal activity. At puberty, gonadotropin levels increase and testosterone secretion occurs; there is an increase in the number of Leydig's cells and spermatogenesis increases. The testes increase in size, there is an increase in penile growth and pubic hair, and linear growth accelerates.

Testosterone also is responsible for the development of secondary sexual characteristics, nitrogen retention with enlargement of muscle mass, increased skeletal structure, and fat mobilization. Testosterone accelerates epiphyseal closure in both men and women. LH, being secreted in pulsations throughout the day, stimulates Leydig's cells to secrete testosterone and other steroids. A negative feedback loop between testosterone and LH modulates hormonal balance.

FSH is required for normal spermatogenesis. Although both FSH and testosterone are required for the maturation of the primordial germ cells at puberty, FSH is not necessary to complete maturation of spermatogonia. The passage of spermatogonia into mature spermatozoa takes approximately 2-½ months. The feedback loop of FSH is thought to be modulated by a product of the germinal epithelium (inhibin), questionably secreted by Sertoli's cells. In cases of oligospermia or azoospermia with patent ducts, there is an elevation of FSH secretion by the pituitary; when spermatogenesis progresses normally, FSH is inhibited.

PRIMARY HYPOGONADISM

Failure of spermatogenesis and Leydig's cell function is referred to as primary hypogonadism. The level of testosterone is low and because of the lack of negative feedback, FSH and/or LH are elevated. There are many causes of testicular failure including toxins, infections, sex chromosome abnormalities, and developmental anomalies.

The most common hypogonadal disorder, other than failure of spermatogenesis, is Klinefelter's syndrome, or dysgenesis of the seminiferous tubules. Patients appear eunuchoid with gynecomastia and small, firm testes. There is decreased facial and body hair, infertility, azoospermia, an increased incidence of mental retardation, and a karyotpye of XXY, although other chromosomal variants may occur. The incidence may be as high as 0.2% of the male population, being even higher in mentally retarded men. Diagnosis is suggested by the above clinical findings, and testicular biopsy reveals clumping of Leydig's cells and hyalinized tubules. Gonadotropins are elevated, with either a low or normal serum testosterone. Although some patients are diagnosed during puberty when they fail to mature normally, others may escape diagnosis until an infertility work-up is pursued or complaints of impotence surface during the second and third decades of life. Treatment rests on androgen replacement; infertility is irreversible.

SECONDARY TESTICULAR FAILURE

Secondary failure of testicular function is due to a disorder of the pituitary or hypothalamus. FSH and LH may be affected either singly or together. Gonadotropin failure before puberty results in sexual infantilism. Failure after sexual maturation results in subtle changes, such as thinning of the facial hair, and reduced muscle mass, libido, and potency. Causes of secondary hypogonadism include pituitary tumor, with or without elevations in prolactin, and isolated gonadotropin deficiency occurring either as a familial entity or sporadically. In Kallmann's syndrome, an X-linked recessive or male-limited autosomal dominant trait, hypogonadism is associated with anosmia and other congenital defects such as a cleft palate and color blindness. Secondary sexual characteristics can be maintained with testosterone therapy; however, induction of spermatogenesis mandates complex therapy with human chorionic gonadotropin (HCG) and human menopausal gonadotropin (HMG) and is best left in the hands of fertility specialists.

ECTOPIC HORMONE PRODUCTION

The production of ectopic hormones by tumor cell lines that normally do not produce that hormone have increasing interest. One of the earliest ectopic hormones recognized was ACTH produced by a bronchogenic carcinoma. The ectopic hormone has both metabolic and systemic effects that resemble those of the physiologic hormone; it is capable of suppressing the endocrine gland that normally produces the hormone. The substance secreted can be identical to an endocrine hormone or may be chemically different but capable of exerting physiologic activity. Failure to recognize that cancer may produce clinical symptoms resembling an endocrine hormone excess may lead to an incorrect diagnosis.

At a certain early stage in development, some cells may have the genetic capability to become other cells with the capacity of synthesizing any protein. Subsequent cellular differentiation results in a mature cell with a single function. Under certain conditions, cancer cells seem capable of transformation with a resultant alteration in function. Studies have linked approximately 24 cell types by common biochemical and ultrastructural features, with the postulate that they originate in a common embryonic tissue, the neural crest. These cells have been labeled APUD (amine precursor uptake and decarboxylation).

When tumors arise in cells of APUD origin, they are capable of excessive secretion of any substance made from the other differentiated cell lines. It is postulated that some embryonic link exists between all ectopic hormone-secreting tumors and their tissue of resemblance, even if not from an APUD cell.

The most common ectopic hormone syndromes include bilateral adrenal hyperplasia, inappropriate antidiuresis, hypercalcemia, spontaneous hypoglycemia, hyperthyroidism, erythrocytosis, precocious puberty, gynecomastia, and gastrin-secreting tumors. Treatment of an underlying malignancy abates the endocrine syndromes.

CARBOHYDRATE METABOLISM

PHYSIOLOGY OF INSULIN

The concentration of glucose in human plasma is maintained in a relatively narrow range. This is brought about by the opposing actions of insulin on one hand and the anti-insulin hormones on the other. Disorders of clinical significance result when the plasma glucose is significantly decreased or markedly elevated.

Insulin is synthesized as preproinsulin (molecular weight 11,500) in the β cells of the pancreatic islets. Proinsulin (molecular weight 9,000) is formed by enzymatic action and transported to the Golgi apparatus, where it is packed into granules. Further enzymatic cleavage converts proinsulin to insulin (molecular weight 6,000) and the C-peptide (molecular weight 3,000), both of which are subsequently secreted in equimolar concentrations in the plasma. The insulin molecule consists of an A chain of 21 amino acids and a B chain of 30 amino acids linked together by two disulfide bridges. The biologic activity of the insulin molecule depends on the integrity of the whole molecule.

Physiologic Actions of Insulin

Insulin is a hormone of energy storage. Its major action is to lower the blood level of glucose, but it also affects protein and fat metabolism. One of its primary actions is to increase the permeability of the cell membrane to glucose (and other monosaccharides), amino acids, and fatty acids. The cell membranes of hepatic and brain cells do not depend on this facilitatory action of insulin, since glucose can enter these cells by simple diffusion. The first step in the action of insulin is its binding to the specific receptors on the cell membrane that, in turn, activates an effector system to bring about the final effects. Although cyclic AMP is recognized as the second messenger for actions of many hormones, the second messenger for actions of insulin has not been clearly defined.

The anabolic effects of insulin involving carbohydrate, protein, and fat metabolism can be summarized as follows:

Insulin promotes

- Plasma membrane transfer of glucose, amino acids, and fatty acids
- Synthesis of glycogen
- Oxidation of glucose
- Uptake of amino acids and synthesis of protein
- Lipogenesis

Insulin inhibits

- Neoglucogenesis
- Lipolysis
- Glycogenolysis
- Proteolysis
- Ketogenesis

Regulation of Secretion of Insulin

The β cells secrete insulin at an estimated basal secretory rate of 0.5 unit/h. The sympathetic nervous system plays a role in modulating the basal secretory rate of the β cell, in that stimulation of α-adrenergic receptors inhibits, and the stimulation of β-adrenergic receptor stimulates, the secretion of insulin. The concentration of glucose in plasma is by far the most important regulator of insulin secretion. When islets are exposed to a concentration of glucose greater than 100 mg/dl, a biphasic insulin release is observed. There is an immediate rise in the level of insulin occurring within 1 minute, which then declines and is followed by a more gradual increase in insulin. This has lead to the suggestion that insulin exists in two metabolic pools: a storage pool for immediate release, and another pool that represents the newly synthesized insulin thought to be responsible for the second phase of insulin release. Other substrates such as amino acids (especially arginine) increase insulin secretion. Fatty acids and ketone bodies are also weak insulin secretagogues. Gastrointestinal hormones such as gastrin, pancreozymin, secretin, and gastric inhibitory polypeptide (GIP) also increase insulin secretion. Growth hormone, estrogens, and progesterone are associated with increased insulin secretion; however, this is accompanied by decreased responsiveness of tissues to insulin, resulting in impaired glucose tolerance in spite of an increased insulin concentration. Decreased tissue responsiveness to insulin is also an important characteristic of obesity. Increased basal secretion of insulin and hyperresponsivness to many insulin secretagogues have been well established in naturally occurring and experimentally induced obesity. Insulin secretion is also influenced by the secretion from other islet cells. Glucagon (α cells) increases, and somatostatin (δ cells) decreases, the secretion of insulin.

Insulin Receptors and Insulin Resistance

As already mentioned, the first step in the action of insulin is its binding to specific receptors present on the cell membrane. These receptors are complex proteins. The concentration and affinity of the receptors are regulated by a variety of factors including diet, concentration of insulin, and other hormones. Insulin resistance may result from a decrease in the number or affinity of insulin receptors (receptor defect), or from an abnormality in the sequence of events that follows after insulin binds to the receptors (postreceptor defect). The insulin resistance of obesity is associated with a decrease in the number of insulin receptors. When calorie-restricted diets are given to obese animals (or patients) the number of insulin receptors increases within a few weeks. Patients with type II diabetes, or noninsulin-dependent diabetes mellitus (NIDDM), also have a decrease in the number of insulin receptors. The decrease in the number of insulin receptors adequately explains the mild insulin resistance encountered in obesity and in NIDDM patients without fasting hyperglycemia. However, in NIDDM patients with marked hyperglycemia and in obese individuals with marked hyperinsulinemia, a post receptor defect is also present and may, in fact, be the major abnormality.

Several nonobese patients with acanthosis nigricans and marked insulin resistance have also been described. These patients are markedly hyperinsulinemic, and may be subdivided into types A and B. Type A patients are young females (12-14 years of age) that have difficulty with sexual maturation hirsutism, virilization and often have polycystic ovaries. Insulin binding to their receptors is markedly dimished, but they have no circulating antibodies or other autoimmune features. Type B patients are older, have other autoimmune features (increased gamma globulins, antinuclear and anti-DNA antibodies), and contain circulating antibodies directed against the insulin receptor. These antireceptor antibodies bind to the receptor and interfere with the binding of insulin to its receptor. A decrease in insulin binding at the receptor sites has also been observed in patients with acromegaly and glucocorticoid excess, and may partly explain the presence of insulin resistance in these disorders. Studies of insulin receptors with the use of sulfonylureas have also resulted in a better understanding of the mechanisms of action of these drugs.

PHYSIOLOGY OF GLUCAGON

Pancreatic glucagon is a 29-amino acid polypeptide (molecular weight, 3,500) secreted by the α cells of the islets. Its actions are mediated via an increased concentration of cyclic AMP as a result of stimulation of the enzyme adenyl cyclase. The effects of glucagon are directly opposite to that of insulin. Glucagon promotes neoglucogenesis, ketogenesis, glycogenolysis, and protein catabolism. It also stimulates lipase activity, resulting in increased lipolysis. Thus, glucagon may be viewed as a hormone of energy need.

Regulation of Secretion of Glucagon

Due to the opposing actions of insulin and glucagon, it has been suggested that the α and β cells of the islets function as a bihormonal unit to maintain the plasma concentrations of glucose in a narrow range. For example, hypoglycemia stimulates, and hyperglycemia inhibits, the secretion of glucagon. Intravenous infusion of amino acids or ingestion of a protein-rich meal stimulates the secretion of both insulin and glucagon. The increased secretion of insulin in this situation directs the amino acids toward protein synthesis, while an increased concentration of glucagon prevents the development of hypoglycemia that would otherwise result from the unopposed action of insulin. Pancreozymin increases, whereas secretin inhibits, the secretion of glucagon. In addition, the sympathetic nervous system also modulates the secretion of glucagon.

PHYSIOLOGY OF SOMATOSTATIN

Somatostatin, the hypothalamic hormone also secreted by the δ cells of the islets, inhibits the secretion of both insulin and glucagon. Glucagon (but not insulin), in turn, stimulates somatostatin release. Although the exact role of somatostatin in the regulation of carbohydrate metabolism has not been clearly established, in short-term experiments it has been shown to lower blood glucose and results in better control of diabetes. These effects may be due to inhibition of glucagon. It has also been shown that somatostatin decreases absorption of carbohydrates from the gastrointestinal tract.

DIABETES MELLITUS

Diabetes mellitus is a syndrome of altered carbohydrate, fat and protein metabolism resulting from an absolute or relative deficiency of insulin. Although accompanied by a relative or absolute excess of glucagon, the role of glucagon excess in the pathogenesis of diabetes remains controversial. The most common biochemical abnormality is hyperglycemia. When long-standing, it is commonly associated with structural abnormalities in a variety of tissues resulting in the so-called complications of diabetes.

The prevalence of diabetes is difficult to estimate accurately partly because of lack of definitive criteria for the diagnosis. The prevalence differs greatly among different races and with environmental conditions. In general, more affluent communities have a higher prevalence. The U.S. National Commission on Diabetes estimates that the disease now affects 5% of the U.S. population, and appears to be increasing at a rate of 6% per year. At this rate, the number of diabetics will double every 15 years! The socioeconomic impact of the disease, therefore, is obviously great.

CLASSIFICATION

In recent years, evidence has accumulated to indicate that diabetes is a heterogeneous disorder, but there has been no general agreement on the classification of the syndrome based on either etiology or clinical manifestation. An international study group convened under the sponsorship of the National Institutes of Health has developed recommendations for classification and diagnosis of diabetes mellitus. The recommendations, given below, are those made by this group. They are based on contemporary knowledge of diabetes and also represent compromises of different points of view.

1. *Type I: Insulin-Dependent Diabetes Mellitus (IDDM).* This type of diabetes is characterized by a sudden onset of symptoms, insulin insufficiency, susceptibility to the development of ketoacidosis, and dependence on insulin for maintenance of life. Classically, this type of diabetes occurs in young subjects and was previously called juvenile diabetes.
2. *Type II: Noninsulin-Dependent Diabetes Mellitus (NIDDM).* The second type of diabetes is characterized by paucity of symptoms, absence of dependence on insulin, and lack of susceptibility to ketoacidosis. Insulin levels may be high, low, or normal in these patients. The onset of this type is frequently after the age of 40 years but may occur in younger age groups. In the past, this type has been referred to as maturity-onset diabetes.

   The above classification emphasizes the fact that either type may occur in any age group and includes the group formerly called maturity onset diabetes of young MODY) in type II.

3. Other types of diabetes (formerly called secondary diabetes) are those where diabetes is a result of know etiologies and includes:
   (a) Pancreatic disease: for example, calcific pancreatitis, hemochromatosis, pancreatectomy
   (b) Hormonal disorder: Cushing's syndrome, acromegaly, Loran dwarfism
   (c) Drugs and chemical agents: chlorothiazide, phenytoin, steroids
   (d) Insulin receptor abnormalities: acanthosis nigricans, congenital lipodystrophy
   (e) Genetic syndrome: ataxia telangiectasia, Prader-Willi syndrome, Turner's syndrome
   (f) Diabetes associated with malnourished populations

DIAGNOSIS

The sine qua non of the diagnosis of diabetes is hyperglycemia. It is usually accompanied by glycosuria but the latter is not pathognomonic of diabetes mellitus. Fasting hyperglycemia (or abnormal glucose tolerance test) remains the most important criteria for the diagnosis of diabetes mellitus. The distribution of fasting plasma glucose levels, and levels achieved after a glucose load, in most population studies has been unimodal. Therefore, in the past, various arbitrary criteria have been used to make a diagnosis of diabetes mellitus (Conn and Fajans, U.S. Public Health, British Diabetes Association, and University Group Diabetes Project criteria) without uniform agreement among experts. Use of different glucose loads by various investigators has resulted in further difficulty in interpretation of the data. An international study group (National Diabetes Data Group) has recommended the following criteria to diagnose diabetes mellitus with the hope that these criteria will become generally accepted. Any one of the following criteria will establish the diagnosis: unequivocal elevation of fasting plasma glucose along with the classic symptoms of diabetes, an elevated fasting plasma glucose concentration on more than one occasion, or an elevated glucose concentration after an oral glucose load. In adults, if fasting plasma glucose is higher than 140 mg/dl on more than one occasion, a glucose tolerance test is not necessary. If a glucose tolerance test is performed, it should be done in the absence of any drugs, in the morning, after an overnight fast (not more than 16 hours). The subjects should have unrestricted physical activity and a minimal intake of 150 g of carbohydrates for 3 days prior to the test. The glucose load to be administered should be 1.75 g/kg ideal body weight up to a maximum of 75 g. During the test, the subject should be seated and smoking prohibited. The interpretation of a glucose tolerance test (after a 75 g glucose load) is summarized in Table 2.

In the past, terms like latent diabetes and chemical diabetes have been applied. It is best to avoid these terms since patients with such abnormalities do not necessarily progress to overt diabetes. It should also be emphasized that one should be careful not to make a diagnosis of diabetes when the data are equivocal, as this may result in higher insurance rates, difficulty in employment, and great personal stress for patients.

ETIOLOGY OF DIABETES

Heredity

It has been known for years that inheritance plays an important role in the etiology of diabetes mellitus. While a strong family history of diabetes is frequently evident, the mode of inheritance is not well known and presently is considered multifactorial.

There is an increased prevalance of HLA B8 and Bw15 antigens in insulin-requiring diabetics. In recent studies, a closer association of the HLA-D antigens with IDDM has also been described.

Autoimmunity

The autoimmune nature of IDDM is suggested by its frequent association with other autoimmune disorders. Insulin-dependent diabetics have also been shown to have anti-islet antibodies and abnormalities of cell-mediated immunity, while these abnormalities have not been demonstrated in patients with NIDDM.

Infections

Many epidemiologic studies have suggested that a temporal relationship exists between onset of certain viral infections, particularly mumps, rubella, and coxsackie viruses, and the subsequent development of juvenile-onset diabetes mellitus. More recently, it has been demonstrated that a coxsackie virus isolated from the pancreas of a child with juvenile diabetes damaged cultured animal and human pancreas cells, and induced diabetes in susceptible mice. This evidence suggests that when certain virus infections occur in individuals with the appropriate genetic predisposition, diabetes mellitus may result.

Environmental Factors

Obesity is a factor most strongly and consistently associated with an increased prevalence of NIDDM. Other nutritional factors that may be involved are excessive iron, and deficiencies of zinc and chromium. The relationships between parity, geographic, and racial factors in diabetes, while perhaps of some importance, have not been clarified.

PATHOLOGY

Pancreas

The histologic examination of the pancreas in diabetes mellitus shows several abnormalities. Many of the changes are quantitative rather than qualitative. Pancreata of diabetics are frequently smaller in weight and contain less insulin than do those of nondiabetics. Early in the course of diabetes, a slight reduction in the β-cell granulation may be observed. This is followed by vacuolation of the β cells. These vacuoles contain glycogen and give a positive periodic acid-Schiff (PAS) reaction. In more advanced cases, hyalinization of the islets is frequently encountered. The hyaline material consists of deposits of homogeneous acidophilic substances. Another pathologic change observed is lymphocytic infiltration in the absence of generalized pancreatic inflammatory disease. This finding is frequently found in young diabetics and has been called insulitis. Fibrosis of the islets is observed in about 25% of the patients. This process may completely replace the functioning islet cells, and may also extend into the exocrine portion of the pancreas.

Blood Vessels

Diabetes affects both the larger and smaller blood vessels. The major arteries are affected by atherosclerotic changes that are indistinguishable from those of nondiabetics. The atherosclerosis, however, occurs at a younger age and is more advanced in patients with diabetes mellitus. The specific lesion in the blood vessels of diabetics is called microangiopathy and affects the smaller blood vessels, namely, the capillaries, the smallest arterioles, and the venules. The basic lesion consists of a thickening of the basement membrane. This thickening has been described in practically every tissue of the body, but has been best studied in the skeletal muscle capillaries and in the renal glomeruli. Although it is generally agreed that most patients with long-standing diabetes have a thickened basement membrane, a great deal of controversy exists as to whether this pathologic feature is a consequence of prolonged hyperglycemia.

Nervous System

Both the peripheral and the central nervous systems are affected by diabetes mellitus. Electron microscopic study of peripheral nerves have shown that early lesions include a thickening of the Schwann's cell basement membrane and a segmental demyelinization. Degeneration of the dorsal root ganglia and associated axons also occur in advanced cases.

CLINICAL FEATURES

The classic triad of symptoms is polyuria, polydipsia, and polyphagia. These symptoms are a result of insulin insufficiency leading to hyperglycemia that, upon exceeding the renal threshold, leads to glycosuria. Glucose, being an osmotic diuretic, causes increased water excretion that leads to polyuria which, in turn, results in polydipsia. Loss of calories results in a sensation of increased hunger and polyphagia. Patients frequently lose weight in spite of increased food intake. These symptoms are classically observed in patients with insulindependent diabetes mellitus. Infection of the skin, vulvovaginitis in women, and balanitis in men may bring the patient to the physician's attention. NIDDM is frequently detected by screening examinations, and by the presence of glycosuria and hyperglycemia as part of routine preemployment physical examinations. Some of these patients may present with symptoms of reactive hypoglycemia. These symptoms commonly occur between 3 and 5 hours after meals. Some patients present only with atherosclerotic complications such as myocardial infarction or evidence of peripheral vascular disease. Others may present with involvement of the microvasculature leading to blurred vision due to retinopathy, and chronic renal failure due to nephropathy. In others, peripheral neuropathy may be the initial complaint. Rarely, patients may present with diabetic ketoacidosis or hyperosmolar coma.

TREATMENT

The aims of treatment are to relieve the symptoms, so that the patient can lead a nearly normal life, and to prevent or delay the onset of chronic vascular complications.

Over several years of experience, it has become evident that it is relatively easy to relieve the symptoms, but the vascular complications have not been prevented. In fact, these chronic vascular complications now account for a majority of the deaths in patients with diabetes mellitus. Controversy still exists if control of diabetes is beneficial in preventing or delaying the onset and progression of vascular complications. This question is discussed in somewhat greater detail at the end of this section.

The treatment of diabetes mellitus includes dietary therapy, insulin administration, and oral hypoglycemic drugs.

Diet

Dietary therapy forms the essential part of the treatment, irrespective of the type of diabetes and whether or not oral hypoglycemic agents or insulin is administered. The principle of dietary therapy is to provide an adequate number of calories to meet energy needs. In general, depending on physical activity, nonobese adults require 25-40 calories per kg of body weight for weight maintenance. Obese individuals should be encouraged to lose weight by prescribing lower-calorie diets. Higher-calorie diets are prescribed for patients who are undernourished. Forty-five to 55 percent of these calories can be provided by carbohydrates. About 15-20% of the calories can be provided by protein. The protein intake is often determined by the socioeconomic status of the patients, but at least 1 g of protein per kilogram of body weight should be provided. Additional calories and protein should be provided for growth in children and pregnant women. The remainder of the calories can be provided by fats. Recent studies have demonstrated that increasing the carbohydrate intake of diabetics does not result in poor control of diabetes, and that an increased fiber content of the diet may result in better control of diabetes. Once the total caloric requirement has been determined, the distribution should be decided after a thorough discussion with the patient to take into account food preferences, work schedule, and other personal factors. Generally, this is prescribed as three major meals with two or three snacks during the 24-hour period. Particularly large meals at any one time and rapidly absorbable sugars should be avoided. It is helpful to give the patient an exchange list such as those provided by the American Diabetes Association. The reader is encouraged to be familiar with these exchange lists. It provides the patient a readily available meal plan, with a variety of foods to choose from and minimal inconvenience.

Insulin Therapy

Insulin has been commercially available for therapeutic use for over 50 years. Since 1972, insulin preparations have been single-peak insulin containing less than 1% impurities. More recently, the monocomponent insulins that are even more purified have also become commercially available. Most insulin preparations are mixtures of beef and pork insulin, although pure pork and pure beef insulins are also available. The regular unmodified or crystalline zinc insulin is a rapidly-acting preparation, the activity of which lasts for a short duration. The other insulin preparations have been modified to prolong the insulin action. The clinical characteristics of these preparations are shown in Table 3. The NPH and lente insulins act for about 24 hours. These insulins are, therefore, well suited for once-a-day administration. These two preparations are clinically interchangeable and may be mixed with regular insulin if required. Protamine zinc and ultralente insulin have a duration of action longer than 24 hours. Dosage adjustments with these preparations are, therefore, more difficult on a daily basis. Addition of crystalline zinc insulin to protamine zinc insulin is not recommended because, due to an excess of protamine, regular insulin is also converted to protamine zinc insulin. Because of these disadvantages, NPH and lente insulin are preferred over the longer-acting preparations. Lente is preferred by many physicians due to its lower potential for insulin allergy. Although the onset and the duration of action given in the table for various insulin preparations are generally useful guidelines, the response of an individual patient to insulin administration is highly variable. There is also no way to predict an exact dose of insulin for an individual patient; this must be arrived at by trial and error. In general, a small dose of an intermediate-acting insulin (10-15 units) is given as an initial dose. Glycosuria or blood sugar is monitored frequently during the day. Urine specimens obtained about 30 minutes after emptying the bladder (second-void specimens) are more useful. These urine specimens reflect more accurately the blood sugar levels during the preceding 30 minutes. The dose of insulin is gradually increased over the next few days to control the glycosuria. Plasma glucose values should be determined before breakfast, before lunch, and before supper. Ideally, these plasma sugars should be kept below 150 mg% without producing symptoms of hypoglycemia. Many patients will require the addition of a small amount of regular insulin to cover the hyperglycemia following breakfast. Most patients are better controlled by two injections of intermediate-acting insulin, or a mixture of intermediate- and short-acting insulin, one in the morning and another in the evening.

An alternative way to arrive at the correct dose of insulin is to give a small dose of short-acting insulin ½ hour before each meal during the day. The amount of insulin is determined by the degree of hyperglycemia or glycosuria. The advantage of initially starting with short-acting insulin is that rapid adjustments can be made and the diabetes brought under control rapidly. Once that is achieved, the patient may be switched to an intermediate-acting insulin. To avoid hypoglycemia, in general, two-thirds, or three-quarters, of the total dose of regular insulin is administered as intermediate-acting insulin. Finer adjustments are made later. On an experimental basis, it has been shown that continuous infusion of insulin results in better control of hyperglycemia. It has also been shown, however, that similar degrees of control can be achieved by multiple injections of regular insulin. Many patients with diabetes, however, may not find it practical to take multiple injections daily. It remains to be proven if either of these methods of insulin administration leading to better control of hyperglycemia will result in fewer chronic complications of diabetes.

Complications of insulin treatment include the development of hypoglycemia. The signs, symptoms, and management of hypoglycemia are described in the next section. Patients may develop local allergic reactions to insulin at the site of injection. These may include itching, redness, or urticaria. Rarely, generalized urticaria or angioneurotic edema may occur. If the patient is insulin dependent and allergic to insulin, desensitization can be performed. After repeated injections, some patients develop atrophy or hypertrophy of the subcutaneous fat in the areas of injections. These complications have become

Table 3. Characteristics of Insulin Preparations

Name	*Onset of Action (h)*	*Maximum Action (h)*	*Duration of Action (h)*
Regular	$\frac{1}{2}$-1	2-4	6-8
NPH (isophane)	1-2	8-12	20-24
Protamine zinc	6-8	14-20	24-36
Lente series			
Semilente	$\frac{1}{2}$-1	4-6	12-16
Lente	1-2	8-12	20-24
Ultralente	5-8	16-18	30-36

less frequent with the use of more purified insulin prapara-tions.

Oral Hypoglycemic Drugs

A number of drugs administered orally have the potential of lowering the blood glucose, but only the sulfonylurea group of drugs have found clinical usefulness. Phenformin (a biguanide) in use for a number of years, has been removed from the market in the United States because of its high incidence of side effects and number of deaths from lactic acidosis. Characteristics of oral hypoglycemic drugs in clinical use are shown in Table 4.

When given over a brief course, the sulfonylurea group of drugs stimulate the secretion of insulin from the pancreatic β cells. After long-term use, even though insulin secretion is not increased, the glucose tolerance remains improved. This suggests that sulfonylureas have extrapancreatic actions. The latter include increased peripheral utilization of glucose and suppression of hepatic glucose production. Recent data suggest that these drugs may exert their effects by increasing the number of insulin receptors.

These drugs can be used only in the management of NIDDM; they should be prescribed for those patients whose blood sugar is not controlled by diet alone and in whom insulin therapy is not practical. They are contraindicated in insulin-dependent, ketosis-prone diabetes and in pregnant women. Side effects of these drugs include gastrointestinal disturbances such as anorexia, nausea, vomiting, diarrhea, and hepatocellular or cholestatic jaundice. Maculopapular eruptions with pruritus, hematologic toxicity including agranulocytosis and pancytopenia have also been reported. Severe and prolonged hypoglycemia may sometimes occur with these drugs especially in those patients who are malnourished, or have impaired liver or kidney functions. Many other drugs such as phenylbutazone, probenecid, salicylates, bishydroxycoumarin, and monoamine oxidase inhibitors may potentiate the effect of these drugs and produce hypoglycemia. About 5% of the patients taking sulfonylurea drugs develop a disulfiram-like reaction upon alcohol intake. Chlorpropamide (rarely tolbutamide) has been associated with hyponatremia and water intoxication due to potentiation of ADH effects.

A multicentric, cooperative, prospective randomized study of oral sulfonylurea drugs in maturity onset diabetes (UGDP study) demonstrated an increased mortality due to cardiovascular causes in a group of patients taking tolbutamide. In this study, about 200 patients in each of the 5 groups were treated with diet in addition to placebo (PLBO), a fixed dose of tolbutamide (TOLB), a fixed dose of insulin (INSTD), a variable dose of insulin (IVAR), or a fixed dose of phenformin (PHEN). The results of the study are highly controversial and are not agreed upon by authorities in the field of diabetes. The detailed reasons for this controversy are many and beyond the scope of this chapter but include the facts that:

1. Patients in the TOLB group had increased cardiovascular risk factors at the time of entry.
2. Some patients transferred from one group to another but were analyzed in the original group.
3. TOLB was used in a fixed dose of 1.5 g daily, contrary to the usual clinical practice.
4. Other factors that may have influenced the final outcome were not adequately controlled for, such as cigarette smoking and weight gain.
5. Follow-up and management of hyperglycemia and hypertension were not adequate. Actually, all groups (except INVAR) experienced a rise of blood sugar after 5 years of follow-up.

In spite of the adverse effects of TOLB shown in this study, these drugs appear to have a place in clinical practice, albeit for a small number of patients who cannot be controlled by diet alone. The decision to prescribe these drugs should be made after an open discussion with the patient. An attempt should be made to control the blood glucose with a minimal dose of the drug. Chlorpropamide, a longer-acting drug, is administered once daily, whereas the others may have to be given more frequently due to their shorter duration of action, in the dose range shown in Table 4.

Patient Education

Education of a patient with diabetes mellitus is the most important part of the treatment of this disease. Patients should be carefully instructed in the signs and symptoms of hyperglycemia as well as hypoglycemia. Some authorities recom-

Table 4. Characteristics of Oral Hypoglycemic Drugs

Name	*Duration of Action*	*Daily Dose Range*	*Metabolism*
Tolbutamide (Orinase)	6-12 h	0.5-2 g	Oxidized in liver, metabolite excreted in the urine
Tolazamide (Tolinase)	10-15 h	0.1-1 g	Metabolized in liver, excreted in the urine
Acetohexamide (Dymelor)	12-24 h	0.25-1.5 g	Reduced in the liver, secreted by renal tubules
Chlorpropamide (Diabinese)	24-72 h	0.1-0.5 g	Metabolism minimal, primarily excreted in the urine

mend that under controlled conditions, a mild hypoglycemic reaction should be induced in the hospital so the patient can recognize the symptoms produced by hypoglycemia. All patients should be taught to test their urine for glucose and acetone. Necessary instructions must be given regarding asepsis and proper technique for the measurement and administration of insulin. Those taking oral hypoglycemic drugs should be informed about the interreactions that can result with other drugs. All patients must be taught how to take care of their feet. These include instructions in appropriate washing and drying of feet and instructions in paring their nails. The patient should also be told to treat infections with respect, and at the earliest signs of infection to report to a physician. It is also a good precaution for all patients taking insulin or oral hypoglycemic agents to carry Medic-Alert or similar disease identifications on their person.

COMPLICATIONS

The complications of diabetes mellitus may be divided into acute and chronic.

Acute Complications—Diabetic Ketoacidosis and Hyperosmolar Coma

The term diabetic coma is loosely applied to these clinical entities since most of the patients are not unconscious and about 20% have no alteration in mental status. These complications are the direct result of insulin deficiency. The distinction between ketoacidosis and nonketotic diabetic coma is not an absolute one, since marked hyperosmolarity is often present in ketoacidosis and ketonemia of a mild degree may be present in patients with hyperosmolar coma. Recent observations have made this distinction less important since similar amounts of insulin can be used for both conditions.

Pathophysiology. The pathophysiology of diabetic ketoacidosis and hyperosmolar coma is summarized in Figure 11. The most important pathogenetic element in the development of the hyperosmolar state and ketoacidosis is an insufficient action of insulin. This is further complicated by the unopposed action of anti-insulin hormones, namely, catecholamines, growth hormones, glucocorticoids, and glucagon. A direct consequence of insufficient insulin action is increased blood glucose due to decreased glucose utilization and increased glucose production. Hyperglycemia, when exceeding the renal threshold, results in glycosuria. The osmotic diuresis produced by glucose results in loss of water and electrolytes leading to hyperosmolarity, dehydration, hypovolemia, and shock.

Insulin inhibits lipolysis by its effect on hormone dependent lipase. This action of insulin is very sensitive and requires amounts less than those needed to maintain euglycemia. It has been suggested that the presence of such small quantities of insulin may allow hyperglycemia to develop but prevents the development of ketosis leading to a hyperosmolar nonketotic state. In the absence of insulin, an increase in lipolysis makes increased amounts of free fatty acids available to the liver. In the liver, the fate of fatty acids is determined by the hormonal milieu. In an insulin-rich state, fatty acids are converted into acyl coenzyme A (acyl CoA). Acyl CoA is then oxidized to acetyl CoA and can be metabolized in one of three ways: condensation with oxaloacetate to form citrate or oxidation in Kreb's cycle, fatty acid synthesis, and condensation of two molecules of acetyl CoA to form acetoacetyl CoA. In the absence of insulin, the first and second pathways are inhibited, so the conversion of acetyl CoA to acetoacetate and its reduction product β-hydroxybutyrate is increased. These ketone bodies can be utilized as a source of energy by the muscles. However, when the ketone body production exceeds the rate at which they can be excreted or oxidized, they begin to accumulate in the blood. Ketone bodies are organic acids that readily dissociate and release hydrogen ions into the body fluids, resulting in a fall in pH. This metabolic state is called ketoacidosis. Because of differences in their clinical presentation and treatment, these two entities are separately discussed below.

Diabetic Ketacidosis

Clinical Features. The onset of diabetic ketoacidosis is characterized by an increase in the symptoms of diabetes, namely polyuria and increased thirst. Patients with previously undiagnosed diabetes may give a history of weight loss. Precipitating events, such as infection, myocardial infarction, or injury may be present but are not always evident. Nausea, vomiting, and pain in the abdomen are common accompaniments. Lethargy and some alteration of consciousness is generally present. Although most patients are not comatose at the time of admission, deep coma may result. Both in patients with a hyperosmolar state and in diabetic ketoacidosis, the depression of consciousness closely parallels hyperglycemia and hyperosmolality. On physical examination, the signs of dehydration are evident, in the form of dry skin, a dry tongue, soft eyeballs, and hypotension. Increasing hydrogen ion concentration at first leads to an increased rate and depth of respiration (Kussmaul's respiration), but in severe acidosis respiration may be inhibited. Death may occur due to hypovolemia and shock.

Diagnosis. The diagnosis of ketoacidosis is established by biochemical criteria. These include marked hyperglycemia and ketonemia with acidosis. Blood glucose generally ranges between 400-800 mg/100 ml. A semiquantitative measure of the concentration of ketone bodies can be obtained by utilizing the Acetest tablet (nitroprusside reaction) with progressive dilutions of plasma. This reaction is sensitive only to acetoacetate (to a lesser extent to acetone), but not to β-hydroxybutyrate. Measurement of arterial blood gases and electrolytes reveal acidosis and anion gap, respecitvely. The anion gap is calculated by the following formula: $(Na^+ + K^+) - (Cl' - HCO_3')$. Normally this difference is about 16 mEq/L and is made up of phosphates, sulfates, and proteins. The increased unmeasured anion gap roughly correlates with the severity of ketoacidosis. It is also a useful guide to follow during the first few hours of treatment of ketoacidosis as a reflection of biochemical recovery. Leukocytosis is usually present. Many enzymes including amylase, SGOT, LDH, and CPK may be elevated, requiring greater reliance on clinical and other criteria for the diagnosis of associated

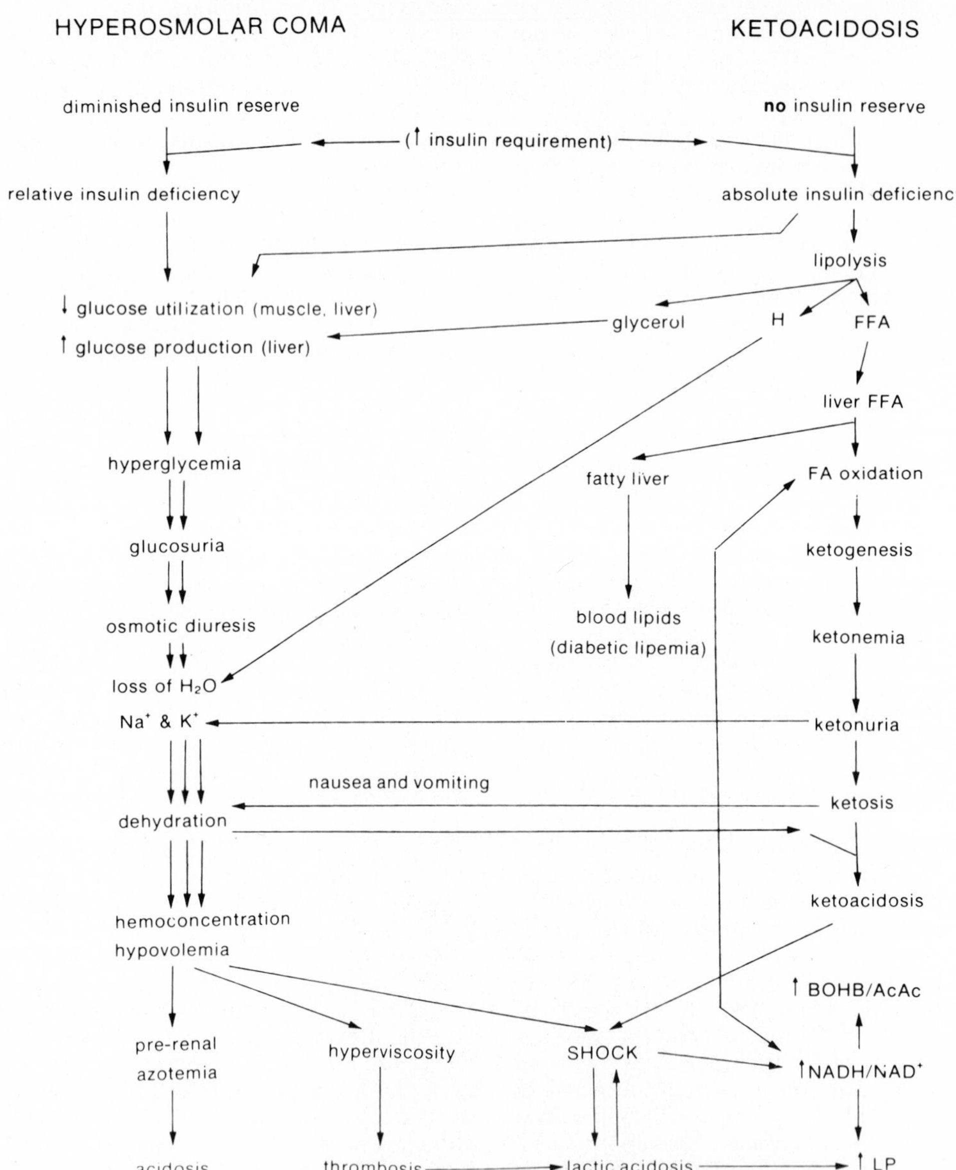

Figure 11. Pathophysiology of diabetic ketoacidosis and hyperosmolar coma.

illnesses such as pancreatitis and myocardial infarction. Urinalysis reveals large amounts of glucose and acetone.

Treatment. The principles of treatment of diabetic ketoacidosis are administration of insulin, replacement of fluid and electrolytes, and management of precipitating events.

Only regular insulin should be used in the treatment of patients with ketoacidosis. Until recently, large doses of insulin were advised on the assumption that a certain degree of insulin resistance existed in patients with diabetic ketoacidosis. Many studies have now shown that much smaller doses of insulin are equally effective in the treatment of these patients. The added advantages of a low-dose insulin regimen compared to high doses of insulin are that the development of late hypoglycemia and hypokalemia are less frequent and less severe.

The preferred mode of administration is a continuous infusion of insulin regulated by an infusion pump. An initial loading dose of 10-20 units of insulin may be given but is not always needed. The infusion is given at the rate of 0.1 unit/kg/h. While some insulin does bind to the bottle and intravenous tubing, it does not seem to influence patient recovery, and the addition of albumin to solutions containing insulin to prevent this binding therefore seems unnecessary. When the plasma glucose concentration reaches approximately 250 mg/dl, the intravenous fluid is changed to 5% glucose. At this time, the dose of insulin infusion is reduced to 2 units/h, or 5 units/IM or subcutaneously every 2 hours until the patient starts eating. One should carefully and frequently monitor the responses of glucose and ketone bodies after treatment is begun. During the first 2-4 hours of the treatment, the ketone bodies as measured by the Acetest tablets may show an increase even though the total ketone bodies are decreasing. This is because β-hydroxybutyrate (BOHB) and acetoacetate (AcAc) normally exist in equilibrium. During the development of ketoacidosis, increased fatty acid oxidation generates large quantities of NADH, acetoacetate, and H^+. This results in an increase in the BOHB:AcAc ratio. During recovery, this process is reversed and is accompanied by a fall in total ketone bodies and a decreased BOHB:AcAc ratio. Since the Acetest tablets only react to AcAc (and not to BOHB) this may be reflected in an increase in ketone bodies. However, this is accompanied by a decrease in the anion gap and serum glucose. If no response to treatment is evident in 2 hours, the insulin infusion rate should be doubled. Occasionally, true insulin resistance may be encountered, in which case large doses of insulin should be administered without hesitation. Hypoglycemia is to be avoided as it may predispose to cerebral edema and brain damage.

The fluid losses in moderate to severe diabetic ketoacidosis have been estimated to range between 5-11 liters. Although the loss of fluid is hypotonic in ketoacidosis, fluid therapy is started with normal saline. This is to achieve a prompt re-expansion of the circulating blood volume. The first liter of normal saline is administered rapidly in 1 hour and should be followed by a liter of half-normal saline given in the next hour. The remainder of the fluids can be given more slowly until the fluid deficit is replaced, usually in 24 hours. In patients with compromised cardiovascular function, measurement of central venous pressure or pulmonary wedge pressure should be performed to guide fluid therapy.

At the time of admission, although the total potassium is depleted, serum K^+ may be normal or even high. Hyperkalemia is the result of a shift of potassium from the intracellular to the extracellular compartment due to acidosis. With administration of glucose and insulin, and correction of acidosis, the development of hypokalemia should be anticipated. Therefore, potassium administration at the rate of 20-30 mEq/L of fluid should begin after an adequate urinary output has been established. Additional potassium usually is required for 3-5 days after recovery and may be given orally. Potassium administration occasionally must be started at initiation of therapy if hypokalemia or low normal serum potassium is present on admission. Hypophosphatemia is common during therapy for ketoacidosis and is most profound after 24 hours of treatment. Administration of potassium phosphate is helpful in correcting both potassium and phosphate deficiencies. In the majority of cases, administration of bicarbonate is not required. However, if the pH is less than 7.1 and bicarbonate is less than 10 mEq/L, sodium bicarbonate may be administered intravenously. In very severe acidosis, 50-100 mEq of sodium bicarbonate may be given IV push or more slowly in those with less severe acidosis.

A diligent search for precipitating causes should be made. If an infection is detected, it should be treated with appropriate antibiotics. A silent myocardial infarction should be suspected unless disproved by serial ECGs and appropriate blood tests. If the patient is semiconscious and gastric dilatation is present, nasogastric aspiration of the stomach contents may be needed. It should be emphasized that diabetic ketoacidosis is a life-threatening situation. Its management requires close observation and careful attention to details to achieve an optimal outcome.

Hyperosmolar Coma

Hyperosmolar coma is about one-sixth as frequent as diabetic ketacidosis; it usually occurs in older patients but has been reported in infants. These patients usually have mild diabetes, or there may be no history of diabetes mellitus. The patients usually present with a history of polyuria, polydipsia, and polyphagia that may be of several days or weeks duration. The coma may be precipitated by an associated illness such as acute infection, myocardial infarction, or exacerbation of an underlying chronic illness. It is estimated that as many as 85% of patients have associated renal or cardiac disease. Many drugs have been implicated in the precipitation of the hyperosmolar state including phenytoin, thiazides, propranolol, immunosuppressive agents, and steroids. Physical examination reveals evidence of dehydration and a clouded sensorium. Focal neurologic signs are frequently encountered and can lead to a misdiagnosis of cerebrovascular accident or organic brain syndrome.

Biochemical determinations are required to establish the diagnosis. These consist of severe hyperglycemia with blood sugar usually ranging around 1000 mg/100 ml. The plasma ketones are usually negative or, if present, exist only in small amounts. The serum osmolarity is significantly increased. This can be measured directly, or can be estimated by the following formula:

$$\text{Serum osmolarity (mOsm/L)} = 2(\text{Na}^+ + \text{K}^+ \text{ in mEq/L}) + \frac{\text{glucose in mg/dl}}{18} + \frac{\text{BUN in mg/dl}}{2.8}$$

The principles of treatment are similar to that of diabetic ketoacidosis with the following differences:

1. The patients are usually more dehydrated and need more fluids. Many of these patients have underlying cardiovascular abnormalities; therefore, caution should be exercised in fluid administration. For reasons stated above, even

though the fluid lost is hypotonic, the first liter of fluid should be normal saline.

2. These patients may be more sensitive to insulin.
3. Administration of alkali is not required.
4. These patients are at increased risk for venous thrombosis; careful consideration should be given to administration of anticoagulants to prevent late deaths from pulmonary emboli.

Chronic Complications

Vascular Complications

With the availability of insulin and potent antibiotics, and the resultant control of diabetic acidosis and infections, the cardiovascular and renal complications of diabetes have become the major causes of death among diabetics, accounting for almost 74% of deaths. Diabetes affects both the large and the small blood vessels.

Large Vessel Lesions–Coronary Artery Disease. Atherosclerosis is the predominant lesion affecting the medium-sized muscular arteries such as the radial, tibial, and coronary arteries. Atherosclerosis occurs more frequently, and with greater severity, in diabetic patients than in normal people. Except for these quantitative differences, the atherosclerosis is qualitatively similar to that noted in the general population. Risk factors such as hypertension, cigarette smoking, and hyperlipidemia seem to be similar for the diabetic and nondiabetic. The cumulative risk for coronary artery disease increases with the duration of diabetes, but whether hyperglycemia (or glucose intolerance) is an independent coronary risk factor still remains controversial. The clinical features, the diagnosis, and the management of coronary artery disease in diabetics is similar to that in nondiabetics.

Peripheral Vascular Disease. Like coronary artery disease, peripheral vascular disease is also more common among diabetics and has probably increased in the past three decades. Involvement of the large or medium-sized blood vessels in the lower limbs can result in gangrene of the feet, a serious and frequent complication of diabetes; it is associated with absent peripheral pulses. Gangrene may also result from neuropathy, superimposed infection or injury, and involvement of small vessels. In these cases, the pedal pulses are not decreased. A diagnosis of arterial insufficiency is suggested by a history of claudication. Physical examination may reveal absent or weak peripheral pulses, pallor on elevation, rubor on dependency, and prolongation of the venous filling time. If the occlusion of a major vessel is suspected, arteriography should be performed. Delineation of such an obstruction is extremely helpful in planning for reconstructive surgery in these patients. If arterial bypass surgery cannot be performed, amputation is the treatment of choice. Since the atherosclerotic process involves the blood vessels diffusely, one-third of the diabetics who require amputation of one leg usually require amputation of the other leg within the next 3 years. Thus, care of the feet and prevention of injury often goes a long way to prevent or delay the onset of diabetic gangrene.

Small Blood Vessel Lesions or Microangiopathy. Diabetic retinopathy is the leading cause of blindness in patients up to the age of 60 in the United States, and the major cause of blindness throughout the world. Some degree of diabetic retinopathy can be detected in more than 90% of patients after they have had diabetes for 20-25 years. Diabetic retinopathy may be divided into two stages: background retinopathy and proliferative retinopathy. The earliest recognizable lesions of background retinopathy consist of dilatation of the veins and microaneurysms. Capillary degeneration with leakage of fluid and edema formation result in the development of exudates. Macular edema or a plaque of hard exudate may result in loss of vision (maculopathy). In some patients with long-standing diabetes, progression of background retinopathy may occur to the proliferative stage. In this phase, new vessels usually arise from the disk or from the periphery of the retina. Traction on these new vessels may lead to hemorrhage in the vitreal space and may cause visual impairment. Organization of these hemorrhages with secondary fibrosis ultimately results in retinal detachment. Mild background retinopathy requires careful follow-up so that if preproliferative changes develop, appropriate treatment is provided without delay. The treatment of diabetic retinopathy consists primarily of photocoagulation. Xenon arc and argon laser beam both have been used for this purpose. The high-intensity light beam produces coagulation and scarring. It is helpful in preventing leaks from abnormally permeable blood vessels, reduction of macular edema, and in the treatment of neovascularization. The rationale of this treatment is based on the theory that new vessel growth is a response to areas of nonperfusion. If these areas were destroyed completely, new blood vessels would cease to grow and might even regress. That such treatment is effective has been shown by the diabetic retinopathy research group. Pituitary ablation for treatment of diabetic retinopathy has been abandoned in favor of photocoagulation. Vitrectomy may be performed in selected patients with long-standing, non-resolving vitreous hemorrhages.

Diabetic Nephropathy

Diabetic nephropathy is frequently present in association with retinopathy and neuropathy. Hypertension is a frequent accompaniment. A specific lesion of diabetic nephropathy is nodular sclerosis, also called a Kimmelstiel-Wilson lesion. It is visible on light microscopy as a rounded hyaline mass at the center of the glomerular lobules. Much more frequent, but not as specific, is the diffuse glomerulosclerosis with thickening of the glomerular basement membrane and an increased mesangial matrix. The first clinical evidence of nephropathy is proteinuria. It is at first intermittent, but later becomes constant. Progressive nephropathy results in heavy proteinuria and the development of the nephrotic syndrome. The latter often progresses to renal failure, usually within 5 years.

The treatment of diabetic nephropathy should be aimed at strictly controlling blood sugar. As renal function declines, the renal threshold for glucose may increase and the urine sugar may lose its value in the adjustment of insulin dosage. Insulin requirements fall as renal failure becomes established, and hypoglycemia may become a frequent event. However, management of chronic renal failure in the diabetic otherwise is not different from management of end-stage renal disease.

Hemodialysis and, more recently, renal transplantation have been employed successfully in the management of end-stage renal disease in the diabetic population.

Diabetic Neuropathy

Diabetic neuropathy is probably the most common of the chronic complications of diabetes. Neuropathy may result primarily from involvement of the vasa nervorum. Thickening of the walls of these vessels occasionally sufficient to produce complete occlusion have been demonstrated. When involvement of the vasa nervorum is not demonstrated, the basis of neuropathy appears to be primarily related to an abnormal sorbitol pathway. Diabetic animals have been shown to have increased sorbitol formation and retention within the nerve fibers. Depletion of myoinositol has also been suggested as an underlying cause for diabetic neuropathy.

Diabetic neuropathy affects both the somatic and the autonomic nervous systems. Somatic neuropathy may present as symmetric peripheral neuropathy. This is by far the most common expression of diabetic neuropathy. It frequently affects patients in the fifth and sixth decades of life. Numbness and tingling usually in the feet and legs is the initial manifestation, but may progress to loss of sensation. Response to sensory stimuli, especially bone vibration, is frequently diminished. Distal weakness and diminished tendon reflexes may be present.

Less commonly, the neuropathy may involve a single peripheral nerve resulting in motor or sensory deficit in the distribution of the nerve involved (Mononeuropathy). Similar impairment of function may involve the oculomotor system especially the third nerve. Other peripheral nerves may be affected either singly or in combination, producing a mononeuritis multiplex. Diabetic amyotrophy is characterized usually by an initial onset of severe pain, rapid onset of proximal muscle weakness, and atrophy. The tendon reflexes are usually decreased or absent. Sensory impairment is minimal or even absent. The symptoms are usually self-limited with spontaneous recovery possible, although occasional residual deficits may persist.

Autonomic neuropathies seldom occur without the presence of somatic neuropathies, but can affect nearly all organ systems. Involvement of the skin results in anhidrosis, dependent edema, increased skin fragility, and neuropathic ulcers.

Involvement of the cardiovascular system results in orthostatic hypotension, and absence of reflex tachycardia. Neurogenic bladder dysfunction, impotence, and retrograde ejaculation are results of involvement of the genitourinary system. Impotence is very common in male diabetics with a prevalence of 75% between the ages of 60 and 65. Signs and symptoms of gastrointestinal autonomic neuropathy are varied and may include delayed emptying of the esophagus and stomach, gastric dilatation, and frequent, profuse, watery, urgent bowel movements occurring especially at night (nocturnal diabetic diarrhea).

Treatment of diabetic neuropathy consists of simple analgesics to help diminish the severity of pain. Phenytoin in doses of 100 mg three times a day can be useful in some patients. More recently carbamazepine (Tegretol), and tricyclic antidepressants have been tried with some success. Some instances of diabetic diarrhea are considerably helped by a broad-spectrum antibiotic, but the majority of treatment is symptomatic. Patients with orthostatic hypotension should be instructed to sleep with the head of the bed elevated, and to rise slowly from a supine or prone position. Leg bindings, and 9 α-fludrocortisone may be useful. Impotence is difficult to treat and is usually not responsive to the administration of testosterone. Penile implants are now available for surgical management of impotence.

Relationship of Control of Diabetes and Chronic Complications

The question of whether strict or tight control of diabetes will prevent or delay the onset of chronic complications has been debated for years, but still remains unanswered. A large number of studies have attempted to answer this question. However, many of these cannot be evaluated because some of them were retrospective studies and others were not well controlled.

Another problem in relating the degree of control to these complications has been the difficulty of monitoring the blood glucose levels. These levels have been measured in the clinic, home, school, or office; however, such sporadic measurements may not accurately reflect the degree of control over the previous several hours or days. Recently, it has been shown that measurement of HbA_{1c} (glycosylated hemoglobin) may be a better measure of diabetic control over a prolonged period than measurement of blood glucose concentration. HbA_{1c} is synthesized in a slow, nearly irreversible reaction throughout the life of the red blood cell. The rate of synthesis is a function of blood glucose concentration. Once synthesized, the HbA_{1c} remains in circulation until the end of the life span of the red blood cells. Thus, a single HbA_{1c} measurement reflects the mean blood glucose concentration over the previous 2-3 months.

In the past few years, numerous animal experiments have shown that the reduction of hyperglycemia by insulin therapy, or by other means, prevents or minimizes formation of diabetes-like lesions in various tissues, but these data cannot be directly applied to humans. Electron microscope studies of capillary basement membranes from diabetic patients have yielded conflicting results. From the available clinical data, the question of whether poorly controlled diabetes leads to greater basement thickening cannot be answered at this time. Biochemical data, however, indicate that hyperglycemia produces alterations in the basement membrane as well as accumulation of glucose-derived substances (e.g., sorbitol) in various tissues.

Kidney biopsies obtained from renal transplants in diabetic patients, received from nondiabetic cadaver kidneys, have shown the development of lesions of diabetic nephropathy in these patients. In a small but prospective study of randomly assigned patients with diabetic retinopathy, it was shown that in diabetics treated with multiple injections of insulin (well controlled), the progress of diabetic retinopathy was significantly less as compared to the group that was treated with single injections (not well controlled). A recent study of 4,400 patients with prolonged follow-up also supports the relationship of higher blood sugar levels and more frequent or more severe complications.

While it must be conceded that these data may not be sufficient to convince all physicians, they are highly suggestive that strict control of hyperglycemia may help delay or even prevent the vascular complications of diabetes. It is therefore recommended that every effort should be made to achieve a normal blood glucose level in patients with diabetes, particularly in young and middleaged patients who are at highest risk for microvascular complications. However, the best possible control should be achieved without producing frequent hypoglycemic reactions and also without significantly compromising the patient's way of life.

SPECIAL PROBLEMS IN MANAGEMENT OF DIABETES

Diabetes and Pregnancy

Diabetes and pregnancy are found to coexist in approximately 1 percent of pregnancies. Pregnancy can be characterized as a state of accelerated starvation, with a tendency to fasting hypoglycemia. At the same time, pregnancy is a diabetogenic stress. Glucose tolerance deteriorates during pregnancy and many women demonstrate an abnormal glucose tolerance test only during the pregnant state, that is, gestational diabetes. The cause of glucose intolerance during pregnancy is not completely clear; but increased secretion of human placental lactogen, an anti-insulin hormone, is believed to play a major role. Estrogens, progesterone, and increased cortisol levels may also contribute to glucose intolerance. Recently, a decrease in the number of insulin receptors in pregnancy has also been described. Because of these metabolic alterations, the criteria for interpretation of a glucose tolerance test in the nonpregnant patient cannot be applied to the pregnant state. The following criteria are widely accepted for making a diagnosis of diabetes during pregnancy. After administration of a 100 gram glucose load, two or more of the following values must be met or exceeded:

	Fasting	1 hour	2 hours	3 hours
Venous plasma glucose (mg/dl)	105	190	165	145
Whole blood glucose (mg/dl)	90	170	145	125

In considering the interaction between pregnancy and diabetes, the effect of pregnancy on the diabetes mellitus and the effect of diabetes on pregnancy should be considered.

Effect of Pregnancy on Diabetes

The tolerance of carbohydrate improves in the first trimester. This improvement is believed to be due to the drain of glucose from the mother to the fetus. In insulin-requiring patients, hypoglycemia may occur frequently in the first trimester. The second trimester is characterized by intensification of maternal diabetes and susceptibility to ketoacidosis. In the third trimester, the insulin requirements increase further. The renal threshold for glucose decreases during pregnancy. The presence of glycosuria, therefore, becomes an unreliable measure for controlling diabetes. Labor is a severe exercise and insulin requirements are significantly decreased during labor. The postpartum period is also characterized by decreasing insulin requirements, and a short remission of diabetes lasting 3-5 days may be encountered.

Effect of Pregnancy on the Complications of Diabetes

Pregnancy is associated with increased infections of skin and the urinary tract. A preexisting neuropathy may worsen. Retinopathy and nephropathy may become evident for the first time or may progress. The eventual course of nephropathy, however, does not appear to be altered unfavorably by pregnancy. The effect of pregnancy on diabetic retinopathy is not well defined, although clinical impressions suggest that background retinopathy is relatively unaffected while proliferative changes tend to worsen. Rarely, and unpredictably during pregnancy, retinopathy and may suddenly intensify and become an indication for termination of pregnancy.

Effect of Diabetes on Pregnancy

The fertility in diabetic women is not decreased. If the duration of diabetes is short, spontaneous abortions occur in 10% of diabetics, a rate similar to the general population; but the rate of spontaneous abortions is increased with longer duration of diabetes. Hydramnios and toxemia of pregnancy occur more commonly in diabetic women, compared to the general population. Eclampsia or the development of ketoacidosis frequently results in intrauterine fetal death, most commonly at 36 weeks of gestation. Hyperglycemia, especially during early pregnancy, may contribute to an increased incidence of congenital abnormalities among offspring of diabetic women.

Management of Pregnant Diabetics

In the initial evaluation of a pregnant patient, an effort should be made to classify the patient according to the severity of the disease. The classification suggested by White is widely accepted for these purposes and is given below.

Class A. Patients with gestational diabetes mellitus. These patients are asymptomatic.

Class B. Age of onset 20 years or older, or duration of diabetes less than 10 years.

Class C. Age of onset between ages of 10 to 19 years, or duration of diabetes between 10 to 19 years.

Class D. Age of onset less than 10 years, or duration of diabetes 20 years or more, or evidence of vascular disease (e.g., retinopathy).

Class E. Pelvic vascular disease.

Class F. Renal disease.

Class R. Retinitis proliferans or vitreous hemorrhages.

To these has been added Class T, which includes patients

who have had renal transplants and subsequent pregnancies. In general, the more severe the diabetes the less favorable is the outcome of pregnancy. In addition, signs suggested by Pederson that indicate a bad prognosis should be sought. These include clinical pyelonephritis, severe acidosis, toxemia, and neglect, that is, noncompliance with the recommended regimen. A combination of White's classification with that of bad prognostic signs of pregnancy improves the possibility of predicting fetal outcome.

While there is some controversy regarding strict control and long-term complications of diabetes, it has been adequately shown that a strict control of diabetes results in better outcome of the pregnancy. Therefore, every effort should be made to achieve the best possible control of diabetes during pregnancy. The principles of management of a pregnant diabetic include:

1. Diet should provide adequate calories. A rough estimate of calories can be determined by providing at least 30 calories per kg of the ideal body weight. For obese individuals, weight reduction programs should not be instituted during pregnancy. At least 150-200 grams of carbohydrate and at least 1-1.5 gram per kg of protein should be provided in the diet. The quantity of the night snack is usually increased.
2. Oral hypoglycemics have no place in the management of diabetic pregnancies. The drugs may be teratogenic, they cross the placental barrier, and may produce significant prolonged hypoglycemia in the newborn.

Insulin is administered as dictated by the levels of blood glucose. Every effort should be made to prevent the development of ketoacidosis since it is associated with a high incidence of intrauterine fetal death. The timing of delivery should be determined for each patient individually in consultation with the obstetrician. For insulin-requiring diabetics, 37-38 weeks is considered the optimal delivery time. Those with renal disease and other evidence of vascular disease may be delivered between 35-36 weeks, but these should serve only as guidelines. Laboratory procedures such as ultrasound examination and determination of the lecithin-sphingomyelin ratio in the amniotic fluid provide a measure of fetal maturity. Urinary estriols may be measured on a daily basis. A sudden fall in the urinary estriol indicates fetal compromise. Oxytocin challenge test and nonstress testing may also provide a measure of fetal well-being. A combination of these measures is helpful in determining the optimal times of delivery in individual patients. The insulin resistance of pregnancy disappears soon after the delivery. Therefore, on the day of delivery, the patient should receive only one-half or one-third of the prepregnancy insulin dose. A five percent glucose infusion is generally started in the morning, with further adjustments of insulin made by frequent monitoring of blood sugar. On the day of delivery, an IV infusion of insulin up to the time of delivery may also be utilized. The continuous infusion is discontinued when the placenta is extruded. Subsequent insulin administration is withheld until hyperglycemia reappears. The use of continuous subcutaneous insulin infusion (by pump) throughout pregnancy is being tried on an experimental basis at several institutions to improve the outcome of pregnancy in diabetic patients.

Surgery in a Diabetic Patient

Surgery represents a definite metabolic stress that can result in increased secretion of anti-insulin hormones leading to hyperglycemia. Even ketoacidosis may be precipitated if this stressful situation is severe and prolonged. If the surgical procedure is an elective one, the patient should be admitted to the hospital in the best metabolic control possible. Not infrequently, diabetes is first diagnosed when a patient is admitted to the hospital for surgery. In such situations, the operation should be delayed until the patient's diabetes is controlled.

On the day of operation, approximately half the patient's usual insulin requirement is administered subcutaneously. Instead of breakfast, a five percent dextrose and water solution is administered intravenously. This infusion is continued during and following surgery. At least 100-150 g of carbohydrate should be administered on the day of surgery. This can be easily accomplished by administering about two to three liters of five percent dextrose and water solution. On return to the recovery room, another blood glucose or urine glucose is obtained and an additional dose of regular insulin administered depending upon the blood sugar level. Later in the day, another estimate of blood glucose is obtained and additional insulin administered, if necessary. During the period of intravenous therapy, a glucose value of 200 mg is considered satisfactory. A continuous infusion of insulin may also be utilized. When the postoperative situation permits, fluids are given by mouth and the diet is gradually resumed.

Those patients receiving oral hypoglycemic agents, if undergoing minor surgical procedures, can be managed without any change in their therapeutic regimen. However, many of these patients require insulin before, during, and a few days after surgery. Usually, small doses of regular insulin in the range of 10-12 units given once or twice daily maintain an adequate glucose control.

In patients brought to the hospital requiring emergency surgery, the management of diabetes can be carried out as described above. On the other hand, if the patient is in ketoacidosis, surgery should be delayed for a few hours to treat the diabetes. During this period a continuous infusion of insulin, administration of fluid and electrolytes, and the close monitoring of the patient may improve the condition significantly to allow the emergency surgery to be performed.

HYPOGLYCEMIA

The term *hypoglycemia* implies blood glucose lower than the lowest limit of normal, taking physiologic fluctuations into account. However, it is difficult to define clinically significant hypoglycemia by a specific blood glucose level. Although symptomatic hypoglycemia usually occurs whenever blood glucose drops to 40 mg/dl (plasma glucose 50 mg/dl or less), many healthy adults can have this blood glucose level and remain asymptomatic.

The symptoms of hypoglycemia result from catecholamine release and neuroglycopenia. The symptoms of catecholamine release predominate when the rate of fall of glucose is rapid and consist of sweating, hunger, tachycardia, and inward trembling. If the fall of blood glucose occurs more slowly, the symptoms occur due to inadequate glucose supply to the brain (neuroglycopenia) and consist of headache, blurred vision, diplopia, mental confusion, incoherent speech, coma, and convulsions. Bizarre neurologic and psychiatric manifestations may be present when significant hypoglycemia persists over long periods of time. Sensory or motor deficit in an extremity or hemiplegia may occur. Permanent brain damage may result from repeated episodes of hypoglycemia. When the decrease of blood glucose is rapid, profound, and persistent, the initial symptoms due to excessive epinephrine release may merge with those of neuroglycopenia.

CLASSIFICATION

Hypoglycemia may be classified in many different ways, but from a clinical standpoint, the following classification is a practical one.

Fasting hypoglycemia occurs after a fast of a few hours or prolonged fasting. The causes include:

Insulin-producing pancreatic tumors (insulinoma)
Nonpancreatic tumors associated with hypoglycemia
Severe liver disease
Hypofunction of anterior pituitary or adrenal cortex
Hypothyroidism
Deficiency of glucagon
Certain inborn errors of metabolism

Reactive hypoglycemia occurs a few hours after intake of food and includes:

Alimentary hypoglycemia
Reactive hypoglycemia of early diabetes
Reactive functional (idiopathic) hypoglycemia

Drug-induced hypoglycemia is caused by:

Insulin or sulfonylurea administration, either therapeutically or factitiously
Alcohol
Other miscellaneous drugs: phenylbutazone, probenecid, salicylate, monoamine oxidase inhibitors

Insulinoma is a rare tumor of the β cell of islets of the pancreas. These tumors are encountered in all age groups. The majority of these tumors are benign and may be extremely small. Symptoms are generally those of neuroglycopenia and are frequently brought about by a missed meal or vigorous physical activity. Whipple's triad, which consists of hypoglycemic attacks precipitated by fasting accompanied by a low blood sugar level and relief of symptoms by administration of glucose, is frequently encountered; however, these symptoms are found in any hypoglycemia, regardless of origin.

The diagnosis of insulinoma is often delayed because the true significance of symptoms are not realized. Many patients learn to avoid symptoms by eating at short intervals with resulting obesity.

DIAGNOSIS

The diagnostic biochemical abnormality in a patient with insulimoma is an inappropriately increased secreation of insulin in association with hypoglycemia in the fasting state. A normal insulin level in association with low blood sugar is inappropriately high and is diagnostic of insulinoma if no insulin has been administered exogenously. To better describe the insulin-glucose relationship, an insulin-glucose ratio has been utilized for diagnosis of insulinoma. The insulin-glucose ratio is calculated as follows:

$$\frac{\text{Insulin } (\mu\text{u/ml}) \times 100}{\text{Glucose (mg/dl)} - 30}$$

Expressed in this manner, normal subjects have values below 30, and patients with insulinoma usually have values higher than 150. The insulin-glucose ratio is obtained after an overnight fast. If it is not diagnostic, the fast may be prolonged for 24-72 hours. The patient must be carefully watched for severe hypoglycemia throughout the fasting period.

Another test frequently used is the tolbutamide test. In this test, 1 gram of tolbutamide is administered intravenously. The normal response consists of a fall of blood glucose that returns to normal in about 2 hours. Marked insulin release and prolonged hypoglycemia with poor recovery is characteristic of patients with insulinoma. With a combination of a prolonged fast and a tolbutamide test, diagnosis can be established in 95% of the patients.

Certain nonpancreatic tumors can cause hypoglycemia. About one-third of these tumors are of mesenchymal origin. Many of these are retroperitoneal and often achieve a large size. The mechanism of hypoglycemia in nonpancreatic tumors is not well understood. In certain cases, ectopic production of insulin or substances with insulin-like activity by the tumors has been reported. Another possibility is that, because of their size and rapid metabolism, these tumors utilize glucose at a rapid rate resulting in hypoglycemia.

The symptoms of *reactive hypoglycemia* are predominantly those of epinephrine release, and neuroglycopenic symptoms generally do not occur. *Alimentary hypoglycemia* is observed almost exclusively in those patients who have had previous gastric surgery. The symptoms of hypoglycemia occur 90-180 minutes after meals. Characteristically, these patients have a rapid absorption of glucose resulting in hyperglycemia usually exceeding 200 mg/dl. Hyperglycemia acts as a powerful stimulus for the rapid release of insulin that precipitously lowers the blood glucose, producing symptoms.

Majority of the individuals with *reactive hypoglycemia of*

early diabetes are obese and have a family history of diabetes mellitus. Symptoms of hypoglycemia occur 3-6 hours after ingestion of food. The mechanism of hypoglycemia appears to be a delayed release of insulin from the β cells, which results in a diabetic glucose tolerance test. In addition 2-4 hours after ingestion of glucose the insulin levels are abnormally high and result in hypoglycemia. As it progresses, glucose intolerance may deteriorate to a frank diabetic state.

Reactive, functional (idiopathic) hypoglycemia is a poorly defined clinical entity. Indeed, the existence of this condition has been questioned following several studies demonstrating that 25-30% of apparently healthy individuals without any hypoglycemic symptoms may exhibit plasma glucose values of 60 mg% or below after a glucose load. These individuals tend to be thin, more often are women, and tend to be emotionally unstable, tense, anxious, and nervous. They may also have somatic manifestations of a hyperactive autonomic nervous system as reflected by gastric hypermotility, excessive nausea and vomiting, and irritable colon. Glucose and insulin response to administration of glucose is normal except for a low blood glucose at 2-4 hours. To make this diagnosis, at least the following criteria should be met:

1. Symptoms occurring in a patient's daily life are associated with hypoglycemia.
2. These symptoms can be reproduced a few hours after administration of glucose or an equivalent mixed meal.
3. They are relieved by administration of glucose.
4. It has been suggested, but not widely accepted, that a rise in serum cortisol and growth hormone levels should be demonstrated in response to the development of hypoglycemia and associated symptoms.

Drug-induced Hypoglycemia

Perhaps the most common cause of hypoglycemia is insulin induced. This may result from an overdose of insulin prescribed by the physician, or by factitious administration of insulin by the patient. The onset of hypoglycemic symptoms depends on the type of insulin the patient is taking. With regular insulin, these symptoms appear in 4-6 hours. Reactions from excessive intermediate insulin given before breakfast usually occur in the late afternoon, and those from long-acting insulin may occur at night or even early the next morning. Symptoms usually consist of an adrenalin response and may become persistent if not treated. These symptoms include headache, night sweats, nausea and vomiting, mental confusion, and drowsiness. Coma may sometimes follow. Factitious administration of insulin can be encountered in patients who have access to the drug. These patients are emotionally disturbed and may require extensive psychiatric evaluation. Presence of insulin antibodies in individuals who have not received insulin is an evidence of exogenous insulin administration. As mentioned previously, C peptide is secreted in equimolar concentrations along with insulin. If hypoglycemia is due to excessive production of insulin, both insulin and C peptide are increased. On the other hand, if hypoglycemia is due to exogenous insulin administration, the C peptide levels are suppressed. Therefore, low blood sugar accompanied by high insulin levels (due to exogenous insulin administration) but a low C peptide level is strong evidence of exogenous administration of insulin.

Because of their ability to increase insulin secretion, sulfonylurea drugs frequently produce hypoglycemia. Malnutrition and the presence of hepatic and renal disease predispose to the development of hypoglycemia, which usually occurs due to these drugs. Hypoglycemia resulting from sulfonylurea drugs may be prolonged and severe.

Seventy percent of all drug-induced hypoglycemias occur due to alcohol alone or its association with insulin or sulfonylurea. Alcohol-induced hypoglycemia occurs in previously fasting individuals and may be severe in alcoholic subjects. The mechanism of action appears to be the inhibition of several reactions responsible for neoglucogenesis.

TREATMENT

The treatment of hypoglycemia depends upon the cause. If an insulinoma is diagnosed, selective celiac angiography may be able to locate the tumor in 30-70% of the cases; in others, the tumors are not visualized due to their small size. Surgery is curative if the tumor is removed. The tumors that cannot be removed or have metastasized may be managed by drug therapy. Both diazoxide and phenytoin have been shown to reduce insulin output from the tumor. Streptozotocin has been tried with some success for malignant insulinomas.

Alimentary hypoglycemia can be managed by small, frequent feedings and carbohydrate restriction. Anticholinergic drugs by delaying stomach emptying, and phenformin by decreasing the rate of absorption of glucose, have been found to be useful. The reactive hypoglycemia of diabetes is treated by a program of diabetic diet and weight reduction. If a diagnosis of idiopathic hypoglycemia is made, carbohydrate restriction and protein-rich snacks at frequent intervals are generally useful for symptomatic relief.

The treatment of drug induced hypoglycemia is directed towards the offending drug, e.g., decrease in insulin dosage, avoidance of alcohol, or discontinuation of a potentiating drug. It should be emphasized that hypoglycemia due to Sulfonylurea drugs may be prolonged. Patients who develop hypoglycemia while on these drugs should be hospitalized and treated with intravenous glucose until stable (as long as 4 to 5 days in some patients).

OBESITY

Obesity, or excess body fat, is the most common nutritional disorder in the population of industrialized and affluent countries. There are several ways to measure body fat. Techniques like isotope dilution are available to directly measure body fat, and indirect measurements are employed to make a diagnosis of massive obesity. Tables of ideal body weight compiled by insurance companies, or measurement of skinfold thickness, can also be employed to determine body fatness. A useful rule to determine ideal body weight is that, at a height of 60 inches, the desirable weight for women and men is 100 and 106 pounds, respectively, For each additional inch of height, five pounds are added for women and six pounds for men. Using these somewhat arbitrary criteria of ideal body weights and skinfold thickness, several studies have attempted to obtain an estimate of obesity. In one study, when obesity was defined as excess weight of 30% of more, 15% of men and 20% of women were found to be obese.

ETIOLOGY

Obesity is a symptom rather than a disease and has multiple etiologies.

1. *Exogenous.* Ingestion of excess calories compared to the calories needed is the most common cause of obesity.
2. *Genetic.* It is a clinical observation that children of obese parents have a ten times greater chance of being obese compared to the children of nonobese parents, suggesting a genetic cause for obesity. However, in obese families it is difficult to separate the genetic influences from the eating habits of the family.
3. *Hypothalamic.* Animal experiments have shown that the ventromedial area of the hypothalamus functions as a satiety center, and injury to this area results in hyperphagia and obesity. A few cases of hypothalamic injury in humans have resulted in obesity, but this is rare. However, it has been suggested that there may be a dysfunction of the satiety center among the obese and their eating habits may be controlled by external factors rather than endogenous satiety.
4. *Endocrine causes.* Hypothyroidism and Cushing's disease are often associated with a slight degree of weight gain. The latter also results in redistribution of body fat and, in the former, other clinical features of hypothyroidism are usually evident. It should be emphasized that these endocrine causes do not result in massive obesity. Only hypothyroid patients lose weight on thyroid; therefore, therapy with thyroid hormone has no place in the treatment of exogenous obesity. Patients with hyperinsulinemia often learn to eat frequently (to avoid hypoglycemia) and become obese. The weight gain, however, is a result of excessive caloric intake rather than hyperinsulinemia.

Morphologically, all human obesity is characterized by an increase in the size of adipocytes (hypertrophic type). Massively obese individuals with an early onset of obesity typically also have hyperplasia of adipocytes (hyperplastic type). The number of adipocytes may also be increased in some individuals with the late onset of obesity.

HEALTH CONSEQUENCES OF OBESITY

Vascular Diseases

Data obtained from insurance companies suggest that the mortality among obese individuals is increased by 1.5 for men, and 1.47 in women, at all ages. Diabetes mellitus, gallbladder disease, and cardiovascular disease are the major causes of excess mortality. Similar data also show that, in patients who lost weight and maintained it, life expectancy improved to a standard risk. In the Framingham study, weight gain was associated with an increase of serum lipids, a rise of blood pressure, impairment of glucose tolerance test, and a slight increase in uric acid. The obese had double the incidence of brain infarction and congestive heart failure and a distinct, but more moderate, increase in the incidence of coronary artery disease. It was also observed that the effect of obesity in increasing cardiovascular disease was greater in women than men; this effect diminished with advancing age. However, much of the effect of obesity may be mediated through other risk factors.

Alterations in Pulmonary Functions

A decrease in expiratory reserve volume along with increased oxygen consumption due to more labored breathing may be observed. Some obese patients also show a decreased sensitivity of the respiratory center that may play a role in the development of the pickwickian syndrome.

Diabetes Mellitus

Diabetes mellitus can be precipitated by an increase in body weight. In one study of 73,000 respondents, less than 1% of normal weight women aged 25-44 had diabetes mellitus, whereas 7% of those who were 100% overweight were diabetic. Even moderate degrees of weight loss result in improvement of carbohydrate tolerance.

Toxemia of Pregnancy

There is an increase in the incidence of toxemia in pregnancy among obese women. The duration of labor is also prolonged. In one study, 5.5% of obese women required cesarean section compared, to only 0.7% in normal women.

Social Implications

Although the medical risks of obesity are apparent, many patients are more concerned about the social stigma attached to obesity. It has been associated with discrimination in social interactions, admission to schools, and in obtaining employment.

HORMONAL ABNORMALITIES

Many hormonal abnormalities have been associated with obesity.

Insulin

Increased plasma insulin levels in the fasting state and in response to insulin secretagogues are present in many patients. Hyperplasia of β cells resulting in an increase in the total β cell mass has been demonstrated.

Obesity is also associated with a decrease in sensitivity to endogenous and exogenous insulin, probably due to a decrease in the number of insulin receptors.

Glucagon

Studies of glucagon have produced conflicting results. Although the basal glucagon levels in most studies are normal, high normal or even low levels after stimulation with various amino acids have been reported. In any event, glucagon does not appear to contribute in a major way to the insulin resistance of obesity.

Growth Hormone

Suppressed basal growth hormone levels that do not stimulate adequately with various stimuli (exercise, arginine) are commonly present in obesity.

Adrenal Corticosteroids

The adrenal function is normal in obesity, although some laboratory tests may indicate aberrations. The total cortisol production and 24-hour excretion of 17-hydroxysteroids is frequently increased. However, when the quantity of 17-hydroxysteroids excreted is related to the body surface area or creatinine excretion, it is in the normal range. The plasma cortisol, excretion of free cortisol, and the response to a standard dexamethasone suppression test are normal.

Reproductive System

Although the menarche in obese females often occurs at a younger age, subsequent menstrual periods are more often irregular. Lower FSH levels in the preovulatory phase, and failure of progesterone to rise normally in the second half of the menstrual cycle, have also been observed in obese women.

It should be mentioned that almost all the hormonal abnormalities appear to be consequences of obesity rather than of pathogenetic significance since these abnormalities revert to normal following weight loss and can be reproduced by induction of experimental obesity.

TREATMENT

Management of obesity is difficult and the results generally poor. Many fad diets for weight reduction have appeared from time to time, most of which have proved no better than previous ones. Some have proved dangerous and have been banned, such as the liquid protein diet. Prior to institution of any therapeutic program, the physician must have a detailed discussion with the patient regarding the patient's need and motivation to lose weight. This should include the patient's eating patterns, especially the circumstances under which the patient tends to eat more, and the previous dietary programs should be discussed. It needs to be pointed out to the patient that no weight change will occur if caloric intake and consumption are kept in balance. A need to decrease caloric intake and an effort to increase consumption by increased physical activity should be discussed. The goals for weight loss should be realistic. These can be determined approximately by determining the negative caloric balance. It takes 10 days to lose 1 kg if the daily negative caloric balance is 900 calories, as each gram of fat provides 9 calories. To encourage patients to follow the prescribed diet, various behavior modification techniques have been tried. For similar reasons, patients in group therapy organized in the clinics or by lay groups may do somewhat better than patients attempting to lose weight on their own. A more rapid weight loss can be achieved by a complete fast, but this is a drastic and dangerous way to lose weight. If it is decided to attempt a complete fast, it should be carried out under careful medical supervision. Patients should be carefully watched for electrolyte depletion, which can have serious consequences. Elevation of uric acid can precipitate acute gout in some patients.

Various anorectic drugs have been tried as adjunctive measures. Although these drugs appear effective in short-term studies, no long-term studies have been performed. A large number of these drugs are amphetamine congeners with substantial potential for abuse. For those patients who fail to lose

For those patients who fail to lose weight on a medical program, a surgical approach has been recommended. These operations consist of anastomosing jejunum to terminal ileum, thus bypassing a large segment of small bowel. Following operation, most patients will lose weight, but the operation is associated with approximately 3% operative morality and a high incidence of complications, which include pulmonary emboli, wound infection, and gastrointestinal hemorrhage. An additional serious complication is the development of liver disease. Rarely, the liver disease may progress to hepatic failure. Almost all patients continue to have diarrhea postoperatively, but the majority tolerate it well. Minor degrees of electrolyte abnormalities and hypoproteinemia are present in 40-80% patients; a few develop severe electrolyte abnormalities and arthritis. Urinary calculi also develop with increased frequency. Approximately 4% of patients require reversal of the operation for management of these complications. The operation should be prescribed only after a careful consideration by the patient, the internist, and the surgeon. In order to avoid the complications of intestinal bypass, gastric bypass has been developed. In this operation, 90% of the stomach is left in continuity with the duodenum, and the remaining 10% is anastomosed to jejunum. In the postoperative period, patients note an early satiety after meals and there is a steady weight loss that averages about 2-2.5 lb/week. Although electrolyte abnormalities and liver disease have not been observed after this operation, marginal ulcers and wound infections have been significant problems.

LIPID METABOLISM

Triglycerides, cholesterol, and phospholipids circulate in the body in a soluble form by binding to proteins. This complex, known as a lipoprotein, contains varying amounts of lipid and protein with resulting alterations in electrical charge and density. Using ultracentrifugation or electrophoresis, lipoproteins can be subdivided into the following classes: chylomicrons, very-low-density lipoproteins (VLDL, or pre-β), low-density lipoproteins (LDL, or β), and high-density lipoproteins (HDL, or α). Chylomicrons consist of 80-95% triglyceride, with the remainder being cholesterol, phospholipid, and protein. These particles are synthesized in the intestinal cells and carry dietary triglycerides into the venous circulation with entry via the thoracic duct. The next largest particles are VLDL, composed of 60-80% endogenous triglycerides synthesized in the liver. Both chylomicrons and VLDL are acted upon by lipoprotein lipase with a resulting free triglyceride that can be hydrolyzed to yield free fatty acids and glycerol, capable of crossing all membranes and being utilized for energy storage for future use.

The removal of triglyceride and some of the protein from VLDL leads to the formation of intermediate-density lipoprotein (IDL). This molecule is further processed, most likely in the liver, to form LDL. LDL contains approximately 50% cholesterol and 25% protein, and constitutes almost one-half of the circulating plasma cholesterol.

HDL is the heaviest lipoprotein by weight and contains 20% cholesterol, 30% phospholipid, and approximately 50% protein. HDL has recently been shown to correlate inversely with atherosclerotic heart disease and increase after alcohol intake and exercise. HDL is secreted by the liver and interacts with the enzyme lecithin-cholesterol acyltransferase (LCAT). HDL has recently been divided, for classification purposes, into two major proteins, Apo A-I and Apo A-II. Apo A-I helps activate LCAT to generate cholesterol esters from free cholesterol and lecithin. Apo B is the major protein of plasma LDL, although it is also found in VLDL and chylomicrons. Apo C-I, Apo C-II, and Apo C-III are low-molecular-weight proteins present in HDL, VLDL, and chylomicrons.

Cholesterol is stored in cells in the form of cholesterol esters and is hydrolyzed to yield free cholesterol. Triglycerides are stored primarily in adipocytes until they are needed for energy production.

LIPID DISORDERS

Lipid disorders can be classified as either primary or secondary. The primary disorders are either inherited or idiopathic. Secondary disorders result from multiple causes including abnormalities in insulin, thyroid, estrogen, and catecholamines. Certain drugs and diet may increase lipid levels. Stress also can alter the lipids, leading to increased triglycerides and decreased cholesterol, a finding often seen for 4-6 weeks after an acute myocardial infarction. The causes of secondary hyperlipidemia are listed in Table 5. The lipid disorders can be classified into five types, based on the specific lipoprotein abnormality. Although there is less emphasis on this classification in recent years, a thorough knowledge of this classification system enables one to understand more fully various clinical pathologic stages. Although normal levels of plasma lipids cannot be precisely defined, a fasting cholesterol is considered to be elevated if over 245 mg/100 ml. A useful rough estimate is 200 mg/100 ml plus age. Fasting triglycerides over 150 mg/100 ml are considered abnormal, although recent data have also shown a linear increase with age.

Table 5. Causes of Secondary Hyperlipidemia

1. Diabetes mellitus
2. Exogenous obesity
3. Alcohol
4. Hypothyroidism
5. Chronic pancreatitis
6. Chronic renal disease (e.g., nephrotic syndrome)
7. Chronic liver disease (e.g., biliary cirrhosis)
8. Dysglobulinemia
9. Contraceptive pills
10. Other endocrinopathies
11. Porphyria
12. Others

Type I

This rare disorder is characterized by an excess in circulating chylomicrons. Chylomicronemia can result from eating, or from an abnormality in the clearance of these lipoproteins. It is imperative that the patient undergo a 16-hour fast prior to determining a lipid profile, since temporary chylomicronemia may occur normally after meals. Chylomicron elevation beyond this period is abnormal and indicates an abnormality in clearance resulting from an inherited deficiency in the enzyme lipoprotein lipase. Because heparin in unaffected patients releases these enzymes from their bound sites in blood vessels, a small intravenous injection of heparin with measurement of this enzyme before and after can serve a diagnostic function.

Type II

This abnormality has been divided into two subgroups: IIa is characterized by elevation of LDL; IIb by elevations of both LDL and VLDL. Perhaps the most common of the primary hyperlipidemias, it is estimated to be present in one of every 200 live births. It has a high association with atherosclerosis and coronary artery disease. It appears that the disorder is inherited as an autosomal dominant trait with variable penetrance. Patients homozygous for the dominant trait develop clinical symptoms early in life with early mortality. The heterozygous form of the disease is usually detected later in life and is less severe. An abnormality in HMG CoA reductase regulations appears to be the key factor in this inherited lipid abnormality.

Type III

Type III hyperlipidemia becomes manifest in adults, with the first presenting symptoms often being angina pectoris. Abnormal carbohydrate tolerance is common. Both cholesterol and triglycerides are elevated. Xanthomas are described as tuberoeruptive, tuberous, and plane. Type III is best diagnosed electrophoretically by noting a broad band in the β region, leading to the name broad-β-band disease. An elevation in total Apo-E concentration, or an absolute absence of Apo E-III, is presently the best way to diagnose Type III hyperlipidemia.

Type IV

This disorder is characterized by elevated VLDL. Because many patients with Type IV are obese and have relative insulin resistance, some feel that fatty acids produced by VLDL breakdown are unable to enter the adipose cells, and are thus transported to the liver by albumin producing even more VLDL. Serum cholesterol is moderately increased and triglycerides are elevated. Patients present with eruptive xanthomas and, occasionally, with abdominal pain if the triglycerides are very high. There is a slight increase in premature vascular disease. Diabetes is very frequently associated.

Type V

This represents a combination of Types I and IV, with high levels of chylomicrons and VLDL. This lipid disorder is rare and the etiology uncertain. Often the patient presents with abdominal pain, although it characteristically occurs in adults and not in children, as does Type I. Both Types I and V exhibit lipemia retinalis. Blood triglyceride levels may reach 5,000 mg/100 ml or more. It appears that this entity results from a deficiency in lipoprotein lipase impeding chylomicron clearance from the plasma. Although the lipase is reportedly absent in Type I, it is present in Type V but appears to function inadequately.

In recent years, it has been shown that elevated HDL may have beneficial effects. There is an inverse relationship between HDL cholesterol and coronary artery disease. Exercise, estrogens, and a small amount of alcohol consumed daily are known to increase HDL levels. Table 6 summarizes the various primary hyperlipoproteinemias.

Polygenic Hypercholesterolemia

Combined hyperlipidemia is commonly found, and the clinician must recognize and treat this disorder appropriately. This disorder is thought to result from multiple genes interacting with environmental factors. Polygenic hypercholesterolemia and sporadic hypertriglyceridemia (see below) are together the most common form of lipid disorder, reportedly occurring in 3-4% of the population. Although atherosclerotic disease is more common in this entity, pathology occurs later than is seen in type II lipid disorders.

Sporadic Hypertriglyceridemia

This disorder is characterized by elevations in plasma triglycerides without any apparent genetic, drug, or disease linkage. Only recently defined, the exact significance and prevalence in the population is still not known.

Table 6. Primary Hyperlipoproteinemias

Type	*I*	*II*	*III*	*IV*	*V*
Elevated level of	Chylomicrons	LDL (β)	Abnormal LDL	VLDL (pre-β)	Chylomicrons and VLDL
Other description	Exogenous (fat-induced) hyperlipemia	Essential hypercholesterolemia	Broad β disease	Endogenous (carbohydrate induced) hyperlipemia	Mixed hyperlipemia
Prevalence	Rare	Relatively common	Relatively uncommon	Most common	Uncommon
Appearance of plasma after overnight refrigeration	Creamy layer over infranate on standing	Clear, or slightly opalescent	Turbid, moderately lactescent	Turbid, lactescent	Creamy layer over milky infranate on standing
Cholesterol elevation	+	+++	++	0-+	+
Triglyceride elevation	+++	0-+	+	++	+++
Clinical features	Abdominal pain; hepatosplenomegaly; eruptive xanthomas; lipemia retinalis; pancreatitis lipoprotein lipase absent	Tendon and tuberous xanthomas; accelerated atherosclerosis	Planar (palms) and tuberous xanthomas; abnormal glucose tolerance; accelerated vascular disease	Abnormal glucose tolerance; accelerated vascular disease; eruptive xanthomas; occasionally, abdominal pain	Abdominal pain; eruptive xanthomas
Treatment	Low-fat diet	Restrict dietary cholesterol and saturated fats; cholestyramine, nicotinic acid	Low saturated fats; clofibrate	Low carbohydrate diet; exercise	Low fat, reducing diet; avoid alcohol; clofibrate, nicotinic acid; plasmaphoresis (?)

TREATMENT

Although it is generally agreed that high levels of circulating cholesterol (LDL) are associated with a higher incidence of atherosclerosis, debate continues as to how and when to treat. Once atherosclerotic heart disease is established, evidence suggests that benefits of lipid reduction are insignificant. Primary attention must therefore be directed toward early detection of monogenic hyperlipidemia. Drug therapy is probably best reserved for persons who have not benefited from diet, who have not already had myocardial infarction, and who are showing developing clinical signs of hyperlipidemia.

Diet

A low-cholesterol, low-saturated fatty acids, low-calorie reducing diet is recommended until ideal body weight is reached; after this, a low-fat maintenance diet is used. These should reduce both plasma cholesterol and triglyceride concentrations. Exercise is a key adjunct, especially for type IV, and persons with hypertriglyceridemia should limit intake of alcohol and simple sugars. Diet therapy has only limited benefit and can be frustrating to both physician and patient.

Lipid-Reducing Drugs

Clofibrate (Atromid-S) primarily is useful to lower plasma triglycerides, although it may lower plasma cholesterol to a lesser degree. It works mainly by decreasing cholesterol synthesis. In addition, it appears to inhibit fructase 1-citrate cleavage enzyme, acetyl CoA carboxylase, 6-diphosphate addolase, and glucose 6-phosphate dehydrogenase, resulting in reduced synthesis of glycerol and fatty acids. It is not useful in type I lipid disorders, or in familial hypercholesterolemia. Side effects include an increased incidence of gallstones.

Nicotinic acid, also known as niacin, lowers both cholesterol and triglyceride levels by decreasing the synthesis of VLDL and consequently LDL, and can be effective in all but type I hyperlipidemia. Given in a dosage of 3-6 grams daily in divided doses after meals, side effects often prevent long-term use. Flushing and pruritis occur 1-2 hours after each dose; however, in most patients, these side effects disappear after several weeks and some advocate starting the drug in a dose of 100 mg three times a day to minimize these early symptoms.

Cholestyramine (Questran), the drug of choice in familial hypercholesterolemia, is the chloride salt of a basic anion-exchange resin that binds bile salts tightly, thus interfering with the enterohepatic circulation to cause the loss of neutral steroids and bile acids. Because of a compensatory increase in HMG CoA reductase, cholestyramine is effective only in large doses that impair the maximal ability to synsynthesize cholesterol. Triglycerides are not appreciably affected by this agent. The recommended dosage is 24-32 grams per day given in two or four doses. Major side effects include cramps, diarrhea, or constipation. Colestipol (Colestid) is very similar to cholestyramine in its action. Probucol (Lorelco) and gemfibrozil (Lopid) are newer agents useful in lowering serum cholesterol and triglycerides, respectively.

QUESTIONS

More than one answer may be correct

1. Administration of 500 μg TRH intravenously to a 25-year-old healthy young man will be expected to cause
   A. increase in serum TSH level
   B. increase in serum estradiol level
   C. increase in serum growth hormone
   D. increase in serum FSH
   E. increase in serum prolactin
2. Administration of somatostatin (growth hormone release inhibiting hormone) has been noted to inhibit release of
   A. growth hormone
   B. insulin
   C. glucagon
   D. gastrin
   E. TSH in response to TRH

3.1. A 34-year-old white woman took oral contraceptives for 6 years. She discontinued taking them about a year ago. She has not had a menstrual period since she stopped taking the oral contraceptive agents. She does not have any other symptoms, and physical examination is entirely normal. Which of the following laboratory tests would you consider appropriate?
   A. serum estradiol, FSH, and LH
   B. serum prolactin
   C. T_4 and T_3 resin uptake
   D. serum cortisol at 8:00 AM and 5:00 PM
   E. serum growth hormone

3.2. All the tests were reported normal, except serum prolactin was elevated to 250 ng/ml (normal 5-22 ng/ml). The most likely diagnosis is
   A. elevated prolactin due to long use of oral contraceptives
   B. elevated prolactin due to occult hypothyroidism; serum TSH should be obtained
   C. patient is taking drugs but she has not informed her physician
   D. prolactin-producing adenoma
   E. laboratory error

4. A 24-year-old white female delivered a full-term, normal infant about 9 months ago. The delivery was complicated by postpartum hermorrhage for which she required several transfusions. She was not able to nurse the infant because of absence of milk in her breasts. Since the delivery, she has been feeling weak, lethargic, and cold. Physical examination showed a pale-appearing, ill-looking woman. Breasts were normal sized. Axillary hair had been shaved. The pubic hair shaved at the time

of delivery had not regrown. Remainder of the physical examination was normal. Laboratory data included a serum T_4 of 1.2 μg/dl (normal 5-11 μg/dl); T_3 resin uptake was 22% (normal 25-35%); serum TSH was 2 mIu/ml (normal up to 10 mIu/ml; serum cortisol at 8:00 AM was 1.0 μg/dl (normal 5-20 μg/dl); serum ACTH was 20 pg/ml (normal up to 80 pg/ml). With ACTH infusion, plasma cortisol increased to 35 μg/dl. These findings are suggestive of

A. primary adrenal insufficiency
B. primary hypothyroidism
C. ACTH deficiency
D. combined primary adrenal, and thyroid insufficiency (Schmidt's syndrome)
E. TSH deficiency

5.1. A 37-year-old white female has been complaining of increased thirst and polyuria. She had previously been in good health. There is no history of head injury or drug ingestion. The patient's brother has insulin-requiring diabetes. The physical examination was normal. The diagnostic possibilities at this time include

A. central diabetes insipidus
B. diabetes mellitus
C. compulsive water drinking
D. nephrogenic diabetes insipidus
E. none of the above

5.2. A fasting blood glucose was 75 mg/dl. Urinalysis revealed a specific gravity of 1001, was free of glucose and protein, and microscopic exam was within normal limits. You would now obtain

A. BUN and creatinine
B. serum and urine osmolality
C. glucose tolerance test
D. intravenous pyelogram
E. serum cortisol

5.3. A water deprivation test was performed and the patient was able to concentrate her urine from a baseline of 150 mOsm/kg to a maximum of 895 mOsm/kg. Administration of vasopressin resulted in no further increase of urine osmolality. You would now conclude that the patient has

A. central diabetes insipidus
B. nephrogenic diabetes insipidus
C. compulsive water drinking
D. the test is inclusive and should be repeated
E. the test results are inconclusive and the patient should have a hypertonic saline test

6.1. A 25-year-old white female presents with enlarged thyroid and increased nervousness, and she also complains of being increasingly warm. She is 8 weeks pregnant. On physical examination, there was diffuse and moderate enlargement of the thyroid. Lab data revealed T_4 = 13.5 μg (4.5-11.5 normal), T_3 resin uptake = 22% (normal 25-35%), and T_3 by RIA = 235 ng/ml (normal 120-200 ng/ml). What is the most likely diagnosis?

A. hyperthyroidism
B. hypothyroidism
C. normal thyroid function test compatible with pregnancy

6.2. Two months after her initial visit (she is now 4 months pregnant) she reports that her symptoms have progressed and she has been told that her eyes are beginning to bulge. At this time you would order

A. repeat T_4 and T_3 resin uptake
B. ^{131}I uptake
C. serum TSH
D. TRH test
E. serum HCG

6.3. Based on the clinical findings and more recent lab data, a diagnosis of hyperthyroidism is made. You will now advise

A. immediate subtotal thyroidectomy
B. treatment with potassium iodide
C. treatment with propylthiouracil
D. treatment with radioactive ^{131}I

6.4. She remained well for 2 years following delivery, when her disease relapsed. She was then treated with radioactive iodine. Three years later she returned with heavy menstrual bleeding and excessive tiredness. On exam she was anemic, her skin was dry. Pulse was 60/mm and reflexes were difficult to elicit. Remainder of the physical exam was normal. Which of the following lab tests would you now order?

A. T_4, T_3 resin uptake
B. T_3 by RIA
C. TSH
D. ^{131}I uptake
E. serum TRH

7. A 20-year-old white male had received external radiation for an enlarged thymus in early infancy. He has remained asymptomatic, but on examination there is a solitary firm nodule about 1 cm × 1 cm in the left lobe of the thyroid. On radioisotope scanning, the nodule appeared as a cold area. The most logical approach at this time would be

A. a needle biopsy
B. ultrasonic study of the nodule
C. surgical excision
D. continued follow-up with no treatment
E. continued follow-up with full suppressive doses of levothyroxine

8. Serum calcium levels are influenced by

A. serum pH

B. serum albumin
C. parathyroid hormone
D. diet
E. all the above

9. Causes of hypercalcemia include:
A. excess parathyroid hormone production
B. thiazide usage
C. sarcoidosis
D. Addison's disease
E. all of the above

10. Vitamin D_3 is converted into more biologically active forms in
A. liver
B. kidney
C. intestine
D. parathyroid glands
E. all of the above

11. Osteomalacia may result from
A. deficient vitamin D
B. hypophosphatemia
C. fluoride intoxication
D. phenytoin
E. all of the above

12. Primary aldosteronism is characterized by
A. elevated blood pressure
B. hypokalemia
C. high plasma renin activity
D. low plasma renin activity
E. hyperkalemia

13. Administration of metyrapone results in increased secretion of ACTH by
A. increased secretion of corticotropin-releasing factor
B. inhibition of the enzyme 11β-hydroxylase
C. inhibition of the enzyme 21β-hydroxylase
D. by increasing peripheral metabolism of cortisol
E. none of the above

14.1. A 30-year-old obese white female was noted to have increased blood pressure about 2 years ago. About a year ago, another physician performed a glucose tolerance test and told her it was abnormal. In spite of the fact that she has gained weight, she complains of being weak and has noted a tendency to bruise easily. You are considering obesity and Cushing's syndrome as possible diagnoses. A useful screening procedure would be to obtain
A. plasma cortisol at 8:00 AM
B. plasma cortisol at 8:00 AM, after 1 mg dexamethasone administration on the previous night
C. plasma cortisol at 8:00 AM, after 2 mg dexamethasone administration on the previous night
D. serum ACTH level
E. plasma electrolytes

14.2. Plasma cortisol level failed to suppress after 1 mg dexamethasone, so a 2 mg dexamethasone suppression test was performed. The results of 24-hour urine 17-hydroxysteroids are as follows:

Baseline–16.0 (normal 3-10 mg/24 hr)
After Dexamethasone–0.5 mg q 6 h for 2 days, 2.0 mg

These results are suggestive of
A. Cushing's syndrome due to adrenal adenoma
B. Cushing's syndrome due to pituitary adenoma
C. Cushing's syndrome has been excluded
D. Cushing's syndrome due to factitious intake of steroids
E. the test is inconclusive and she should now have an 8-mg dexamethasone suppression test

15.1. A 22-year-old male had been complaining of not feeling well for the last 2-3 months. He complained of being tired, and he had a decreased appetite. He had two wisdom teeth extracted, following which he developed an abscess and was being treated with antibiotics. He returned to his dentist for extraction of another tooth and nearly fainted after administration of local anesthetic. He was given a liter of 5% glucose and transferred to the hospital. On examination the patient was afebrile but appeared ill and slightly dehydrated. His blood pressure lying down was 90/70 and dropped to 60/? on standing. His skin appeared well-tanned and he stated that he had developed the tan about 6 months ago and had not lost it like he usually did. Serum glucose was 75 mg/dl; Na was 128; K was 5.3; Cl 90 mEq/L; BUN 40 mg/dl. The most likely diagnosis is
A. primary adrenal insufficiency
B. allergic reaction to local anesthetic
C. inappropriate ADH syndrome
D. renal impairment due to use of antibiotics
E. septic shock

15.2. It was suggested that the patient had adrenal insufficiency. To confirm this diagnosis, a blood sample was obtained for assay of cortisol, ACTH, and antiadrenal antibodies. He was then given intravenous fluids and hydrocortisone, and he made an uneventful recovery. Serum cortisol was <1.0 μg/dl; serum ACTH was 350 pg/ml (normal up to 80 pg/ml), obtained before treatment was begun. The results of the antiadrenal antibodies were lost. Based on this information, you will conclude that
A. the patient has primary adrenal insufficiency
B. the patient has secondary adrenal insufficiency
C. the data is inconclusive to make a distinction between primary and secondary adrenal insufficiency
D. results of antiadrenal antibodies are required to

make the distinction between primary and secondary adrenal insufficiency

E. it is necessary to do an ACTH infusion test to make the distinction between primary and secondary adrenal insufficiency

16. The ovum is released from the mature graofian follicle at midcycle
   A. due to FSH release
   B. because of an LH surge from the pituitary
   C. never
   D. twice monthly

17. In men, which of the following serves as a negative feedback to FSH production by the pituitary?
   A. inhibin
   B. testosterone
   C. estrogen
   D. LH

18. Normal spermatogenesis requires
   A. testosterone
   B. FSH
   C. LH
   D. all

19. Insulin inhibits (true or false)
   A. neoglucogenesis
   B. lipolysis
   C. proteolysis
   D. glycogenolysis
   E. peripheral metabolism of glucose

20. Glucagon promotes (true or false)
   A. synthesis of glycogen
   B. lipolysis
   C. neoglucogenesis
   D. insulin secretion
   E. ketogenesis

21. The National Diabetes Data Group recommendations suggest that the diagnosis of diabetes mellitus can be made if one or more of the following are present: (true or false)
   A. a fasting plasma glucose of 140 mg/dl or more, on more than one occasion
   B. unequivocal elevations of fasting plasma glucose along with classical symptoms of diabetes
   C. elevated glucose concentration after an oral glucose load
   D. history of having delivered heavy babies
   E. presence of glucose in the urine

22.1. A 50-year-old executive with a strong family history of diabetes, had a glucose tolerance test performed as part of his annual physical examination. His usual diet was estimated to contain 250 g of carbohydrates. He received a 75 g glucose load, and the results of the glucose tolerance test are as follows (values are plasma glucose in mg/dl):

Fasting	½ hour	1 hour	2 hour
130	180	220	250

Based on the criteria suggested by the National Diabetes Data Group, you will classify this glucose tolerance test as
   A. normal
   B. diabetic
   C. impaired
   D. nondiagnostic

22.2. Two years later, this patient began to complain of polyuria and polydipsia. He had gained 25 lb in the interim. His fasting blood glucose was 215 mg/dl. Which of the following statements are true?
   A. He has type I diabetes mellitus.
   B. He should be started on a weight reduction diet.
   C. He should be given 10 units regular insulin and hospitalized.
   D. He should begin taking oral hypoglycemic agents, otherwise his disease will progress.
   E. With continued weight reduction, his glucose levels may decrease sufficiently so that he will only require dietary therapy for his management.

23. Which of the following is true for the sulfonylurea group of drugs?
   A. They may be used in selected patients with type II diabetes.
   B. Given acutely, they increase the secretion of insulin.
   C. They have been shown to increase the number of insulin receptors.
   D. Some of these agents may produce hyponatremia.
   E. Some of these agents may have an antabuse-like effect.

24. Match the following. The statements may be true for both (A) and (B).
   A. diabetic ketoacidosis
   B. hyperosmolar coma
      1. usually seen in older patients, often with no prior history of diabetes
      2. elevated blood glucose
      3. pH <7.2
      4. serum ketones–none to 1+
      5. plasma insulin–none detected

25. Which of the following statements regarding diabetic ketoacidosis are true?
   A. Low-dose continuous infusion is as effective as large doses of insulin.

B. All patients should receive sodium bicarbonate soon after admission.
C. Kussmaul's breathing is pathognomonic of this diagnosis
D. serum K^+ is always low
E. an anion gap is always present

26. A 28-year-old woman with insulin-requiring diabetes is scheduled for elective cesarean section. She was taking 48 units of Lente insulin in the AM and 12 units in the PM until the previous day. Her prepregnancy insulin requirements were 25 units daily. A fasting plasma glucose is 98 mg/dl on the morning of surgery. She should receive on the morning of surgery
A. no insulin
B. same dose of insulin as on the previous day
C. double the dose of insulin as she received on the previous day
D. $\frac{1}{2}$ to $\frac{2}{3}$ the amount of insulin she received before pregnancy
E. double the amount of insulin she received before pregnancy

27. Which of the following statements regarding pregnancy in the diabetic patient is/are true?
A. There is a prompt fall in insulin requirements immediately postpartum.
B. The renal threshold for glucose is decreased in pregnancy.
C. Insulin requirements increase during the second and third trimesters of pregnancy.
D. Transient maternal hypoglycemia does not appear to affect fetal survival.
E. Insulin requirements usually decrease during early pregnancy.

28. A 23-year-old white female nurse came to the Emergency Room complaining of palpitation, nervousness, and excessive perspiration. An electrocardiogram was normal except for frequent PVCs. She was given intravenous glucose, and the symptoms improved. She had two similar episodes at work during the next week. She could not identify any precipitating factors, and there was no relationship with food intake. She was hospitalized and, after a 60-hour fast, developed similar symptoms. A blood sample obtained at that time showed

Plasma glucose	23 mg/dl	(60-120 mg/dl)[a]
Serum insulin	245 μu/ml	(<20 μu/ml)[a]
Serum C peptide	<0.05 ng/ml	(0.5 to 2ng/ml)
Serum growth hormone	20 ng/ml	(5-20, depending on the time of the day)[a]
Serum cortisol	22 μg/dl	(up to 10 in women)[a]

[a]Values in parenthesis indicate normal range.

Which of the following is the most likely diagnosis?
A. insulinoma
B. factitious administration of insulin
C. reactive hypoglycemia of early diabetes
D. hypoglycemia due to adrenal insufficiency
E. idiopathic reactive hypoglycemia

29. Obesity has been associated with many endocrine abnormalities. Which of the following are true?
A. low plasma insulin levels
B. low growth hormone levels
C. high plasma insulin levels
D. decreased T_4 and T_3 resin uptake
E. decreased excretion of 17-hydroxysteroids in 24-hour urine

30. The rate-limiting enzyme in cholesterol synthesis is
A. HMG CoA reductase
B. Apo-A-I
C. Apo C-II
D. lipoprotein lipase
E. lipase

31. Side-effects of nicotinic acid include
A. flushing
B. pruritus
C. anemia
D. constipation
E. diarrhea

32. An elevation in total Apo-E concentration helps diagnose
A. type I hyperlipidemia
B. type II hyperlipidemia
C. type III hyperlipidemia
D. type IV hyperlipidemia
E. pancreatitis

ANSWERS

1. A, E
2. All are correct
3.1. A and B are correct.
3.2. D
4. C, E
5.1. A, B, C, D
5.2. B
5.3. C
6.1. C
6.2. A
6.3. C
6.4. A, C
7. C
8. E
9. E
10. A, B
11. E
12. A, B, D
13. B
14.1. B
14.2. C
15.1. A

15.2. A
16. B
17. A
18. B
19. A: T
B: T
C: T
D: T
E: F
20. A: F
B: T
C: T
D: T
E: T
21. A: T
B: T
C: T
D: F
E: F

22.1. B
22.2. B, E
23. All are correct
24. 1: B
2: A, B
3: A
4: B
5: A
25. A, E
26. D
27. All are correct
28. B
29. B, C
30. A
31. A, B
32. C

BIBLIOGRAPHY

TEXTBOOKS

Bondy PK, Rosenberg LE (eds): *Metabolic Control & Disease*, ed. 8. Philadelphia, WB Saunders Co, 1980.

Marble A, White P, Bradley RF, Krall LP: Joslin's *Diabetes Mellitus*, ed. 11. Lea & Febiger, 1971.

Rasmussen H, Bordier P: *The Physiological and Cellular Basis of Metabolic Bone Disease.* Baltimore, The Williams & Wilkins Co, 1974.

Rifkin H, Raskin P, Bowie MD (eds): *Diabetes Mellitus*, vol V. Robert J Brady Co, 1981.

Williams RH (ed): *Textbook of Endocrinology*, ed. 5. Philadelphia: WB Saunders, 1974.

Yen SS, Jaffe RB (eds): *Reproductive Endocrinology*. Philadelphia: WB Saunders, 1978.

ARTICLES AND MONOGRAPHS

Pituitary Gland and Hypothalamus

Cobb WE, Spare S, Reichlin S: Neurogenic diabetes insipidus: Management with DDAVP (1-desamino-8-D arginine vasopressin). *Ann Intern Med* 88(2):183-188, 1978.

Geheb M, Cox M: Renal effects of demeclocycline. Editorial *JAMA* 243(24):2519-2520, 1980.

Guillemin R, Gerich JE: Somatostatin: Physiological and clinical significance. *Ann Rev Med* 27:379-388, 1976.

Kleinberg DL, Noel GL, Rantz AG: Galactorrhea: A study of 235 cases, including 48 with pituitary tumors. *N Engl J Med* 296(11):589-600, 1977.

Krieger DT, Martin JB: Brain peptides. *N Engl J Med* 304(15-16):876-885, 944-951, 1981.

Miller M, Dalakos T, Moses AM, et al: Recognition of partial defects in antidiuretic hormone secretion. *Ann Intern Med* 73:721-729, 1970.

Moses AM, Miller M, Streeten DHP: Pathophysiologic and pharmacologic alterations in the release and action of ADH. *Metabolism* 25(6):697-721, 1976.

Wilson CB, Dempsey LC: Transsphenoidal microsurgical removal of 250 pituitary adenomas. *J Neurosurg* 48(1):13-22, 1978.

Thyroid Gland

Brown J, Chopra IJ, Cornell JS, Hershman JM, Solomon DH, Uller RP, Van Herle AJ: Thyroid physiology in health and disease. *Ann Int Med* 81:68-81, 1974.

Burrow GN: Hyperthyroidism during pregnancy. *N Engl J Med* 298(3): 150-153, 1978.

Evered D, Hall R (eds): Hypothyroidism and goiter. *Clin Endocrinol Metab* 8(1):1-245, 1979.

Mazzaferri EL, Young RL, Oertel JE, Kemmerer WT, Page CP: Papillary thyroid carcinoma: The impact of therapy in 576 patients. *Medicine* (Baltimore) 56(3):171-196, 1977.

Schneider AB, Favus MJ, Stachura ME, Arnold J, Arnold MJ, Frohman LA: Incidence, prevalence and characteristics of radiation-induced thyroid tumors. *Am J Med* 64(2):243-252, 1978.

Volpe R (ed): Thyrotoxicosis. *Clin Endocrinol Metab* 7(1):3-29, 1978.

Walfish PG, Hazani E, Strawbridge HTG, Miskin M, Rosen IB: Combined ultrasound and needle aspiration cytology in the management of hypofunctioning thyroid nodule. *Ann Intern Med* 87(3):270-274, 1977.

Parathyroid Gland and Calcium Metabolism

Aurbach GD, Keutman HT, Niall HD, Tregear GW, O'Riordan JLH, Marcus R, Marx SJ, Potts JT Jr: Structure, synthesis and mechanism of action of parathyroid hormone. *Recent Prog Horm Res* 28:353-398, 1972.

DeLuca HF: Parathyroid hormone as a trophic hormone for 1,25-dihydroxy-vitamin D_3, the metabolically active form of vitamin D. *N Engl J Med* 287:250-251, 1972.

Mallette LE, Bilezikian JP, Heath DA, Aurbach GD: Primary hyperparathyroidism: Clinical and biochemical features. *Medicine* 53(2): 127-146, 1974.

Nusynowitz ML, Frame B, Kalb FO: The spectrum of the hypoparathyroid states; a classification based on physiologic principles. *Medicine* 55(2):105-119, 1976.

Adrenal Cortex and Medulla

Axelrod L: Glucocorticoid therapy. *Medicine* (Baltimore) 55(1):39-65, 1976.

Engelman K: Phaeochromocytoma. *Clin Endocrinol Metab* 6(3):769-797, 1977.

Gwinup G, Johnson B: Clinical testing of hypothalamic-pituitary-adrenocrotical system in states of hypo- and hypercortisolism. *Metabolism* 24(6):777-791, 1975.

Knochel JP: The syndrome of hypereninemic hypoaldosteronism. *Ann Rev Med* 30:145-53, 1979.

Mitchell JR, Taylor AA, Pool JL, Lake CR, et al: Renin aldosterone profiling in hypertension. *Ann Intern Med* 87(5):596-612, 1977.

Nelson DH: The adrenal cortex: Physiological function and disease. *Major Probl Intern Med* 18:iii-xii, 1-281, 1980.

Scott HW Jr, Liddle GW, Mulherin JL Jr, et al: Surgical experience with Cushing's disease. *Ann Surg* 185(5):524-534, 1977.

Ovary

Abraham GE, Odell WD, Swerdloff RS, Hopper K: Simultaneous radioimmunoassay of plasma FSH, LH, progesterone, 17-hydroxyprogesterone, and estradiol-17 beta during the menstrual cycle. *J Clin Endocrinol Metab* 34(2):312-318, 1972.

Besser GM, Edwards CRW: Hirsuitism and virilism. *Clin Endocrii Metab* 1:491-501, 1972.

Gilson MD, Knab DR: Primary amenorrhea: A simplified approach to diagnosis. *Am J Obstet Gynecol* 117:400-406, 1973.

Moghissi KS, Syner FN, Evans TN: Composite picture of the menstrual cycle. *Am J Obstet Gynecol* 114:405-418, 1972.

Testis

Baker HWG, Bremner WJ, Burger HG, De Kretser DM, Dulmanis A, Eddie LW, Hudson B, Keogh EJ, Lee VWK, Rennie GC: Testicular control of follicle-stimulating hormone secretion. *Recent Prog Horm Res* 32:429-476, 1976.

Perez-Palacios G, Jaffe RB: The syndrome of testicular feminization. *Pediatr Clin North Am* 19:653-667, 1972.

Carbohydrate Metabolism and Diabetes Mellitus

Bar RS, Roth J: Insulin receptor status in disease states of man. *Arch Intern Med* 137(4):474-481, 1977.

Fajans SS, Floyd JC Jr: Fasting hypoglycemia in adults. *N Engl J Med* 294(14):766-772, 1976.

Fajans SS, Floyd JC Jr: Heterogeneity in diabetes mellitus. in Freinkel, NE (ed): *Contemporary Metabolism*, vol. 1, pp 235-245. New York: Plenum, 1979.

Gossain VV, Matute ML, Kalkoff RK: Relative influence of obesity and diabetes on plasma alpha cell glucagon. *J Clin Endocrinol Metab* 38: 238-443, 1974.

Jarrett RJ, Keen H, Grabauskas V: The W.H.O multinational study of vascular disease in diabetes: 1. General discription. *Diab Care* 2(2): 175-186, 1979.

Jarrett RJ, Keen H: The W.H.O. multinational study of vascular disease in diabetes: 3. Microvascular disease. *Diab Care* 2(2):196-201, 1979.

Keen H, Jarrett J: The W.H.O. multinational study of vascular disease in diabetes: 2. Macrovascular disease prevalence. *Diab Care* 2(2): 187-195, 1979.

Kreisberg RA: Diabetic ketoacidosis: New concepts and trends in pathogenesis and treatment. *Ann Intern Med* 88(5):681-695, 1978.

Liang JC, Goldberg MF: Treatment of diabetic retinopathy. *Diabetes* 29(10):841-851, 1980.

National Diabetes Data Group: Classification and diagnosis of diabetes mellitus and other categories of glucose intolerance. *Diabetes* 28(12):1039-1057, 1979.

Pirart J: Diabetes mellitus and its degenerative complications: A prospective study of 4,400 patients observed between 1947-1973. *Diab Care* 1(3):168-188, 1978.

Pyörälä K: Relationship of glucose tolerance and plasma insulin to the incidence of coronary heart disease. Results from two population studies in Finland. *Diab Care* 2(2):131-141, 1979.

Raskin P, Unger RH: Glucagon and diabetes. *Med Clin North Am* 62(4):713-722, 1978.

Rifkin H: Why control diabetes? *Med Clin North Am* 62(4):747-752, 1978.

Seltzer HS: Drug-induced hypoglycemia. *Diabetes* 21(9):955-966, 1972.

Statement on hypoglycemia. *Arch Intern Med* 31(4):591, 1973.

Obesity

Bray GA: *The Obese Patient*. Philadelphia: WB Saunders, 1976.

Gordon T, Kannel WB: Obesity and cardiovascular diseases: The Framingham Study. *Clin Endocrinol Metab* 5(2):367-375, 1976.

Hirsch J, Batchelor B: Adipose tissue cellularity in human obesity. *Clin Endocrinol Metab* 5(2):299-311, 1976.

Lipid Metabolism

Bierman EL, Porte D Jr: Carbohydrate intolerance and lipemia. *Ann Intern Med* 68:926-933, 1968.

Fogelman AM, Edmond J, Seager J, Popjak G: Abnormal induction of 3-hydroxy-3-methylglutaryl coenzyme A reductase in leukocytes from subjects with heterozygous familial hypercholesterolemia. *J Biol Chem* 250(6):2045-2055, 1975.

Hazzard WR, O'Donnell TF, Lee YL: Broad-β disease (type III hyperlipoproteinemia) in a large kindred. *Ann Intern Med* 82(2):141-149, 1975.

Levy RI (moderator), Fredrickson DS, Shulman R, Bilheimer DW, Breslow JL, Stone NJ, Lux SE, Sloan HR, Krauss RM, Herbert PN (discussants): Dietary and drug treatment of primary hyperlipoproteinemia. *Ann Intern Med* 74(2):267-294, 1972.

Dr. Gossain contributed the following sections: Pituitary, Thyroid, Adrenals, Carbohydrate Metabolism, Diabetes, Hypoglycemia, and Obesity.

Dr. Gambert contributed the following sections: Parathyroid and Calcium Metabolism, Ovary, Testis, Ectopic Hormones and Lipid Metabolism.

CHAPTER 6
GASTROENTEROLOGY

Harry N. Hoffman, II

THE ESOPHAGUS

ANATOMY OF THE PHARYNX AND ESOPHAGUS

The esophagus is a hollow, muscular conduit that conveys swallowed material from the oropharynx to the stomach, and prevents the reflux of gastric contents. The cricopharyngeus muscle, a part of the inferior pharyngeal constrictor muscle, functions as the superior esophageal sphincter and marks the proximal end of the esophagus. The body of the esophagus, approximately 25 cm in length, lies for a short distance in the neck and the remainder within the posterior mediastinum. It passes through the esophageal hiatus of the diaphragm and joins the gastric cardia immediately inferior to it. The esophageal lumen is lined with squamous epithelium. The submucosa contains a few cells, some sparse mucus-secreting glands, blood vessels, and nerve fibers. The muscularis in the upper one-third of the esophagus is composed of striated muscle, both striated and smooth muscle in the middle third, and only smooth muscle in the lower third. It consists of inner circular and outer longitudinal layers. At the level of the esophageal hiatus of the diaphragm is the lower esophageal sphincter (LES), which has no distinctive anatomic characteristics but does have important functional properties. The esophagus has no serosa (Fig. 1).

Innervation of the pharynx is by parasympathetic fibers from the pharyngeal plexus, the laryngeal branches of the vagus nerves, the glossopharyngeal nerves, and by sympathetic fibers from the cervical sympathetic ganglia. Vagal branches innervate the thoracic esophagus. Intrinsic autonomic (para-

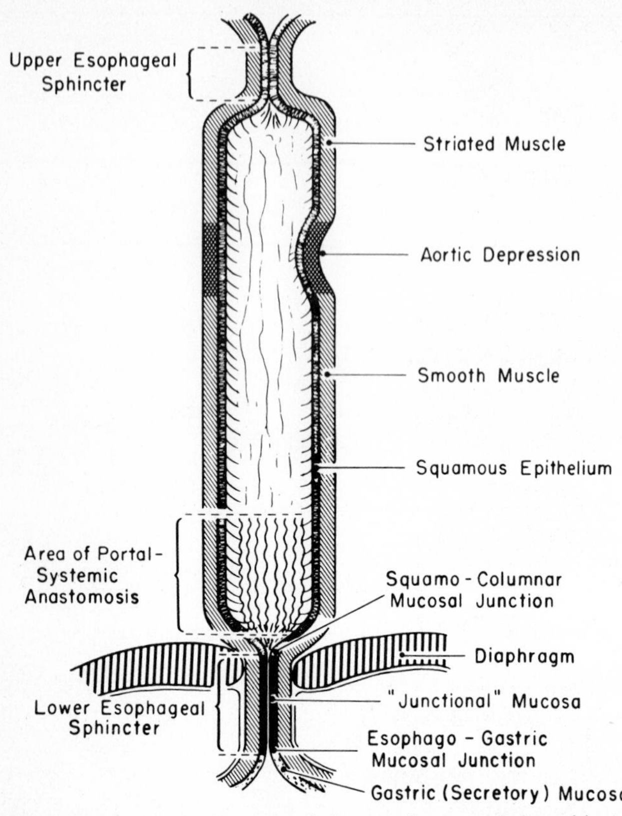

Figure 1. Anatomic features of the esophagus and its sphincters. (From *Disorders of the Gastrointestinal Tract*, edited by J. Dietschy. Copyright 1976, Grune & Stratton, Inc. Used by permission.)

sympathetic) innervation consists of Auerbach's (myenteric) plexus lying between the longitudinal and circular muscle layers, and of Meissner's (submucosal) plexus.

The blood supply of the esophagus comes from branches from the descending aorta and the left gastric artery, as well as from branches of the bronchial arteries. Submucosally located esophageal veins normally drain to the azygos and gastric veins. In the presence of portal hypertension, flow in the gastric veins reverses in the direction of the esophageal and azygos veins, resulting in distended, dilated varices in the distal esophagus.

PHYSIOLOGY OF THE ESOPHAGUS

The act of swallowing is initiated voluntarily by pressing the tip of the tongue against the hard palate, after which the tongue rises against the hard palate, propelling the bolus back into the pharynx. Thereafter, swallowing is a reflex act. The muscles of the soft palate and nasopharynx contract, shutting off the posterior opening to the nose. The larynx is pulled upward and forward under the base of the tongue, shutting off the lower airway, as the epiglottis retroverts to occlude the laryngeal orifice. Pharyngeal contractions move the bolus toward the esophageal introitus, where the superior sphincter has relaxed its tone, allowing entry into the esophagus, after which the sphincter again contracts. In the body of the esophagus, the muscular contraction waves continue downward while the LES relaxes to allow the bolus to pass when it arrives at that point. Fluid may be shot downward ahead of the wave, but solids are propelled by peristalsis. After the bolus has passed through the distal esophagus into the stomach, the LES contracts more strongly for a few moments, then reverts to its resting tone. Except when its tone is reduced in advance of an approaching peristaltic wave, the LES is closed by contraction of the circular muscle fibers, producing an intraluminal pressure (15-30 mm of mercury) above intra-abdominal pressure, thus preventing gastroesophageal reflux. The tone of the LES is not fixed but has been shown to vary in response to changes in intra-abdominal pressure; it is also influenced by gastrointestinal hormones. Of the latter, gastrin seems to be of major importance since it increases LES strength and may well be the mediator for rises in tone following antacids and protein meals. (Fig. 2)

It is currently held that prevention of gastroesophageal reflux is due entirely to LES tone and competence and that

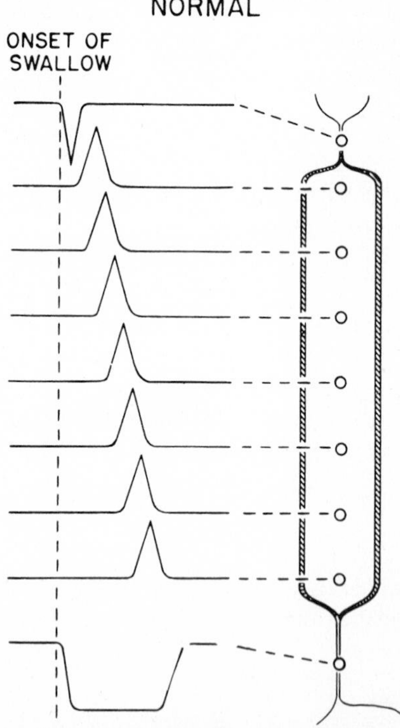

Figure 2. Normal esophageal motility sequence initiated by swallow. Pressure recordings from upper and lower sphincters and within the body of esophagus. (From *Disorders of the Gastrointestinal Tract*, edited by J. Dietschy. Copyright 1976, Grune & Stratton, Inc. Used by permission.)

the diaphragm, the angle of His, and other mechanical or anatomic factors do not play significant roles.

DIFFERENTIAL APPROACH TO SYMPTOMS OF ESOPHAGEAL DISEASE

The two functions of the esophagus are transport of material from mouth to stomach and prevention of gastroesophageal reflux; therefore, disease and disturbances that interfere with these functions usually produce the following symptoms.

Dysphagia
Difficulty in swallowing, or the awareness that swallowed material is impeded in its orderly transport from mouth to stomach. This symptom must be distinguished from the sensation of a lump in the throat without actual difficulty swallowing, known as globus hystericus. In skeletal muscle diseases and in disorders affecting the brain stem, the patient may be unable to propel the bolus from the mouth and pharynx into the esophagus, resulting in aspiration of material into the larynx and trachea, or reflux of material into the nasopharynx and nasal passages. This arises most commonly in brainstem vascular accidents, bulbar palsy, and neurologic disorders such as amyotrophic lateral sclerosis, multiple sclerosis, and myasthenia gravis. The dysphagia and aspiration produced by Zenker's diverticulum and, occasionally, by cricopharyngeal muscle dysfunction may closely resemble that of neuromuscular disorders.

In the body of the esophagus, dysphagia can be broadly attributed either to ineffective peristalsis or to obstruction of the lumen. Hence, patients with esophageal motor weakness note difficulty swallowing both liquids and solids, whereas a narrowed lumen typically produces dysphagia for solids. Patients with motor dysfunction usually describe little or no progression in their dysphagia, in contrast to the progressive obstruction caused by a neoplasm of the esophagus. Intermittent, sporadic dysphagia only for solids is characteristic of a lower esophageal ring.

Pain
Pain of esophageal origin arising from esophageal mucosal disease typically occurs while swallowing (odynophagia). Such pain is fairly well localized by the patient to the level of mucosal disease, is usually substernal, but commonly also radiates to the neck. Esophagitis from gastroesophageal reflux, swallowed corrosives, or from infections of the mucosa most commonly produces this type of pain. Another type of esophageal pain arises from motility disorders, presumably from spasms of esophageal muscle, and is a deeper, more severe oppressive pain, usually substernal though tending to radiate in a pattern resembling angina.

The most common type of esophageal pain is heartburn, a retrosternal burning or acid type discomfort that most people have experienced. It typically responds promptly to alkalis and antacids, and is closely correlated with the reflux of material from the stomach into the esophagus. However, evidence is conflicting as to whether the pain arises from esophageal mucosal inflammation or from muscle spasm.

PROCEDURES IN DIAGNOSIS OF ESOPHAGEAL DISORDERS

X-ray
Roentgenographic and fluoroscopic examination employing barium sulfate is the single most valuable procedure in the diagnosis of esophageal disorders. A radiologist may vary the consistency of the medium, or employ barium-filled capsules to assess motility or the caliber of a stricture. The examination is usually done in the supine position to better observe motor activity without gravity. Although the radiologist may tilt the patient's head downward or use manual pressure on the abdomen to assess gastroesophageal reflux, these techniques correlate poorly with other methods for measuring reflux and with clinical estimates of reflux. On occasion, cineradiography is useful in studying esophageal motor disorders.

Esophageal Manometry
Recording of intraluminal pressure transmitted via fluid-filled, open-tipped catheters to transducers is a valuable method of studying motor function of the esophagus and its sphincters. An assembled set of three water-filled polyethylene tubes (internal diameter 0.76 cm) is attached to strain gauges. The tubes have lateral orifices spaced 5 cm apart in their distal portions. Some laboratories incorporate a fourth tube, at the distal end of which is placed a 5 mm balloon that serves as the most distal pressure sensor. All tubing, the balloon, and the external strain gauges are filled with water. The intraluminal esophageal pressure changes are reflected as changes in current in the strain gauges or transducers, and are graphed on a multichannel recorder. The set of pressure detectors is passed via the mouth into the stomach, after which the patient is placed in the supine position, asked to breathe normally, and to refrain from swallowing. After recording the resting profile of the gastroesophageal junction, the tube assembly is withdrawn at 0.5-1.0 cm intervals until the most distal sensor is in the lower esophagus above the sphincter. The pressure sensors again are placed in the stomach and then the sphincter's response to 0.5 ml water swallows while withdrawing the sensors in 0.5 cm sequences through the junction, and then in 2-3 cm intervals through the body of the esophagus and cricopharyngeal sphincter, is recorded (Fig. 2).

Potential Difference Recordings
Since a significant transmural potential difference (PD) is present in the stomach compared to the nearly negligible PD across the esophageal mucosa, one of the pressure-detecting tubes of the manometry assembly may be used as a salt bridge to record the sharp change in PD detected at the mucosal junction of stomach and esophagus. This is an accurate means of determining this landmark in conjunction with other data recorded during the manometric study.

pH Determination
Small intraluminal electrodes in the esophagus have been employed in the diagnosis and investigation of gastroesophageal reflux, with or without hydrochloric acid infusion into the stomach, and to test the ability of the esophagus to clear acid from the lumen.

Scintiscanning
This technique employs a 300 ml gastric load of saline containing 100 μCi of technetium-labeled sulfur colloid, after which the stomach and esophagus are scanned to determine reflux. If no spontaneous reflux is observed, an abdominal binder is applied and the esophageal region reexamined. A high correlation of patient's reflux symptoms with pH probe studies has been reported.

The Bernstein Test
(Esophageal Acid Perfusion)
This test is used to determine if the patient's distress is due to reflux. It is also regarded by some as a useful tool in the elucidation of the cause of some types of chest pain. The study consists of placing a tube in the middle portion of the esophagus, the external end of which is connected to a Y tube, whose other ends are connected to bottles of 0.1N hydrochloric acid and normal saline. After initial instillation of saline at a rate of 7 ml/min for 5 minutes, the flow is switched to 0.1N hydrochloric acid at the same rate and without the patient's knowledge. Acid is perfused until the patient's symptoms appear, or for up to 30 minutes. If the patients says that the distress produced by the acid infusion is the same as his usual symptoms, the flow is switched to saline, which should make the symptoms disappear in 3 or 4 minutes. Then reinfusion of acid is usually done in order to confirm the acid-induced symptoms. All tests are not conclusive, since both or neither infusion may produce symptoms, or those that arise may be entirely different sensations or distress. The test may be negative in the presence of esophagitis or stricture that has arisen without symptoms. The test is useful in pursuing the possible esophageal origin of a patient's distress.

Esophagoscopy
The use of flexible fiberoptic esophagogastroscopes has made esophagoscopy a low-risk, important diagnostic procedure. It is usually done using topical anesthesia, with the patient awake but premedicated with intravenous diazepam. The examination is of particular value in the appraisal of dysphagia, upper gastrointestinal hemorrhage, esophagitis, and obstructing lesions (including biopsy and cytology examination from direct brushing of a lesion). Rigid esophagoscopy is used in the removal of foreign bodies from the esophagus.

DISEASES OF THE ESOPHAGUS

Achalasia

Etiology
This motor disorder is characterized by aperistalsis in the body of the esophagus, failure of the LES to relax, and an elevated resting tone of the sphincter. The dominant symptom is dysphagia. The disease is worldwide and affects both sexes equally. The etiology is unknown, but defects in the neural pathway have been proposed at various sites from the dorsal vagal nucleus and the vagal nerves to the intramural neurons or in synaptic or neuromuscular transmission. An inhibitory role has been proposed for vagal influence on LES function, and impairment on this inhibition could theoretically lead to an unopposed excitatory effect, or failure to relax. In achalasia, the LES has been shown to be supersensitive to circulating gastrin. In Brazil, patients with Chagas' disease have esophageal dysfunction indistinguishable from achalasia, and have lesions of myenteric neurons produced by the parasite *Trypanosoma cruzi*. In idiopathic achalasia a neurotoxic virus, ischemia, or an autoimmune process have also been proposed as possible causes.

Clinical Features
The disease most commonly presents in the third and fourth decades, though in some cases early symptoms can be traced back many years. Typically, patients describe dysphagia to liquids and solids that may be mild and sporadic. Regurgitation of food and swallowed saliva that is not sour, bitter, or bile-colored is especially apt to occur bending over and at night, leading to nocturnal coughing paroxysms and a risk of tracheal aspiration that may result in pneumonitis, lung abscess, and bronchiectasis. Some patients overcome the dysphagia for solids by drinking water, which forces solids into the stomach. However, others induce emesis to relieve the discomfort, after which they may be able to eat. In general, the problems of overflow, spillage, and aspiration into the airway are symptoms of more advanced disease. In the early stages, patients may experience not only dysphagia but significant acute chest pains radiating to the neck, jaws, or arms that has been termed vigorous achalasia. In such cases, the distinction between diffuse esophageal spasm and achalasia can be difficult without manometry, and the progression of diffuse esophageal spasm to achalasia has been reported. Caution is called for in the appraisal of patients whose achalasia-like symptoms, x-ray, and manometric pictures develop beyond the fourth decade, as some neoplasms involving the LES or infiltrating the esophageal wall and presumably damaging the myenteric plexus may closely mimic true achalasia. Such neoplasms are most often adenocarcinoma of the gastric fundus, bronchogenic carcinoma, or lymphoma.

Diagnosis
Diagnosis of achalasia should be initially suspected from the dysphagia for solids and liquids. Weight loss may be present. The chest x-ray may show a widened mediastinum due to a dilated, distended esophagus. An air-fluid level behind the heart is seen at times, and the absence of a gastric air bubble has also been considered highly suggestive of this disorder. Lastly, chest x-ray may show the pulmonary complications mentioned above.

Barium swallow shows weak or absent peristalis in the body of the esophagus that may be almost normal to greatly dilated and tortuous, with retained food and fluid. The distal esophagus near the lower esophageal sphincter typically tapers to a beaklike ending.

Esophagoscopy is advisable to exclude organic obstructing lesions in the distal esophagus, especially in patients whose symptoms begin after the age of 40 and appear to be of short duration. Manometric studies reveal absent peristalsis in the body of the esophagus; there may be weak repetitive or spontaneous contractions that are not peristaltic. Occasionally, in early cases there may be aperistaltic contractions of greater than normal amplitude. The LES when assessed with open-tipped infused catheters is shown to have an elevated resting pressure, and does not relax to normal (intragastric) levels on swallowing (Fig. 3). Patients with achalasia show denervation sensitivity to an intravenous injection of 5-10 mg of methacholine (Mecholyl), consisting of a rise in baseline pressure over 50%, vigorous, nonperistaltic contractions, and relaxation of the LES. The test may produce severe chest pain and other side effects, and is falling into disuse.

Treatment

Therapy aimed at reducing the resistance at the lower esophageal sphincter thus allowing the esophagus to empty, may be accomplished by two methods. For initial treatment, forced pneumatic dilatation of the sphincter is widely favored. It carries a 2.5% risk of perforation and produces excellent to good results in about 70% of patients. Repeated dilatations over the years may be necessary. A modified Heller esophagocardiomyotomy to surgically disrupt the lower esophageal sphincter has been favored by some centers. Excellent to good results are achieved in 75-85% of cases. However, symptomatic reflux esophagitis, at times resulting in peptic stricture, is a known late development after myotomy. A late complication of achalasia (occurring in 5-10%) is carcinoma of the esophagus.

Scleroderma

Esophageal dysfunction resulting in dysphagia and esophageal reflux occurs in 75% of patients with scleroderma (systemic sclerosis). The most characteristic histologic change is smooth muscle atrophy with fibrosis. The pathogenesis of the muscle abnormality is uncertain, though some evidence supports neurologic damage as a primary event. Most scleroderma patients with esophageal involvement also have Raynaud's phenomenon, suggesting a common pathogenesis for the autonomic dysfunction. Both these features of systemic sclerosis may precede the development of the characteristic skin changes.

The symptoms of esophageal involvement consist of dysphagia to liquids and solids, plus persistent and progressive

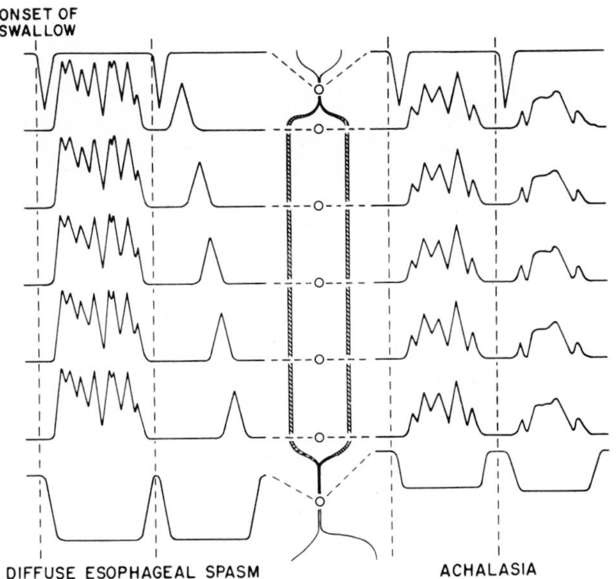

Figure 3. Esophageal manometry patterns in diffuse esophageal spasm (left) and achlasia (right). Note elevated resting pressure and partial relaxation of lower sphincter in achalasia. In the body of the esophagus in both conditions, contractions are aperistaltic, repetitive; higher amplitude contractions are characteristic of DES. (From *Disorders of the Gastrointestinal Tract*, edited by J. Dietschy. Copyright 1976, Grune & Stratton, Inc. Used by permission.)

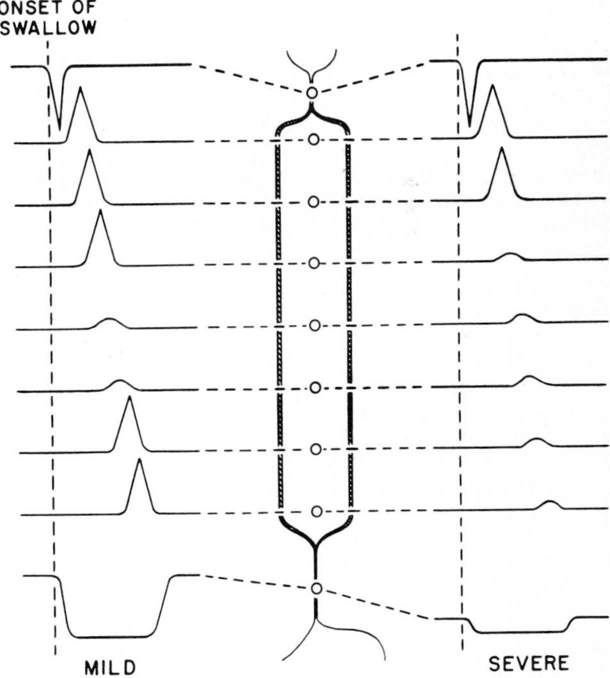

Figure 4. Esophageal manometric findings in mild and severe scleroderma. Diminished to absent peristaltic activity and reduced lower esophageal sphincter pressure develop as the disease progresses. (From *Disorders of the Gastrointestinal Tract*, edited by J. Dietschy. Copyright 1976, Grune & Stratton, Inc. Used by permission.)

reflux, resulting in esophagitis that may lead to stricture formation and more severe dysphagia. X-ray examination shows loss of peristaltic activity, impaired emptying, and gastroesophageal reflux. Manometric changes consist of a marked diminution or loss of peristalsis in the distal one-half to two-thirds of the body of the esophagus, and hypotension of the LES (Fig. 4). Similar esophageal dysfunction and Raynaud's phenomenon occur frequently in mixed connective tissue disease and less frequently with other collagen diseases; regardless of the type of underlying collagen disease, patients with esophageal dysfunction nearly always have Raynaud's phenomenon. Prognosis of the esophageal dysfunction in systemic sclerosis is that of the primary disease and its systemic manifestations. Treatment consists of frequent antacids and/or cimetidine, head-up bed, and dilatation of esophageal strictures. Although antireflux operations involving fundoplication may give symptomatic relief and heal esophagitis, fundoplication carries the risk of worsening the dysphagia.

Diffuse Esophageal Spasm (DES)

Clinical Features and Diagnosis

DES is an uncommon disorder of esophageal peristalsis, appearing most often in midlife. Its clinical picture varies, but most typically consists of dysphagia and chest pain. The dysphagia is not constant, and pain tends to be the most common symptom. It may closely mimic angina pectoris in character, including referral to the neck, jaws, shoulders, and arms, as well as its reported relief by nitroglycerin. However, the pain of DES is not induced by exercise nor relieved by rest. Attacks of pain often seem to occur with emotional stress and drinking hot or cold liquids. If the spasm episode occurs during a meal, the patient notes dysphagia. Esophagitis and regurgitation are uncommon. It is sometimes difficult to distinguish DES from early achalasia, as an occasional patient may have clinical and manometric features of both disorders (that is, dysphagia, chest pain, and regurgitation), and it is likely that an occasional case of DES progresses to achalasia. Roentgenographically, barium swallow studies may reveal diffuse irregular spasm, diffuse constant narrowing, or pseudodiverticulosis but may be normal. Manometric studies if recorded during symptoms are diagnostic, with simultaneous repetitive, prolonged, high amplitude contractions in the smooth muscle portion of the esophagus. Between episodes, normal peristalsis is seen, in contrast to achalasia. Upper and lower sphincter resting pressures are usually normal, though the LES in 30 percent of patients is hypertensive or contracts prematurely or excessively. It relaxes normally in response to swallowing, and the mecholyl test is negative (Fig. 3).

Treatment

Management of patients with DES may be difficult. In some, the symptoms may be averted by reducing stress at mealtimes and avoiding cold liquids. As mentioned earlier, in some patients nitroglycerin relieves attacks of pain, though long-acting nitrates are rarely helpful. An occasional patient may obtain long-term benefit from pneumatic dilatation; in sufferers with frequent, severe, and intractable symptoms, a long esophagomyotomy has given excellent to good results in about 65% of cases.

Esophageal Webs and Rings

A mucosal web projecting into the lumen from the anterior wall at the upper end of the esophagus in the region of the cricopharyngeus muscle is known variously as the Plummer-Vinson syndrome, the Patterson-Kelly syndrome, or sideropenic dysphagia because of the common association of iron deficiency anemia. It is seen principally in middle-aged and elderly women, and is usually noted roentgenographically during swallowing. Esophagoscopy is advisable to exclude carcinoma if the period of symptoms is short; furthermore, it is said that carcinoma of the cervical esophagus may occur more frequently in patients with this syndrome than in the general population. Esophagoscopy for the purpose of diagnosing the web is not always successful, for the web may be missed or disrupted during the procedure. Treatment of the anemia with iron may relieve the web, but endoscopic rupture of the web is the most direct method of relieving the dysphagia.

Lower Esophageal Ring (Schatzki's Ring)

A persistent, annular, thin, ringlike narrowing of the lower esophagus may be a cause of episodic dysphagia. Rings with a luminal diameter greater than 12-14 mm usually cause no symptoms and are not rare on roentgenographic study of the esophagus. Most such rings are mucosal, constant, and of uncertain etiology; a congenital etiology is favored by some authorities, although others link it to the diaphragmatic hernia with which it frequently coexists. Reflux symptoms and esophagitis are rare; the primary symptom is dysphagia that is characteristically intermittent and only for solids. The frequency with which it occurs when eating steak or eating with haste has led to the term steak-house syndrome. The ring almost always occurs just proximal to the LES, and has been shown to be lined with squamous epithelium on its upper surface and gastric mucosa on its distal side. Treatment consists of advice to eat slowly, and careful chewing of solid foods that should be swallowed in small amounts at a time. Patients who have frequent and severe dysphagia with tight rings may need repeated forceful dilatations, but only rarely need surgical treatment.

Gastroesophageal Reflux

Etiology

Gastroesophageal reflux is a syndrome characterized primarily by heartburn due to the passage of acid and other material such as bile from the stomach into the esophagus; at times also by the sequelae of reflux esophagitis including stricture, esophageal ulcer, bleeding, and Barrett's (columnar-lined epithelium) esophagus. Present thinking discounts the importance of anatomic properties of the diaphragm and the gastroesophageal junction as important barriers to reflux, and holds that the LES is the major antireflux barrier. Although the common association of hiatal hernia previously led many physicians to conclude that reflux was secondary to this anatomic defect, most current data support the position that LES pressure per se is the important barrier to gastroesophageal reflux. Patients with LES pressures of less than 10 mm of mercury frequently have reflux, whereas pressures greater than 15 mm of mercury are rarely associated with reflux. Although the association with diaphragmatic hernia has been largely discounted in the causation of reflux, the pathogenesis of reflux remains poorly understood.

However, a closer look at the clinical settings in which reflux occurs has shown that incompetent LES has different mechanical properties that may account for its dysfunction; 24-hour pH monitoring also has shown that spontaneous reflux episodes occur in normal people, resulting from inappropriate LES relaxation (i.e., without motor activity such as swallowing, or during sleep). The importance of this mechanism in patients with reflux esophagitis is unknown at present; a decreased muscle responsiveness of the LES due to female hormones probably accounts for the reduced lower esophageal sphincter pressure during pregancy, which reverts to normal after delivery. In neural and muscular disease, especially systemic sclerosis, there is marked hypotension of the LES as part of the esophageal involvement seen in this disease and in other connective tissue diseases. Hormonal influence on the LES also may be at fault. A decreased gastrin effect on the sphincter has been observed in patients with gastroesophageal sphincter incompetence. Inappropriate LES relaxation has been shown to occur spontaneously with or without peristalsis; clearance of refluxed material from the esophagus is delayed in patients with esophagitis, and this poor clearance has been correlated with decreased swallowing episodes after reflux.

Symptoms

Heartburn is the most prominent symptom of gastroesophageal reflux, although an occasional patient may be encountered with a complication of reflux who has been essentially asymptomatic. Frequently, heartburn is induced or worsened by bending, squatting, and lying down. Some patients also experience regurgitation of sour, bitter gastric contents into the pharynx or mouth. Esophageal ulceration may occur in association with chronic reflux symptoms, producing more persistent retrosternal and interscapular pain, odynophagia, or bleeding. Chronic reflux has been implicated in asthma symptoms in some patients. Progressive dysphagia for solids in a patient with a history of significant heartburn suggests a stricture. As the luminal narrowing and dysphagia increase, heartburn often lessens.

Diagnosis

Heartburn with or without regurgitation should suggest gastroesophageal reflux. Roentgenographic demonstration of reflux of barium from the stomach into the esophagus with the patient in the supine position is a valid but imprecise procedure. Monitoring of intraesophageal pH by a luminal pH electrode is a reliable indicator of reflux; when combined with manometric study of the distal esophagus and lower esophageal sphincter, sphincter pressure and competence can be measured, as well as its functional correlation with reflux. Occasionally, the Bernstein test of acid perfusion of the esophagus may help by inducing the symptoms of reflux, and in differentiating various types of chest pain. If the patient has had recent intensive antacid therapy, the acid perfusion may not produce any pain.

Esophagoscopy is often useful in the appraisal of the heartburn patient. However, the mucosa may appear grossly normal in the presence of definite symptoms of reflux. Suction capsule biopsies of the esophageal mucosa in such patients have shown thickening of the basal layer and extension of dermal pegs near, or to, the surface. These changes are said to correlate better with objective evidence of reflux than does the endoscopic finding of esophagitis, which is regarded as a complication of reflux, not the cause. Esophagoscopy is additionally helpful in the appraisal of stricture, ulceration, or to exclude carcinoma.

Treatment

Medical measures suffice for the majority of patients with gastroesophageal reflux. Antacids after meals and at bedtime control or improve symptoms in most patients by their acid-neutralizing effect and also the resultant increase in LES pressure, thereby decreasing reflux. Diet plays no significant role, though an increased protein, low-fat diet and avoiding alcohol, coffee and spices might enhance LES tone. Bethanechol has been shown to increase resting LES tone, to decrease reflux, and to facilitate acid clearance from the esophagus in reflux, and has been of significant benefit in clinical trials. Alginic acid (combined with sodium bicarbonate) has proven as effective as antacids for gastroesophageal reflux symptoms. Metoclopramide, a dopamine antagonist, appears to hold promise in the treatment of reflux via its action in increasing LES pressure and improving abnormal gastric emptying. Its role, however, must await further clinical trials and assessment of the frequency and magnitude of side effects. Cimetidine has been shown in several trials to offer relief of reflux symptoms superior to antacids, and to suggest a trend toward healing of esophagitis.

Surgery is reserved for those patients in whom vigorous or intensive medical therapy has failed to relieve symptoms or in whom complications of reflux arise, such as stricture, hemorrhage, ulceration, Barrett's mucosal metaplasia, and so on. Currently effective antireflux surgical procedures that prevent reflux by wrapping the stomach around the esophagus and fixing these structures to the diaphragm are the Belsey transthoracic fundoplication, the Hill transabdominal gastropexy, or the Nissen transabdominal fundoplication. Most strictures of the esophagus can be dilated to 40-50F and dysphagia overcome; many patients can continue to be treated in this fashion, especially if vigorous antireflux measures are also initiated. However, many authorities consider the development of a stricture to be an indication for surgery to restore gastroesophageal competence.

Neoplasms of the Esophagus

Benign tumors and cysts are uncommon. The most frequent is leiomyoma that, when small, is asymptomatic but eventually may cause dysphagia, retrosternal pressure, and fullness. Less common benign lesions are lipomas, hemangiomas, and cysts.

Carcinoma

Carcinoma of the esophagus occurs predominantly in older men. Commonly associated or implicated factors include achalasia, Plummer-Vinson syndrome, lye burns of the esophagus, tylosis, and chronic alcoholism. The vast majority of esophageal carcinomas arise from squamous mucosa; the remainder are adenocarcinomas occurring in the esophagogastric region and are considered to arise in the gastric cardia, extending proximally into the lower esophagus.

Clinical Features

The most common clinical presentation is that of dysphagia for solids that progresses in a short time to soft foods and liquids. Odynophagia is also common. Regurgitation of swallowed food and secretions often occurs, and weight loss is progressive. Hoarseness due to recurrent laryngeal nerve involvement, cough, tracheoesophageal fistula, pneumonitis, and pulmonary abscess may also occur.

Diagnosis

Diagnosis is made by history, roentgenographic examination of the esophagus with barium, and by esophagoscopy with biopsy and cytologic examination. It must be emphasized that any patient with recurrent, persistent, or progressive dysphagia requires x-ray examination, and even if this is unrevealing, esophagoscopy should be done. Manometric studies do not reveal a characteristic pattern in esophageal neoplasm; in some instances of distal carcinoma, an abnormal sphincter resting profile and impaired relaxation can simulate achalasia, and warrants esophagoscopy. Prognosis is poor, with an overall 5 year survival rate of less than 5-8% despite surgery and radiation therapy.

Treatment

Only about 50-60% of patients with esophageal carcinoma are operable, and of those operated on, less than half are resectable. Surgical mortality is high (10-15%) and overall postoperative survival at 5 years is discouragingly low (5%). Tumors of the cervical esophagus and upper thoracic esophagus tend to be treated by radiation or by preoperative radiotherapy. Lesions of the mid- and distal esophagus are more often resected.

Congenital Anomalies

The rare embryologic defects of the esophagus arise from abnormal development and separation of the respiratory and proximal alimentary tracts from their common origin. Atresia of the esophagus with tracheoesophageal fistula is the most common anomaly seen in infants and is treated by early surgical closure of the fistula and reanastomosis of the esophagus. Of the five main categories of congenital fistulas, in the most common form the proximal esophagus ends blindly, and the distal esophagus communicates with the trachea. Excessive salivation (often frothy), difficulty in nursing followed by choking, dyspnea, and cyanosis in the newborn suggest the diagnosis. Roentgenograms of the chest and abdomen, posteroanterior (PA) and lateral, with a previously passed catheter in place if obstruction is encountered, may be sufficient to make the diagnosis. Complete absence of gas in the abdomen is diagnostic of the most common type of fistula.

Diverticula of the Esophagus

Three sites of predilection are known for the development of esophageal diverticula. The first, at the level of the cricopharyngeus muscle, is known as a Zenker's, or pharyngeoesophageal, diverticulum. It consists of an out-pouching of mucosa posteriorly between the oblique fibers of the inferior pharyngeal constrictor muscle and the transverse fibers of the cricopharyngeus muscle. Evidence favors incoordination between pharyngeal contraction and relaxation of the superior esophageal sphincter such that the sphincter contracts prematurely before pharyngeal contraction is complete, resulting in the generation of a transmural pressure gradient sufficient to encourage mucosal herniation through an anatomically weak point in the posterior wall above the cricopharyngeus muscle. As the diverticulum enlarges, the sac may lie in the midline and deflect the esophagus anteriorly, producing dysphagia. If the diverticulum projects laterally, a soft cervical mass may be noted. Most pharyngeoesophageal diverticula give rise to progressive symptoms consisting of high dysphagia and spontaneous regurgitation, episodes of coughing and choking, foul breath, and occasional noisy deglutition. Weight loss and pulmonary complications may result in long-standing cases. Diagnosis is best made by roentgenography. Treatment is by surgical diverticulectomy for larger sacs, and cricopharyngeal myotomy for small ones.

Midesophageal diverticula are considered to result from traction on the esophageal wall arising from inflammatory mediastinal lymph nodes, and are seldom of clinical importance because of their broad mouths and conical configuration.

In the lower esophagus, diverticula may develop by pulsion as a consequence of obstruction (functional or mechanical) at the level of the sphincter. Their epiphrenic or supradiaphragmatic location correlates with the fact that the majority of such diverticula appear associated with lesions such as hiatal hernia, achalasia, diffuse esophageal spasm, and so on. Most patients have no symptoms referrable to the diverticulum, although some may experience dysphagia and regurgitation. Roentgenographic study of the esophagus is the best means of diagnosis. Endoscopy is seldom necessary, except for better appraisal of associated pathology. No treatment is needed for the majority of cases. Surgical extirpation of the diverticulum is usually carried out only when surgery is done for an associated condition.

Lacerations and Perforations

Mallory-Weiss Syndrome

This syndrome must be considered among the causes of upper gastrointestinal hemorrhage. It consists of postemetic mucosal and submucosal laceration of the gastric cardia, followed by hematemesis and/or melena. Increased gastric pressure related to the force of vomiting is responsible for the laceration. Blunt trauma has rarely produced the syndrome. Although alcoholic debauche is the most common clinical setting, one or more episodes of vomiting and retching of any cause may induce the laceration that can also involve the lower esophageal mucosa. Endoscopy is probably the best means of confirming the diagnosis, though the lesion may be missed. Celiac angiography is helpful in localizing the site of bleeding. However, roentgenographic barium study is not helpful and may obscure the area if angiographic study is done subsequently. Surgery is occasionally necessary to establish a diagnosis and to control hemorrhage. Initial treatment of Mallory-Weiss syndrome consists of supportive measures such as restoration and maintenance of blood volume, close monitoring, and esophagogastric suction. In the majority of instances, bleeding stops spontaneously. Surgical exploration is infrequently needed for uncontrolled massive hemorrhage.

Esophageal Perforation

Etiology and Pathology. The most common cause of perforation of the esophagus is instrumentation (endoscopy, bougienage, or intubation), and sites of predilection from instrumentation are the proximal cervical and lower thoracic esophagus. Postemetic perforations occur in the distal thoracic esophagus or the adjacent intra-abdominal segment. Traumatic rupture of the esophagus is rare, and usually associated with other neck, chest, or mediastinal injury. The pathophysiologic consequences of perforation relate to the contamination of the fascial spaces of the mediastinum, neck, and peritoneal cavity. Respiratory movements and the negative intrathoracic pressure help disseminate contaminated material into the mediastinum and pleural spaces. Gastric and oral contents containing air, saliva, food, acid, bile, enzymes, and bacteria may promptly lead to a putrid necrotizing infection that can involve not only the mediastinum but also adjacent pleural and pericardial tissues and spaces.

Clinical Features

The clinical picture following perforation depends on the level of esophagus injured, and the nature and extent of the leakage of bacteria and chemically irritating contents into adjacent tissues. Pain accompanies almost all perforations and generally reflects the level of adjacent tissue involvement. Neck and upper anterior chest pain are seen with lesions at these levels, whereas lower esophageal perforations usually produce left chest, epigastric, and infrascapular pain. Fever is common and respiratory distress may indicate pleural involvement; dysphagia is usually a sign of adjacent inflammation, the level of distress often indicating the level of perforation.

Pain with neck motions, tenderness to palpation, and cervical crepitus are characteristic of perforations of the cervical esophagus; a lower esophageal perforation may simulate an acute upper abdominal catastrophe.

Diagnosis

Lateral x-ray examination of the cervical spine and chest may show free air in the neck or mediastinum, mediastinal widening; pleural effusions, and so forth. Water-soluble x-ray contrast medium studies are especially valuable in detecting intrathoracic perforations (but not in cervical perforations). Esophagoscopy is not generally used or considered advisable for diagnosis.

Treatment

Although careful observation may be justified when there is uncertainty as to the existence of cervical perforation, such expectant medical treatment should include antibiotics, avoidance of swallowing, and parenteral nutrition; in most cases, it is best to proceed with cervical mediastinotomy for drainage to avoid suppuration and a protracted convalescence. Distal esophageal perforation should be surgically closed, with the establishment of adequate drainage and other underlying or associated obstruction corrected also. Postemetic perforations of the distal esophagus necessitate early surgical closure of the perforation, plus debridement and drainage. Delayed recognition and treatment of esophageal perforations beyond 24 hours results in a high mortality from consequences of infection, and complications involving septic or hypovolemic shock, and hypotension.

Esophageal Hiatal Hernia

Definition and Pathology

An esophageal hiatal hernia is any abnormal protrusion of the stomach through the esophageal hiatus of the diaphragm into the thorax, and may be classified as either sliding or paraesophageal. The most common type is the sliding hernia in which the esophagastric junction and a portion of the proximal stomach are displaced upward through the hiatus into the posterior mediastinum. In most instances the esophagus is of normal length. The so-called short esophagus reported by radiologists with some hernias is thought to represent longitudinal shortening of the tube consequent to reflux esophagitis, rather than a congenitally short esophagus. The paraesophageal hiatal hernia, in its early stages, is a protrusion of the gastric fundus through the hiatus alongside the esophagus, with the esophagogastric junction remaining below the diaphragm. Later, there may be herniation of increasing amounts of greater curvature, sometimes resulting in an entire upside-down intrathoracic stomach, along with herniation of other abdominal viscera. Since the esophagogastric junction remains fixed below the diaphragm, reflux is not usually encountered. Combined forms of sliding and paraesophageal hernias are not uncommon.

Etiology

The etiology of hernias is unknown but developmental factors, including an abnormally large esophageal hiatus and delayed descent of the esophagogastric junction during embryonic development, have been proposed as causes. More likely, the diaphragmatic attachments of the esophagus are weakened and stretched by such events and factors as pregnancy, obesity, tight abdominal garments, abdominal trauma, and excessive straining. Others have felt that repeated and prolonged contraction of the longitudinal musculature of the esophagus may pull the esophagogastric junction above the diaphragm.

Incidence

Depending on the techniques applied, hiatal hernias have been identified in up to 50% of the adult population. By careful x-ray study alone, approximately 10% of subjects examined are found to have hiatal hernias.

Symptoms

Most sliding diaphragmatic hiatal hernias are asymptomatic. Sporadic substernal pain of an aching, squeezing nature resembling angina may occur and is attributed to esophagospasm. Occasionally dysphagia is experienced, most typically for solid food or cold liquids with the first swallow or two of a meal, and when eating in haste or under stress. Probably lower esophageal spasm causes this type of discomfort.

Diagnosis

Roentgenographic study with barium is the most common means of diagnosis. Large hiatal hernias may be apparent on standard chest x-ray as air-fluid levels behind the heart. Esophagoscopy is not necessary for diagnosis although it may be valuable in assessing the presence and degree of an associated esophagitis, and the location and mobility of the esophagogastric junction, to help in decisions regarding surgery. Esophageal manometry can detect even small hiatal hernias (although such diagnostic testing is best directed at assessing the functional state of the gastroesophageal sphincter).

Treatment

In the absence of symptoms attributable to a sliding hernia, no treatment is indicated. A radiologic diagnosis of hiatal hernia should be carefully viewed in the clinical perspective of the patient's symptoms that are often attributable to other disorders. Medical treatment should be aimed at management of reflux and esophagitis, if these exist. Weight reduction helps lower intra-abdominal pressure. The avoidance of tight abdominal garments and of positions such as stooping and straining that also raise intra-abdominal pressure should be emphasized. If reflux symptoms are present, antacids are used after meals and at bedtime; elevating the head of the bed by blocks placed under the legs at the head of the bed, 4 to 6 inches in height, helps to keep gastric contents in the stomach. Anticholinergic drugs should be avoided because they tend to promote reflux and delay gastric emptying.

Paraesophageal Hernia

Many patients with paraesophageal hernia have no symptoms, or may note only vague postprandial dyspepsia or retrosternal fullness; reflux symptoms and esophagitis are not seen. Probably the most common manifestation of paraesophageal hernia is asymptomatic blood loss anemia, attributable to edema and congestion of the mucosa of the herniated portion of the stomach, sometimes with erosions or frank ulcer formation. Gastric volvulus is the most serious complication of paraesophageal hernia, since delayed recognition and decompression by nasogastric intubation may result in incarceration and strangulation of the stomach. Complete inability to swallow, retching with production of saliva only, and severe progressive chest pain suggest incarceration.

No effective medical treatment is available. Antacids and iron therapy seldom significantly improve the anemia. Because of the risk of serious complications that may arise without warning, all paraesophageal hiatal hernias should be considered for surgical repair; it has a low mortality (less than 1%) and successfully corrects the defect.

Acute Esophagitis

Although specific forms of esophagitis may occur in tuberculosis, syphilis, and herpes simplex, the most common form of infectious esophagitis is due to the *Candida albicans* or monilia that is usually associated with oropharyngeal infection. The patient is usually aware of painful swallowing and, at times, dysphagia. Esophagoscopy discloses a white membrane with inflamed mucosa. Roentgenographically, a shaggy, ulcerated mucosa is seen. Moniliasis of the esophagus is encountered most frequently in patients receiving corticosteroids or immunosuppressive drugs, in diabetes, and sometimes following broad-spectrum antibiotic therapy. Diagnosis is made by demonstrating the pseudohyphae on smear or biopsy. Treatment consisting of swallows of nystatin suspension; sucking on tablets of nystatin is usually sufficient. Rarely, a course of intravenous amphotericin B is necessary.

STOMACH AND DUODENUM

ANATOMY OF THE STOMACH AND DUODENUM

The stomach serves as a reservoir (with a capacity of 1,000-1,500 ml) for swallowed food, as well as a mixing and digestive organ. It lies entirely within the abdominal cavity, with all surfaces covered by peritoneum. The *cardia* is that portion of the proximal stomach surrounding the esophagogastric junction. The dome-shaped portion to the left of the cardia and lying beneath the left hemidiaphragm is the *fundus*. Extending downward and to the right from the fundus is the *corpus, or body*, the main portion of the stomach. The narrower distal stomach, the *antrum*, terminates in the *pylorus*, a narrow channel that connects with the first portion of the duodenum known as the bulb. The smooth muscle of the stomach consists of the usual outer longitudinal and inner circular layers, but in addition there is an innermost oblique muscle layer that is most prominently developed in the fundus and dwindles out in the distal stomach.

The mucosa may be divided into two major areas and histologic types, the larger of which is the acid-secreting *oxyntic gland area* of the fundus and body that is approximately 800 sq cm (four-fifths of the gastric mucosa). The mucosa of this area consists of tall, columnar epithelial cells that extend into the small pits leading to underlying glands. Mucous cells line the necks of the glands extending away from the surface. In the midportion of the glands, the epithelium is comprised of chief cells that produce pepsinogen, and parietal cells that produce hydrochloric acid and intrinsic factor. The second area consists of the 120 sq cm of *pyloric glands* of the distal stomach or antrum. In this region, the mucosa is lined by columnar epithelium and contains the shorter pyloric glands lined only by mucous neck cells and gastrin-producing cells, as well as some argentaffin cells.

The paired vagus nerves that enter the abdomen via the esophageal hiatus constitute the parasympathetic nerve supply to the stomach. The left, or anterior, vagus gives off the hepatic branch and branches to the fundus and corpus of the stomach, as well as a branch to the pyloric region. The right, or posterior, vagus branch gives off branches to the celiac plexus and branches to the posterior portion of the gastric corpus. The axons of the vagi terminate in the myenteric and submucosal plexuses of the stomach, where they synapse with ganglion cells whose axons are the postganglionic parasympathetics. Sympathetic postganglionic efferent fibers to the stomach arise in the prevertebral celiac ganglion, and travel with the blood vessels to terminate in the intrinsic nerve plexuses of the stomach wall. The sympathetic afferents return to the cord without synapsing with the ganglion cells of the intrinsic plexuses or the prevertebral ganglia. The blood supply of the stomach arises from the celiac axis, although anastomotic connections exist via the inferior pancreatoduodenal branch of the superior mesenteric artery. Venous drainage of the stomach is by way of the portal vein to the liver.

PHYSIOLOGY OF THE STOMACH AND DUODENUM

Motility

Gastric motor functions include storage and volume adaptation, mixing of contents, and propulsion or emptying. The stomach has two distinct motor regions, each with a different functional role. The proximal stomach, consisting of the fundus and upper body, acts as the gastric reservoir and is capable of receptive relaxation, by which the gastric volume may increase without a corresponding increase in intragastric pressure. The proximal stomach exerts slow, sustained, or tonal contractions that, by steady pressure on its contents, gradually press them toward the distal stomach. This mechanism is largely responsible for emptying of liquids from stomach to duodenum. The distal stomach is the site of mixing and grinding, and has a major regulatory role in the gastric emptying of solids. The motor activity of this part of the stomach is under the control of the gastric pacemaker, located in the smooth muscle cells of the greater curvature in the midbody of the stomach. Electrical cycles, known as the basic electric rhythm or pacesetter potentials, are generated from this site at a rate of 3 per minute. These are propagated from the pacemaker distally to the pylorus, and phase the timing of action potentials that, in turn, give rise to peristaltic contractions. The pacesetter potentials determine the frequency, direction, and velocity of muscle contractions, whereas the amplitude of the action potentials determines the force of contractions. Vagal fibers stimulate contractions, although some vagal efferents, as well as the sympathetics, inhibit contractions. Liquids are advanced to the distal stomach by the tonic contractions of the proximal stomach and pass readily into the duodenum. Solids are retained in the antrum where they are propelled against the pylorus, ground by the peristaltic contractions of the antrum, and then retropelled into the orad of the stomach. This process is repeated over and over until the solids are reduced to a particle size of less than 1 mm, at which point they are allowed to enter the duodenum. In the small intestine, gastric contents initiate and influence neurohumoral signals that govern the subsequent rate of gastric emptying. Such elements of gastric contents as osmolality, pH, hydrochloric acid, and fatty acids are known stimuli for small intestinal feedback signals.

Gastric Secretion

The principal constituents of gastric juice are hydrochloric acid, electrolytes (Na^+, Cl^+, K^+), mucus, digestive enzymes, and intrinsic factor. It is generally held that pure parietal cell secretion of hydrogen ion occurs at a concentration of 160-170 mEq/L and that the acid is then diluted by nonparietal secretions. Hence, variability in the electrolyte composition of gastric juice is due mainly to the hydrogen ion content that, in turn, is a function of the number of parietal cells secreting at a given time. Gastric mucus consists of a variety of mucoproteins and mucopolysaccharides including intrinsic factor and blood group substances. Their precise physiologic roles (excluding intrinsic factor) are uncertain. The major enzyme present is pepsinogen that is produced by chief cells, and in man has been shown to contain at least 7 fractions. Pepsin has a pH activity range from 1.8-3.5, but does not appear to be an important proteolytic enzyme in human digestion.

Regulation of Gastric Secretion

Gastric secretion is regulated during digestion of food, as well as in the interdigestive period, by the interplay of stimulatory and inhibitory mechanisms. The two major pathways for stimulation of gastric acid are neural and hormonal, both of which act via long extragastric routes; that is, the vagus nerves, and the systemic circulation via the celiac axis. In addition, the paracrine pathway acts at a local level but interacts with neural and hormonal stimuli. The vagus pathway transmitter at the level of the parietal cell is acetylcholine, whereas the humoral influence is mediated by gastrin, and the paracrine via histamine. It is thought that there is potentiating interaction between the three separate parietal cell receptors, all requiring the presence of histamine that is released by mast cells in the vicinity of parietal cells by acetylcholine stimulus discharged at nerve terminals, as well as by gastrin. This would explain the potent inhibitory action of the H_2-receptor antagonist cimetidine on gastric acid secretion.

Hormonal Regulation

Gastrin is the main hormone stimulating gastric secretion under physiologic circumstances. Two major forms of gastrin, G_{17} with 17 amino acid residues and G_{34} with 34 amino acids, account for more than 90% of the total activity of this hormone in the antrum and plasma. Gastrin is produced by specialized cells (G cells) located mainly in the antrum but also present in the duodenum and pancreas. Antral gastrin is released into the blood by food contact with antral mucosa, mainly partially digested protein containing specific peptides and amino acids. Gastrin is also released by distention of the antrum and by vagal impulses. Most stimulatory and inhibitory impulses for antral gastrin release are mediated via a cholinergic system in the antral mucosa. Intragastric pH also influences gastrin release, facilitating it at a neutral pH, and inhibiting it when the acidity of antral contents falls below pH 3.5. Basal antral gastrin release is not suppressed by acid, and alkali alone does not stimulate gastrin release, but acid and alkali modulate gastrin release where a stimulus for gastrin release is operating.

Neural Regulation
Neural mechanisms consist mainly of vagal afferents and efferents in a long reflex arc to the brain and spinal cord; this vagal system is closely linked to local reflex pathways within the intrinsic plexuses of the stomach wall that, in turn, can be activated by short reflexes completed within the wall of the stomach. Finally, there are also vagal and intramural connections of the gastric mucosa to the gastrin release system.

In the process of eating a meal, neural stimulation is triggered at different levels. Anticipation, sight, smell, and so forth constitute the cephalic phase. The tasting, chewing, and swallowing of food, and the presence of food in the stomach, probably by causing distention, all cause acid secretion through neural reflexes; this also result in release of gastrin that, in turn, contributes to parietal cell stimulation to produce hydrochloric acid. Direct stimulation of parietal cells by protein has also been demonstrated. Calcium, in the lumen or as hypercalcemia, stimulates acid production in part by gastrin release, as well as by direct parietal cell stimulation. Caffeine directly stimulates parietal cell secretion of acid.

Inhibitory mechanisms are located mainly distal to the pylorus and are stimulated by acid and also by digestive products, acting as a feedback regulatory mechanism on gastric acid secretion. Secretin is released into the blood stream from the duodenal mucosa in response to acid in the lumen, and noncompetitively inhibits gastric acid secretion. Cholecystokinin, also released from duodenal mucosa by protein and fat entering the duodenum, competitively inhibits gastrin-stimulated acid secretion. Gastric inhibitory peptide (GIP) is liberated by small intestinal mucosa in response to fat and glucose, and also inhibits gastric acid secretion. Other peptides have been isolated from intestinal mucosa with inhibitory effects on gastric acid secretion, but their structures and physiologic roles have not been well-characterized. Neural reflexes (bulb-fundic reflex) inhibiting acid secretion have been shown to originate in the duodenal bulb stimulated by acid. Hence, neuroendocrine control of gastric secretion is an integrated autoregulatory system, with stimulatory and inhibitory influences acting to modulate and adjust gastric secretion to specific needs after food intake, as well as during the interdigestive period.

Pepsin and Intrinsic Factor
Pepsinogen, especially pepsinogen I fraction, originates in chief cells and correlates well with acid secretory capacity. Stimuli that increase acid output raise gastric juice enzyme concentrations as well. Secreted in the inactive precursor form of pepsinogen, the enzyme is converted to pepsin by gastric acid and by pepsins. Its peak proteolytic activity is at a pH of 2, and is inactivated above a pH of 5.5.

Intrinsic factor is a product of the parietal cell but does not depend on stimuli for gastric acid secretion for its elaboration or secretion. It firmly binds dietary vitamin B_{12}, facilitating its active absorption in the distal ileum. It is the only component of gastric secretion essential to life, due to its critical role in vitamin B_{12} absorption from food.

DIAGNOSTIC PROCEDURES FOR GASTRODUODENAL DISORDERS

Radiographic Examination
An upper gastrointestinal examination includes not only the pharynx and esophagus described earlier, but also the stomach and duodenum. It is performed with the patient in the fasting state, employing barium sulfate suspension. Such studies provide information about position abnormalities as produced by displacement due to adjacent masses and organ enlargement, or the presence of hernias. Abnormal gastric motility may be noted as in diabetic gastroparesis, outlet obstruction, and infiltrating gastric neoplasm. Ulcerations, diverticula, neoplasms, fistulas, gastric polyps, foreign bodies, and bezoars may be recognized by barium contrast study. Double-contrast barium examination, of increasing importance, employs high-density barium sulfate suspension to coat the stomach, effervescent tablets for gastric distention, and simethicone to disperse or reduce the size of gas bubbles within the stomach. This examination gives better mucosal detail in the appreciation of polyps and Menetrier's disease. Gastritis and superficial erosions are better detected by direct endoscopic visualization, as are problems in the postoperative stomach.

Endoscopy
Fiberoptic gastroduodenoscopy is the current standard form of endoscopic examination of the upper gastrointestinal tract. These flexible instruments are easier to introduce, less hazardous to the patient, and permit gastric biopsy and brushings for cytology. They also afford better visualization of the cardia and pyloric areas, as well as visual access to the proximal duodenum for examination and instrumentation. Gastroscopy indications include assessment of the patient with upper gastrointestinal bleeding, and further evaluation and biopsy of roentgenographic findings such as ulcerations, masses, and abnormal folds. Gastroscopy is especially useful in the evaluation of postgastrectomy problems such as pain, vomiting, and bleeding, when stomal ulceration or bile reflux is suspected.

Measurement of Gastric Secretory Capacity
Modern techniques for measurement of gastric acidity include titration of gastric juice with sodium hydroxide to an end point of pH 7.0 (hydrogen ion concentration). The acidity of gastric juice should be expressed in milliequivalents per liter, and gastric acid output in mEq secreted in a given time. The current approach to measurement of gastric secretory rates consists of:

1. *Basal acid output* (BAO)—performed on the fasting stomach, after first aspirating or removing any fasting residual contents, and without any secretory stimulation. The period of collection is one hour, and normal basal acid secretory rate varies from 0-6 mEq/hour.
2. *Maximal acid output* (MAO)—the acid secretion rate in the sum of four consecutive 15-minute periods following stimulation with a maximal dose of pentagastrin or betazole; normal subjects secrete approximately 25 mEq/hour.
3. *Peak acid output* (PAO)—calculated by combining the two 15-minute periods of highest secretion, and multiplying by two.

There is considerable interpersonal variation in basal secretory rate, as well as within the individual when studied repeatedly over hours, days, or weeks. In healthy persons, basal acid secretion ranges from 0-6 mEq/hour, with a mean rate of 2.5 mEq/h for men. The basal acid secretory rate for duodenal ulcer patients ranges from 0-15 mEq/h with a mean rate for duodenal ulcer males of 6.0 mEq/hour. As a group, patients with duodenal ulcers have secretory rates greater than normal controls, with approximately 50% of duodenal ulcer subjects having significantly greater rates than normal. Gastric ulcer patients as a group have secretory rates of approximately 60% of those for normal individuals. Patients with gastrinomas and the Zollinger-Ellison syndrome usually have marked basal hypersecretion with basal secretory rates exceeding 15 mEq/h.

Owing to the wide overlap in secretory rates between normals and patients with duodenal ulcers and gastric ulcer, gastric secretory assessment in the diagnosis of peptic ulcer probably has no value. Gastric acid secretion should be measured in patients suspected of having Zollinger-Ellison syndrome; some authors advise that acid secretion measurement be carried out on all gastric ulcer patients, as achlorhydria would signify a presumptive diagnosis of malignancy. Patients with abdominal pain or gastrointestinal bleeding after peptic ulcer surgery, suggesting recurrent ulcer due to inadequate control of gastric acid output after resection or vagotomy, should have testing of gastric secretory capacity before further operation is undertaken. BAO in the postoperative stomach exceeding 5 mEq/h, or MAO exceeding 15 mEq/h, are associated with a high incidence of recurrent ulcer. The Hollander test, in which the gastric secretory rate is measured following insulin-induced hypoglycemia, is used to assess the completeness of vagotomy, and hence the chance of recurrent ulcer. Several criteria have been proposed by various users of this test. The procedure carries some risk of side effects, namely hypoglycemia, and the precipitation of angina pectoris or cerebrovascular ischemia symptoms in susceptible patients. The test should be performed with these precautions clearly in mind; some centers have abandoned this test.

Serum Gastrin

Radioimmunoassay has made feasible the clinical measurement of serum gastrin, as well as a growing number of other serum polypeptide gastrointestinal hormones. Methods and normal values vary between laboratories and must be known to the clinician for accurate evaluation of the results of serum gastrin measurement. Currently, serum gastrin determination is not considered a necessary part of the diagnostic work-up of an ordinary duodenal ulcer. Its greatest value is the diagnosis of the Zollinger-Ellison syndrome and related ulcer disease, but serum gastrin should also be determined in every patient with active ulcer disease associated with diarrhea or multiple endocrine adenomatosis, with virulent ulcer disease, and in every candidate considered for surgical treatment of duodenal ulcer. Other causes of hypergastrinemia must be kept in mind. Patients with pernicious anemia have raised serum gastrin levels, presumably because the achlorhydria represents failure of the feedback mechanism governing antral gastrin release. Carcinoma of the stomach is frequently associated with increased gastrin levels due to low or absent acid secretion. Hypergastrinemia occurs in some patients with renal insufficiency, probably due to impaired renal degradation of gastrin. Raised serum gastrin levels and acid hypersecretion are apt to follow massive small bowel resection, though the mechanism is uncertain. The retention of antral mucosa in continuity with the duodenum following partial gastric resection and Billroth II anastomosis has resulted in hypergastrinemia and stomal ulcer. The mechanism here is the exclusion of the antral gastrin cells from gastric acid, or other inhibitory factors in the feedback regulation of antral gastrin release. Antral G-cell hyperplasia is associated with gastric hypersecretion.

Occasionally, it is necessary to differentiate various clinical problems characterized by gastric hypersecretion and hypergastrinemia. Patients with gastrinomas and the Zollinger-Ellison syndrome exhibit a substantial increase in serum gastrin level following intravenous calcium infusion that significantly exceeds that noted in common duodenal ulcer disease. Intravenous secretin infusion also produces a substantial further elevation in serum gastrin in gastrinomas, whereas in duodenal ulcer patients secretin may decrease the gastrin level. In the presence of retained antrum, secretin infusion does not produce a paradoxical increase in serum gastrin. Following a protein meal, serum gastrin is essentially unchanged in gastrinoma patients. In antral G-cell hyperplasia, the meal produces a marked increase in serum gastrin, whereas it barely increases in response to calcium or secretin.

Biopsy and Cytology

Gastroscopically performed biopsies of discrete stomach lesions are of practical value in distinguishing an ulcer from gastric carcinoma, and in assessing the histologic character of gastric polyps (hyperplastic vs. adenomatous polyps). Biopsy is less useful in the clinical diagnosis of most forms of acute and chronic gastritis. In practice, multiple biopsies (at least 6), as well as brushings for cytologic study, should be obtained from around the inner margins of ulcerating gastric lesions.

DISEASES OF THE STOMACH

Peptic Ulcer Disease

Peptic ulcer is a mucosal ulceration (usually well-demarcated) occurring in the upper gastrointestinal tract, and characterized by discrete margins, loss of mucosa and submucosa, and often extending into the muscularis. It has a necrotic base covered with inflammatory debris. Peptic ulcers have an implied pathogenetic association with acid and pepsin, and are found only in the presence of gastric acid secretion. They are nearly always located in areas of the gastrointestinal tract exposed to acid; the lower esophagus, stomach, duodenum, at sites of ectopic gastric mucosa, and in the jejunum after gastrojejunostomy or in the Zollinger-Ellison syndrome.

Duodenal Ulcer

Duodenal ulcer, the predominant form of peptic ulcer, is nearly always located in the first portion of the duodenum, and usually within 2 cm of the pylorus. Most are small (less than 2 cm in diameter), but giant duodenal ulcers occur rarely, and paradoxically may be difficult to recognize radiographically. More diffuse inflammation without ulcer but with superficial patchy loss of mucosal layers, or duodenitis, is considered by many to be part of the spectrum of duodenal ulcer disease.

Epidemiology

Peptic ulcer disease afflicts approximately 10% of the American population at one time in their lives. Peak incidence of duodenal ulcer is at the age of 55-65 years, with male predominance.

Etiology and Pathogenesis

As implied by its name, the pathogenesis of peptic ulcer is considered to be intimately associated with abnormalities in the interrelationship between gastric acid, pepsin, and the mucosa of the proximal alimentary tract. However, despite knowledge of the regulation of acid secretion and investigations into mucosal resistance and mucosal barriers, there currently is no satisfactory explanation of the development of peptic ulcer or the roles played by gastric acid and pepsin. Peptic ulcers occur only in the presence of hydrochloric acid (no acid–no ulcer). Duodenal ulcer patients as a group secrete more acid than normal, but there is appreciable overlap with normal persons. Parietal cell counts in duodenal ulcer subjects are double the number for patients without ulcer. Higher basal, maximal, and nocturnal secretion rates have also been measured in duodenal ulcer subjects. Although serum gastrin levels are normal in duodenal ulcer, increased parietal cell sensitivity to a given dose of gastrin, and increased liberation of gastrin into the serum following a protein meal, have been observed. These phenomena contribute to the hypothesis that a defect in the feedback inhibition of gastrin may exist in duodenal ulcer patients.

Mucosal resistance seems to figure less prominently in the pathogenesis of duodenal ulcer than gastric ulcer, but it is uncertain whether local or regional factors exist at sites where peptic ulcer is most common. Both duodenal ulcer and gastric ulcer occur with greater frequency in smokers than nonsmokers. There is no proven effect of smoking on acid secretion, although pancreatic bicarbonate output has been shown to be reduced by smoking, perhaps resulting in less buffering of acid in the duodenum. There is no evidence that diet contributes to the pathogenesis of duodenal ulcer. Similarly, there is no conclusive evidence that psychiatric factors play a role in causing peptic ulcer, though clinical experience holds that exacerbations of ulcer commonly occur in settings of emotional stress. Ulcer disease incidence also is not related to socioeconomic class or occupation. Peptic ulcer is more common among first-degree relatives of patients with duodenal ulcer. Blood group O carries a slightly increased incidence of duodenal ulcer, as does nonsecretion of ABO antigens in saliva.

Natural History of Duodenal Ulcer. Duodenal ulcer death rates rise logarithmically with increasing age. Fifty-one percent of deaths from duodenal ulcer are due to bleeding, 31 percent from perforation, and 18 percent from other ulcer-related problems. The incidence of major complications is less than 1% per year.

Natural History of Duodenal Ulcer

Duodenal ulcer death rates rise logarithmically with increasing age. Fifty-one percent of deaths from duodenal ulcer are due to bleeding, 31 percent from perforation, and 18 percent from other ulcer-related problems. The incidence of major complications is less than 1% per year.

Clinical Picture

The prime symptom of duodenal ulcer is epigastric pain. Classically, the clinical picture is that of non-radiating epigastric pain that occurs on an empty stomach (from 1-3 hours after meals), and is relieved by food, antacids, or emesis. It typically awakens the patient from sleep at night, and is seldom present in the morning before breakfast. Such a picture occurs in daily episodes for a few days to a few weeks, with symptom-free intervals of weeks to months. However, a significant percentage of ulcer patients have atypical symptoms and patterns, and duodenal ulcer may be found in essentially asymptomatic individuals. The pain is often described as gnawing or burning but may be noted more as heartburn, a dull ache, or merely vague discomfort. Other symptoms and patterns of pain are usually related to unusual location of the ulcer, or to complications of the disease or its treatment; for example, back pain due to penetration of the ulcer into the pancreas; nausea and vomiting with pyloric obstruction; or hematemesis and melena as manifestations of bleeding. Physical examination may be negative or disclose only epigastric tenderness to palpation. A succussion splash is often elicited in the presence of gastric retention due to pyloric obstruction.

Diagnosis

The clinical history taken alone is an imprecise tool. Some asymptomatic ulcers are found at autopsy, and it is well-recognized that many patients with ulcerlike symptoms have negative x-rays and endoscopic examinations. Roentgenographic examination of the esophagus, stomach, and duodenum with barium sulfate has been the standard diagnostic measure; in expert hands, it has an 80-90% diagnostic accuracy. Endoscopy is capable of detecting perhaps a further 5-10% of ulcers but should be performed mainly in patients with negative x-rays and significant symptoms. Once the diagnosis of duodenal ulcer is established, it is probably sufficient to empirically reinstitute treatment at times of recurrence unless there are atypical features, or surgery is being considered.

Laboratory Studies

Routine laboratory tests should be performed, including the hemoglobin or hematocrit, serum calcium, and a stool examination for occult blood. Serum gastrin assay is not indicated in routine diagnosis of duodenal ulcer, but should be performed when Zollinger-Ellison syndrome is suspected. It is also indicated in duodenal ulcer associated with hyperparathyroidism, in ulcer patients with a family history of endocrine neoplasia, in patients who are soon to undergo elective ulcer surgery, and in the assessment of patients with recurrent ulcer after ulcer surgery.

Medical Treatment

The objectives of ulcer therapy are to relieve pain, to promote ulcer healing, to minimize recurrences, and to avoid ulcer complications. To accomplish these goals, therapy is aimed at the reduction of acid secretion or its more effective neutralization. Controlled studies have not demonstrated that any form of diet therapy contributes to ulcer healing or prevention of recurrence. Patients should be allowed a regular diet, but told to avoid those foods that seem to cause abdominal distress. Many physicians restrict caffeine-containing beverages, owing to their weak acid-stimulating potential. Although the ability of alcohol to increase gastric acid secretion is in some doubt, it is best proscribed during treatment of active ulcer since its ability to contribute to mucosal injury and bleeding is significant. Smoking should be stopped. Frequent between-meal milk feedings offer little acid-buffering, probably stimulate more acid secretion, and in long-term use are atherogenic.

Antacids are the mainstay in routine medical management of duodenal ulcer. The goal of such therapy is to effect an intragastric pH of 5 or higher, in order to minimize mucosal damage due to acid and to inactivate pepsin. The number of antacid preparations available and their variability in composition, cost, palatability, and acid-neutralizing capacity is great (Tables 1, 2). Absorbable antacids such as sodium bicarbonate may cause alkalosis, and hence should be avoided. Prolonged use of absorbable antacids and milk carries a significant risk of the milk-alkali syndrome that is characterized by hypercalcemia, alkalosis, azotemia, and nephrocalcinosis. In general, aluminum and magnesium combination antacids are preferred, and it is better to employ liquid preparations in view of their greater acid-neutralizing capacity. All antacids may cause toxicity related to their metallic cations in patients with advanced renal impairment, and phosphate depletion has also been produced by aluminum hydroxide, giving rise to such symptoms as tetany, weakness, and apnea. Magnesium antacids tend to cause diarrhea, and aluminum antacids are often constipating. Antacids low in sodium content are preferred in ulcer management of patients with congestive heart failure and other sodium-retaining disorders. Calcium antacids, although effective acid neutralizers, are currently in disfavor owing to the risk of hypercalcemia and rebound stimulation of gastric acid. For the management of the symptomatic ulcer patient, liquid antacid therapy taken 1 and 3 hours after meals and at bedtime is advised, in a dose calculated to contain at least 100 mEq of acid-neutralizing capacity. Patients should be advised to use additional doses of antacids at other times of the day, or night, if distress occurs. Most patients become asymptomatic within 1 week, and have been shown to have healed ulcers in 6 weeks. At times, it may be necessary to use hourly antacids to gain initial control of acute or severe ulcer symptoms. Until the advent of H_2-receptor blocking agents, anticholinergic drugs were used by many physicians for their inhibitory effect on vagal stimulation of parietal cells, and also to reduce vagal release of gastrin. Despite their proven ability to reduce gastric acid secretion by 30-50%, conclusive evidence that they promote duodenal ulcer healing was lacking in many studies. Undesirable systemic side effects occur including dry mouth, visual blurring, constipation, and urinary retention. When pyloric obstruction is imminent or present, they should not be used. Glaucoma and prostate hypertrophy are also contraindications. Patients prone to gastroesophageal reflux are likely to have increased reflux symptoms, owing to delayed gastric emptying. Some physicians employ anticholinergic agents only at bedtime to help reduce nocturnal gastric secretion.

It is unnecessary to reexamine the patient by stomach x-ray or endoscopy to confirm or assess duodenal ulcer healing, after a suitable period of treatment (4-6 weeks) and disappearance of symptoms. Most physicians liberalize antacid treatment, and then discontinue medication in 2 or 3 months.

Patients must be taught and reminded that duodenal ulcer tends to be a chronic, recurring disease and that active medical therapy should be resumed at the first sign of recurrent symptoms. Physical and mental rest are important components of ulcer therapy, although routine use of sedatives or tranquilizers is inadvisable.

Knowledge of the natural history of duodenal ulcer is still growing, with new observations recently derived from the closer scrutiny (including periodic endoscopy) of patients participating in long-term randomized trials of cimetidine treatment. Endoscopy demonstrates that symptoms are not reliable indicators of ulcer recurrence, since 20-30% of patients with endoscopically documented recurrences were virtually asymptomatic. It has also shown that symptomatic relief appears to be a poor indicator of healing. Furthermore, spontaneous healing has been noted to take place at 4 weeks in a significant percentage of ulcer patients on placebo treatment.

Cimetidine Therapy. The place of this H_2-receptor antagonist in routine management of duodenal ulcer and its role relative to traditional antacid use are unsettled issues. Although antacids have been shown in experimental trials to be more effective than a placebo, this superiority required approximately 1,000 mEq of antacid daily. Low compliance for antacid use (30-45%) has been documented among ulcer patients, perhaps accounted for by the inconvenient frequency of prescribed doses, the volume required to be kept at hand and consumed, and altered bowel behavior. When the added

Table 1. Neutralizing Capacity, Sodium Content, and Cost Effectiveness of Liquid Antacids

Antacid	*Acid Neutralizing Capacity*	*Volume Containing 140 meq*	*Sodium Content*	*Monthly Cost of Therapy*	*Composition*	*Manufacturer*
	meq mL	*mL*	*mg/5 mL*	*$*		
Maalox TC	4.2	33	1.2	44	Aluminum hydroxide, magnesium hydroxide	W. H. Rorer, Inc., Fort Washington, Pennsylvania
Titralac	4.2	33	11.0	35	Calcium carbonate, glycine	Riker Laboratories, Inc., Northridge, California
Delcid	4.1	34	1.5	57	Aluminum hydroxide, magnesium hydroxide	Merrell-National Laboratories, Cincinnati, Ohio
Mylanta II	3.6	39	1.1	63	Aluminum hydroxide, magnesium hydroxide, simethicone	Stuart Pharmaceuticals, Wilmington, Delaware
Camalox	3.2	44	2.5	55	Aluminum hydroxide, magnesium hydroxide, calcium carbonate	W. H. Rorer, Inc., Fort Washington, Pennsylvania
Gelusil II	3.0	47	1.3	74	Aluminum hydroxide, magnesium hydroxide, simethicone	Parke-Davis, Morris Plains, New Jersey
Basaljel ES	2.9	48	23.0	101	Aluminum carbonate	Wyeth Laboratories, Philadelphia, Pennsylvania
Maalox Plus	2.3	61	2.5	68	Aluminum hydroxide, magnesium hydroxide, simethicone	W. H. Rorer, Inc., Fort Washington, Pennsylvania
Gelusil	2.2	64	0.7	80	Aluminum hydroxide, magnesium hydroxide, simethicone	Parke-Davis, Morris Plains, New Jersey
Riopan Plus	1.8	78	0.7	78	Aluminum hydroxide, magnesium hydroxide, simethicone	Ayerst Laboratories, New York, New York
Amphojel	1.4	100	7.0	114	Aluminum hydroxide	Wyeth Laboratories, Philadelphia, Pennsylvania
Phosphaljel	0.3	466	12.5	498	Aluminum phosphate	Wyeth Laboratories, Philadelphia, Pennsylvania

From Drake and Hollander, *Anals of Internal Medicine* 94:215, 1981. Reprinted by permission.

potential for more serious side effects, toxicity, and the long-term cost are considered, cimetidine emerges in the minds of many physicians as safer, no more expensive, comparably effective, and more apt to be properly used by the ulcer patient.

Some physicians initiate treatment with a conventional antacid program and reserve cimetidine for resistant symptoms, poor surgical risks, and for patients with chronically recurring disease. There is growing use of cimetidine as initial therapy in place of antacids, employing full doses (300 mg four times daily) for 6 to 8 weeks, then reassessing the case. Longer use of cimetidine in the above doses, or in a schedule such as 300 mg once or twice daily, has been shown to reduce the incidence of recurrence while on therapy. Prophylactic use of cimetidine in selected cases might be carried out for a year or two, or indefinitely in more complicated cases and poor surgical risks. However, duration of treatment of up to 2 years does not influence the recurrence rate once the drug is stopped.

Sucralfate Therapy. Sucralfate, a nonabsorbable aluminum salt of sucrose sulfate, has been shown to work locally on peptic ulcer by protectively binding to ulcerated mucosa; it also buffers acid, inhibits pepsin action, and adsorbs bile salts. This comprehensive protective barrier effect has been shown in clinical trials to provide symptomatic relief of ulcer pain and to enhance ulcer healing at a rate comparable to antacids and cimetidine, when doses of 1 gram four times daily were used. It is well tolerated and apparently free of serious side effects.

Surgical Treatment

Indications for surgery in management of duodenal ulcer are perforation, gastric outlet obstruction, hemorrhage, and intractable pain. These are considered complications of the disease that lead to surgery in 10-15% of duodenal ulcer patients.

Perforation. Duodenal ulcer perforation, an acute emergency occurring in about 2% of ulcer patients and almost always requiring surgical treatment, may appear without prior

Table 2. Neutralizing Capacity, Sodium Content, and Cost Effectiveness of Tablet Antacids

Antacid	*Acid Neutralizing Capacity*	*Dose Containing 140 meq*	*Sodium Content*	*Monthly Cost of Therapy*	*Composition*	*Manufacturer*
	meq tablet	*tablets*	*mg/tablet*	*$*		
Camalox	16.7	8	1.5	54	Aluminum hydroxide, magnesium hydroxide	W. H. Rorer, Inc., Fort Washington, Pennsylvania
Basaljel	15.4	9	2.0	68	Aluminum carbonate	Wyeth Laboratories, Philadelphia, Pennsylvania
Mylanta II	11.0	13	1.3	85	Aluminum hydroxide, magnesium hydroxide, simethicone	Stuart Pharmaceuticals, Wilmington, Delaware
Tums	10.5	13	2.7	56	Calcium carbonate	Norcliff Thayer, Inc., Tuckahoe, New York
Alka II	10.5	13	2.0	58	Calcium carbonate	Miles Laboratories, Inc., Elkhart, Indiana
Riopan Plus	10.0	14	0.3	76	Aluminum hydroxide, magnesium hydroxide, simethicone	Ayerst Laboratories, New York, New York
Titralac	9.5	15	0.3	57	Calcium carbonate, glycine	Riker Laboratories, Inc., Northridge, California
Gelusil II	8.2	17	2.1	107	Aluminum hydroxide, magnesium hydroxide, simethicone	Parke-Davis, Morris Plains, New Jersey
Rolaids	6.9	20	53.0	86	Aluminum carbonate	Warner Lambert Company, Morris Plains, New Jersey
Maalox Plus	5.7	25	1.4	106	Aluminum hydroxide. magnesium hydroxide; simethicone	W. H. Rorer, Inc., Fort Washington, Pennsylvania
Digel	4.7	30	10.6	101	Aluminum hydroxide, magnesium hydroxide, simethicone, magnesium carbonate	Plough, Inc., Memphis, Tennessee
Amphojel	2.0	70	7.0	360	Aluminum hydroxide	Wyeth Laboratories, Philadelphia, Pennsylvania

From Drake and Hollander, Annals of Internal Medicine 94:215, 1981. Reprinted by permission.

ulcer symptoms. It is usually marked by the dramatically sudden onset of severe pain, most typically epigastric or right upper quadrant in location, that is constant and steady in nature. The patient usually lies quietly, avoiding movement and straining. There is marked tenderness to palpation, and boardlike rigidity of the abdominal wall. Bowel sounds are usually absent. Shock features may appear if diagnosis and treatment are delayed. Diagnosis rests on the clinical picture, leukocytosis, and the presence of free air beneath the diaphragm on plain roentgenograms of the abdomen taken in the supine and upright positions, or in the lateral decubitus positions. Free air is seen in 85% of cases. Occasionally, hemorrhage accompanies the perforation. A small percentage of patients show progressive clinical improvement after several hours, owing to sealing of the perforation. Treatment of acute perforation of duodenal ulcer is by gastric intubation and suction, and fluid loss replacement followed promptly by surgery. Simple closure of the perforation is often performed, but many surgeons prefer to carry out a more definitive ulcer operation to avert future ulcer troubles that have been shown to develop in 20-30% of cases.

Obstruction. Although most commonly caused by cicatricial narrowing of the pyloric channel consequent to chronically recurring ulcer attacks, gastric outlet obstruction may be due to inflammatory edema and reduced gastric motility, aggravated at times by anticholinergic therapy. Owing to the insidious development of obstruction, and the concurrent atony and dilatation of the stomach, the clinical picture at times evolves over many weeks, with the symptoms varied and less dramatic. The patient may vomit only once a day or less, and complain of a vague fullness with declining appetite and weight loss. Weakness, lethargy, muscle cramps, headaches, and confusion occur as hypokalemic alkalosis develops. Emesis is typically voluminous, foul smelling, and contains evidence of retained food. The patient may appear dehydrated and wasted, and abdominal inspection may reveal the outlines of a distended stomach. A succussion splash is a common and valuable sign. Hemoconcentration, alkalosis, and hypokalemia are the main laboratory features. Acute pyloric obstruction may remit on a regimen of gastric decompression by nasogastric suction of stomach secretions for a few days, plus intravenous fluids and electrolytes to correct the dehydration and metabolic hypokalemic alkalosis. Anticholinergic medication must be stopped. However, if the symptoms do not improve or soon recur, or if other features such as pain or intractability color the clinical picture, surgery should be performed when the patient is in optimal condition.

Hemorrhage. Acute hemorrhage may be the presenting manifestation of duodenal ulcer. Significant hemorrhage occurs in the course of ulcer disease in about 20% of patients, is responsible for nearly half the deaths from duodenal ulcer, and is also the main indication for surgery in one-third of patients operated upon for peptic ulcer. Patients with acute hemorrhage from ulcer are managed by prompt assessment of cardiovascular status, including estimation of the magnitude of blood loss. A large caliber intravenous needle is inserted to draw blood for hemoglobin or hematocrit, blood typing and cross matching, and for measuring creatinine, blood sugar, liver enzymes, and prothrombin time. Intravenous fluid replacement is then started until blood is available. Meanwhile, a large-bore stomach tube is passed to empty the stomach, to gauge the rate of continued bleeding and, perhaps, to irrigate the stomach with iced saline solution. A central venous pressure monitoring line is also placed while blood and fluids are administered. As soon as the stomach is evacuated of clots, endoscopy is performed to define the source of bleeding. Most commonly, bleeding ceases and the nasogastric tube can be removed, after which medical therapy for duodenal ulcer can be pursued. However, when active bleeding persists, emergency surgery should be considered if the rate of bleeding requires rapid blood administration and fails to correct signs of shock. Persistent bleeding at a rate requiring more than 3 units of blood in the first 24 hours carries a worsening prognosis, especially in older patients, and should force a decision for emergency surgery despite concerns about age and other medical problems unless they pose clearly prohibitive risks or contraindications. Recurrence of bleeding following an initial hemorrhage during the same hospitalization is also generally considered an indication for emergency surgery. Recent studies suggest that visible vessels in the bleeding ulcer seen endoscopically are associated with a higher rate of rebleeding during hospitalization.

In a nonemergency situation, hemorrhage as an indication for elective duodenal ulcer surgery is less well agreed upon. However, there is evidence that massive hemorrhage from peptic ulcer recurs in 25-30% of cases and, given the 15-20% mortality from recurrent massive hemorrhage in patients over 60 years of age versus the lower mortality from elective ulcer surgery in patients of the same age range who are in reasonably good health, it is appropriate to advise elective gastric surgery following one massive hemorrhage in these patients. In younger patients who have had one massive hemorrhage, the risks of surgery or death from recurrent hemorrhage approximate each other. Therefore, hemorrhage should be regarded as one indication for elective surgery, but weighed along with other complications and indications.

Intractability. Intractability connotes social and/or economic incapacitation of the patient by severe or frequent refractory pain despite adequate treatment. Although it represents the most frequent indication for ulcer surgery (40-50% of duodenal ulcer surgery), intractable pain is the most difficult of all indications to define and apply, owing to its subjective nature. It implies certainty of ulcer diagnosis, critical appraisal of the adequacy of medical treatment, and even the need for a trial of hospital treatment in some cases. Also relevant to intractability as a surgical indication are age of onset below 20 or over 60, possible postbulbar or channel location of the ulcer, and an associated serious personality disturbance or emotional illness, making patient cooperation in effective medical treatment difficult or impossible.

Surgery as Elective Therapy of Duodenal Ulcer. The objectives of surgery for duodenal ulcer are threefold: to cure the ulcer, to avoid mortality, and to minimize adverse postoperative sequelae. Subtotal (60-75%) gastrectomy, the most common procedure before the advent of vagotomy, was aimed at reducing the parietal cell mass, and in good hands achieved a 5% ulcer recurrence rate. However, the frequency and severity of postoperative sequelae (20%) such as rapid gastric emptying with resultant maldigestion, malabsorption, and the dumping syndrome, in addition to alkaline reflux gastritis, anemia, and osteoporosis, led surgeons to explore other procedures.

The advent of truncal vagotomy offered a comparably effective ulcer-curing operation (5-15% recurrence rate) with lower mortality by surgically removing the parasympathetic drive to the parietal cells, as well as to the gastrin-producing antrum. However, truncal vagotomy often resulted in diarrhea as well as impaired gastric emptying, leading to stasis and an increased risk of gastric ulceration. Pyloroplasty or gastrojejunostomy, added to truncal vagotomy to deal with stasis, increased the incidence of dumping symptoms and bile reflux. Antrectomy combined with vagotomy, physiologically aimed at removing both vagal and humoral stimuli to acid secretion, has given perhaps the lowest ulcer recurrence rate (less than 1%) but has also yielded a 20% rate of significant postoperative sequelae. The most recent surgical procedure accruing favorable results is proximal gastric vagotomy. In this operation, the vagus branches to the parietal cell-bearing fundus and corpus of the stomach are selectively divided, greatly reducing acid and pepsin secretion. Vagal branches to the antrum, the small intestine, and liver are preserved in order to minimally affect gastric emptying of solids and reduce the incidence of diarrhea. No drainage operation is incorporated. No, or minimal, operative mortality has been noted, and a low (less than 5%) incidence of postoperative sequelae has thus far been observed. However, the ulcer recurrence rate after proximal gastric vagotomy in most series (5% at 5 years) appears to be higher than that following vagotomy and antrectomy. Hence, for elective surgical management of duodenal ulcer, vagotomy and antrectomy, or proximal gastric vagotomy, would seem the operations of choice. Patients with well-established pyloric obstruction, gastric dilatation, and edema may be a special group who deserve the incorporation of some sort of drainage procedure such as pyloroplasty, or vagotomy and antrectomy, or simple gastroenterostomy in older, poor risk patients.

Syndromes Following Gastric Surgery: Early Dumping Syndrome. This combination of vasomotor and gastrointestinal symptoms usually becomes apparent soon after surgery, and is most frequent following gastric resection or pyloroplasty. Patients experience sweating, giddiness, lightheadedness, tachycardia, and often hypotension, along with a vague, sick, miserable feeling. All the above symptoms usually respond to lying down for a short time. Concurrently, most patients also experience cramping and diarrhea, at times with nausea and vomiting. It is thought that accelerated entry of the hyperosmolar gastric contents into the proximal jejunum induces a contraction of effective circulating blood volume and also brings about release of several humoral substances; serotonin, bradykinin, and other gut peptides. However, thus far there has been no convincing induction of an experimental dumping syndrome by infusion of several of these peptides. Although a high percentage of patients experience these symptoms soon after surgery, they tend to abate in severity in many, but remain significantly troublesome in 5-15% of patients. The avoidance of large meals, restricting the intake of liquids during or near meals, and the avoidance of large amounts of simple sugars and milk help minimize dumping symptoms. In a small percentage of postgastrectomy patients who are physically and economically incapacitated by severe intractable dumping, the surgical interposition of a short antiperistaltic jejunal segment between stomach and duodenum has given significant benefit.

Reactive Hypoglycemia. Sometimes called the late dumping syndrome, significant hypoglycemia arises 2-3 hours after a meal in a modest number of cases, producing typical symptoms of diaphoresis, weakness, and faintness. It usually follows the intake of sugars and other carbohydrates that results in an abnormally high postprandial blood sugar level, causing release of excessive insulin, and giving rise to hypoglycemia.

Postvagotomy Diarrhea. Diarrhea is observed by more than half the patients following vagotomy, though it tends to gradually diminish in severity. Its cause is not understood. Low sugar intake is helpful in some patients; anticholinergics, however, are of little benefit. Diphenoxylate and tetracycline in intermittent courses have helped some patients. Cholestyramine has produced conflicting results, but may be worth a trial. A reversed antiperistaltic jejunal segment 10 cm in length performed 90-100 cm distal to the ligament of Treitz was reported by Herrington to improve the status of severely symptomatic subjects.

Afferent Loop Syndrome. Following gastric operations incorporating a gastrojejunal anastomosis, partial or complete obstruction of the afferent loop may occur. Causes are varied but adhesions, internal hernias, and intussusception have been noted. One form of the syndrome has been termed bilious vomiting owing to the forceful emesis of bilious fluid, usually containing no food, that occurs following the postprandial onset of epigastric fullness, pressure, and nausea. Relief follows emesis until another meal. In some instances, the afferent loop obstruction does not result in the above clinical picture, but consists of the consequences of stasis and bacterial overgrowth with megaloblastic anemia due to vitamin B_{12} deficiency, and steatorrhea due to bacterial deconjugation of bile acids. Relief of these syndromes requires surgical correction of the obstructed afferent loop.

Alkaline Reflux Gastritis. The reflux of bile and duodenal contents into the stomach is common after operations that bypass, alter, or remove the pyloric sphincter mechanism. In 5-35% of patients undergoing such surgery, a clinical syndrome of varying severity develops characterized by epigastric pain and burning, vomiting of bile, weight loss, and often an iron deficiency anemia. The pain is more or less continuous, and not significantly affected by food or relieved by vomiting.

The pathogenesis of this lesion is thought to involve the removal or stripping of protective mucus from the gastric mucosa, and disruption of the mucosal barrier by refluxed bile acids and duodenal contents, allowing back-diffusion of hydrogen ions and eventual inflammation, erosion, and even ulceration of the mucosa.

Diagnosis is suggested by the clinical setting and symptoms, and the endoscopic appearance of a red, friable, granular gastric mucosa, most marked in the peristomal area. Bile refluxing into the stomach is often noted. Biopsy of the involved area shows inflammation, atrophy, and intestinal metaplasia. Gastric analysis usually shows hypochlorhydria, or achlorhydria. Treatment consists of surgical diversion of duodenal contents from the gastric pouch by the Roux-en-Y procedure. If vagotomy or antrectomy were not previously done both should be carried out, as gastric acid secretory capability will be restored as the mucosa reverts toward normal following the Roux-en-Y procedure, and marginal ulcer may result.

Medical treatment using cholestyramine or bile-binding aluminum antacids has not given satisfactory results.

Other Postoperative Sequelae. Chronic anemia due to low intake or impaired absorption of iron following gastric resection has been shown to develop in a significant percentage of patients studied over a 10-year period following surgery. In some patients, chronic gastritis, leading to atrophic gastritis and loss of intrinsic factor production, may develop after gastric resection, resulting in a megaloblastic anemia due to vitamin B_{12} deficiency. Impaired vitamin D absorption and calcium malabsorption are known to occur after gastric resections, and osteomalacia has been noted in 5% of such patients. Supplemental dietary or medical calcium, or vitamin D, should be given. Finally, cancer of the stomach has been shown to occur in the gastric remnant following partial gastric resection.

Zollinger-Ellison Syndrome

The Zollinger-Ellison syndrome is an uncommon syndrome of hypergastrinemia, hyperchlorhydria, often virulent ulcerative disease of the proximal gastrointestinal tract, and diarrhea, caused by the elaboration and autonomous release of gastrin by a non-β cell tumor of the pancreas (termed a gastrinoma).

Epidemiology

This disorder has been described from the first to the tenth decades of life, and is slightly more common in men.

Gastrinomas may occur sporadically or be associated with other endocrine tumors, most commonly of the parathyroid, pituitary, or adrenal glands, constituting the so-called multiple endocrine adenomatosis type I syndrome, an autosomal dominant familial disorder.

Pathology
Gastrinomas are most commonly located in the head and tail of the pancreas, but are not uncommonly encountered in the wall of the stomach or duodenum, or in the hilus of the spleen. Sixty percent of the tumors are malignant, and the majority have metastasized at the time of diagnosis. Metastases occur to regional lymph nodes, liver, peritoneal surfaces, bone, and skin. Hyperplasia or multiple tumors are found in 20-25 percent of cases. Immunofluorescence techniques have demonstrated immunoreactive gastrin within the cells of gastrinomas. The exact identity and nomenclature of the islet cells producing gastrin is a matter of some dispute. Patients with Zollinger-Ellison syndrome have large parietal cell masses, probably due to the chronic stimulatory effect of gastrin. Brunner's glands of the duodenum may be unusually prominent in number and size. Superficial erosions and ulcerations of the proximal small intestinal mucosa, with associated hyperemia and inflammatory cell infiltration, are quite common.

Clinical Features
The Zollinger-Ellison syndrome, as originally described, consisted of peptic ulcer disease that presented clinically in a severe and often dramatic fashion, with multiple ulcers in atypical locations, uncontrollable symptoms, and a high tendency to recur following peptic ulcer surgery. However, it has been increasingly recognized that patients with hypergastrinemic, hypersecretory duodenal ulcer disease often present with clinical, radiologic, and endoscopic features indistinguishable from ordinary duodenal ulcer. Nevertheless, 90-95 percent of patients with the Zollinger-Ellison syndrome have ulcers at some stage of their disease.

Although many patients will have had symptoms or proven ulcer disease for up to several years, persistent symptoms and reduced responsiveness to conventional ulcer therapy may hint at the Zollinger-Ellison syndrome. Most ulcers are single in number, and located in the first part of the duodenum. Should they be multiple, or be located beyond the bulb in the second to the fourth portion of the duodenum, one should suspect the Zollinger-Ellison syndrome. The gastric folds are usually prominent, and increased secretions in the stomach may be noted by the radiologist. The small bowel x-ray not uncommonly shows coarse folds of the proximal bowel and increased fluid in the lumen. Diarrhea has been noted in 36-80 percent of cases and, in 7-10 percent of cases, is the presenting feature without ulcer. The diarrhea is thought to be due to the hypersecretion of a large volume of acid that produces irritating effects on the proximal small bowel mucosa. The diarrhea stops during chronic or continuous gastric aspiration, or during treatment with antisecretory drugs. Steatorrhea is common. It has also been shown that the large volume of acid in the proximal small intestine produces a low ph that inactivates pancreatic lipase and trypsin and reduces the solubility of bile acids, thereby making them unavailable for micelle formation.

The moribidty and mortality from this syndrome relate principally to the gastric hypersecretion and aggressive ulcer features, not to the malignant nature of the gastrinoma or its metastases, which are slow-growing.

Diagnosis
The diagnosis of Zollinger-Ellison syndrome should be based upon the following: a compatible clinical history, fasting hypergastrinemia on several occasions (occasional normal values do not exclude the Zollinger-Ellison syndrome), and either basal acid output exceeding 15 mEq/H or >5 mEq/h after gastric surgery, or histologically proven non-β cell tumor in patients with proven peptic ulcer disease. The recent emergence of a similar but rare syndrome of hypergastrinemia and duodenal ulcer attributed to excessive gastrin elaboration by hyperplastic G cells of the gastric antrum has made it important to differentiate between this entity and the Zollinger-Ellison syndrome because of potentially important differences in management. This is usually possible employing gastrin challenge tests that show the following: In antral G-cell hyperplasia, a protein meal produces a significant further increase in serum gastrin level. This does not occur in the Zollinger-Ellison syndrome. Intravenous secretin infusion or intravenous calcium infusion does not produce further elevations of serum gastrin in antral G-cell hyperplasia, whereas very significant further increases occur in the Zollinger-Ellison syndrome.

Treatment
Until the advent of pharmacologic control of gastric secretion by cimetidine, the management of the Zollinger-Ellison syndrome was almost inevitably total gastrectomy to remove the target organ of gastrin and thus abolish acid secretion. The only exception was the occasionally successful excision of a single gastrinoma in the pancreas or, more commonly, in the wall of the duodenum or stomach. However, cimetidine has now been shown to be effective in maintaining many patients clinically compensated for several years. Antacids and anticholinergics are usually added to cimetidine. Currently, the role of surgery is to resect localized tumors, as has been possible in some duodenal wall tumors, resulting in prolonged remissions or complete cures. Medical failure may necessitate total gastrectomy to control the ulcer disease, but if antral G-cell hyperplasia appears to be the basic underlying abnormality, antrectomy is preferable since it has been successful in controlling the disorder.

Gastric Ulcer

Etiology
Ulceration of the gastric mucosa is more diverse in its etiology, pathogenesis, and clinical manifestations than is duodenal ulcer. Acute gastric ulcerations occur frequently in the antrum, are usually multiple and superficial (those limited to the mucosa are called erosions), and commonly arise in clinical settings differing from chronic peptic ulcer. They are most frequently encountered following exposure of the gastric mucosa to alcohol and aspirin, or to other drugs known to injure or disrupt the mucosal barrier to back diffusion of

hydrogen ions. They also arise in situations of stress such as trauma, sepsis, or other serious medical or surgical illnesses, accompanied by shock in which ischemia of the gastric mucosa may occur. The presence of gastric acid seems to be necessary as an additional causative factor. Such acute gastric mucosal lesions, perhaps best termed stress-induced acute hemorrhagic gastritis, have no proven role in the pathogenesis of chronic gastric ulcer.

The etiology and pathogenesis of chronic gastric ulcers are less certain. As a group, patients with gastric ulcer secrete less acid than normal people, but the presence of acid still appears necessary for ulcer formation. Several hypotheses incorporating other possible etiologic factors have been proposed. Antral stasis from various causes was thought to result in antral distention that, in turn, stimulated gastrin release, producing gastric acid secretion leading to gastric ulcer formation. However, the evidence against this theory is that most gastric ulcer patients have normal gastric emptying, and tend to have low acid secretion. Moreover, the elevated serum gastrin levels appear to be consequent to low acid secretion, not a cause of hypersecretion. Diffuse gastritis has been noted in most gastric ulcer patients, and usually is more severe in the antral and pyloric regions; most evidence suggests it is not secondary to gastric ulceration, but a more basic and perhaps predisposing lesion. A third hypothesis presumes an abnormality in the gastric mucosal barrier, permitting sufficient back diffusion of hydrogen ions to produce ulceration. Although the barrier has been shown vulnerable to salicylates, bile salts, and alcohol, sufficient data are lacking to define how frequently these factors are at work in chronic gastric ulcer. Chronic aspirin ingestion has been associated with an increased incidence of gastric ulcer, at least in women. Defective antroduodenal motility has been proposed to account for the higher than normal stomach concentrations of bile acids noted in some gastric ulcer subjects.

The majority of gastric ulcers occur in the antrum near the junction of the parietal and antral mucosa, and more commonly on the lesser curve. Male incidence predominates, but less so than in duodenal ulcers. The peak incidence for gastric ulcer is a decade later than for duodenal ulcer.

Symptoms and Manifestations

Not uncommonly, gastric ulcer is asymptomatic, or may be discovered only at the time of hemorrhage or perforation. Though the typical pain-food-relief pattern may occur, it is often less distinct and the picture may be dominated by vague, diffuse upper-abdominal pain, fullness, and nausea, along with anorexia and perhaps weight loss. All these symptoms may resemble or suggest the picture of gastric cancer. Nocturnal pain is said to be less common in gastric than duodenal ulcer.

Diagnosis

Radiographic examination with barium can detect 85-90% of gastric ulcers. Gastric cancer may be misinterpreted as a benign gastric ulcer in 3-7% of cases. Roentgenographic signs associated with a benign gastric ulcer are the extension of the crater beyond the projected wall of the stomach, the more or less round or oval configuration of the defect with the absence of mass at the periphery of the crater, the presence of normal-appearing gastric folds reaching the margins of the crater defect, and the movement of normal wall peristaltic contractions though the lesion. However, the added diagnostic accuracy derived from endoscopic visualization of the ulcer, plus multiple biopsies within the ulcer margins and brushings for cytologic examination, explain the almost universal combined use of x-ray and endoscopy in the diagnosis of gastric ulcer. It must be emphasized that a biopsy diagnosis of benignity does not exclude carcinoma, which proves to be the ultimate nature of 5-7% of gastric ulcers. Cytologic examination of gastric juice in expert hands produces a diagnostic accuracy of about 90% with rare false positives, but it is not widely practiced. Gastric acid secretion measurement is not indicated in all gastric ulcer patients, despite the fact that histamine-fast achlorhydria means that gastric malignancy cannot be excluded. Only 20% of gastric cancers are achlorhydric, and these usually are large lesions.

Treatment

If all the above measures have not produced evidence of malignancy, it is reasonable to start medical treatment. Physical rest, frequent antacids, stopping smoking, and avoiding coffee, alcohol, and drugs such as aspirin and other anti-inflammatory agents are the main elements of treatment for the first 3 weeks. The goals are to reduce gastric acid, relieve pain, and to remove agents known to damage gastric mucosa. Although not universally practiced, it has been shown that hospitalization for medical treatment of gastric ulcer results in a higher incidence of healing. Antacids should be taken 1 and 3 hours after meals and at bedtime in doses of 80-100 mEq of antacid. The diet may be of the patient's own choosing, but not eating at bedtime is recommended. Many physicians also use cimetidine, 300 mg four times daily for 2-3 months.

At the end of 3-4 weeks from the time of diagnosis and initiation of therapy, the stomach is reexamined by barium x-ray or endoscopy. If the ulcer is healed, reexamination should be done in 2 or 3 months. If healing is felt to be progressing satisfactorily on the first reexamination (50% reduction of crater size), reexamination in another 3 or 4 weeks is indicated. If, at that time, the ulcer is not 80-90% reduced from its original size, gastric surgery should be considered. Should progress seem satisfactory, however, further medical treatment is appropriate, with reexamination in another 6 weeks (12 weeks from the time of diagnosis). If the ulcer is not 100% healed, surgery is usually recommended at this point. An exception should be made for large gastric ulcers measuring 3 cm or more in diameter since, even with a normal rate of healing, such ulcers may not be completely healed, and continuation of medical therapy for another 3 or 4 weeks is justified. Once complete healing has been demonstrated, a follow-up x-ray or endoscopic examination is indicated in 3-6 months, or at any time sooner should symptoms recur. Thirty to 40 percent of gastric ulcers recur in 2 years, and up to more than 50 percent in 5 years. The recurrence is usually in the same region of the stomach as the original ulcer. Recurrent ulcers have been shown to heal as readily as initial gastric ulcers, and therefore justify another course of medical therapy. A coexistent duodenal ulcer, past or present, has been noted in 30-40% of cases of gastric ulcer, and is thought to indicate a reduced likelihood of malignant gastric ulcer.

Complications of Gastric Ulcer
These are essentially the same as those for duodenal ulcer; that is, hemorrhage, perforation, and pyloric obstruction (See the section on duodenal ulcer).

Polyps and Neoplasms of the Stomach

Polyps

Gastric polyps are uncommon. The majority (75-80%) are hyperplastic polyps that have no malignant potential. Approximately 95% of gastric polyps occur in stomachs with absolute achlorhydria. Adenomatous polyps are potentially malignant. They are most frequently seen in patients with pernicious anemia, are usually located in the antrum, and often are 2 cm or larger. In most instances, multiple gastric polyps are of the hyperplastic variety and are randomly distributed throughout the stomach. Five percent of gastric cancers have associated polyps. Most patients with gastric polyps are asymptomatic, or have vague upper abdominal symptoms. Overt bleeding is rare, but occult blood loss is not uncommon. Physical examination is usually noncontributory. Roentogenographic examination is capable of detecting most polyps, and double-contrast examination is of particular value. Gastroscopy is used to confirm the presence of polyps and to perform biopsy and brushing, although the small samples may not always give the true nature of the polyp. Small size (less than 2 cm in diameter) usually indicate benignity.

Therapy
All gastric polyps do not require removal. If the lesions are shown by biopsy to be hyperplastic and are not thought symptomatic, they may be observed. It is possible to remove polyps through the gastroscope employing snare and cautery. The prognosis, in general, is excellent. Periodic x-ray or endoscopic inspection, biopsy, and cytology are considered adequate follow-up measures, and should be done at approximately yearly intervals.

Other benign tumors of the stomach include leiomyoma, lipomas, neurofibromas, fibromas, and pancreatic rests. As a group, they are rare and often asymptomatic, although leiomyomas may bleed. Surgical removal is done most commonly when malignancy cannot be excluded, or for significant bleeding.

Cancer

Adenocarcinoma represents 95% of all malignant tumors of the stomach. For reasons that are unclear, gastric cancer incidence has decreased strikingly in the United States in the past 30-50 years, although it remains a major type of malignancy in many countries.

Etiology
Familial occurrence of gastric cancer has been noted, along with an increased incidence in blood group A. The relationship to gastric adenomatous polyps has already been mentioned. Polyps have been noted in the stomachs of 5% of gastric cancer victims. Chronic gastritis and atrophic gastritis are found commonly in stomachs harboring polyps and cancer, but the relationship is uncertain. However, in pernicious anemia, gastric cancer incidence is said to approximate 10%. It has been recognized that many years after gastric resection for ulcer disease, gastric cancer may arise in the remaining stomach. A small number of stomach cancers have been reported in hypertrophic gastropathy (most are achlorhydric). Dietary factors such as smoked fish, aflatoxins, and hot foods have been suggested as contributing factors. Men exceed women in the incidence of gastric cancer.

Clinical Features
Early gastric cancer is often asymptomatic, and discovery at this stage comes about not uncommonly by chance. Peptic ulcerlike symptoms are noted by some patients, but are of variable duration even up to a few years, with or without a recent change in the character of the symptoms.

It is unlikely that more early gastric cancers will be discovered without some sort of mass screening program (as in Japan); this is probably not justified in the United States.

Anorexia, vague fullness, peptic ulcerlike pain, or any change in digestive function in a middle-aged man should prompt consideration of gastric cancer and a stomach x-ray examination. Endoscopy with biopsy and cytology are often necessary if uncertainty and suspicion remain.

Physical examination may be entirely negative in early cases. However, in advanced gastric cancer signs of cachexia, a palpable epigastric mass, an enlarged liver, anemia, or a palpable left supraclavicular node, a rectal shelf, or ascites may be noted.

Roentgenography
An overall accuracy of 90-95% in diagnosing gastric cancer by roentgenographic examination has been achieved, especially employing double contrast techniques that have given excellent mucosal detail and permit detection of small and superficial lesions. The radiographic features suggesting gastric cancer are: a polypoid mass; a mass with ulceration within it; diffusely infiltrating tumor that produces areas of rigidity or narrowing, and absent peristalsis; superficial spreading plaque; and an ulcer surrounded by mass that erases the mucosal folds from its margins. Malignant ulcers may appear benign by x-ray criteria; appropriate and careful follow-up of medically treated gastric ulceration is of utmost importance.

Endoscopy
When gastroscopy with biopsy and cytologic examination are added to roentgenographic examination of the stomach, the diagnostic accuracy of gastric cancer approaches 100%. Gross

endoscopic appearance of ulcers is not sufficiently sensitive, and linitis plastica may produce only some lack of distensibility and ironing out of mucosal folds. At least six biopsies, including the margins of ulcers, are recommended. Lavage cytology in centers experienced in this technique is a highly accurate diagnostic tool in gastric cancer.

Treatment
Surgery remains the only means of accomplishing a cure, and should be offered to all patients without evidence of metastatic disease. However, some patients may need palliative surgical treatment to relieve obstruction or control hemorrhage. Although surgery for early superficial spreading cancer has yielded a high (80-90%) 5-year survival in Japan, nearly all these lesions have been found by chance or by screening programs. Over 50% of all gastric cancer patients are not surgically curable when they come to operation, and the overall 5-year survival rate for all patients undergoing surgery is 10-20%. In most instances, limited or subtotal gastrectomy is the operation chosen. There appears to be no place for total gastrectomy in treating this lesion.

Lymphoma
This neoplasm involves the stomach in 20-25% of cases with systemic lymphoma, but also occurs as a primary gastric lesion. Symptoms are not specific or distinctive but usually include pain, weight loss, fullness, and, perhaps, nausea and vomiting. Physical examination is often negative. With systemic disease, hepatosplenomegaly or lymphadenopathy are often noted. No characteristic laboratory abnormalities are seen in gastric lymphoma.

Roentgenography. Gastric lymphomas appear as ulcerating lesions, polypoid tumors, or more diffuse infiltrative lesions. Hence, it is often difficult to distinguish a lymphoma from adenocarcinoma, but the most suggestive type of lesion is one with enlarged rugal folds and submucosal mass. Endoscopic examination is usually unable to distinguish carcinoma from a lymphoma, but biopsy and cytology are helpful.

Treatment. Surgical resection followed by radiation therapy is standard treatment, even if it appears that no disease was left by the surgeon. However, in disseminated lymphoma chemotherapy is indicated.

Leiomyosarcoma
This tumor represents 1-2% of all gastric neoplasms. It has no characteristic symptoms, but vague or ulcerlike epigastric pain, fullness, weight loss, or occasional nausea and vomiting may occur. Leiomyosarcomas bleed more often than other gastric neoplasms, due to central ulceration or cavitation. Roentgenography confirms the extramucosal, intramural nature of this tumor that often appears as a spherical mass with central ulceration. Gastroscopy confirms the above features, but biopsies are rarely diagnostic owing to the submucosal location of the tumor. Surgery is the only means of cure. There is no effective chemotherapy or radiation therapy program. Approximately 50% of patients are cured by surgical extirpation of the tumor.

Gastritis
Although this term has suffered from a looseness of definition and application, current tools of investigation such as endoscopy, mucosal biopsy, acid secretory studies, and perhaps immunologic studies, have improved our understanding of the various mucosal lesions known as gastritis.

Acute Gastritis
Synonyms for this entity are acute erosive gastritis, acute hemorrhagic gastritis, and acute stress erosion. This lesion may be focal or diffuse and occurs in a variety of settings, including following the ingestion of aspirin and alcohol, and as a consequence of such stress situations as sepsis, trauma, or surgery in which shock is superimposed. Chemotherapy, abdominal radiation, and staphylococcal food poisoning are also known to produce acute gastritis. The lesion appears to be the end result of a variety of exogenous agents and influences that directly injure mucosa or increase its permeability, allowing back diffusion of hydrogen ions and resulting in inflammation, necrosis of surface cells, and damaged blood vessels in the lamina propria. The only means of diagnosis is by gastroscopic examination that reveals edema and hyperemia with superficial erosions and mucosal hemorrhage.

Clinically, acute gastrointestinal hemorrhage is the principal manifestation and probably accounts for 30-40% of instances of upper gastrointestinal hemorrhage seen on admission to the hospital. In the majority of instances, the injurious factors and predisposing settings are transient, and bleeding stops spontaneously soon after hospitalization. Continued bleeding may respond to ice water gastric lavage, followed by antacids given at a rate and frequency to keep the gastric pH near 7, but may require intra-arterial vasopressin infusion. Rarely, unresponsive massive bleeding requires surgery. Cimetidine is also widely used in treatment of hemorrhage from acute gastritis.

Chronic Gastritis
The etiology of this form is unknown. Although some authorities distinguish two types, one that involves mainly the corpus and fundus leading to hyposecretion and hypergastrinemia, and the other type involving the pyloric gland area of the antrum, this distinction seems to have little clinical value at present. Also, there is little evidence linking the etiologic factors responsible for acute gastritis to the development of chronic gastritis, although many clinicians believe that repeated attacks of acute gastritis as induced by aspirin, and alcohol may be a cause of chronic gastritis. Bile acid reflux through the pylorus or via the anastomosis after gastrojejunostomy has received much recent attention in the context of the pathogenesis of gastric ulcer, as well as the chronic gastritis often seen in association with ulcer. Several studies have documented pyloric dysfunction in gastric ulcer patients, which allows increased bile acid reflux into the stomach. Varying

degrees of chronic gastritis are thought to appear as part of normal aging. Gastric polyps, achlorhydria, pernicious anemia, almost all types of thyroid disease, gastric ulcer, gastric carcinoma, pituitary and adrenal insufficiency, and diabetes are other settings in which chronic gastritis (chronic atrophic gastritis) is encountered. Antibodies to parietal cells have been demonstrated in 60% of patients with atrophic gastritis, and in 90% of patients with pernicious anemia, as well as 30% of patients with thyroid disease. Antibodies against intrinsic factor have been noted only in pernicious anemia. Whether the autoimmune process is primary or secondary is a matter of dispute.

Chronic superficial gastritis appears to be an early, and sometimes self-limited, form of chronic gastritis. More advanced injury is known as chronic atrophic gastritis, which leads to complete atrophy with a thin mucosa, loss of gastric glands, chief cells, and parietal cells, and often intestinal metaplasia of the surface epithelium. Lymphocytes and plasma cells infiltrate the lamina propria. The gastroscopic appearance may be unremarkable in lesser degrees of chronic atrophic gastritis, but later a dull, gray-blue mucosa with readily apparent submucosal vessels and perhaps gastric polyps are commonly seen.

There is a poor correlation between the morphologic picture on biopsy and the clinical status. Chronic gastritis is essentially asymptomatic.

Hypertrophic Gastritis

Also termed Menetrier's disease, this form of gastritis is characterized by marked hypertrophy of the mucosa with tortuous, pseudopolypoid, thickened rugal folds. Microscopic examination shows elongated, tortuous, branched, and dilated gastric pits lined mainly by hypertrophic surface epithelium. The process may be diffuse, or localized to the greater curvature. Patients may have epigastric pain, emesis, or edema due to hypoproteinemia; bleeding occasionally occurs. Radiographically, enlarged folds are the characteristic feature. The gastroscopic appearance may be suggestive, but accurate diagnosis depends upon a full-thickness biopsy. Acid secretory capacity may be normal, but there is often achlorhydria. In most instances, patients are hypoproteinemic, and it is possible to demonstrate exudative protein loss across the gastric mucosa by suitable isotope studies. There is no good symptomatic treatment. It may be necessary to replace serum proteins, and surgery may be required for bleeding or severe protein loss. At times, resection is curative if the process is sufficiently localized.

Eosinophilic Gastritis

This unusual condition may be confined to the mucosa, but not uncommonly involves mainly the muscular layer and the serosa. It may be asymptomatic, but when the antrum and pyloric region are involved, enlarged antral folds and a clinical picture of pyloric obstruction result. It is sometimes associated with exudative protein loss into the gastrointestinal lumen and, in rare instances when serosal involvement is prominent, the patient may present with a clinical picture of peritoneal irritation and ascites. Peripheral eosinophilia is common. The condition usually responds to steroids.

Granulomatous Gastritis

The stomach may be involved with the granulomatous tissue reaction of sarcoidosis, but it rarely produces symptoms.

Corrosive Gastritis

This unusual lesion results from the ingestion of strong acids. Usually the cardia and pyloric regions are most commonly affected. Occasionally, perforation may occur during the acute stages, or extensive gastric scarring and possible pyloric obstruction may result after healing.

THE PANCREAS

EMBRYOLOGY

The pancreas evolves from dorsal and ventral buds of entodermal cells that arise from the foregut in the third and fourth weeks. The dorsal bud grows into the dorsal mesentery, whereas the ventral bud arises in common with the hepatic bud. By the sixth to seventh week, the dorsal pancreas has grown into an elongated nodular structure, while the smaller ventral bud is carried away from the duodenum by elongation of the common bile duct. During the seventh week, growth of the duodenal wall results in a shifting of the ventral bud and common bile duct to a position dorsal to the duodenum, and soon the two primordia fuse. The dorsal pancreas becomes the upper head, body, and tail, whereas the ventral bud becomes the lower head and uncinate process. The duct of the ventral bud taps the long dorsal duct to become the main pancreatic duct (of Wirsung), which enters the second portion of the duodenum in conjunction with the common bile duct. The proximal segment of the dorsal duct becomes the accessory duct (of Santorini), and empties into the duodenum 2 cm proximal to the main duct. In a small percentage of cases, there may be failure of fusion of the two anlage, or failure of union of the two duct systems known as pancreas divisum. Annular pancreas results from failure of the ventral bud to migrate dorsally and to the left of the duodenum, resulting in pancreatic tissue surrounding the duodenum.

ANATOMY

The pancreas is entirely retroperitoneal in location. The head of the pancreas and uncinate process lie within the curve of the duodenum, and rest on the inferior vena cava, aorta, and common bile duct. The body and tail lie in the posterior abdomen, extending obliquely to the hilus of the spleen. The splenic vein courses along the posterior surface of the pancreas and joins the superior mesenteric vein behind the neck of the gland to become the portal vein. The splenic artery usually lies on the superior border of the body and tail. The superior mesenteric artery arises from the aorta posterior to the neck of the pancreas and emerges from the inferior border of the gland.

The arterial blood supply of the pancreas arises from branches of the celiac axis and superior mesenteric artery; the gastroduodenal artery branch of the celiac artery gives off anterior and posterior superior pancreatoduodenal arteries, and the superior mesenteric artery gives off anterior and posterior inferior pancreaticoduodenal artery branches. The splenic artery also supplies the pancreas with several branches as it passes along the superior border of the gland. Venous drainage is into the portal vein. Lymphatic drainage terminates in nodes near the duodenum, in preaortic nodes, and also in nodes near the splenic hilus. Parasympathetic preganglionic efferent fibers from the vagi terminate in ganglia within the substance of the pancreas, synapsing with postganglionic fibers that innervate acinar cells and smooth muscle cells of the ducts. Preganglionic sympathetic fibers synapse within the celiac ganglion with postganglionic fibers that innervate only blood vessels.

Microscopic Anatomy

The pancreas is a tubuloacinar gland, much like the parotid, consisting of exocrine acini, intercalated ducts, and intralobular ducts. The acinus is a rounded or short tubular structure comprised of a single row of epithelial (zymogen) cells, the bases of which converge on a lumen that drains into an intercalated duct. The latter unite to form intralobular ducts that converge into interlobular ducts, and lead to the main pancreatic duct. The ducts are lined by low columnar epithelium. Acinar cells contain secretory particles (proenzymes, or zymogens) and a Golgi apparatus that functions in intracellular transport of newly synthesized exportable protein in the form of zymogen granules that are discharged into the lumen of the acinus by an energy-dependent, hormone-responsive process.

PHYSIOLOGY

Pancreatic juice is composed of water and electrolytes that transport a mixture of approximately 20 enzymes and proenzymes. Pancreatic juice is isotonic with plasma; the osmolality is independent of flow rate. The principal anions are chloride and bicarbonate. With increasing flow rates, bicarbonate increases and chloride decreases. The main cations are sodium and potassium, whose concentrations are independent of flow rate. The acinus secretes a chloride-rich, low-bicarbonate fluid in which the enzymes are dispersed. Active bicarbonate secretion takes place along the entire duct system, and water moves passively to follow the active secretion of ions.

Some of the acinar cell's enzyme products are secreted in proenzyme forms (also known as zymogens): trypsinogen, chymotrypsinogen, proelastase, and procarboxypeptidases A and B. Ribonuclease and deoxyribonuclease, amylase, lipase, phospholipase, and cholesterol esterase are secreted as the active enzymes.

Trypsinogen is activated to trypsin in the duodenum by enterokinase, an enzyme from duodenal mucosa; trypsin, in turn, activates all other zymogen proteases. Vagal (parasympathetic) stimuli induce enzyme-rich secretion either directly (sight, smell, taste of food), or indirectly by the medium of vagally stimulated gastric acid secretion, resulting in pancreatic enzyme secretion. Splanchnic sympathetic stimuli inhibit pancreatic secretion.

Humoral influences on pancreatic secretion include the stimulation of enzyme-rich secretion by cholecystokinin (CCK) and gastrin, the depression of enzyme output by pancreatic glucagon, depression of water and bicarbonate secretion by enteroglucagon, and the predominant water and bicarbonate-rich secretion induced by secretin. Secretin and CCK represent duodenal intraluminal stimuli, the former being released by acid in the duodenal lumen lowering the pH below 3, and the latter by the presence of amino acids and fatty acids in the duodenum.

DIAGNOSTIC PROCEDURES

Enzyme Levels in Blood and Body Fluids

The secretion of pancreatic juice into a duct system obstructed by inflammation, tumor, a stone, or disrupted by trauma causes some regurgitation of enzymes into the blood, resulting in raised serum amylase and lipase values. This is encountered most typically in acute pancreatitis in the first 24 hours after onset, and usually returns to normal within 3-4 days. Approximately 40% of serum amylase is normally excreted by the kidney, and in acute pancreatitis, renal clearance of amylase is especially increased. Abnormal amounts of amylase may be measured in the urine for several days after raised serum amylase levels have returned to normal. Persistently raised serum enzyme levels in the absence of pancreatic disease, and with low or normal amylase values, indicates macroamylasemia, a benign condition that results from the complexing of amylase with immunoglobulin, forming an aggregate too large for renal excretion. No clinical picture or significant disease associations are linked with macroamylasemia, and the importance of its recognition lies mainly in avoiding a mistaken diagnosis of pancreatic disease. Column chromatography and isoelectric focusing can fractionate amylase into pancreatic (P type) and non-pancreatic (S type) isoenzymes, adding specificity to the serum amylase. A new radioimmunoassay of serum trypsinelike activity also appears promising.

Tests of Pancreatic Exocrine Function and Disease

Quantitative measurement of fecal fat is the best means to document steatorrhea. This study should ideally comprise a 72-hour stool collection while the patient is consuming 80-100 g of fat per day. Steatorrhea may be due to small intestinal mucosal disease or other disorders; thus, jejunal mucosal biopsy and small intestine barium x-ray study are usually performed to exclude these possibilities.

Another test involves the duodenal aspiration of pancreatic secretions after stimulation with intravenous cholecystokinin.

A double-lumen tube is passed into the duodenum, with gastric contents aspirated from a proximal port to avoid mixing with the duodenal contents. After a maximal stimulating dose of CCK is given intravenously, duodenal and pancreatic juice are aspirated and the enzyme concentrations of trypsin and lipase measured. This study is most useful in the diagnosis of pancreatic exocrine insufficiency as caused by chronic pancreatitis or pancreatic duct obstruction.

Ultrasonography
This noninvasive procedure is useful in the diagnosis of pancreatic tumors, pseudocysts, and some cases of acute and chronic pancreatitis. It may also give evidence of common bile duct dilatation, gallstones, pancreatic duct dilatation, and pancreatic calculi.

Computed Tomography (CT Scan)
The role of CT is roughly equivalent to ultrasound; however, it is more expensive and involves radiation. CT is less compromised by intestinal gas, allows the use of oral contrast in the study, and yields a higher percentage of technically satisfactory examinations than ultrasonography. It also permits nonoperative scan-directed pancreatic biopsy.

Roentgenography
Plain abdominal films may demonstrate calcifications in the region of the pancreas indicative of chronic pancreatitis. Localized areas of ileus, such as the sentinel loop of jejunum or the colon cutoff sign, are occasionally seen in acute pancreatitis. Pleural effusions secondary to pancreatitis are noted on chest x-rays.

Roentgenographic barium study of the stomach may reveal anterior displacement by a pancreatic pseudocyst, duodenal loop widened by tumor, or invasion of the duodenal wall or stomach by neoplasm of the head of the pancreas.

Endoscopic Retrograde Cholangiopancreatography (ERCP)
Visualization of the pancreatic duct system by this technique is useful in looking for obstruction by carcinoma of the pancreas, or duct abnormalities such as strictures, dilatations, and calculi seen in chronic pancreatitis, where it may be of aid in surgical planning. ERCP should not be done during, or soon after, an episode of acute pancreatitis or when a known pseudocyst is present, because contrast medium entering a pseudocyst may cause acute pain, fever, and other symptoms. The procedure has a complication rate of 3% for acute pancreatitis, and 5% for acute cholangitis if jaundice is present.

Angiography
This study is mainly of value in detecting pancreatic carcinoma and islet cell tumor, but is less accurate than CT scan and ultrasonography. Carcinoma is usually hypovascular, and often the arteries are observed to deviate around the tumor or show evidence of encasement or cutoffs. Sometimes tumor encasement or encroachment upon the portal, splenic, or superior mesenteric veins are noted; the study also may show evidence of metastases in the liver. It is difficult to differentiate some of the changes seen in chronic pancreatitis from those associated with neoplasm. Islet cell tumors are usually hypervascular.

Biopsy
Nonoperative CAT-guided needle biopsy has recently been introduced, and is of particular value in obtaining histologic evidence of pancreatic carcinoma.

DISEASES OF THE PANCREAS

Acute Pancreatitis

Etiology and Pathogenesis
No universally applicable hypothesis or experimental model of pancreatitis fits all human acute pancreatitis. The common-channel theory, the duodenal regurgitation concept, and the obstruction-secretion theory all invoke some activation of proteolytic and lipolytic enzymes within the pancreas, or presume the presence of biliary and duodenal contents in the pancreatic duct that may be directly injurious (e.g., bile acid and bacteria), activate pancreatic enzymes, or release kinins and other vasoactive peptides.

In human acute pancreatitis, several clinical conditions are commonly associated with acute pancreatitis; biliary tract disease (especially choledocholithiasis), alcohol, hypercalcemia, trauma, hyperlipidemia, vascular disease, heredity, drugs, and peptic ulcer. Some of these conditions are obvious triggers, while others remain mysteries as to the mechanisms by which acute pancreatitis results. Yet, probably the essential components necessary for pancreatitis are the disruption of the integrity of the duct system or the acini, the leakage of pancreatic secretions into the parenchymal spaces, and inappropriate activation of pancreatic enzymes.

In addition to the direct tissue damage from the proteolytic activity of trypsin, the latter also activates the other proteases whose actions and predilections may explain at least some of the features of acute pancreatitis. For example, elastase may cause the digestion of the elastic lamina of blood vessels. Toxic lysolecithin, formed from lecithin by phospholipase A, may contribute to tissue damage in other organs such as the lung by its action on surfactant. The liberation of vasoactive peptides such as kallikrein may also be responsible for the vascular permeability defects of pancreatitis.

Pathology
Acute pancreatitis in its milder, reversible form is characterized histologically by congestion, interstitial edema, and foci of polymorphonuclear leukocyte infiltration. More severe injury consists of foci of tissue destruction and hemorrhage, along with adjacent tissue digestion and fat necrosis. Severe acute pancreatitis is marked by large areas of glandular necrosis and interstitial hemorrhage, with more extensive mesenchymal fat necrosis, and by retroperitoneal edema and hemorrhage.

Clinical Manifestations
The cardinal presenting feature is pain in the epigastrium and midabdomen. It is usually steady, boring, and severe, and

commonly radiates to the back. The pain is often hard to alleviate, lasts for many hours, and forces the patient to lie quietly in the fetal position or to sit leaning forward. Nausea, vomiting, and low-grade fever are common. The abdomen is tender to palpation, but rigidity and rebound are usually not present. Bowel sounds are subdued or absent. Severe attacks may produce a shocklike picture with hypotension, tachycardia, cyanosis, or air hunger. In such cases, the pain is usually more severe; the abdomen is more distended and silent, with greater tenderness and guarding. The hypotension and shocklike picture are due to hypovolemia, resulting from the extravasation of blood and plasma into the retroperitoneal spaces, and the activation of vasoactive peptides that enhance not only local changes but have systemic effects on myocardial function, vascular permeability and so on. A variety of pulmonary complications may accompany severe pancreatitis, including basilar atelectasis from diaphragmatic elevation due to abdominal distention; pleural effusions rich in amylase and other pancreatic enzymes; or a form of adult respiratory distress syndrome (pancreatitis lung) characterized by hypoxemia and pulmonary edema. The pathologic changes in the lung consist of interstitial and alveolar edema, hemorrhages, and microemboli. Causative factors that have been considered include fat emboli, surfactant damage from lecithinase, vasoactive and other unidentified peptides, disseminated intravascular coagulation, and microembolization. Renal failure, due to decreased perfusion and perhaps also to vasoactive substances, may complicate severe pancreatitis. Tetany is sometimes seen in the presence of profound hypocalcemia. Ecchymotic skin discoloration in the flanks or around the umbilicus may be noted but is rare.

Laboratory Diagnosis
The most characteristic and reliable laboratory finding is a raised serum amylase concentration that usually develops within 2-12 hours of the onset of the attack, and returns to normal within 3-4 days. Increased urine amylase occurs almost as promptly as raised serum amylase, and may persist after serum amylase has returned to normal. It is best measured in a two-hour urine collection and expressed as units/h. Serum lipase is commonly raised also, and serves to complement the amylase.

Calculation of the ratio of amylase to creatinine clearance may occasionally be of added value, since in acute pancreatitis amylase has been shown to be cleared by the kidney at a particularly greater (three times normal) rate than creatinine, as opposed to most other causes of hyperamylasemia. This temporary proximal renal tubular malfunction is not pathognomonic for acute pancreatitis, but has been noted also in diabetic acidosis, malignant myeloma, postoperative states, thermal burns, and other serious illnesses.

Hyperglycemia in the nondiabetic patient is often noted in severe acute pancreatitis. Similarly, hypocalcemia when present helps corroborate the diagnosis of acute pancreatitis; the degree of serum calcium depression tends to correlate with the severity of the pancreatitis. A value below 8 mg/dl has been regarded as a poor prognostic sign. Serum bilirubin, alkaline phosphatase, and SGOT may be raised, due to either common duct narrowing by pancreatic edema or to duct obstruction by a gallstone. It has recently been claimed that the higher the degree of acute elevation of these enzymes, the greater the likelihood of pancreatitis due to biliary tract stone. Hypertriglyceridemia is noted in 10-15% of patients with acute pancreatitis and may be primary or secondary. High serum lipids may inhibit amylase activity in the laboratory measurement of serum amylase, giving a falsely normal value.

Roentgenography
Although a number of positive signs have been claimed to occur in acute pancreatitis, abdominal plain films are of greatest value in excluding other acute intra-abdominal conditions such as a perforated viscus or intestinal obstruction. The reported forms of ileus, at times largely confined to the dilated sentinel loop of jejunum or to the colon proximal to the splenic flexure (colon cutoff sign), are relatively infrequent and, in the author's experience, unreliable. Opaque gallstones and pancreatic calcification may also be noted on plain films. Ultrasound examination may reveal enlargement of the pancreas due to inflammation and edema, and also may detect cholelithiasis or choledocholithiasis. Contrast studies of the gallbladder and biliary tree are best delayed for 2-4 weeks after the acute attack has subsided, as they usually yield inconclusive or false-negative results when done during the acute phase. Barium studies are not necessary during acute pancreatitis. At the present time, endoscopic retrograde cholangiopancreatography has no place in the evaluation or diagnosis of acute pancreatitis; most physicians regard that condition as a contraindication to the procedure.

Medical Management
In recent years, controlled clinical trials have cast doubt on several of the standard elements of medical management aimed at putting the pancreas at rest. These include anticholinergics and nasogastric suction to reduce the amount of gastric acid entering the duodenum, thereby diminishing the humoral stimulation to pancreatic secretion by secretin release.

The currently realistic goals of nonoperative treatment are relief of pain, maintenance of intravascular volume, nasogastric suction to help in relieving pain and preventing ileus, and the alert detection and management of complications such as the respiratory distress syndrome, hypocalcemia, and so on. Antibiotics have not been shown to affect the course of acute pancreatitis in the absence of complications such as pancreatic abscess or cholangitis. Antisecretory agents such as glucagon, or large doses of anticholinergics or inhibitors of hydrolytic enzymes or kallikrein (such as aprotinin), have not been of proven value. Most (90-95%) cases of acute pancreatitis subside spontaneously after a few days of conservative treatment. Less than 5% of acute pancreatitis cases pursue a fulminant course dominated by hypotension, renal failure, respiratory insufficiency, hypocalcemia, and cardiovascular collapse. Management of these desperately ill patients is difficult. Ranson has shown that surgical resuscitation of an appreciable percentage of such patients is possible by surgical drainage and then peritoneal lavage of toxic peritoneal exudate by acute percutaneous dialysis catheter. Favorable response usually occurs within a few hours, and failure to respond may be an indication for laparotomy to establish better drainage, and to deal with any possible cholangitis due to biliary stone obstruction.

Surgery in Acute Pancreatitis
Recent evidence suggests that surgery in the presence of acute pancreatitis is not intrinsically dangerous, and in some instances may improve the prognosis. Surgery indeed may be indicated when there is doubt as to the diagnosis, or when there is evidence of infection in the biliary tract, especially cholangitis, for which relief of biliary obstruction and drainage are necessary. Early surgical consultation is advisable in severe acute pancreatitis, particularly when very high amylase levels are present.

Complications possibly requiring surgery also include deterioration despite apparent adequate vigorous medical treatment. At laparotomy, it is possible to drain an abscess or cyst, to assess the biliary tract, or to drain a hemorrhagic necrotic pancreas. Surgery for pancreatic pseudocyst per se is not mandatory; many will spontaneously resorb, and some spontaneously rupture into the gut. Most surgeons allow a pseudocyst to ripen for several (4-6) weeks.

Peritoneal Lavage
A clinical appraisal by Ranson of the objective findings in acute pancreatitis identified several that were associated with high morbidity and mortality. These hospital admission criteria were age greater than 55, leukocytosis above 16,000, blood glucose over 200 mg/dl, and SGOT over 250 U. Included during the first 48 hours of hospitalization were: drop in hematocrit greater than 10%, BUN rise greater than 5 mg/dl, serum calcium below 8 mg, PO_2 below 60 mm mercury, base deficit over 4 mEq/L, and estimated fluid sequestration over 6 L. Patients with three or more of these signs treated by Ranson with nonoperative peritoneal lavage have had a reduced early mortality from the cardiovascular and respiratory complications of severe pancreatitis.

Investigations for underlying biliary tract disease, cholelithiasis, or of the cause of hypercalcemia are best deferred for a few weeks after the acute attack in order to avoid the problems of interpretation of borderline or abnormal results.

Another complication of acute pancreatitis is ascites, which is thought to be due to a leak from a pseudocyst or from disrupted continuity in the pancreatic duct system, allowing pancreatic secretions to accumulate in the peritoneal cavity. A very high amylase content of the ascitic fluid is characteristic. Management of this complication is difficult, as the ascites does not often resorb even with hyperalimentation, diuretics, and prolonged observation. Surgical approach is also difficult, although careful retrograde pancreatography may demonstrate the site of leakage and other duct pathology, thus aiding in the surgical decision.

Chronic Pancreatitis

The spectrum of clinical features of chronic pancreatitis is broad and varied, but this term refers to the presence of irreversible sequelae rather than the duration or number of attacks. Some patients present with attacks resembling acute pancreatitis. These are often rather mild, and their recurrent nature may evolve insidiously. Other patients may have a persistent form of chronic abdominal and back pain without acute exacerbations. A small percentage of patients have manifestations of pancreatic exocrine insufficiency and diabetes without pain.

Etiology and Pathogenesis
The majority of cases of chronic pancreatitis are associated with chronic alcoholism. Pancreatic exocrine insufficiency due to alcohol-induced chronic pancreatitis has been shown to correlate well with a history of at least 10 years of alcohol consumption. Based upon histologic studies of the pancreas in animal models, and in patients with alcohol-related chronic pancreatitis that have shown deposits of proteinaceous material in the lumens of pancreatic ducts along with other changes, it is assumed that chronic alcohol consumption leads to precipitation of proteins of pancreatic secretions producing duct obstruction, with ensuing local parenchymal damage that may become more advanced and widespread with time.

Pathology
In the early stages of chronic pancreatitis there may be patchy inflammation and fibrosis, the main features of which are the above-mentioned proteinaceous, occasionally calcified plugs in pancreatic ducts, plus focal inflammation and destruction of acinar cells, and fibrosis. Glandular destruction progresses with more deposits, more acinar destruction and fibrosis, metaplasia of duct epithelium, calcium carbonate calculi in the ducts, and multiple sites of stenosis and dilatation of the ducts, eventually resulting in a small, hard, fibrotic, atrophic gland.

Clinical Manifestations
As mentioned earlier, the majority of patients have abdominal pain that is often intermittent in the early stages but may become persistent or almost constant. It is usually periumbilical or epigastric in location, often spreading to the back; the patient often seeks a measure of relief by leaning forward to assuming a hands-knees position. Pain attacks usually last 24 hours or more and require narcotics or strong analgesics, which may eventually lead to addiction. Between pain episodes, patients may be asymptomatic, but often complain of vague dyspepsia. Some patients do not experience pain but may develop clinical manifestations of exocrine insufficiency. Steatorrheal diarrhea is characterized by bulky, pale, foul-smelling, floating, oily stools, and weight loss. Unlike celiac disease, clinical signs of widespread nutritional deficiency such as tetany, purpura, and edema, are uncommon. Diabetes occurs in 10-15% of cases of chronic pancreatitis, but abnormal glucose tolerance test results are noted more frequently. Physical examination often shows only the effects of weight loss; however, the patient may be jaundiced, have epigastric tenderness or a palpable mass due to a pseudocyst.

Laboratory Findings
During a bout of acute abdominal pain, raised serum amylase

and lipase and urine amylase are often noted, but the degree of enzyme elevation diminishes as the disease progresses with more glandular destruction. Steatorrhea and azotorrhea are best documented by quantitative fecal fat and nitrogen measurements on a 72-hour stool collection. Primary small intestinal mucosal disease as a possible cause for malabsorption and steatorrhea should be excluded by small intestine x-ray study and mucosal biopsy. Then, a test of pancreatic exocrine function should follow, such as the CCK stimulation test, or the Lundh test meal. In these pancreatic function testing circumstances, exocrine insufficiency causing steatorrhea signifies that enzyme output is reduced below 10% of normal levels.

Plain roentgenograms of the abdomen, including oblique and lateral views of the pancreatic area, often show calcification in the parenchyma or pancreatic duct calculi, especially in alcoholic chronic pancreatitis. Such calcification, even in the absence of clinical evidence of pancreatic disease, almost always means chronic pancreatitis.

Ultrasound and computed tomography scanning are useful in some circumstances; in searching for gallstones, to look for tumor of the pancreas, and for the identification of pseudocysts. Endoscopic retrograde pancreatography can provide valuable information regarding the pancreatic duct system, such as a possible pancreatic tumor, or major duct distortion due to calculi or strictures that might aid the surgeon in deciding whether surgically correctable lesions are present.

Medical Management

For many patients with chronic relapsing pancreatitis, there is little to offer that will alter the course of the disease, although obviously it is important that underlying or associated causative factors for pancreatitis be recognized and eliminated. These include the total elimination of alcohol, consideration of hyperparathyroidism, and the search for biliary tract disease especially for cholelithiasis, for appropriate surgical treatment early in the course of chronic relapsing pancreatitis may have a beneficial effect on the prognosis. Too often, patients slowly become worse, with more frequent abdominal pain, often intensified by food intake that may also induce nausea and vomiting. Weight loss and malnourishment ensue as steatorrhea and azotorrhea appear from progressive loss of pancreatic enzyme secretion. Possible common bile duct obstruction due to inflammatory and fibrotic changes in the pancreatic head may produce jaundice. Occasionally, splenic or portal vein thrombosis complicates chronic pancreatitis, leading to portal hypertension. A sensible supervised program for pain management is necessary to avoid narcotic addiction. Sometimes the avoidance of large meals, reduction of dietary fat, and abstinence from alcohol provide some subjective improvement. If exocrine insufficiency is present, pancreatic enzyme replacement therapy should be started, along with a low-fat diet (25 g/meal). Pancreatin (Viokase) or pancrelipase (Ilozyme), six to eight tablets given during and after each meal, will usually abolish azotorrhea but not steatorrhea, although improvement in nutritional status and reduction in symptoms is accomplished. For some patients who do not appear to benefit from enzyme therapy, further reduction in dietary fat or the addition of cimetidine to the pancreatin or pancrelipase usually corrects the steatorrhea and diarrhea. An enteric-coated enzyme preparation usually is not necessary and is more expensive.

Surgical Management

Indications for surgery in chronic pancreatitis include pain (chronic severe pain or frequent recurrent acute attacks), bile duct or duodenal obstruction, and pancreatic duct disruption (pseudocyst, ascites, or chronic pleural effusions). Ultrasonography and ERCP are valuable in aiding decisions for surgery aimed directly at the pancreas, such as for decompression of pancreatic duct obstruction with pain, drainage of pseudocysts or abscesses, or by resection of a portion of the gland that cannot be decompressed or shows advanced destruction. The ultimate choice of surgical procedure depends not only upon endoscopic retrograde pancreatography, but also on careful evaluation of the gland at surgery. Internal drainage of pseudocysts, caudal gland resection combined with ductal-intestinal anastomosis, midductal decompression with or without resection and, occasionally, extensive (90-95%) pancreatic resection are potential surgical approaches, depending upon the site and degree of ductal obstruction, the amount of gland damage, and the severity of pain. Continued alcohol abuse is a major factor that may limit the effectiveness of any surgical procedure. Diabetes is to be expected in the majority of patients with chronic pancreatitis, and is even more likely following surgery on the gland.

CYSTIC FIBROSIS

This systemic disorder of mucus-producing exocrine glands affects the pancreas in addition to the bronchi, intestine, and liver. It is an autosomal recessive disease manifested by malabsorption due to pancreatic achylia, and by recurring pulmonary infections secondary to bronchial obstruction by inspissated mucus, and to bronchiectasis. Lastly, there is a diagnostically abnormal sodium and chloride content of sweat.

Etiology

The cause of this disease is essentially unknown, although recent studies of cultured skin fibroblasts from cystic fibrosis patients have shown structural and biochemical abnormalities suggesting that somatic cells other than exocrine gland cells are affected. Additionally, serum factors inhibitory to ciliary activity have been demonstrated.

Pathophysiology

Although the mechanism is not understood, it has been proposed that the defective mucus leads to blockage of bronchial and pancreatic ducts, resulting in pancreatic damage and septic obstructive pulmonary disease. In the liver, focal biliary fibrosis produced by obstruction of intrahepatic bile ducts may lead to a form of biliary cirrhosis.

Symptoms and Clinical Manifestations

The typical triad of malabsorption, recurrent pulmonary infections, plus an abnormally high sweat sodium or chloride is not a common mode of presentation, and the clinical picture may be dominated by either the pulmonary features or by the gastrointestinal elements of steatorrhea and weight loss. The increasing mean survival of cystic fibrosis patients (now 16-18 years), owing to improved management especially of pulmonary sepsis, means that some patients may pass beyond childhood without diagnosis or may present with a form of biliary cirrhosis, or so-called meconium ileus equivalent. The latter represents the accumulation of semisolid fecal material and abnormal mucus most commonly in the lumen of the terminal ileum. The resulting obstruction may be transient or cause few symptoms. A palpable painless mass in the right lower quadrant is characteristic, though some patients may present with full-blown obstruction. The mass has led to ileocolic intussusception, or to volvulus.

Diagnosis
In addition to the clinical features mentioned above, the sweat chloride test is the most specific diagnostic procedure. Sweat electrolyte concentration increases with age, and therefore results must be compared with those of controls of a similar age. Pancreatic exocrine insufficiency is best assessed by the IV CCK test of enzyme content and activity. Pulmonary radiographic and function studies define the pulmonary status. Plain films of the abdomen and barium enemas in patients with symptoms suggesting the meconium ileus equivalent may show signs of obstruction plus a mass of bubbling intestinal contents.

Treatment
Management consists of pancreatic enzyme replacement, control, prevention of respiratory infections with long-term antibiotics, inhalation therapy to reduce bronchial secretions, and postural drainage. In the absence of complications, efforts to relieve intestinal obstructing masses with increased doses of pancreatic enzymes, oral doses of *N*-acetylcysteine (100-200 ml of 10% solution) and docusate sodium, and *N*-acetylcysteine by retention enema may be successful and avert surgery.

TUMORS OF THE PANCREAS

Adenocarcinoma

Nonendocrine pancreatic cancer is the fourth most common cancer as a cause of death (behind lung, colorectal, and breast), and has a 5-year survival rate of only 1 to 2%, one of the lowest of all cancers. Furthermore, its incidence has nearly tripled in the last 40 years, but the reasons for its increased occurrence are uncertain. Cancer of the pancreas accounts for more than 10% of all gastrointestinal system malignancies (behind colorectal cancer).

Epidemiology
The cause of pancreatic cancer is not known, but associations have been noted with cigarette smoking, coffee, and certain industrial carcinogens. Other etiologic factors have been implied, including chronic alcoholism, chronic pancreatitis, and preexistent diabetes. At the present time, epidemiologic data are too inconclusive to allow identification of population groups clearly at risk, or to be of aid in diagnosis.

Pathology
Various studies have identified 75-90% of pancreatic cancer as duct cell adenocarcinoma that is multicentric in up to 35% in some series. The remainder of malignancies are composed of acinar cell cancer, ampullary carcinomas, cystadenocarcinomas, and so forth.

Symptoms and Clinical Manifestations
Early diagnosis of pancreatic cancer is rare; most patients have reached a surgically incurable stage by the time diagnosis is definitively established. Weight loss and abdominal pain, often present for several months and noted in up to 75% of patients, are the most common symptoms. Anorexia, exocrine insufficiency, and diabetes contribute to the weight loss. Pain from carcinoma of the head of the pancreas is usually located in the epigastrium, or right upper quadrant, with penetration to the back. Lesions in the body and tail more often produce mid-abdominal to left upper quadrant pain, sometimes radiating to the left flank and left back. The pain is usually steady and boring, and patients seem to gain some amelioration by leaning forward, or assuming a hands and knees position.

Jaundice with liver enlargement and tenderness occurs in 80-90% of malignancies of the head of the pancreas, but less frequently with lesions of the body (5-10%). A palpable gallbladder is noted in about one-third of cases. The jaundice results from obstruction of the intrapancreatic portion of the distal common bile duct. Rarely, splenic artery narrowing by tumor produces a periumbilical bruit. Invasion of the wall and mucosa of the duodenum, occasionally appreciated by contrast study of the stomach and duodenum, may cause nausea, vomiting, or upper gastrointestinal bleeding. Occasionally, carcinoma of the pancreas presents as an episode of acute pancreatitis. Mental depression has been noted not infrequently, at times preceding other manifestations of the disease. Migratory thrombophlebitis and marantic endocarditis have also been identified as features of pancreatic carcinoma. Examination may reveal only an anxious or depressed individual manifesting abdominal pain and weight loss, and perhaps jaundice with pruritus. An enlarged gallbladder should be sought by inspection of the right upper quadrant, as well as by palpation. Enlargement of the liver may occur as biliary obstruction becomes complete, or may signify metastases. Splenomegaly may be secondary to occlusion of the splenic vein. Infrequently, an abdominal mass or bruit may be noted.

Diagnosis
Raised serum amylase and lipase occur in only 10-20% of patients, though increased urine amylase values are seen more frequently. Other blood tests in the absence of jaundice are often normal or may show only mild anemia. With common duct involvement and jaundice, hyperbilirubinemia and a cholestatic profile (predominantly alkaline phosphatase elevation) are noted. Plasma carcinoembryonic agent was noted in

a minority of cases when it was prospectively assayed; in these, advanced disease was usually present. Radiographic examination of the upper gastrointestinal tract may show widening of the duodenal loop, displacement of the stomach or duodenum, or mucosal ulceration, but these findings signify advanced disease. Tests of exocrine function (maximal dose secretin or CCK stimulation with measurement of bicarbonate or enzyme output in duodenal juice) are abnormal in a high percentage of cases of cancer of the head of the pancreas, less often in lesions of the body and tail. Cytologic examination of pancreatic juice after secretin or CCK stimulation, or obtained from the pancreatic duct after cannulation for endoscopic retrograde pancreatography, has been found to yield malignant cells in the majority of cases of cancer of the head of the pancreas.

Ultrasonography (US)

Ultrasonography yields a diagnostic accuracy of 75-90%, and is appealing as an early procedure owing to its noninvasive and harmless nature. Computerized tomography is of comparable or superior value with a higher percentage of technically satisfactory studies and fewer false negatives than US. Both techniques are increasing in accuracy as equipment and examiner skills improve, but their relative value has not been definitively settled. Selective angiography has been reported to have a diagnostic accuracy approaching 90% in pancreatic cancer. It may help in identifying vessel involvement or liver metastases, clues to the resectability of the tumor relative to regional spread. Endoscopic retrograde pancreatography allows the examiner an opportunity to inspect the duodenal mucosa and papilla, as well as to cannulate the pancreatic duct for contrast studies. The main clues of ductal cancer on retrograde study are in the form of blockage or stenosis with proximal dilatation of the duct. In some cases, differentiation of patterns of duct obstruction and dilatation from those seen in pancreatitis is difficult. Nonoperative biopsy of the pancreas, using a thin needle aspiration technique guided by ultrasonography or computed tomography, has become increasingly popular and yields a positive diagnosis in 80% of cases with a low complication rate. The technique would seem of value when evidence of regional or distant spread is present or suspected, or in patients who are poor surgical risks for pancreatic surgery.

It does not seem appropriate to perform a biopsy in a patient for whom resective surgery is planned, or for whom operation is indicated to relieve biliary or gastrointestinal obstruction. The diagnostic approach to pancreatic cancer beyond routine laboratory tests would be ultrasonography; if this reveals a pancreatic lesion, and liver metastases are seen on ultrasonography or radionuclide liver scan, liver biopsy (percutaneous or at peritoneoscopy) should follow to confirm the diagnosis and avoid laparotomy. If ultrasonography shows a pancreatic tumor and there are no evident liver metastases, CT scanning or arteriography could be done to assess operability, or by proceeding directly to laparotomy for diagnosis and possible resection of the tumor. If the initial ultrasound study does not show a lesion or is indeterminate, a CT scan should be done. If this is negative and clinical suspicion of pancreatic neoplasm is still high, endoscopic retrograde pancreatography or pancreatic exocrine function testing, or both, should be done. If these are negative, pancreatic cancer is excluded with 90-95% accuracy.

Surgery

The objectives are palliation and attempt to cure. If the need for palliation is obvious (biliary obstruction, duodenal obstruction, etc.), excessive testing should be avoided in favor of confirming the diagnosis at surgery. If attempted curative resection seems feasible, further efforts to define the extent of the tumor are reasonable, including searching for local or distant spread and metastases by imaging techniques, peritoneoscopy, and biopsy.

Only about 15-20% of patients with cancer of the head of the pancreas have a resectable lesion at exploration; at best, 25% of these are cured. Pancreatic cancer surgery is perhaps best confined to centers where there is interest and expertise in this problem. The best operation for cure is probably total pancreatectomy with regional node removal, rather than the Whipple operation that is preferable for ampullary cancer. This operation involves removal of the gallbladder, common bile duct, duodenum, and proximal jejunum with or without gastric resection. Meticulous node removal and dissection of the pancreas off the portal vein and superior mesenteric vessels are required. For palliation, cholecystojejunostomy or choledochoduodenoscopy to relieve jaundice and pruritus are reasonable operations with very low morbidity and mortality. Intraoperative irradiation for localized disease is being assessed in several centers.

Debilitating, chronic progressive abdominal and back pain in advanced pancreatic cancer may be relieved or significantly lessened by percutaneous splanchnic nerve block.

Islet Cell Tumors

Tumors of the islets of Langerhans represent a variety of neoplasms that may be benign or malignant. Nearly all benign islet cell tumors and 75-80% of malignant islet cell tumors are associated with clinical syndromes due to hormonal hypersecretion. The hormones are either indigenous to the cells of the pancreatic islets, or may be ectopic in nature. Tumors may secrete more than one hormone. Of the 20% of nonfunctioning tumors, it is possible that future methods will identify hormone production and secretion not presently recognized.

Insulinoma is the commonest islet cell tumor. It arises from the β cell, producing symptoms caused by hypoglycemia, although malignant insulinomas may present with abdominal mass, metastases, or jaundice. Eighty percent of insulinomas are single and benign, and therefore are amenable to resection. Ten percent are multiple or islet cell hyperplasia, and 10 percent are malignant.

Gastrinoma is the next most common islet cell tumor and produces a syndrome resembling peptic ulcer (see section on Zollinger-Ellison syndrome). Sixty percent of gastrinomas are malignant, the majority of which have metastasized at the time of diagnosis. Twenty percent of gastrinomas are multiple or due to islet cell hyperplasia. Hence, less than 25% of these tumors are single and amenable to resection. Twenty to 50 percent of patients with Zollinger-Ellison syndrome have multiple endocrine adenomatosis (MEA) type I syndrome; 50 percent of MEA type I patients have peptic ulcer.

The diarrheogenic non-β islet cell tumor produces a clinical complex of watery diarrhea, achlorhydria, hypovolemia, and hypokalemia known as the WDHA syndrome, VIPoma, or the Verner-Morrison syndrome. In many, but not all, patients with this syndrome, increased plasma concentrations of vasoactive intestinal peptide (VIP) have been measured. Diarrhea is the most common symptom; it may be daily or episodic, and has the features of a secretory diarrhea. Daily stool volume may exceed four liters per day and contains large amounts of potassium and bicarbonate, resulting in hypokalemia and metabolic acidosis. Basal achlorhydria is present in the majority of patients. Diarrhea persists with fasting. Most pancreatic tumors in WDHA are single, the great majority in the body and tail, and most are benign. All these factors favor surgical removal of the tumors as the treatment of choice.

Glucagonoma is the least frequent islet cell tumor secreting an endogenous hormone. The majority are malignant and occur in women. The clinical picture consists of diabetes, weight loss, skin rash or migratory necrolytic erythema, and glossitis or stomatitis. Some islet cell tumors produce ectopic hormones; ACTH, secretinlike material, serotoninlike material, melanophore-stimulating hormone, VIP, and somatostatin.

SMALL INTESTINE

ANATOMY

The small intestine extends from the pylorus to the ileocecal valve. Its length, as measured by intubation in vivo, is 250-300 cm. The first 10 inches, the duodenum, are retroperitoneal but the remainder of the small intestine lies free, being attached to its mesentery that runs from the ligament of Treitz in the left upper quadrant to the right lower quadrant. Through this mesentery pass the arterial and venous vessels, the nerve supply, and lymphatic drainage. The proximal two-fifths of the small intestine from the ligament of Treitz are arbitrarily designated as jejunum, and the distal three-fifths are considered ileum. The reader is referred to the standard textbooks for further details regarding gross anatomy and anatomic relationships.

The arterial blood supply of the duodenum is derived from pancreaticoduodenal artery branches originating from the celiac artery and the superior mesenteric artery. Important collateral anastomotic branches between these arteries can be demonstrated in the region of the duodenum and head of the pancreas. The remainder of the small intestine is supplied by a series of intestinal branches of the superior mesenteric artery. Collateral branches of major clinical importance also exist between the middle colic branch of the superior mesenteric artery and the left colic artery branch of the inferior mesenteric artery, known as the marginal artery of Drummond.

The parasympathetic nerve supply to the small intestine is from the vagus nerves that terminate in the myenteric and submucosal plexuses of the bowel wall. Sympathetic efferents are postganglionic fibers from the celiac and superior mesenteric ganglia.

Many features of the small intestine's gross and microscopic structure underscore the digestive and absorptive activities peculiar to this segment of the gut. The diameter of the proximal intestine is greater than that of the distal ileum. The mucosa is thrown up into many transverse folds that are most prominent in the proximal small intestine, and become sparse or almost absent in the distal ileum. The mucosal surface of the folds is studded with innumerable slender villi whose height diminishes progressively toward the ileocecal valve. Pit-like crypts encircle the villi around their bases. The crypts and villi are lined with a continuous sheet of a single layer of columnar absorptive epithelial cells, the luminal surfaces of which are lined by a brush border of microvilli that further increase the digestive/absorptive surface area manyfold. A glycoprotein coat covers the outer surface of the microvillus membrane. All the above anatomic surface features create a total small intestinal surface area of 20-40 m^2, approximately equal to the area of a tennis court.

The main function of the crypt epithelium is cell renewal, arising from the undifferentiated crypt cells where mitoses are commonly seen. These newly formed cells migrate up the walls of the crypts and onto the villi, where they undergo biochemical and enzymatic differentiation into mature absorptive cells. After they have migrated up the villi and reach the extreme villus tips, they are sloughed off into the intestinal lumen. This process of cell migration and maturation from crypt to villus tip takes place in 3-5 days.

The lamina propria, the loose cellular connective tissue lying beneath the epithelium, contains the capillaries, venules, and lymphatics serving the absorptive epithelium. In both the stomach and intestine, the lamina propria also contains a population of lymphocytes and plasma cells that function as important elements of the local and systemic immune system. The lymphocytes may be found wedged between the columnar epithelial absorptive cells, in the lamina propria beneath the epithelium, and in focal aggregates called lymphoid follicles and Peyer's patches. The lymphocytes are of both T and B types, and appear to interact with antigens that gain entry through the epithelium to reach associated lymphoid elements. It is thought that the antigen-sensitized B lymphocytes migrate to the lamina propria where they evolve into immunoglobulin-synthesizing plasma cells.

Immunofluorescence techniques have shown that 80-90 percent of the plasma cells synthesize and contain IgA, and the remainder contain IgM (12-16 percent) and IgG (2-4 percent). The locally synthesized IgA is secreted into the gut lumen, and contains antibodies developed in response to exposure to antigens within the lumen. IgA in the gut lumen, termed secretory IgA, is essentially all in dimer form, the two IgA molecules joined by a locally synthesized J-piece to which a glycoprotein, secretory component, is added. The secretory component is believed to be synthesized by the epithelial cells and attached to the IgA before it enters the lumen. Secretory component probably protects IgA from intraluminal enzymatic digestion. Small amounts of gut-synthesized IgA also appear in the general circulation as 7S protein.

Secretory IgA is thought to play an important role in regulating gut bacterial flora, in preventing and controlling tissue invasion by enteric viruses, and in preventing the absorption of undesirable antigenic material by the gut.

CONGENITAL ABNORMALITIES

Most clinical disorders resulting from congenital anomalies are encountered during infancy and childhood, although occasional asymptomatic anomalies may be discovered in the adult. The following are the major anomalies:

Atresia and Stenosis

This rare anomaly may vary from complete separation of the proximal bowel by an atretic segment, to lesser degrees of stenotic narrowing that sometimes takes the form of an intraluminal diaphragm. This anomaly is usually discovered in the first week or two of life, and attention to this possibility should be aroused by persistent bile vomiting, abdominal distention, lack of stool, and air-filled loops of bowel. Occasionally, contrast studies are needed. Surgery is mandatory after decompression of the proximal gastrointestinal tract.

Duplications

These tubular or spherical cystlike structures attached to the mesenteric side of the gut occur most often in the ileum, and may or may not communicate with the true intestine. Large cysts may cause obstructive symptoms, or they may be encountered incidentally at surgery later in life for an unrelated problem.

Meckel's Diverticulum

This is the most frequent congenital anomaly of the intestine. Although it usually remains asymptomatic through life, problems resulting from the diverticulum tend to be encountered most commonly within the first two years of life. This anomaly arises from incomplete obliteration of the vitelline duct at the intestinal end, leaving a sac or diverticulum that arises from the antimesenteric border of the ileum about 80-100 cm proximal to the ileocecal valve. Gastric, duodenal, colonic, and pancreatic ectopic mucosa have been found in these diverticula, the most common being gastric. Hemorrhage, diverticulitis, perforation, and intestinal obstruction may be encountered as complications, the most common of which is bleeding from ulceration of ileal mucosa adjacent to the ectopic gastric mucosa. This anomaly accounts for nearly half of all lower gastrointestinal bleeding in children. Diverticulitis produces a clinical picture often indistinguishable from acute appendicitis. Nonsurgical diagnosis of Meckel's diverticulum is difficult because it seldom fills with barium. Isotope scanning with radioactive pertechnetate may demonstrate those diverticula containing gastric mucosa, but false negative reports have occurred. Occasionally, mesenteric angiography may be helpful in the presence of significant bleeding.

Anomalies of Rotation and Fixation

These predispose to anomalous positioning of the small and large intestines, and to internal herniation and volvulus. The latter two are the only reliable symptoms attributable to these anomalies.

PHYSIOLOGY

Motor Activity

Motility of the small intestine is controlled by the rhythmic electrical activity of the smooth muscle cells and is modulated by the intrinsic nerve supply and hormonal substances. Small intestinal smooth muscle cells have an inherent, rhythmically fluctuating membrane potential known variously as the basic electrical rhythm, slow-wave activity, or the pacesetter potential. These slow waves occur continuously and in synchrony in adjacent cells of the longitudinal layer of muscle. There is a descending gradient of slow-wave frequency, declining from 12 cycles per minute in the duodenum to about 8 in the terminal ileum. Multiple recordings from electrodes placed along the small intestine show that slow-wave activity does not occur simultaneously at all points but, rather, takes place in a proximal to distal phasing that resembles a distally migrating signal. Muscle contractions of the small intestine smooth muscle occur only in relation to a second electrical phenomenon, the spike potential, a burst of one or two more spikes that are superimposed on the slow waves. This phase relationship between slow waves and spike potentials is constant, and the frequency of spike potentials and muscle contractions varies in time and in relationship to food intake, as well as in response to neural and hormonal stimuli. Meanwhile, basic electrical rhythm or slow wave activity goes on constantly, influenced little by fasting or feeding, or by hormonal or nervous stimuli.

The most common form of motor activity in the small intestine is the segmental contraction, a localized ringlike contraction usually less than 1-2 cm in length and lasting only a few seconds. These disappear and recur, often adjacent to previous contractions in a rhythmic fashion that seem ideal for the movement of intestinal contents back and forth for mixing and better exposure to the mucosal surface. True peristalsis in the small intestine is an uncommon event. The aborally declining frequency gradient of electrical slow wave activity with its regulatory effect on motor activity is the basis for the aboral movement of intestinal contents.

The Epithelial Cell and Absorptive Mechanisms

Material to be absorbed from the lumen of the small intestine is passed through the absorptive surface of the epithelial cell or through the tight junctions, the spaces between cells. Absorbed material that enters the cell then passes out of the cell and into the lateral intercellular space from where it enters the lacteal vessels (lymphatic system), or into the venous end of the capillaries and hence via the portal venous system to the liver.

Several basic mechanisms are known by which molecules move from the gut across the epithelial cell into the lymphatics or mesenteric venous circulation. First, materials may leave the lumen and cross the semipermeable epithelial membrane by passive diffusion, diffusing through the lipid membrane or through aqueous pores in the membrane in compliance with the Fick equation, meaning that transport is linear with respect to concentration. Other substances interact with the membrane in a chemical sense, that is, by active transport that is nonlinear with respect to concentration differences, an energy-requiring process with saturable kinetics that is presumably carrier-mediated. A few materials are transported by a third process known as facilitated diffusion, in which a carrier is required but transport is not active or is against electrochemical gradients. Lastly, there is evidence for coupling of movement processes by which two molecules are linked in movement in the same direction, or are coupled with movements in opposite directions.

Absorption of Specific Nutrients

Carbohydrates. Although dietary carbohydrate is entirely dispensable, it makes up approximately 50% of the total daily calories. The principal carbohydrates in the diet are starch (60%), sucrose (30%), and lactose (10%). Intraluminal digestion is initiated by salivary and pancreatic amylases, producing short-chain carbohydrates, mainly disaccharides. Enzymatic hydrolysis of disaccharides to monosaccharides by specific disaccharidases (lactase, sucrase, maltase, isomaltase) located on the surface of the microvilli is necessary for small bowel absorption. The greatest enzymatic concentration and activity occur in the jejunum, with a gradient of decreasing enzymatic activity in the distal small intestine. The resultant monosaccharides—glucose, galactose, and fructose—are then transported into the epithelial cell by a carrier-mediated, sodium-dependent active process that, under normal circumstances, is completed in the duodenum and jejunum. Fructose appears to be absorbed by the process of facilitated diffusion.

Fat Absorption. Dietary fat is nearly all long-chain triglycerides, the major fatty acids being palmitic, stearic, oleic, and linoleic. The remaining 5% of dietary lipid is comprised of medium-chain triglycerides, structural lipids (phospholipids, sphingolipids, glycolipids, etc.), cholesterol, lipovitamins, and so forth. Several intraluminal events and processes are necessary before fat absorption can take place. Emulsification of dietary fat into smaller particles occurs in the stomach and proximal small intestine, providing greater surface area for lipase activity. Conjugated bile acids entering the duodenum act as detergents, helping to stabilize the emulsion. Pancreatic lipase, acting at neutral pH, cleaves the 1-ester and 3-ester bonds of the triglyceride, forming two fatty acids and 2-monoglyceride. The constant removal of fatty acids and monoglyceride by bile acids and their incorporation into micelles facilitates further triglyceride hydrolysis. Other lipids (cholesterol, phospholipids, lipovitamins) are also solubilized by incorporation in these mixed micelles, and move through the solution of intestinal contents and the unstirred layer to the surface of the absorptive cell membrane. Transport into the cell is by passive diffusion, but the bile acid of the micelle is not absorbed. Within the absorptive epithelial cell the long chain fatty acids are reesterified to triglycerides by two pathways. The newly synthesized triglycerides are combined with cholesterol, cholesterol esters, and phospholipid, along with an outer protein surface coat in particles known as chylomicrons, a necessary process for newly absorbed fat to leave the epithelial cell and enter the mesenteric lymphatics. Medium-chain triglycerides are also hydrolyzed by pancreatic lipase but the resultant fatty acids and monoglyceride are absorbed without the intermediary step of micelle formation and intraluminal transport. These fatty acids are not reesterified within the cell, and pass from the cell into the portal blood. Fat-soluble vitamins A, D, E, and K also require micelle solubilization for absorption and are incorporated in chylomicrons.

Protein Absorption

Dietary protein averages 70 g/day (the recommended minimum for adults is 0.8 g/kg). Daily intake of protein is nearly equaled by endogenous protein in the gut lumen, derived from intestinal secretions, desquamated intestinal cells, and daily loss of 1-2 g of plasma protein into the gut.

Intraluminal digestion makes a modest beginning in the stomach via gastric pepsin, a nonessential protease. Pancreatic proteases comprise a group of substrate-specific enzymes secreted in inactive (zymogen) form, activated within the duodenal lumen by the transformation of trypsinogen to trypsin by enterokinase, a brush-border enzyme of the duodenum. The remainder of the proteases are activated by trypsin. The resultant two- to six-amino acid peptides are further hydrolyzed to free amino acids, dipeptides, and tripeptides. Amino acids formed within the lumen and by the brush border peptidases are actively transported by several structurally specific, carrier-mediated mechanisms. Di- and tripeptides can be transported into the absorptive cell intact, where they encounter the intracellular peptidases. Small amounts of intact peptides pass through the intestinal cell without hydrolysis. The vast majority of dietary protein is hydrolyzed, and absorbed in the duodenum and jejunum.

A brief overview of the absorptive processes of additional substances is as follows: bile acids, special active transport mechanism in the ileum; vitamin B_{12}, special transport process in the ileum, requires intrinsic factor from the stomach; sodium, active sodium pump, most prominent in the distal bowel (ileum and colon); potassium, probably mainly passive; polyvalent ions (calcium, magnesium), may have specialized acceptor proteins; water, probably simply a passive movement, determined osmotically by transfer of solutes.

METHODS OF DIAGNOSIS AND ASSESSMENT

Quantitative Stool Fat

The measurement of fat in a 72-hour stool collection while the subject consumes 80-100 g of fat/day, basically a fat-balance study, is the most reliable standard by which fat maldigestion and malabsorption are appraised. Under conditions of total fasting, fecal fat excretion is 2-3 g/day, derived from biliary lipids, bacterial lipids, and desquamated intestinal cells. The average diet in the United States contains 80-100 g of fat, and stool fat is approximately 5 g/day. The coefficient of fat absorption remains at .95 for dietary fat consumptions as high as 300 g/day.

^{14}C Triolein Breath Test

The ^{14}C triolein breath test can detect moderate but not mild steatorrhea. A low excretion of $^{14}CO_2$ after ingestion of ^{14}C triolein is indicative of steatorrhea. The test is completed in a few hours, but is expensive, exposes the patient to radioactivity and is not quantitative. Falsely low values can be seen in hyperlipidemia, hyperthyroidism, diabetes or chronic obstructive lung disease.

D-Xylose Absorption Test

This pentose has a low affinity for the carrier system for glucose and galactose, and therefore is relatively inefficiently absorbed and little metabolized, so that measurement of urinary d-xylose has been shown to correlate with the functional integrity of the proximal small bowel mucosa. The usual test dose is 25 g taken orally. Normal urinary excretion over the next 5 hours is 5 g or greater. It is also possible to assess absorption by measurement of blood xylose levels 1 and 2 hours after the test dose. Emesis, ascites, significant renal impairment, and bacterial overgrowth in the proximal small bowel may give falsely low values.

Roentgenographic Examination

Plain films are of limited value in diagnosis of small intestinal disease beyond giving evidence of mechanical obstruction or perhaps of motility disorders. They may reveal pancreatic calcification, and thus indicate possible pancreatic exocrine insufficiency. Barium sulfate examination of the small intestine is often of great value, as it may show obstructing mass lesions or strictures, mucosal ulcerations of an inflammatory or neoplastic nature, multiple diverticula, sinus tracts and fistulae, altered motility from a variety of causes, and the malabsorption pattern of mild dilatation, increased secretions, coarse folds, and flocculation, as seen in celiac disease.

Mucosal Biopsy

Small intestinal biopsy is the most definitive means for diagnosing diffuse mucosal disease. Employing any of a variety of capsule or suction biopsy instruments, the procedure is a painless, safe, and efficient means of obtaining jejunal mucosal tissue. Several disorders show characteristic and diagnostic changes (abetalipoproteinemia, celiac sprue, agammaglobulinemia, Whipple's disease). Others may show suggestive or typical abnormalities (lymphangiectasia, lymphoma, IgA deficiency, amyloidosis, hypogammaglobulinemia, giardiasis, eosinophilic enteritis). Biochemical assay of mucosal biopsy specimens for disaccharidase activity is an accurate means of diagnosing these deficiencies.

Vitamin B_{12} Absorption Test

The simultaneous oral administration of radiolabeled vitamin B_{12} as two different isotopic forms of the vitamin, each of which is labeled with a different isotope with one form also complexed to intrinsic factor, has shortened the test from 2 days to 1 day without compromising accuracy and interpretation. Inasmuch as the study incorporates both free and intrinsic factor-complexed vitamin B_{12} forms, it can yield information regarding gastric production of intrinsic factor, as well as intestinal absorption that depends upon the functional integrity of the specialized ileal absorptive site. Massive bacterial overgrowth states of the small intestine, or fish tapeworm infestation, can also produce abnormal test results that are corrected by appropriate treatment.

Serum Proteins

Total serum protein concentration may be abnormally low in diseases of the small intestine characterized by significant impairment of protein digestion and absorption as in celiac disease. Vitamin K-dependent coagulation factor proteins may be low in malabsorptive disorders such as celiac sprue, but this deficiency is easily corrected by parenteral administration of vitamin K. Protein loss into the gastrointestinal tract resulting in hypoproteinemia may be detected by employing radiolabeled proteins such as chromium 51-labeled albumin. After intravenous administration of such a substance, it is possible to measure stool protein loss and to estimate the quantity of plasma lost into the gastrointestinal tract per day. It is also possible to calculate plasma pool size, fractional catabolic rate, and the synthesis rate of plasma protein.

Breath Tests of Carbohydrate and Bileacid Malabsorption

Breath tests rest on the measurement of the breath excretion of a byproduct of bacterial action upon a disaccharide or a bile acid. In the case of lactase deficiency, undigested and malabsorbed lactose reaches the distal ileum and colon, where fermentation of the disaccharide by bacterial enzymes produces hydrogen. It is then absorbed into the portal venous system and transported to the lungs, exhaled, and measured by gas chromotography in the expired breath. Another version of the test uses carbon 14-labeled lactose, and the expiration of C14-carbon dioxide is measured by a liquid scintillation counter. These two tests are noninvasive, and sampling at half-hour intervals for 2-3 hours can give prompt, accurate, and reliable estimates of the total ability of the small intestinal mucosa to digest lactose and absorb its monosaccharide components.

The bile acid breath test measures the rate of bacterial deconjugation of cholylglycine-C14. Like the lactose breath test, it is simple to perform, noninvasive, and presents no radiation hazard; it also does not require professional personnel. The fasting patient is given a liquid meal containing a 5 μCi dose of N-cholylglycine labeled in the carboxyl atom of the glycine moiety. The breath is sampled at hourly intervals, and the specific activity of the expired carbon dioxide is calculated. The rate of appearance of carbon dioxide in the breath is a semiquantitative measure of the rate of bacterial deconjugation of endogenous cholylglycine in the gut, because once the glycine is split from the cholic acid, it is rapidly decarboxylated and absorbed. An increase in the rate of carbon dioxide in the breath signifies that either there is small bowel overgrowth of deconjugating bacteria, or that bile acids are not being absorbed with normal efficiency in the small intestine, and are passing into the colon. If simultaneous fecal collection of ring-labeled bile acid is conducted, it is possible to identify and quantify bile acid malabsorption as well.

Serum Carotene and Prothrombin Time
These are rough but useful screening tests for fat malabsorption. Serum carotene reflects not only the efficiency of intestinal absorption of this dietary, fat-soluble precursor of vitamin A, but also the recent and current nutritional status of the patient; thus, a low serum carotene level may be noted in the patient who has not eaten lately owing to a variety of reasons. A prolonged prothrombin time due to vitamin K malabsorption corrects promptly with a very modest dose of intramuscularly administered vitamin K, whereas the hypoprothrombinemia of liver disease is not responsive to vitamin K. Similarly, serum calcium and serum iron are quite frequently low in malabsorption due to diffuse intestinal mucosal dysfunction as in celiac disease, but not in pancreatic deficiency maldigestion. All these tests are fairly useful screening tests for malabsorption, but they provide little help in the differential diagnosis.

5-Hydroxyindoleacetic Acid (5-HIAA)
Determination of 5-HIAA in urine is the most reliable screening test for the presence of carcinoid tumor that has metastasized to the liver or involves the foregut.

Bacterial Cultures
Bacterial cultures of duodenal or jejunal contents obtained by intubation and aspiration give valuable and specific indication of overgrowth of colonic flora in the proximal small intestine, such as bacteroides, *Bifidobacterium*, and *E. coli* in concentrations greater than 10^5 microorganisms/ml. Stool examinations for ova and parasites, and examination of duodenal aspirate for *Giardia*, are also useful tests for diagnosis of small intestinal disease produced by parasites.

DISORDERS OF ABSORPTION (MALABSORPTION SYNDROMES)

Any classification that must involve both anatomic and functional abnormalities will risk imperfections owing to the multiple mechanisms operative in numerous disorders and diseases characterized by malabsorption.

Inadequate Digestion

1. Steatorrhea after gastric resection. This disorder is thought to be due to rapid emptying of food from the stomach, or to asynchrony between emptying and the arrival of bile acids and pancreatic secretions at the site of entry of food into the small intestine. Bacterial overgrowth may also play a role.
2. Deficiency or inactivation of pancreatic enzymes. Pancreatic exocrine insufficiency as a consequence of chronic pancreatitis, pancreatic carcinoma, or cystic fibrosis has already been discussed. In the Zollinger-Ellison syndrome, the low pH in the proximal small intestine from gastric acid hypersecretion irreversibly inactivates pancreatic lipase and also precipitates glycine-conjugated bile acids, thus impairing micelle formation and dispersion of dietary lipid. Probably the excess acid load also causes some mucosal structural damage, contributing to malabsorption.
3. Bile salt deficiency. Hepatic and chronic biliary diseases with cholestasis at times result in impaired bile acid formation and/or biliary secretion. Bacterial overgrowth with colonic flora that deconjugate bile acids in the lumen, resulting in defective micelle formation, is encountered in small bowel multiple diverticula, hypomotility states such as scleroderma or idiopathic pseudo-obstruction, blind loops, and strictures. Disease, or surgical resection of the ileum, can disrupt the enterohepatic circulation of bile acids and result in a contraction of the bile acid pool such that critical micelle concentrations of bile acids in the proximal small intestine are not achieved. Some drugs, such as neomycin or cholestyramine, can precipitate or sequester bile acids.

Inadequate absorptive surface
Short bowel syndromes resulting from massive resection or jejunoileal bypass surgery for obesity are commonly associated with moderate or severe malabsorption. Infrequently, inadvertent gastroileostomy may be performed as part of gastric resection for peptic ulcer disease.

Lymphatic obstruction
Intestinal lymphangiectasia, a congenital or developmental disorder in which distorted and dilated villus lacteals leak newly absorbed dietary fat and lymph into the gut lumen, is commonly associated with steatorrhea and hypoproteinemia from exudative loss of plasma proteins. Neoplasms and inflammatory diseases of the abdominal lymphatics such as lymphoma and Whipple's disease also interfere with the lymphatic transport of absorbed dietary fat, resulting in steatorrhea.

Primary mucosal absorptive defects
A number of inflammatory and infiltrative diseases produce significant damage or disruption of the small intestinal mucosa, resulting in defective absorption of dietary fat and other nutrients. Examples are celiac sprue, regional enteritis, amyloidosis, lymphoma, eosinophilic enteritis, and mastocytosis.

Celiac sprue is the outstanding clinical example of a mucosal absorptive defect responsible for malabsorption. The pathogenesis of the mucosal damage is intimately linked to a poorly understood sensitivity to, or inability to metabolize, gluten, a protein component of wheat, rye, oats, and barley. A higher than normal frequency of HLA-B_8 histocompatibility antigen occurs in sprue patients. There is accumulating evidence to support the concept that gluten or its metabolites may induce an immunologically mediated injury to the intestinal mucosa. The histologic alterations are sufficiently characteristic to play an important part in the diagnosis of celiac disease by mucosal biopsy. The untreated celiac disease mucosa reveals blunting, shortening, and flattening of the surface with loss of villi, elongation of the crypts, and alterations of the epithelial cells that are changed from columnar to cuboidal cells with some loss of brush border microvilli. There is also dense infiltration of the lamina propria with lymphocytes and plasma cells. These changes revert to a nearly normal state after institution of a gluten-free diet, and can be reproduced by reexposure to gluten.

Clinical manifestations vary widely. Classically, steatorrheal diarrhea and weight loss are noted, along with some abdominal distention, cramps, and mild malaise. However, at times the clinical picture is dominated by signs of a nutritional deficiency state resulting from impaired absorption of iron, calcium, vitamin D, vitamin B_{12}, vitamin K, dietary protein, or other nutrients. Occasionally, celiac disease first becomes apparent following gastric surgery. The disease may appear in infancy or childhood and, not infrequently, remits in adolescence only to reappear later. Physical examination may be normal or show signs of weight loss, decreased muscle mass, or signs of specific nutritional deficiency such as easy bruising, dependent edema, tetany, glossitis, and so forth. Laboratory findings may be normal, or may reflect any of the deficiencies mentioned above. The diagnosis is best established by quantitative fecal fat measurement followed by mucosal biopsy, and then proving clinical, biochemical, and morphologic remission by dietary gluten exclusion.

The prognosis is generally excellent on a gluten-free diet. Several complications of celiac disease have been described, however. These include lymphoma that may appear many years after the existence of celiac disease has been established. Avoidance of dietary gluten does not appear to offer any protection. Cancer of the esophagus and colon are said to occur with greater than normal frequency. An unusual complication is that of ulcerative jejunitis, associated with an adverse clinical course in terms of worsening diarrhea and malabsorption, weight loss, and occasional bleeding. So-called collagenous sprue has been noted in a few patients while on gluten-free programs. On jejunal biopsy, a collagenous infiltrate has been noted beneath the basement membrane of the epithelium extending for variable distances into the lamina propria. Patients with this histologic picture show clinical deterioration with weight loss, increasing malabsorption and diarrhea, hypoproteinemia, and anemia, which are unresponsive to steroids and other agents.

Biochemical defects of small intestine mucosa

Defects associated with malabsorption include disaccharidase deficiency, hypogammaglobulinemia, and abetalipoproteinemia. Primary lactase deficiency due to a deficiency of brush border lactase is noted in up to 80% of Orientals, black Americans and Indians, but is found in less than 5% of white Americans. A history of milk intolerance causing abdominal pain, cramps, flatulence, and diarrhea is most characteristic. The diarrhea results from the passage of unhydrolyzed lactose through the small intestine into the colon where bacterial fermentation produces volatile fatty acids (propionic, acetic, and lactic acids) that induce increased motility and osmotic influx of water resulting in cramps and watery diarrhea. An oral lactose load (1 g/kg) should reproduce the patient's symptoms and result in a rise in plasma glucose of less than 20 mg/dl. The diagnosis also may be made by breath tests (see section on diagnostic procedures). Secondary lactose intolerance may occur in a variety of small intestinal diseases in which widespread mucosal damage results in decreased brush border lactase.

DISORDERS OF THE SMALL INTESTINE

Regional Enteritis (Crohn's Disease of the Small Intestine)

Etiology

Regional enteritis or Crohn's disease is a chronic, progressive, granulomatous, inflammatory disorder of unknown cause, which can involve the gastrointestinal tract from mouth to anus with secondary involvement of regional lymph nodes, liver, skin, eyes, and joints. Small intestinal disease is stressed here.

Pathology

The cellular reaction in the intestine extends through all layers of the gut wall and is composed of acute and chronic inflammatory cells (lymphocytes and plasma cells), as well as the aggregation of mononuclear cells that tend to form giant cells and noncaseating granulomas. A chronic inflammatory reaction with edema and fibrosis involves all layers of the gut wall. Mucosal ulceration and deep fissures extending into the submucosa and muscularis are commonly seen. There is generally good preservation of the epithelium and its goblet cell population. Macroscopically, Crohn's disease of the small intestine is characterized by anatomic discontinuity, skip lesions, a tendency to fistula formation, and a high incidence of recurrence after surgery. The bowel wall is thick and stiff, with hypertrophy of the mesentery in the involved segments and so-called normal skip areas between diseased segments. The disease process is thought to involve initially the submucosa with lymphatic inflammation and edema that then progresses to transmural inflammation and fibrosis.

The small bowel is the only site of involvement in 20% of cases. In 60%, there is evidence of ileocolitis; 20% of cases of Crohn's disease involve only the colon. Duodenal involvement is noted in 1-3% of cases. More proximal involvement is very rare. In 1-3% of cases, the disease is confined to the anal area.

Clinical Features

The clinical picture depends upon the area or site of gastrointestinal involvement. Esophageal disease usually produces dysphagia. Gastric antrum or duodenal involvement most often produces ulcerlike distress that may progress to pyloric or duodenal obstruction. In small intestinal disease, the most common symptom is abdominal pain that may vary from a steady ache, often localized to the right lower quadrant, to crampy, colicky, obstructionlike pains with relief following bowel movements. Nonbloody diarrhea is also a common feature. There may be steatorrhea due to extensive disease, or from ileal damage that causes bile salt malabsorption. Weight loss is common, and may be due to anorexia with fear of inducing pain, or from steatorrhea or septic complications. Perianal disease in the form of fistulas, anal ulcers (often with large edematous, dusky skin tags), perianal or ischiorectal abscesses, and anorectal stricture can be severe. Rectal bleeding is most often occult, although minor rectal bleeding may occur with anorectal disease. Fever and growth retardation are common systemic symptoms.

Physical examination often reveals localized abdominal tenderness. With ileal or ileocolonic disease, a palpable tender mass is common, which may signify thickened terminal ileum, an inflammatory mass, and/or enteroenteric fistulas. There may also be physical signs of partial intestinal obstruction. Perianal disease, rectovaginal, or enterocutaneous fistulae may be noted. There are occasionally signs of extracolonic complications such as arthritis, uveitis, and oral aphthous ulcers.

Diagnosis

Sigmoidoscopy is normal in at least 50% of cases of Crohn's disease but may show perianal lesions as described above, or spotty involvement of the rectal mucosa with isolated ulcers and intervening normal mucosa. Roentgenographic barium study of the small intestine is the best means of detecting disease. Barium enema examination of the colon is an essential study for revealing large bowel involvement; it usually provides information about the distal ileum as well. Plain films of the abdomen are indicated in the presence of symptoms suggesting intestinal obstruction. Laboratory abnormalities commonly include microcytic anemia, hypoalbuminemia, low serum vitamin B_{12} and folate levels, and increased fecal fat. They are usually the result of multiple mechanisms such as extensive active disease of the small bowel, extensive resection of diseased small intestine, bile acid deficiency from an interrupted enterohepatic circulation due to extensive ileal disease or ileal resection, or bacterial overgrowth in the small intestine secondary to stasis from strictures and blind loops.

Management

There is no specific treatment for regional enteritis. Management is made difficult by the natural history of this disease, including the high recurrence rate after surgical resection of all detectable disease. Recurrences are most common at sites of anastomosis. The goals of medical management are to control symptoms, to expedite a remission, to provide nutritional support, to correct anemia, and to resolve emergencies. In the active phase of the disease, physical rest including bed rest is important. Relief of diarrhea and pain may be provided by codeine and other agents such as diphenoxylate. Severe abdominal pain often indicates a complication such as impending intestinal obstruction or an intra-abdominal abscess. Nutritional support involves the replacement of vitamin and mineral deficiencies mentioned above, and a low-fat, high-calorie diet. Chemically defined or elemental diets are advantageous in some cases. Intravenous hyperalimentation may be necessary in preparation for surgery, or as part of therapy to induce a remission, but it is not of proven benefit in long-term management except in patients who are nutritional cripples due to extensive disease or surgical resection. In this group, home parenteral alimentation programs have enabled patients to survive out of the hospital and to lead useful lives.

Steroids are of value in inducing clinical remission, and are superior to sulfasalazine in this regard. The general objective is to discontinue steroids once the disease is under control, but some pat ents require long-term maintenance therapy at a dose that sho ıld be kept as low as possible. Steroids are of no value in the management of complications such as abscesses and fistulas, and there is no evidence of prophylactic benefit from steroids in reducing or averting recurrences. Benefit from azathioprine and metronidazole has been claimed by some investigators, but other studies have not confirmed this. Surgery in the management of regional enteritis is limited to dealing with complications that cannot be handled medically. These include intra-abdominal abscesses, enteroenteric and enterocutaneous fistulas, intestinal obstruction, and severe hemorrhage (which occurs infrequently). Surgical resection of diseased intestine is sometimes undertaken in patients whose disease is incapacitating and unresponsive to medical measures, even though the risk of recurrence is acknowledged. (Other aspects of Crohn's disease are discussed in the section on the colon.)

Whipple's Disease

Whipple's disease is a chronic, progressive, multisystem disease predominantly encountered in middle-aged men, and is considered an antibiotic-responsive bacterial infection.

Etiology and Pathogenesis

In all untreated patients, jejunal biopsies and electron microscopy reveal PAS-positive macrophages, and intracellular and extracellular rod-shaped organisms approximately half the size of *E. coli* in the lamina propria of the jejunal villi, even in the absence of diarrhea and malabsorption. Stool and blood cultures are negative, and thus far no organism has been isolated consistently from cultures. There may be a host defect as well, since the organisms phagocytized by the macrophages are not destroyed. Other bacteria lie free in various organs, including the brain, without evoking a prominent inflammatory cell response. PAS-positive macrophages have been found in lymph nodes, liver, pancreas, spleen, heart valves, lung, myocardium, and brain.

Clinical Features

Episodic arthralgias and arthritis, especially in large joints and without deformities, may antedate gastrointestinal symptoms by several years. Pneumonia, cough, pleurisy, and other serositides are also seen along with occasional low-grade fever, anorexia, nausea, and vomiting. Gastrointestinal manifestations are typically late features. Steatorrheal diarrhea, edema, and ascites are common. A variety of central nervous system symptoms have also been described, including headache, mild and progressive dementia, myoclonus, ataxia, and supranuclear ophthalmoplegia. On examination, the patient often appears cachectic and is febrile. There may be ascites, lymphadenopathy, and progressive hyperpigmentation of the skin.

Diagnosis

Diagnosis depends upon the demonstration of PAS-positive macrophages that are most readily seen on jejunal biopsy. Intestinal villi also are commonly swollen and distorted, the lamina propria packed with PAS-positive macrophages, and the lacteal vessels in the lamina propria often dilated. Patients commonly have excess fecal fat and other laboratory manifestations of malabsorption. Small intestine x-rays usually show dilated loops of small intestine with coarse, irregular folds.

Therapy

Clinical response has been favorable to an empirical regimen consisting of penicillin, 1.2 million units, and streptomycin, 1 g per day administered daily for the first 10 to 14 days, followed by tetracycline administered orally, 1 g daily for a year.

Prognosis

Complete remissions are regularly achieved on the above regimen, but some patients relapse. Central nervous system involvement is less responsive to treatment, and has been noted to occur in the absence of gastrointestinal symptoms or histologic abnormalities.

Diverticulosis

Diverticula of the duodenum are relatively common, usually single, and most often occur on the medial surface of the second or third portion of the duodenum. They are usually innocuous and asymptomatic but, in rare instances, have been the site of diverticulitis or hemorrhage. Very rarely, they appear to exert sufficient pressure on the pancreatic and common bile ducts to cause symptoms of pancreatitis or obstructive jaundice. Jejunal diverticula are often multiple, and are relatively asymptomatic. However, diverticula may harbor colonic bacterial flora in large numbers, producing bacterial deconjugation of bile acids with resultant steatorrheal diarrhea, and a macrocytic or megaloblastic anemia due to bacterial competition for dietary vitamin B_{12}. Infrequently, acute diverticular inflammation leading to hemorrhage, or to suppuration and peritonitis, has been noted. The Schilling test of vitamin B_{12} absorption is abnormal, both with and without intrinsic factor in the presence of bacterial overgrowth, but reverts to normal after antibiotic therapy. Surgery is usually infeasible due to the multiple and widespread distribution of diverticula that would require extensive resection. Repeated courses of antibiotics such as tetracycline are indicated in symptomatic diverticulosis.

Protein-Losing Enteropathy

This term is used in reference to a clinical syndrome of a pathophysiologic mechanism in which plasma protein is lost by leakage into the gastrointestinal tract in excess of the modest amount (1-1.5 g/day) that regularly undergoes intestinal degradation. A number of clinical disorders are associated with protein-losing enteropathy, but the mechanisms responsible can be categorized as: extensive mucosal inflammation or ulceration; increased lymphatic pressure from right heart failure, or inflammation or neoplastic disease of the lymphatics; dilated and deformed lacteals and lymphatics as seen in idiopathic intestinal lymphangiectasia; and disordered epithelial cell structure and function, as in celiac disease. Clinical conditions associated with protein-losing enteropathy include giant rugal hypertrophy of the stomach, celiac disease, allergic enteritis, viral and bacterial enteritis, and diseases producing increased pressure in the intestinal lymphatic drainage system, such as obstruction of the inferior vena cava, constrictive pericarditis of the right side of the heart, congestive right heart failure, tricuspid valvular disease, and so forth. In some cases, dependent edema or anasarca is the primary presenting manifestation. In others, the clinical picture is basically that of the underlying gastrointestinal or cardiac disease. In lymphangiectasia, and in some other forms of protein-losing enteropathy, lymphocytopenia in the peripheral blood is characteristic. In such patients, there may be inadequate numbers of immunologically competent lymphocytes, leading to reduced delayed hypersensitivity. The diagnosis of enteric protein loss is made by administering radioactive chromium-labeled serum albumin intravenously and collecting the stools for 96 hours, measuring the radioactive label. It is possible by this study, and the use of other isotopes, to perform plasma decay curves and to estimate the amounts of albumin lost from the plasma per day.

Mesenteric Vascular Disease and Insufficiency

Mesenteric arterial insufficiency is a formidable problem for the clinician, the surgeon, and the radiologist. The arterial circulation of the gastrointestinal tract, especially the collateral interconnecting arteries between the celiac, superior mesenteric, and inferior mesenteric arteries, endows the gut with a significant degree of protection from ischemia. However, intestinal ischemia does occur, and can give rise to acute or chronic clinical pictures.

Chronic intestinal ischemia, also known as abdominal angina, has been associated with atherosclerotic stenosis or occlusion of two of the three major arteries to the gut, often at, or near, their origins from the aorta. It is most commonly described as producing midabdominal or generalized pain, usually steady and often severe, and occurring 20-30 minutes after meals in older individuals. At times, gradual weight loss occurs due to fear of pain on eating. It rarely evolves to a malabsorption syndrome attributable to mucosal or muscular deterioration from ischemia. Angiography has been the major diagnostic tool, yet this technique shows that comparable stenosis may be observed in patients free of the above symptoms. Physical examination is usually unrevealing, although an abdominal bruit is common. Unfortunately, the incidence of bruits in this age group is rather high, and commonly unassociated with any clinical picture. It is most important to eliminate the more common causes of chronic abdominal pain before arriving at a diagnosis of intestinal angina or considering surgical attempts at revascularization.

Acute mesenteric ischemia is a more common and life-threatening intra-abdominal catastrophe, arising from sudden compromise of the intestinal blood supply due to arterial or venous thrombosis, arterial embolus, or vasoconstriction. The condition tends to afflict ischemia-prone patients with serious cardiovascular, renal, or other systemic diseases. A dissecting aneurysm of the aorta, or vasculitis, may also produce this complication.

In recent years, with more aggressive use of angiography and wider recognition of acute mesenteric insufficiency, several series have shown that nonocclusive acute ischemia accounts for at least half of the cases. Arterial embolism and thrombosis comprise an added 35%, and vasculitis, aortic dissection, and venous thrombosis make up the remainder. It is claimed that the critical event in hypoperfusion states is a persistent splanchnic vasoconstriction that often perseveres after the acute and primary cause has been reversed or corrected. Patients at greatest risk are those above 50 with chronic congestive heart failure despite therapy with digitalis and diuretics, cardiac arrhythmias, recent myocardial infarction, hypotension or hypovolemia secondary to trauma, gastrointestinal hemorrhage, pancreatitis, and so on.

Clinical Picture

Abdominal pain is the most common initial symptom, at times associated with the urge to defecate. Early on, there are usually few, if any, abdominal findings accompanying the pain; some patients may have little or no pain. Occult blood in the stools may be noted and, as the process progresses, there may be nausea, vomiting, back pain, signs of peritonitis, leukocytosis, fever, and blood-tinged peritoneal fluid that denote progressive intestinal necrosis.

Diagnosis

It is imperative to consider the diagnosis of acute mesenteric ischemia in any patient who complains of persistent, acute, severe abdominal pain without other abdominal findings or plain film abnormalities, especially since this often indicates that the process is an early stage of preinfarction ischemia. In this setting, rapid assessment of the cardiovascular status and prompt resuscitative measures to alleviate or correct any congestive heart failure, pulmonary edema, or arrhythmias should be carried out. Abdominal plain films are then obtained to rule out other acute abdominal processes and to look for signs of ischemic bowel. Angiography is subsequently performed, to find the type and severity of mesenteric ischemia and assess the state of the splanchnic vasculature, and to then infuse a vasodilator. Nonocclusive mesenteric ischemia is suggested by narrowing at the takeoff point of the major branches of the superior mesenteric artery, intermittent narrowing and dilatation of the branches, or absence of the arcades and intramural vessels. A flush aortogram is first done to exclude an aneurysm, emboli, or occlusions of the major vessels, and to assess the collateral circulation between the superior, celiac, and inferior mesenteric arteries. Selective angiography is then carried out. Papaverine infusion at this point has been advocated to overcome the persistent splanchnic vasoconstriction, either as potentially definitive treatment for nonocclusive ischemia in the absence of peritoneal signs, or as a preoperative measure before laparotomy is done for resection, embolectomy, or arterial reconstruction.

Other forms of vascular disease may cause ischemia of the small intestine. These include allergic or hypersensitivity angiitis, necrotizing angiitis, Henoch-Schönlein purpura, polyarteritis nodosa, and rheumatoid arthritis. In these disorders, mesenteric involvement producing ischemia usually causes abdominal pain, often chronic and without local or impressive findings. Mucosal ulceration usually leads to gastrointestinal bleeding. Intussusception is rather common in children with Henoch-Schönlein purpura.

Tumors

Neoplasms of this segment of the gut occur infrequently. The majority are benign tumors, and are quiescent or found incidentally. They include lipomas, leiomyomas, hemangiomas, and hamartomas. Leiomyomas, like their malignant counterpart, may cause obstruction but more commonly undergo central ulceration or cavitation with hemorrhage. Hemangiomas are usually a necropsy finding that may bleed, in which case angiography may be the only means of detecting them. Hamartomas are notable principally as multiple polypoid lesions of the Peutz-Jeghers syndrome, and may cause recurrent melena or intussusception. The clinical features of this syndrome include melanotic pigmentation of the lips, fingers, and oral mucosa, and hamartomatous polyps of the small intestine, colon, and stomach. The small intestine lesions have no malignant potential, but adenocarcinomas of the duodenum, stomach, and colon have been noted in 3-5% of patients with this syndrome. The precise origin of these cancers is uncertain.

Adenocarcinoma

Adenocarcinoma is the most common malignant tumor and produces symptoms due to obstruction of the lumen, to ulceration and bleeding, and occasionally to intussusception or perforation. Adenocarcinoma in the region of the papilla of Vater may produce ulcerlike symptoms but also commonly causes obstruction of the common bile duct or ampulla, giving rise to a clinical picture resembling pancreatic carcinoma.

Carcinoid

Carcinoid tumors arise from enterochromaffin cells that belong to the amine precursor uptake and decarboxylation (APUD) cell line distributed throughout the intestinal tract in the mucosal crypts. Tumors may arise in the wall of the stomach, the duodenum, or in the rectum, but are most common in the terminal ileum and appendix. They appear grossly as yellow, nodular, submucosal lesions. The great majority of carcinoid tumors are small, asymptomatic, and incidentally encountered at surgery or autopsy. Approximately half of carcinoid tumors are malignant, but malignant potential cannot be discerned from the histologic appearance. Metastases, which are found in 20-30% of cases, appear to correlate best with size. Carcinoid tumors are slow-growing neoplasms that produce a desmoplastic reaction in the adjacent mesentery and nodes, often resulting in a thickened mass that can produce considerable distortion and kinking of the bowel or mesentery with symptoms of partial obstruction. Carcinoid tumors that have metastasized to the liver may produce a syndrome characterized by intestinal hyperactivity with cramps and watery diarrhea, cutaneous flushing, bronchial constriction with asthma, telangiectases, and right heart valvular lesions. Many of the clinical features appear related to biochemical properties of the carcinoid tumor cells that hydroxylate and decarboxylate tryptophan to serotonin, which is subsequently metabolized to 5-hydroxyindoleacetic acid (5-HIAA) and excreted in large amounts in the urine. Although increased urinary content of 5-HIAA is a diagnostic hallmark of the syndrome, and although concentrations of serotonin in tumor tissue may be high, the pathogenesis of the cutaneous flush and cardiac valvular lesions as well as the diarrhea are unclear. Tumor release of kallikrein, resulting in increased circulating bradykinin, may be responsible for the flush. Foregut carcinoids also produce and liberate excessive histamine, but its role in the clinical syndrome is not clear. Food intake may precipitate flushing in tumors of the foregut, and some observers have described differences in the pattern of the flush from tumors arising in the ileum. Carcinoid tumors bear a close histologic resemblance to islet cell tumors; this may account for some of the reported cases in which carcinoids appear associated with multiple endocrine adenomas and peptic ulceration.

Surgical resection of the tumor should be considered, even though hepatic metastases are present, in order that intestinal obstruction and bleeding may be prevented. Resection of tumor masses in the liver, if confined to one lobe, has been performed to reduce the load of functioning tumor tissue. Carcinoid tumors and their metastases have an uncommonly slow rate of growth, with many patients surviving 5-10 years. In the presence of hepatic metastases, almost 25% of patients survive 5 years. Widespread metastases are rare. Death usually is attributable to hepatic or cardiac failure.

Pharmacologic control of the humoral effects of the tumor is difficult although methysergide may help control diarrhea, and *p*-cholorphenylalanine, a tryptophan hydroxylase inhibitor, has also been said to diminish the diarrhea. Chemotherapy with combined 5-fluorouracil and streptozotocin has shown initial promising results. Surgical ligation of the hepatic artery has resulted in reduction of liver metastases and the urinary secretion of 5-HIAA.

Lymphoma

Primary lymphoma of the small intestine occurs most commonly in the ileum and may take several forms. A polypoid or localized, infiltrative and ulcerative form produces a radiographic picture resembling regional ileitis. Involvement may be multifocal and nodular, affecting several segments. At times, diffuse lymphomatous involvement of much of the small intestine may mimic celiac disease, including the radiographic and biopsy features, as well as a clinical picture of malabsorption. Fever, abdominal pain, and anorexia in this setting are suggestive of diffuse lymphoma, which is further characterized by an abnormal immunoglobulin of the IgA type, devoid of light chains, and composed of heavy chains of the α-1 subclass. This form of lymphoma has been called α-chain disease, or α-chain lymphoma, and has been described largely among adolescents and young adults of Middle Eastern countries. More recently, however, it has been observed in Europe, Asia, South America, and the United States. Symptoms of lymphoma include abdominal pain, weight loss, diarrhea with malabsorption, fever, and bleeding. If these symptoms appear as new features in a patient with long-standing celiac disease, or should they appear in a patient suspected of celiac disease but without response to a gluten-restricted diet, lymphoma of the small intestine should be suspected. Current techniques have shown that the great majority of gastrointestinal lymphomas are derived from monoclonal proliferation of B lymphocytes in the intestine. Treatment and prognosis depend upon the extent of intestinal involvement, and the presence or absence of extraintestinal lymphoma. Localized or small segment disease is best treated by surgery, with postoperative radiotherapy and/or chemotherapy employed if adjacent extension is noted at surgery. Management of patients with primary diffuse lymphoma involving a long segment of intestine is less satisfactory because surgery is usually out of the question; in these cases, radiotherapy and chemotherapy must be relied upon.

Acute Intestinal Obstruction

This syndrome, although not a disease, is characterized by failure to pass or to advance intestinal contents, and may be caused by mechanical obstruction or by generalized hypomotility of intestinal smooth muscle (paralytic ileus).

The etiology varies, with mechanical obstruction due either to intraluminal blockage (as by tumors, foreign bodies, gallstones, worms, etc.) or to extrinsic compression and obstruction of the bowel resulting from adhesions, tumors, herniations, or volvulus. Paralytic ileus is usually a secondary reaction to some underlying disorder that results in an imbalance in the autonomic nervous system input to the gut, such that sympathetic function predominates. Trauma, peritoneal inflammation (bacterial, chemical, or enzymatic) and metabolic abnormalities such as uremia, hypocalcemia, or hypokalemia may be the underlying derangements. Sometimes, these underlying causes are systemic in nature such as: toxic—uremia and sepsis; neurogenic—trauma, postoperative atony from manipulation of abdominal viscera at surgery, or from pelvic, rib, and spinal fractures; metabolic—hypokalemia and hypocalcemia; pharmacologic—ganglionic blocking drugs and narcotics.

Common clinical manifestations of mechanical obstruction are crampy or colicky abdominal pain, nausea, vomiting, distention, and constipation or obstipation. Pain is generalized or midabdominal, and occurs in rhythmic cramps that reach a peak, causing the patient to writhe, and which then recede. Pain is usually synchronized with audible bowel sounds early in the course of the obstruction. The more proximal the site of obstruction, the more prompt and severe the appearance of symptoms, including vomiting. The appearance of peritonitis causes more steady pain and a decrease in bowel sounds. There is often a local maximal tenderness if strangulated intestine is present, along with the usual physical signs of peritonitis. Abdominal distention is usually present, unless obstruction is very high in the small intestine, with frequent emesis. Obstipation occurs later in small bowel obstruction, after the distal bowel is emptied; but early on, spontaneous stools or satisfactory evacuation of an enema may occur. However, if obstruction is complete, obstipation and failure to pass flatus appear earlier. In paralytic ileus, pain is usually absent and discomfort results from significant abdominal distention. Obstipation is also usually present. Dyspnea and tachypnea may be noted secondary to the distention. The clinical picture may evolve insidiously and be overshadowed by the accompanying or underlying pathologic state. Physical examination in mechanical obstruction reveals distention as the most common finding, unless the obstruction is proximal, with frequent early vomiting. The abdomen is usually soft and tympanitic, and visible dilated intestinal loops may be noted. The paroxysms of small intestinal contractions are accompanied by exaggerrated, often high-pitched, or hollow, bowel sounds. The abdomen may be equally distended in paralytic ileus but is characteristically silent, as may also be noted with advanced mechanical obstruction with peritonitis. Emesis at first may contain bile and food, but later becomes brown and has a fecal odor and appearance.

Dehydration from repeated emesis and from sequestration of fluid in the bowel lumen, and perhaps in the abdominal cavity as well, develops as the obstruction continues. If strangulation, infarction, or peritonitis develops, the physical signs of shock and sepsis including disorientation or obtundation are also noted. Unrelieved mechanical obstruction evolves to a clinical picture of continued dehydration, and diminishing cramps and bowel sounds with signs of peritoneal irritation, shock, sepsis, disorientation, and death. Paralytic ileus fortunately is often self-limiting or responsive to correction of the underlying disease state or pathophysiology by intestinal decompression, correction of fluid, and electrolyte derangement. At times, paralytic ileus may evolve to mechanical obstruction, owing to kinking and angulation of edematous, fluid-filled bowel loops. Laboratory abnormalities are not specific. Alkalosis develops with high proximal small bowel intestinal obstruction with frequent emesis. In lower intestinal obstruction, alkalosis may occur. Leukocytosis and hemoconcentration are noted with peritoneal irritation and loss of vascular fluid. Serum amylase may be elevated.

Plain films of the abdomen with the patient in the supine, as well as the upright or lateral decubitus, position should be taken as soon as the diagnosis is suspected and if evidence is inconclusive, they should be repeated in a few hours. Multiple or single loops of distended small bowel with air-fluid levels (in the upright film) are the most frequent and reliable signs of mechanical obstruction. Ileus is most characteristically depicted as generalized distended gas-filled small and large intestinal loops, with gas in the lower colon and rectum also. Evidence should be sought for patterns of bowel gas distribution that might suggest inguinal or other internal hernias, as well as cecal or sigmoid volvulus. The right upper quadrant should be carefully examined on the films to search for air in the biliary tree (suggesting gallstone ileus) or gas in the portal vein (suggesting bowel infarction). If the clinical and radiographic pictures are those of a mechanical obstruction in the colon, a cautiously performed colon x-ray using barium or a water-soluble contrast medium often demonstrates the level of obstruction and the nature of the obstructing lesion. If small intestinal obstruction is suspected and an intestinal decompression tube is placed, contrast material may be injected via the tube to better define the point of obstruction. Treatment consists of correction of fluid and electrolyte balance, alleviating emesis, and decompressing the small intestine of its fluid and swallowed air by a nasogastric tube. It may be necessary to start treatment for peritonitis and shock. If mechanical obstruction is suspected, early operative intervention should be considered of greatest importance as soon as efforts to achieve biochemical and vascular stability are under way.

Colon obstruction is most commonly due to carcinoma, and presents a clinical picture that may include a recent history of bowel habit change, rectal bleeding, or recurrent abdominal pain. The latter may signify either partial bowel obstruction, or be more localized and related to the neoplasm. The whole clinical picture tends to evolve more gradually in terms of distention, nausea, and vomiting, but obstipation appears earlier than in small intestinal obstruction. If the ileocecal valve is competent, a gas-filled colon may be noted on abdominal examination and plain films. The latter often shows a point in the colon distal to which gas is not visible. Cecal volvulus usually produces a large abdominal or left upper quadrant gas-filled viscus with a paucity of gas in the colon distal to the cecum, whereas sigmoid volvulus shows a large dilated loop of colon arising from the pelvis. A barium enema shows a normal rectum and distal sigmoid tapering to a bird's beak at the site of the volvulus. At times, sigmoidoscopy or barium enema have been successful in reducing sigmoid volvulus.

Appendicitis

Appendicitis is the most common abdominal disease necessitating surgical intervention. It can occur at any age, but the incidence is highest in young adults. It is rare below the age of 2, but not uncommon in elderly persons.

Pathogenesis

Although obstruction of the lumen by a fecalith with secondary infection resulting from stasis, ischemia, and erosion with mucosal ulceration is a commonly described sequence, in many cases no obstruction or foreign body is found and the associating event or agent is not known. The histologic chain of events with luminal obstruction usually leads to local ischemia, vascular thrombosis, infarction, and perforation. Undoubtedly, some of the acute events described above stop short of perforation or gangrene, and the process subsides. Usually the clinical picture evolves within 24 hours and may be followed soon thereafter by perforation or rupture.

Clinical Picture
The clinical picture has many variations, but the classic history is that of acute epigastric or periumbilical pain that is followed by anorexia, nausea, and vomiting. Pain in the early stages is presumably due to distention of the lumen of the appendix, and contractions of its musculature. As the serosa and adjacent peritoneal surfaces become involved, the pain shifts to the right lower quadrant and fever, tenderness to palpation of that region, plus muscle spasm and rebound tenderness become apparent. If the inflamed appendix is retrocecal, abdominal signs may be absent but pain may be elicited by iliopsoas muscle stretching.

Differential Diagnosis
Acute gastroenteritis may simulate acute appendicitis; but initial emesis or diarrhea before abdominal pain, and other concurrent cases, may be helpful distinguishing points. Referred abdominal pain from pneumonia, mesenteric lymphadenitis, right renal stone or pyelonephritis, ruptured right ovarian follicle or right tubal pregnancy, and right-sided chronic diverticulitis all need consideration.

Intestinal Pseudo-Obstruction

Intestinal pseudo-obstruction is a syndrome in which there are symptoms and signs of intestinal obstruction without evidence for an actual lesion that obstructs the intestinal lumen. The syndrome may be chronic or recurrent; cases of chronic intestinal pseudo-obstruction are classified on clinical grounds as primary or secondary.

Secondary Chronic
Intestinal Pseudo-Obstruction
In this category, the syndrome appears to be caused by coexistent systemic disease or by some pharmacologic agent. The causes may be broadly divided as follows: diseases involving intestinal smooth muscle, such as collagen-vascular diseases and muscular dystrophies; neurologic diseases such as Parkinson's disease, Hirschsprung's disease, and Chagas' disease; endocrine disorders such as myxedema, diabetes, and hypoparathyroidism; pharmacologic causes, such as the use of phenothiazines, tricyclic antidepressants, and ganglionic blockers; and miscellaneous causes, such as celiac disease, jejunoileal bypass, porphyria, and eosinophilic gastroenteritis. The most common causes of secondary chronic intestinal pseudo-obstruction are scleroderma, the muscular dystrophies, and diabetes. Treatment of disorders such as hypoparathyroidism, myxedema, and pheochromocytoma can improve the obstructive symptoms.

Primary (Idiopathic) Chronic
Intestinal Pseudo-Obstruction
Patients in this category have no associated systemic diseases that appear causative; the syndrome can occur either sporadically or as a familial entity.

Familial Primary Chronic
Intestinal Pseudo-Obstruction
To date, nine families have been studied in detail and reported in the literature, but the pattern of inheritance remains unclear.

In some of the families, the disease appears to be a myopathy. Ten to 20 percent of patients with objective evidence of the disorder may be symptomatic. Recurrent postprandial upper abdominal pain is the most common symptom, followed by nausea and vomiting, and less frequently by abdominal distention, diarrhea, constipation, urinary retention, and dysphagia. The diarrhea in some cases is due to malabsorption secondary to bacterial overgrowth in the small intestine. Weight loss and malnourishment may result from reduced nutrient intake to avoid postprandial abdominal pain. Full-blown attacks of pseudo-obstruction are characterized by severe abdominal pain, distention, and vomiting, with radiographic evidence of dilated loops of small bowel and colon with air-fluid levels. Many patients have milder and less specific symptoms preceding and between recurrent attacks.

Although esophageal dilatation and impaired peristalsis have been seen in some instances, x-ray studies of the esophagus are usually normal. Similarly, the stomach is usually normal, and delayed gastric emptying is seldom seen. Megaduodenum is the most common finding, plus multiple dilated loops of small bowel or dilatation of all the small intestine. The colon may appear dilated and redundant. Although megacystis often has been found, no evidence of involvement of the gallbladder has been noted.

Esophageal manometric examinations have been few but, in the majority of instances, there are abnormalities such as low pressure in the LES with or without impaired or absent peristalsis in the lower half of the esophagus. The proximal esophagus and upper esophageal sphincter function normally. Duodenal motility has been found to be quite inactive in the fasting state but can be stimulated by drugs such as bethanechol, neostygmine, and cholecystokinin. Small bowel myoelectric activity has been inadequately studied.

Medical management is difficult since agents such as bethanechol and metoclopramide have not been helpful. Repeated courses of antibiotics have usually improved symptoms resulting from bacterial overgrowth of the small intestine. A home parenteral hyperalimentation approach has been lifesaving in severe cases. Surgical drainage of megaduodenum or, less frequently, surgical excision of a limited dilated segment, may be beneficial but should be avoided as long as possible. Full-thickness biopsies taken from dilated segments are important for histologic diagnosis. Urinary retention in men may require prostatic resection.

Sporadic Primary Chronic
Intestinal Pseudo-Obstruction
The pathology observations in these cases have been varied. Degeneration and atrophy of the smooth muscle and degenera-

tion of intramural nerves have been noted most commonly, although some patients have apparently normal smooth muscle and myenteric nerve elements. The clinical symptoms resemble those already described in the familial syndrome, but the symptoms often occur in younger patients, and medical management poses the same difficulties and disappointments. The drugs already mentioned, and a variety of others, have been unsuccessful in relieving symptoms, and surgical treatment has helped less often because the small intestinal involvement is more often diffuse or may be total. Total parenteral nutrition appears to help in severe cases.

COLON

ANATOMY

The colon begins at the ileocecal valve and, approximately 150 cm further, ends at the anus. Its length is divided into the cecum with the appendix, the ascending, transverse, descending, and sigmoid portions of the colon, and the rectum and anus. The cecum extends below the ileocecal valve and usually lies free in the right iliac fossa, being entirely covered by peritoneum. The appendix, 2-20 cm in length, opens into the posteromedial wall of the cecum. It has a short mesenteric fold in which runs the appendiceal artery. Approximately 60% of appendices are retrocecal or retrocolic; the remainder are pelvic. The ascending colon that runs from the cecum at the ileocecal valve to the hepatic flexure beneath the right lobe of the liver is without a mesentery, and is covered by peritoneum on its front and sides. At the hepatic flexure it becomes the transverse colon that hangs suspended by its mesentery, the transverse mesocolon, which contains the vascular, nerve, and lymphatic supplies. The splenic flexure lies beneath the left diaphragm adjacent to the left kidney and spleen, and represents the junction of the transverse and the descending colon. The latter, like the ascending colon, is covered by peritoneum only on its front and side surfaces. The descending colon distally curves medially at the brim of the pelvis to become the sigmoid that is enfolded in its mesentery and thus mobile and variably convoluted. The sigmoid rests on the bladder or uterus, and becomes the rectum in the midline at the level of the third sacral segment. The rectum descends through the posterior pelvis covered by peritoneum until it passes through the pelvic floor or diaphragm composed of the levator ani muscles and the peritoneal reflection, after which it becomes the anal canal and anus, which is approximately 4 cm in length. The walls of the anal canal are thrown into longitudinal folds that converge distally as anal valves at the pectinate line. At this point, entodermal gut mucosa ends, and the anus is lined distally by squamous epithelium. The external anal sphincter surrounds the anus and is composed of skeletal muscle. The upper anal canal is encircled by its thickened transverse muscle layer as the internal anal sphincter.

The arterial blood supply to the proximal colon comes from the ileocolic, right colic, and middle colic branches of the superior mesenteric artery that anastomose near the splenic flexure with the left colic branches of the inferior mesenteric artery. This continuous vessel lying near the colic wall is known as the marginal artery of Drummond. The descending and sigmoid colons, and the rectum, are supplied by branches of the inferior mesenteric artery. Distally, blood is supplied to the rectum by branches of the median sacral and internal pudendal arteries. Veins accompanying the arteries flow into the portal vein except for the venous drainage of the distal anal canal, which is by way of the iliac veins. Lymph nodes lie near the marginal artery, and in the mesentery and its root. Lymphatic drainage from most of the colon is directed to the cisterna chyli, but that of the distal anal canal is to the inguinal nodes. The vagus nerves supply parasympathetic efferents and afferents to the colon down to the splenic flexure. Distal to that point, parasympathetic innervation comes from the pelvic splanchnic nerves derived from the second, third, and fourth sacral segments of the cord. The fibers to the colon from both the vagi and pelvic splanchnics are preganglionic, and synapse with the nerve cell bodies of the myenteric and submucosal plexuses in the wall of the colon. Sympathetic innervation (postganglionic efferent and afferent) to most of the colon is via fibers from the superior and inferior mesenteric ganglia. The rectum and anus receive sympathetic nerve fibers from the hypogastric plexus. The striated muscle of the external anal sphincter is supplied by the somatic pudendal nerves.

PHYSIOLOGY

Motility

Evidence exists for a sphincteric mechanism at the ileocecal valve in the form of an intermittently sustained zone of elevated pressure at that site, with ileal contents entering the colon during periods of relaxation. Like small intestine musculature, the muscles of the colon are autorhythmic, but there appears to be two separate rhythms. The predominant rhythm is 6-9 slow waves per minute; the other is 3 per minute. Spike potentials that initiate and regulate the contractile process also occur. The primary motor activity of the colon is the regularly spaced ringlike segmental or haustral contractions lasting 60 seconds, which are thought to be partly responsible for the haustrations of the colon. These movements occur in adjacent segments in an independent, nonpropulsive fashion and appear to effect a limited to-and-fro movement of contents designed to expose them to the mucosa for absorption of water and electrolytes. Occasional coordinated organization of contractions occurs in a propulsive aboral direction, sometimes amounting to a mass movement that sweeps intraluminal contents over a considerable distance toward the rectum. Thereafter, haustrations and segmental shuttling resume. Segmental contractions are more frequent in the descending and sigmoid colon than in the proximal colon, but here they are regarded as acting to retard flow of contents into the rectum. Propulsive mass movements do occur in this area also, and advance material into the rectum. The rectum is usually empty of contents, probably because segmental contractions occur frequently in the upper rectum. When fecal material is passed into the rectum distending its lumen, there is a sense of fullness that signals an urge to defecate. At this time, reflex relaxation of the internal anal sphincter and contraction of the external sphincter occur (the rectosphincteric reflex). The internal sphincter relaxation is transient, due to accommodation of the sphincter to distention, and the rectum is able to accommodate and store rather large volumes of material. Defecation is accomplished by relaxation of both the internal sphincter and the voluntary relaxation of the external sphincter. Voluntary straining aids propulsion of the fecal bolus from the rectum by raising intra-abdominal pressure.

Gastrointestinal hormones released by eating are thought to physiologically modulate colonic movements. Cholecystokinin, gastrin, and motilin stimulate colonic smooth muscle, whereas secretin, glucagon, and VIP are inhibitory. Epinephrine inhibits all contractile activity while prostaglandins of the E type diminish segmental activity and increase propulsions.

Fluid and Electrolyte Transport in the Colon

Colonic epithelium differs functionally from that of the small intestine, where much of the water and electrolyte absorption in the proximal small bowel occurs by solvent drag, which is the entrapment of solute in the stream of absorbed fluid that follows nutrient absorption. However, in the ileum and to a more prominent extent in the colon, there is evidence of what has been termed a tight membrane with higher electrical resistance and transmucosal potential difference, low effective pore size, low osmotic permeability for water, limited permeability to inert hydrophilic solutes, and the ability of the colon to absorb sodium and chloride actively against electrochemical gradients. Bicarbonate ion is secreted by an anion-exchange mechanism to balance chloride absorption in excess of sodium. Aldosterone increases sodium absorption in vivo. Potassium is absorbed if luminal concentration is high, but secreted if lower concentrations are perfused. Water is thought to be absorbed by the colon along osmotic gradients secondary to electrolyte transport; however, the colon can absorb water in the face of an osmotic gradient up to 50 mOsm/L. Perfusion studies have also shown regional differences in the colon, with more rapid absorption occurring in the proximal colon.

Estimates of normal colonic function are best made by comparing the composition of what enters the cecum with normal stool composition. Ileal flow into the colon in a healthy person measures approximately 1,500 ml, containing 250 mEq of sodium per day. Stool output contains 100-200 ml of water with 5-10 mEq of sodium per day.

Bacteriology of the Colon

Distal to the ileocecal valve there is a luxuriant metabolically active bacterial population averaging 10^{11}/ml, composed mainly of (99%) strict anaerobes such as bacteroides and bifidobacteria. Their activities alter intraluminal contents in a variety of ways such as the fermentation of carbohydrate to short-chain fatty acids; deamination and decarboxylation of proteins and amino acids; formation of ammonia from urea; hydroxylation of fatty acids; degradation of bilirubin to urobilins; deconjugation and dehydroxylation of bile acids; and the synthesis of vitamin K and folate. Bacteria also act on foreign compounds and drugs, such as the deconjugation of glucuronide conjugates, or the conversion of inert compounds to pharmacologically active metabolites such as cascara sagrada, and the splitting of sulfasalazine into 5-aminosalicylic acid and sulfapyridine.

PROCEDURES IN THE DIAGNOSIS OF COLON DISORDERS

Radiography

Plain films of the abdomen are useful in the detection of toxic colonic dilatation (as in inflammatory bowel disease), and large bowel mechanical obstruction from neoplasms or volvulus of the sigmoid or cecum. Contrast study in the form of a barium enema is the most widely used and practical means for detecting most intraluminal and mural neoplasms, inflammatory bowel disease, diverticulosis, ischemic colitis, and motility disorders such as Hirschsprung's disease. Sometimes mucosal detail, including detection of polyps, is better appreciated by double-contrast x-ray.

Sigmoidoscopy

Sigmoidoscopy is indicated in patients with bowel habit changes, rectal bleeding, and anorectal pain. It is an examination of low cost, extremely low morbidity, and potentially high yield. In addition to observing the appearance of the mucosa and the vascular pattern, and looking for gross lesions such as polyps and tumors, it is possible to biopsy and to take specimens for parasitologic examination and bacterial culture.

Stool Examination

Stool obtained on digital examination should be inspected and tested for blood. Microscopic examination of stool or fecal exudate for erythrocytes and leukocytes in patients with diarrhea is diagnostically helpful. Proper collection and handling of fecal specimens for bacteriologic and parasitologic examination is essential to success, and guidelines established by the clinical laboratory must be observed. These examinations should be performed before antibiotic therapy, and prior to the administration of oily laxatives or before barium radiographic studies. Freshly obtained and promptly examined purged stools yield a higher percentage of positive results than normally passed stools.

Colonoscopy

Colonoscopy is a valuable complement to radiography in the further evaluation of abnormalities such as the detection, biopsy, and removal of colon polyps, and further evaluation of the nature and extent of mucosal diseases such as inflammatory bowel disease. It has also been helpful in the investigation of cryptogenic rectal bleeding.

DISEASES OF THE COLON

Congenital Motility Disorders

Aganglionic Megacolon (Hirschsprung's Disease)
This is a familial congenital disease thought to result from failure of the intramural ganglion cells (which derive from the neural crest) to migrate into all parts of the gastrointestinal tract. Most commonly, a variable length of the distal colon, involving the internal sphincter and adjacent rectum in nearly all cases, is devoid of myenteric ganglion cells. Rarely, more extensive portions or all of the colon are devoid of ganglion cells. The aganglionic segment is unable to transport fecal contents through it, causing constipation and progressive dilatation of the normal proximal bowel that eventually results in abdominal distention. The clinical history consists of obstipation dating from birth. Some newborns and infants develop a severe enterocolitis. On digital examination of the rectum, the ampulla is usually empty. Barium radiographic examination reveals a narrowed distal colon, and dilatation of the remainder of the bowel. Manometric study of the internal and external anal sphincters reveals an inability of the internal sphincter to relax in response to rectal distention. Diagnosis is established by the demonstration of the absence of myenteric ganglion cells on deep or full thickness biopsy of the rectal wall in the narrowed segment. Treatment consists of resection of the aganglionic segment, employing the Swenson pull-through or the Duhamel procedure. It may be necessary to perform a temporary colostomy in some patients before definitive surgical correction.

Acquired Motility Disorders

Idiopathic Megacolon
This form of colon enlargement and constipation is not associated with any known neurologic or other anatomic defect, and its cause is uncertain. It may appear in childhood due to psychogenic factors related to toilet training and parental attitudes towards bowel behavior. In adults, causative factors are more obscure. In either case, there is no contracted segment, and the rectum is full of feces. Treatment with patient reeducational tactics, aided for a time by judicious use of enemas and laxatives, is often successful. Infrequently in adults, abdominal colectomy and ileorectostomy has been performed.

Cathartic Abuse Colon
In some adults, a form of colon motility disorder results from the chronic abuse of cathartics. The colon may show neuromuscular changes presumably induced by the laxatives; radiographically, the colon often appears as a smooth, featureless, sometimes contracted tube due to pseudostrictures, a picture that can resemble long-standing ulcerative colitis. Electrolyte abnormalities in the form of hypokalemia, dehydration, and secondary hyperaldosteronism have been noted. Sigmoidoscopy often shows melanosis coli if anthraquinone laxatives have been abused. Symptomatically, the patient may conceal or deny laxative use and complain of diarrhea, abdominal pain and weakness, and not mention constipation. Alkalinization of the stool will produce a pink-purple color in the presence of phenolphthalein agents. Management of surreptitious laxative abuse is difficult and should involve the proposal for psychiatric assistance (that may be declined).

Irritable Bowel Syndrome

Etiology
Irritable bowel syndrome (IBS) is a common sympton complex considered to be a motility disorder of uncertain cause. Abnormalities in the interaction between myogenic, hormonal, and neural influences on the colon have been observed in IBS and may be the basis of the symptoms. These observations include an increase in three-cycle-per-minute slow wave activity. This activity pattern has not been observed in other colonic diseases and is present during symptomatic and quiescent phases. There is also a delay in the appearance of increased spike potentials following meals in IBS, as well as reduced numbers of long spike bursts, the correlates of peristalsis. Cholecystokinin administration produces abdominal pain in patients with IBS and stimulates three-cycle-per-minute contractile activity only in IBS patients. The postmeal gastrocolic reflex is abnormal in IBS patients, that is, delayed, and this delay can be inhibited by anticholinergics, suggesting an abnormality in neural control. Patients with IBS have increased discomfort sensations from rectal balloon distention, followed by increased slow wave activity. An increased incidence of psychoneurosis has been shown in IBS. Conventional wisdom has convinced most physicians that psychologic factors are important, and that symptoms often correlate with periods of psychologic and physiologic stress and fatigue. Acute gastrointestinal illnesses such as gastroenteritis, dysentery, or amebiasis are prone to be followed by symptoms of IBS that may persist for months.

Clinical Picture
Symptoms commonly begin in the second or third decade. They seldom appear initially above the age of 50; thus, one should suspect and carefully search out organic disease in that age group. Symptomatology is quite variable among patients and from time to time in an individual; but irregular bowel habits, alternating constipation and diarrhea, often with lower abdominal pain of colonic distribution, are the most common symptoms. Crampy or dull pain, flatulence, and a sense of distention are frequent. Stools vary from narrow ribbons to pellets. A common bowel pattern is the passage of three to four loose, watery, urgent stools with mucus in the morning. All the above symptoms seem to be exacerbated by environmental stresses, depression, dysenteric illnesses, and are not uncommonly linked by the sufferer to certain foods. Nocturnal stools do not occur with IBS and should caution the physician against this diagnosis.

Physical examination is unrewarding, except that there may be tenderness to palpation on the right and left colons. Sigmoidoscopy, stool examination for blood and parasites, bacterial culture, and colon barium roentgenographic examination should be done but are normal in this disease; the diagnosis of IBS is reached by excluding organic disease.

Treatment
A recent survey revealed at least transient functional bowel symptoms of IBS in almost one-third of a population of apparently healthy people; such patients might be expected to seek help only during symptom flare-ups, and to respond favorably to medical treatment. A small group with persistent classic IBS may try the physician's patience and ingenuity, and never be restored to normality.

Treatment should be comprised of: measures to relieve acute symptoms—rest, pain relief with nonnarcotic analgesics or tranquilizers; relief from diarrhea with nonnarcotic agents, reduced carbohydrate diet; relief of constipation with increased dietary fiber, hydrophilic colloid, and abstinence from haphazard cathartics.Correction of possible secondary factors such as removal of suspected food intolerances, eliminating coffee, dealing with any enteric pathogens (e.g., *Giardia*) should be tried. The patient should be counseled on changing or adapting to a stressful environment. Also, an explanation of symptoms should be made in terms of the body expression and consequences of stress and emotions, reassurance that serious organic disease is not present, plus encouraging physical exercise and activities on a regular basis. Psychiatric referral such as biofeedback may also be considered.

Prognosis
The prognosis is excellent, although patients experience many ups and downs through the years. There is no evidence to hint that IBS predisposes patients to diverticular disease, inflammatory bowel disease, or neoplasm. The symptoms usually diminish as the years pass.

Diarrhea

Diarrhea is an increase in the frequency, fluidity, or volume of stool. It is a symptomatic manifestation of decreased absorption or increased intestinal secretion of fluid into the lumen, not a disease. Although normal bowel frequency varies from three stools per day to three stools per week, a definition of diarrhea must include a change in stool habits or characteristics for that individual. Because of considerable overlap in the proportion of water in solid stools (60-80%) and liquid stools (70-90%), water content of stools is not a good criterion on which to base a definition of diarrhea. In modern urban societies, daily stool weight is less than 200 g. The 24-hour total fecal weight is a good index of diarrhea, although obviously in many diarrheas the increased weight is comprised mainly of water. However, small volume diarrhea does occur in distal colon disease, with frequent urgent passages of blood and mucus in small amounts.

Normal Fluid Secretion and Absorption
From dietary intake (2 liters) and endogenous secretions (7 liters composed of salivary, gastric, biliary, pancreatic, and small intestinal input), 9 liters of isotonic fluid are delivered to the proximal small intestine daily. Normally efficient reabsorption from the bowel varies in character at different levels of the gut. In the duodenum and jejunum most of the water and electrolyte reabsorption occurs by solvent drag, following nutrient absorption. In the ileum, an efficient sodium pump and a tight mucosa result in effective reabsorption of sodium. Chloride conservation at this level is also efficient, via an exchange mechanism for bicarbonate. The daily volume of intestinal fluid entering the colon is up to 1,500 ml, yet average daily fecal water is only 150 ml. Net colonic absorption of sodium changes the ileal sodium concentration of 125 mEq/L to stool sodium of 40 mEq/L. Ileal potassium is 9.0 mEq/L, stool potassium 40 mEq/L. Colonic absorption of chloride reduces the ileal concentration of 60 mEq/L to fecal chloride of 15 mEq/L.

Pathophysiology of Diarrhea
Diarrhea may be classified on the basis of one or more of the following mechanisms. Osmotic diarrhea results from osmotic retention of water in the lumen by a sufficient content of unabsorbable or poorly absorbable water-soluble molecules. Among disease states and conditions causing osmotic diarrhea are carbohydrate malabsorption such as primary or secondary disaccharidase deficiencies and rare monosaccharidase deficiencies. Saline laxatives (polyvalent ions such as magnesium sulfate and phosphate) also induce osmotic diarrhea. When malabsorbed carbohydrate enters the colon, osmolar load is further increased by bacterial fermentation of carbohydrate to short-chain fatty acids that may also compromise colon absorption by reducing pH in the lumen to values as low as 5. Osmotic diarrhea characteristically abates during fasting. The diarrhea fluid contains a greater sodium than potassium content, and since some of the content is the unabsorbed osmotically active solute, the sum of fecal Na^+ plus K^+ cations is less than half the total fecal osmolality

$$\left(\mathrm{Na} + \mathrm{K} \ll \frac{\mathrm{m0sm/kg}}{2}\right); \text{stool pH} \sim 5$$

In secretory diarrhea, the diarrhea is caused by excessive secretion by the digestive glands and/or intestinal mucosa, and decreased absorption by the small bowel. The stool volume usually exceeds 1 L/day. The hallmark of this form of diarrhea is its persistence despite fasting. Except for bile acids and fatty acids, there is little evidence for abnormal colonic function in secretory diarrhea. Normal colon activity in these patients compensates for sodium and water loss and accelerates potassium loss. Hence, Na and K and their anions account for nearly all the osmolality of stool water. (Na + K)/2 = 250 – 280; stool pH is approximately 7. This category of diarrhea can be subdivided into: infections, in which injury caused by direct mucosal invasion (*Giardia, Shigella, Salmonella*) or by bacterial enterotoxins (cholera, staphylococcal, and clostridial food poisoning, and *E. coli* diarrhea) induce secretion in association with an increase in intracellular cyclic AMP. Hormonal agents can cause diarrhea, as in medullary thyroid cancer, islet cell tumors producing the Zollinger-Ellison syndrome, or the WDHA syndrome. Steatorrhea can occur that gives rise to secretagogue effects of hydroxylated long chain fatty acids on the small and large bowel mucosa. Diarrhea caused by bile acid malabsorption, since bile acids in the colon act as mucosal secretagogues. Inflammatory bowel disease and intestinal neoplasms can cause diarrhea associated with exudative loss of serum protein, blood, and mucus. Villous adenomas may secrete excess fluid and mucus. Disordered contact between chyme and the absorptive surface, as from altered motility producing rapid transit, or a decrease in absorptive surface as from intestinal resection, bypass, or internal fistulas may cause diarrhea, and intestinal obstruction may result in impaired absorption and excessive secretion into the lumen above the obstruction.

In many diarrheal disorders there are multiple pathophysiologic mechanisms at work, but from a clinical standpoint, the following categories are proposed:

1. Malabsorption—fat malabsorption, bile acid diarrhea, and perhaps also an osmotic effect of unabsorbed carbohydrate
2. Intestinal secretion—same as above
3. Infections, infestations, and viral illnesses
4. Other major causes—inflammatory bowel disease, obstruction, metabolic disease, drug-induced diarrhea, and functional diarrhea

Inflammatory Bowel Disease of the Colon

Two disease entities, ulcerative colitis and Crohn's disease, are considered under this terminology. The features of Crohn's disease of the small intestine were discussed earlier (see the section on regional enteritis), including theories as to etiology, epidemiology, and pathology. Only so-called Crohn's colitis and ulcerative colitis will be covered below.

Ulcerative Colitis

Ulcerative colitis is a chronic inflammatory disease of the mucosal surface of the colon, of unknown cause.

Epidemiology. The incidence of chronic ulcerative colitis is higher in whites than blacks, and in Jews than non-Jews. The annual incidence rate is 5-10/100,000. Prevalence in the United States is 45-80/100,000. There appear to be two incidence peaks, one at ages 20-30, and again about age 60. Five to 10 percent of patients have a family history of inflammatory bowel disease.

Etiology

The cause of ulcerative colitis is unknown. No satisfactory hypothesis or solid evidence favoring an infectious, allergic, immunologic, or psychologic etiology has held up under careful evaluation. Genetic factors may be contributory in view of multiple cases in families, and the association between HLA-B27 phenotype incidence in colitis patients with spondylitis.

Pathology

The disease process is an inflammatory reaction confined to the colonic mucosa and submucosa. Inflammation always involves the mucosal epithelial cells, including those of the crypts. In acute and early stages, inflammatory cells are neutrophils and eosinophils, but in advanced and chronic stages, plasma cells and lymphocytes are seen throughout the lamina propria. The mucosa is diffusely involved with inflammation and ulceration. The above changes almost always involve the rectum and usually begin there. There is also usually continuous involvement of mucosa extending proximally from the rectum. In two-thirds of cases, the left colon is involved, and in one-third all colonic mucosa is diseased. The persistent and recurrent inflammation results in shortening of the colon due to retraction and thickening of the muscular layers. Strictures of a gradual tapering configuration may develop. The rectum is usually contracted. There is thinning of the mucosa as it becomes destroyed or denuded, but often islands of hyperplastic regenerating mucosa in the form of pseudopolyps develop. In severe, acute, or fulminating disease, the ulceration and inflammatory reaction extend into the muscle layers, with vasculitis and probable intramural plexus damage, resulting in dilatation and impaired motor function.

Clinical Features

Most commonly, ulcerative colitis appears in the second to fourth decades, and may vary in severity from a mild form in which local bowel or rectal symptoms are present but without disability, to a fulminating form in which acute, explosive, devastating, systemic, and abdominal symptoms appear in life-threatening severity. The most common or characteristic symptoms are diarrhea with blood, abdominal pain, weight loss, and fever. Bleeding results from the ulcerations, hyperemia, and vascular engorgement producing a friable, inflamed, and granular mucosal surface. Diarrhea is secondary to damaged mucosa with resultant impaired absorption of water, electrolytes, and serum protein exudation, although small volume diarrhea may represent frequency caused by rectal irritability due to localized rectal involvement. Cramps usually precede bowel movements. Occasionally, extracolonic manifestations are the presenting features, or they may overshadow symptoms from the bowel.

Clinical Course

In approximately two-thirds of cases, there are intermittent exacerbations with complete asymptomatic remissions, although objective evidence of disease persists on sigmoidoscopy and colon x-ray. In 10-15% of cases, the disease is continuously active without remission. Approximately 5-10% have an initial acute attack and then go into complete remission.

Physical Examination

Examination may be essentially normal, but often patients look ill, pale, and anxious, with evidence of weight loss; they may also be febrile. Abdominal examination commonly shows tenderness over the involved area of the colon. Abdominal distention, tympany, and increased tenderness in acutely ill patients should suggest toxic megacolon. Extracolonic manifestations should be sought for pyoderma gangrenosum, erythema nodosum, arthritis, and aphthous ulcers. Digital rectal examination often reveals the mucosa to have a slightly granular wet sandpaper texture, and bloody mucus often is seen on the glove.

Laboratory Features

There are no diagnostic laboratory abnormalities, but testing should be used for the exclusion of other diseases and evaluation of the status of the patient. Anemia is common and usually reflects blood loss, but in chronic cases may be the anemia of chronic disease. Leukocytosis is common in acute, active, and severe disease. The sedimentation rate is usually raised with disease activity. Hypokalemia is often seen with severe diarrhea. Hypoproteinemia (especially hypoalbuminemia) is common. Leukocytes are present on fresh smears of rectal exudate. Parasite examinations and stool cultures should be done on new cases to exclude specific causes of diarrhea (amebiasis, shigellosis, *Campylobacter*, etc.).

Sigmoidoscopy

Virtually all (95%) patients with chronic ulcerative colitis have rectal involvement beginning at the dentate line, with a uniformly friable, hyperemic, finely ulcerated or granular mucosa, and edema that obscures the usual fine tracery of vessels beneath the mucosa. In a comparatively mild form of the disease confined to the rectum, ulcerative proctosigmoiditis, the changes described above fade away proximally to normal mucosa within the viewing range of the proctoscope.

Roentgenography

A plain film of the abdomen is of value in assessing the diameter of the colon in suspected toxic megacolon. In this severe transmural form of the disease, the portion of the colon most prominently distended on AP films in the supine position is the transverse colon. Erect or left lateral decubitus views should also be done in this clinical setting to look for free air in the abdomen. Often the air-filled dilated transverse colon will show few or no haustrations and have a shaggy, thickened mucosal profile due to pseudopolyps, or may even show air-filled mucosal crevices thought to be due to deep ulcers.

Barium enema roentgenographic study is used to supplement the findings on sigmoidoscopy, especially to determine the extent of the disease and to better define its nature. It may appear normal or nearly so in early or mild disease. In the acute stage, spasm and irritability are more prominent, and there may be more luminal secretions of mucus and blood. Ulcerations are tiny and difficult to see, often appearing as fuzzy serrations or fine spiculations in contour. Air-contrast studies may bring out these fine details more clearly. In less-active and continued inflammatory stages, the colon mucosal surface may be more nodular or finely polypoid in a rather uniform symmetrical way, with some lessening and irregularity of haustra. In the chronic stages, the radiographic features are due to attempts at epithelial regeneration, fibrosis, and pseudopolyposis. Hence, the colon is shortened, and the lumen is tubular and narrowed, with absent haustra. The flexures are often depressed and may be contracted. In addition to the above features, other important diagnostic points are that the disease is continuous rather than segmental in distribution and extends proximally for varying distances from the rectum, which is almost always (95%) involved. Strictures of variable lengths and usually with smoothly tapered ends are occasionally seen. When the entire colon is involved, backwash ileitis changes in a short segment of the terminal ileum are not uncommon. This ileal segment is dilated and the mucosa is smooth. Furthermore, the absence of sinus tracts, fistulas, and skip areas of the ileum help in differentiating this from regional ileitis.

Barium examination of the colon is not without dangers, and should not be done in acute severe colitis owing to risk of perforation or inducing toxic megacolon. It is best to avoid harsh laxatives in preparing for the examination, relying on a liquid diet for 24 hours, a tapwater enema, and perhaps a saline cathartic.

Differential Diagnosis

The differential diagnosis of ulcerative colitis includes amebiasis, shigellosis, salmonellosis, *Campylobacter* infection, ischemic colitis, laxative abuse colonic changes, postantibiotic colitis, and Crohn's disease of the colon.

Medical Management

The goals of medical management are to terminate the acute attack, to prevent recurrences, and to correct nutritional, fluid, and electrolyte deficiencies, all of which may minimize the disability. Mild disease with local (rectal) symptoms can usually be managed while the patient is ambulatory. Sulfasalazine, 0.5-1.0 g four times daily, and perhaps added steroid enemas or suppositories nightly for 4-6 weeks, may suffice. Antispasmodics, antidiarrheal drugs, and bulk-forming agents, as well as physical and mental rest, may hasten improvement.

In more severe active disease, patients are best managed in the hospital, although bed rest at home may suffice. Sulfasalazine, 1.0 g four times daily, and oral prednisone, 40-60 mg per day as an initial dose, are started. Blood cultures should be done if the patient is febrile. Fluid and electrolyte losses are replaced intravenously, and blood is given to correct anemia. Parenteral alimentation may be necessary. The patient is watched closely for ominous physical signs such as abdominal distention, persistent tachycardia, and unremitting diarrhea. An important aspect of medical management is the early identification of the acutely ill colitis patient who is a potential treatment failure or who may be developing toxic dilatation, and hence require emergency colectomy.

As the acute disease comes under control, prednisone should be reduced by 5.0 mg every 3-5 days with the goal of terminating steroids within 3 months, as steroids have not been shown effective in preventing acute recurrences. Sulfasalazine, however, is useful in maintaining clinical remissions and reducing the frequency of recurrences, and should be continued for perhaps 1 or 2 years in daily dosage of 2-4 g. Sulfasalazine carries with it a risk of several dose-related effects, including nausea, vomiting, and headache during the first few days of use. Other potential side effects include skin rash, Heinz-body anemia, and reversible impaired male fertility.

Patients with fulminating disease should be promptly hospitalized and treated with intravenous steroids (40-60 mg/day) or ACTH. Nutrition should be by parenteral hyperalimentation. Blood cultures should be done. Antibiotics have a disputed role in this setting but are often used. Efforts to correct fluid and electrolyte deficiencies with saline, plasma and blood should be undertaken forthwith. Lack of significant improvement in 5-7 days on intravenous steroids and bowel rest should prompt serious consideration of colectomy. However, if the patient is young and physiologically strong, it may be safe and reasonable to persist longer, with continued careful and frequent assessment, including a close watch for signs of deterioration. If improvement occurs, the patient may be gradually started on oral feedings and steroids.

Special Considerations

Ulcerative proctitis is colitis confined to the distal 10-15 cm of the anal canal, with visible evidence of normal mucosa proximally, and normal colon seen on barium enema above the distal rectal disease. Symptoms in this form of the disease are usually restricted to small volume diarrhea with bloody mucus, or rectal bleeding without diarrhea. Ambulatory treatment consists of sulfasalazine, and nightly steroid enemas (100 mg of hydrocortisone, or 20 mg prednisone in 100 ml of saline) retained as long as possible. There is evidence of 35-45% absorption of steroids administered by this route. This form of colitis carries an especially favorable prognosis, since disability is minimal and the disease remains confined to the rectum in one-half to two-thirds of cases. Furthermore, if more extensive ulcerative colitis is going to evolve, it usually does so within the first 2 years of symptoms.

Ulcerative colitis in children has the same general clinical features as in adults. However, in this group, growth retardation and delayed maturation are special and not uncommon considerations, not only from the colon disease but also as a possible consequence of long-term steroid use. Steroids should be employed in full but weight-related doses, although courses longer than 3 months should be avoided owing to their adverse effects on growth. Special efforts to correct protein and calorie malnourishment are helpful in promoting growth and in enhancing the response to steroids. However, if the patient shows evidence of growth retardation and inability to fare well off steroids as puberty approaches, total colectomy should be seriously considered. Children adapt well to ileostomies. Recently, favorable experience in this age group has been reported with total colectomy with rectal mucosectomy plus ileoanal anastomosis.

Colonic Complications

Toxic Megacolon. This serious complication generally develops during acute and fulminating attacks of colitis when bowel wall inflammation extends into the muscular layers and mural nerve plexuses following severe mucosal destruction. Precipitating factors include the use of opiates and anticholinergic drugs, hypokalemia, or the performance of a barium enema during acute severe colitis. The bowel is atonic and hypomotile, and on plain films of the abdomen the transverse colon is 8 cm or more in diameter, often thick-walled, and may show a shaggy mucosa. It signifies potentially impending perforation and calls for intensive efforts to correct fluid and electrolyte abnormalities and stopping certain medications, but if definite improvement is not apparent in 24-36 hours, emergency total colectomy should be done.

Strictures. These lesions are noted in more than 10% of patients with ulcerative colitis, and probably arise from fibromuscular hyperplasia. They may be long or short in length, tend to be smooth, and tapered in form. They need to be distinguished from carcinoma, which in ulcerative colitis may occasionally take the form of a filiform stricture.

Cancer. In some cases, carcinoma in the colon affected by ulcerative colitis may appear as a typical colonic malignancy. However, carcinoma tends to be multifocal in 25% of cases, and can appear as a persistent irregularity in contour, or an infiltrative stricture. Cancer in ulcerative colitis does not have the same predilection for the rectosigmoid, is frequently of high-grade malignancy, and occurs at an earlier age than in the normal population. In several western countries, including the United States, patients with ulcerative colitis have a 7-11 times greater risk of developing a colonic malignancy than the general population. Risk seems related to the duration of disease, increasing exponentially after 10 years of colitis. It is also related to a severe initial attack, total colon involvement, continuous activity of disease, and onset before age 20. In the first 10 years, there is a 3% incidence of cancer; after 10 years, there is a 20% incidence per decade in colitis patients. The diagnosis of cancer in ulcerative colitis may be difficult since the symptoms are often quite similar to those of the underlying colitis. X-ray diagnosis is more difficult, and less accurate, than in otherwise normal colons. Mucosal biopsies obtained at sigmoidoscopy and colonoscopy may show precancerous and severe dysplastic changes. Probably all patients should be under annual or semiannual surveillance, employing colonoscopic biopsies and x-ray after 10 years of disease. The measurement of serum carcinoembryonic antigen (CEA) is not helpful, as one-third of patients with ulcerative colitis have elevated CEA levels with or without cancer. Probably only very high values are meaningful.

Massive Hemorrhage. Severe or exsanguinating hemorrhage is uncommon and occurs only in the presence of severe disease. If the patient cannot be kept physiologically stable by transfusions, colectomy may be necessary.

Pseudopolyps. This is discussed under neoplasms of the colon and rectum. They have no malignant potential.

Extracolonic Manifestations

Arthritis. A characteristic form of arthritis accompanies ulcerative colitis in 20-25% of cases. It appears to favor involvement of large joints such as knees, ankles, hips, elbows, and shoulders, and usually affects one or two joints at a time. It rarely precedes the clinical appearance of the underlying bowel disease. Activity of the arthritis tends to parallel the activity of the bowel disease. Rheumatoid factor is negative. The joint involvement is nondeforming, and is cured by colectomy. There also appears to be an increased incidence of rheumatoid arthritis in patients with ulcerative colitis, but the course of the joint disease is unrelated to the colitis.

Ankylosing spondylitis and sacroiliitis may precede the onset of ulcerative colitis for years, and tends to persist or may even first appear after colectomy. The sex incidence is equal, and all patients with ulcerative colitis and ankylosing spondylitis have the HLA-B27 antigen.

Skin and Mucous Membranes. Lesions involving skin and mucous membranes complicate colitis, including erythema nodosum, pyoderma gangrenosum, and aphthous ulcers of the mouth.

Liver. Fatty infiltration is the most common histologic abnormality, and is at times associated with midly abnormal liver tests. Pericholangitis is the most characteristic hepatic abnormality, and consists of a mononuclear infiltrate of the portal tracts with preservation of the limiting plate. It may later evolve to progressive fibrosis, chronic active hepatitis, and cirrhosis. The most common laboratory abnormality accompanying pericholangitis is a raised alkaline phosphatase. Sclerosing cholangitis is noted in 1-3% of ulcerative colitis patients. It consists of irregular narrowing of the extrahepatic bile ducts (and, at times, the intrahepatic ducts as well) by fibrosis and chronic inflammation. In several series of so-called primary sclerosing cholangitis, patients with inflammatory bowel disease, particularly ulcerative colitis, comprised approximately half the cases. Laboratory abnormalities are those of cholestasis; the major symptoms are pruritus, jaundice, recurring cholangitis, and, eventually, secondary biliary cirrhosis and liver failure. The diagnosis is best made by endoscopic retrograde cholangiography. Bile duct carcinoma and gallstones are also increased in incidence.

Kidney. The most common renal complication is nephrolithiasis, which results mainly from chronic dehydration secondary to diarrhea. The incidence of kidney stones is approximately twice that of normal individuals. After total colectomy and the establishment of ileostomy, the incidence of kidney stones also rises. Uric acid stones are most common, followed by calcium-magnesium phosphate stones.

Blood. Hematologic abnormalities are mainly those of chronic iron deficiency due to blood loss, and thrombocytosis. A hemolytic anemia may result from sulfasalazine therapy.

Crohn's Disease of the Colon

The incidence of Crohn's disease of the colon in the United States is 6/100,000 population per year. Etiologic factors are probably the same as those for ulcerative colitis and regional enteritis, but essentially no cause is known for this disorder. (The reader is referred to the discussion of Crohn's disease of the small intestine).

Pathology

Twenty percent of Crohn's disease affects the colon. As in the small intestine, the changes are those of a transmural, predominantly submucosal, inflammatory process with edema, and intense lymphocytic infiltration, ultimately resulting in thickening and fibrosis of the bowel wall, as well as patchy serpiginous mucosal ulcerations and deep fissures. Epithelioid cell granulomas are found in 50-75% of cases. Involvement of the colon is characteristically segmental. The rectum is spared in 50% of cases.

Clinical Features

The onset is often more insidious than that of ulcerative colitis, with more subtle symptoms. Most patients have diarrhea, abdominal pain, and weight loss. Rectal bleeding is infrequent. Fever and anemia are common.

Sigmoidoscopy

Abnormal findings are noted on sigmoidoscopy in only 50% of cases. They include mucosal edema producing a cobblestone pattern, plus discrete and, at times, large ulcers with nearly normal intervening mucosa. The anal canal is often thickened, and there may be edematous tags with a dusky cyanotic hue, as well as fissure/ulcer of the anus. Perianal abscesses and fistulas are also seen. Anal lesions may precede intestinal lesions by months or years.

Radiographic Findings

In only 10-15% of cases of Crohn's disease of the colon is there universal involvement, and then usually with ileal disease also. The most frequent pattern of distribution of Crohn's disease of the colon is from the ileocecal valve to the distal segment, with rectal sparing. The roentgenographic features include segmental distribution, a cobblestonelike mucosal pattern, eccentric or asymmetric anal involvement, and longitudinal and transverse ulcers that contribute to the cobblestone appearance of the mucosa. Deep fissures are also occasionally seen, as well as sinus tracts and enteroenteric fistulas. There is marked thickening and rigidity of the bowel due to fibrotic changes, giving rise to irregular stenoses and strictures.

Medical Management

There is, in fact, no treatment for the disease as such, but only treatment for the patient. The goals of such empirical, palliative treatment are to contain symptoms, to expedite remissions, to provide nutritional support, and to resolve emergencies. Medical management should be the first approach until such time or events arise as to make the risks of perseverence exceed those of surgical intervention. There are certain basic disease differences that influence the medical management of Crohn's disease of the colon as opposed to ulcerative colitis. In Crohn's disease, there is a tendency to recurrence after surgery, a different pathology picture that may explain why response to treatment is slower, as well as the possible coexistence of small intestinal disease. Bed rest is an important but understressed element of treatment. The matters of diet, steroid therapy, and the use of sulfasalazine are the same as in medical management of chronic ulcerative colitis.

Surgical Treatment

Surgery should be delayed as long as possible, and reserved for intractable symptoms or the treatment of complications. It may occasionally be necessary to operate for emergency treatment of bowel perforation, toxic megacolon, or severe hemorrhage. Colectomy is the most common operation, but the decision to preserve the rectum depends upon the presence and extent of rectal involvement or perianal complications. Where reasonable, later ileoanal anastomosis should be considered. Surgery is done for colon obstruction in approximately 25% of cases. In 35% of cases, palliation of severe, disabling, and unresponsive symptoms such as anemia, diarrhea, and pain are the indications for surgery. Abscess and fistula account for 20% of cases. Recurrence of disease after surgery is most common at, or just proximal to, the site of anastomosis.

Results of Medical Management

Spontaneous healing is rare, although temporary remissions do occur. After the surgical resection of all detectable disease, there is a 45% recurrence in 2 years, 68% at 5 years, and 78% at 10 years. When disease was restricted to the ileum, a 33% recurrence rate at 5 years and 50% recurrence in 10 years was reported. Approximately half of each group required further surgery.

Prognosis

A recent Mayo Clinic study reported that for a group of patients with Crohn's disease with onset below the age of 20, 76% were alive 20 years later, compared to a control population survival of 98%. Survival appeared independent of the site of the original disease.

Complications

Intestinal obstruction due to stricture is more common than in ulcerative colitis. Not uncommonly, fistulas form in Crohn's disease and may be internal such as enteroenteric, enterovesical, or enterosigmoidal. External fistulas include perianal, rectovaginal, and enterocutaneous types. Perforation of the bowel occurs in less than 3%. The risk of carcinoma in Crohn's disease is less than that of chronic ulcerative colitis, but in patients with disease beginning below the age of 20, the incidence appears to be several times that of a comparable normal population. Several cases of adenocarcinoma occurring in surgically bypassed ileum have been reported. Protein-losing enteropathy also occurs in Crohn's disease.

Systemic Complications. Arthritis with large joint involvement occurs, similar to that seen in chronic ulcerative colitis. Ankylosing spondylitis differs from that of colitis, in that the joint involvement precedes the bowel disease in the majority of cases.

Calcium oxalate renal stones occur with increased frequency in Crohn's disease with ileal involvement or after ileal resection. The pathogenesis is thought to be due to increased absorption of oxalate from dietary sources by the colon. Liver changes similar to those described in chronic ulcerative colitis occur but with less frequency. An increased incidence of gallstones occurs with ileal Crohn's disease.

Diverticular Disease of the Colon

Diverticulosis is a disorder of the colon characterized by small herniations of colonic mucosa through the muscular layer of the colon wall.

Etiopathogenesis

The etiology is unknown, but the pathogenesis is thought to involve a pressure gradient between the colonic lumen and the serosa, as well as points of weakness in the colon wall. The most common site for the appearance of diverticula is the sigmoid colon, though they may occur in any portion of the colon. Motility is particularly active in the sigmoid segment of the colon. Diverticular herniations commonly occur at points of penetration of the colonic wall by intramural vessels through the circular muscle layer. However, a recent careful review of studies relating sigmoid pressures, motility index data, coloinic wall strength analyses, and so forth, reached the conclusion that none of the above could be convincingly shown to explain the formation of diverticula, or to give rise to complications. Diverticulosis is common in western nations, and prevalence rates in autopsy series in those countries have risen from 5% in 1910, to 50% in the 1970's. The prevalence rises rapidly with age. Although diverticulosis is rare below the age of 35, two-thirds of patients have diverticula by age 85. Patients with diverticular disease also have significantly increased frequencies of gallstones, ischemic heart disease, varicose veins, hiatal hernias, and hemorrhoids, but not colon carcinoma or appendicitis.

Natural History

Most people with diverticulosis remain asymptomatic throughout life. In some, the diverticula are found on investigation of recurring left lower quadrant pain, when radiographic examination may show muscular thickening of the wall of the sigmoid (mychosis) with or without diverticula, producing an irregular sawtooth appearance. In other patients, the radiographic appearance is that of massed, or multiple, diverticula involving the descending colon and sigmoid without evidence of muscle hypertrophy or spasm. Perhaps 10-20% of patients with known diverticula show clinical signs of diverticulitis when followed over a period of 5-10 years. A second recurrence of diverticulitis occurs in one-third of cases treated medically, most commonly within 5 years.

Diagnosis

Diverticula are most commonly diagnosed by barium enema radiographic examination. However, the radiographic distinction between diverticulosis and diverticulitis is often difficult and at times in error. Muscle spasm of the sigmoid may be mistaken for diverticulosis. Radiographic evidence of fistulas and abscesses are the most reliable signs of diverticulitis, although they are not pathognomonic. Barium enema examination is contraindicated in severe acute diverticulitis. A rather common problem is the differentiation of carcinoma with perforation or obstruction from diverticulitis with spasm or stricture. Colonoscopy may at times be helpful in this regard, although it has its hazards and is relatively contraindicated in acute diverticulitis. Crohn's disease, occasionally chronic ulcerative colitis, and gynecologic pelvic mass lesions may mimic the clinical picture of diverticulitis.

Acute Diverticulitis

The pathogenesis of this complication is now thought not to be diverticular obstruction or fecal impaction, but rather the result of perforation of one or more diverticula, resulting in inflammation and suppuration of the wall and the serosa, producing peridiverticular abscess, a mural sinus tract, or free perforation. The diagnosis is assisted by the presence of fever, leukocytosis, abdominal tenderness, and occasionally signs of peritonitis, usually in the left lower quadrant. Plain films of the abdomen should be done to exclude colon obstruction and to look for free air. Careful sigmoidoscopy may help exclude other diseases. Barium contrast radiographic examination should be delayed until the acute process subsides. Colonoscopy may be performed after the acute inflammatory stage is passed.

Treatment

Asymptomatic diverticular disease may require no treatment, but it is currently popular to advise a diet high in fiber as an empirical measure. It is felt by some physicians that this may help correct constipation, relieve abdominal discomfort, and possibly prevent attacks of diverticulitis.

In the treatment of acute diverticulitis, bed rest and a liquid diet or parenteral fluids are commonly used. Antibiotics are widely employed, although controlled trials are lacking. The presumption is that bacteroides and other anaerobes are the organisms most likely responsible for the inflammation, and thus gentamicin plus clindamycin or cefoxitin are commonly used. Most episodes of diverticulitis subside spontaneously or with antibiotic treatment. However, abscess formation, bacteremia, bowel perforation, fistula formation to the bladder or vagina, or obstruction require surgical intervention in 15-30% of patients hospitalized for diverticulitis. Surgery should be advised for recurrent attacks or the above-mentioned complications. Sigmoid colectomy is the most common operation. In the presence of active diverticulitis, a three-stage surgical procedure is often necessary: a proximal colostomy with drainage of any abscess found, later resection of the diseased bowel, and closure of the colostomy with restoration of continuity by end-to-end anastomosis. Elective resection of the abnormal segment with end-to-end anastomosis is usually possible during a quiescent interval.

Rectal bleeding is a frequent complication of diverticular disease and usually occurs in the absence of inflammation. Its course is usually benign, with bleeding occurring at a steady, moderate rate for one to several days, but without life-threatening loss of blood. Bleeding stops spontaneously in 75-90% of cases managed conservatively, but occasionally emergency angiography and a decision for surgery may be necessary.

Acute Inflammatory Diseases of the Colon

Acute inflammatory diseases of the colon such as shigellosis, amebic colitis, salmonellosis, *Campylobacter* infection, and pseudomembranous colitis give rise to cramps and tenesmus, watery or bloody stools, fever, and at times, nausea and vomiting. They are most often due to tissue invasion by parasites, bacteria, or, occasionally viruses (lymphopathia venereum).

Stool examinations for blood, leukocytes, parasites and ova, and bacterial cultures should be done before other gastrointestinal diagnostic procedures are initiated. Sigmoidoscopy should then follow, but it is best conducted without cleansing preparation of the bowel. The mucosa should be inspected for hyperemia, edema, friability, and the presence of exudates, membranes, and ulceration. Wet smears obtained at sigmoidoscopy should be examined for amebae, and biopsies taken from ulcerated areas should be stained for amebic trophozoites. Serology testing is useful in the diagnosis of amebiasis (indirect hemagglutination) and Salmonella infection (H and O agglutinin titers). Salmonella seldom produces much actue colonic inflammation.

Pseudomembranous colitis (antibiotic-associated colitis) may arise in patients receiving broad-spectrum antibiotics (especially clindamycin and lincomycin), or after a course of such treatment has been completed. Symptoms of this acute colitis include watery diarrhea (90-95%), bloody diarrhea (5-10%), abdominal cramps (80-90%), fever (80%), leukocytosis, and rebound tenderness (10-20%). Sigmoidoscopy usually discloses erythema, edema, and erosions plus cream-colored pseudomembranes. Occasionally, sigmoidoscopy has been negative, but typical changes were seen on colonoscopy. Some patients develop diarrhea and rectal bleeding with segmental proximal erythema and friable mucosa seen on colonoscopic examination, most commonly after ampicillin treatment. The disorder is presently considered to be caused by the presence of *Clostridium difficile* and its cytopathic exotoxin in the colon and feces. Two clinical patterns of pseudomembranous colitis have been noted. If symptoms arise during antibiotic treatment, and if the drugs are stopped immediately, the clinical illness is milder and resolves in 4-14 days. If antibiotic treatment is continued, or if the symptoms appear after a course of antibiotics, the illness is usually more severe, with fluid and electrolyte imbalance and hypoalbuminemia. Treatment of pseudomembranous colitis consists of the prompt cessation of antibiotics and, in severe cases, the administration of Vancomycin, 0.5 to 2.0 g/day for 7-14 days. This usually produces a favorable resolution of symptoms in 48 hours, with improvement in proctoscopic findings in 5-10 days. Relapse after treatment has occurred in 10-15% of cases, but responds to retreatment. Treatment trials with bacitracin and metronidazole suggest these drugs may be beneficial also.

In recent years, *Campylobacter fetus* ssp. *jejuni* has emerged as an important pathogen capable of causing diarrhea, and indeed perhaps may be the most commonly identified bacterial agent causing diarrhea among children and adults. Clinical features often include a prodome of malaise followed by abdominal cramps, diarrhea, anorexia, fever, nausea, and vomiting. Diarrhea is often grossly bloody. Proctoscopic findings may be similar to those seen in inflammatory bowel disease or pseudomembranous colitis, and lead to misdiagnosis. The epidemiology of *C. fetus* ssp. *jejuni* has not been worked out but the organism exists widely in the animal kingdom, and has been isolated in water, raw milk, poultry, and diarrheic puppies. Clinical microbiology laboratories should include studies to identify this organism in all cases of diarrhea. Treatment with erythromycin should be instituted in all cases of proven *C. fetus* diarrhea to prevent fecal carriage and relapses.

Ischemic Colitis

Colonic ischemia occurs most commonly in patients over 50 years of age who have evidence of atherosclerotic disease. Colonic ischemia may also occur as part of the syndrome of acute mesenteric insufficiency, involving other parts of the gut, in patients with heart failure and other hypoperfusion states. It occasionally results from acute interruption of the blood supply to the colon during intra-abdominal aneurysm or bowel surgery. Occasionally, it is associated with vasculitis, amyloidosis, and the use of oral contraceptive pills. The precise relationship between the latter and segmental colon ischemia is not well understood.

This disorder usually presents with acute onset of lower abdominal pain and cramps, rectal bleeding, and perhaps fever and vomiting. Tenderness, guarding, and leukocytosis are common, and may suggest acute diverticulitis. Although life-threatening infarction, perforation, and gangrene may occasionally result, more commonly the disorder is less severe and characteristically segmental, particularly affecting the splenic flexure and the rectosigmoid area. Sometimes patients are seen after the acute episode has subsided, or they give a history of similar prior symptoms. If the acute episode is not too severe, and if the physical findings are not sufficiently suggestive of acute peritoneal irritation to justify laparotomy, the patient may be observed closely while managed with parenteral fluids and antibiotics. Sigmoidoscopy is characteristically negative because the rectum is usually spared from ischemia. A barium enema examination usually shows thumbprinting due to intramural edema and bleeding, also producing some narrowing of the involved segment. Usually the process and the radiographic changes subside completely, although occasionally residual stricturing is noted.

Radiation Colitis

Acute radiation colitis is usually encountered in patients during or after radiotherapy for a colonic or (more often) a pelvic neoplasm. When the syndrome arises during therapy, the patients are usually experiencing nausea and vomiting and may develop cramping, tenesmus, lower abdominal pain, and rectal bleeding. Sigmoidoscopy often shows a hyperemic, edematous mucosa with variable friability, and perhaps ulcers as well.

There is also a chronic form of radiation colitis that may be encountered months or years after therapy. Patients may still complain of crampy abdominal pain, tenesmus, stools with blood and mucus, and they occasionally gradually develop obstruction due to stricture. Sigmoidoscopy may show a granular, friable membrane, variably sized ulcers, and prominent telangiectases. Rectal strictures may be encountered in, or proximal to, areas of ulceration.

Neoplasms of the Colon and Rectum

Cancer

Cancer of the colon is the most common visceral malignancy in the United States, accounting for nearly 20% of all deaths due to malignancy. Among gastrointestinal malignancies, colon cancer represents 45% of deaths, twice the death rate from stomach cancer. The estimated mortality for 1979 for colorectal cancer was 98,000 patients. Five-year survival has not changed significantly in the last 20 years.

Etiology

The relationship of colon polyps to cancer is an area of controversy. There is little understanding of the pathogenetic factors in colon polyp development, and poor understanding of cancer development in colons with and without polyps. Much evidence, however, suggests that most colorectal cancers go through a transitional polypoid stage (Table 3).

Certain types of polyps are recognized as having malignant potential. The following is a classification of epithelial colonic, polyps:

1. Neoplastic
   a. Tubular adenoma
   b. Villous adenoma
   c. Tubulovillous adenoma
2. Hyperplastic (metaplastic)
3. Hamartomatous
   a. Juvenile (retention)
   b. Peutz-Jeghers
4. Inflammatory (pseudopolyps)
5. Colitis cystica profunda
6. Endometriosis
7. Heterotopia (gastric)

The only neoplastic epithelial colonic polyp with indisputable malignant potential is the adenoma. Most (75%) are tubular adenomas, 10% are villous adenomas, and the remainder are of a mixed tubulovillous pattern. Only 5% of tubular adenomas, but up to 40% of villous adenomas, show malignant change. Potential increased prevalence of colorectal cancer is thought to be associated with the presence of multiple polyps, polyps greater than 2 cm in diameter, sessile polyps, and past history of colon cancer. Twenty percent of patients with benign or malignant colonic lesions have multiple synchronous lesions, and 7-10% will develop a subsequent metachronous lesion (benign or malignant). Of patients with a resected colon cancer, 3.5% will develop a second colon cancer within 8 years. If there were benign adenomatous polyps in the resected specimen, the frequency is doubled. Certain types of polyps occurring in the heredofamilial polyposis syndromes (familial polyposis, Gardner's syndrome, and perhaps Turcot's syndrome) have a very high incidence of malignant transformation (see Table 3). Furthermore, atypia or dysplasia in a given polyp correlates with an increased risk for malignant change.

Table 3. Hereditary Polyposis Syndromes of the Gastrointestinal Tract

Syndrome	*Polyp Type*	*Location*	*Malignant Potential*	*Inheritance*	*Associated Manifestations*
Familial polyposis	Adenoma	Colon	+	Autosomal dominant (A.D.)	0
Polyposis of entire GI tract	Adenoma		+	A.D.	0
Gardner's syndrome	Adenoma	Colon	+	A.D.	Osteomas, epidermoid cysts, fibrous tumors
Peutz-Jeghers syndrome	Hamartomas	Stomach, SB, Colon	0	A.D.	Buccal & cutaneous pigmentation. Recurrent SB obstruction.
Juvenile polyposis of colon	Hamartomas (retention or juvenile polyps)	Colon	0	?	0
Generalized gastro-intestinal juvenile polyposis	Retention or juvenile polyps	Stomach, SB, Colon	0	A.D.	Increased incidence of colon CA not from polyps.
Cronkhite-Canada	Juvenile	Stomach, SB, Colon	0	?	Alopecia, nail dystrophy, hyper-pigmentation, protein-losing enteropathy.
Turcot	Adenoma	Colon	Probably	A.R.?	CNS tumors

Biopsies of polyps via the sigmoidoscope or colonoscope are of value in determining the type of colonic polyp, but are too small and superficial to exclude a diagnosis of malignancy, which requires histological examination of the submucosa (the stalk core) of the polyp to establish a diagnosis of invasive carcinoma.

Hamartomatous polyps are composed of elements of normal colonic epithelium but in disorganized array. Histologically, they show prominent cystic dilatation of glands with mucus, hence, they are also known as retention polyps. Their surfaces may ulcerate, leading to inflammation or hemorrhage. They occur mainly in the rectum in children usually less than 10 years of age, giving rise to their other name, juvenile polyps. Clinical presentation is usually by bleeding, or anal protrusion. They may twist and self-amputate. In rare instances, retention polyps are multiple and scattered throughout the colon, and may involve the small bowel as well. They have no malignant potential, although there is an increased incidence of colon cancer in families of patients with juvenile polyps. Occasionally, hamartomas of the colon are seen in the Peutz-Jeghers syndrome but do not give rise to colon cancer.

Risk Factors in Colorectal Cancer

The evidence facoring the adenoma-carcinoma sequence has been presented. Removal of benign polyps at yearly sigmoidoscopy over a 25-year period in a cancer detection clinic resulted in reduction of rectosigmoid cancer to 15% of the anticipated frequency. Other risk factors already mentioned are heredity and inflammatory bowel disease. Reference has already been made to the increased incidence of colon cancer in patients with long-standing ulcerative colitis. Studies to date suggest that severe epithelial dysplasia in rectal and colonic mucosal biopsies of such patients may be a valuable indicator of the patient at risk for cancer.

Pathology

Adenocarcinoma is the predominant type, although several histologic variations of little clinical significance have been described. A shift in the distribution of colon cancer from the rectum to the proximal colon has been occurring in the United States. Approximately half of all cancers of the rectum lie within the distal 25 cm. The cecum and right colon harbor 15% of cancers, and the remainder are scattered throughout the rest of the colon.

Symptoms

The clinical presentation of colorectal cancer depends on the site. Right colon cancers often grow to large size before symptoms develop; this is probably attributable to the liquid nature of the luminal contents of the right colon. The most common picture is that of chronic blood loss anemia with symptoms of dyspnea, lassitude, angina, weight loss, and occasionally fever, with or without right abdominal pain. Lesions encroaching upon the ileocecal valve may produce symptoms of partial small bowel obstruction. Tumors in the left colon, and especially the sigmoid, are apt to give rise to early symptoms of constipation and colon obstruction; rectal lesions may cause tenesmus. A change in bowel habits and rectal bleeding are the most common symptoms. The nature of the bleeding often correlates with the location of the tumor. Occult blood is characteristic of right colon cancer. Blood mixed with the stool is seen in other locations, whereas blood streaking or coating the surface of the stool usually characterizes a cancer of the rectum and sigmoid. Rectal tumors may produce blood separate from the stool.

Physical Examination

In early cases, examination is often unrevealing. Pallor and wasting may signify anemia and advanced disease. Digital examination reveals the neoplasm in 15-20% of cases. A mass may be palpated anywhere in the colon, but is most common in right colon lesions. With obstructing neoplasms of the left colon, there may be evidence of proximal colon distention. Sign of advanced disease includes an enlarged liver, but there are no diagnostically specific laboratory abnormalities. Detection of occult or gross blood in the stool is important. A microcytic or iron deficiency anemia, raised erythrocyte sedimentation rate, and leukocytosis are not uncommonly seen.

Diagnosis
Colorectal cancer should be considered in evaluating the complaints of any individual reporting a change of bowel habits, and in all types of rectal bleeding. Sigmoidoscopy with biopsy should lead to a positive diagnosis in approximately 50% of cases. Radiographic examination of the colon with barium, or an air-contrast study, usually discloses a filling defect that may be polypoid or annular, or may show wall infiltration with mucosal destruction. Barium enema should not be relied upon to detect all rectal neoplasms.

Carcinoembryonic antigen testing is of no value as a cancer screening tool. However, there is much current interest in the use of guaiac-impregnated paper slides to detect occult blood in asymptomatic persons. Approximately 1-2% of persons over 40 years of age will have positive tests; and, when further investigated by sigmoidoscopy, barium enema and colonoscopy, about half of these have been found to harbor a colon polyp or cancer. Furthermore, most of the malignancies thus detected tended to be localized.

Treatment
Surgery remains the currently preferable approach for rectal lesions below the peritoneal reflection. Combined abdominoperineal resection with colostomy is generally performed. Right hemicolectomy is done for lesions in the cecum and ascending colon, and segmental resections are performed for tumors in other parts of the bowel. The importance of early diagnosis is underscored by the fact that only 41% of colorectal cancers are in a localized stage without lymph node involvement when diagnosed. Five-year survival rate for patients with localized disease is 70%; for those with lymph node or distant spread, 5-year survival is 40%. If asymptomatic when detected by screening surveys, 5-year survival rates approaching 85-90% have been noted. In some patients with regional or distant metastases, surgical palliation may be indicated for symptomatic relief of bleeding or obstruction.

Lymphoma
Primary lymphomas of the colon and rectum are uncommon neoplasms, but may produce a change in bowel habits, abdominal pain, and rectal bleeding. Radiographic examination often shows multiple polypoid lesions over a segment of colon; at times these are coarse and nodular, suggestive of segmental Crohn's disease or ischemic colitis. Diagnosis is best made by sigmoidoscopic or colonoscopic biopsy. Surgical excision is preferable and should be followed by radiation therapy.

Carcinoid
Carcinoid tumors of the colon occur most commonly in the rectum, where they are noted as small, smooth, submucosal rounded yellow nodules. Nearly all patients with rectal carcinoids are asymptomatic, and the lesions may be treated by local excision or fulguration. Only if the lesion is invasive or very large should radical excision be done. The carcinoid syndrome has rarely arisen from a rectal tumor.

THE LIVER

EMBRYOLOGY

In the third or fourth week, a diverticulum that will give rise to the liver and biliary tract buds from the duodenal segment of the foregut. Soon thereafter a maze of liver cell cords extends ventrally, the proximal portions of which become the hepatic ducts. At the confluence of the hepatic ducts, a bud gives rise to the gallbladder which elongates into a saccular distal end and a narrow proximal cystic duct; that portion nearest the duodenum becomes the common bile duct. The distal liver tubules or cords develop into the parenchymal cells of the liver that encompass and break up the omphalomesenteric veins draining the gut, thus forming the vascular sinusoids within the liver. The original trunks of the omphalic vein anastomose to form the portal vein. The umbilical vein carrying placental blood develops into a large direct channel, the ductus venosus, within the liver and drains into the inferior vena cava along with the hepatic veins.

At birth, umbilical vein flow ceases and the vein withers to a fibrous cord, the ligamentum teres, which lies in the falciform ligament connecting the umbilicus to the liver. The ductus venosus becomes the ligamentum venosum, which divides the liver into its classic right and left lobes.

ANATOMY

The liver is the largest organ in the body, normally weighing 1.2 to 1.5 kg. It lies in the right upper abdominal quadrant immediately inferior to the diaphragm and behind the right lower ribs. The liver is entirely enclosed by peritoneum except for the bare area on its superior surface where it is in direct contact with the diaphragm, and in the gallbladder fossa. As classically described, the liver is externally divided into a larger right lobe and a smaller left lobe by the falciform ligament anteriorly, and the fissures for the ligamentum teres inferiorly and ligamentum venosum posteriorly. The right lobe is further marked by lesser segments, the caudate lobe posteriorly and the quadrate lobe on the visceral (inferior) surface. However, the above anatomic characterization has limited surgical relevance because it is knowledge of the arrangement of blood vessels and bile ducts entering and within the liver substance that is vital to the operative management of hepatic trauma and the removal of portions of the liver involved by tumors. Hence, a division of the liver according to blood supply and branching biliary ducts should be fixed in mind. In this scheme, the division is based on the primary branching of hepatic arterial and venous afferents close to the porta hepatis; the two lobes are nearly equal in weight. The interlobar plane extends between the gallbladder fossa and the fossa for the inferior vena cava. Each lobe receives a separate blood supply with essentially no collateral circulation between them. The right lobe is subdivided into anterior and posterior segments relating to secondary branches of the right hepatic artery, portal vien, and bile ducts. The left lobe is subdivided into medial and lateral segments with a plane of division marked by the attachment of the falciform ligament on its parietal surface and the fossa of the ligamentum venosum on the inferior surface. Thus, the left lobe of classic description is only the lateral segment of the anatomic left lobe, and the quadrate lobe is the medial segment of the left hepatic lobe. The caudate lobe has an independent circulation. The venous drainage is not so conveniently distributed.

Vascular Supply and Innervation

The liver has a dual blood supply. The hepatic artery from the celiac axis supplies only 30% of liver blood flow at rest. The remainder is provided by the portal vein that brings venous blood from the intestinal tract and spleen. Both afferents terminate in the hepatic sinusoids. The liver straddles the inferior vena cava, which receives many small direct veins from the liver substance, particularly from the caudate lobe, in addition to three major hepatic veins from the right and left lobes. Normal hepatic blood flow is 1,100-1,500 ml/minute and is decreased by exercise, sympathetic stimulation, and the upright posture; it is increased by fever, alcohol, and food intake. Oxygen supply to the liver is derived about equally from each afferent system. Pressure in the portal vein is 6 to 7 mm of mercury.

Lymphatic drainage from the liver accounts for 25-50% of total thoracic duct flow and is characterized by high protein content. Presumably, lymph is formed in the spaces of Disse (between sinusoids and parenchymal cells). Lymphatics draining the liver are subcapsular as well as deep. They pass through the diaphragm, and also travel with the hepatic vein.

Innervation of the liver and biliary tract is from the vagal nerves, the right phrenic nerve, and the celiac plexus. Nerves travel with the blood vessels into the portal spaces. The parenchymal cells are probably not directly innervated. Sensory fibers from the gallbladder and extrahepatic bile ducts enter the cord at the sixth through ninth thoracic segments. Sensory fibers from the liver capsule are derived from the sixth through the ninth thoracic segments, and the third to fifth cervical segments.

Microanatomy

Parenchymal cells (hepatocytes) constitute most of the liver mass. They are arranged in a continuum of single cell plates or sheets separated by a labyrinth of sinusoids that anastomose freely, but have a directional flow orientation from hepatic artery and portal vein to the central (or terminal hepatic) vein. Each hepatocyte is bathed by sinusoidal blood on two surfaces. The terminal afferent portal veins and hepatic arteries lie in the mass of liver cells in tunnels called portal tracts, each surrounded by a limiting plate of hepatic cells. Terminal hepatic (central) veins and portal tracts interdigitate at right angles to each other, and communicate with each other via the interposed sinusoids. The latter are lined by a fenestrated network of endothelial cells and phagocytic Kupffer cells that are permeable to all except large molecules (greater than 250,000) and formed blood elements. The space of Disse between the endothelial lining of the sinusoids and the hepatocyte surfaces contains hepatic interstitial fluid that drains via the lymphatics.

Two conceptualized structural subunits should be mentioned and understood in terms of the liver's microvasculature. The classic lobule is based on the regular four-, five-, or six-sided geometric interrelationships between several portal tracts and a central vein, radiating toward which are the sinusoids. The hepatic acinus of Rappaport is perhaps functionally the more credible schema, since it is centered upon the terminal portal vein, the hepatic artery, and the parenchyma surrounding them. Blood flows from the portal vein and hepatic artery toward either of two terminal hepatic (central) veins located at the apices of the acinus. The acinar concept is validated by experimental and clinical evidence that hepatocytes located peripherally (near the terminal hepatic vein) are more vulnerable to ischemia than those with a more favorable microenvironment near the point of inflow of blood. Furthermore, differences in hepatocyte structure and enzyme content are noted in different zones of the acinus (see below). The parenchymal cell surfaces facing the sinusoids are lined by microvilli that lie in the space of Disse adjacent to sinusoidal endothelium. Interposed between nonsinusoidal surfaces of adjoining liver cells are bile canaliculi, the terminal radicles of the biliary system. Canaliculi are bound by the microvilli-studded parenchymal cell membranes and sealed by tight junctions. Bile canalicular flow is toward the portal tracts, where it drains into interlobular bile ducts.

Study of ultrastructural anatomy of the liver cell has given us insights into its functions. Mention has already been made of the differing morphologic and biochemical characteristics of hepatocytes located in different areas of the acinus. Cells in zone 1 (adjacent to the rich afferent blood supply) have abundant mitochondria, the major source of cellular energy and rich in enzymes of the citric acid cycle and those involved with fatty acid oxidation. Oxidative phosphorylation, ADP formation, and heme synthesis also take place in mitochondria. Cells in zone 3 adjacent to venous outflow are more remote from nutrient and oxygen input. They contain more rough endoplasmic reticulum, the site of protein, triglyceride, and lipoprotein formation, as well as smooth endoplasmic reticulum that contains the enzymes employed in bilirubin and drug conjugation and detoxification, and steroid synthesis (including cholesterol and bile acids). Lysosomes located adjacent to bile canaliculi contain hydrolytic enzymes, and act as an intercellular digestive system for disposing of worn-out organelles and other intracellular substances via biliary secretion. The Golgi apparatus, also lying near bile canaliculi, is regarded as a packaging apparatus for preparing materials for biliary secretion. Actinlike microtubules and microfilaments provide a supporting cytoskeleton and may play a role in secretion as well.

PHYSIOLOGIC FUNCTIONS OF THE LIVER

Bilirubin Metabolism

Bilirubin is a waste product with no known physiologic function. Approximately 250 mg are formed daily by the catabolism of hemoglobin from senescent erythrocytes in the reticuloendothelial system (spleen, bone marrow, and liver). In this process, the iron and globin are reutilized by the body, and the macrophages' heme oxygenase splits the tetrapyrrole ring to form biliverdin and carbon monoxide. Biliverdin reductase transforms biliverdin to bilirubin, which then is transported to the liver bound to serum albumin. At the sinusoidal surface of the hepatocyte, the albumin is detached and bilirubin is transported inside the cell by a carrier-mediated mechanism. It is bound within the cell mainly to a cytosol product protein known as Y protein or ligandin that also has affinity for other organic anions. Within the hepatocyte, bilirubin undergoes conjugation with glucuronic acid and other sugar derivatives, forming mono- and diglucuronides, a process catalyzed by bilirubin glucuronyl transferase. Conjugated bilirubin is transported across the canalicular membrane into the bile against a concentration gradient, presumably an active process that is shared with other organic ions. This is the rate-limiting step in moving bilirubin from plasma into bile. Conjugated bilirubin in bile and in the proximal gastrointestinal tract undergoes little or no reabsorption. Colonic bacteria, however, deconjugate and transform bilirubin to a family of reduced nonpigmented urobilins, most of which are excreted in the stool although there is some enterohepatic recirculation and a modest urinary excretion of urobilinogen. Fifteen percent of bilirubin is derived from heme proteins such as cytochromes, and heme from red cell precursors due to inefficient erythropoiesis.

Protein Synthesis

The liver is the source of synthesis of all plasma proteins except gamma globulin. These proteins are formed in the rough endoplasmic reticulum of the hepatocyte for export. They function as transport proteins (carriers of drugs, bilirubin, copper, iron, lipids, etc.), provide osmotic equilibrium, and clotting factors. The liver also synthesizes intracellular proteins necessary for normal hepatocellular functions such as detoxification and excretion. These proteins incude enzymes, ligandins, and storage proteins. Furthermore, the liver is capable of utilizing endogenous and exogenous amino acids for carbohydrate and fat metabolism. It also excretes nitrogenous waste by the conversion of ammonia to urea, and purines into uric acid.

Albumin is the major serum protein synthesized by the liver. The average daily synthesis rate is 12-14 g/day, but the normal liver is capable of increasing its rate threefold. The amino acids necessary for albumin formation are derived from dietary sources under normal circumstances, although in starvation the liver uses its own hepatic protein. Insulin is necessary for maximum synthesis. Osmotic pressure in hepatic interstitial fluid is a sensitive regulatory mechanism of albumin synthesis. Sites and mechanisms for albumin degradation are poorly understood. Ten to 15 percent occurs in the liver, and only 10 percent in the gastrointestinal tract. Insignificant degradation occurs in the normal kidney. The rate of degradation equals the synthesis rate.

Albumin is distributed to two pools in dynamic equilibrium, with a total exchangeable pool (TEP) of 250 g. The intravascular pool constitutes 35-40% of the TEP, and the extravascular pool 60-65%. Skin is the major component of the extravascular pool. The most prominent abnormality of hepatic protein metabolism in acute viral hepatitis is hypoprothrombinemia, owing to the short half-life of prothrombin. Albumin synthesis and content are little affected in the acute situation. In chronic liver disease such as cirrhosis, albumin synthesis is impaired and hypoalbuminemia is common along with increased serum gamma globulin, the latter perhaps as some sort of osmotic compensation. Ammonia transformation to urea is also impaired in severe liver disease.

Carbohydrate Metabolism and the Liver

The liver has a central role in maintaining a stable serum glucose concentration, at the same time providing a continuous fuel supply for itself and other vital organs, especially central nervous system, red cell mass, skeletal muscle, kidneys, and skin. Its role in carbohydrate metabolism is mediated by hormonal and neural factors. Liver uptake of dietary monosaccharides from the portal blood is regulated by the serum glucose concentration. Any excess is converted via phosphorylation and polymerization to glycogen, and some is also converted to triglycerides. The liver is also able on demand to supply glucose from glycogen by glycogenolysis, and to convert noncarbohydrates to glucose via gluconeogenesis, a more chronic adaptation to free glucose deprivation. Synthetic processes by the liver involving carbohydrate incude glucuronate formation for conjugation of organic anions, the hexose monophosphate shunt by which pentoses are formed for nucleic acid synthesis, and reduced NADPH for fatty acid synthesis. Nonglycogen sources of glucose acted upon by the liver are amino acids, lactate from erythrocytes and skeletal muscle, glycerol from adipose tissue lipolysis of triglycerides, and from diet. Glucose metabolism by the liver is under hormonal regulation by insulin, glucagon, epinephrine, adrenal glucocorticosteroids, and growth hormone.

Liver disease manifests many abnormalities of carbohydrate metabolism. Hypoglycemia may occur in severe viral hepatitis or acute ethanol intoxication. Hyperglycemia is common in cirrhosis, owing to insulin resistance and raised plasma glucagon. Hypoglycemia associated with increased hepatic glycogen accumulation is seen in genetic deficiencies of enzymes necessary for glycogenolysis.

Fat Metabolism by the Liver

Normal hepatic lipid content is approximately 5% of total liver weight, and consists of triglycerides, phospholipids, fatty acids, cholesterol, and cholesterol esters. Hepatic lipid arises from dietary fat, adipose tissue, and by synthesis within the liver from acetate and NADPH. Most fatty acids entering the liver are converted to triglycerides, cholesterol, and phospholipids. The triglycerides are exported as lipoproteins. Cholesterol is secreted in bile as cholesterol or as newly synthesized bile acids, or exported from the liver to the blood as part of lipoproteins. Phospholipid is excreted in bile or used by the liver as structural lipid. However, considerable amounts of fatty acid in the liver are oxidized in that organ to carbon dioxide as a major energy source for the liver, or partially metabolized to ketones, which are then released as an energy source for skeletal and cardiac muscle.

LIVER FUNCTION TESTS

It has been said that the many functions of the liver are exceeded only by the number of biochemical methods designed to test them (Sherlock). However, in recent years with the introduction and proven value of a growing number of other diagnostic procedures, a reduced number of more rational and specific blood tests has evolved. Standard liver function tests currently include serum bilirubin, alkaline phosphatase, aspartate aminotransferase (AST), alanine aminotransferase (ALT), gamma-glutamyl transpeptidase, prothrombin time, serum albumin and globulin concentrations, and several immunologic tests, including smooth muscle antibody, antimitochondrial antibody, and viral hepatitis markers.

Serum Bilirubin

Bilirubin metabolism has already been discussed. Serum bilirubin measurement is by Ehrlich's diazo reaction or van den Bergh's test, whereby conjugated (direct) and total bilirubin concentrations are calculated. The unconjugated (indirect) fraction is calculated by subtracting the conjugated bilirubin value from the total bilirubin concentration figure. Normally up to 1.5 mg total bilirubin/100 ml (essentially all unconjugated) is present. Raised total serum bilirubin concentrations may indicate either excess formation of bilirubin as in hemolysis, or hepatobiliary disease in which bilirubin uptake, conjugation, or biliary excretion are impaired. Elevated values for unconjugated bilirubin may indicate overproduction as in hemolysis, impaired hepatic uptake, or defective conjugation in the hepatocyte. Isolated unconjugated hyperbilirubinemia probably indicates Gilbert's disease, the most common form of hyperbilirubinemia. Raised conjugated bilirubin concentrations are indicative of hepatic or biliary tract disease, but are not otherwise specific as to type or site of lesion (Tables 4, 5).

Normally there is no bilirubin in urine, as only conjugated bilirubin appears in urine; hence bilirubinuria indicates liver or biliary tract disease, not excess production. Urine urobilinogen in excess indicates hepatocellular dysfunction and may be an early and sensitive test. It is detected employing a dipstick. Urine and fecal urobilinogens are rarely performed now.

Serum Alkaline Phosphatase

The alkaline phosphatase normally present in serum represents fractions from bone, liver, and intestine. These may be identified by measuring isoenzyme fractions. Liver alkaline phosphatase synthesis and serum concentrations are most prominently and consistently raised in biliary obstruction as well as in infiltrative diseases of the liver, where serum values greater than three times normal are commonly found, and are the hallmark of cholestatic jaundice, whethere extrahepatic or intrahepatic. In place of isoenzyme fractionation, measurement of serum 5′-nucleotidase or gamma-glutamyl transpeptidase may be helpful in identifying the source of a raised serum alkaline phosphatase. These enzymes are more specifically hepatic in origin, and if their levels are also raised, a high serum alkaline phosphatase likely signifies hepatobiliary disease.

Serum Aminotransferases (Transaminases)

Acute hepatic parenchymal damage is characterized by a

Table 4. Disorders with Unconjugated Hyperbilirubinemia

Disorder	*Mechanism*	*Comment*
Hemolysis: drug-induced spherocytosis	Increased production	May have minor (<20%) conjugated bilirubin
Abnormal or ineffective erythropoiesis	Increased production of early-labelled bilirubin	Shunt hyperbilirubinemia. Pernicious anemia. Congenital erythroporphyria. Thalassemia
Gilbert's syndrome (constitutional hepatic dysfunction)	Decreased hepatic uptake; probably also decreased bilirubin conjugation. May also 50% have associated hemolysis	Bilirubin increases >50% with fasting stress. Other liver tests normal. Bilirubin ↓ by phenobarb
Crigler-Najjar syndrome	Decreased conjugation due to low (II) or absent (I) bilirubin glucuronyl transferase	Type I—no glucuronyl transferase. Serum bilirubin 15-50 mg.% Phenobarb. no help. Autosomal recessive. Bile colorless. Kernicterus usual Type II—decreased glucuronyl transferase. Serum bilirubin 5-25 mg.% Phenobarb. helps. ? Autosomal dominant. Bile yellow
Lucy-Driscoll syndrome	? Decreased conjugation	Neonatal jaundice. Probably related to a steroid from maternal blood
Breast milk jaundice	Inhibition of UDP-transferase	Breast milk contains an inhibitory steroid

Table 5. Disorders with Conjugated Hyperbilirubinemia

Disorder	*Mechanism*	*Comment*
Dubin-Johnson Syndrome	Decreased biliary excretion of organic anions	Yellow-brown pigment in hepatocytes. Normal liver tests. Oral cholecystogram nonvisualized. Retained conjugated BSP. Pregnancy, oral contraceptives may accentuate jaundice.
Rotor syndrome	Decreased uptake (?) and excretion of organic anions	Probable variant of D-J. No pigment in liver cells. Oral cholecystogram usually visualized
Benign recurrent cholestasis	Unknown	Recurrent cholestasis, usually since childhood; occasionally familial; normal liver biochemically and clinically between episodes; cholestasis only morphol. abnormality; Phenobarb. may help

striking rise in serum transaminase levels. Aspartate transaminase is most commonly used, and there is no clearcut advantage in measuring alanine transaminase (ALT) or both enzymes routinely. Some clinicians regard a high AST/ALT ratio as a useful indicator of alcoholic liver injury. Very high transaminase levels are found in viral and drug hepatitis but may also be seen in severe right heart failure with low cardiac output and liver hypoperfusion. Alcoholic hepatitis and cholestasis are associated with modestly raised transaminase values. Cirrhosis and metastatic involvement of the liver usually produce trivial or modest elevations.

Serum Proteins

Since the half-life of albumin is 20-25 days, acute liver disease, unless severe and protracted, does not produce hypoalbuminemia. A low serum albumin is suggestive of chronic liver disease such as cirrhosis, although in many such patients the value is normal. Maldistribution of albumin within the extravascular pool, as in edema or ascites, may explain a low serum albumin more accurately than reduced synthesis.

In view of the short half-life and rapid turnover of many coagulation factors synthesized by the liver, clotting studies may be abnormal in both acute and chronic liver disease. Furthermore, since many of these factors (II, VII, IX, X) are vitamin K dependent, impaired blood coagulation in patients with chronic cholestatic jaundice may be due to vitamin K malabsorption rather than liver disease. The prompt correction of an abnormal prothrombin time by parenteral vitamin K is compatible with obstructive jaundice rather than parenchymal cell disease.

Immunologic Serum Tests and Other Proteins

Smooth muscle antibody is positive in a small percentage of patients with chronic active hepatitis. Antimitochondrial antibody is present in significant titers in the great majority (90-95%) of patients with the syndrome of primary biliary cirrhosis. Viral hepatitis and serologic markers will be discussed under that entity. Other serum proteins of clinical laboratory significance include the serum α-1 antitrypsin level, which is very low in homozygous deficiency states often associated with a form of cirrhosis; serum ceruloplasmin, which is low in homozygous deficiency associated with the clinical picture of Wilson's disease; and serum ferritin, which may be useful in the diagnosis of iron overload states such as hemochromatosis.

Non-Invasive Imaging

Radionuclide Scintiscanning

Currently, the most frequently used isotopically labeled compound is 99^{m} technetium sulfur colloid that produces an image of the uptake by the Kupffer cells of the liver. A good depiction of liver size and configuration is provided by the anterior, posterior, and lateral views, and filling defects as small as 2 cm in diameter may be detected. Caution must be employed in interpreting abnormalities noted in the margins of the liver. Primary liver cancer, metastases, cysts, hemangiomas, and abscesses appear as filling defects. Cirrhosis, severe steatosis, and hepatitis often show a generally reduced uptake but may also show inhomogeneous or variable irregularities of isotope uptake that may resemble multiple metastases. In chronic hepatic disease, however, there is often increased uptake by the spleen and bone marrow not seen with hepatic metastases. Gallium scintiscanning is useful in detecting liver abscesses and hepatocellular cancer, as this isotope accumulates in tissues and cells that actively synthesize protein.

Ultrasound

High-frequency sound beam reflections from tissue planes and junctions between areas of differing density have been converted into electrical charges and recorded on a television monitor or on film. Employed in the study of the liver and biliary system, ultrasound is capable of recording solid and cystic liver lesions as small as 1-2 cm, as well as bile ducts, gallbladder, portal and hepatic veins, hepatic artery, and the vena cava. The relative low cost, noninvasive nature, and lack of radiation make it a useful technique. Its use in biliary tract disease will be detailed later, but assessment of the size of intrahepatic and extrahepatic ducts is currently an essential part of the investigation of cholestatic jaundice.

Computerized Tomography (CT)

CT of the liver provides a series of cross-sectional images of the liver and other intra-abdominal organs and structures. Size, shape, density, and mass of liver are usually accurately noted. It is highly accurate in detecting and characterizing solid and cystic lesions, abscesses, and hemangiomas in the liver, more so than radionuclide scanning. It can also suggest hepatic steatosis and hemochromatosis by lesser and greater liver densities. The accuracy of CT in detection of dilated bile ducts is at best comparable to ultrasound, but is additionally valuable in defining structures and lesions outside the liver, including pancreatic tumors causing biliary obstruction. It is less accurate than ultrasound in detecting gallstones.

Invasive Tests

Needle Biopsy of the Liver

The reader should refer to other sources for details of the technique of liver biopsy, and of the care of patients undergoing biopsy. A list of more common diseases and conditions in which needle biopsy may be indicated includes metastatic tumors, cirrhosis and chronic hepatitis, alcoholic liver disease, jaundice (acute and chronic), and infiltrative diseases. Most diffuse inflammatory disorders (such as acute hepatitis), steatosis, and infiltrative processes (such as amyloid and myeloproliferative disorders) are also detected by biopsy. Needle biopsy is usually a hospital procedure but favorable outpatient experience has been reported with good risk patients, close post-biopsy observation, and the availability of an adjacent hospital with medical and surgical support. The coagulation status must be determined, with prothrombin time and platelet count measurements in normal or near normal range before biopsy is performed. Patients must be alert and cooperative. Ascites and deep jaundice are considered contraindications to needle biopsy. Intercostal biopsy is preferable to the subcostal approach, though with enlarged livers and a specific palpable lesion below the costal margin, the latter approach may be employed. Mild postbiopsy pain at the site of needle entry or in the right shoulder is not uncommon but soon disappears spontaneously. Hemorrhage, bile leak, and hypotension are infrequent complications, and when encountered are noted usually within 3 hours of the biopsy. Multiple passes of the biopsy needle increase the incidence of complications.

Peritoneoscopy

This procedure, often combined with directed biopsy, is occasionally valuable in diagnosis of suspected liver disease in patients with hepatomegaly, abnormal liver function tests, and ascites when other and simpler tests have not yielded explanation. Suspected cirrhosis, primary and secondary tumors, and the assessment of unexplained ascites are additional indications. Contraindications are more or less the same as for liver biopsy.

Endoscopic Retrograde Cholangiopancreatography (ERCP)

This procedure will be discussed in the section on biliary tract disease, along with percutaneous transhepatic cholangiography.

DISEASES OF THE LIVER

Disorders of Bilirubin Metabolism

Jaundice

It is logical to consider jaundice as due to one of three mechanisms: prehepatic–disturbances of bilirubin metabolism before bilirubin enters the liver; hepatic–referring to diseases of the liver; post-hepatic–where the flow of bile is impeded, within the liver or in the extrahepatic bile channels. In the pathogenetic spectrum of liver diseases associated with jaundice, there may be two or three mechanisms operating simultaneously, making any classification artificial though still useful for conceptual thinking and diagnostic work-up.

In considering jaundice from the standpoint of the pathway of bilirubin metabolism, a classification may be offered as follows:

1. Conditions associated with unconjugated hyperbilirubinemia (Table 4):
   - (a) Overproduction of bilirubin–absolute, or relative to the liver's ability to handle the load. Examples include hemolysis, ineffective erythropoiesis, and shunt hyperbilirubinemia.
   - (b) Impaired bilirubin uptake by the hepatic cell–drug-induced, Gilbert's disease, post-hepatitic hyperbilirubinemia, etc.
   - (c) Impaired conjugation by the liver cell–as due to deficiency of glucuronyl transferase. Examples include physiologic jaundice of the newborn, Lucey-Driscoll syndrome, breast milk jaundice, and congenital non-hemolytic jaundice (Crigler-Najjar syndrome, types I and II).
2. Conditions in which there are both unconjugated bilirubin and conjugated bilirubin in the serum (Table 5):
   - (a) Disturbances in excretion of bilirubin and/or bile salts. The location of the defect can be anywhere from the conjugating site within the liver cell to the duodenum, and is covered by the term cholestasis. The defect may be biochemical or mechanical.

Viral Hepatitis

Although jaundice occurring in epidemics has been noted for over 2,000 years, the past 15 years have seen immense strides in our knowledge of the epidemiology, immunology, and clinical aspects of viral hepatitis. Two distinct hepatitis viruses have been identified and isolated, hepatitis A virus (HAV) and hepatitis B virus (HBV). Serologic evidence is firm that other viruses produce the same clinical illness, and these are referred to as non-A, non-B (NANB), pending the identification of specific organisms or their serologic markers (acute hepatitis may also be produced by the Epstein-Barr virus, herpes simplex virus, and the cytomegalovirus).

Hepatitis A

Type A hepatitis previously known as infectious hepatitis (IH) is caused by an RNA enterovirus 27 nm in diamter transmitted by the fecal-oral route. The virus appears in the feces of patients 2 weeks prior to jaundice and clinical illness, and for about 1 week thereafter. The incubation period is 14-50 days. In the blood, the HAV appears only for a matter of a few days days early in the infection. Therefore, parenteral transmission rarely occurs. The greatest incidence occurs in the first two decades of life, but serum antibodies to HAV are found in variably higher (30-95%) percentages of adult populations around the world. The incidence is falling with improved hygiene and sanitation. Sporadic cases result from person-to-person transmission but epidemics are usually from a point source, as from water or food contamination. No chronic viremia, chronic hepatitis, or carrier state has been identified. The first antibody to HAV, of the IgM class, appears in infected humans by the time clinical symptoms and abnormal liver tests appear, at about the same time that fecal shedding stops. The IgM antibody rises abruptly, peaks in 1-2 weeks, and then gradually declines. IgG anti-HA rises more gradually, peaks in 1-2 months, and persists for years as serologic evidence of past infection and immunity. Thus, our ability to measure IgM-specific anti-HA can identify recent acute infection of probably not more than 8 weeks' duration, whereas IgG anti-HA alone signifies infection at some earlier time (Fig. 5).

Type A hepatitis is usually benign; histologic damage tends to be mild, and does not result in a carrier state, chronic active liver disease, cirrhosis, or death. Since the period of viremia is so brief, type A hepatitis rarely results from blood transfusion. Precautions regarding stool and blood are unnecessary after the first week or two of illness.

Hepatitis B

The hepatitis B virus (HBV) is a DNA virus composed of an inner core of 25-29 nm in diameter (containing core antigen

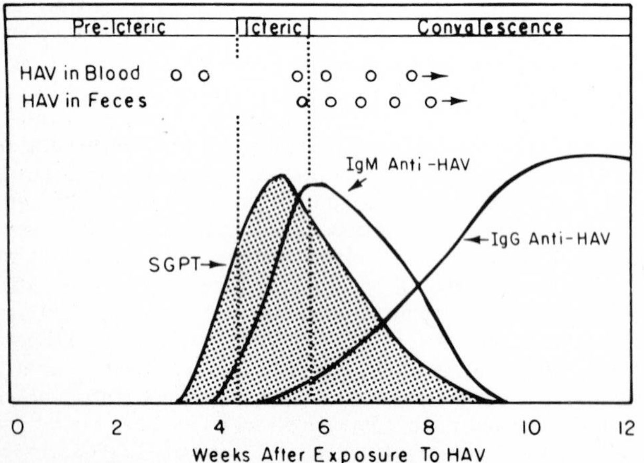

Figure 5. Diagram of the serologic and immunologic markers of hepatitis A infection. Their relationships to serum transaminase elevation, viremia, and fecal excretion of hepatitis A virus are also shown. (From *Viral Hepatitis*, by R. Koff. Copyright 1979. Used by permission.)

(HB_cAg), DNA, and DNA polymerase), and an outer envelope of lipoprotein containing the surface antigen, HB_sAg. The complete virus, the Dane particle, is 42 nm in diameter. Within the infected liver cell, the core particle is found only in the nucleus. The DNA polymerase of the core is so closely associated with HB_cAg that it may be used as a biochemical marker for the core of the virus or for HBV itself. HB_cAg is distinct from HB_sAg and connotes active viral infection and replication. It is usually present in conjunction with HB_sAg. HB_cAg essentially never appears in serum as a free particle, and the liver is the sole site of replication. It is consistently present in chronically infected patients, and elicits a specific antibody, HB_cAb, in the course of type B hepatitis.

The 17-25 nm outer envelope of the intact Dane particle is comprised largely of the lipoprotein HB_sAg. This antigenically and structurally specific material is not the etiologic agent of HBV, is not infectious per se, but rather is a viral product resulting from infection. It is synthesized in the cytoplasm of the infected hepatocyte in greater amounts than required for assembly of the complete virus. These surplus particles of HB_sAg appear in the serum in several forms: tubules, round particles, and tadpole-shaped pieces. HB_sAg shares antigens with the envelope of the intact Dane particle, and therefore persons with HB_sAg immunity are protected against HBV infection. Another antigenic component of the HBV, HB_eAg, is less well understood but seems associated with the complete HBV and specifically with the core of the HBV. It is serologically unrelated to HB_sAg and HB_cAg. Virtually all type B hepatitis patients become transiently positive for this antigen, but only for a few days. Failure of HB_eAg to disappear as the acute hepatitis is resolving carries a guarded prognosis and connotes the likelihood of a chronic carrier state, chronic hepatitis, and also implies infectivity. The appearance of anti-HB_e suggests that the patient is no longer highly infectious (Fig. 6).

HBV itself or its HB_sAg marker has been demonstrated in numerous body fluids, secretions, and excretions—feces, sweat, semen, vaginal secretions, bile, pancreatic juice, and blood. It is prudent to treat all biologic fluids as potentially infectious, though trasmissibility varies considerably. Blood probably contains the highest concentrations of virus, next to the liver. Fecal excretion and fecal-oral transmission of HBV are not well documented, and it is assumed that fecal antigens are somewhat inactivated or destroyed.

Viremia exists for 1-4 weeks after exposure, well before the onset of symptoms, and for variable periods thereafter. Human transmission studies have shown that the appearance of HB_sAg is the first sign of HBV infection; the incubation period and the appearance time of the HB_sAg depend on the route of infection and the size of the inoculum—2 weeks after administration of infected blood, 2 months after intramuscular transmission, and 3 months after oral transmission. HB_s antigenemia persists during the acute clinical illness, and disappears 1-13 weeks after onset of laboratory abnormalities. Persistence beyond this time occurs in only 4-5% (that is, a carrier state), may be indefinite, and is commonly associated with clinical and biochemical signs of chronic hepatitis. Anti-

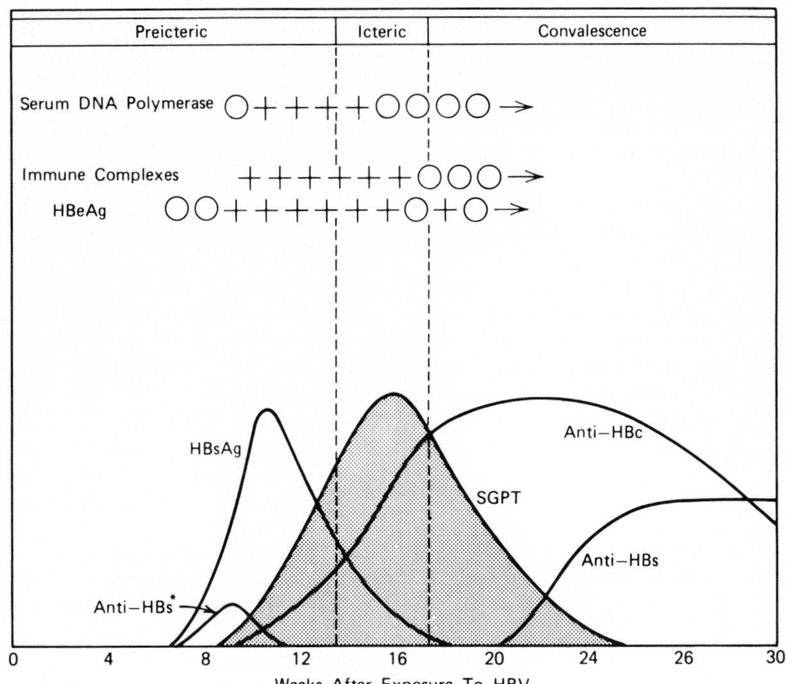

Figure 6. Diagram of seroimmunologic markers of hepatitis B infection in relationship to serum transaminase elevation and time of exposure. (From *Viral Hepatitis*, by R. Koff. Copyright 1979. Used by permission.)

HB_c appears while HB_sAg is still detectable, even before or at the time of onset of clinical symptoms, persists for many months, and occasionally for years. Numerous studies have shown that after circulating HB_sAg disappears and before anti-HB_s appears, anti-HB_c may be the only serologic marker of recently acquired infection. Anti-HB_c believed to be a marker of HB viral replication, or an indicator of the presence of HBV in infected hepatocytes. In chronic carriers and in many patients with chronic hepatitis associated with persistent HB_s antigenemia, anti-HB_c is characteristically found in serum; in fact, a small number of such chronic hepatitis patients lacking HB_sAg have anti-HB_c. Individuals who develop chronic hepatitis or who become carriers of HB_sAg rarely show anti-HB_s.

Type B hepatitis is propagated from person to person by a variety of mechanisms, including close contact, percutaneous or parenteral introduction of human tissue derivatives, and by contaminated instruments. The virus occurs throughout the world as both actue and chronic infections, and in some areas and populations there is a high prevalence of carriers. In the United States, surface antigenemia has a prevalence of 0.25%. Antibody to HB virus is found in 11% of the general U.S. population. About 10% of acute type B hepatitis infections become chronic, lasting from several years to the remainder of some individuals' lives.

Type B hepatitis has an incubation period ranging from 2 to 6 months, the majority being 60-110 days. In 10-20% of patients a prodromal syndrome occurs, involving an erythematous maculopapular rash, urticaria, or angioedema, complicated by polyarthralgias or arthritis. This transient serum sicknesslike syndrome is thought to be somehow related to immune complex formation, including HB_sAg, anti-HB_s, and often complement components, occurring at a time of HB_s antigen excess. Extrahepatic deposition of these complexes may occur in vessels of the skin and joints, as well as in glomerular basement membranes. In more chronic HBV infections, other manifestations related to immune complex formation have been described, including forms of necrotizing vasculitis, polyarteritis nodosa, and a syndrome of mixed cryoglobulinemia comprising vasculitis, purpura, arthralgias, Raynaud's phenomenon, and progressive renal disease with some liver involvement.

Non-A, Non-B (NANB) Hepatitis

Evidence for NANB hepatitis derives from studies of human hepatitis in which both types A and B hepatitis have been shown not to be present. One line of evidence results from the occurrence of multiple episodes of acute hepatitis in parenteral drug users, since reinfections with HAV and HBV probably do not occur. Secondly, despite increasingly effective screening of donor blood for HBV during the 1970's, the incidence of post-transfusion hepatitis has not been markedly reduced. Furthermore, most post-transfusion hepatitis appears to have a unimodal incubation period peak of 45-49 days, which is between A and B. Hence, in the absence of an identifiable agent and without serologic markers, NANB hepatitis is a diagnosis of exclusion, defined by the absence of HAV, HBV, Epstein Barr virus, cytomegalovirus and herpes simplex virus. There is ample evidence of a chronic carrier state for NANB lasting at least several years. NANB hepatitis is responsible for more than 90% of post-transfusion hepatitis in the United States. It is worldwide in distribution, and is probably responsible for 25-30% of cases of sporadic hepatitis in adults. The epidemiologic and clinical patterns of NANB hepatitis resemble type B hepatitis, including transfusion- and needle-associated disease, and other examples of parenteral transmission, the lack of fecal-oral transmission, ample evidence of a chronic carrier state, and the propensity to progress to chronic liver disease. It appears that a large proportion of patients with acute fulminant hepatitis lack serologic markers for HAV and HBV.

Clinical Aspects

Probably 50% of patients with all forms of acute viral hepatitis remain asymptomatic. Of symptomatic patients, only one-third become jaundiced. One to 3 percent of patients develop fulminant hepatitis. There are no major clinical distinctions between types of acute viral hepatitis as to symptoms, laboratory and other tests, pathology, major aspects of diagnosis, and treatment.

Pathology

In the liver, the essential morphologic lesions are the same whether due to HAV, HBV, or NANB. They consist of combinations of portal mononuclear cell inflammation, some edema, periportal hepatitis that may merge with the portal inflammatory exudate across and, at times, destroying the limiting plate, and lobular hepatitis consisting of randomly distributed spotty cell injury and necrosis with Kupffer's cells at sites of cell damage and loss. Cholestasis is variably present.

Two morphologic lesions of special significance are seen in some cases of acute hepatitis, so-called bridging necrosis, and multilobular submassive necrosis. In the former, parenchymal cell necrosis affects substantial groups of hepatocytes so that collapse and condensation of the reticulum fibers form a septum bridging portal tracts or central veins. When such confluent necrosis and bridging involves adjacent lobules or larger areas, multilobular submassive necrosis is said to be present. Although such cases may not be distinguished from typical viral hepatitis on the basis of any laboratory or clinical feature and are dependent on biopsy for detection, these lesions probably occur in 10-30% of acute hepatitis cases, may be more common in B hepatitis, and in 15-30% of cases progress to chronic hepatitis or cirrhosis.

Chronic Hepatitis

Chronic hepatitis connotes ongoing liver inflammation initiated by viral, drug, or unknown factors, perpetuated beyond the expected period of resolution, and capable of progression to cirrhosis or liver failure. Opinions differ as to the time period part of the definition. Some investigators maintain that continuation of the disease process for 10 weeks without clinical or laboratory improvement excludes most self-limited hepatitis and implies chronicity. Others have defined a 3- or 6-month minimum period, feeling that resolution in some cases of protracted acute hepatitis is possible during that period.

Chronic hepatitis has been divided into various forms. Chronic persistent hepatitis (CPH) is characterized by mononuclear cell inflammation and some fibrosis of the portal zones, absence of piecemeal necrosis of liver cells, and confinement of the inflammation to the portal tract, the limiting plate of liver cells between portal zones and lobule remaining intact. Chronic active hepatitis (CAH) shows the above portal changes, but also periportal and limiting plate piecemeal necrosis. In a small percentage of cases, so-called unresolved acute hepatitis is noted, with histologic features resembling acute viral hepatitis consisting mainly of intralobular inflammation and necrosis, but without piecemeal necrosis or bridging necrosis. Cirrhosis on biopsy denotes chronicity and aggressiveness of the inflammatory process. Bridging or multilobular necrosis on liver biopsy indicates more severe disease and greater likelihood of a fatal outcome or cirrhosis. Bridging necrosis probably leads to cirrhosis in 30-40% of cases.

The etiology of CAH is multifactorial and includes some drugs (see below), but a viral etiology is well documented and probably accounts for the majority of cases. Only 25% or less of patients in various series with CAH have HB_s antigen. Thus, the majority of patients have no identifiable etiology, and may represent NANB infection. Only 40% of chronic hepatitis patients give a history of acute onset of symptoms resembling hepatitis. As stated earlier, type A hepatitis has never been associated with chronic liver disease or a carrier state. CAH may be divided into mild or severe forms on the basis of histologic and laboratory abnormalities, with differences in prognosis. Severe CAH as defined by Mayo Clinic investigators incorporated patients who had at least tenfold elevations in serum transaminase levels, or at least a fivefold rise in conjunction with at least a twice-normal serum gamma globulin over a period longer than 10 weeks. A high rate of death was noted in such patients within 3 years, only 6% surviving 10 years. Patients may be entirely asymptomatic and remain well indefinitely, the diagnosis being made incidentally as a result of laboratory tests. Many patients insidiously develop fatigue, lassitude, vague abdominal discomfort, or extrahepatic features such as arthralgias, arthritis, low-grade fever, amenorrhea, and so forth. Laboratory tests may be entirely normal, or show variable rises in bilirubin, transaminases, gamma globulin, and alkaline phosphatase. There is much ongoing interest and investigation of immunologic mechanisms that many feel are responsible for the perpetuation of the liver cell injury in CAH.

The prognosis of CAH in patients with less severe biochemical and clinical disease is not known, but no doubt the disease may progress to cirrhosis and liver failure in some patients. It is not known how often bridging and multilobular necrosis occur in the presence of mild to moderate clinical and biochemical disease. No clinically controlled trial of steroids or other treatment has been conducted in mild to moderate CAH.

As mentioned earlier, virtually the entire clinical and histologic picture can be caused by reactions to such drugs as α-methyldopa, isoniazid, oxyphenisatin, and nitrofurantoin, and may progress to cirrhosis.

Treatment

The agents used most frequently in the treatment of severe CAH as defined above have been corticosteroids, with or without azathioprine. Several prospective controlled trials have shown that treatment with the above agents has ameliorated symptoms, improved biochemical parameters, and induced histologic remission with enhancement of life expectancy. Such treatment does not prevent progression to cirrhosis and carries a significant incidence of drug-related side effects, depending upon dose and duration of treatment. Trials combining lower dose prednisone with azathioprine have shown the same efficacy as prednisone alone, but with a gratifying reduction in the incidence of side effects. The decision to start treatment is difficult in patients with only mild or modest symptoms and laboratory abnormalities, and in some instances several months' observation without treatment may be best. Liver biopsy should precede each treatment decision, and should be repeated at the time clinical and laboratory remission have been achieved; a decision is then made to taper or to stop medication.

Prophylaxis of Hepatitis

Passive immunization with immune serum globulin (ISG) in doses as low as 0.01 ml/kg is effective in either preventing type A hepatitis or suppressing the disease and its clinical manifestations. ISG is indicated for prophylaxis of type A hepatitis in a variety of pre- and postexposure circumstances. It gives effective prophylaxis in postexposure contact in the household and in institutional settings, but is not usually indicated in casual contact circumstances at school and work. In household contacts, secondary type A hepatitis attack rates of up to 45% among children and 5-20% among adults have been observed, so prophylaxis in households is clearly indicated. It is best given soon after exposure, and efficacy is clearly reduced if given more than 2 weeks after exposure. It is not thought justified to immunize all classmates or office workers. Inmates of institutions in which there is a high rate of sporadic type A hepatitis, and medical and paramedical personnel exposed to environments with excessive fecal soiling, if they have no anti-HA, deserve protection. Preexposure ISG probably should be given persons planning to reside or work abroad in areas with a high incidence of hepatitis. The period of passive immunity is 6 months. No human active anti-A vaccine is yet available.

Passive immunization against type B hepatitis with ISG or hyperimmune serum globulin is of value in certain circumstances. With sensitive screening of blood donors for HB_sAg, it now seems unnecessary to use ISG or hepatitis B immune globulin (HBIG) except when contaminated blood has been accidentally administered. Current, HBIG is approved only for those exposed to materials containing HB_sAg by accidental needle stick or oral ingestion, as might occur in a laboratory accident. The initial dose is given as soon as possible after exposure, and should be followed by a second dose 1 month later. Personnel in settings of chronic exposure to HBV, if treated with HBIG, probably should receive doses every 3 to 5 months. Unfortunately, despite several sizeable studies of the efficacy of both ISG and HBIG, clearcut conclusions as to effectiveness and use are not available. Variable titers of anti-HB_s in ISG, some very low, make data comparison impossible. The use of ISG seems to provide some protection and results in passive-active immunity though at some risk of clinically inapparent hepatitis B. It also appears that HBIG but not ISG is probably effective in preventing maternal-fetal transmission of type B hepatitis.

Active Immunization

The vast excess of HBV surface coat proteins synthesized by infected hepatocytes means that the serum of such individuals is full of immunogenic material. Such material from the plasma of HBV carriers containing HB_sAg particles has been selectively purified and concentrated, and any residual live virus inactivated with formalin. Testing in chimpanzees and marmosets has confirmed its safety and immunogenicity. Broad scale trials of such a vaccine have been conducted in homosexual men, who had previously been shown to have a prevalence of HBV markers ten times greater than a male blood donor population in the same city. In this homosexual group, there was moreover an annual seroconversion rate from HB_sAg negative to positive of 7.6%, and anti-HB_s negative to positive of 11.6%. The subjects were given three doses of vaccine over 6 months. Ninety percent developed anti-HB_s after two doses, and 96% after the third dose. A second study involving hemodialysis patients resulted in an 89% incidence of serum HB_s antibodies after three doses given over 6 months. Vaccination is recommended in persons 3 months of age or older, especially those who are at increased risk of infection with hepatitis B virus.

Drug Hepatotoxicity

Drug-induced hepatic injury accounts for approximately 5% of instances of jaundice in hospitalized patients. Many of these reactions are minor, but some are quite serious. Hepatic drug reaction injury may be divided into two types: predictable (type I)—dose- and time-dependent, and reproducible in animals, nonpredictable (type II)—independent of dose and time; sporadic, occurring in a minority of individuals; may have associated allergic manifestations. Both types may be manifest as acute or chronic hepatitis with cholestasis. Cirrhosis may complicate either type.

In type I drug hepatotoxicity, the initiating event is thought to be the metabolic activation by the liver of chemically stable drugs to potent alkylating, arylating, or acylating agents that are toxic. The central role of the liver in drug metabolism may account for its susceptibility to drug injury. Toxic metabolites produced by hepatic metabolism have been implicated as mediators of hepatic necrosis from acetaminophen, phenacetin, furosemide, and isoniazid.

An example of a type I drug hepatotoxic reaction is that of acetaminophen, which is normally metabolized by the liver to sulfate and glucuronide conjugates. Usually a minor pathway of metabolism is via the mixed function oxidase system of the smooth reticulum. In this pathway a reactive, potentially toxic electrophilic intermediate is produced that is then conjugated with glutathione. However,when glutathione supplies are depleted by large doses of acetaminophen, the reactive electrophilic metabolite arylates macromolecules, causing hepatic necrosis. Treatment with glutathione precursors and glutathionelike substances that can penetrate the liver cells, such as *N*-acetylcysteine which is rapid hydrolyzed to cysteine, have been shown to be effective in preventing severe liver damage and death if administered within 8 hours of the ingestion of the drug.

Type II drug reactions are less well understood as to mechanism. Small molecules such as a drug are not generally immunogenic but may first combine covalently with macromolecules to serve as antigens and thereby induce an immunologic hepatic lesions. Usually only a small percentage of individuals taking a drug have type II or hypersensitivity -type hepatic injury, which is unrelated to dose. Examples of this type of drug-induced liver injury include halothane hepatitis, cholestatic jaundice from chlorpromazine, hepatitis from alphamethyldopa, oxyphenisatin, erythromycin, sulfonamides, and hepatic reactions to sex hormones.

Liver Reactions to Sex Hormones

Oral contraceptives are capable of producing several unique liver reactions.

Cholestasis

Sex hormones as used in oral contraceptives are capable of inducing cholestasis, which is probably related to an effect of estrogen on the bile canalicular membrane. Cholestasis is rare in relation to the numbers of birth control pill users, and raises the question of some genetic component.

Hepatic Tumors

Liver cell adenomas were considered rare until the recognition of their association with oral contraceptives within the past 10 years. The incidence of adenomas relates directly to the dose and duration of oral contraceptive use, and does not appear to increase significantly with less than 4 or 5 years of drug use. Focal nodular hyperplasia of the liver is probably unrelated to oral contraceptive use, but must be carefully differentiated by the clinician and pathologist. Peliosis hepatis is an uncommon excessive dilatation of vascular spaces in liver lobules lined or unlined by endothelium. It has been most consistently associated with androgens and anabolic steroids. Hepatocellular carcinoma is a rare association with oral contraceptives and requires further study.

Patients with liver cell adenomas may be asymptomatic; some present with a right upper quadrant mass that may be either painless or tender, and may be observed to enlarge over a relatively short period of time. Spontaneous rupture and intra-abdominal hemorrhage, or hemorrhage within the tumor itself, have both been noted to occur.

Alcohol and the Liver

Alcohol is one of the most widely used drugs, as well as a food that yields 7.1 kilocalories/g. Its effects on the liver may be: metabolic—related to its oxidation and the resulting high ratio of NADH to NAD, adaptive—by enzyme induction, or the direct toxic effects.

Alcohol is promptly absorbed from the stomach and small intestine, and is metabolized almost entirely in the liver that has no feedback system by which the rate of metabolism of alcohol can be controlled; hence, alcohol must be preferentially metabolized by the liver. Within the liver cell, alcohol is oxidized by alcohol dehydrogenase to acetaldehyde. This reaction is coupled with the conversion of NAD to NADH. Many of the toxic effects of ethanol appear to be the result of the liver cell's efforts to restore the normal ratio of NADH to NAD. Ethanol is also oxidized in the endoplasmic reticulum by the microsomal ethanol-oxidizing system (MEOS), in which NADP is the acceptor. The biochemical consequences of alcohol metabolism in the liver are:

1. increase in liver fat
2. elevated blood lipids, chiefly the triglyceride and cholesterol fractions, producing a type IV hyperlipidemia
3. lactic acidemia
4. increased gluconeogenesis, which may lead to hypoglycemia
5. hyperuricemia
6. albumin and other protein synthesis by the liver may be impaired
7. inhibition of the citric acid cycle of mitochondria, resulting in impaired drug metabolism
8. MEOS induction

Alcoholic Fatty Liver

Fatty infiltration of the liver is the most common liver abnormality associated with alcohol. The normal fat content of the liver constitutes 5% of the organ's total weight. Fat accumulation is the result of multiple biochemical effects: increased mobilization of fat from peripheral fat stores, increased formation of triglycerides in the liver, decreased fatty acid oxidation by the liver, and increased synthesis but reduced lipoprotein release by the liver. Histologically, the increased fat deposition involves all parts of the lobule but is more prominent in the central and midzones. Fat may occupy the entire interior of the cytoplasm of the hepatocyte, displacing the nucleus to one side. Hepatocytes appear to merge to produce fat cysts.

The patient may be asymptomatic and physical examination may be unremarkable, although usually the liver is enlarged. Laboratory studies may be normal, or show only a mild rise in serum transaminase or type IV hyperlipidemia. Fatty infiltration of the liver usually clears after alcohol is stopped.

Alcoholic Hepatitis
Alcoholic hepatitis is a syndrome that has both morphologic and functional components. Morphologically, there is not only fatty infiltration but also a polymorphonuclear cellular infiltrate around areas of spotty necrosis of hepatocytes and in the portal tracts, plus the presence of alcoholic hyalin or Mallory's bodies, seen as clumps of intracellular eosinophilic material in hepatocytes. Sclerosing central hyaline necrosis often occurs around the central veins, and may then radiate out into the lobule, along with variable fibrosis that appears in areas of cell necrosis. Early there is preservation of lobular architecture, but the histologic picture may evolve to a micronodular cirrhosis. Furthermore, a patient with established alcoholic cirrhosis may have episodes of acute alcoholic hepatitis related to spells of heavy alcohol ingestion. Clinically, patients with alcoholic hepatitis may vary from an asymptomatic state to a severe illness with marked jaundice, fever, and fatal outcome. Even in patients who appear healthy, an enlarged, tender liver is often noted. In the more acute or florid cases, jaundice, fever, and right upper quadrant tenderness, guarding, and mild rebound may suggest acute cholecystitis to the unwary diagnostician. In some cases, cholestasis may be intense. Signs of chronic liver disease such as arterial spider angiomas, edema, ascites, and encephalopathy may be noted. Leukocytosis is common and, at times, may be impressively high. Hematologic studies may also show macrocytosis with round macrocytes, and occasionally a hemolytic anemia with hyperlipidemia. There usually are moderate elevations of alkaline phosphatase, transaminases, and GGT. Prothrombin time is often prolonged and unresponsive to vitamin K. There may be raised serum creatinine, oliguria, hyponatremia, and hypokalemia.

The clinical picture and setting may make the diagnosis apparent, but histologic confirmation is desirable although not essential, and at times may not be possible owing to unresponsive hypoprothrombinemia. If the clinical picture suggests acute cholecystitis, ultrasound may be useful to look for gallstones or evidence of dilated bile ducts. Patients with acute alcoholic hepatitis are at risk for serious infections, gastrointestinal bleeding, and coma.

Patients are best observed in the hospital in the early stages to be certain that progress is favorable. A low sodium diet, diuretics, and even parenteral nutrients may be necessary. Patients with jaundice, encephalopathy, and hypoprothrombinemia have a mortality exceeding 50%. Several clinical trials employing steroids have failed to produce good evidence that they favorably affect the prognosis of alcoholic hepatitis.

Cirrhosis

Cirrhosis is a general term that characterizes a variety of chronic diffuse liver diseases in which widespread loss of hepatocytes results in fibrosis and collapse of the network of reticulum fibers, with consequent distortion of the vascular bed of the liver and nodular regeneration of the residual viable mass of liver cells.

The clinical counterpart of the above morphologic picture is highly variable and does not always reflect the severity of the tissue damage. Patients may be essentially free of symptoms, or they may present a picture of advancing liver decompensation marked by jaundice, ascites, edema, renal failure, and encephalopathy.

For purposes of further discussion, cirrhosis will be classified and discussed as Laennec's cirrhosis, postnecrotic cirrhosis, biliary cirrhosis, cardiac cirrhosis, hemochromatosis, and a group of rare or uncommon forms.

Laennec's Cirrhosis (Alcoholic, Portal, or Micronodular Cirrhosis)
This form of cirrhosis, as the synonyms imply, is linked to alcohol as the most common etiologic factor, and morphologically to predominant and initial portal tract orientation of the fibrosis and scarring. A more uniformly small regenerative nodularity is seen on cut sections and on the surface of the liver.

Pathology. Further detailed histologic features include cytoplasmic fat vacuoles and cysts (they may disappear with therapy and alcohol avoidance), the frequent presence of alcoholic hyalin, and inflammatory cell infiltration varying from polymorphonuclear cells in the presence of associated or superimposed alcoholic hepatitis to a bland scattering of mononuclear cells in the portal tracts. The fibrosis is dispersed quite uniformly as connective tissue septa extending from portal tracts to central veins with intervening nodules of regenerating liver tissue, but without maintenance or preservation of intrahepatic afferent and efferent vessels and lymphatics. These abnormalities of intrahepatic vasculature underlie the pathogenesis of portal hypertension and ascites.

Etiology. All evidence implicates alcohol as the dominant cause of this form of cirrhosis. It is not understood why only 12-15% of alcoholics develop cirrhosis, but clearly individual susceptibility varies in ways not understood. However, from excellent German studies there appears to be a definite correlation between cirrhosis and the duration and quantity of alcohol consumed. The recent production of alcoholic hepatitis and subsequent cirrhosis in baboons fed ethanol while maintained on a nutritionally adequate diet further emphasizes the role of alcohol. Alcoholic hepatitis in humans is now regarded as a precirrhotic lesion, especially if central sclerosing hyalin necrosis with increased collagen formation is present. The current view is that nutritional factors are clearly less important in the development of cirrhosis than previously believed.

Clinical Manifestations. Well-established cirrhosis may be clinically silent. More commonly, patients experience fatigue, weakness, and may have edema or abdominal enlargement due to ascites. There may be abdominal wall venous collaterals, splenomegaly, enlarged parotids, reduced muscle mass, and Dupuytren's contractures of the hands. Abdominal and inguinal hernias may be accentuated with ascites. Jaundice, spiders, testicular atrophy, gynecomastia, sparse body hair, and purpura are commonly seen. Patients may have superimposed episodes of more active disease or alcoholic hepatitis, with more rapid progression of the downhill course perhaps leading to coma, renal failure, gastrointestinal bleeding from esophageal varices, or peptic ulcer. Serious bacterial infections and spontaneous bacterial peritonitis also may occur.

Laboratory Diagnosis. A variety of hematologic abnormalities can occur. Macrocytosis is common. Anemia may be due to bleeding varices or to hemolysis that is not uncommon in cirrhosis. Leukopenia and thrombocytopenia are frequently present when splenomegaly and portal hypertension exist. Hypoprothrombinemia refractory to vitamin K is common. Hypoalbuminemia may be present, due to decreased albumin synthesis and altered distribution in the extravascular pool. Hypergammaglobulinemia of a broad-based or polyclonal nature is common. The serum bilirubin is often normal but may be raised due to increased conjugated and unconjugated bilirubin components. Serum transaminases may be normal to modestly elevated. A high serum gamma-glutamyl transpeptidase level is often noted, and attributed to chronic alcohol ingestion. Furthermore, it is widely held that a serum aspartate transaminase level more than twice the level of alanine transaminase is characteristic of alcoholic liver injury. Serum alkaline phosphatase is usually normal or modestly raised. Hyponatremia caused by dilution, and hypokalemia due to renal loss, are often seen with advanced cirrhosis, along with a slowly rising creatinine due to functional renal failure. Urinary sodium excretion is commonly reduced to less than 10 mEq/24 hours. Radionuclide liver scanning characteristically shows reduced isotope uptake that may be so inhomogeneous as to suggest metastases. However, ancillary scan features such as the overall reduction in liver mass and increased radionuclide uptake in the reticuloendothelial cells of the vertebral column and in an enlarged spleen are not seen in liver metastases. One or more large areas of reduced uptake may raise the question of hepatocellular carcinoma and prompt consideration of additional tests such as a gallium scan or arteriography. Barium studies of the esophagus and endoscopy may show varices. It is desirable but not imperative to confirm the diagnosis by needle biopsy if the prothrombin time and platelet count make the procedure safe and if ascites is minimal. Sometimes, peritoneoscopy is helpful in establishing the diagnosis.

Prognosis. With abstention from alcohol, the course may be more favorable. Jaundice, ascites, a serum albumin value less than 2.5 g, hyponatremia, hypoprothrombinemia, and spontaneous bacterial peritonitis, as well as signs of encephalopathy, are unfavorable prognostic signs. Management of uncomplicated cirrhosis consists of the complete avoidance of alcohol, an adequately balanced diet, limitation of sodium intake if edema and ascites are present, and the possible use of diuretics. It may be necessary to restrict dietary protein to control or prevent encephalopathy.

Postnecrotic Cirrhosis

This form of cirrhosis is said to be the most common form worldwide. Morphologically, it is characterized by a confluent loss of liver cells with fibrous septa surrounding larger irregular nodules of remaining and regenerating hepatocytes. Synonyms are posthepatitic cirrhosis and coarsely nodular cirrhosis. The clinical features, laboratory diagnosis, and management are essentially the same as in Laennec's cirrhosis.

Cryptogenic Cirrhosis

This term comprises what is regarded as a heterogeneous group of cases of cirrhosis without any apparent etiology. They do not represent any unique clinical or morphologic subset. It is likely that, with the advent of new knowledge, cases under this heading will be moved to more specific etiologic categories, as was the case of patients who in recent years have been found to be harboring serologic markers of viral hepatitis and have been placed in the category of postnecrotic cirrhosis.

Primary Biliary Cirrhosis (PBC)

This is a chronic cholestatic syndrome of unknown etiology, in which progressive destruction of intrahepatic bile ducts eventuates in a form of cirrhosis. It is predominantly a disease of women (90%), and most commonly presents initially in the fifth and sixth decades. Etiologic theories include an immunologic association (its association with collagen diseases, the presence of granulomas in liver lesions, and evidence of anergy), and some genetic factors such as family clustering, and positive serologic markers in other family members.

Clinical Manifestations. The disease may be first established following investigation of an asymptomatic woman who is found on routine laboratory tests to have an elevated serum alkaline phosphatase. Pruritus with or without jaundice is the most common initial symptom. Patients often show mild pigmentation, excoriations, and enlargement of the liver and spleen. They may remain anicteric or have a more or less stable level of serum bilirubin for several years. Many patients also remain asymptomatic or minimally symptomatic for several years, but the eventual development of xanthomas, steatorrhea, bone pain, osteomalacia, esophageal varices, and liver failure is a common clinical course. PBC may be associated clinically with a symptom combination comprised of Raynaud's phenomenon, esophageal motor abnormalities, sclerodactyly, telangiectasia, and calcinosis cutis (CREST); other patients may have the sicca syndrome. There are also associations with pigmented gallstones, thyroiditis, and an uncommon association with celiac disease. Histologically, the liver abnormalities may be divided into evolutionary stages: in stage I, portal hepatitis with florid duct lesions are characteristic. These lesions are also referred to as chronic nonsuppurative destructive cholangitis, and consist of inflammatory destruction of the interlobular bile ducts, with lymphocyte and plasma cell infiltration of the portal spaces, accompanied by a few eosinophils and occasional epithelioid granulomas. Usually no cholestasis is seen. In stage II, the stage of ductular proliferation, there is an extension of the inflammatory process into the periportal parenchyma with liver cell necrosis, further destruction of the interlobular ducts, and fibrosis. Cholestasis may be present. Stage III shows scarring; often the inflammatory infiltrate appears to be subsiding, and fibrous septa are seen extending from the portal tracts into the lobules, along with lymphocytic infiltration. In stage IV, the stage of regenerative nodules or cirrhosis, there is further loss of interlobular bile ducts, and usually peripheral cholestasis.

Laboratory Diagnosis. Evidence of cholestasis is most characteristic, with serum alkaline phosphatase usually raised more than threefold. The serum bilirubin may be normal to high. Increased serum IgM is seen in a high percentage of cases. The antimitochondrial antibody test is positive in 95% of cases of PBC. It may also be present in 10-15% of patients with chronic active hepatitis. Serum cholesterol levels usually rise as the disease progresses.

Diagnosis. The sex and age of the patient, the insidious clinical picture and course, and the accompanying laboratory evidence of cholestasis and antimitochondrial antibodies, make the diagnosis likely; liver biopsy should be confirmatory. It is necessary to exclude chronic drug jaundice, primary sclerosing cholangitis, carcinoma of the bile ducts, and inflammatory bowel disease with associated liver abnormalities. In these instances, intravenous cholangiography is occasionally helpful, but ultrasound or endoscopic retrograde cholangiography may by necessary and are more reliable.

Prognosis. The course is usually slow and insidious, with gradually progressive evidence of cholestasis and liver impairment. Most patients die of the disease or its complications within 5 to 10 years.

Management. The disease is incurable at present. Pruritus may be controlled or lessened with the use of cholestyramine, a bile acid-binding resin. Vitamin D and supplemental calcium may be necessary to help combat osteomalacia. A low-fat diet and, perhaps, medium-chain triglycerides are helpful in reducing steatorrheal diarrhea. The use of D-penicillamine is currently receiving close attention. Its actions include removal of the excess hepatic copper stores that accumulate in this disease. It also blocks immune reactions, and has been shown to inhibit cross-linkage between collagen molecules. Side effects of the drug are not uncommon and include nausea and vomiting, loss of taste, proteinuria, renal functional impairment, and bone marrow suppression with neutropenia. Some patients may need portal-systemic shunts for bleeding varices.

Complications of Cirrhosis

Portal Hypertension

As stated earlier, the portal vein is the final common channel for blood from the alimentary tract from stomach to sigmoid, as well as from the spleen, pancreas, and gallbladder. Approximately 1,000-1,500 ml of blood per minute flow via the portal vein into the liver at a pressure of 7 mm of mercury, contributing 70% of the oxygen supply to the liver in the fasting state. Flow in the portal vein increases in the digestive period, but oxygen content is diminished. Collateral circulation of the portal venous system consists of anastomotic flow via the left gastric and short gastric veins to the esophageal and azygous veins; via the umbilical vein remnant to the abdominal wall; via the superior hemorrhoidal vein to the inferior hemorrhoidal veins, and thence to the inferior vena cava; and via mesenteric and visceral veins to the retroperitoneal spaces and abdominal wall, the splenorenal ligament, and so forth. Total collateral flow may carry the great majority of blood entering the portal venous system in the presence of portal hypertension.

Clinical Aspects. The history should be carefully perused for evidence of neonatal umbilical vein infection, a history of prior hepatitis, or alcohol abuse. Any past history of gastrointestinal bleeding or episodes of encephalopathy should also be noted. Physical examination usually reveals signs of chronic liver disease and splenomegaly. There may be prominent abdominal wall veins radiating from the umbilicus (caput medusae) where a venous hum may be heard.

Laboratory Manifestations. With portal hypertension and splenomegaly, leukopenia and thrombocytopenia are often present. Other laboratory data are those of the underlying cirrhosis or the state of the liver. Endoscopy or barium swallow examination of the esophagus are used to demonstrate esophageal varices. Visualization of the portal venous system may be achieved by a variety of approaches and methods: percutaneous transsplenic contrast injection; cannulation of the umbilical vein; transhepatic portography; and venous phase filming of the superior mesenteric arteriogram. Currently, venous phase arteriography is the most commonly employed method. Computed tomography and ultrasound may also give information on the patency of the portal and splenic veins, but not of the extent and distribution of collateral circulation. Portal pressure may be measured via umbilical vein cannulation, percutaneous splenic pulp pressure, by cannulation of tributaries of the portal vein at surgery, and via hepatic vein cannulation, in which the catheter is advanced to a wedged position that records sinusoidal venous pressure (normal wedged hepatic venous pressure equals 5-6 mm of mercury). The catheter is then withdrawn slightly to also measure free hepatic vein plus vena cava pressures.

A classification of portal hypertension based upon the site of flow resistance is as follows: presinusoidal–extrahepatic or intrahepatic; intrahepatic (sinusoidal and post-sinusoidal); post-hepatic and suprahepatic.

Extrahepatic portal vein obstruction results from intra-abdominal infections, thrombosis as in trauma or pregnancy, occlusion by tumors, and hematologic diseases. Clinically, patients with this form of portal hypertension lack the stigmata of chronic liver disease, have relatively normal liver function, and are not vulnerable to encephalopathy with hemorrhage from varices. Furthermore, this form is at times seen in children who may have asymptomatic splenomegaly and pancytopenia before bleeding occurs. Management of this form of portal hypertension is often difficult, for effective surgical shunting is frequently not possible owing to the lack of adequate vessels due to thrombosis and their small size. Direct surgery on the esophagus is sometimes necessary as the only option. Intrahepatic presinusoidal portal hypertension is observed in congenital hepatic fibrosis, schistosomiasis, in myeloproliferative diseases where there is cellular infiltration of the portal tracts, and in sarcoidosis. In presinusoidal portal hypertension, direct measurements of portal vein pressure or intrasplenic pulp pressure show increased values, while wedged hepatic venous pressure is normal. Cirrhosis is the most common example of intrahepatic portal hypertension, in which there is obstruction of flow from portal tracts into the hepatic venous outflow system (sinusoidal and postsinusoidal) by nodular regeneration, fibrous septa, and so on. Other examples are partial nodular transformation, and veno-occlusive disease (occlusion of small hepatic venous radicles by phlebitis and inflammation), which is discussed later. Post-hepatic and suprahepatic portal hypertension include hepatic venous outflow occlusion (Budd-Chiari syndrome), which is discussed later.

Bleeding Esophageal Varices

Hemorrhage often occurs in a spontaneous fashion without any precipitating event or setting. There appears to be good general correlation with the level of portal venous pressure. However, the role of acid reflux into the esophagus, and gastroesophageal erosions, is unsettled. Bleeding may be slow and gradual, or abrupt and of significant volume, with hematemesis and melena. Endoscopy is the most valuable means of confirming the site of bleeding and should be performed promptly. Patients with cirrhosis not uncommonly bleed from peptic ulcer, gastritis, and stress erosions. The clinical state of the underlying liver disease often undergoes deterioration, with increasing jaundice, ascites, and encephalopathy. Patients with suspected bleeding esophageal varices should be promptly hospitalized, and active medical and surgical collaboration in management should be the rule from the time of admission. Blood replacement with fresh blood or frozen plasma is preferable, and supplemental vitamin K should be given promptly. Cimetidine, 300 mg four times daily, should be administered. The gastrointestinal tract should be emptied with enemas and the oral administration of lactulose. Neomycin, 1 g orally four times daily, often is added. Vasopressin, 20 U in 100 ml of 5% dextrose solution, should be administered over a 10-15-minute period, and this may be repeated in 1 or 2 hours, or may be given as a continuous venous drip over a 1-2-hour period. If active bleeding continues, a four-lumen Sengstaken-Blakemore or Minnesota esophageal tamponade tube should be placed in the esophagus with both gastric and esophageal balloons inflated for 24-36 hours, after which the esophgeal balloon is usually deflated and traction somewhat eased. If rebleeding occurs in the next 24 hours, the esophageal balloon should be reinflated and traction reestablished. Dangers of the Sengstaken-Blakemore tube include possible aspiration of secretions accumulated above the esophageal balloon, rupture or ulceration of the esophagus, as well as the risk of asphyxia if the tube is displaced proximally, occluding the airway. Sclerotherapy, utilizing injections of ethanolamine into the varices via the esophagoscope is a new and promising approach that has controlled bleeding in a high percentage of cases. The procedure may be repeated every few weeks in an effort to obliterate all visible varices and provide long-term protection from future bleeding. Elective portal-systemic surgical shunting has been a major management technique, with the goal of reducing portal venous pressure while at the same time striving not to greatly reduce portal blood flow to the liver. However, some decline in hepatic function usually follows all forms of surgical shunting. Surgery is indicated if at least one proven episode of variceal bleeding has taken place. Additional indications are the presence of a vein suitable for shunting, age less than 50, serum bilirubin less than 2.5 mg/dl, and serum albumin greater than 3.0 g/dl. Additional positive selection factors are the absence of ascites, and no prior history of episodes of encephalopathy. Portacaval anastomoses with the inferior vena cava may be either end to side with ligation of the portal vein, or side to side, maintaining the continuity of the portal vein. There appears to be a lower incidence of encephalopathy following end-to-side anastomoses. The results of portal-systemic surgery include an operative mortality ranging from 5-10% for good risks, to as high as 50% for poor risks. Encephalopathy occurs in 20-40% of cases postoperatively.

The more recent introduction of the selective distal splenorenal shunt, with the objective of decompressing gastroesophageal varices while maintaining portal blood flow to the liver has, in experienced surgical hands, shown promise. Comparable prevention of further variceal bleeding, and a significantly lower incidence of post-shunt encephalopathy than follows total portal-systemic shunts, have been reported.

All shunt operations appear capable of preventing further bleeding but do not materially prolong life.

Ascites

Chronic liver disease accounts for the great majority of instances of ascites encountered in hospital populations. Other causes of ascites include pancreatitis, chronic congestive failure, nephrotic syndrome, lymphoma, and other intra-abdominal neoplasms. When due to liver disease, it implies seriously defective hepatocellular function, but usually several factors are operating in concert. Albumin synthesis is often reduced due to hepatocellular disease, resulting in lowered plasma oncotic pressure, while at the same time cirrhosis with portal hypertension produces increased portal capillary pressure. There is also increased formation of hepatic lymph, some of which exudes into the abdominal cavity. Continuous and significant exchange of fluid occurs between the plasma compartment and ascites, with perhaps half the volume of ascitic fluid entering and leaving the peritoneal cavity hourly. Cirrhotic patients with ascites show avid sodium retention by the kidneys with urinary sodium output as low as 5 mEq or less per day. There is usually dilutional hyponatremia and a reduced effective intravascular volume that signals the kidney to retain sodium. The reduced blood perfusion of the renal cortex increases production of renin, leading to increased aldosterone secretion and sodium retention.

Ascites usually develops insidiously, often associated with a sensation of bloating and flatulence. It may appear more acutely on the heels of decompensation of liver function following an episode of hemorrhage, an alcoholic spree, or some other illness. Patients with ascites almost always show numerous other features of advanced liver disease. When lying supine, the flanks bulge and there is percussion dullness in the flanks that shifts if the patient then assumes a lateral decubitus position. Ventral and inguinal hernias may be induced or accentuated. Respiratory embarrassment occurs with tense large volumes of ascites, and there may be associated pleural effusions. In cirrhosis, the ascitic fluid protein concentration is usually low, less than 2 g/dl. The cell count is usually less than 100 leukocytes with less than 25% polys. Spontaneous bacterial peritonitis occasionally develops in patients with advanced liver disease and ascites, manifested by fever, abdominal pain, jaundice, and sudden further decompensation in liver function. Ascitic fluid cell counts in this condition are greater than 500/cu mm, of which more than 75% are neutrophils. The most common organisms are streptococci or gram negative coliforms. Ascitic fluid pH of less than 5 is said to be diagnostic.

Mild to moderate ascites is a cosmetic problem and does not require treatment, although usually it will respond to appropriate diuretics. Conservative measures, including bed rest, more rigid control of dietary sodium intake to less than 22 mEq of sodium per day, and limitation of fluid intake to 1,000-1,500 ml often initiate diuresis. However, if diuretics are felt indicated, it is best to start with a combination of spironolactone and a thiazide agent. It has been shown that ascitic fluid mobilization and renal excretion is limited to about 900 ml/day. Larger urinary outputs than this come from other fluid spaces, and there is a danger of inducing hypovolemia leading to further impairment of renal perfusion, and a risk of precipitating the hepatorenal syndrome. Vigorous diuretic therapy may also induce encephalopathy, very possibly due to hypovolemia. Long-term diuretic use is often necessary in some combination such as 100-200 mg of spironolactone daily, plus a thiazide or furosemide. Obviously, dietary sodium restriction is necessary, and the patient should be advised to monitor progress with a daily weighing.

The recently introduced peritoneal-venous shunt (the LeVeen shunt) has proven of value in the small number of patients with severe, resistant ascites. The shunt is based upon the presence of a pressure-sensitive valve that permits one-way flow from the peritoneal cavity via a subcutaneous tube connecting the peritoneum with the superior vena cava. Respiratory motions trigger the opening and closing of the valve to encourage the flow of ascitic fluid to the vena cava. Disseminated intravascular coagulation has complicated the use of this shunt in a significant percentage of cases. In extremely rare cases, a portacaval side-to-side anastomosis has been employed in the management of ascites, inasmuch as this type of shunt relieves hepatic outflow obstruction and encourages ascites reabsorption. Unfortunately, encephalopathy is a common sequela to this procedure.

Hepatorenal Syndrome

This term applies to a clinical state that usually develops in severe or far advanced chronic liver disease, and is characterized by oliguria and uremia without renal morphologic abnormalities. The syndrome may develop spontaneously, or result from changes in blood volume and liver blood flow often related to vigorous diuresis therapy, or paracentesis. It commonly appears in the setting of other signs of hepatic decompensation such as ascites, jaundice, and so forth. The patient usually complains of weakness and loss of appetite, and may develop nausea, vomiting, and drowsiness. Laboratory studies characteristically show rising blood creatinine and urea concentrations, along with hyponatremia that may fall below 120 mEq/L. The pathogenesis appears to be related to reduced effective renal blood flow, and particularly to redistribution of blood reaching the kidney, such that cortical blood flow is diminished. Management consists principally of efforts to correct or compensate for any precipitating factor such as gastrointestinal bleeding, superimposed infection, or electrolyte disturbances. There is no satisfactory therapy for the syndrome.

Hepatic Encephalopathy

Also known as portal-systemic encephalopathy, this is a neuropsychiatric syndrome occurring in a variety of liver diseases, both acute and chronic. Hence, it may be encountered in acute fulminant hepatitis, in cirrhosis, and may follow portal-systemic shunt surgery.

Pathogenesis. The pathogenesis of hepatic encephalopathy is multifactoral. Although many toxins including ammonia, fatty acids, mercaptans, and weak neurotransmitters have been incriminated as a specific cause of hepatic coma at various times, not one of these alone readily accounts for the development of this disorder in all patients studied. Likewise, no critical protective substance normally elaborated by the healthy liver has been identified as lacking in patients with hepatic coma. These observations in patients, and the findings of synergistic toxins in laboratory animals, have led to the hypothesis that hepatic coma in humans is caused by the combined effect of various cerebral toxins, whose individual contributions in any one patient may differ. Finally, although the molecular basis and cerebral anatomic landmarks for impaired consciousness in hepatic encephalopathy have yet to be defined, attention has focused on three cerebral processes as likely mechanisms for the induction of hepatic coma: impaired synaptic transmission resulting from deranged neurotransmitter balance, a disturbance of the neuronal membranes, and altered brain energy metabolism. These mechanisms, of course, are not mutually exclusive, and different toxins may exert their effect on the brain by one or several of these mechanisms.

Several putative toxins have been associated with hepatic encephalopathy. Among these are ammonia, whose concentrations in spinal fluid and blood are elevated in patients with encephalopathy, and are higher during encephalopathy than during the recovery period in the same patients. Therapeutic measures to reduce ammonia concentrations usually improve encephalopathy. Also, encephalopathy can be precipitated in cirrhotic patients by administration of ammonium chloride, foods high in ammonia, or the administration of ammonia precursors. Against the primacy of ammonia as a toxin is the recognized discrepancy between the degree of encephalopathy and blood ammonia levels. Also, short-chain fatty acids have been shown to interfere with ammonia detoxification by impairment of urea synthesis and glutamate formation. Thus, a synergistic role has been suggested for fatty acids in precipitating encephalopathy. Mercaptan levels have been demonstrated to be elevated in nearly all patients with encephalopathy and there is evidence for an interaction between mercaptans, fatty acids, and ammonia, as each can amplify the toxic effect of the other in animals. Mercaptans are also felt to interfere with ammonia detoxification and to affect directly neuronal/synaptic membranes. The breath excretion of mercaptans is probably responsible for fetor hepaticus, commonly noted in patients with encephalopathy. Alterations in plasma amino acids have been noted in patients with hepatic encephalopathy, marked by increased levels of aromatic amino acids (phenylalanine, tyrosine, methionine), and decreased levels of branched-chain amino acids. These alterations are thought to result in depletion of some true neurotransmitters and to cause the accumulation of weak or false neurotransmitters, thus altering normal cerebral function. Evidence favoring the role of altered amino acids includes the precursor relationship of phenylalanine and tyrosine to the synthesis of cerebral catecholamines, and of tryptophan to the synthesis of serotonin; the formation of false neurotransmitters as a result of imbalance of these aromatic amino acids in the brain; the possible enhancement of aromatic amino acid transport into the brain due to decreased competition by reduced plasma branch chain amino acids; and coma induction in dogs by infusion of tryptophan and phenylalanine.

The precise mechanism of the altered plasma amino acid profile in hepatic encephalopathy is unclear, although the hypercatabolic state of these patients, including altered insulin and glucagon homeostasis with subsequent changes in peripheral utilization of amino acids, may contribute.

Clinical Features. Hepatic encephalopathy can be grouped into four stages on the basis of intellectual function, psychometric testing, altered state of consciousness, and decerebrate or decorticate posturing. In stage I, the patient may be confused or show altered motor behavior. Psychometric defects are detectable. In stage II, the patient may appear agitated, drowsy or confused, and show asterixis, as well as inappropriate behavior. In stage III, the patient may be stuporous or comatose but arousable, and able to obey simple commands. The patient is severely confused, with inarticulate speech. In stage IV, coma is present without response to pain, and decerebrate-decorticate signs are noted. Seizure activity may be noted in stages III and IV.

Other clinical features include: fetor hepaticus, a sweetish or musty breath odor noted in most subjects with encephalopathy; and asterixis (flapping tremor). This probably most characteristic neurologic sign is best demonstrated with the patient's arms outstretched, wrists hyperextended, and fingers separated. The flapping tremor tends to occur in bursts at a rate of 1/1-2s. Asterixis is not specific for hepatic encephalopathy and may be noted in uremia, hypokalemia, pulmonary insufficiency, and sedative overdose. Other neurologic abnormalities may be detected, especially spasticity with hyperreflexia and extensor-plantar responses.

Laboratory Features. Blood ammonia is elevated in the majority of patients, but there is imperfect correlation with the degree of coma. Sequential measurements in the same patient are helpful in following the course of the process.

Liver function tests reflect the severity of the underlying liver disease.

Spinal fluid pressure and protein content are usually normal. Spinal fluid glutamine is usually normal.

The encephalogram in hepatic coma shows a slowing of cerebral electrical activity with large, bilaterally synchronous slow waves, maximal in the frontal and central regions.

Simple but important bedside tests of cerebral function help in the diagnosis of very early encephalopathy and are useful in following the response of therapy. These include tests of handwriting, the Reitan trail-making test, and simple manual construction tests such as drawing or constructing five-pointed stars.

Precipitating Causes of Encephalopathy. Hepatic encephalopathy may develop spontaneously in a cirrhotic patient, a point of prognostic importance. Such patients are poor candidates for shunt surgery, with a high risk of severe postoperative encephalopathy. Precipitating causes of encephalopathy include the use of sedatives, tranquilizers, and analgesics; gastrointestinal bleeding; metabolic alkalosis; bacterial infections; and electrolyte disturbances producing metabolic alkalosis.

Treatment. (1) Identify and correct precipitating factors (i.e. gastrointestinal bleeding, electrolyte imbalance, etc.) (2) Reduce blood levels of ammonia (a) Dietary protein restriction to less than 20 g protein/day (b) Bowel cleansing to reduce ammonia production, using enemas and laxatives (c) Antibiotics—neomycin given orally, to reduce bacterial urease activity in the colon (d) Lactulose—this carbohydrate passes through the small bowel undigested to the ileum and colon, where it is hydrolyzed by bacterial action, forming lactic and acetic acids. The lower colonic pH reduces absorption of ammonia. Lactulose also decreases urea production by altering gut flora, and lowers intestinal transit time. (3) Newer and unproven measures include treatment with levodopa, a precursor of normal neuro-transmitters, and Bromocriptine, a dopamine agonist. (4) Infusion of branched chain amino acids—Early trials with infusions of branched-chain amino acid mixtures have produced encouraging results. (5) Alpha-keto analogs—These are nitrogen-free compounds having the structure of the corresponding amino acid without an amino group. Intravenous or oral administration of these substances to cirrhotic patients has shown that they may be aminated into the corresponding amino acids. Neuropsychiatric improvement and lowered plasma glutamine and ammonia concentrations have been noted.

Hemochromatosis

Hemochromatosis is a disease of iron storage characterized by failure to control iron absorption by the intestine. There is a generalized increase in body iron stores with resultant tissue damage. Clinically, hemochromatosis is characterized by the triad of hepatomegaly evolving to cirrhosis with eventual liver failure, skin pigmentation, and diabetes mellitus. Additional features include the development of congestive heart failure, evidence of endocrine failure in addition to diabetes mellitus, and pseudogout or chondrocalcinosis. There is persuasive evidence for autosomal recessive transmission in hemochromatosis, with associations with HLA-A3 and HLA-B14 phenotypes, both of which occur with a frequency in hemochromatosis considerably higher than in normal people.

Pathology Early in hemochromatosis, the liver shows only portal fibrosis and iron deposition in periportal hepatocytes and Kupffer's cells. Ultimately, cirrhosis develops without fat and with little inflammatory reaction. Iron accumulates progressively in the hepatocytes, Kupffer's cells, and bile duct epithelium. In the pancreas, fibrosis and acinar cell iron deposition and injury occur. Increased iron deposition also occurs in gut epithelium, kidneys, and particularly in heart muscle. Iron deposition and fibrosis are noted in a wide variety of endocrine tissues including the pituitary gland, adrenal cortex, and thyroid. Testicular atrophy is common, but there is no excess iron.

Etiology. The process seems closely related to a lifelong history of increased iron absorption from the small intestine. However, when iron stores are high, as in fully developed disease, intestinal absorption may revert to normal.

Clinical features. The disease is more common in men who characteristically show a grayish skin pigmentation, hepatomegaly, testicular atrophy, reduced body hair, and some decrease in muscle mass. An occasional patient presents with cardiac failure, although 30-40% of patients eventually develop cardiac dysfunction. Arthropathy occurs in two-thirds of the cases, usually beginning in the small joints of the hands and progressing to larger joints. Not uncommonly, acute arthritis occurs involving the knees, due to calcium pyrophosphate-related acute synovitis that may be diagnosed by microscopic examination of synovial fluid. There is often x-ray evidence of chondrocalcinosis, most typically noted on knee joint x-rays.

Laboratory. Serum levels of hepatic enzymes are often normal. The serum iron is characteristically elevated with a high degree of saturation (85-90%) of transferrin iron-binding capacity. Serum ferritin concentrations are raised in proportion to body iron stores, although the ferritin level may be normal early in the course of the disease before cirrhosis develops. The d-ferroxamine test is a useful means of estimating total body iron stores but is not essential to diagnosis. Liver biopsy should be performed for diagnosis and for comparison with later post-treatment stages.

Treatment. Current management is based upon venisection therapy in which weekly phlebotomies of 500 ml are performed to deplete the iron stores. Hemoglobin production can be increased five- to sevenfold under these circumstances, and patients tolerate regular phlebotomies as above for 1 to 2 years without a progressive drop in hemoglobin. The consequences of such treatment include a reversion toward normal of liver function abnormalities, an improvement in diabetes mellitus, a reduction in skin pigmentation, and, in a few cases, a reversal of cirrhosis or reduction of the amount of hepatic fibrosis. Cardiac dysfunction may improve, but it does not appear that joint abnormalities or endocrine derangements are benefited. Thus, it may be necessary to include replacement endocrine therapy to contribute to the improved well-being experienced by most people on a phlebotomy program. It is probably best to perform a liver biopsy when it appears that a therapeutic end point is being reached, to confirm the depletion of iron deposition in the liver.

Liver cell cancer appears in 15% of patients with hemochromatosis; it may be suggested by the development of pain, liver enlargement, or other signs of clinical deterioration.

Hepatic iron overload is seen in other conditions, including disorders of erythropoiesis, chronic oral or parenteral iron administration, following portal-systemic shunt surgery, and alcoholism. In the latter instance, liver biopsies usually show histologic features diagnostic of alcoholic disease, as well as increased iron deposition.

Wilson's Disease

Originally termed progressive hepatolenticular degeneration, Wilson's disease is a rare autosomal recessive disorder characterized by excessive copper storage in the brain, liver, kidneys, and corneas, with resultant degeneration of basal ganglia of the brain, cirrhosis of the liver, renal tubular lesions, and Kayser-Fleischer rings in the corneas. The precise etiology is still undetermined although some investigators hold that Wilson's disease is caused solely by a lack of ceruloplasmin, a serum α-2 globulin responsible for transport of copper in the plasma. Ceruloplasmin concentration is seriously depressed in 90-95% of patients with Wilson's disease, but normal levels have been conclusively demonstrated in the remainder, and no structural or functional defect in the protein has been noted in these few patients. Furthermore, some heterozygotes have very low ceruloplasmin levels, yet do not develop full-blown disease. Lastly, it is possible that a defective copper-associated protein (a metallothionein) with a high copper affinity is present in Wilson's disease, resulting in impaired transfer to ceruloplasmin.

Pathology. Liver changes vary from mild portal and periportal inflammation and fibrosis to cirrhosis. The histologic picture may resemble alcoholic hepatitis, with considerable fatty infiltration, parenchymal cell necrosis, and alcoholic hyalin, but usually with less neutrophil and inflammatory infiltrate. Special stains for copper may at times be helpful in demonstrating periportal granules thought to be copper-binding protein, but the correlation with other diagnostic parameters is not good.

Clinical Manifestations. Although the disease was initially described by Wilson as a degenerative central nervous system disorder, we now recognize the great variability of expression with clinical manifestations in the blood, joints, kidneys, and eyes, as well as in the liver and brain.

Although the most common form of presentation of Wilson's disease is as subtle neurologic dysfunction, the most common mode of presentation in childhood is liver disease with the age of onset of hepatic symptoms given as 6-14 years in one series, and a mean age of 15 years in another. Most commonly the liver disease begins insidiously and runs a chronic progressive course with fatigue, weakness, anorexia, mild jaundice, hepatosplenomegaly, and may clinically resemble non-A non-B chronic active hepatitis. However, acute and even fulminant hepatitis, chronic active hepatitis, or cirrhosis with portal hypertension, ascites, and so forth, may be seen. The diagnosis of Wilson's disease should always be considered in patients under the age of 30 years with hepatitis antigen-negative liver disease, acute or chronic, since it is one of the forms of liver disease for which there is specific and effective treatment.

An acute hemolytic anemia may be the presenting episode, or it may appear concurrent with the onset of liver disease. Sometimes the disease presents in young people as a psychiatric syndrome.

Diagnosis. Liver function abnormalities are like those of acute and chronic active hepatitis with elevated serum bilirubin, high transaminase values, and hypergammaglobulinemia. Serum ceruloplasmin and serum copper levels are usually low, and urinary copper excretion is increased. In the event of a normal range serum ceruloplasmin, or when there is reason to suspect that defective ceruloplasmin synthesis may be on the basis of chronic liver disease, or if liver biopsy is contraindicated, radiocopper incorporation studies are helpful. In Wilson's disease, an oral dose of copper-64 is followed in 1-2 hours by an initially high serum peak of nonceruloplasmin-bound radioactivity, but no secondary rise in serum radioactivity. In normal people, a higher secondary rise is observed over the next 1-2 days as the copper is incorporated in ceruloplasmin. Slit lamp examination should be done by an ophthalmologist to search for Kayser-Fleischer rings. Liver biopsy should be done on all patients both for histologic examination and for measurement of copper content. It should be remembered that hepatic copper accumulates in all forms of chronic cholestasis.

Treatment. Patients with all forms of Wilson's disease should be treated with D-penicillamine, although neuropsychiatric dysfunction responds better than the liver disease. Patients with portal hypertension and variceal bleeding should be managed as with other forms of liver disease.

Screening for asymptomatic Wilson's disease should be conducted in all siblings of established cases of Wilson's disease, as the disorder is inherited as an autosomal recessive and most patients are the product of the marriage of two heterozygotes. Hence, the disease will manifest itself in the siblings of patients with Wilson's disease. Approximately 25% of the children of two heterozygotes will have the disease, 50% will be carriers, and 25% will be normal. Screening should include the search for Kayser-Fleischer rings, ceruloplasmin, and urine copper determinations; liver biopsy should be done for measurement of copper content. Homozygotes have more than 250 μg/g of wet liver weight, and heterozygotes have values below this.

Other Forms of Chronic Liver Disease

Liver and Cardiac Disease

Hypoperfusion, as in prolonged shock or acute heart failure with splanchnic vasoconstriction, results in reduced hepatic artery and portal vein blood flow to the liver. Centrilobular hypoxic necrosis occurs, usually with high transaminase values, jaundice, and hypoprothrombinemia.

In chronic congestive heart failure, and particularly with tricuspid and mitral valvular disease, raised right-sided pressures are transmitted to the liver that grossly appears enlarged enlarged, congested, and tender. Microscopically, there are central vein dilatation, sinusoidal congestion, and occasional hemorrhages around the central vein. Liver cell necrosis also is seen in the central part of the lobule. Depending upon chronicity, collagen formation and fibrosis evolve from the region of central veins, producing cardiac cirrhosis. Patients often have tender hepatomegaly, although with well-developed cardiac cirrhosis the liver is small. Ascites is commonly present, and jaundice is also common. Alkaline phosphatase is usually normal to slightly elevated, and serum transaminases are mildly to moderately raised.

In constrictive pericarditis, cardiac cirrhosis with liver enlargement, ascites, and mild abnormalities of liver function in terms of elevated serum transaminases, but not jaundice, are seen. Diagnostic clues include paradoxical pulse, electrocardiographic abnormalities, and finding seen on echocardiography and right heart catheterization.

Postoperative Jaundice

In the immediate postoperative period, jaundice may develop as a consequence of several factors. Blood transfusions, especially of stored blood, may yield a load of bilirubin several times greater than normal daily production. Hemorrhage into body spaces and tissues adds to the bilirubin load. Shock, anesthesia, and surgical stress may impair liver function and, at times, produce a clinical and laboratory picture with elements of parenchymal cell damage and cholestasis lasting 7-10 days. All the above clinical features may be seen with greater prominence and frequency after open heart surgery owing to larger volumes of blood, more mechanical trauma to blood, and, frequently, an element of cardiac failure. Liver dysfunction appearing later following surgery may be due to post-transfusion viral hepatitis (most commonly NANB) or cytomegalovirus hepatitis.

Hepatic Vein Occlusion

Obstruction of the major hepatic veins producing occlusion of hepatic venous outflow results in right upper quadrant pain, hepatomegaly, and ascites with high protein content. It is most commonly seen as a result of occlusion by malignant disease (metastatic or primary liver cancer), thrombosis as in polycythemia vera, paroxysmal nocturnal hemoglobinuria, and with the use of oral contraceptives. The same picture may result from impedance of hepatic venous outflow in the vena cava from invading tumor, thrombus formation, webs, trauma, and constrictive pericarditis. Histologically, central vein dilatation, sinusoidal congestion and hemorrhage, as well as centrilobular liver cell necrosis, occur. Clinically, the picture most commonly develops with variable abruptness in a patient with one of the underlying predisposing diseases mentioned above. Commonly, the course is one of progressive liver failure leading to coma and death. Laboratory studies show elevations of serum alkaline phosphatase and transaminases, often hypoalbuminemia, and hypoprothrombinemia. A liver biopsy shows characteristic centrilobular congestion. The diagnosis may be substantiated by hepatic venography, showing occluded or narrowed veins, and the inability to measure a true hepatic vein wedge pressure. Radionuclide liver scanning may show reduced liver isotope uptake, with relatively normal isotope concentration in the caudate lobe. Ultrasonography will probably prove an accurate means of assessing hepatic vein patency.

Veno-Occlusive Disease

This inflammatory and thrombotic occlusion of smaller hepatic venous radicles may be seen following the use of azathioprine, in graft-versus-host disease, irradiation of the liver, and as a result of toxic injury produced by certain alkaloids ingested as herbal teas, and so forth. As a consequence of the occlusion and fibrosis of the hepatic vein radicles, massive centrilobular congestion and loss of liver cells result in fibrosis and a form of cirrhosis in which portal hypertension may arise. Liver biopsy and the clinical history are the most important diagnostic aids. In most cases treatment is symptomatic, but occasionally portocaval shunt surgery may be necessary to relieve the portal hypertension.

Tumors of the Liver

Liver cell tumors may be classified as benign or simple tumors, and malignant neoplasms. Similarly, they may be categorized as primary and metastatic.

Primary tumors arise from parenchymal cells, blood vessels, bile ducts, and connective tissue.

Hemangioma

Hemangiomas are the commonest form of benign tumor. They may be single, small, multiple, or large. They are found in 3-5% of all autopsies. Most hemangiomas are cavernous, tend to be solitary, and may be recognized at surgery or peritoneoscopy as a dark, red subcapsular lesion. Nuclear scanning shows reduced uptake by the tumor. Rupture, and severe or fatal hemorrhage, have occasionally been noted. Needle biopsy should not be undertaken if the diagnosis is suspected. Selective hepatic arteriography and computed tomography are capable of establishing a correct diagnosis. The appearance is that of cotton wool pooling in the tumor. Occasionally, calcification of the capsule or speckled calcification in the lesion are seen. Ultrasound may suggest a cystic lesion, or multiple internal echos may be noted, suggesting trabeculations within the lesion. Blood pool imaging is helpful if it is positive but may not be definitive, perhaps due to sluggish blood flow within the vascular lakes of the lesion.

Liver Cell Adenoma

Prior to the advent of oral contraceptives, hepatic adenoma was considered a rare tumor. However, several hundred liver tumors have been reported in women who were prolonged users of oral contraceptives (greater than 4 or 5 years), the majority being benign liver cell adenomas. The estimated incidence of this lesion in oral contraceptive users is 3-4/100,000. Adenomas may be single or multiple, and are usually subcapsular with a smooth surface overlying them. Histologically, they consist of thickened trabeculae or small sheets of hepatocytes without bile ducts, protal tracts, or central veins. They may, or may not be, encapsulated. The latter often show little or no demarcation from adjacent normal liver tissue. The lesions may be asymptomatic and discovered at the time of physical examination as a right upper quadrant mass, at laparotomy, at autopsy, or at the time of rupture or bleeding within the lesion.

Diagnosis. Ultrasound and CT scan are helpful in localization, but are not diagnostic. Nuclide scanning usually shows areas of decreased uptake. On angiography, the lesions are hypervascular, but differentiation of liver cell adenomas and focal nodular hyperplasia is not always certain.

Treatment. If the diagnosis can be reasonably certain, it is best to stop the oral contraceptives and observe the patient with CT scanning or ultrasonography every few months. If hemorrhage and other symptoms develop, laparotomy may be necessary to perform local resection or lobectomy. It is best to perform angiography before surgery to aid the surgeon in his procedure.

Focal Nodular Hyperplasia (FNH)

This benign, tumorlike liver lesion, not a true neoplasm, bears an uncertain relationship to oral contraceptives. Attention has been drawn to this abnormality by recent interest and awareness of liver tumors in young women using oral contraceptives. These tumors often appear as lobulated discrete masses but are not encapsulated. Histologically, focal nodular hyperplasia consists of liver cell cords and sinusoids that look normal. The margins are usually demarcated from the adjacent normal liver tissue. Typically, there is a stellate scar near the center of the lesion, from which fibrous septa radiate into the mass. There also are bile ducts and some inflammatory cells in the lesion. Clinically, patients with FNH infrequently have symptoms attributable to the mass. Rupture or bleeding are rare, and surgical excision is not necessary.

Peliosis hepatis is a focal vascular lesion that, at times, accompanies liver cell adenomas or may appear alone in patients receiving oral contraceptives, and androgenic or anabolic steroids. It consists of blood-filled spaces or ectatic blood vessels, often lined with endothelium. Intrahepatic or peritoneal bleeding may result from this lesion. Its clinical course is otherwise not well understood.

Hepatocellular Carcinoma

Hepatocellular carcinoma comprises 80-90% of primary liver malignancies, the remainder being cholangiocarcinomas. Geography, race, and environment have emerged as important determinants of the etiology and prevalence of this tumor. In Africa and Asia, where hepatocellular carcinomas are common and almost always associated with cirrhosis, a strong correlation exists between the prevalence of hepatitis B_sAg and the mortality from liver cell cancer. Industrial carcinogens, aflatoxin consumption, alcoholism, anabolic, androgenic, or estrogenic steroids, and hemochromatosis are associated with an increased incidence of hepatocellular carcinoma.

Clinical Manifestations. There is a 4:1 predominance in men. Abdominal pain, anorexia, and weight loss are common early symptoms. In the presence of cirrhosis, unexplained deterioration, or a change in the size and configuration of the liver, may suggest liver cell cancer. A friction rub or a systolic bruit are quite often heard over the lesion. Ascites may occasionally develop, although jaundice is not common as an early sign. Hepatic venous outflow block may be produced by the tumor, resulting in the appearance of ascites, jaundice, and accelerated deterioration. Sometimes, acute pain and tenderness may develop if hemorrhage occurs in the tumor. Erythrocytosis, hypercalcemia, and hypoglycemia may be noted. Hepatocellular cancer is associated with an increased incidence of pulmonary embolism. There are no specific diagnostic tests. Some liver cell cancers are associated with high plasma cholesterol values. A disproportionate elevation of serum alkaline phosphatase is rather commonly seen. Alpha-fetoprotein, as measured by immunoassay, may be present in very high levels in hepatocellular carcinoma, and has been considered strongly diagnostic of this tumor. Further experience is needed, as the protein has also been detected in normal people, during pregnancy, and in a variety of chronic liver diseases. Radionuclide liver scanning with technetium sulfur colloid shows liver cell cancer as a filling defect. Gallium scanning shows increased uptake by the lesion. Ultrasonography and CT scanning may demonstrate the tumor, but are not further diagnostic. Selective hepatic angiography is a valuable means of localizing the tumor and determining the extent and operability of the lesion, and should be considered a necessary preoperative study. The lesion usually shows stretching and displacement of vessels around it, and pooling of blood within the tumor. Although needle biopsy usually confirms the diagnosis, some surgeons prefer to withhold biopsy if surgery is to be done.

Treatment. If no evidence of spread beyond the liver is noted, and if hepatic angiography shows resection is feasible, surgery is usually attempted. Only a small percentage of hepatocellular carcinomas are resectable.

Other Primary Liver Malignancies

Cholangiocarcinoma

This malignant neoplasm of biliary epithelium may arise within the liver. Since the clinical picture is usually that of cholestasis, it is discussed later in the section on diseases of the bile ducts.

Angiosarcoma

Hepatic angiosarcoma is a rare, highly malignant tumor that has been causally associated with occupational exposures to vinyl chloride, inorganic arsenic, and Thorotrast (thorium dioxide), as well as androgenic and anabolic steroids.

Metastatic Tumors of the Liver

It has been stated that the liver is more frequently invaded by tumor metastases than any other organ, whether or not the primary tumor arises within the drainage system of the portal vein. Alimentary tract, pancreas, breast, and lung are the most common primary sites. Most malignant cells are thought to reach the liver via the blood stream. When seen on the liver surface, metastases are characteristically round, white, and often show umbilicated centers. The size and number of metastases vary greatly from one or two tiny nodules to countless larger lesions.

Clinical Manifestations. The patient usually notes the gradual but progressive development of right upper quadrant dull ache, fullness, anorexia, malaise, and nausea. The patient may have fever, and occasionally experiences sharp, acute colicky pains. The liver may be normal in size and configuration, but more often gross hepatomegaly with occasionally palpable hard nodules are noted. Sometimes a friction rub is heard over a surface lesion. Ascites may develop, at times with edema of the lower extremities due to hepatic vein and inferior vena cave compression by tumor.

Laboratory. Elevation of serum alkaline phosphatase is the predominant abnormality. At times, there is slight elevation of serum transaminases and mild hyperbilirubinemia, as well as leukocytosis. Diagnosis may be suggested by single or multiple, variably sized uptake defects on radionuclide liver scanning, or may be detected by ultrasonography or CT scanning. Needle biopsy should be performed using scan films as a guide. Subcostal biopsy may be attempted if an obvious palpable nodule is present. Peritoneoscopy combined with needle biopsy significantly increases the yield of positive tissue diagnosis.

Fatty Liver (Steatohepatitis)

Macrovesicular fatty infiltration of the liver is commonly noted in chronic alcoholic liver disease, adult-onset diabetes mellitus, obesity, corticosteroid-treated patients, or those who have undergone intestinal bypass surgery for obesity. Lobular inflammatory cell infiltration, fat cysts, and Mallory's bodies (alcoholic hyalin), plus macrovesicular fat, characterize the histologic picture of alcoholic hepatitis or alcoholic steatohepatitis. However, drug-related hepatic changes similar to the above have been noted from the use of methotrexate, corticosteroids, and perhexiline maleate. The liver disorder encountered in patients who have undergone intestinal bypass surgery may be morphologically indistinguishable from alcoholic hepatitis.

The same histologic picture (striking fatty changes with evidence of lobular hepatitis, focal necroses, with mixed inflammatory infiltrates and, in most instances, Mallory's bodies) has been reported in 20 patients who did not use alcohol, and has been termed nonalcoholic steatohepatitis. The disorder appears capable of progressing to cirrhosis. Most patients were moderately obese, or had obesity-related diseases (for instance, diabetes, gallstones). Common clinical findings were hepatomegaly and mild abnormalities of liver function tests.

Microvesicular fatty liver is the major morphologic change seen in some unusual disorders associated with fulminant hepatic failure: Reye's syndrome, tetracycline-induced liver failure, and the acute fatty liver of pregnancy. Reye's syndrome is a complex of post-viral acute encephalopathy and panlobular microvesicular fatty accumulation in the liver and other viscera (the kidneys and heart). Electron microscopy reveals swollen and distorted mitochondria. Hepatocellular necrosis and inflammatory infiltration, if present, are not prominent. Serum transaminase is elevated, but the serum bilirubin is usually normal, or only slightly raised. The prothrombin time is prolonged. Clinical evidence of liver dysfunction is minimal and overshadowed by the cerebral symptoms.

Acute fatty liver of pregnancy typically occurs with the first pregnancy in a young woman in her third trimester, and presents as acute liver failure with associated renal failure. Vomiting, epigastric discomfort, jaundice, encephalopathy, and renal failure are the usual clinical picture. Hypoglycemia may be present, but serum bilirubin and transaminases are only slightly raised. Serum uric acid is usually very high. Histologically, the liver shows multiple intracellular fine droplets of fat without necrosis or inflammation. This form of liver failure carries a high mortality, and death usually results from encephalopathy with cerebral edema and infection.

A small number of cases of fulminant hepatic failure have been noted with marked microvesicular fatty liver, following large doses of intravenous tetracycline given for urinary tract infections in pregnant women. Most of these cases terminated in hepatorenal failure.

GALLBLADDER AND BILIARY TRACT

ANATOMY

For a discussion of the embryology of the gallbladder and bile ducts, the reader should refer to the section on the pancreas.

The biliary system originates within the liver as bile canaliculae, tiny, groovelike channels that run between liver cells and transport bile secreted by the liver cells to the portal spaces. where they empty into the interlobular bile ducts. The canaliculae are walled bv the microvillus-studded surfaces of the cell membranes of adjacent liver cells. Their margins are bound by the junctional complexes. Interlobular bile ducts merge into larger ducts until the right and left main hepatic ducts emerge from the liver at the porta hepatis, and form the common hepatic duct. The cystic duct from the gallbladder joins the common hepatic duct, which then becomes the common bile duct. It lies in the hepatoduodenal ligament at the free edge of the lesser omentum, along with the hepatic artery and portal vein. The common bile duct passes posterior to the second portion of the duodenum, penetrates the back of the head of the pancreas, and enters the posteromedial wall of the second portion of the duodenum, where it joins the main pancreatic duct to form the ampulla of Vater before opening into the duodenum at the papilla. Thickened circular and longitudinal smooth muscle fibers surround the terminal common bile duct within the duodenal wall to form Oddi's sphincter.

The pear-shaped gallbladder lies against the visceral surface of the liver to the right of the quadrate lobe and near the anterior margin of the liver. It has a fundus, body, and a tapering neck that merges into the cystic duct. The upper surface of the gallbladder is in direct contact with the liver, but peritoneum covers the other surfaces of the gallbladder. The fundus lies at, or near, the lower anterior border of the liver.

PHYSIOLOGY OF BILE FORMATION AND SECRETION

The gallbladder serves as a reservoir for bile, and can hold 20-50 ml when full. It concentrates hepatic bile with a subsequent 80-90% reduction of volume. It also regulates the pressure within the biliary system, along with Oddi's sphincter. Contraction of the gallbladder occurs in response to cholecystokinin, as well as vagal stimuli. The gallbladder also alters relative bile composition by active sodium transport, which is tightly coupled to chloride or bicarbonate transport. Water movement is passively dependent on sodium absorption. Ions such as calcium and potassium become more concentrated. Concentrations of bilirubin, cholesterol, and bile acids increase but cholesterol saturation does not change. The presence of bile acid micelles permits the high concentration of electrolytes, bile acids, phospholipids, and cholesterol to be isotonic in gallbladder bile.

Little bile enters the duodenum between meals. Soon after food intake, cholecystokinin released from the duodenal mucosa humorally stimulates gallbladder contraction. Bile flow via the common duct is influenced by Oddi's sphincter, which functionally represents a zone of basal pressure 6 mm of mercury above the common duct and pancreatic duct pressures, and shows phasic wave contractions with a mean frequency of 4 per minute.

Bile Acids

Approximately 0.5 g/day of primary bile acids, cholic acid, and chenodeoxycholic acid, are synthesized in the liver from cholesterol, conjugated with glycine and taurine, and excreted by active transport into the bile where they are stored in the gallbladder in the fasting state. Postprandially, they enter the duodenum where they promote intraluminal fat digestion and absorption. More than 95% of the bile acids are absorbed in the terminal ileum by an active transport mechanism, and returned via the portal blood to the liver for reexcretion into the bile. The small percentage of bile acids that enters the colon undergoes two major changes, bacterial deconjugation, or the splitting off of the glycine and taurine moieties, and 7-α dehydroxylation, by which cholic acid is converted to deoxycholic acid, and chenodeoxycholic acid is converted to lithocholic acid. Some of these free secondary bile acids are excreted in the feces (0.5 g/day), the remainder (especially deoxycholic acid) being returned to the liver via the portal blood. Some lithocholic acid is absorbed and returned to the liver where it is sulfated and reexcreted into the bile, and, being water-soluble, is excreted in the feces. Thus the total body pool of bile acids is a mass of primary (cholic and chenodeoxycholic) and secondary (deoxycholic and small amounts of lithocholic) bile acids that total 2-3 g. It is essentially constant in size, since fecal loss is balanced by hepatic synthesis. The pool has been shown to cycle twice with each meal, thus making a functionally effective pool of 12-18 g. Bile acid synthesis is governed by its own negative feedback. Bile acids returning to the liver suppress the rate-limiting enzyme for synthesis of cholesterol, HMGCoA reductase, and the rate-limiting enzyme for bile acid synthesis, 7-α hydroxylase. If the return of bile acids to the liver is eliminated, hepatic synthesis of bile acids can increase five- to tenfold. Feeding bile acids reduces hepatic synthesis.

Bile Formation and Secretion
Hepatic bile secretion totals 500-1,000 ml/24 hours, 96% of which is water. Bile solids consist of bile acids, lecithin, cholesterol, bilirubin, calcium, sodium, potassium, and chloride. Bile also serves as the main route of excretion of numerous endogenous substances such as cholesterol, bilirubin, porphyrins, steroid hormones, and so on, as well as many exogenous organic ions including radiopaque media, conjugated drugs, or copper and iron. Bile formation and secretion have been divided into bile acid dependent and independent components. The primary controlling factor of bile volume ($\frac{2}{3}$ of human bile) and flow rate is the active secretion of bile acids into the canalicular lumen, thus producing osmotic and electrical gradients with a resultant solvent drag of solutes, water, bile pigments, organic ions, and so forth. A small component of canalicular bile flow is independent of bile acid transport, and is thought to be driven by active sodium transport. Ductular bile secretion is less well understood, but appears at least partly under hormonal control in that secretin stimulates active secretion of bicarbonate by duct epithelium.

DISEASES OF THE GALL BLADDER AND BILIARY TRACT

Cholestasis

Cholestasis is defined as altered secretion or some reduction of bile flow between the interior of the liver cell and the duodenum. It does not imply mechanical obstruction as the basic mechanism, although some examples of cholestasis are due to blockage. Cholestasis is not synonymous with jaundice, but includes altered excretion of all substances normally carried in bile.

Cholestasis has been divided into intra- and extrahepatic forms based upon the site of impairment of bile flow. Another conceptual scheme classifies cholestasis according to more specific sites, including:

1. Intrahepatic cholestasis at the hepatocellular level, exemplified by the infrequent cholestatic forms of alcoholic hepatitis and viral hepatitis, and by cholestasis caused by drugs such as chlorpromazine and sulfonamides
2. Cholestasis due to lesions at the bile canalicular membrane, including those caused by sex hormones, the cholestasis occasionally seen with Hodgkin's disease, the cholestatic jaundice of pregnancy encountered in the third trimester, and the unusual syndrome known as benign recurrent intrahepatic cholestasis, a familial disorder characterized by multiple episodes of cholestatic jaundice with resolution of the biochemical process between episodes
3. Cholestasis due to lesions of the interlobular intrahepatic bile ducts, which includes that due to primary biliary cirrhosis, the pericholangitis seen in inflammatory bowel disease, and sarcoid granulomas of the liver
4. Cholestasis due to lesions of the macrointrahepatic bile ducts such as Caroli's disease, the Klatskin tumor (adenocarcinoma at the bifurcation of the common hepatic duct), primary sclerosing cholangitis, and cholangiocarcinoma
5. Cholestatic jaundice due to obstructing lesions of the extrahepatic bile ducts, including that caused by choledocholithiasis, bile duct carcinoma, benign stricture, primary sclerosing cholangitis, choledochal cyst, and stenosis of the distal common duct due to pancreatic tumor or inflammation

Laboratory Abnormalities
In cholestasis, there is usually some degree of conjugated hyperbilirubinemia. With complete bile duct obstruction, the serum bilirubin rises to 15-20 mg/dl, but usually then stabilizes, presumably due to other disposal mechanisms for bilirubin. Serum alkaline phosphatase rises, usually greater than threefold, due to increased synthesis in the obstructed liver. Gamma-glutamyl transpeptidase usually rises several-fold also. Total cholesterol and phospholipid concentrations increase in serum, and there is often the appearance of a unique lipoprotein X, thought to be a low-density lipoprotein. Bile acid concentrations rise in all forms of cholestasis, even before the appearance of jaundice. Serum transaminases are normal, or only modestly elevated.

General Diagnostic Approach to Cholestasis
A careful history is essential, including a thorough inquiry as to current and recent drug use, prior abdominal or biliary tract surgery, the possible existence of diseases clinically associated with cholestasis, the family history, and an inquiry about fever, chills, pain, and colic.

Physical examination should include careful palpation of the liver and spleen, a search for an enlarged, palpable gallbladder, and signs of scleroderma, Raynaud's, lipomas, xanthomas, and so forth.

Laboratory tests should include measurements of bilirubin, alkaline phosphatase, transaminases, and prothrombin time. The first imaging procedure for further investigation of clinical and laboratory evidence of cholestasis should be an ultrasound examination of the liver, bile ducts, and pancreas to determine whether there is dilatation of the intra- and/or extrahepatic bile ducts. If the bile ducts appear dilated, percutaneous transhepatic cholangiography is the next step, employing a thin needle. If the site and nature of the lesion causing cholestasis is demonstrated by cholangiography, the next step is either surgery to relieve the obstruction and correct the basic process, or the radiographer may cannulate the obstructed biliary tree to externally decompress it. If the ultrasound examination fails to demonstrate any bile duct dilatation, the next step is often endoscopic retrograde cholangiography although, in some instances, it may be preferable to perform a needle biopsy of the liver at this point. Biopsy would be particularly indicated if the clinical picture strongly supported alcoholic hepatitis, use of drugs capable of producing cholestasis, or if the antimitochondrial antibody test were positive in significant titer. Liver histology in intrahepatic cholestasis shows bile stasis, but no dilatation of bile ducts or edema of the portal tracts. In extrahepatic biliary obstruction, histologic changes consist of ductular proliferation, bile lakes and infarcts, edema of the portal tracts; often, there is polymorphonuclear cellular infiltration of the portal tracts if cholangitis is present.

Clinical Features

The most common clinical features are jaundice with conjugated hyperbilirubinemia, and pruritis which may precede the appearance of jaundice. The precise cause is unknown; it is often assumed to be due to the skin accumulation of bile acids, but clinical studies have not fully established this. Xanthomas and xanthelasmas also are seen on the trunk and creases of the hands and feet as flat deposits, or tuberous lesions over the extensor surfaces of joints and the buttocks. Xanthoma formation is related to the level of total serum lipids and of cholesterol. Other clinical manifestations of cholestasis are: acholic stools owing to the lack of bile reaching the duodenum; steatorrhea due to the absence of bile acids in the small intestine; dark urine from bilirubinuria; osteomalacia and osteoporosis, probably due to several factors such as impaired vitamin D and calcium absorption from the gut; easy bruising or hemorrhage due to vitamin K malabsorption, resulting in hypoprothrombinemia; copper accumulation in the liver and, rarely, corneal rings resembling Kayser-Fleischer rings.

Histology

There are many histologic features in the liver common to cholestasis, regardless of the cause. Some that may give a clue as to the pathogenesis will be discussed below. Bile stasis is most prominent in the centrilobular regions, with only minimal cellular necrosis and foci of mononuclear cells. In prolonged cholestasis, portal fibrosis and round cell infiltration develop, with fibrous strands connecting adjacent portal tracts, plus ductal proliferation. With further prolonged cholestasis, portal fibrosis becomes more extensive, with septa running between portal tracts and hepatic veins, leading to nodular regeneration and the picture of secondary biliary cirrhosis. The liver is enlarged, green, and nodular.

Gallstones

Bile contains three lipids that are polar amphipaths; cholesterol, lecithin, and bile acids. Cholesterol, with only one hydroxyl group, is practically water-insoluble; lecithin can interact with water, and forms liquid crystalline complexes with it; bile acids have a major hydrophilic side, and thus have detergent properties and form micelles. Bile is 90-95% water. Bile acids in water form micelles and incorporate lecithin, greatly increasing the capacity to incorporate cholesterol in the hydrophilic interior of the micelle.

Several methods for expressing the solubility relationships of the three biliary lipids have been devised. In common, they illustrate that there are limits to the solubility of cholesterol, and that bile with insufficient bile acids and lecithin to dissolve all the cholesterol in micellar solution is supersaturated with cholesterol. Such bile is termed lithogenic, in that cholesterol nucleation and crystal formation occur, resulting in crystal growth and gallstone formation.

Patients with cholesterol gallstones have been shown to have lithogenic bile, containing relatively more biliary cholesterol than lecithin and bile acids. Mechanisms for which there is evidence to explain this abnormality include:

1. Decreased biliary secretion of solubilizing lipids
   (a) Diminished hepatic secretion of bile acids and a reduced body pool
   (b) Possibly, an oversensitive feedback inhibition of bile acid synthesis by the liver
2. Increased biliary secretion of cholesterol
   (a) Increased activity of HMGCoA reductase, the rate-limiting enzyme in hepatic synthesis of cholesterol
   (b) Diminished activity of 7-α-hydroxylase, the rate-limiting enzyme in hepatic conversion of cholesterol to bile acids

Gallstone disease afflicts 10% of Americans; it increases with age, occurring in 30% of the population over 65. Gallstones are more prevalent in women than in men at an early age, but in middle age the incidence of gallstones increases equally according to sex. Associated factors relating to an increased incidence of gallstones include diabetes mellitus, obesity, prior vagotomy, and the use of oral contraceptives or other estrogens. Data are mixed regarding the association of gallstones with pregnancy. Also associated with an increased incidence of gallstones are ileal resection or disease, and the prolonged use of cholestyramine or clofibrate. Bile pigment stones constitute approximately 20% of all gallstones. They contain less than 25% cholesterol. Most of them are radiopaque and are seen in chronic hemolysis, cirrhosis, and other disorders.

Radiology

Only 10 percent of gallstones are radiopaque (most of them are pigment stones). Some are lucent but have rings of calcium near the surface. Oral cholecystography will demonstrate most gallstones, but a successful examination requires reliable ingestion and normal absorption of the contrast medium, a healthy liver, and a patent cystic duct. Ultrasonography is a highly reliable and accurate imaging technique for demonstrating gallstones. Endoscopic retrograde cholangiography also may be used to demonstrate common duct and gallbladder stones.

Natural History of Gallstones

Most gallstones are silent and asymptomatic. There are insufficient prospective data concerning long-term follow-up, but probably modest numbers of patients with cholelithiasis become symptomatic and require cholecystectomy. Symptomatic cholelithiasis includes biliary colic, acute and chronic cholecystitis, and occasional pancreatitis. Rarely, fistula formation between gallbladder and duodenum, or colon, occur. Gallstone ileus is a rare complication producing lower small bowel obstruction, most typically in elderly persons, caused by a stone that has eroded from the gallbladder or biliary tree into the duodenum and become impacted in the lower distal ileum. Cholangitis and liver abscess are additional features in symptomatic gallstone disease. Lastly, cancer of the gallbladder, a rare neoplasm, is almost always associated with stones in the gallbladder.

Treatment of Cholelithiasis

In the United States, cholecystectomy is the only available treatment for cholelithiasis. As stated earlier, the natural history of gallstones is relatively benign, and asymptomatic gallstones probably may be observed until symptoms or complications appear. There is considerable support for the position that a small percentage of patients with silent gallstones become symptomatic each year; usually, they begin with warning signals rather than severe or catastrophic complications.

The recent discovery that patients with cholesterol gallstones have a small bile acid pool with bile that is saturated with cholesterol was followed by the demonstration that oral administration of chenodeoxycholic (chenic) acid produced unsaturated bile. Soon thereafter, it was shown that partial or complete dissolution of radiolucent gallstones was accomplished by oral chenic acid intake for 1 year. Extensive, but mostly uncontrolled, experience from several countries has confirmed the efficacy of chenic acid dissolution of stones. Doses of 12-15 mg/kg/day have been effective in desaturating bile and dissolving stones over periods up to 2 years or more. Hence, medical therapy would appear unsuitable for patients with acute cholecystitis, colic, or cholangitis, and most effective in patients with mild symptoms, a functioning gallbladder, and an unobstructed biliary tract. The only common side effect is diarrhea, which is dose related.

The epimer of chenodeoxycholic acid, ursodeoxycholic acid, has been shown comparably effective with fewer side effects.

Once stones are dissolved, recurrence takes place in 30-40% of cases and long-term therapy may be necessary but has not been prospectively determined.

Acute Cholecystitis

In the great majority of instances (90-95%), acute cholecystitis is associated with a gallstone impacted in the cystic duct. The clinical picture usually consists initially of epigastric and right upper quadrant pain of a deep, dull, visceral nature, rather often associated with nausea and emesis, and not aggravated by movements or respiration. It is thought that this pain is caused by distention of the gallbladder. Usually, the pain later shifts to the right upper quadrant with radiation to the right shoulder and often to the right scapular region, as well as in the right subcostal area. There is tenderness to palpation, respiratory blunting, and Murphy's sign is often positive. Muscle guarding, rebound, fever, and leukocytosis are common. Often, there is a palpable, tender mass in the right subcostal region. This pain is thought to be due to inflammation of the gallbladder wall extending through to the peritoneal surfaces. The serum bilirubin may be slightly to moderately raised, along with a modest elevation of the alkaline phosphatase. The diagnosis depends largely on the history and physical findings, and is further suggested if similar episodes in the past have been experienced. Differential diagnosis must include perforation or penetration of peptic ulcer, myocardial infarction, acute pancreatitis, pneumonia, drug-induced hepatitis, and acute pyelonephritis of the right kidney. Therefore, plain films of the chest and abdomen, electrocardiogram, measurements of serum amylase and lipase, and urinalysis should be performed early in the course of the acute illness. Plain films of the abdomen may disclose gallstones in the region of the gallbladder. Rarely, gas within the gallbladder can be seen in emphysematous cholecystitis, a form of acute cholecystitis noted most commonly in diabetics. Intravenous cholangiography is being replaced by ultrasonography of the gallbladder, which is entirely without risk and detects gallstones in the gallbladder with a high degree of accuracy. Technetium-99^m labeled iminodiacetic acid (HIDA) for scanning of the gallbladder has proved an important tool in the detection of acute cholecystitis, in which the common bile duct is visualized but not the gallbladder, owing to obstruction of the cystic duct. HIDA scans are safer, less expensive, and involve less exposure to radiation than intravenous cholangiography, and are rapidly replacing cholangiography in the diagnosis of acute cholecystitis.

Treatment

The patient should be treated with narcotics to relieve pain, and with parenteral fluids. At least half of the patients with acute cholecystitis are found to have positive bacterial cultures of the gallbladder and bile at surgery, the most common organisms being aerobic coliforms, streptococci, *Clostridium*, and bacteroides; hence, it is best that antibiotic coverage with a regimen such as gentamycin and clindamycin be started early. Surgical consultation should be obtained promptly when the patient enters medical treatment. The majority of patients with acute cholecystitis respond satisfactorily within 3 or 4 days, but if clinical deterioration occurs, and if the patient is medically fit, early cholecystectomy that should include operative cholangiography should be performed. Some surgeons prefer to wait several weeks before proceeding with elective cholecystectomy. However, complications such as gangrene, perforation, and empyema of the gallbladder are probably reduced by early surgery within the same hospitalization.

Chronic Cholecystitis

Some patients have recurrent attacks of mild to severe acute cholecystitis, although the condition usually develops rather insidiously over many months or years. Ninety-five percent of such patients have gallstones, and cholecystectomy is indicated. Caution should be taken in the patient with gallstones and a nonfunctioning gallbladder who complains of less specific symptoms such as fatty food intolerance, postprandial discomfort, and flatulence, since chronic cholecystitis may not be responsible for the symptoms and may not be relieved by cholecystectomy.

Acalculous Cholecystitis

This relatively rare form of cholecystitis that develops in the absence of gallstones has been observed largely in patients with recent trauma, burns, sepsis, and in those patients with polyarteritis or undergoing steroid treatment.

Choledocholithiasis

Nearly all common duct stones arise in the gallbladder, and usually produce biliary colic, nausea, vomiting, and jaundice. The upper abdominal pain often radiates to the right scapular region, and jaundice usually develops 24-48 hours after the onset of the acute attack; it is mild and often transient, with the serum bilirubin usually less than 5 mg/dl. Fever and shaking chills, nausea, and vomiting occur in the majority of patients. However, 20 percent of patients with choledocholithiasis have no pain, and 25-30 percent of patients have no jaundice.

Diagnosis

Elevation of serum alkaline phosphatase and mild hyperbilirubinemia are the most characteristic abnormalities. The former may be noted in the absence of pain or other symptoms, and without jaundice. If the gallstone produces partial obstruction of the pancreatic duct, hyperamylasemia may occur with the acute attack. Leukocytosis is common, and bacteremia due to enteric organisms may be present. Plain films of the abdomen may show stones in the gallbladder, and perhaps in the common duct as well. Ultrasonography may show dilatation of the intrahepatic bile ducts. Endoscopic retrograde cholangiography usually confirms the presence of stones, but should be done under cover of antibiotics and after surgical consultation. Biliary obstruction is rarely complete.

Complications

Choledocholithiasis can be complicated by bacterial cholangitis, pancreatitis, secondary biliary cirrhosis, and liver abscess.

Treatment

Common duct stones should be removed soon after diagnosis, to avert complications. Surgical exploration of the common duct is the best treatment, combined with cholecystectomy, if the gallbladder is not removed.

Retained Common Duct Stones

The incidence of common duct stones at the time of cholecystectomy has been reported to vary from 10-25%. Operative cholangiography should be included in all cholecystectomies, and common duct exploration at the time of cholecystectomy should be done if there is a past history of jaundice, a dilated common bile duct, or palpable stones within it. T-tube cholangiography should be repeated during the postoperative period before the tube is removed; residual duct stones are suggested by pain or jaundice experienced during the postoperative period when the T-tube is occluded.

Treatment

If retained stones are demonstrated at postoperative cholangiography, the T-tube may be left in place for 3 or 4 weeks, and then passage of a steerable catheter with a Dormia basket may be performed to extract the stones. Small stones may pass into the duodenum. An alternative approach is to perform an endoscopic sphincterotomy of Oddi's sphincter, which usually allows stones to pass spontaneously, or for larger stones to be extracted. Mono-octanoin, a medium-chain triglyceride capable of dissolving gallstones, may be perfused into the common duct through a T-tube, or into the distal common duct after a catheter has been placed through the papilla by retrograde endoscopy.

Internal Bile Fistulas

Biliary-enteric fistulas may form as a consequence of long-standing cholelithiasis, probably as a result of chronic inflammation and adhesions of the duodenum or hepatic flexure to the gallbladder. No specific clinical picture is associated with biliary enteric fistulas, but patients may continue to have symptoms of biliary colic or chronic cholecystitis, and sometimes have associated cholangitis. Gallstone ileus may follow erosion of a gallstone into the intestinal tract, with mechanical obstruction most commonly resulting from gallstone impaction in the terminal ileum. Rarely, large bowel obstruction has resulted from a large gallstone that has eroded into the colon, and pyloric obstruction has been observed from a stone in the stomach. Gallstone ileus is most commonly seen in elderly patients.

Hemobilia

Hemorrhage into the biliary tree may result from needle biopsy of the liver, upper abdominal trauma, aneurysms of the hepatic artery or its branches, tumors of the liver or biliary tree, and so forth. The clinical picture is comprised of acute biliary pain due to partial obstruction and passage of blood clots, jaundice, and gastrointestinal bleeding manifested by hematemesis and melena. Elective hepatic angiography provides the most precise diagnosis, although retrograde cholangiography may demonstrate blood clots in the bile ducts.

Benign Stricture of the Bile Ducts

Most (95% or greater) benign strictures arise in the common bile duct from operative trauma at the time of biliary tract surgery. Less commonly, they may result from choledocholithiasis or chronic pancreatitis. The clinical picture is most commonly that of insidious jaundice developing a few weeks or months following surgery, often with recurring episodes of abdominal pain, fever, chills, and pruritus. Bile pigment stones may form above the stricture in more chronic cases. Unrelieved obstruction leads to secondary biliary cirrhosis, and complications of cholangitis such as bacteremia and hepatic abscess. The laboratory picture is that of variable but chronic cholestasis. Ultrasonography often shows dilatation of the intrahepatic bile ducts. Intravenous cholangiography may fail if significant jaundice and liver dysfunction are present. Percutaneous transhepatic or retrograde cholangiography are usually successful in defining the problem.

Treatment

Surgical correction or bypass of the stricture is the only treatment offering hope of halting an otherwise tragic chain of events, and should be undertaken only by experts. Satisfactory end-to-end anastomosis after excision of the stricture is rarely possible or successful. Choledochojejunostomy, hepaticojejunostomy, or other procedures are more commonly applicable.

Primary Sclerosing Cholangitis

This uncommon entity is characterized by obliterative inflammatory fibrosis of the extrahepatic bile ducts, with or without involvement of the intrahepatic ducts. The etiology is not known. There is a slight male predominance, and the mean age at onset of clinical features is less than 40. The disorder is associated with inflammatory bowel disease (usually chronic ulcerative colitis) in 50% of cases. The clinical picture is usually one of insidious onset of malaise, jaundice, and pruritus with varying right upper quadrant pain. Some patients have acute attacks of pain, nausea, vomiting, and fever simulating acute cholecystitis or cholangitis. The disease generally follows a slowly progressive course, eventually leading to cirrhosis, portal hypertension, and death from liver failure. In those cases with associated chronic ulcerative colitis, the bowel disease antedates the biliary tract disorder and is often mild. The laboratory picture is that of cholestasis with elevated bilirubin, alkaline phosphatase, and cholesterol, with minimal or modestly elevated transaminase levels. The diagnosis is best established by endoscopic retrograde cholangiography, which discloses areas of irregular stricturing, narrowing, and dilatation (beading) of the extrahepatic biliary tree, the area of involvement in essentially all cases. Intrahepatic biliary radicles may also be involved and, very rarely, the process may be confined to the intrahepatic biliary tree. Differential diagnosis is mainly a problem of distinguishing bile duct carcinoma. Indeed, there may be an increased incidence of bile duct carcinoma in the natural history of this disorder. No medical treatment is effective, and specifically no beneficial effect from steroids has been conclusively demonstrated. Surgical decompression of the biliary tree is infrequently possible. The role of colectomy in those cases with associated colitis is unclear.

Fibrocystic Diseases of the Liver and Biliary Tree

This term embraces a group of hamartomatous conditions (mostly genetic) involving the liver and kidneys. Although features of individual cases may overlap, a satisfactory classification is as follows:

1. *Solitary cyst of the liver*—lined by cuboidal epithelium
2. *Adult polycystic disease*—an uncommon, benign, autosomal dominant disorder that consists of cuboidal epithelium-lined cysts of the liver and kidneys, filled with clear fluid. The liver cysts are believed to be due to a congenital malformation of the bile ductules, but do not involve the biliary tree. The cysts in the liver may vary from few to many in number, and from tiny to huge. In the uninvolved liver, so-called Meyenberg complexes, tiny spheres of loose connective tissue containing collections of undilated intralobular bile ducts, are often seen. Patients may be asymptomatic, or experience dull discomfort in the right upper quadrant, along with variable fullness or a palpable liver. About 50% of the patients with liver cysts have polycystic disease of the kidneys; however, in patients with polycystic kidney disease, liver cysts are found in 25-30%. Hepatic function is almost always normal, even with massive involvement of the liver. The prognosis is excellent, and is determined by the natural history of coexistent polycystic kidney disease.
3. *Congenital hepatic fibrosis*—a condition occuring both sporadically and in familial form. It may be diagnosed in children or adolescents who present with hepatomegaly or bleeding from esophageal varices, but may not become manifest until 9 or 10 years of age. The disease is characterized by broad fibrous bands containing bile ducts in large numbers, surrounding normal hepatic lobules in which there is no inflammation or cellular necrosis. Hepatosplenomegaly is usually present, but liver function is almost always normal. The diagnosis is usually firmly established by liver biopsy. The clinical course is dominated by hemorrhage by esophageal varices in otherwise healthy young people. The portal hypertension is of the intrahepatic presinusoidal type. Portacaval shunt surgery and variceal bleeding are well tolerated from the standpoint of liver function. The disorder is often associated with renal tubular ectasia (medullary sponge kidney) or with renal cysts, and the prognosis is often dependent on the severity of renal dysfunction.
4. *Choledochal cysts*—congenital localized or aneurysmal dilatations of the common duct, single or multiple, are usually encountered in children or adolescents, more often women. Jaundice, pain, fever, and the possibility of a palpable mass or fullness in the right upper quadrant, cystic in nature, should suggest this disorder. The jaundice is variable, or intermittent and of a cholestatic nature. There may be associated congenital hepatic fibrosis. Diagnosis is most accurately achieved by ultrasonography, or by percutaneous or retrograde cholangiography. Barium studies of the stomach may show displacement of the stomach and duodenum, and of the right transverse colon. Treatment by surgical excision of the cyst is desirable if possible, but in many instances anastomosis of the cyst to some portion of the proximal gut is necessary.
5. *Caroli's disease* (congenital intrahepatic bile duct dilatations)—saccular dilatations of the intrahepatic bile ducts, usually multiple, are seen in this condition which has no known hereditary basis, but is occasionally associated with congenital hepatic fibrosis and medullary sponge kidney. Attacks of right upper quadrant pain, chills, fever from biliary tract infection but seldom with jaundice, and an increased incidence of stones are the usual clinical features. Recurring episodes of bacteremia, and an increased incidence of liver abscesses, add to the seriousness of this disorder. Sometimes, the bile duct abnormalities may be seen by ultrasonography, but percutaneous or retrograde chol-

angiography are the best diagnostic procedures. Surgery offers no cure for the disease, but may be necessary to deal with the biliary calculi. Antibiotics are necessary to deal with the episodes of cholangitis. Death is usually related to infection or liver failure.

Neoplasms of the Biliary Tree and Gallbladder

Cancer of the Gallbladder

Cancer of the gallbladder is predominantly seen in elderly women. It carries a strong association with gallstones and chronic cholecystitis, although the causal relationship is uncertain. It is an uncommon form of cancer with an insidious clinical picture of dull but persistent right upper quadrant pain, often with anorexia, nausea, and weight loss. A hard mass associated with the liver is noted in more than half of the patients but the diagnosis is seldom made before surgery, although ultrasonography or CAT scan may suggest the tumor. The neoplasm is usually advanced, with local or regional extension at the time of surgery. Five-year survival is 1-5%.

Carcinoma of the Bile Ducts

Carcinoma arising from the intrahepatic ducts (cholangiocarcinoma) presents a clinical picture not unlike hepatocellular carcinoma. There appears to be an increased incidence in congenital hepatic fibrosis and other congenital biliary tract malformations, but there is no association between cholangiocarcinoma and any form of cirrhosis. The diagnosis and management are essentially the same as for hepatocellular carcinoma.

Adenocarcinoma at the junction of the right and left main hepatic ducts at the porta hepatis is a common site for bile duct carcinoma with local extension into the liver (so-called Klatskin tumor). Slow and insidious growth of the lesion producing a gradually evolving clinical picture of cholestasis may simulate a non-neoplastic cholestatic disorder. A collapsed gallbladder, and dilatation of the intrahepatic bile ducts as detected by ultrasonography and confirmed by percutaneous transhepatic cholangiography, usually establish the diagnosis. However, the surgeon may be unable to feel or appreciate the presence of the lesion.

Primary cancers of the common bile duct may be polypoid, but are more commonly scirrhous, and produce a spreading stricture that may simulate a benign stricture or sclerosing cholangitis. Jaundice, progressing to complete obstruction, and pruritus are the most common presenting features. Significant pain is uncommon early in the disease. Secondary bacterial cholangitis is rarely seen in malignant biliary obstruction. The liver is usually enlarged and rounded. A nontender, enlarged, palpable gallbladder is a useful sign of malignant biliary obstruction, but does not exclude this diagnosis if not palpated. Laboratory findings are those of cholestatic jaundice, and diagnosis is best established by percutaneous transhepatic cholangiography.

Surgical exploration may not reveal porta hepatis tumors, but distal common bile duct neoplasms are usually palpated, or at least suggested, by a dilated common bile duct. Surgery may be necessary to establish the diagnosis. Operability is low, and often it is necessary to decompress the obstructed biliary tree by cholecystojejunostomy or choledochoenterostomy.

Experience is growing in the technique of biliary decompression by percutaneous transhepatic cannulation of the biliary tree, which will then permit dilatation of the obstructing lesion followed by passage of an endoprosthesis through the lesions, with its tip beyond the tumor or in the duodenum. If the lesion cannot be passed, external biliary drainage can be established. Relief from jaundice and pruritus, and an improved quality of life, have been provided for an increasing number of sufferers.

QUESTIONS

Select the *one* lettered answer or completion that is BEST in each case.

1. An 18-year-old white woman in the third trimester of pregnancy has pruritus. She has no abdominal pain, chills, or fever. She had previously experienced episodes of pruritus while taking oral contraceptives. Physical examination discloses no abnormalities. Laboratory studies showed the following:

Leukocyte count	7500/mm^3 with normal differential
Serum bilirubin	1.8 mg/dl
Serum alkaline phosphatase	300 IU
Serum glutamic oxalo-acetic transaminase (SGOT)	35 IU
Antimitochondrial antibody test	negative

The most likely diagnosis is

A. benign recurrent cholestasis of pregnancy
B. primary biliary cirrhosis
C. acute fatty liver of pregnancy
D. calculous biliary tract disease
E. Dubin-Johnson syndrome

2. A 60-year-old man has had gradual onset of jaundice, fatigue, and weight loss of 4.5 kg (10 lb) over the past 6 months. Right upper quadrant discomfort, unrelated to meals or body position, has been observed. There has been some nausea, but no vomiting. The patient has ingested alcohol (5 oz whiskey per day) for many years, and has recently been given chlorpromazine for treatment of nervousness. There is no history of chills or fever. His temperature and vital signs are within normal limits. Scleral

These questions are from Part III, *Medical Knowledge Self-Assessment Program V*, copyrighted 1980 by the American College of Physicians and Annals of Internal Medicine. Used by permission.

icterus and a firm, nontender liver enlarged to 15 cm below the coastal margin in the midclavicular line are found on physical examination. Laboratory studies showed the following:

Hematocrit	38%
Leukocyte count	10,000/cu mm with normal differential
Serum bilirubin	10.0 mg/dl (total), 6.0 mg/dl (direct-reacting)
Serum alkaline phosphatase	300 IU
SGOT	100 IU
Serum albumin	3.8 g/dl

Of the following, the most valuable initial procedure for this patient would be

A. oral cholecystography
B. percutaneous biopsy of the liver
C. abdominal ultrasonography
D. endoscopic retrograde cholangiography
E. percutaneous cholangiography

3. Ricinoleic acid (castor oil) is most likely to cause diarrhea by

A. an osmotic effect
B. damaging the small bowel mucosa
C. producing a disaccharidase deficiency
D. stimulating intestinal secretion
E. altering the flora in the colon

4. A 34-year-old man was admitted to the hospital for evaluation of watery diarrhea that he has had for the past 9 months. A roentgenographic series of the bowel showed edematous and blunted duodenal and jejunal folds. Laboratory studies showed the following:

Serum gastrin	greater than 1000 pg/ml on three occasions
Basal gastric acid output	22 mEq/h

Findings on upper gastrointestinal endoscopy, computed tomography (CT scan) of the abdomen, celiac arteriography, liver scan, and liver function tests were all normal. The most appropriate treatment for this patient is to

A. perform a laparotomy to look for a resectable tumor, and, if none is found, resect the distal half of the pancreas
B. perform a laparotomy to look for a resectable tumor, if none is found, carry out total gastrectomy
C. start him on a course of streptozocin
D. start him on a course of cimetidine
E. start him on a course of propantheline bromide

5. A 32-year-old man was admitted to the hospital with dysphagia (to liquids as well as solids) that was localized in the neck region. Swallowing of liquids frequently caused choking and coughing. He was found to have marked cardiomegaly with an irregular cardiac rhythm. Examination of his extremities revealed marked muscle weakness.

This patient's dysphagia is most likely caused by

A. myotonic dystrophy
B. esophageal compression due to an enlarged left atrium
C. dysphagia lusoria
D. amyotrophic lateral sclerosis
E. midesophageal stricture

6. A 26-year-old woman has had profuse watery diarrhea for the past 6 weeks. She has lost 4.5 kg (10 lb) in weight and is clinically dehydrated. She denies any occurrence of nausea or vomiting, hematemesis, or melena. Laboratory studies show the following:

Serum sodium	140 mEq/L
Serum potassium	3.2 mEq/L
Sodium concentration of stool water	46 mEq/L
Potassium concentration of stool water	94 mEq/L
Osmolality of stool water	280 mOsm/kg water

This patient's clinical condition most likely represents

A. celiac disease
B. lactose intolerance
C. ingestion of large amounts of milk of magnesia
D. pancreatic islet cell adenoma
E. giardiasis

7. True statements regarding screening cancer of the colon in patients with chronic ulcerative colitis include each of the following EXCEPT:

A. The appearance of a strictured segment is an uncommon complication, and should heighten the concern for the presence of cancer.
B. Serum assays for carcinoembryonic antigen are of limited value.
C. The symptoms occurring secondary to cancer of the colon may be indistinguishable from those associated with a relapse of ulcerative colitis.
D. The finding of precancer on examination of biopsy material from the rectum indicates cancer elsewhere in the colon.
E. The incidence of cancer of the colon is markedly increased in patients with active disease of greater than 10 years' duration.

8. In a patient with inflammatory bowel disease involving the entire colon, Crohn's disease is most likely to be differentiated from ulcerative colitis by the presence of

A. associated arthritis
B. colonic ulcerations
C. an erythrocyte sedimentation rate of 80 mm/h
D. roentgenographic evidence of renal calculi
E. a subserosal sinus tract in the sigmoid colon

In questions 9-31, respond to each of the alternatives A to E with either YES or NO.

9. Hyperamylasemia has been shown to be associated with
   A. parotitis
   B. esophageal carcinoma
   C. ovarian neoplasm
   D. diabetic ketoacidosis
   E. renal failure

10. A 36-year-old woman has had dyspepsia and duodenal ulcer disease for the past 6 months. Determination of serum gastrin levels on three occasions were 750, 500, and 350 pg/ml, respectively.
   Appropriate steps in the evaluation of this patient's condition include
   A. a secretin test with serial measurements of serum gastrin levels
   B. determination of serum calcium levels
   C. upper gastrointestinal endoscopy
   D. computed tomography (CT scan) of the abdomen
   E. celiac arteriography

11. A 45-year-old woman has had gradual onset of pruritus over the past year, and a darkening of her urine during the past 3 months. There is no history of alcoholism, exposure to drugs known to induce cholestasis, abdominal pain, or fever. A tinge of scleral icterus, scratch marks, and mild hepatosplenomegaly were observed. Laboratory studies showed the following:

Serum bilirubin	2.0 mg/dl (total); 1.3 mg/dl (direct-reacting)
Serum alkaline phosphatase	500 IU
SGOT	100 IU
Serum cholesterol	450 mg/dl
Serum IgM	600 mg/dl

   Faint visualization of a normal-appearing gallbladder was achieved on oral cholecystography. Ultrasound studies showed a normal-appearing gallbladder, with no dilatation of intrahepatic bile ducts.
   True statements regarding this patient's clinical condition include:
   A. results of an antimitochondrial antibody test are likely to be positive in high titer
   B. corticosteroid therapy is likely to be beneficial
   C. excess copper may be deposited in the liver
   D. there is an increased risk of developing biliary tract calculi
   E. there is an increased risk of developing telangiectasia, sclerodactyly, and Raynaud's phenomenon

12. In patients with primary (idiopathic) hemochromatosis
   A. the diagnosis is most confidently made by finding liver damage and increased iron deposits on percutaneous liver biopsy
   B. a finding of normal serum ferritin levels in an asymptomatic patient excludes the presence of excess hepatic iron store
   C. associated liver failure is the commonest cause of death in young patients
   D. there is an approximately 20% incidence of hepatoma
   E. impotence is due to primary testicular damage by iron deposition

13. Acetaminophen-induced liver damage
   A. causes hepatic cholestasis
   B. is enhanced by a concomitant decrease in caloric intake
   C. will usually produce jaundice and stupor within 24 h of drug intake
   D. is lessened after ingestion of toxic doses of the drug if cysteamine or acetylcysteine is given within 12 h
   E. is likely to lead to chronic liver disease if massive liver necrosis occurs

14. Lactulose (Cephulac) is preferred to neomycin in the treatment of hepatic encephalopathy in cirrhotic patients who
   A. have a lack of prior response to neomycin
   B. have renal disease
   C. have electroencephalographic abnormalities
   D. have hearing impairments
   E. are receiving long-term therapeutic regimens

15. Established causes of chronic liver disease include
   A. hepatitis A virus
   B. hepatitis B virus
   C. non-A, non-B hepatitis virus(es)
   D. methyldopa
   E. tetracycline

16. Features of Gilbert's syndrome include
   A. unconjugated hyperbilirubinemia with onset usually in early youth
   B. an excellent prognosis
   C. need for a percutaneous biopsy of the liver to establish a diagnosis
   D. impaired bilirubin uptake by the liver
   E. a doubling of the serum bilirubin level when the patient fasts over a 48-h period

17. Measuring the urinary excretion of D-xylose following an oral dose is commonly used to screen for intestinal malabsorption. Other conditions that may also reduce the excretion of D-xylose through the urine include
   A. bacterial overgrowth of the small intestine
   B. ulcerative colitis
   C. cirrhosis of the liver with ascites
   D. pancreatic insufficiency and steatorrhea
   E. hypothyroidism

18. Primary lactase deficiency is likely to be associated with
    A. increased intestinal secretory activity
    B. stool pH of less than 6
    C. abnormal histologic findings on examination of jejunal biopsy specimens
    D. abnormal findings on a hydrogen breath test after ingestion of 50 g of lactose
    E. a rise of 30 mg/dl or more in the serum glucose level after the ingestion of 50 g of lactose
19. Incompetence of the lower esophageal sphincter often results from
    A. scleroderma
    B. hiatal hernia
    C. ingestion of oral contraceptives
    D. hypergastrinemia
    E. polymyositis
20. Indications for endoscopy of the upper gastrointestinal tract include
    A. duodenal ulcer disease in a 23-year-old medical student who has had dyspepsia for 1 month and black stools for 5 days
    B. cirrhosis of the liver, esophageal varices, and prior bouts of hematemesis in a 46-year-old man; he has been admitted to the hospital because of retching, vomiting, and one episode of hematemesis
    C. a vagotomy and pyloroplasty performed 12 months ago in a 50-year-old woman for treatment of duodenal ulcer disease; she is now admitted to the hospital for evaluation of dyspepsia and anemia
    D. a gastric ulcer that was completely healed 6 months ago in a 45-year-old woman; she is currently asymptomatic and has come to your office for a routine follow-up examination
    E. A Billroth II subtotal gastrectomy in a 62-year-old man; he returns for a check-up after having been lost to follow-up for 15 years
21. Patients with duodenal ulcer disease
    A. have an increased sensitivity of the parietal cells to pentagastrin, meals, and secretagogues
    B. respond to food ingestion by releasing larger amounts of gastrin than normal persons
    C. have an accelerated gastric emptying time that delivers acid to the duodenum at an above-normal rate
    D. have a lower than normal output of bicarbonate by the pancreas in response to duodenal instillation of acid
    E. secrete more acid than normal subjects in about 50% of cases
22. A diagnosis of uncomplicated reflux esophagitis is likely to be established by
    A. a biopsy of the mucosa showing basal cell hyperplasia and elongation of papillae from the distal 2 cm of the esophagus
    B. findings of round cell infiltration on examination of mucosal biopsy specimens
    C. findings of polymorphonuclear neutrophil infiltration on examination of mucosal biopsy specimens
    D. an esophageal motility study
    E. roentgenographic examination of the esophagus with barium
23. In scleroderma of the gastrointestinal tract,
    A. malabsorption can occur, even in the absence of skin involvement
    B. peptic strictures of the esophagus occur
    C. abnormal esophageal motility and dysphagia are common
    D. biopsy of the small bowel can establish the diagnosis if the small bowel is involved
    E. wide-mouth colonic diverticula are characteristic
24. True statements concerning candidal esophagitis include:
    A. Culture of *Candida albicans* from a smear of mucosal tissue is necessary to make the diagnosis.
    B. Severe heartburn frequently occurs.
    C. The demonstration of mycelial forms, by smear, on examination of plaque or mucosal biopsy material is the best way to establish the diagnosis.
    D. Roentgenograms of the esophagus with barium usually reveal abnormalities.
    E. Stricture formation is a common complication.
25. In patients with acute pancreatitis, pseudocysts
    A. occur less frequently when the patients are treated with nongastric suction
    B. routinely require surgical drainage
    C. are most reliably detected by sonography
    D. are almost always present when pleural effusion and ascites appear
    E. indicate that alcohol is the cause of the pancreatitis
26. A 33-year-old obese woman has acute abdominal pain and lipemic serum. Her serum amylase activity is within normal limits.

    True statements associated with such a clinical condition include:
    A. A normal serum amylase activity excludes a diagnosis of pancreatitis.
    B. Amylase activity should be determined on serial dilutions of serum.
    C. Determination of serum lipase activity may be helpful in establishing a diagnosis.
    D. Urinary amylase activity will be clearly elevated if the patient has pancreatitis.
    E. The ingestion of oral contraceptive agents may precipi-

tate hypertriglyceridemia and acute pancreatitis in predisposed persons.

27. The amylase/creatinine clearance ratio (C_{am}/C_{cr})
    A. is usually increased in patients with acute pancreatitis with hyperamylasemia
    B. when increased, appears to represent a reversible renal tubular defect and resultant decreased renal tubular amylase reabsorption
    C. is helpful in establishing the diagnosis of hemorrhagic pancreatitis
    D. is helpful in establishing the diagnosis of acute pancreatitis in the presence of renal failure
    E. is increased when macroamylasemia exists
28. True statements about patients with chronic pancreatitis with exocrine insufficiency and steatorrhea include:
    A. lipase output is reduced to less than 10% of normal
    B. pancreatic bicarbonate secretion is uniformly decreased
    C. the administration of cimetidine is a useful adjunct to pancreatic enzyme replacement therapy in ameliorating steatorrhea
    D. there is an increased incidence of abnormal findings on a Schilling test for vitamin B12 absorption
    E. findings on endoscopic retrograde cholangiopancreatography are usually abnormal in such patients
29. Characteristic features of pseudomembranous enterocolitis include
    A. bloody diarrhea
    B. toxic megacolon
    C. diagnostic findings on sigmoidoscopic examination
    D. presence in feces of *Clostridium difficile* toxin in high titer
    E. development only in patients currently receiving antibiotic treatment
30. Fecal leukocytes are found in increased numbers in patients with
    A. giardiasis
    B. infection due to toxogenic *Escherichia coli*
    C. clindamycin-associated colitis
    D. shigellosis
    E. idiopathic ulcerative colitis
31. In patients with the irritable bowel syndrome,
    A. there is an increased risk of development of colonic diverticulosis
    B. symptoms may be indistinguishable from those of painful colonic diverticular disease
    C. there is often an increase in slow-wave activity (i.e., a higher percentage of 3 cycle/min waves) as the basic electrical rhythm of sigmoid and rectal smooth muscle
    D. diarrhea commonly awakens the patient from sleep
    E. during periods of diarrhea, stools contain a modest increase in the number of leukocytes

ANSWERS

1. A
2. C
3. D
4. D
5. A
6. D
7. D
8. E
9. yes, no, yes, yes, yes
10. yes, yes, no, no, no
11. yes, no, yes, yes, yes
12. yes, no, no, yes, yes
13. no, yes, no, yes, no
14. yes, yes, no, yes, yes
15. no, yes, yes, yes, no
16. yes, yes, no, yes, yes
17. yes, no, yes, no, yes
18. no, yes, no, yes, no
19. yes, no, yes, no, no
20. yes, yes, yes, no, yes
21. yes, yes, yes, no, yes
22. yes, no, yes, no, no
23. yes, yes, yes, no, yes
24. no, no, yes, no, no
25. no, no, yes, yes, no
26. no, yes, yes, yes, yes
27. yes, yes, no, no, no
28. yes, yes, yes, yes, yes
29. no, no, yes, yes, no
30. yes, no, yes, yes, yes
31. yes, yes, yes, no, no

BIBLIOGRAPHY

TEXTBOOKS

Banks PA: *Pancreatitis*. New York: Plenum, 1979.

Baron JH: *Clinical Tests of Gastric Secretion*. New York: Oxford University Press, 1979.

Brooke BN (ed): *Crohn's Disease*. London: Macmillan Publishing Co Inc, 1977.

Brooks FP (ed): *Gastrointestinal Pathophysiology*, ed 2. New York: Oxford University Press, 1978.

Conn HO, Lieberthal MM: *The Hepatic Coma Syndromes and Lactulose*. Baltimore: Williams & Wilkins, 1979.

Gitnick G (ed): *Current Gastroenterology and Hepatology*. Boston: Houghton Mifflin Co, 1979.

Goodman MJ, Sparberg M: Ulcerative Colitis. New York: John Wiley & Sons, 1978.

Henderson RD: *The Esophagus: Reflux and Primary Motor Disorders*. Baltimore: Williams & Wilkins, 1980.

Johnson LR: *Gastrointestinal Physiology*, ed 2. St. Louis: C.V. Mosby, 1981.

Kirsner JB, Shorter RG (eds): *Inflammatory Bowel Disease*, ed 2. Philadelphia: Lea & Febiger, 1980.

Koff RS: *Viral Hepatitis*. New York: John Wiley & Sons, 1978.

Payne WS, Olsen AM: *The Esophagus*. Philadelphia: Lea & Febiger, 1974.

Scheuer PJ: *Liver Biopsy Interpretation*, ed 3. London: Bailliere Tindall, 1980.

Sleisenger MH, Fordtran JS (eds): *Gastrointestinal Disease*, ed 2. Philadelphia: WB Saunders Co, 1978.

Shoenfield LJ: *Diseases of the Gallbladder and Biliary System.* New York: John Wiley & Sons, 1977.

Sherlock S: *Diseases of the Liver and Biliary System*, ed. 6. St. Louis: C. V. Mosby, 1981.

Wright R (ed): *Liver and Biliary Disease*. Philadelphia: WB Saunders Co, 1979.

ARTICLES AND MONOGRAPHS

Esophagus

Code CF, Schlegel JF: Motor action of the esophagus and its sphincters, in Code CF (ed): *Handbook of Physiology*, Section 6: Alimentary canal. Vol. 4: Motility. Washington, D.C.: American Physiological Society, 1968, pp. 1821-1839.

Cohen S: Motor disorders of the esophagus. *N Engl J Med* 301:184-192, 1979.

Earlam R, Cunha-Melo JR: Oesophageal squamous cell cancer: I–A critical review of surgery. *Br J Surg* 67:381-390, 1980.

Stomach

Fordtran JS: Acid-pepsin secretion, in Sleisenger MH, Fordtran JS (eds): *Gastrointestinal Disease*, ed 2. Philadelphia: WB Saunders Co, 1978, pp. 794-796.

Grossman MI: Peptic ulcer: New therapies, new diseases. *Ann Intern Med* 95:609-627, 1981.

Kelly KA: The mobility of the stomach and gastroduodenal region. In Johnson LR, Christensen J (eds): *Physiology of the Gastrointestinal Tract*. New York: Raven Press, 1981.

McCarthy DM: Peptic ulcer: Antacids or cimetidine? *Hosp Pract.* 14: 52-64, 1979.

Silen W: The prevention and management of stress ulcers. *Hosp Pract.* 15:93-100, 1980.

Small Intestine

Bayless TM, Knox DL: Whipple's disease: A multisystem infection. (Editorial) *N Engl J Med* 300:920-921, 1979.

Gray GM: Carbohydrate digestion and absorption. *N Engl J Med* 292: 1225-1230, 1975.

Hendrix TR, Bayless TM: Malabsorption, in Harvey AM, Johns RJ, Owens Jr AH, Ross RS (eds): *The Principles and Practices of Medicine*, ed 19. New York: Appleton-Century-Crofts, 1976, pp. 841-863.

Senior JR: Celiac disease, in Brooks FP (ed): *Gastrointestinal Pathophysiology*, ed 2. New York: Oxford University Press, 1978, p. 275.

Sleisenger MH, Kim YS: Protein digestion and absorption. *N Engl J Med* 300:659-663, 1979.

Waldman TA: Protein-losing gastroenteropathies, in Bockus HL (ed): *Gastroenterology*, ed 3, vol. 2. Philadelphia: WB Saunders Co, 1974, p. 361.

Colon

Dobbins WO 3d: Current status of the precancer lesion in ulcerative colitis. *Gastroenterology* 73:1431-1433, 1977.

Drake AA, Gilchrist MJR, Washington JA, Huizenga KA, Van Scoy RE: Diarrhea due to Campylobacter fetus subspecies jejuni. *Mayo Clin Proc* ty:414-423, 1981.

Drossman DA, Powell DW, Session JT Jr: The irritable bowel syndrome. *Gastroenterology* 73:811-822, 1977.

Huizenga KA: Colonic cancer in inflammatory bowel disease (Editorial). *Mayo Clin Proc* 53:474-475, 1978.

Larson DM, Masters SS, Spiro HM: Medical and surgical therapy in diverticular disease: A comparative study. *Gastroenterology* 71: 734-737, 1976.

Phillips SF, Devroede GJ: Functions of the large intestine, in Crane RK (ed): *Gastrointestinal Physiology* III, Chapter 7 (International Reviews of Physiology, Vol. 19). Baltimore: University Park Press, 1979.

Phillips SF: Diarrhea: Pathogenesis and Diagnostic Techniques. *Postgrad Med* 57:65-71, 1975.

Sachar DB, Greenstein AJ: Cancer in ulcerative colitis: Good news and bad news. *Ann Intern Med* 95:642-643, 1981.

Thompson WG, Heaton KW: Functional bowel disorders in apparently healthy people. *Gastroenterology* 79:283-288, 1980.

Pancreas

DiMagno EP, Malagelada JR, Taylor WF, Go VL: A prospective comparison of current diagnostic tests for pancreatic cancer. *N Engl J Med* 297:737-742, 1977.

Ettien JT, Webster PD III: The management of acute pancreatitis. *Adv Intern Med* 25:169-198, 1980.

Kimura T, Toung JK, Margolis S, Permutt S, Cameron JL: Respiratory failure in acute pancreatitis: A possible role for triglycerides. *Ann Surg* 189:509-514, 1979.

Lamers CB, Stadil F, Van Tongeren JH: Prevalence of endocrine abnormalities in patients with the Zollinger-Ellison syndrome and in their families. *Am J Med* 64:607-612, 1978.

Levitt MD, Johnson SG: Is the amylase/creatinine ratio of value for the diagnosis of pancreatitis? *Gastroenterology* 75:118-119, 1978.

Ranson JHC: Acute pancreatitis. *Curr Probl Surg* 11:1-84, 1979.

Schein PS (Moderator): Islet cell tumors: Current concepts and management. *Ann Intern Med* 79:239-257, 1973.

Winship D (Moderator): Pancreatitis: Pancreatic pseudocysts and their complications. *Gastroenterology* 73:593-603, 1977.

Liver

Czaja AJ: Current problems in the diagnosis and management of chronic active hepatitis. *Mayo Clin Proc* 56:311-323, 1981.

Galambos JT: Ascites in cirrhosis, in Galambos JT (ed): Cirrhosis (Major Medicine, Vol. 17). Philadelphia: WB Saunders CO, 1979, p. 335.

Galambos JT: Evaluation and therapy of encephalopathy in cirrhosis, in Galambos JT (ed): Cirrhosis (Major Problems in Internal Medicine, Vol. 17). Philadelphia: WB Saunders Co, 1979, p. 288.

Hoyumpa AM, Desmond PV, Avant GR, Roberts RK, Schenker S: Hepatic encephalopathy. *Gastroenterology* 76:184-195, 1979.

Isselbacher KJ: Metabolic and hepatic effects of alcohol. *N Engl J Med* 296:612-616, 1977.

Rojkind M, Dunn MA: Hepatic fibrosis. *Gastroenterology* 76:849-863, 1979.

Schmid R: Bilirubin metabolism: State of the art. *Gastroenterology* 74: 1307-1312, 1978.

Schoenfield LJ, Lachin JM: Chenodiol (chenodeoxycholic acid) for dissolution of gallstones: The National Cooperative Gallstone Study. *Ann Intern Med* 95:257-282, 1981.

Thistle JL, Hofmann AF, Ott BJ, Stephens DH: Chemotherapy for gallstone dissolution. I. Efficacy and safety. *JAMA* 239:1041-1046, 1978.

CHAPTER 7

GERIATRIC MEDICINE

Steven R. Gambert

Edmund H. Duthie

More people are living to a maximal life span than ever before, resulting in an increasing number of elderly people. Persons aged 65 and older constituted 4% of the United States population in 1900 and presently comprise approximately 12%. By the year 2020, however, estimates place the population over 65 at 20%. This change in demographic structure will require physicians to be thoroughly skilled in those aspects of health care specific to the elderly. An apparent awareness of this problem has hastened the development of gerontology and geriatrics in the United States.

Gerontology is the study of the aging process as it affects the psychologic, sociologic, and biologic functioning. Geriatric medicine is that aspect of gerontology that deals with the diagnosis and treatment of diseases affecting the aged.

Morphologic and physiologic changes occur on a continuum from young adulthood through senescence and affect organ systems at different rates and at different times during the life span. This chapter is an attempt to introduce the health professional to some of the problems specific to the elderly.

A physician dealing with the problems of the elderly must be able to tell whether findings obtained from history-taking, physical examination, and laboratory evaluation are due to the normal aging process, a disease state, or to a combination of the two. This differentiation may alter both diagnostic and therapeutic management. The physician must be aware of how increasing age can alter disease presentation. A standard textbook on internal medicine describes bacterial pneumonia as presenting with a sudden onset of shaking chills, production of rust-colored sputum, pleuritic chest pain, and a high fever and white blood cell count. In elderly patients, however, pneumonia does not necessarily present in this way. An acute confusional state or minor change in mental status accompanied by a rise in pulse and respiratory rate may be all that is present. Once a diagnosis is made, treatment must be modified. Priority must be given to the prevention of dehydration and bedsores, and postural drainage and cupping must be individually designed to meet the needs of the elderly patient.

Other common diseases with unusual presentation in the elderly include myocardial infarction, hyponatremia, and hyperthyroidism.

In caring for the ill elderly, one must consider the multiple medical and psychiatric illnesses frequently seen. Economy of diagnosis does not necessarily apply as it does in a younger population. One must also consider quality of life and whether medical treatment will actually be of benefit. The geriatrician must be able to maximize a patient's potential despite chronic illnesses and disabilities. Most elderly people have at least one chronic disease and those institutionalized tend to have between three and six. Adverse drug effects occur commonly in the elderly. Working knowledge of drug side effects, interactions, and alterations of kinetics with aging is essential to all physicians caring for the complex and multifaceted illnesses affecting the elderly.

THEORIES AND PHYSIOLOGY OF AGING

Although scientific discoveries have done much to improve the quality of life, there has been little change of the maximal human life span (100-110 years). More and more people, however, are approaching this maximal life span than ever before. The human life span can be divided into three periods of development: embryonic life, maturation, and senescence.

There are numerous definitions for aging. Webster's Dictionary defines aging as "showing signs of growing old." Others define it as "anything after birth." Realizing, however, that the maximal number of brain cells is present in the first trimester in utero, even birth represents an advancement in aging. Aging is a process with an eventual end point, that is, 100% mortality; mathematicians tell us that as one approaches 30 years of age, the attainment of each successive 8 years doubles the chance of reaching this end point. Gerontologists define the aging process as something occurring in all members of the population (i.e., is universal) and is progressive and irreversible, at least as it is known today.

There are numerous theories on the aging process; however, chapter restraints do not permit a thorough review. In observing nature, it is apparent that there exist species differences in maximal life span. The mayfly lives only 1 day, the fruit fly 1 month, the shrew 1 year, the rabbit 10 years, and humans 100-110 years.

The Hayflick theory proposes that species differences in life span are due to differences in the ability of cell populations to multiply. It was observed that fibroblasts grown in tissue culture from long-lived species had a greater potential to double than fibroblasts grown in tissue culture from short-lived species. Martin et al. demonstrated a 20% decrement in population doublings of fibroblasts grown in culture for each year of life of the donor after maturity. It has been pointed out, however, that fibroblasts grown in tissue culture require fetal calf serum, making the model perhaps less than physiologic. In addition, not all species fit linearly into the pattern for population doubling described.

Another theory attempting to explain differences in maximal life span between species is the "hit theory." This theory states that ultraviolet irradiation causes damage to cells every day. Species better able to repair this cell damage live longer than those with less repair capability. Studies of skin fibroblasts grown in tissue culture provide evidence for this theory. The most active repairs of DNA are found in cells from humans, elephants, and cows, nearly five times as active as the cells from mice, rats, or shrews. However, although the hamster's life span is similar to that of the latter group its repair capability is intermediate, causing skeptics to question the validity of the theory. In addition, repair capability and life span are not proportional: humans live approximately 25 times longer than the rat, not five times as suggested by repair capability.

Another molecular theory proposes that aging is related to changes in the oxidation-reduction ratio of enzyme systems. These changes may result in altered cellular and organ function. The latter theory has been used by some to argue for the administration of antioxidants in an attempt to prolong life's processes.

In the 1930s, Cornell University biologist Clive McCay fed rats a diet low in fats and carbohydrate with a resultant decrease in age-related diseases and a prolonged life span for some of the group. Dietary influences on the endocrine and immune system continue to be studied and may lead to a better understanding of the aging process.

Other theories have focused on the endocrine system. For years, gerontologists have reported an age-related decline in human basal metabolic rate. Only recently has this decline been questionably associated with a decline in lean muscle mass. To make things more confusing, in the rat there is an approximate 60% decrease in oxygen consumption during the life span after corrections are made for lean muscle mass, changes in core body temperature, and analeptic stimulation. This parameter, minimal oxygen consumption (MOC), has been shown by W. Donner Denckla to have thyroid and athyroid components; the former is reduced with increasing age. Denckla also reported that thyroid hormone administration to older rats exerted a less stimulatory effect on MOC, implying some degree of tissue insensitivity to thyroid hormone. For years, gerontologists have noted similarities between senescence and thyroid hormone deficiencies. Both may present clinically with constipation, cardiomegaly, changes in mental status, and hypothermia, among other things. In an attempt to investigate this relationship, numerous studies on thyroid function and aging have been undertaken. Although it now appears that age-related changes in circulating thyroid hormone levels are negligible, data suggest that aging may be accompanied by a peripheral tissue insensitivity to thyroid hormone. More work needs to be done to better define this relationship.

Other endocrine theories on aging have included relationships to the thymus, pancreas, male and female gonads, and the pituitary. In the early 1970s, Denckla described a pituitary aging hormone named DECO (decreasing oxygen consumption hormone). Rats who had their pituitaries removed and were given back all hormones except a crude extract containing

DECO failed to exhibit the normal age-related decline in MOC. In addition, these rats did not grow old when the ability to reject grafts, grow hair, and respond to certain drugs was studied.

Whatever the actual cause of the aging process, no one theory presently is the accepted one. Only by further investigation and continued inquiry will a better understanding of senescence become a reality; perhaps then advances will be made to improve the quality and duration of life.

NUTRITIONAL ASSESSMENT AND REQUIREMENTS OF THE ELDERLY

Nutritional disorders are more frequently found among the elderly who are particularly prone to social isolation and mental and physical impairment compared to their middle-aged counterparts. Although all agree that the incidence of nutritional deficiencies is high among the hospitalized elderly, surveys from England and the United States imply that the general nutritional state of an overwhelming majority of the elderly at home is normal. In one study, only 3% of the elderly visited were considered to be malnourished, with the most common causes being prolonged illness, limited mobility, mental dysfunction, and domestic difficulties. It is important to remember, however, that nutritional inadequacy can exist before clinical signs become apparent.

PHYSIOLOGIC ALTERATIONS AFFECTING NUTRITIONAL STATUS

A number of age-related physiologic changes occur that can influence the nutritional state. The most important of these changes relate to the gastrointestinal, renal, and neuromuscular systems. Dental problems may result in an inability to properly chew foods; age-related changes in bone and soft tissue often cause dentures to fit improperly.

In humans, the ability of parietal cells to secrete hydrochloric acid declines with increasing age. There is also a general reduction in the secretory ability of the digestive glands. In addition, the ability to absorb calcium in the small intestine decreases after age 65. Despite these changes, xylose absorption remains normal until the ninth decade. It is apparent that aging can affect a large number of processes essential to the normal mastication, digestion, and absorption of nutrients.

Renal blood flow, glomerular filtration rate, Tm (tubular absorption) for glucose and PAH (para-aminohippuric acid) all decrease with age. The ability to form concentrated urine also decreases with age, and there is an age-related decline in the total number of nephrons. Although controversial, these data have been used by some to argue that certain minerals and proteins in the diet of the elderly should be restricted to avoid the accumulation of toxic degradation products.

The motor function of humans also declines with age. A decrease in the number of functioning muscle fibers and contractile elements may lead to declining strength. In both men and women, bone mass begins to decrease by the fifth decade, progressing at least twice as fast in women. Body composition studies in the elderly show a decrease in extracellular fluid and a loss of lean body mass; current evidence suggests, however, that persons with reduced lean body mass live longer. Recently, it has been shown that aged animals can actually increase adipocyte cells late in life, implying that obesity in the aged may be due not only to cellular hypertrophy but also to an actual hyperplasia within the adipose tissue. These age-related changes in body composition may affect nutritional assessment as well as requirements and food utilization.

DIETARY REQUIREMENTS

Although age-related physiologic changes suggest that nutritional requirements be modified in the elderly (Table 1), it is generally agreed that the same nutrients are required throughout life and only the amount of each may change in relation to health, sex, and age. A decreased muscle mass would suggest that protein and amino acid requirements may change with age. Renal impairment causes some investigators to question the soundness of high-protein diets. Changes in calcium absorption and bone mass cause concern over calcium and phosphorus intake. Decreased gastric acid production suggests an increased requirement of iron and, perhaps, vitamin B_{12}. It appears that total caloric requirements decline throughout life, though absolute amounts vary greatly between individuals, dependent largely on exercise, genetic makeup, and

Table 1. Recommended Daily Dietary Allowance for Adults 51 Years of Age or Older

	Men	*Women*
Energy (kcal, average)	2,400	1,800
Protein (g), average, 0.8 g/kg body weight)	56	46
Vitamins		
Vitamin A (RE)[a]	1,000	800
(IU)	5,000	4,000
Vitamin E	15	12
Ascorbic acid (mg)	45	45
Folic acid (μg)	400	400
Niacin (mg)	16	12
Riboflavin (mg)	1.5	1.1
Thiamine (mg)	1.2	1.0
Vitamin B_6 (mg)	2.0	2.0
Vitamin B_{12} (μg)	3.0	3.0
Minerals		
Calcium (mg)	800	800
Phosphorus (mg)	800	800
Iodine (μg)	110	80
Iron (mg)	10	10
Magnesium (mg)	350	300
Zinc (mg)	15	15

[a]Retinal equivalents.

environment. Despite these findings, recent studies suggest that protein requirements do not change with aging.

The current recommendation for daily protein intake is 0.8 g/kg ideal body weight, regardless of age. In addition, preliminary data suggest no age-related change in the requirement of the amino acids tryptophan and threonine.

Vitamin and Minerals

The estimated daily needs are vitamin C (50 mg), vitamin D (250 IU), vitamin A (5,000 IU), B_1 (0.8 mg), B_2 (1.3 mg), B_{12} (3 μg), and folic acid (400 μg). Vitamin deficiency in high-risk patients can be avoided by a daily supplement. Deficiency states are varied in presentation. A vitamin B_1 deficiency can lead to congestive heart failure, cramps, paresthesias, and memory impairment. A vitamin C deficiency can result in abnormalities in wound healing, fatigue, bleeding problems, hyperkeratosis of hair follicles, angular stomatitis, and atrophic changes in the mucosa of the mouth and tongue. Anemia can result from atrophic gastritis through iron and B_{12} deficiency. Trace mineral requirements are still being investigated. Calcium requirements will be discussed later.

CLINICAL CONSIDERATIONS OF MALNUTRITION

Although florid malnutrition is easily recognized, it is rare and frequently results from intentional nutritional neglect. The more common and more easily treated borderline or subclinical nutritional deficiencies seen in the aged are frequently difficult to identify; the physician can improve clinical care by applying a high index of suspicion to the elderly patient at risk. The physician must consider multiple factors in nutritional maintenance, that is, infirmity, economics, dental problems, depression, loneliness, poor housing, distance from stores, and/or a loss of interest in preparing a variety of foods. The "Meals-on-Wheels" program is not the cure-all. Frequently, on visiting the home of an elderly patient the refrigerator is found to be filled with well-balanced meals that have never been touched. One solution is to ensure that the elderly can afford to purchase and prepare food of the quality necessary to provide daily nutritional requirements. Anorexia must be specifically addressed. It is important to remember that normal physiologic changes accompanying aging may alter the nutritional state, despite adequate nutritional intake. Freedom of choice frequently provides incentive to eat.

PREVENTION OF MALNUTRITION

Prevention is the key to the treatment of nutritional deficiencies in the aged. The elderly should be informed as to which foods provide what nutrients and also the foods that are most beneficial. Protein is best provided from fish, soft cheese, lean meats, and fowl, as well as certain vegetables. Red meat, liver, and fortified cereals are rich in iron and vitamin B_{12}. When necessary, local dietary services should be used for counseling. At least 3 pints of fluid intake daily, including 1 pint of milk, should be encouraged.

There is much to learn about nutrition and aging; however, there are certain practical things that can be done to improve the nutritional status of the elderly such as to encourage eating a balanced diet high in fiber, adequate in calcium, iron, vitamin B_{12}, and low in saturated fats.

CLINICAL APPROACH TO THE GERIATRIC PATIENT

In approaching the elderly patient, the history and physical examination must be modified. Knowledge of home circumstances, optimally obtained from a home visit or an unbiased report of a home visit, is a necessary prerequisite to proper patient assessment. Through this mechanism, standards of living and support available at home, factors contributing to an illness such as malnutrition, poor habits and self neglect, relationships with relatives and friends, environmental impediments to normal function such as stairs for stroke victims or life in a high crime area, can be assessed. A geriatric team consisting of a geriatrician, physiatrist, nurse, geropsychiatrist, and social worker are often required to accomplish a total assessment of the elderly patient. Other disciplines, such as nutrition, audiology, ophthalmology, neurology, podiatry, dentistry, and recreational therapy, may be called upon frequently for assistance.

Knowledge of geriatric medicine derived only from hospital experience gives a distorted view of the aging process. Approximately 5% of the total elderly population are cared for by institutions, including hospitals, nursing homes, and extended care facilities. The vast majority of elderly individuals are either self-sufficient or provided for in private homes. Geriatric medicine should be community and not hospital oriented.

Although the world population will double in the next 35 years, the number of people 60 years of age or older is expected to double in only 30 years, with those over 80 increasing by more than 120% in this same time period. Increasing age is accompanied by an increased rate of illness and morbidity. The three leading causes of death in the elderly in the United States include cardiovascular disease, neoplasia, and stroke. Early detection of risk factors with appropriate intervention may lead to a better quality of life, perhaps with prolonged longevity.

The incidence of unreported disabling illnesses is high among the elderly. Although obvious complaints receive consideration, attention is rarely given to incapacitating but less dramatic conditions such as anemia, urinary incontinence, painful feet, musculoskeletal complaints with or without falls, and/or dementia.

Other factors to be considered when approaching the elderly patient include alteration in pain perception, altered pharmacology, and response to stress (homeostasis). The threshold of pain increases with aging, causing further diagnostic confusion. Conditions that cause intense discomfort early in life (pleurisy, peritonitis, fractures, myocardial infarction) may escape recognition. Altered handling of drugs due to changes in absorption, distribution, metabolism, and excretion must always be considered in treating the elderly. Recovery from an illness is frequently prolonged due to altered wound healing, predisposing malnutrition, and/or immunologic changes.

A clinician treating the aged must remember that diseases frequently have an insidious onset and that the elderly often have an altered response to a given illness. The routine physical examination usually reveals several pathologic conditions requiring medical attention. Cerebrovascular insufficiency and peripheral vascular diseases are common findings, as are arthritis, visual disorders, auditory disorders, cancer, neuromuscular disorders, and respiratory ailments. It is hoped that, as medical knowledge increases, the prevalence of these conditions will decrease. In the elderly, defining the cause for change in mental status presents a challenging task in that organic causes must be differentiated from the nonorganic. Geriatric medicine involves practicing the art of medicine to its fullest, an art requiring time and patience, consideration, gentleness, and tact.

MULTISYSTEM CHANGES DUE TO AGING

A full description of both the normal morphologic changes and the clinical pathologic trends that accompany aging is beyond the scope of this chapter. A brief discussion of a few of the age-related changes in key organ systems follows.

SKIN

Aging skin is classically thin, wrinkled, dry, and fragile, Senile purpura as well as Campbell-Morgan spots are prevalent. Nails are frequently deformed or atrophic, and greying of the hair occurs with increasing frequency. Morphologically, there are thickened blood vessels and degeneration of elastin. Skin pigmentation is increased, with atrophy of the hair follicles and sweat glands. Subcutaneous fat declines with aging.

CENTRAL NERVOUS SYSTEM

Eye

Due to decreased retro-orbital fat, the eyes of elderly people frequently appear recessed. Ptosis is common secondary to changes in soft tissue structures. Due to degenerative changes leading to lipid deposits in the cornea, an arcus senilis is seen that is probably of no consequence. Muscles of accommodation degenerate, leading to presbyopia. Visual acuity is decreased, as is the tolerance of glare, visual fields, and color vision. Pupils respond sluggishly to light and floating objects (muscae voitantes) are commonly reported. Stenosis of the lacrimal duct can lead to excessive tearing, while atrophy of the lacrimal gland may lead to corneal drying.

Ear

Presbycusis with impaired sound localization, cortical sound discrimination, perception, and tone sensitivity results from alterations in the elasticity of the basilar membrane, otosclerosis of ossicles in the middle ear, loss of cochlear nerves and temporal cortex, and degeneration of cells in the organ of Corti, respectively. Cerumen accumulation increases. Instability and potential falls can result from age-related degeneration of the hair cells in the semicircular canals.

Brain and Spinal Cord

Brain weight is reduced approximately 10% between the ages of 30 and 70, despite increased deposits of lipofuscin. Neuron numbers are also diminished. Neurofibrillary tangles, senile plaques, and vascular changes are common. Clinically, there is diminished perception and mental agility, and short-term memory as well as learning ability may be impaired. Performance as judged by standardized tests implies slower sensorimotor action. Nerve conduction velocity is reduced 10% by age 75, and impaired sensory awareness is almost universal with alteration in pain, touch, temperature, and position senses.

LOCOMOTOR SYSTEM

Aging is associated with a decline in size of muscle fibers, a decrease in muscle mass, and decline in physical strength, range, and speed of movement. Osteoporosis and osteomalacia are seen more frequently. Posture becomes stooped, and height decreases due to spinal column compression. Joints suffer from years of use with loss of elasticity in ligaments, cartilage, and periarticular tissues. Calcification of the joint capsule and cartilage frequently lead to disability.

GASTROINTESTINAL SYSTEM

Caries in teeth, periosteal bone resorption, and abnormalities of the gingiva lead to loss of dentition and may result in altered eating habits. There is a decrease in the total number of taste buds. Alterations in secretion, mobility, and absorption are due to atrophy of the gastric mucosa and intestinal glands and degenerative changes in the muscularis. Achlorhydria may result in defective absorption of iron. Achlorhydria is also associated with pernicious anemia and vitamin B_{12} deficiency. Digestive enzymes may be less efficient.

RESPIRATORY SYSTEM

Osteoporosis of the rib cage and vertebrae may cause kyphosis and increased chest wall rigidity. Reduced elasticity and calcification of the costal cartilage can lead to a weakness of the intercostal and accessory muscles of respiration, causing impaired functional reserve capacity, especially during stress. There is sclerosis of the bronchi and supporting tissues and degeneration of the mucous glands and bronchial epithelium. This entire process may result in decreased vital capacity and oxygen diffusion, leaving total lung volume unchanged. Due to a balance between diminished elastic recoil, increased lung stiffness, and decreased chest wall flexibility, little change in compliance is seen. Alveoli are often found to be coalescent due to atrophy and loss of septa elasticity. The aged have an increased incidence of pneumonia, pulmonary tuberculosis, bronchogenic carcinoma, and pulmonary embolism.

CARDIOVASCULAR SYSTEM

Aging is accompanied by intimal hyperplasia and loss of elasticity in the media of the aorta. Degeneration of the aortic valve cusps is commonly seen, frequently associated with nodular sclerosis and calcifications that may extend into the septum. The media may atrophy and the coronary arteries may show intimal hyperplasia. The incidence of atheroma in the coronary arteries increases with age, although it clearly begins early in life. The myocardium has deposits of lipofuscin, and myocardial fibrosis and amyloidosis are more commonly seen. In states of severe debilitation, brown atrophy may occur.

Clinically, the aorta is dilated and unfolded. Due to abnormalities in the bony thorax, the apical beat is frequently difficult to localize. Valve changes may result in murmurs, most commonly of the aortic and mitral valves. Cardiac output declines secondary to a decrease in stroke volume with a resultant decrease in exercise capability. For a given amount of work, blood pressure may rise more than in youth; however, the elderly may not be able to increase the heart rate in relation to need for increased cardiac output. Changes in mental status are often the best indicator of heart disease in the elderly. The incidence of arrhythmias, conduction defects, aortic stenosis, cor pulmonale, orthostatic hypotension, and ischemic heart disease increase with age. Ischemic heart disease is the most common cause of heart failure in the elderly.

GENITOURINARY SYSTEM

Age-related morphologic changes affecting this system include atrophy and a reduced number of nephrons, tubular degenerative changes, and thickening of the basement membrane of Bowman's capsule with resultant changes in permeability. There is a decrease in renal blood flow, glomerular filtration rate, and maximum excretory capacity, resulting in a less efficient kidney. This decline approaches 0.6% per year throughout life. One must remember that in the elderly even minor degrees of dehydration, obstruction, or changes in cardiac output may precipitate renal insufficiency with azotemia. Due to an age-related decline in lean muscle mass, a normal serum creatinine in the sixth decade of life may well represent a 50% decline in creatinine clearance from young adulthood, a finding that must always be remembered in clinical practice. Prostatic hypertrophy is almost universal; benign nodular hyperplasia approaches 70% in males 70 years of age, and histologic evidence of prostatic carcinoma is almost certain in males over 90, although clinical disease is less common.

There is an increased incidence in the elderly of gynecologic disorders, urinary retention, incontinence, renal infections, and calculi.

ENDOCRINE SYSTEM

Endocrine deficiency states are more commonly seen due to degeneration of the secretory systems, autoantibody production, and, perhaps, peripheral resistance to hormones. Although controversial, secretory capacity of the pancreatic β cell may decrease. This, and an apparent reduction in insulin receptors, may account for the increased glucose intolerance in the elderly. Criteria for the diagnosis of diabetes mellitus must take age into consideration.

The thyroid gland is less efficient. In laboratory animals, a decreased response of Na^+, K^+-ATPase, malic enzyme, and α-glycerophosphate dehydrogenase to T_3 stimulation imply a degree of peripheral tissue resistance. There is a decrease in minimal oxygen consumption in rats; in humans, basal metabolic rate decreases, although this may be due to a decline in total lean muscle mass. Little change is seen in serum T_4, although T_3 declines slightly. Myxedema is three to four times more common than thyrotoxicosis; thyroid hormone excess in the elderly frequently presents as apathetic hyperthyroidism, with minimal classic symptoms other than that of cardiac arrhythmias. Thyroid-stimulating hormone is significantly elevated in approximately 6% of patients over 60 years of age despite a clinical impression of euthyroidism by the primary care physician. In animals, pituitary adrenocorticotropic hormone (ACTH) shows a slight decline with age, while β-endorphin declines with age in the hypothalamus and corpus striatum. This may relate to the decreased ACTH secretion seen during severe stress and the altered thermoregulation accompanying aging.

COMMON PRESENTING SYMPTOMS IN THE ELDERLY

SYNCOPE

The differential diagnosis for syncope should include all the causes brought to mind in a younger person, such as metabolic, cardiovascular, or neurologic causes.

Metabolic causes for syncope are many, although predominantly due to hypoglycemia. Elderly patients being treated for diabetes with hypoglycemic agents are particularly prone to this disorder. Autonomic responses to hypoglycemia may be impaired, not only by age but also by other active disease processes or other drugs (e.g., propranolol) affecting the patient.

Cerebrovascular disease is a cause of fainting in the elderly. Decreased flow of blood to the brain can result from partial occlusion of the vertebral arteries with changes in neck position compromising blood flow. Emboli from blood vessels or the heart must be ruled out as a cause of transient ischemic attacks and syncope. A hypersensitive carotid is also known to cause faints.

Syncope can be the only symptom of acute blood loss. Myocardial malfunction from arrhythmias associated with conduction abnormalities or acute infarction may present with syncope. Cardiac valve abnormalities, especially aortic stenosis, are associated with syncope and should be ruled out.

Postural hypotension is commonly seen in the elderly. This is thought to be due to vascular rigidity and abnormalities in the baroreceptors and autonomic nervous system. Drugs resulting in autonomic dysfunction should be recognized and diabetes mellitus should be considered as a possible etiology. Falls with or without syncope may result from these defects in blood pressure regulation.

Primary central nervous system disease with or without seizure activity can result in syncope. Seizures are worrisome in the elderly since these may imply presence of space-occupying lesions such as a hematoma or tumor; most frequently, however, they are the result of a prior vascular insult.

CONSTIPATION

There are multiple reasons for constipation in the elderly; the most common are relaxation of the pelvic floor, insufficient intake of fluids and bulk-producing foods, immobility, and loss of abdominal muscle tone. As the patient becomes more concerned about constipation, laxative abuse leads to further bowel problems.

Since colonic carcinoma has an increased incidence in the elderly, an obstructing lesion must be considered upon initial complaint. Annual testing of stool for the presence of occult blood is advocated because it may lead to the early detection of malignancy. Other differential diagnoses include depression, metabolic disorders such as hypercalcemia, diabetic autonomic neuropathy, neurologic lesions of the spinal cord, and local anal pathology. Dietary changes with an increase in bulk foods and fluids may prevent constipation in the aged. Exercise is another nonpharmacologic measure that is thought to relieve constipation. Stool softners and bulk preparations are preferred over stimulants or mineral oil preparations in treatment of uncomplicated cases. A sympathetic approach with appropriate reassurance is underestimated but essential.

WEAKNESS AND FATIGUE

Frequently, the physician is faced with a decision as to whether complaints are significant. The elderly are no different from other groups and complaints should not be ignored. The physician must determine if symptoms are of recent onset or if they have been present for some time. Weakness or fatigue in an elderly patient who has always been active and vigorous may be the first indication of acute illness. Myocardial infarction may be painless, and fatigue that is occasionally associated with heart failure may be the only symptom of this cardiac disorder. Fatigue may be the only sign of anemia, infections, malignancy, hypoxia, hypokalemia, or other electrolyte abnormalities. Drug interactions and side effects must be considered. Anemia is more common in the elderly. What constitutes a normal hemoglobin is debated; however, it seems reasonable to say that a hemoglobin less than 12 g/dl in women and 13 g/dl in men is abnormal, regardless of age. The approach to this problem is the same as it would be for any group. To attribute anemia to old age is without scientific foundation and is poor medical practice. Depression and loneliness are also common causes of fatigue and are not infrequent in the elderly.

A distinction between generalized lassitude and true muscular weakness is essential. Although muscle strength declines with age, these changes should not affect the activities of daily living. Due to proximal muscle weakness, it may be impossible to rise from a chair. Inability to stand on the toes or to hold the hands extended for any length of time is also evidence of organic disease. The inability to perform because of pain must be distinguished from the inability to perform because of motor abnormality. A thorough neurologic evaluation may reveal a central or peripheral abnormality in the nervous system or a primary myopathy. Electromyography is one tool useful in distinguishing neurogenic from primary muscular disorders.

Hormonal imbalance must also be considered in evaluating fatigue. Hypothyroidism in the elderly may have an insidious onset with mental changes, apathy, cold intolerance, and alterations in skin, hair, and nails, all too commonly being recognized retrospectively. Anemia and muscle and joint pain are also commonly seen in this entity. Hyperthyroidism in the elderly may also present insidiously with insensitivity to the effects of thyroid hormone being common. The patient is frequently apathetic and appears depressed. Atrial fibrillation and congestive heart failure are common, as well as proximal muscle weakness. The thyroid is usually multinodular and only slightly enlarged.

Only after thorough questioning and physical and laboratory assessment can the common complaints of the elderly be properly evaluated. Attributing symptoms to the aging process without the proper knowledge of that process nor proper investigation of the complaint is a disservice to the patient. In addition, attributing too much to the aging process will give the patient a sense of helplessness and hopelessness that is unnecessary. The elderly as a group desire to be independent and healthy; they expect health professionals to take their complaints seriously. Using age to inappropriately explain a symptom weakens the patient's confidence in the health provider.

ANOREXIA

Often not a complaint, a history of anorexia may be elicited upon thorough questioning. Loss of appetite in the elderly may result from depression or organic causes. Once again, drug effects cannot be overlooked and toxicity from digoxin, sedatives, and other agents may result in reduced appetite. Dementia in its end stages is associated with a disinterest in food. Hepatic and renal insufficiency and cardiac cachexia are accompanied by anorexia and are usually clinically apparent.

Aging is associated with decreased sensations of taste and smell and, often, with a decreasing interest in food. Pain on swallowing, peptic ulcer disease, or abnormalities in the stomach due to tumor or atrophic gastritis must also be considered. A search for acute illnesses such as pneumonia or urinary tract infection is indicated and may provide a reason for the anorexia.

INSOMNIA

Insomnia is a common complaint in the geriatric population. Sleep deprivation may result in an impaired mental and physical state with diminished tolerance to pain, noise, and daily situations. In most cases, insomnia results from anxiety, pain, mental disturbance, and/or illnesses in which anxiety and fear are prominent symptoms. It is important to distinguish those patients with true insomnia from those who are seeking an unattainable quantity or quality of sleep, or sleep hypochondriacs. A specific diagnosis is important and illnesses that may be contributing to the pain, discomfort, and anxiety should be treated accordingly.

A number of agents are available to treat insomnia. Barbiturates should be avoided in the elderly because of cumulative effects with resulting confusion or paradoxical restlessness. Analgesics frequently provide relief of pain, the cause for insomnia. Chloral hydrate is a relatively safe agent and may be helpful. Major tranquilizers in low doses may be extremely useful in limiting the confusion, anxiety, and delusional problems that accompany dementia. Nonpharmacologic methods are preferred since any of the hypnotics can lead to psychologic dependence and may have hangover effects as well. Side effects may lead to falls at night, with subsequent fractures, or accidental hypothermia. Warm milk, possibly through the central effect of tryptophan increasing serotonin production, has long been a favored remedy for insomnia. Alcohol in small amounts may also be beneficial in this regard. Biofeedback, relaxation techniques, and sexual activity have all been employed in promoting sleep.

DEMENTIA

Dementia is the syndrome of progressive intellectual decline, and the differential diagnosis is quite large (Table 2). It is important for the physician to distinguish reversible from irreversible causes. It is estimated that as many as 4.4% of the 23 million people over the age of 65 in the United States have some degree of intellectual impairment. Some feel that senile dementia and related organic brain disorders reduce life expectancy, not to mention the effect on quality of life. Mental deterioration is a sad and frightening process for both patient and family.

The leading cause of dementia in the elderly is primary degenerative dementia, also known as presenile dementia or Alzheimer's disease. This accounts for 50-60% of cases of dementia in the elderly. The cause of this disorder is unknown and is the target of intense investigation. Cerebrovascular disease by itself is estimated to account for another 20% of cases of dementia and is distinguished at autopsy by multiple cerebral infarctions. When presented with a case of dementia, it is important to rule out treatable or reversible causes. Estimates vary as to the percentage of patients with dementia who have pseudodementia. Investigators argue that anywhere from 5%-40% of patients with dementia fall in this category. Causes of pseudodementia include depression or other emotional disturbances, drug effects, vitamin and nutritional deficiencies, or endocrinopathies, to name a few.

The approach to the patient requires a good history. Since the patient may be incapable of providing this information, family and friends also should be consulted. A rapid onset with an explosive course suggests an acute problem such as head trauma, infection, or drug reaction. An insidious onset with gradual memory deterioration followed by lapses in the social graces, personality change, and, finally, self-neglect is

Table 2. Causes of Dementia

Degenerative
Presenile
Parkinson's disease
Senile dementia
Cerebrovascular
Atherosclerosis
Arteritis
Lacunar infarcts
Nutritional
Malnutrition
Pernicious anemia
Vitamin B deficiency
Toxic
Drug reaction
Carbon monoxide
Alcohol
Heavy metal poisoning
Metabolic
Myxedema
Hypoglycemia
Hyperglycemia
Electrolyte imbalance
Hypercalcemia
Infection
Syphilis
Abscess
Mechanical
Tumor
Subdural hematoma
Normal-pressure hydrocephalus
Hydrocephalus
Miscellaneous
Hypoxia
Anemia
Trauma

more compatible with a degenerative disease. A history of symptoms similar to those just described but marked by periods of sharp decline, followed by a plateau phase with or without clear-cut neurologic deficit, is more compatible with a multi-infarct picture.

Physical examination is directed primarily toward the nervous system. Mental status examination is paramount in estimating the degree of disability. In addition, it is of major importance in distinguishing depression from dementia. Frontal release signs such as the palmomental reflex, snout reflex, and glabellar reflex are compatible with the diagnosis of primary degenerative dementia, but are not specific (i.e., they may be seen in healthy older people). Other findings may include resistance to passive movement, inability to follow commands (must be differentiated from aphasia), and a paucity of voluntary movement. Focal neurologic findings suggest a multi-infarct disorder or degenerative process such as Huntington's chorea or Parkinson's disease.

Dementia is a serious disorder. The diagnosis has profound medical and social implications and cannot be taken lightly. It is not an inevitable outcome of the aging process and requires a well-thought out diagnostic approach. Treatment is difficult and is directed at both the patient and family; the latter may benefit more from therapeutic efforts than the patient.

FALLS

One problem that is common in the geriatric population, but often goes unreported, is falling episodes. Falls are a serious health hazard for the elderly. They number in the top ten causes of death in the elderly; of all fatal falls in the United States, three-quarters occur in the elderly population. Too often, the medical approach to a fall is to check for injury and dismiss the patient. This approach is insufficient since it does not recognize that the fall is a symptom of some other problem that requires identification and possible treatment. Causes for falls include anything that impairs safe ambulation (i.e., visual acuity problems, neuromuscular disease, drugs, joint problems, etc.), environmental hazards, drop attacks, and anything that can cause syncope. Treatment depends upon the underlying problem. Efforts to improve safety in ambulation are best provided by physiatrists, physical therapists, and occupational therapists.

INCONTINENCE

Urinary incontinence is estimated to be present in 20% of the community-dwelling elderly. It is most commonly due to an uninhibited neurogenic bladder (detrussor hypersensitivity) and is frequently associated with abnormalities in mentation. It is often underreported because patients feel ashamed or feel that there is no hope for treatment, especially if they attribute this symptom to old age.

The evaluation and differential diagnosis involves knowledge of the process of micturition and age-related changes of the lower genitourinary system. For example, trigonitis may be due to estrogen withdrawal and can result in incontinence. Treatment involves a course of estrogen. With increasing age, it is known that bladder capacity declines and that detrussor contraction begins close to the time when the sensation of bladder fullness is first noted (unlike the situation in youth, where bladder capacity is greater and there is a lag between the time bladder fullness is sensed and detrussor contractions begin). The elderly individual may have urgency and precipitancy. At home, the patient allows for this by not taking fluids at night and arranging the home so that easy access to a bathroom or commode is possible. Acute illness with hospitalization results in a change in environment and less ability to cope with the urgency (e.g., how does one get out of a restraining jacket and overcome bed rails to get to a bathroom halfway down the hall in the hospital?). Therefore, transient incontinence in the sick hospitalized elderly is common and should never be assumed to be permanent until properly investigated. Indiscriminant use of catheters is to be condemned.

The effects of drugs that alter the cholinergic or adrenergic nervous system should always be considered in evaluating incontinence. Diuretics can lead to large urine flow and incontinence. Sedatives can alter the conscious perception that the bladder is full and therefore result in incontinence. Local factors, such as sacral spinal cord disease, autonomic nervous dysfunction (e.g., diabetes or tabes), prostatic hypertrophy, gynecologic abnormalities (lax pelvic floor, cystocele, urethrocele, uterine prolapse), and fecal impaction, can result in incontinence and are amenable to therapy.

PREVENTIVE GERIATRIC HEALTH CARE

Physician-patient contacts can be classified as either initial, interval, or episodic. The initial visit is the first planned visit and should include a comprehensive history and physical examination. Frequently, a multidisciplinary evaluation is necessary for the numerous problems of the geriatric patient. Interval visits are planned and include a limited history and complete or regional physical examination as indicated. Episodic visits for the evaluation of a specific concern are unplanned; these include either a comprehensive or limited history and a complete or regional physical examination as indicated.

GOALS

The goals of health maintenance as outlined by Breslow and Somers vary with age. In the young aged (60-75 years of age), it is important to faciliate prolongation of mature mental, social, and physical function. Attempts should be made to detect incipient disease and/or degenerative processes and to minimize disability from already established conditions. The physician must also begin preparing the geriatric patient for death. One must be especially aware of the following: hypertension; hyperlipidemia; hematological and immunological insufficiency; diabetes mellitus; chronic obstructive pulmonary disease, vascular insufficiency; renal insufficiency; malignancies; usage of tobacco, alcohol, and drugs; iatrogenic drug reactions; social and physical dependence; death of spouse or friends; decreasing physical or mental vigor; and neglect of diet, exercise, and estate planning.

In the older elderly (75 or older) an attempt should be made to facilitate independence in social, mental, and physical functions as well as detect diseases and degenerative processes. Help is needed to adjust to disability and dependence; often a multidisciplinary approach is necessary to accomplish these goals.

PHYSICAL EXAMINATION

An emphasis is placed upon the complete physical examination as the most reliable method for detecting existing and/or incipient disease. Only selected laboratory tests are recommended on a routine basis.

To accommodate differing goals, the frequency of a physical examination varies with age. Most feel a complete examination every 5 years, with a regional rectal and/or gynecologic examination annually, is sufficient in those 40-59 years of age. In the 60- to 74-year-old age group, complete examination every 2 years with annual rectal and/or gynecologic examination is recommended. Patients over 75 years of age deserve a complete physical examination annually. This is based on the prediction that each additional complaint between physicals will be individually evaluated as they surface.

Consistent with the concept of total health maintenance, regularly planned preventive dental and ophthalmologic evaluations are encouraged.

LABORATORY EVALUATION

Age-related recommendations for preventive laboratory testing have been provided by Olson et al. (1976).

Regardless of the presence or absence of symptoms, some argue that a urine culture should be done at the time of urinalysis for women patients. Although this may lead to a diagnosis of an asymptomatic urinary tract infection, it has not been demonstrated that treating this entity is beneficial to the overall health status of the elderly female patient; more data is needed in this regard. Stool for occult blood should be routinely obtained at the time of each rectal examination and patients over the age of 60 should have three stools tested annually for occult blood as an early indicator of occult colonic neoplasm. Yearly mammograms are recommended for women over 50 by the American Cancer Society. In females over age 70, the Pap test may be painful and have limited value due to the low incidence of cervical carcinoma in this age group. The pelvic examination, however, must always be done to rule out primary ovarian or vulvar pathology.

Patients either over 50 years of age or who are debilitated or suffering from an immunologic ailment should have an annual influenza inoculation. The recent introduction of a vaccine against pneumococcus (Pneumovax) is presently being evaluated by multiple centers, although data suggests that patients over 50 should receive this vaccine every 3 years. If not inoculated within recommended intervals, tetanus toxoid should be administered at the time of lacerations and puncture wounds. This is often overlooked and results in a relatively high incidence of tetanus in the elderly.

DEATH AND DYING

ATTITUDES

Every living thing, be it a plant, an animal, or even bacteria, shares the inevitability of death. Accidental death due to trauma is usually quick and without prolonged physical or mental suffering. Although some deaths due to natural causes can be equally as swift, some illnesses lead to prolonged pain, suffering, depression, and anxiety. Physicians and paramedical personnel working with the elderly must be particularly skilled in ensuring minimal suffering and maximal dignity with dying.

In many respects, the dying patient has medical needs similar to those of other ill patients but also has special needs. Terminal care begins when it has been decided that there is nothing to gain from efforts to prolong life. Treatment is aimed at symptom control and making dying a peaceful experience. Pain is frequently present, and its management provides a continuing challenge. A combination of drugs and varied administration schedules are indicated to keep the patient pain free while preserving mental alertness.

The patient must be assured of basic necessities such as warmth, fluids, food, and companionship. Fever may be associated with decreased diet and fluid intake leading to dehydration, constipation, fecal impaction, and severe discomfort. Electrolyte abnormalities may result in weakness and changes in mental status. Vitamin replacement is needed if diets are restricted.

Patients' questions must be answered completely by the appropriate person, be it physician, nurse, chaplain, social worker, or others. Thrusting information on a dying patient and providing empty reassurances must be avoided, although it is necessary to assure the patient that pain and fear can and will be managed when necessary.

Maintenance of the highest quality of life possible should be sought. The patient should be as symptom free as possible so that energy can be best utilized. A skilled health professional can provide relief of unpleasant symptoms to keep the patient and family comfortable. Approaching death upsets the equilibrium of the family unit, and attempts should be made to maintain the status quo regarding life style and life philosophies.

Care must be available 24 hours a day for both patient and family. Isolation and loneliness are significant sources of frustration to dying patients and problems may arise at any time. Education and counseling often help in making decisions since a physician cannot attempt to be all things to all people. A multidisciplinary approach should be utilized to encompass all the aspects of dying: legal, social, physiologic, spiritual, economic, or personal.

Frequently, patients and their families have difficulty dealing with the realities of death. It is important that this be recognized and that decisions to place the dying member in a hospice or other extended-care facility be supported. The elderly patient should be an active participant in decisions; infantilization must be avoided. The family should not be made to feel guilty or that they are abandoning their loved one. The physician skilled in geriatric health care must assume a coordinative function in providing a peaceful life-termination experience for both the dying patient and the grieving family.

SEDATION AND PAIN CONTROL

Every effort must be made to evaluate a complaint of sleeplessness or restlessness and to resolve any possible causes of anxiety or discomfort. Frequently, merely an encouraging word will prevent the need for medication.

Tranquilizers or hypnotics should not be given for anxiety or insomnia due to pain. Although elderly patients frequently have a higher pain threshold, complaints often are vague and poorly localized. When drugs are necessary, the physician should be aware of side effects and drug interactions, as well as what adjustments are necessary due to the aging process. Barbiturates should be avoided in the aged due to frequent paradoxical restlessness and confusion. Chloral hydrate (250-500 mg at bedtime) in the patient without severe liver impairment will provide adequate sedation in most cases, although it should be used only when needed.

Agitation can be treated with multiple agents, all with side effects. The most commonly used drugs in the aged include thioridazine, haloperidol, perphenazine, and chlorpromazine. The physician should be familiar with each drug and its side effects before prescribing it for a patient.

Pain thresholds vary from person to person and response to analgesics is unpredictable. The dose must be titrated on an individual basis. The physician must maintain patient confidence and aim to ensure a pain-free state, without necessarily worrying over drug addiction; however, as the pain lessens, dosage reduction is indicated. It is important to remember that anxiety over pain helps defeat the analgesic action of drugs.

Although the list of pain medications is great, the physician should use whatever he is most comfortable with, titrating dosage to need. Brompton's cocktail is an effective oral analgesic that is widely utilized in terminal care. The dose is 5-10 ml every 3-6 hours, as needed, and the ingredients are as follows:

Morphine sulfate	300 mg
Cocaine	200 mg
Gin (or pure ethanol)	100 ml
Honey (or simple syrup)	100 ml
Chloroform water (or distilled water) q.s. ad	400 ml

It is the physician's role to make dying less difficult, to know the prescribed drug, its effects and side effects, to titrate dosage on an individual basis, and use it regularly to assure a pain-free existence. It must be remembered that the aged frequently have paradoxical effects to drugs and often require only pediatric doses.

DRUG THERAPY IN THE AGED

Numerous physiologic changes accompanying the normal aging process must be considered to utilize drugs properly in the elderly.

For a drug to exert an effect, it must be absorbed from the site of administration and reach its site of action. Since aging is associated with changes in the gastrointestinal tract, including decreased arterial blood supply, the oral route may be theoretically compromised; however, studies have not shown this to be true to any great extent.

A drug must be distributed within the organism. Body composition changes with age: total body fat may increase twofold between the third and ninth decades. There is a decrease in extracellular body water. Circulating plasma albumin, a major source of drug binding, is decreased, although a marked decline probably reflects chronic illness. All these changes affect drug distribution. Fat-soluble drugs may actually accumulate to a greater extent, leading to a more pronounced and longer duration of action. Those that are protein bound may show less binding with age, allowing a more unbound drug to exert an effect. Warfarin, salicylate, phenylbutazone, and phenytoin are examples of drugs that are largely protein bound. Although a bioassay of drug levels ideally should be monitored, drug dosage generally should be reduced in the elderly.

All drugs are excreted; some are metabolized and then excreted. The kidney is largely responsible for excretion, either as a result of passive filtration at the glomerulus or by active secretion into the filtrate. Since renal blood flow and glomerular filtration decrease in the elderly, the elimination of a number of drugs, especially digoxin and antibiotics, are delayed and lead to higher plasma drug levels. Altered drug metabolism by the liver with increasing age has also been shown. Considerable attention has been directed toward alterations in receptor sites in the elderly. With aging, there is a decrease in the number of viable and active cells in various body tissues. In this regard, alterations in the central nervous system may result in a toxic confused state or hypotension following doses of anticholinergic drugs that are well tolerated by younger persons. The ability of amphetamines in aged rats to increase spontaneous motor activity is markedly depressed compared to young rats; however, its ability to suppress appetite is enhanced. A decrease in the number of cells with aging theoretically results in a greater effect merely on the basis of increased dose per milligram of active tissue. Thus, alloxan induces diabetes more readily in aged animals having fewer pancreatic β cells. It has also been demonstrated that the number of β receptors in various tissues also declines with age, leading to less stimulation by catecholamines. More investigation is required to clarify these concepts.

DRUG PRESCRIBING PRINCIPLES

The following principles may provide a useful foundation for drug usage in the elderly.

1. Determine whether the patient actually needs drug therapy. Weigh the risks of drug usage against the possible benefits.
2. Limit the amount of drugs used as much as possible. Drug interactions become a major concern as the number of medications grows, including those self-prescribed.
3. Choose the form of drug most easily administered, be it pill, syrup, or parenteral.
4. Titrate drugs depending on individual needs and not according to predecided dose recommendations.
5. Keep dosage schedules simple.
6. Inform the patient why the drug is being recommended, what side effects may occur, and what to do when side effects occur or the drug is not effective.
7. All prescriptions should be clearly labeled.
8. Be cautious of child-proof containers in the aged as they frequently are difficult for a patient with deformed or weak hands to open; all drugs should be kept out of the reach of children.
9. Instruct patients as to what should be done if a dose is missed in order to avoid taking all the missed doses at once.

MAJOR DRUG CLASSES COMMONLY USED IN THE ELDERLY

Psychotherapeutic Agents

Regardless of age, phenothiazines produce depression of the central nervous system and result in decreased excitement, anxiety, and tension. There appears to be no age-related change in the absorption, distribution, metabolism, or excretion of these agents; however, caution in the elderly is warranted. Associated hypotension occurs more frequently in the aged and it may be necessary to begin with a reduced dose, with dosage increases as side effects lessen. Phenothiazine usage in the elderly is also associated with an increased incidence of extrapyramidal signs and liver toxicity as compared to younger adults. Milder tranquilizing drugs, such as meprobamate and diazepam, may be useful adjuncts in the elderly and have minimal side effects when used in proper dosage; however, they tend to be sedating and possess muscle-relaxing properties. Haloperidol and thioridazine are often prescribed as antianxiety agents. The physician must be familiar with the individual drug side effects and use these drugs cautiously in the geriatric population.

Hypnotics and Sedatives

These drugs are frequently used in the elderly to reduce anxiety, tension, and insomnia. Although they produce a nonselective relief of anxiety, they have some of the characteristic side effects of the major tranquilizers. Older people may exhibit increased sensitivity to barbiturates, at times resulting in apprehension, disorientation, and even delirium. This has been questionably attributed to impaired renal function with resultant drug accumulation, reduced drug metabolism, and direct changes in the central nervous system. It is mandatory to individualize the dose and regimen. Flurazepam is perhaps the most useful nonbarbiturate sedative, although it may accumulate. Chloral hydrate (250-500 mg) is extremely effective in providing sedation with minimal side effects, but tolerance does develop and drug interactions can occur.

Antidepressants

Although both imipramine and amitriptyline appear to be equally effective in treating depression, imipramine appears to be less effective in the elderly than in the young.

Thyrotropin-releasing hormone, thyroid-stimulating hormone, and thyroid hormone have all been used in an attempt to treat depression and to synergize the actions of imipramine; however, data is generally inconclusive. In the elderly, it must be particularly remembered that thyroid hormone administration may cause severe cardiovascular complications and is generally contraindicated for this use alone in a nonhypothyroid patient. Tricyclic antidepressants frequently have multiple side effects including cardiac arrhythmias and hypotension, and extreme caution must be utilized in the use of all antidepressants in the aged. Monoamine oxidase inhibitors have decreased therapeutic efficacy in the aged and are capable of potentiating the action of a number of drugs. For these reasons, extreme caution should be exercised.

Narcotics

Potent narcotics must be used with caution in the elderly. There appears to be an increased sensitivity to the depressant action of morphine; respiratory depression and gastrointestinal and genitourinary difficulties also appear to be more common, mandating dose adjustments. Meperidine has serious side effects, notably hypotension, nausea, and dizziness. Methadone is considered by many as the drug of choice in the elderly requiring significant analgesia due to its low level of sedation or respiratory depression.

Antihypertensive Agents

When a decision is made to treat the elderly for high blood pressure, caution must be taken to prevent too rapid a reduction in blood pressure with resultant coronary and cerebral insufficiency. Sustained diastolic hypertension requires therapy in all age groups. The treatment of isolated systolic hypertension in the elderly is the subject of much controversy and current investigation.

Thiazide diuretics are frequently the drug of choice; side effects include hyponatremia, hypokalemia, hypercalcemia, hyperglycemia, and hyperuricemia. The physician must be aware of these side effects and treat accordingly. A low dosage should be employed initially.

Reserpine has limited usage because of a tendency to cause depression. Agents such as α-methyldopa and beta blockers should be reserved for patients with high blood pressure who fail to respond to salt restriction and diuretics and in whom a change in blood pressure is considered mandatory. Data suggests that ganglionic-blocking drugs may be less effective in the elderly, with a higher incidence of urinary retention and dizziness. Orthostatic hypotension is almost certain and patients should be made aware of this.

Propranolol can be utilized in the aged, although compromise in cardiac function and effects on limiting insulin secretion may provide enough negative benefit to prevent its usage.

Diuretics

Most studies indicate little change in the therapeutic efficacy of these agents; however, some feel that ethacrynic acid and furosemide are less effective in the elderly. Side effects relating to renal function are increased in the elderly, especially hypokalemia. Potassium-sparing diuretics such as triamterene and spironolactone can result in hyperkalemia in the aged with renal impairment. Dehydration must be avoided to assure adequate blood flow to body organs.

Digitalis and Digoxin

These agents continue to be the mainstay of treatment for atrial tachyarrhythmias and control of ventricular response. Despite a long history of use to promote inotropism, there is now some question as to whether tolerance develops and if indefinite treatment is indicated. The margin of safety is narrow and monitoring for toxicity must be ongoing. Prophylactic digitalization in the preoperative elderly patient has been recommended but it remains to be proven that this is of significant benefit. The risk of toxicity is well known. Changes in liver and renal function can result in increased side effects from digitalis and digoxin, respectively.

QUESTIONS

1. Elderly people represent what percent of the current total population in America?
   A. 3%
   B. 7%
   C. 12%
   D. 18%
   E. 25%
2. Dietary protein requirements in the elderly as compared to the young are:
   A. Greater
   B. Less
   C. No change
3. All of the following are popular theories on the aging process except:
   A. Finite cell population doubling
   B. Oxidation-reduction
   C. UV induced DNA damage
   D. Tissue insensitivity to hormones
   E. Chronic infections
4. The leading cause of dementia in the elderly (65+) is:
   A. Multiple infarcts
   B. Primary degenerative
   C. Normal pressure Hydrocephalus
   D. Syphilis
   E. Depression
5. The three leading causes of death in the elderly are:
   A. Arteriosclerotic heart disease
   B. Stroke
   C. Accidents
   D. Malignancy
   E. Suicide
6. All of the following can be used with impunity as hypnotics in the elderly.
   A. Barbiturates
   B. Chloral hydrate
   C. Flurazepam
   D. Diazepam
   E. None of the above
7. What percentage of the elderly (65+) are institutionalized?
   A. 1%
   B. 5%
   C. 8%
   D. 10%
8. As regards immunization in the elderly:
   A. Tetanus toxoid is not indicated since all old people are immune to tetanus.
   B. Influenza vaccine should be given annually.
   C. Pneumovax is recommended annually.
9. Brompton's cocktail is:
   A. Useful as a daily hypnotic
   B. A combination of gin, lime juice, and vodka
   C. A vitamin preparation
   D. A potent analgesic useful in terminal pain management
10. Causes of anorexia in the elderly include:
    A. Drug effects
    B. Age-related loss of taste buds
    C. Age-related loss of olfaction
    D. Presence of acute illness
    E. Depression

ANSWERS

1. C
2. C
3. E
4. B
5. A, B, D
6. E

7. B
8. B
9. D
10. All correct

BIBLIOGRAPHY

TEXTBOOKS AND MONOGRAPHS

Annual Review of Gerontology and Geriatrics, Vol. 1, 1980-. New York, Springer Publishing Co Inc, 1980.

Brocklehurst JC (ed): *Textbook of Geriatric Medicine and Gerontology*, ed. 2. New York, Churchill Livingstone Inc, 1978.

Butler RN: *Why Survive? Being Old in America*. New York, Harper & Row Publishers, Inc, 1975.

Caird FI, Judge TG: *Assessment of the Elderly Patient*, ed. 2. Tunbridge Wells, Eng., Pitman Medical, 1979.

Cape R: *Aging: Its Complex Management*. Hagerstown, Md., Harper & Row Publishers Inc, 1978.

Crooks JE, Stevenson IH (eds): *Drugs and the Elderly: Perspectives in Geriatric Clinical Pharmacology*. Baltimore, University Park Press, 1979.

Finch CE, Hayflick L (eds): *Handbook of the Biology of Aging*. New York, Van Nostrand Reinholdt Co, 1977.

Gambert SR (ed): *Contemporary Geriatrics*. New York, Plenum Press, 1983.

Kubler-Ross E: *On Death and Dying*. New York, Macmillan Publishing Co Inc, 1969.

Natow A, Heslin J: *Geriatric Nutrition*. Boston, CBI Publishing Co Inc, 1980.

Rossman I (ed): Clinical Geriatrics, 2nd Edition. Philadelphia: J. B. Lippincott Co., 1979.

ARTICLES

Breslow L, Somers A: Lifetime health monitoring: A practical approach to preventive medicine. *N Engl J Med* 296:601-8, 1977.

Gambert SR, Guansing AR: Protein-calorie malnutrition in the elderly. *J Am Geriatr Soc* 28:272-5, 1980.

Olson DM, Kane RL, Proctor PH: A controlled trial of multiphasic screening. *N Engl J Med* 294:925-30, 1976.

CHAPTER 8
HEMATOLOGY

Ashok K. Patel

R. Mala Vohra

GENERAL HEMATOLOGY

STRUCTURE AND FUNCTION OF BONE MARROW

Hematopoiesis occurs in the bone marrow, liver, and spleen in the fetus. During postnatal life, the bone marrow remains the principal hematopoietic organ in the body. In adults, active blood cell formation is confined to the vertebrae, ribs, skull, pelvis, and the proximal ends of the femur and the humerus; the marrow cavity of the remaining peripheral bones is occupied by fat. Active marrow is estimated to weigh about 2,600 g in adults.

The basic structure of marrow consists of islands of hematopoietic cells around a rich network of blood vessels within a framework of bony trabeculae. Branches of the central nutrient artery terminate into the venous sinuses. These channels are connected to the tributaries of the venous system that drains blood into general circulation. The venous sinuses are lined by a single layer of endothelial cells supported by discontinuous layers of basement membrane and adventitial cells. The latter are large reticular cells with fine branches extending into the perivascular space. Cords of hematopoietic cells are located in the extrasinusoidal space. Clusters of normoblasts and megakaryocytes are located close to the sinusoidal walls, whereas myeloid precursors are found in the deeper parts of the cell cords. Developing lymphocytes and monocytes have a tendency to lie close to the central portion of the hematopoietic cords near the central arteries.

In addition, the hematopoietic cords contain scattered, morphologically indistinct stem cells. Their presence is inferred from functional studies in lethally irradiated mice. These primitive cells comprise a compartment capable of self-renewal and maintenance of morphologically identifiable elements of the bone marrow. The normal marrow contains multipotential as well as unipotential stem cells.

On the basis of morphology, identifiable forms of normoblastic erythropoiesis include the proerythroblast, basophilic erythroblast, polychromatophilic erythroblast, orthochromatic erythroblast, and the reticulocyte and erythrocyte stage. On the average, three mitotic cell divisions occur between the proerythroblast and the orthochromatic erythroblast stages. Acquisition of a critical amount of hemoglobin is believed to be one of the factors causing extrusion of the nucleus from the orthochromatic erythroblast. The latter, along with the anucleated reticulocyte and erythrocyte, are incapable of cell division. Accumulation of hemoglobin in the cytoplasm continues up to the reticulocyte stage, during which about 35% of hemoglobin synthesis may occur.

Morphologically identifiable stages of granulopoiesis include the myeloblast, promyelocyte, myelocyte, metamyelocyte, and granulocyte (band and segmented) forms. Mitotic cell division occurs up to the myelocyte stage. In normal bone marrow, later forms of development predominate over the earlier stages. Depending on their cytoplasmic granules, myelocytes, metamyelocytes, and granulocytes are classified as neutrophilic, eosinophilic, or basophilic cells.

Maturation of the megakaryocytes is morphologically manifested by loss of basophilic staining of cytoplasm, accumulation of cytoplasmic granules, and increased lobulation of the nucleus resulting in polyploidy. Platelets are generated by fragmentation of the cytoplasm of megakaryocytes.

Mechanisms of release of mature cells from the extrasinusoidal location into the venous channels are incompletely understood. Increased deformability of reticulocytes, erythrocytes, and granulocytes may be one of the factors leading to a selective release of these elements into the circulation. Diapedesis in the case of granulocytes and mechanical factors in the case of erythrocytes and platelets may be additional factors governing the release of mature cells into the blood.

STRUCTURE AND FUNCTION OF THE LYMPHORETICULAR SYSTEM

The lymphoreticular system is the functional unit responsible for maintenance of the body's integrity and defense. Its cellular elements are composed of phagocytic cells such as granulocytes, monocytes, and macrophages, and lymphocytes that are involved in immune responses. Mobile components of the system are widely distributed throughout the body. The fixed portion of the system consists of bone marrow, spleen, Kupffer's cells of the liver, the thymus, lymph nodes, and numerous lymph follicles. The structure of the bone marrow has been described above.

The thymus is located in the anterior mediastinum. Dense aggregates of lymphocytes make up the cortex surrounding the medullary portion, which is composed of blood vessels, epithelial cells, lymphocytes, and macrophages. Thymus-derived lymphocytes (T lymphocytes) have an important role in cell-mediated immune responses.

The lymph node is a bean-shaped structure within the lymphatic system. It is covered by a fibrous capsule from which septa project inward to provide support for internal structures. Afferent lymphatic vessels perforate the convex surface of the capsule to empty into the subcapsular sinus. Septal extensions from the latter surround the lymph follicles. The cortex is made up of aggregates of lymphocytes with germinal centers supported by reticulin fibers. Central extensions of lymphocytes form medullary cords that converge onto the hilum. Ultimately, lymph drains through the efferent lymphatic at the hilum. The bone marrow-derived lymphocytes (B lymphocytes) are located in the follicles and medullary cords, whereas the T lymphocytes are located in the paracortical region of the node. In addition, clusters of lymphocytes are found in the mucosa of the gastrointestinal and respiratory tracts. These drain into the lymphatic system. The mucosal lymphocyte follicles play an important role in the host defense through immunoglobulin A secretion.

While granulocytes, monocytes, and lymphocytes are derived from pluripotential stem cells in the marrow, each cell line is maintained by a clone of unipotential stem cells. Granulocytes are actively phagocytic cells performing a variety of scavenging functions in the tissues following a brief sojourn in the bloodstream. Their kinetics in the tissues are largely unknown. Neutrophilic granulocytes react to a wide variety of stimuli and participate in the initial inflammatory reaction. They are capable of phagocytosis of invading organisms, destroying them by lysozymes. Eosinophils are known to participate in allergic tissue reactions. While the participation of eosinophils and basophils in chronic tissue reactions has been documented, their precise role is unclear. The monocytic macrophage series of cells have phagocytic and antimicrobial properties. These cells are also involved in initiation of the immune response and removal of senescent cells.

Lymphocytes can be divided into two principal groups: T lymphocytes and B lymphocytes. Their life span is brief but some cells (memory cells) survive for months to several years. Lymphocytes are involved in host defense through initiation and maintenance of humoral (B lymphocytes) and cell-mediated (T lymphocytes) immune responses. The lymphocyte, a phylogenetically recent innovation, has come to be recognized as the critical cell for immune defense throughout life. Through its subpopulations and derivative cells, the lymphocyte is involved in recognition of self and nonself at the biochemical level, tolerance of normal tissues, recognition of and immunologic reaction to a wide variety of antigens, immunologic recall and accelerated reaction on repeat antigenic encounter, and mobilization of an appropriate defense of cellular components whenever and wherever needed.

STRUCTURE AND FUNCTION OF THE SPLEEN

The normal adult spleen is covered with a layer of peritoneum, except at the hilum, and is held into position in the left hypochondrium by means of lienorenal and gastrosplenic ligaments. Its posterosuperior surface is apposed to the diaphragm; the anteromedial surface is in contact with the stomach, left kidney, left colic flexure, and the pancreas. The hilum, located on the visceral surface, allows passage of blood vessels, efferent lymphatic channels, and nerves. The normal spleen is clinically nonpalpable. It is estimated to weigh 100-250 g and contains 140 billion cells; its blood flow approaches 300 ml/min.

The spleen consists of a framework of connective tissue supporting specialized vasculature and lymphoreticular cells. The human spleen is covered by a thick, fibrous capsule that prevents active contractility. Internal extensions from the capsule form the trabeculae that support the blood vessels, lymphatics, and autonomic nerves. The trabeculae, in turn, are continuous with the reticulin framework of the splenic pulp. Branches of the splenic artery arborize along the trabeculae; arterial vessels in the pulp carry a dense cylindrical and nodular covering of lymphocytes (white pulp). The terminal branches of the arteries are devoid of adventitial and muscular coating. Some of them connect to the sinuses lined by fenestrated endothelial cells, while others end in the splenic cords. The latter surround the splenic sinuses and consist of reticuloendothelial cells, erythrocytes, granulocytes, lymphocytes, monocytes, plasma cells, and platelets (red pulp). The blood from the splenic cords passes readily into the sinuses that drain into venules and ultimately into the splenic vein via trabecular veins. Blood flow through the spleen is variable and largely controlled through the influence of the autonomic nerves on the arterial smooth muscle.

The spleen performs several functions including reservoir function, hematopoiesis, phagocytosis, iron storage, antibody formation, and storage of factor VIII. Approximately 30% of circulating platelets are reversibly sequestered in the normal spleen. These platelets can be mobilized by endogenous or exogenous epinephrine. There is no significant pool of mobilizable erythrocytes or granulocytes. During fetal life, the spleen is an active site of hematopoiesis. This function ceases in postnatal life. However, in pathologic conditions (chronic hemolytic anemia, myeloproliferative disorders) hematopoiesis may occur in the spleen. Splenic macrophages with phagocytic capability remove particulate foreign material as well as senescent and damaged blood cells from the circulation. These cells are also capable of removing intraerythrocytic inclusions (pitting function). The reticuloendothelial cells of the spleen contain a significant amount of usable iron stores in the body. The spleen participates in immunologic responses through removal and processing of intravenous antigens, interaction of macrophages and lymphocytes, and production of IgM antibody. The spleen also serves as a site of production and storage of factor VIII.

COMPOSITION OF BLOOD

Blood is a fluid tissue consisting of erythrocytes, leukocytes, and platelets suspended in plasma. In addition to performing the vital function of gas transport through erythrocytes, blood serves as a transport system for a wide variety of metabolic functions in the body, the sampling of which has led to the widespread use of blood examination in clinical medicine. Normal values for the formed elements are indicated in Table 1. It is important to recognize that the erythrocyte is fully functional within the circulation. The main function of platelets and leukocytes, however, is performed outside the vascular system, that is, at sites of vascular injury for platelets and extravascular tissues for leukocytes.

Table 1. Normal Values of Formed Blood Elements

Hematocrit	*Mean*	*Range*
Men	46	40-50%
Women	41	35-47%
Hemoglobin		
Men	15.5	13.3-17.7 g/dl
Women	13.7	11.7-15.7 g/dl
Cell Counts		
Red blood cell:		
Men	5.1	4.4-5.9 million/mm^3
Women	4.5	3.8-5.2 million/mm^3
Total leukocyte	7,250	3,500-11,000/mm^3
Platelet	275,000	150,000-400,000/mm^3
Reticulocyte	50,000	25,000-75,000/mm^3

APPROACH TO A PATIENT WITH A HEMATOLOGIC DISORDER

Care of a patient with a hematologic problem involves principles common to all clinical medicine, namely, accurate diagnosis followed by proper treatment. Alterations in the cellular elements of the blood are common clinical phenomena. These are far more commonly caused by disorders of other organ systems than primary hematologic disorders.

Pursuit of the diagnosis begins with a thorough history and physical examination and is followed by carefully selected laboratory examination. This may be supplemented by clinical observation periods depending on the nature of complaints. Success of the diagnostic search depends heavily on completeness and proper interpretation of the data base obtained from observations of the symptoms, signs, and laboratory abnormalities in light of the natural history of hematologic diseases.

Constitutional symptoms commonly encountered in hematologic practice include generalized weakness, malaise, fatigue, fever, weight loss, night sweats, and pruritus. Weakness, malaise, and fatigue are frequently caused by anemia, iron deficiency, and hematologic malignancies. Fever may occur in lymphoma and leukemia, although it is more frequently caused by a secondary infection than by the disease. Night sweats usually indicate low-grade fever due to infection or hematologic malignancy. Significant weight loss (10% of body weight) frequently accompanies advanced lymphoma, leukemia, disseminated carcinoma, and tuberculosis.

Neurologic symptoms include headache in anemia, polycythemia, intracranial infection, or hemorrhage, and meningeal involvement with lymphoma and leukemia. Paresthesia may accompany vitamin B_{12} deficiency, hematologic malignancy, and amyloidosis. Diplopia and impaired consciousness may be caused by intracranial bleeding, infection, and leukemic or lymphomatous infiltration. Jaundice may be seen in hemolytic anemia and megaloblastic anemia. Epistaxis and bleeding gums often accompany bleeding disorders, while dysphagia may reflect iron deficiency or pharyngeal ulceration and infection in agranulocytosis or leukemia. Painless cervical swelling from enlarged lymph nodes frequently accompanies lymphoma, infectious mononucleosis, and tuberculosis. Common cardiovascular findings include palpitations, exertional dyspnea, and leg edema in anemic patients. Localized chest pain frequently accompanies myeloma, leukemia, or herpes zoster. Bruising tendency, hemoptysis, hematemesis, and hematuria may be seen in bleeding disorders. Abdominal pain and discomfort may be an indication of pathologic enlargement of the spleen or liver. Back pain and paraplegia are occasionally seen in multiple myeloma and malignant lymphoma. Painful joint swelling, particularly of the knees, occurs frequently in hemophilia. Attention must be given to previous history of drug ingestion, radiation exposure, and amount of bleeding after surgical procedures; careful family history may yield important information on inheritance pattern of disease in patients suspected to have congenital spherocytosis, sickle cell anemia, and hemophilia.

Physical examination must be complete and must include attention to clues obtained during history-taking. Findings commonly encountered in patients with hematologic disease include pallor of mucous membranes and nails in anemia and flushing in polycythemia. Cyanosis may be found in methemoglobinemia, sulfhemoglobinemia, certain hemoglobinopathies, and excessive deoxyhemoglobinemia ($\geqslant$5 g/dl). Hemorrhagic skin lesions (petechiae, ecchymoses, hematomas) may provide valuable clues to bleeding disorders. Telangiectatic skin lesions may be helpful in the diagnosis of Osler-Weber-Rendu disease. Palpable enlargement of cervical, axillary, epitrochlear, supraclavicular, or inguinal lymph nodes may point to a diagnosis of lymphoma, leukemia, or certain chronic infections. Detection of enlargement of the liver and spleen may be important in the diagnosis of hemoglobinopathies, leukemia, lymphoma, myelofibrosis, and certain chronic infections. Signs of posterolateral spinal column degeneration may be found in pernicious anemia; partial or complete spinal cord compression may be seen occasionally in patients with myeloma and malignant lymphoma.

On the basis of information accumulated, it is possible to determine appropriate laboratory examination such as blood counts, blood smear examination, sedimentation rate, reticulocyte count, bone marrow examination, lymph node biopsy, radiologic studies and chemical and bioassay studies on plasma, serum, and urine as well as radioisotopic studies to arrive at the diagnosis.

Accurate diagnosis leads to appropriate therapeutic decisions and assessment of prognosis. In some cases (e.g., Hodgkin's disease), however, additional studies aimed at establishing the extent of the disease may be needed for proper therapy. A compassionate and humane approach with consideration for a patient's hopes and fears is essential for optimal patient care.

DISORDERS OF ERYTHROCYTES

PHYSIOLOGY OF ERYTHROCYTES

The main function of erythrocytes is transport of oxygen from the lungs to the tissues of the body. Under normal conditions, the intravascular red cell mass is precisely regulated to meet the oxygen requirements of the body through the erythropoietin mechanism and reserve generation capacity in the bone marrow. The concept of the erythron consisting of erythroid precursors in the marrow, and reticulocytes and erythrocytes in the blood, is useful in understanding the red cell physiology in health and disease. Development from proerythroblast to erythrocyte stage (7 days) involves cytoplasmic maturation leading to accumulation of hemoglobin and nuclear maturation resulting in mitotic cell division and progressive clumping of nuclear chromatin. Normally, intramedullary destruction of erythroid cells (ineffective erythropoiesis) amounts to less than 10%. Retardation in cytoplasmic or nuclear maturation may cause low erythrocyte production, with microcytic hypochromic or macrocytic normochromic red blood cells appearing in the peripheral blood.

The red blood cell is composed of 65% water and 34% hemoglobin, the remaining portion comprising electrolytes, stroma, lipids, enzymes, and organic and inorganic substances. The cell membrane is composed of 10% carbohydrate, 40% lipids, and 50% proteins. Its functions are to maintain cellular integrity through mechanical support as well as selective permeability and active ionic transport. Surface protein molecules of the membrane confer antigenic specificity to the erythrocyte. These antigens are important in blood transfusion.

Easily identifiable changes in red blood cell morphology on stained blood smears include microcytosis, macrocytosis, hypochromia, anisocytosis, poikilocytosis, acanthocytosis, spherocytosis, schistocytosis, ovalocytosis, stomatocytosis, burr cells, target cells, sickle cells, and teardrop cells. Occasionally, one may find intraerythrocytic inclusions such as Howell-Jolly bodies (nuclear remnants), siderotic granules (hemosiderin), blunt hemoglobin crystals (hemoglobin C), Heinz bodies (precipitated hemoglobin), and malarial parasites. The proerythroblasts and basophilic and polychromatic erythroblasts contain protein-producing machinery made up of DNA, RNA, ribosomes, and mitochondria, thus allowing production of all the necessary proteins for cell division and maturation. Mitotic cell division is preceded by a doubling of the DNA complement. An adequate supply of amino acids, enzymes, iron, vitamin B_{12}, and folic acid is necessary for normoblastic erythropoiesis. Deficiency of vitamin B_{12}, or folic acid may lead to defective DNA synthesis, resulting in abnormal nuclear maturation. Extrusion of the nucleus results in loss of DNA and the ability to synthesize RNA. Cellular RNA and protein synthetic capacity are lost as the reticulocyte matures into an erythrocyte. The erythrocyte can survive and function in the circulation for approximately 120 days. Inability to replace critical protiens leads to its destruction under physiologic conditions; in certain pathologic conditions, this natural destruction may be accelerated.

Hemoglobin is the major cytoplasmic protein produced during erythropoiesis. Progressive hemoglobinization of the cell is a useful morphologic indicator of cytoplasmic maturation. Adequate supplies of iron, protoporphyrin, and globin are necessary for normal hemoglobin production. Transferrin-bound serum iron serves as the immediate source of iron for the developing erythroblast. Iron absorbed from the bowel and reticuloendothelial iron stores replenishes the serum iron. Hemoglobin synthesis may be limited by iron deficiency, or a block in the release of iron from reticuloendothelial stores may occur, as in certain chronic infections. Protoporphyrin is a tetrapyrrole compound produced in the mitochondria from glycine and succinylcoenzyme A. It combines with ferrous iron to form heme. One binding site of heme iron is firmly attached to globin, while the other binds reversibly with oxygen. Conversion of ferrous to ferric iron leads to formation of methemoglobin and loss of oxygen-carrying capacity. In sideroblastic anemia, abnormal mitochondrial metabolism results in hemoglobin synthetic defect caused by insufficient heme production. Mitochondrial iron accumulation gives rise to the characteristic ringed sideroblasts. Globin, the protein component of hemoglobin, is made up of a pair of α and a pair of non-α polypeptide chains. In postnatal life, erythrocytes contain three types of hemoglobin, that is, hemoglobin A ($\alpha_2\beta_2$), hemoglobin F ($\alpha_2\gamma_2$), and hemoglobin A_2 ($\alpha_2\delta_2$). Individual genes control the synthesis of each of the polypeptides. During fetal life, γ chains are produced in abundance so that fetal hemoglobin makes up the major hemoglobin. During infancy, a switch to predominately β chain production leads to a preponderance of hemoglobin A in children and adults. Genetic abnormalities may cause structural changes in the globin chains and lead to formation of hemoglobins with altered physical and physiologic characteristics. Diseases resulting from such genetic anomalies are called hemoglobinopathies. Abnormal genes may occasionally cause a quantitative defect in globin chain production leading to thalassemia. The syntheses of globin and heme are closely coordinated. Impaired globin synthesis (thalassemia) leads to a decrease in heme synthesis. Thus, an iron, heme, or globin deficit may lead to a hemoglobin synthesis defect resulting in the production of microcytic hypochromic erythrocytes.

Energy requirements for oxygen transport are negligible. A continuous source of energy, however, is needed to maintain the integrity of the cell membrane and hemoglobin and enzyme systems as well as constancy of intracellular electrolyte composition. Almost 90% of the energy is derived from anaerobic glycolysis (Embden-Meyerhof pathway). Three supplementary pathways (hexose monophosphate shunt, Rapapport-Luebering shunt, and methemoglobin reduction pathway) help maintain hemoglobin in a functional state and provide a small amount of metabolic energy. Breakdown of each molecule of glucose results in a net gain of two molecules of high-energy phosphate (ATP) and helps to maintain pyrimidine nucleotides in a reduced form. The hexose monophosphate shunt requires utilization of oxygen, provides metabolic energy, and maintains adequate amounts of reduced glutathione, thus diminishing oxidant stress on functioning hemoglobin. Impaired activity of this metabolic pathway (e.g., glucose-6-phosphate dehydrogenase deficiency) leads to increased vulnerability of erythrocytes to oxidant stress and hemolysis. The Rapapport-Luebering pathway permits the generation of 2,3-diphosphoglycerate at the expense of generation of ATP. The former has the capacity to bind to deoxyhemoglobin and promote oxygen delivery to the tissues by shifting the oxygen dissociation curve to the right. The methemoglobin reductase pathway is important in enzymatic reduction of methemoglobin and maintenance of ferrous iron in heme. Abnormalities in this pathway can lead to methemoglobinemia. A complex molecular configuration of hemoglobin is responsible for the heme-heme interaction, changing oxygen affinity and the Bohr effect. Packaging of hemoglobin into erythrocytes (as opposed to hemoglobin dissolved in plasma), the tertiary and quaternary structure of hemoglobin, intraerythrocytic 2,3-diphosphoglycerate, and the ability of deoxyhemoglobin to bind to 2,3-diphosphoglycerate have important roles in normal oxygen delivery. In clinical practice, alterations in oxygen-delivering capacity because of changes in the 2,3-diphosphoglycerate content of erythrocytes are more common than changes in pH or temperature.

After an average normal life span of 120 days, the senescent erythrocytes are destroyed by the splenic macrophages (extravascular hemolysis). The hemoglobin is broken down to heme and globin. The amino acids from the latter enter the amino acid pool. The protoporphyrin ring is broken at the α-methane bridge, with generation of carbon monoxide and bilirubin. Iron stored in the macrophages in the form of hemosiderin is reutilized for erythropoiesis. Bilirubin is conjugated with glucuronide, excreted into bile, and converted to urobilinogen in the bowel. A fraction of the conjugated bilirubin is absorbed in the gut and reexcreted through the liver, a small amount appearing in the urine. In conditions accompanied by predominantly extravascular hemolysis, there are increased amounts of products of hemoglobin breakdown. In some conditions, the breakdown of erythrocytes occurs in the vascular compartment. In these circumstances, the tetrameric hemoglobin breaks down into dimeric form and is initially bound to haptoglobin. When the serum haptoglobin is saturated, hemoglobinemia and hemoglobinuria ensue. In chronic intravascular hemolysis, filtered hemoglobin is processed by the renal tubular cells and excreted in the urine as hemosiderin. Small amounts of methemalbumin are also found in the blood.

The mass of circulating red cells is precisely regulated by appropriate adjustments in erythropoiesis, so that in both the normal and abnormal steady state, the rate of erythrocyte production equals the rate of destruction. Thus, the static indices of the erythron (e.g., hemoglobin concentration, RBC count) may be supplemented by kinetic parameters of red blood cell production and destruction. The production rate (effective erythropoiesis) is estimated from the reticulocyte count. Since reticulocytes normally survive for 1 day in the circulation, the number of circulating reticulocytes represents red blood cell production for 1 day. Under normal circumstances (production index, 1), the average reticulocyte count is 1% (reference range, 0.5-1.5%). In pathologic conditions, the actual reticulocyte count has to be corrected for the absolute number of red blood cells and erythropoientin-induced shift reticulocytosis. At hematocrit values of 45, 35, 25, and 15, the correction factors for the latter are 1, 1.5, 2, and 2.5, respectively. Rarely, ferrokinetic studies may be needed to estimate total and ineffective erythropoiesis.

Hemolysis is defined as shortening of red blood cell survival. The destruction rate of erythrocytes may be determined by direct (e.g., ^{51}Cr tagged red blood cell survival) or indirect (e.g., serum bilirubin, lactic dehydrogenasc, urine urobilinogen, endogenous carbon monoxide production) tests. In practice, indirect tests suffice for most clinical problems and direct erythrocyte survival studies are rarely needed.

ANEMIAS

Anemia is defined as a reduction in the circulating red blood cell mass. In practice, the erythrocyte count, the hemoglobin concentration, or the packed cell volume are used as estimates of the presence and degree of anemia. The importance of recognition of and systematic approach to anemia lies in the fact that it may be an early sign of disease in a variety of organ systems and that it may be improved in some cases by therapy with iron, folic acid, vitamin B_{12}, or red blood cell transfusions.

From the viewpoint of erythrokinetics, anemia is the result of a negative balance between red cell production and loss. On the basis of etiology, anemia can be classified into:

1. Hypoproliferative anemias
   a. Iron deficiency
   b. Sideroblastic anemia
   c. Megaloblastic
   d. Anemias from disturbed stem cell function
      i. anemia of chronic disease
      ii. aplastic anemia
2. Hemolytic anemias
   a. Congenital
   b. Acquired
3. Blood loss anemias
   a. Acute
   b. Chronic

Another useful classification of anemia, based on morphology of erythrocytes, is:

1. Macrocytic normochromic
   a. Megaloblastic (folate or vitamin B_{12} deficiency)
   b. Miscellaneous (liver disease, hypothyroidism, temporarily macrocytic due to reticulocytosis)
2. Normocytic normochromic
   a. Acute blood loss
   b. Hemolytic anemia
   c. Anemia caused by bone marrow failure
3. Microcytic hypochromic
   a. Iron deficiency
   b. Thalassemia
   c. Sideroblastic anemia

Hypoproliferative Anemias

Iron Deficiency Anemia

Iron deficiency anemia is caused by an impairment in erythropoiesis resulting from insufficient supply of iron for hemoglobin synthesis. Most of the body's iron (90%) is contained in hemoglobin and storage iron such as hemosiderin and ferritin. Small but functionally significant forms of iron include myoglobin, heme enzymes, and transferrin-bound iron. Iron balance is regulated through control of iron absorption. In normal adult males, 1 mg elemental iron is absorbed to replace daily losses. In pathologic conditions, loss of iron in the form of chronic blood loss may be the principal cause of negative iron balance. In the developed countries, chronic bleeding from the gastrointestinal and the female genital tracts are the commonest cause of iron deficiency. Chronic blood loss from hookworm infestation is a frequent cause of chronic blood loss in many developing countries. Unusual causes of iron loss include paroxysmal nocturnal hemoglobinuria, pulmonary hemosiderosis, and repeated blood donations. Dietary deficiency and malabsorption are relatively uncommon causes of iron deficiency in clinical practice. Physiologically, increased requirement of iron occurs during infancy, puberty, pregnancy, and the childbearing years in women. These patients are prone to iron deficiency despite normal dietary iron intake.

Manifestations of iron deficiency anemia depend on its duration and severity. In mild cases, there may be only abnormal laboratory findings. More severe cases may present with tiredness, malaise, easy fatigability, headache, palpitation, exertional dyspnea, or pica (a craving for unnatural foods). Pallor of mucous membranes is a common sign. Occasionally there may be papillary atrophy of the tongue, cheilosis, jugular venous distention, cardiac enlargement, edema of the feet, and koilonychia.

Laboratory diagnosis of iron deficiency depends upon demonstration of anemia, hypochromic and microcytic erythrocytes in more severe cases, low red blood cell production index, decreased serum iron with increased transferrin, and a low serum ferritin level. Absence of stainable iron stores in bone marrow aspirates is presently the most reliable marker of iron deficiency.

Other causes of microcytic and hypochromic anemia include thalassemia, sideroblastic anemia, chronic lead intoxication, and hemoglobin C disease. They can be distinguished from iron deficiency by high serum iron, increased transferrin saturation, elevated ferritin, increased bone marrow hemosiderin, and characteristic findings of the individual conditions.

Objectives of management of iron deficiency anemia include correction of anemia and replenishment of iron stores, and identification of the cause of iron deficiency and its treatment.

Oral ferrous sulfate therapy (300 mg t.i.d.) is the least expensive and the best way to achieve the first objective in most patients. Rarely, it may be necessary to administer iron parenterally because of a malabsorption syndrome or gastrointestinal upset due to ferrous sulfate. Success of the treatment is manifested by reticulocytosis around the sixth day, rising hemoglobin level around the ninth day, and correction of anemia in 4 to 8 weeks. Replenishment of iron stores may require an additional 3 months of treatment. This sequence of events and the duration of iron therapy would, of course, be modified by the degree of success in achieving the second objective of treatment.

Identification and treatment of the primary cause of the iron deficiency are essential to the total care of the patient. Duration of iron therapy is related to whether the primary bleeding lesion can be controlled. For example, definitive surgical treatment of colon carcinoma may stop further bleeding and limit the duration of iron treatment. On the other hand, a patient with Osler-Weber-Rendu disease may require indefinite iron therapy because the lesions may not be surgically resectable. For individuals prone to iron deficiency anemia (e.g., infants, pregnant women), preventive iron therapy is recommended.

Sideroblastic Anemia

Sideroblastic anemia is a heterogenous group of disorders characterized by microcytic hypochromic or dimorphic anemia, elevated serum iron, increased transferrin saturation, high serum ferritin level and ringed sideroblasts in the bone marrow. Impairment of mitochondrial iron metabolism results in accumulation of hemosiderin in the mitochondria. Since the latter are distributed in the perinuclear zone, hemosiderin accumulation in the erythroblasts leads to the development of ringed sideroblasts.

Most cases are attributable to alcoholism, lead intoxication, isoniazid and other antituberculous drugs and certain hematologic conditions such as megaloblastic anemia, thalassemia, leukemia, lymphoma (secondary sideroblastic anemia). Rarely sideroblastic anemia is a manifestation of a myeloproliferative disorder (primary sideroblastic anemia). The treatment of secondary sideroblastic anemia consists of withdrawal of the offending drug or alcohol and the treatment of the associated disease. Primary sidroblastic anemia is managed with supportive red blood cell transfusions. These patients may eventually develop acute non-lymphoblastic leukemia which responds poorly to chemotherapy. In some patients sideroblastic anemia is hereditary; some of these and a few patients with acquired sideroblastic anemia show partial response to large doses of pyridoxine.

Megaloblastic Anemia

Megaloblastic anemias are a group of disorders characterized by retardation of DNA synthesis leading to defective nuclear maturation. The effects of the biochemical abnormality are most pronounced on rapidly dividing cell systems throughout the body (e.g., bone marrow, bowel mucosa). Morphologic abnormalities occur in the erythrocyte, granulocyte, and platelet precursors in the marrow. Since RNA synthesis and protein synthesis are relatively unimpaired, hemoglobin synthesis proceeds normally in the developing erythroblasts. Asynchrony of nuclear and cytoplasmic maturation gives rise to large cells with fine nuclear chromatin and advanced hemoglobinization (megaloblasts). The end product of megaloblastic erythropoiesis consists of macrocytes and macro-ovalocytes with normal mean corpuscular hemoglobin concentration; myeloid cell abnormalities consist of giant metamyelocytes and hypersegmented neutrophils. Ineffective erythropoiesis, myelopoiesis, and thrombopoiesis are frequently seen in these patients. More than 90% of cases of megaloblastic anemia are caused by vitamin B_{12} or folic acid deficiency. Derivatives of these vitamins are essential cofactors in the conversion of uridylate to thymidilate, which is critical in DNA synthesis. Patients with Di Guglielmo's disease, certain congenital enzyme deficiencies, and drug-induced megaloblastosis account for the remainder of cases. Common causes of megaloblastic anemia are listed in Table 2.

Clinical manifestations of megaloblastic anemia depend on the cause and severity of the process. Symptoms of slowly progressive anemia, such as fatigability, malaise, tiredness, headache, irritability, are common. Occasionally, the patient may present with bleeding or infection because of pancytopenia. Soreness of the tongue from papillary atrophy is a common finding. In patients with vitamin B_{12} deficiency, there may be paresthesias, unsteadiness of gait, paraparesis, loss of sensation in the legs, loss of ankle jerks, or extensor plantar reflexes. These are caused by various degrees of peripheral neuropathy and degeneration of the posterolateral columns of the spinal cord. Neurologic findings are usually seen in patients with severe macrocytic anemia; however, in some cases the anemia may be disproportionately mild. In alcoholic or diabetic patients with peripheral neuropathy and folic acid deficiency, the neurologic findings may mimic those seen in vitamin B_{12} deficiency.

Table 2. Common Causes of Megaloblastic Anemia

1. Vitamin B_{12} deficiency
   - A. Pernicious anemia
   - B. Total gastrectomy
   - C. Fish tapeworm infestation
   - D. Malabsorption syndromes
   - E. Blind loop syndrome
2. Folic acid deficiency
   - A. Dietary deficiency
   - B. Chronic alcoholism
   - C. Pregnancy
   - D. Malabsorption syndrome
   - E. Drugs (e.g., phenytoin, oral contraceptives)
3. Refractory megaloblastic anemia
   - A. Di Guglielmo's disease
   - B. Congenital enzyme deficiencies (orotic aciduria)
   - C. Cytotoxic drugs (e.g., Ara-C, 6-thioguanine)

Diagnosis depends primarily on the presence of macrocytic normochromic anemia, hypersegmentation of neutrophils, varying degrees of leukopenia and thrombocytopenia, and megaloblastic changes in the marrow. Low serum levels of vitamin B_{12} (<100 pg/ml) and folic acid (<3 ng/ml) are good screening tests for vitamin B_{12} or folic acid deficiency. In vitamin B_{12} deficiency, it is necessary to perform a ^{57}Co-labeled vitamin B_{12} absorption test (Schilling test) for distinction of gastric from intestinal causes of vitamin B_{12} malabsorption. Rarely, therapeutic trials using physiologic amounts of vitamin B_{12} (1 μg) and folic acid (75 μg) may be necessary to determine the primary cause of megaloblastic anemia. The diagnostic search should not be considered complete until the cause of the vitamin deficiency (e.g., pernicious anemia, total gastrectomy, dietary deficiency, pregnancy) is identified.

Pernicious anemia is characterized by megaloblastic anemia, gastric achlorhydria, and neurologic damage (subacute combined degeneration, peripheral neuropathy and long tract and posterior column degeneration). There is a lack or deficiency of intrinsic factor and a thermolabile glycoprotein secreted by the parietal cells of the stomach, leading to insufficient absorption of vitamin B_{12}. Antibodies directed against gastric parietal cells are found in 84% of patients with pernicious anemia. There is an increased incidence of Hashimoto's thyroiditis, adrenal atrophy, hypoparathyroidism, and gastric cancer in patients with pernicious anemia.

Management consists of administration of pharmacologic doses of vitamin B_{12} (1000 μg/day) or folic acid (1 mg/day). After an initial period of intensive treatment, monthly maintenance treatment with vitamin B_{12} (100 μg) is needed in cases where there is permanent impairment of vitamin B_{12} absorption. Appropriate measures are initiated for the treatment of the primary cause of the vitamin deficiency. In patients presenting with severe anemia (hematocrit below 15%) or with anemia and congestive cardiac failure, use of packed red blood cell transfusion is recommended for symptomatic relief. Success of the treatment is indicated by subjective improvement and reticulocytosis by the fourth day, followed by a steady rise in the hemoglobin during the following 4 to 6 weeks. Recovery of the neurologic deficit is slow. Residual neurologic changes after 18 months are likely to be permanent. With appropriate management, correction of the anemia can be brought about in all cases of megaloblastic anemia with vitamin deficiency.

In the remaining few cases, treatment is directed at the cause of megaloblastic anemia. In drug induced megaloblastosis, spontaneous improvement occurs after withdrawal of the drug. Administration of uridylic acid corrects the megaloblastic anemia in orotic aciduria.

Anemias Related to Disturbance of Stem Cell Function

Anemia of Chronic Disease. This is the most common form of anemia seen in clinical practice. The anemia is usually not severe enough to require treatment. It may serve as an early signal and lead to a proper diagnosis of and care for the primary disease. The anemia is associated with low serum iron, low iron-binding capacity, increased marrow iron stores, increased serum ferritin, and relative bone marrow failure.

This form of anemia is seen in association with chronic infections, malignancy, chronic liver disease, chronic renal failure, collagen diseases, and endocrine disorders. Shortened erythrocyte survival in association with inadequate compensatory erythropoiesis leads to anemia. Iron metabolism is found to be abnormal. A relative block in the transfer of iron from the reticuloendothelial stores into the transferrin-bound pool leads to low serum iron hemosiderosis with decreased sideroblasts in the marrow and compromises the erythropoietic capacity. Occasionally, the iron metabolism may be sufficiently deranged to give rise to hypochromic red blood cells in the presence of increased iron stores.

Clinical manifestations of anemia are mild nonspecific symptoms such as malaise, tiredness, and easy fatigability. These are usually overshadowed by the symptoms of the primary disease. Diagnosis is made primarily on the basis of normocytic normochromic anemia, hypoferremia, low transferrin saturation, and a low red blood cell production index with increased iron stores. As mentioned above, occasionally the red blood cells may be hypochromic and microcytic. Distinction from iron deficiency anemia in such cases may be aided by the elevated serum ferritin level and the demonstration of increased hemosiderin in the marrow. Other conditions giving rise to normocytic normochromic anemia such as aplastic anemia, drug-induced marrow suppression, anemia of blood loss, and metastatic replacement of the marrow should be excluded by appropriate tests. Treatment of anemia of chronic disorders is aimed at the underlying disease. However, if a specific substrate deficiency (e.g., iron, folic acid) complicating the disease is identified, appropriate therapy will improve the anemia to some extent. Control of the primary disease frequently leads to an improvement of the anemia.

Aplastic Anemia. Aplastic anemia is a bone marrow disorder characterized by stem cell failure resulting in subnormal hematopoiesis and varying degrees of pancytopenia. Marked hypocellularity of the marrow is a characteristic finding. In about 50% of the cases, no cause of the disease can be found. The remainder can be attributed to marrow damage by prior exposure to drugs, chemicals, radiation, or a variety of associated diseases (e.g., viral hepatitis, miliary tuberculosis, pancreatitis). Whether the disease affects primarily the stem cells or the microenvironment of the marrow is uncertain. Among the agents known to cause aplastic anemia, some produce marrow damage consistently if the dose and duration of exposure are sufficiently large. These include x-rays and a number of cytotoxic drugs, such as nitrogen mustard, cyclophosphamide, busulfan, melphalan, methotrexate, 6-mercaptopurine, cytosine arabinoside, daunomycin, adriamycin, carmustine (BCNU), lomustine (CCNU), and chlorambucil. In other cases, pancytopenia is idiosyncratic, as in the case of drug exposure to chloramphenicol, phenylbutazone, and gold compounds.

Clinical manifestations of aplastic anemia are related to the extent of decrease of erythrocytes, leukocytes, and platelets. Severe anemia may result from underproduction of the red blood cells and hemorrhagic complications may result from thrombocytopenia. Some patients may present with fever and other manifestations of infection as a consequence of granulocytopenia. Findings on physical examination may include pallor, tachycardia, cardiac enlargement, hepatomegaly, edema of the feet, fever, oral ulcerations, petechiae, or ecchymoses.

Diagnosis of aplastic anemia is based on demonstration of pancytopenia in association with a hypocellular bone marrow. Erythrocytes are usually normocytic and normochromic but may be macrocytic occasionally. The reticulocyte count is consistently low for the degree of anemia. The bone marrow aspirate usually reveals marked hypoplasia with a relative increase in lymphocytes, plasma cells, reticulum cells, and mast cells.

Treatment of aplastic anemia consists of general supportive measures depending on the degree of pancytopenia. These include erythrocyte transfusions for severe anemia, platelet transfusions for bleeding thrombocytopenic patients, and, rarely, leukocyte transfusions for patients with severe granulocytopenia and documented infection. Androgen therapy may bring about a partial or complete remission of anemia; however, improvement in granulocytes and platelets is often not as satisfactory. In patients with severe aplastic anemia (reticulocyte count, $<1\%$; granulocyte count, $<500/mm^3$; platelet count, $<20{,}000/mm^3$) bone marrow transplantation from an HLA-compatible donor should be given serious consideration. With proper selection of the donor and immunosuppressive treatment of the recipient, the risk of graft rejection and graft-versus-host disease can be minimized. In patients with severe aplastic anemia treated with supportive measure only, the median survival is approximately 4 months. Protected environment, such as reverse isolation, can prolong survival. Patients with less severe pancytopenia may survive for several years with supportive treatment and androgens.

Hemolytic Anemias

Hemolytic anemias are a group of disorders characterized by a shortened red blood cell life span. They can be classified as congenital or acquired (Table 3). The former are associated with an intracorpuscular defect. The acquired causes of hemolysis are accompanied by extracorpuscular abnormalities such as antibodies, toxins, altered metabolites, or abnormal hemodynamics.

Clinical manifestations in hemolytic anemia are related to the degree of anemia and the cause of hemolysis. Physical findings may include pallor, tachycardia, signs of congestive cardiac failure, jaundice, and splenomegaly. Normocytic normochromic anemia with an increased production index is an important laboratory sign. Examination of the blood smear may reveal abnormalities that are quite distinctive for certain hemolytic anemias such as sickle cells, spherocytes, ovalocytes, and fragmented cells. Other laboratory findings may include elevated unconjugated serum bilirubin, increased urine urobilinogen, increased serum lactic dehydrogenase, low haptoglobin, high serum iron with increased transferrin saturation, and a high serum ferritin level. Although demonstration of shortened red blood cell life span by measurement of ^{51}Cr-tagged erythrocyte survival provides the most direct evidence for hemolysis, it is rarely needed in clinical practice.

Table 3. Classification of Hemolytic Anemia

- I. Congenital
  - A. Membrane defects
    1. Spherocytosis
    2. Ovalocytosis
    3. Stomatocytosis
  - B. Enzyme deficiencies
    1. Glucose-6-phosphate dehydrogenase
    2. Pyruvate kinase
  - C. Hemoglobinopathies
    1. Sickle cell disease
    2. Hemoglobin C disease
  - D. Thalassemias
- II. Acquired
  - A. Immune hemolysis
  - B. Mechanical hemolysis
  - C. Infectious agents
  - D. Mismatched transfusion and Rh incompatibility
  - E. Liver diseases
  - F. Renal diseases
  - G. Drugs, toxins, venoms, and physical injuries
  - H. Hypersplenism

Congenital Hemolytic Anemias

Congenital hemolytic anemias are characterized by chronic hemolysis with onset at an early age. Family history, ethnic background, and the presence of characteristic red blood cell abnormalities are helpful in determining the cause of congenital hemolytic anemia. Spherocytosis, ovalocytosis, and stomatocytosis are transmitted as mendelian dominant traits; each is accompanied by a characteristic morphologic red blood cell abnormality. Patients with hereditary spherocytosis may have splenomegaly and elevated mean corpuscular hemoglobin concentration levels; the osmotic fragility of the red cells is characteristically reduced. Splenectomy results in remission of the hemolytic anemia, even though the morphologic abnormality persists. Hereditary ovalocytosis is infrequently associated with severe hemolytic anemia. Splenectomy leads to improvement in hemolysis in these patients. In rare cases of hereditary stomatocytosis with severe hemolytic anemia, splenectomy leads to partial remission of hemolysis.

The severity of hemolytic anemia caused by glucose-6-phosphate dehydrogenase (G-6-PD) deficiency varies in different ethnic groups. The abnormality is inherited as an X-linked recessive trait and occurs in approximately 10% of American blacks and more rarely in other racial groups. These patients have normal red blood cell survival under ordinary circumstances. Oxidant stress, such as bacterial infection or exposure to certain drugs (antimalarials, sulfonamides, dapsone, >10 g/day aspirin, nitrofurantoin, and water-soluble vitamin K, menadiol), may produce episodic acute hemolysis. The

Mediterranean variety of G-6-PD deficiency is usually more severe and results in chronic hemolytic anemia. Pyruvate kinase deficiency is the most common erythrocyte glycolytic enzyme deficiency. The pattern of inheritance is autosomal recessive. This enzyme deficiency leads to chronic hemolytic anemia and splenomegaly. Splenectomy results in only partial remission of hemolysis.

Structural abnormalities of the hemoglobin molecule can bring about alterations in chemical and physical properties of hemoglobin and lead to chronic hemolytic anemia. Homozygosity for HbS (sickle hemoglobin) causes a severe hemolytic disease characterized by recurrent episodes of pain and shortened life expectancy. Deoxyhemoglobin S has a tendency to form crystals and give rise to the rigid deformed red blood cells (sickle cells). Obstruction of the microvasculature by the sickle cells leads to multiple organ damage from microinfarctions; hence, the protean manifestations of the disease.

The sickle crisis is a painful and dramatic experience. A PO_2 of 35 to 45 mm Hg may not uncommonly occur in the liver and kidneys, and usually suffices to produce deoxygenated hemoglobin S. On the other hand, in chronic hemolysis the clinical signs relate to anemia and jaundice. Recurrent thrombosis of splenic arterioles and venules leads to hyposplenism and red blood cells with Howell-Jolly bodies. Hepatomegaly and hepatic dysfunction may result from intrahepatic vascular occlusions or from hepatitis arising from multiple transfusions. Pigment gallstones may require cholecystectomy. After repeated episodes of pulmonary thrombosis and infection, cor pulmonale can occur. Cardiac auscultation frequently reveals systolic flow murmurs. Occlusion of cerebral arteries and dural sinuses can produce varying neurologic signs. Renal papillary necrosis leads to hematuria and impaired renal concentrating ability. In patients with sickle cell anemia, there is a high incidence of salmonella osteomyelitis and pneumococcal meningitis. Pregnancy can be hazardous, as hypoxemia and sickling can lead to fetal-maternal complications. Diagnosis is based upon the demonstration of normocytic normochromic anemia, a high red blood cell production index, sickle cells in peripheral blood, the presence of hemoglobin S, and absence of hemoglobin A. No specific therapy is available. Folic acid is prescribed because of increased requirements of the vitamin in these patients. Management of painful crises consists of treatment of precipitating events such as infection. Analgesics, adequate hydration, and, occasionally, partial exchange transfusions may be helpful palliative measures. Aplastic crises are treated with red blood cell transfusions. Chronic leg ulcers tend to heal with simple local measures; however, repeated blood transfusions may occasionally be needed to promote healing.

Homozygous hemoglobin C disease is an uncommon disorder characterized by splenomegaly and mild chronic hemolytic anemia. Heterozygous sickling disorders such as sickle cell thalassemia and sickle cell hemoglobin C disease usually cause mild chronic hemolytic anemia and are frequently associated with splenomegaly.

The thalassemia syndromes are a heterogeneous group of inherited disorders characterized by retarded production of structurally normal globin chains of hemoglobin. Two major categories are recognized: β-thalassemia and α-thalassemia corresponding to the underproduction of the respective β and α globin chains. Homozygous β thalassemia causes a severe chronic hemolytic anemia requiring blood transfusion therapy, hepatosplenomegaly, and death in early adult life. Heterozygous β thalassemia is usually accompanied by mild hemolysis and is compatible with a normal life expectancy. Homozygous α thalassemia is usually found in the Orient and invariably results in stillbirth with hydrops fetalis. Other forms of α thalassemia result in mild or no hemolysis and usually require no treatment.

Acquired Hemolytic Anemias

These acquired disorders can be subclassified according to the extracorpuscular abnormality responsible for hemolysis. Antibody-mediated hemolytic anemias can be divided into those caused by warm antibodies (usually γG) and cold antibodies (usually γM). The former group of hemolytic anemias are characterized by a positive direct antiglobulin (Coombs') test and antibodies (γG) directed against red blood cell antigens. Immune hemolysis may be encountered in patients with systemic lupus erythematosus, chronic lymphocytic leukemia, malignant lymphoma, or after sensitization to certain drugs, such as penicillin, methyldopa, or quinidine; in some cases, no apparent cause of antibody formation is found (idiopathic). The clinical severity of hemolysis is variable. Diagnosis is based on the presence of normocytic normochromic anemia with spherocytes and increased production index, unconjugated hyperbilirubinemia, elevated serum lactic dehydrogenase, and positive direct Coombs' test. Withdrawal of the offending drug is effective in controlling hemolysis in drug-induced hemolytic anemia. In most of the remaining cases, corticosteroid therapy is effective in inducing a remission of hemolysis. For patients who fail to respond to steroids or require prolonged high doses, splenectomy may be needed to control hemolysis. Rare cases of failure of splenectomy may be controlled by immunosuppressive therapy with cyclophosphamide or azathioprine.

Occasionally, hemolytic anemia may be caused by a cold-reactive antibody (cold agglutinin). The most frequent form is a self-limited hemolytic anemia in association with mycoplasmal infection. It may also be seen in association with systemic lupus erythematosus and malignant lymphoma. Corticosteroids and splenectomy do not improve hemolysis due to cold agglutinins.

Mechanical hemolytic anemia results from conditions in which excessive shear stress leads to fragmentation of erythrocytes. Disseminated intravascular coagulation from a variety of causes, turbulent blood flow around abnormal cardiac valves, and giant cavernous hemangioma may be accompanied by such hemolysis. Diagnosis depends on the demonstration of fragmented red blood cells (schistocytes) and hemosiderinuria from intravascular hemolysis in the peripheral blood. Management consists of the treatment of the primary disease. Iron supplementation may be needed when there is chronic iron loss from hemosiderinuria.

Hemolytic anemia may be seen in association with infections. Malarial parasites invade the red cells and bring about hemolysis. Similarly, hemolytic anemia may be found in infections with *Bartonella* and *Clostridium* spp. Treatment of the infection leads to an improvement of hemolysis. Other causes of hemolysis include mismatched transfusion, rhesus incompatibility, liver diseases such as alcoholic liver disease and viral hepatitis, uremia, drugs (Azulfidine, dapsone, phenacetine, sodium percholate, and vitamin K analogs), heavy metals (lead), snake venom and drowning, accidental intravenous administration of sterile water, and burns.

The term hypersplenism refers to the varying degrees of hemolytic anemia, leukopenia, and thrombocytopenia because of an enlargement of the spleen that may result from a wide variety of conditions such as hepatic cirrhosis lymphoproliferative and myeloproliferative disorders connective tissue disorders, tuberculosis, sarcoidosis, Felty's syndrome, and other infectious diseases. Diagnosis is established by the demonstration of normocytic normochromic anemia with an increased production index and splenomegaly. Splenectomy leads to a correction of the hemolytic anemias as well as leukopenia and thrombocytopenia.

Blood Loss Anemias

Acute Hemorrhagic Anemia

Anemia related to acute blood loss is normocytic normochromic morphologically. Besides trauma and surgery, the gastrointestinal and female genital tracts are frequent sites of acute overt blood loss. Significant occult bleeding can occur in the large muscle compartments and body cavities. Clinical manifestations depend upon the degree and rate of blood loss, site of bleeding, and the general condition of the patient. Loss of as much as 10-20% of blood volume over a short period (as in blood donation) does not produce any significant circulatory disturbance in previously healthy individuals. Acute loss of 30-40% of blood volume causes marked circulatory impairment and a loss of half the blood volume is usually fatal. Blood loss is not manifested by a fall in the hematocrit immediately because of the associated loss of plasma volume, but there may be immediate reactive thrombocytosis and leukocytosis. It can take up to 3 days for the hematocrit to reach the nadir. In uncomplicated situations, the platelet count and the leukocyte count return to normal within a few days and the hematocrit starts to rise. The mean corpuscular volume may be increased because of reticulocytosis. Management during the hypovolemic phase consists of immediate restoration of blood volume with intravenous fluids and red blood cell transfusions. When the bleeding is caused by thrombocytopenia or coagulopathy, additional blood components should be administered.

Chronic Blood Loss

Chronic blood loss causes iron deficiency anemia, which is discussed in a previous section.

POLYCYTHEMIAS

Polycythemia is a condition characterized by an elevated hemoglobin level. Polycythemia may be an incidental finding on a routine laboratory test or the patient may present with complaints related to a markedly elevated hematocrit. A single laboratory value of elevated hemoglobin or hematocrit should be rechecked and, if confirmed, investigated. The first step in evaluating such a patient is the documentation of elevated red cell mass as the hematocrit may be spuriously elevated due to contracted plasma volume. In general, a red blood cell mass of more than 32 ml/kg in women and 36 ml/kg in men is considered abnormal. Polycythemia may result from a myeloproliferative disorder (polycythemia vera), or may be secondary to elevated erthropoietin levels (secondary polycythemia). The latter may be elevated either appropriately in response to tissue hypoxia or inappropriately as in patients with certain neoplastic and renal disorders (Table 4).

Polycythemia Vera

Polycythemia vera (P. vera) is a myeloproliferative disorder resulting in overproduction of not only red blood cells but also keukocytes and platelets. Polycythemia vera usually has an insidious onset. Clinical manifestations are caused by increased blood volume and blood viscosity because of expanded red blood cell mass, and thrombotic and hemorrhagic tendencies related to platelet abnormalities. Nonspecific neurologic symptoms, such as headache, dizziness, and vertigo, are the most frequent presenting symptoms. Generalized pruritus, especially after a warm bath, may occur in about 50% of the patients. An important physical finding is splenomegaly in approximately 75% of the patients. The disease runs a chronic course over a number of years and may terminate in myelofibrosis with myeloid metaplasia (spent phase) or acute myeloblastic leukemia. Whether the development of acute leukemia is a part of the natural history of the disease or related to therapy is presently uncertain, but it seems likely that both factors play a role. Diagnostic criteria for P. vera, as used by the National Institutes of Health-sponsored Polycythemia Vera Study Group, have been categorized into two groups according to their significance.

Category A

A_1: Increased red blood cell mass: Female ⩾32 ml/kg
Male ⩾36 ml/kg

Table 4. Causes of Polycythemia

I. Primary: Polycythemia Vera
II. Secondary
  A. Decreased tissue oxygenation
    1. Pulmonary diseases
    2. Congenital heart disease
    3. Hypoventilation syndromes
    4. Abnormal hemoglobins
  B. Inappropriate erythropoietin production
    1. Neoplasms
    2. Renal cyst
    3. Hydronephrosis

A_2: Normal arterial oxygen saturation: 92%

A_3: Splenomegaly

Category B

B_1: Thrombocytosis: Platelets $\geqslant$400,000/mm^3

B_2: Leukocytosis: Leukocytosis $\geqslant$12,000/mm^3 (in absence of fever or infection)

B_3: Elevated leukocyte alkaline phosphatase score: >100 (in absence of fever or infection)

B_4: Elevated serum vitamin B_{12} or unbound vitamin B_{12} binding capacity: B_{12} $\geqslant$900 pg/ml, UB_{12} BC $\geqslant$2,200 pg/ml

All three cateogry A features, or A_1 and A_2 in the presence of two parameters of the B category, are necessary to establish the diagnosis.

Once the diagnoisis of P. vera is established, repeated phlebotomies are effective in restoration to normal red blood cell mass and plasma volume along with immediate symptomatic improvement. For patients requiring more than four phlebotomies every 3 months to maintain near-normal hematocrit, other measures aimed at control of basic myeloproliferative disorders are required. Irradiation in the form of radioactive phosphorus or alkylating agents like chlorambucil (Leukeran) and busulfan (Myleran) are quite effective in controlling the disease. For older or unreliable patients, ^{32}P is preferred because of its ease of administration, fewer side effects, and prolonged effect. Chlorambucil or busulfan has been used intermittently to keep the blood counts near normal levels. Because of the unacceptably high risk of acute leukemia associated with chlorambucil, it should not be used in this disease. Elective surgery should be undertaken only when the disease has been under effective control for at least four months to avoid surgical complications. Treatment has resulted in prolongation of survival in this disease.

Secondary Polycythemia

Secondary polycythemia is associated with elevated amounts of erythropoietin, which is appropriate in situations associated with tissue hypoxia as occurs in congenital cyanotic heart disease, chronic obstructive pulmonary disease, and alveolar hypoventilation. It can also occur as a compensatory phenomenon due to low atmospheric pressure, and in situations with defective oxygen transport as occurs in certain hemoglobin variants and following toxic exposure to coal tar derivatives and carbon monoxide from heavy smoking that cause tissue hypoxia. Hypernephroma, hepatoma, leiomyoma of the uterus, cerebellar hemangioblastoma, and pheochromocytoma may occasionally produce ectopic erythropoietin and result in erythrocytosis. In addition to renal tumors, hydronephrosis, cystic disease, renal artery stenosis, and other renal disorders occasionally may be associated with erythrocytosis. Management consists of treatment of the primary disease. Occasionally, signs and symptoms related to hyperviscosity may require phlebotomy.

DISORDERS OF LEUKOCYTES

PHYSIOLOGY OF WHITE BLOOD CELLS

The white cells in the blood constitute a compartment in dynamic equilibrium with the bone marrow (production site) and the tissue leukocyte pool. There is a unidirectional movement of leukocytes from the marrow into the blood and then into the tissues. Approximately one-half of the blood leukocytes circulate freely while the remainder are sequestered in the marginal pool from which they can be recruited by a variety of physiologic, pharmacologic, and pathologic stimuli. In the steady state, the circulating leukocyte count is a fair measure of the leukocyte production. The half-life of the circulating granulocyte is 7 hours. The life span of the granulocyte in the tissue compartment and the size of the tissue compartment are largely unknown. A wide variety of physiologic and pathologic conditions may change the flux between the various leukocyte compartments resulting in an altered circulating leukocyte count for short periods. Significant changes in the rate of leukocyte production result in a sustained change in the circulating leukocyte count. The normal values for leukocyte count are listed in Table 5.

Table 5. Normal Leukocyte Values in Peripheral Blood

	Total Number (cells/mm³)		
Cell Type	*Mean*	*95% Confidence Limits*	*Percent of Total Leukocyte Count*
Leukocytes	7,250	3,500-11,000	100
Neutrophils	4,300	1,870-6,730	55
Band neutrophils	600	100-2,000	10
Segmented neutrophils	3,700	1,000-6,000	45
Lymphocytes	2,700	1,490-3,930	36
Monocytes	500	140-860	6
Eosinophils	230	0-570	2
Basophils	40	0-120	1

DISORDERS OF GRANULOCYTES

The disorders involving leukocytes are caused by quantitative and qualitative abnormalities (Table 6).

Granulocytopenia

Leukopenia is defined as a white blood cell count of less than $3500/mm^3$; neutropenia refers to a neutrophil count of less than $1800/mm^3$. The differential white blood cell count in conjunction with the total leukocyte count is helpful in distinguishing relative neutropenia from true neutropenia. There are numerous causes of leukopenia (Table 6); neutropenia accounts for the vast majority of clinically significant leukopenias and the risk of infection is markedly increased when the absolute granulocyte count is less than $500/mm^3$. The patient's history, as in many other fields of medicine, is tremendously important in the clinical evaluation of the neutropenic patient. Drugs are the most common cause of neutropenia. Physical examination may reveal fever, bone tenderness, lymphadenopathy, splenomegaly, arthritis, and other features suggestive of rheumatoid arthritis, collagen disease, or malignancy. Examination of the blood smear may show a decrease in the white blood cells along with platelet and erythrocyte abnormalities in some cases. In patients with persistent neutropenia, bone marrow examination may provide valuable diagnostic information. Drug-related marrow suppression usually improves with discontinuation of the drug. Treatment of the primary disease usually leads to an improvement of leukopenia related to infection and megaloblastic anemia. Leukopenia secondary to hypersplenism is usually well tolerated and rarely requires splenectomy.

Leukocytosis and Leukemoid Reactions

Neutrophilic leukocytosis associated with a left shift (a greater rise of band neutrophils than of segmented neutrophils) is frequently seen in patients with bacterial infections. Leukocytosis is also seen in patients with severe burns, after major surgery, in patients with myocardial infarction, in certain metabolic disorders like diabetic ketoacidosis, in poisoning by various chemicals as a consequence of drug exposure, or malignant disorders. Effective treatment of the primary disease leads to a restoration of the leukocyte count to a normal level. Leukemoid reactions are characterized by leukocytosis and the presence of immature cells of the

Table 6. Classification of Granulocyte Disorders

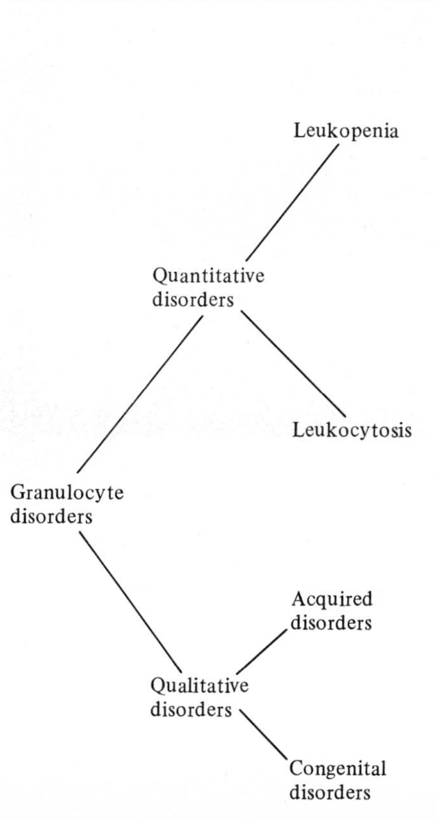

Leukopenia:

1. Marrow suppression
2. Marrow infiltration
3. Ineffective granulopoiesis
4. Infections
5. Cyclic neutropenia
6. Hypersplenism
7. Immune neutropenia
8. Preleukemia, PNH
9. Idiopathic neutropenia

Leukocytosis:

1. Leukemoid reactions (neutrophilic, eosinophilic, monocytic)
   a. Infections
   b. Inflammatory conditions
   c. Malignant disorders
2. Myeloproliferative diseases
   a. Chronic myeloproliferative disorders
   b. Acute myeloid leukemias

Acquired disorders:

1. Myeloproliferative disorders
2. Diabetes mellitus
3. Alcoholism
4. SLE

Congenital disorders:

1. Chronic granulomatous disease and variants
2. Myeloperoxidase deficiency
3. Chediak-Higashi syndrome
4. Complement deficiency

Table 7. Differences Between CGL and Leukemoid Reaction

	CGL	*Leukemoid Reaction*
Splenomegaly	Present	Absent
Sternal tenderness	Present	Absent
Basophilia	Present	Absent
Eosinophilia	Present	Absent
Thrombocytosis	Present	Absent
Leukocyte alkaline phosphatase	Low	High/normal
Philadelphia chromosome	Present	Absent

myeloid series in the blood. Leukemoid reactions should be differentiated from chronic granulocytic leukemia (CGL); the two conditions have a similar appearance in blood smears (Table 7). Leukocyte alkaline phosphatase is important in distinguishing the two conditions as it is increased in leukemoid reactions and markedly reduced in chronic granulocytic leukemia. While the bone marrow morphology can be quite similar in the two conditions, a cytogenetic abnormality (Philadelphia chromosome) is present in the vast majority of patients with CGL. Marrow metastases from solid tumors may be accompanied by leukemoid reactions. Occasionally, leukocytosis may be due to eosinophilia, as may occur in allergic disorders, parasitic infection, Löffler's syndrome, pulmonary infiltrates with eosinophilia, hypereosinophilic syndromes where absolute eosinophil count is greater than $1500/mm^3$, as a part of CGL, and in a variety of other hematologic malignancies. Eosinophilia is most commonly caused by allergic disorders. Monocytic leukemoid reactions are rare but may be seen in association with chronic infections, malignant diseases, and chronic monocytic leukemia. Disseminated tuberculosis may cause myeloid, lymphoid, or monocytic leukemoid reaction with or without anemia and/or thrombocytopenia. Besides the treatment of the primary disease, no additional treatment is needed for leukemoid reactions.

Chronic Myeloproliferative Disorders

Myeloproliferative disorders are characterized by a relentless proliferation of one or more marrow cell lines without any known provocative stimulus. On the basis of the proliferation of the predominant cell line, they can be divided into P. vera, CGL, myelofibrosis and myeloid metaplasia, and thrombocythemia. All these diseases may transform into acute myeloblastic leukemia. Increased nucleic acid turnover leads to hyperuricemia and vitamin B_{12} values are elevated because of increased levels of serum vitamin B_{12} binders. Leukocyte alkaline phosphatase is generally reduced in patients with CGL, and increased or normal in other myeloproliferative diseases. Philadelphia chromosome (translocation 22/9) is found in about 90% of the patients with CGL.

Chronic Granulocytic Leukemia

Chronic granulocytic leukemia is characterized by a progressively rising white blood cell count, immature myeloid cells in the peripheral blood, increase of myeloid precursors in the bone marrow, and progressive splenomegaly. The proliferation of the myeloid series is accompanied by varying degrees of failure of erythropoiesis and thrombopoiesis. The patient may present with nonspecific complaints of generalized weakness, weight loss, abdominal fullness, abdominal pain, or easy bruisability. Splenomegaly is a consistent physical finding. Sternal tenderness and hepatomegaly are frequently seen. Petechiae, purpura, and retinal hemorrhage may be seen in a few patients. The blood examination at the time of diagnosis usually shows normocytic normochromic anemia and thrombocytosis. The white blood cell count is above $100{,}000/mm^3$ in the majority of the patients. Characteristic findings in the differential white blood cell count include basophilia, eosinophilia and the presence of metamyelocytes, myelocytes, promyelocytes, and occasional myeloblasts. Leukocytic alkaline phosphatase is reduced in the majority of patients. Philadelphia chromosome, an acquired cytogenetic abnormality, has been demonstrated in the myeloid as well as erythoid precursors and the megakaryocytes. The presence of the Philadelphia chromosome is useful in establishing the diagnosis. The disease runs a chronic course for several months and terminates in acute leukemia with rapid progression and death from bleeding, infection, or, rarely, leukostatic thrombi. The terminal acute leukemia is non-lymphoblastic (70%) or lymphoblastic (30%).

Chronic granulocytic leukemia can be controlled effectively with chemotherapy before the blastic crisis supervenes. Since the majority of the patients have hyperuricemia, allopurinol (Zyloprim) 300 mg/day orally is started along with specific measures. Patients with anemia and bleeding from thrombocytopenia may require supportive red cell and platelet transfusions. In the chronic phase, busulfan (Myleran) is the drug of choice. The patient can be started on 4 mg of busulfan daily orally; the dose is then tailored according to weekly white blood cell counts and should be discontinued when the total white blood cell count is around $10{,}000/mm^3$. Patients with CGL rarely achieve a complete remission since the cytogenetic abnormalities persist even when hematologic control is achieved. Side effects of busulfan include marrow hypoplasia, skin pigmentation, and pulmonary fibrosis. Under certain special situations, splenic irradiation, leukophoresis, and drugs like hydroxyurea are used. With supportive measures and chemotherapy, the median survival from diagnosis is approximately 3 years. While the addition of chemotherapy has improved the quality of life for these patients, there is no increase in survival time. The blastic crisis is treated with drug combinations effective in the treatment of acute myeloid and lymphoblastic leukemia with very few responses.

Myelofibrosis and Myeloid Metaplasia

Myelofibrosis with myeloid metaplasia is a chronic myeloproliferative disorder characterized by prominent splenomegaly, anemia, thrombocytosis, teardrop cells, a few immature erythroid and myeıoid elements in the blood, and fibrosis of the bone marrow. The presenting manifestations may include nonspecific complaints of weakness, fatigability, bleeding, and gouty arthritis. Physical examination reveals massive splenomegaly; hepatomegaly is seen in about 50% of the patients and generalized lymphadenopathy is rare. Varying degrees of normocytic normochromic anemia, reticulocytosis, marked poikilocytosis of red cells with tear drop cells, a leukoerythroblastic blood picture, giant platelets and fragments of megakaryocytes may also be seen on the blood smear. Associated platelet dysfunction may result in clinical bleeding with a normal or elevated platelet count. Leukocyte alkaline phosphatase, serum uric acid, and lactic dehydrogenase are elevated. Skeletal x-rays may reveal osteosclerosis. Foci of extramedullary hematopoiesis account for the enlarged spleen and liver. This disease must be distinguished from secondary forms of myelofibrosis seen in association with lymphoma, leukemia, metastatic carcinoma, and miliary tuberculosis. There is no specific treatment. Supportive treatment consists of androgens and erythrocyte transfusions for anemia, alkylating agents for the control of marked thrombocytosis, and allopurinol for hyperuricemia. Occasionally, splenectomy may be needed for the control of hypersplenism. After a median survival of about 4 years, the patients succumb to the disease because of infection, bleeding, or thrombotic complications.

Acute non-Lymphoblastic Leukemia

Acute non-lymphoblastic leukemia (ANLL) includes a group of disorders (Table 8) characterized by an aggressive clinical course and failure of myeloid precursors to differentiate into mature cells. The bone marrow is hypercellular and replaced by abnormal cellular elements and normal hematopoiesis is markedly compromised. Varying degrees of anemia, granulocytopenia, and thrombocytopenia account for most of the complications of the disease and eventually lead to the death of these patients. The cause of acute myeloid leukemia is unknown; patients with chronic granulocytic leukemia, Down's syndrome, as well as people with exposure to high-dose irradiation and benzene are predisposed to acute myeloid leukemia. The symptoms include fatigue presenting as weakness, bleeding tendency, fever, weight loss, and bone pain. Physical examination may reveal petechiae, ecchymoses, signs of infection, sternal tenderness, lymph node enlargement, and hepatosplenomegaly. Infiltration of the skin and the gums is commonly found in patients with monoblastic leukemia. Bleeding manifestations related to disseminated intravascular coagulation are common in promyelocytic leukemia. Characteristic laboratory findings include variable degrees of normocytic normochromic anemia, granulocytopenia, and thrombocytopenia; immature myeloid precursors are found in the blood in the majority of these patients. Auer bodies (pink, rodlike cytoplasmic inclusions), when present, are pathognominic for acute non-lymphoblastic leukemia. Patients with acute promyelocytic leukemia may have multiple Auer rods in the promyelocytes. The presence of blast cells and granulocytes with the absence of intermediate myeloid precursors in the blood (a condition termed the leukemic hiatus) is considered a characteristic of acute leukemia. Other laboratory abnormalities may include an elevated muramidase, lactic dehydrogenase and ferritin levels in the serum.

Table 8. Variants of Acute Non-Lymphoblastic Leukemia

1. Acute myeloblastic leukemia
2. Acute promyelocytic leukemia
3. Acute myelomonocytic leukemia
4. Acute monocytic leukemia
5. Erythroleukemia

Treatment of acute non-lymphoblastic leukemias is quite complex and should be attempted only at centers where adequate supportive and laboratory help is available. The patient and the family must receive adequate information about the nature of the disease since their constant cooperation is required. Treatment consists primarily of supportive measures and specific measures. In patients who present with fever and neutropenia, empiric broad-spectrum antibiotic therapy is started after appropriate cultures have been obtained. Since these patients usually are neutropenic, urinary tract infection may be present without pus cells in the urine, and pneumonia may be present without sputum production or even an abnormal chest x-ray film. Metabolic abnormalities are not uncommon and need to be corrected. Supportive red blood cell transfusions are given as required. Platelet transfusions are given for the prevention and control of bleeding from thrombocytopenia.

Two major goals of specific antileukemic therapy are the induction of a complete remission and the maintenance of the remission as long as possible. The most active drugs available for remission induction are cytosine arabinoside (Ara-C) and daunomycin. Other useful drugs include thioguanine, cyclophosphamide, vincristine, prednisone, and Adriamycin. Combination chemotherapy has been found to be superior to single-agent treatment. About 75% of the patients achieve a complete remission that may last for about 6-14 months. Once complete remission is attained consolidation therapy is given. For remission maintenance, various drug combinations are used utilizing Ara-C, thioguanine, 6-mercaptopurine, methotrexate, cyclophosphamide, vincristine, and prednisone. An effective maintenance regimen used at the Cook County Hospital is a combination of Ara-C and thioguanine. Bone marrow aspiration is done every 3 months to look for early signs of leukemic relapse. The value of maintenance therapy in this disease has been questioned in recent studies. In selected patients in remission, bone marrow transplantation from a histocompatible sibling donor has shown promising results. Modern chemotherapy and supportive treatment have improved the outlook for these patients so that a few may be cured and a majority of them can have prolongation of survival. Advanced age (>60 years), infection at the time of diagnosis, chromosomal abnormalities and leukemia developing after chemotherapy are associated with a poor prognosis. Appropriate supportive measures, reverse isolation, and treatment of cardiorespiratory emergencies when they arise are other therapeutic measures that are often necessary.

Qualitative Granulocyte Disorders

Qualitative granulocytic disorders may be acquired or congenital. Among congenital causes of qualitative granulocyte disorders is chronic granulomatous disease, which is a rare X-linked recessive disease characterized by repeated skin infections by organisms of low-grade pathogenicity. Granulomatous lymphadenopathy and hepatosplenomegaly are concomitant physical findings. Morphologic appearance and phagocytic function of the granulocytes are normal. However, the granulocyte bactericidal function is defective. In spite of modern antibiotic therapy, the prognosis for these patients remains poor. Myeloperoxidase deficiency is an autosomal recessive disease with defective intracellular killing, but the frequency of infections is not increased in these patients. The Chediak-Higashi syndrome is an autosomal recessive disorder characterized by large abnormal granules in the leukocytes. These patients have increased susceptibility to infection and partial ocular and cutaneous albinism. Acquired abnormalities in the form of impaired chemotactic response to various stimuli have been reported in alcoholism, diabetes mellitus, and systemic lupus erythematosus; but their clinical consequences are not well defined.

Lymphoproliferative Disorders

Lymphoproliferative disorders include a wide variety of diseases characterized by proliferation of the lymphoid tissue. There may be peripheral lymphocytosis. Lymphomas and myelomas are disorders usually without associated peripheral lymphocytosis and are discussed elsewhere. A classification of the clinically important diseases with peripheral lymphocytosis is shown in Table 9. In adults, lymphocytosis is defined as an absolute lymphocyte count of more than $4500/mm^3$. The absolute lymphocyte count is to be distinguished from the relative lymphocytosis that occurs in patients with neutropenia. Characteristic morphologic changes in lymphocytes may be seen in viral infections such as infectious mononucleosis. Benign disorders are associated with transient lymphocytosis; but in malignant disorders the increase is persistent and progressive.

Reactive Lymphocytosis

Reactive lymphocytosis is commonly seen in a variety of acute and chronic infections. Among the acute infections causing lymphocytosis, viral infections such as infectious mononucleosis, infectious hepatitis, cytomegalovirus disease, and measles account for most cases. Bacterial etiology includes *Bordetella* pertussis infection, brucellosis, tuberculosis, and syphilis. The parasite *Toxoplasma gondii* may be associated with lymphocytosis. Acute infectious lymphocytosis is a benign entity of unknown etiology with transient lymphocytosis of morphologically normal-appearing cells. Lymphocytes appear morphologically normal in pertussis also; but in other reactive disorders lymphocytes are morphologically atypical (they are larger; there may be nuclear or cytoplasmic distortion; nuclear chromatin may be open with vacuolated, foamy, nongranular cytoplasm). Lymphocytosis persists from a few weeks to a few months.

Table 9. Lymphoproliferative Disorders with Peripheral Lymphocytosis

Benign (Transient)	*Malignant (Persistent)*
Reactive lymphocytosis	Chronic lymphocytic leukemia
Infectious mononucleosis	Acute lymphocytic leukemia
	Others: Hairy cell leukemia
	Lymphosarcoma cell leukemia
	Sézary syndrome
	Prolymphocytic leukemia

Infectious Mononucleosis

Infectious mononucleosis is an acute viral disorder caused by Epstein-Barr (EB) virus affecting young adults and characterized by fever, pharyngitis, lymphadenopathy, splenomegaly, and absolute lymphocytosis with many atypical cells. Development of transient heterophil antibodies and persistent EB virus antibodies is characteristic. In the presence of the typical clinical and hematologic picture, elevated heterophil antibody titer is considered diagnostic. Presence of sheep red cell agglutinins is not specific for infectious mononucleosis; in atypical cases, differential absorption of antibody shows that infectious mononucleosis antibodies are completely absorbed by beef red cells but not by guinea pig kidney cells. IgG antibodies to EB virus viral capsid antigen are present early and persist for several years. Cold agglutinins, although increased frequently, are rarely accompanied by clinical hemolysis. Liver function test abnormalities are not uncommon. Palatal enanthem in the form of red petechiae at the junction of the hard and the soft palates, although not diagnostic, is quite characteristic. There is an increased incidence of macular skin rash when these patients are treated with ampicillin. Complications are extremely rare; a few deaths have been reported from splenic rupture, severe hepatitis, and toxic encephalopathy. Other complications involve the cardiovascular system. Coombs' positive hemolytic anemia is the most frequent hematologic complication. In uncomplicated cases, the treatment is symptomatic. For patients with hemolytic anemia, thrombocytopenia, neurologic complications, and respiratory problems, steroids are indicated. Recovery is the rule in nearly 100% of the patients.

Chronic Lymphocytic Leukemia

Chronic lymphocytic leukemia, a predominantly B-lymphocyte disorder, is characterized by a progressive accumulation of mature lymphocytes. Proliferation of lymphocytes results in a marked lymphocytosis, lymph node enlargement, and varying degrees of hepatosplenomegaly. These lymphocytes have an impaired mitogenic response. Lymphocyte circulation between the blood, the bone marrow, and the lymph nodes is unimpaired. The cause of the disease is not known. The disease usually affects the elderly, and a significant proportion of patients may be asymptomatic with accidental discovery of lymphocytosis. The clinical manifestations are insidious in onset and consist of fatigue and weakness from anemia or relate to the enlarged lymph nodes, spleen, or liver. An occasional patient may present with plaquelike or nodular infiltrative skin lesions or bleeding problems related to thrombo-

Table 10. Staging of Chronic Lymphocytic Leukemia

Stage 0: Absolute lymphocytosis >15,000/mm^3
Stage I: Absolute lymphocytosis and lymphadenopathy
Stage II: Absolute lymphocytosis, enlarged liver and/or spleen
Stage III: Absolute lymphocytosis, anemia (<11 g%)
Stage IV: Absolute lymphocytosis, thrombocytopenia (<100,000/mm^3)

cytopenia. Table 10 shows the various stages of the disease depending on clinical findings at presentation.

Diagnosis is usually made on the basis of a persistently high total leukocyte count with predominance of mature lymphocytes. Bone marrow examination reveals hypercellularity and infiltration with mature lymphocytes. The remaining marrow elements are morphologically normal. Lymph node biopsy shows diffuse infiltration of mature lymphocytes and a loss of the normal architecture. Blood and marrow findings are sufficient for a diagnosis and the lymph node biopsy is not needed. Patients with advanced disease may have normocytic normochromic anemia and thrombocytopenia. Immunologic abnormalities are common among these patients. Most of the patients develop hypogammaglobulinemia; monoclonal gammopathy is found in about 5% of the patients. Approximately one-third of the patients develop autoimmune hemolytic anemia with a positive Coombs' test. In addition, some patients may have immune thrombocytopenia.

Management depends upon the stage in which the disease is diagnosed and varies from careful observation in asymptomatic patients to immediate intervention; if disease-related symptoms are present the main goal being to make the patient asymptomatic. Patients can be treated with alkylating agents (chlorambucil and cyclophosphamide). Steroids and cyclophosphamide are also indicated for autoimmune hemolytic anemia or thrombocytopenia. Whole-body radiation therapy has been used under special circumstances with good results. Complete remissions are rare in this disease and, so far, prolongation of survival related to therapy has not been achieved. Patients with Stage 0 disease have a median survival of about 10 years, those with stages I and II have a median survival of 4-8 years, whereas stage III and IV patients have only 1-3 year median survival.

Acute Lymphoblastic Leukemia

Acute lymphoblastic leukemia (ALL) is the most common malignant neoplastic disorder in pediatric patients with a peak incidence between 2-4 years; there is a progressive decrease in incidence with increasing age until the age of 40 years, when the incidence rises with advancing age. The incidence is higher in whites than in blacks, but the former have a better prognosis. Children between the ages of 1-10 do better than younger or older children. Acute lymphoblastic leukemia is a neoplastic disorder of bone marrow lymphocytes which, if untreated, runs a rapidly fatal course. The etiology of the disease is unknown. The child may present with non-specific symptoms of fatigue, fever, or bleeding, or there may be bone or joint pains. Physical examination may show lymphadenopathy and hepatosplenomegaly, but they are not very prominent. Bony tenderness may be quite striking. Other significant findings may include testicular enlargement, skin nodules, petechiae, ecchymoses, and cranial nerve palsy from meningeal infiltration.

Characteristic hematologic abnormalities are present in almost all patients, and establishment of a diagnosis of acute leukemia is not difficult. A normocytic normochromic anemia is usually present and is related to bone marrow failure and bleeding from concomitant thrombocytopenia. Neutropenia and monocytopenia are usually present. The total leukocyte count is elevated in the majority of the patients; in approximately one-third of the patients, the leukocyte count is normal or low. Differential white blood cell count shows a significant number of lymphoblasts. The bone marrow is characteristically hypercellular and infiltrated by a large number of lymphoblasts. The blast cells are about 10-15 microns in diameter and contain large round nuclei with scanty cytoplasm devoid of granules. The nuclei have a finely granular chromatin pattern and one or two nucleoli. Other hematopoietic cells in the marrow are markedly decreased and their morphology is usually normal. A great majority of cases of ALL can be distinguished from ANLL on the basis of morphologic differences visualized with Romanovsky's stain. Auer bodies are never seen in leukemic lymphoblasts. In approximately 5-10% of cases, peroxidase and periodic acid-Schiff staining of the blastic cells may be needed to separate ALL from ANLL. The blastic cells in ALL usually contain PAS-staining material, but no peroxidase granules. Biochemical abnormalities at the time of diagnosis include elevated serum lactic dehydrogenase, hyperuricemia, and, occasionally, azotemia. Recent studies have shown the prognostic significance of lymphoblast surface markers in ALL. Most of the patients with ALL have neither B-nor T-lymphocyte markers. Few ALL patients with T-lymphocyte markers on the blastic cells present a characteristic clinical picture, as seen in adolescent males with mediastinal lymph node enlargement and a poor response to therapy. For a discussion of lymphoblastic lymphoma, see the chapter on oncology.

Management of ALL involves supportive measures, specific antileukemic therapy, and treatment of complications with attention to the social circumstances of the patient. The main supportive measures consist of prevention and treatment of hemorrhage, correction of anemia, and appropriate treatment of infections. Specific therapy for ALL can be divided into three important phases; remission induction, prophylaxis for central nervous system (CNS) leukemia, and maintenance of remission. Vincristine in combination with prednisone has been shown to induce complete remission in approximately 90% of the patients. The addition of adriamycin or asparaginase to the induction regimen appears to prolong the duration of induced remission. Once a complete remission is achieved, 2,400 rad of whole brain irradiation and five injections of intrathecal methotrexate are given to reduce the risk of leukemic relapse in the CNS. The third phase of specific treatment consists of maintenance of remission with administration of weekly intravenous methotrexate and daily oral

6-mercaptopurine. Marrow aspiration is repeated at 3-month intervals to detect signs of early leukemic relapse. If the patient continues to remain in complete remission for 3 years, the maintenance therapy can be stopped. In selected patients in second remission, bone marrow transplantation from a histocompatible sibling donor has shown promising results.

Treatment of the complications depends on the nature of the problems. With modern antibiotic and blood component therapy, infection and bleeding can be effectively controlled. CNS leukemia is an uncommon but serious complication. Although it can be temporarily controlled, long-term control is rarely achieved, emphasizing the importance of the CNS prophylactic therapy discussed above.

The prognosis of children with ALL has been markedly improved with current therapeutic modalities. Approximately 50% of such patients can be expected to survive for 5 years and a significant number of them are cured.

DISORDERS OF HEMOSTASIS

APPROACH TO A PATIENT WITH A BLEEDING DISORDER

A thorough history and physical examination are essential in the evaluation of bleeding disorders because they provide the rational basis for proper laboratory tests. Occasionally, a presumptive diagnosis can be made from the clinical findings; laboratory tests are used to confirm the diagnosis. History of onset of bleeding in relation to trauma is important, as bleeding related to certain coagulation problems may have a delayed onset. Persistent bleeding following superficial cuts is seen in platelet disorders but is minimal in coagulation disorders. Assessment of the magnitude of bleeding in relation to accidental or surgical trauma is important in estimating the severity of the bleeding disorder. Hemarthrosis and deep dissecting hematomas are characteristic of coagulation disorders but are rarely seen in platelet-related problems. Age of onset is another important feature; most of the congenital coagulation disorders are clinically manifest during childhood. Newborn children with hypofibrinogenemia and factor XIII deficiency may have bleeding from the umbilical stump and circumcision and delayed wound healing. The most common cause of bleeding in neonates is vitamin K deficiency. Bleeding diathesis may not be diagnosed until a hemophilic child starts crawling and walking around, when exposure to minor trauma brings out the characteristic bleeding diathesis. Classic hemophilia is an X-linked recessive disorder that occurs almost exclusively in males. A positive family history is important but is not necessary for the diagnosis since in as many as 40% of cases of hemophilia A, family history may be negative. A history of drug and alcohol ingestion should always be obtained in any patient with a bleeding diathesis. A generalized bleeding diathesis is most frequently caused by acquired hemostatic disorders associated with uremia, liver disease, disseminated intravascular coagulation, malignancy, or infection. Petechiae and purpura are suggestive of platelet disorders, whereas large ecchymoses, hemarthroses, and deep dissecting hematomas are characteristic of coagulation disorders.

Laboratory tests are useful in the evaluation of the major components of the hemostatic mechanism, namely, blood coagulation, platelet number and function, and vascular integrity. Platelet count and bleeding time are helpful screening tests for platelet-related problems. The coagulation function is tested with prothrombin time, partial thromboplastin time, and thrombin time. If preliminary tests are normal, factor XIII screening and platelet function tests should be performed. When the preliminary tests are abnormal, correlation with other laboratory findings, coagulation factor assays, or bone marrow examination may be necessary to establish the correct diagnosis. If all the platelet and coagulation tests are normal, the bleeding diathesis is probably related to congenital or acquired vascular disorders. Hereditary hemorrhagic telangiectasia is the most frequent congenital vascular disorder; vascular purpura associated with infections and various immunologic disorders make up most of the acquired vascular disorders.

DISORDERS OF PLATELETS

Platelets are formed in the bone marrow by the fragmentation of the cytoplasm of megakaryocytes. Normal platelet count is 140,000-440,000/mm^3. One-third of the circulating platelets are pooled in the spleen. Young platelets are larger than old ones and are hemostatically more active. The normal life span of platelets is about 10 days.

Thrombocytopenia

Thrombocytopenia is defined as a decrease in the number of circulating platelets in the blood. A deficiency in the number of platelets leads to a bleeding diathesis because of impaired platelet plug formation. The severity of the hemorrhagic tendency correlates with the degree of thrombocytopenia. No significant hemostatic abnormalities are seen in association with platelet counts above 100,000/mm^3. In uncomplicated thrombocytopenia, spontaneous bleeding usually does not occur with platelet counts above 40,000/mm^3. Thrombocytopenia may result from decreased production, increased destruction, and increased pooling of platelets (Table 11).

Table 11. Pathogenesis of Thrombocytopenia

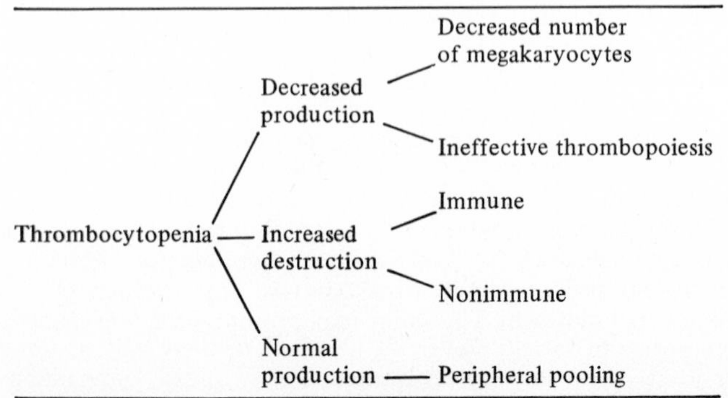

Decreased production of megakaryocytes and platelets results from damage to the marrow by toxins, myelosuppressive drugs, radiation, or as a part of idiopathic aplastic anemia. Suppression of the megakaryocytes may also occur in certain infections. Replacement of the marrow by leukemic and neoplastic cells is another cause of thrombocytopenia. Megaloblastic anemias are associated frequently with ineffective thrombopoiesis, which is also seen in myeloproliferative disorders and certain hereditary disorders (e.g., Wiskott-Aldrich syndrome and May-Hegglin anomaly). Accelerated platelet destruction is a frequent cause of thrombocytopenia. Increased destruction may be brought about by an autoantibody, or the platelets may be consumed by intravascular thrombosis as may occur in disseminated intravascular coagulation and microangiopathic processes. The bone marrow in these instances usually shows an increase in megakaryocytes.

Immune thrombocytopenia may be either primary (idiopathic) or secondarily associated with drugs and diseases such as systemic lupus erythematosus (SLE) or lymphoproliferative disorders (Table 12). Idiopathic immune thrombocytopenia occurs in the acute form most commonly in children between the ages of 2 and 6 years, and the chronic form is seen most frequently in young women. Platelets are coated with platelet autoantibodies; their rapid sequestration in the spleen leads to thrombocytopenia. Patients usually present with petechiae or mucosal bleeding. There is no lymphadenopathy or splenomegaly in idiopathic thrombocytopenic purpura. Clinical findings of the associated disease are seen in other cases. The platelet count is low and the bleeding time is prolonged; the blood smear shows a reduced number of platelets, some of which may be large. Bone marrow examination reveals an increased or normal number of megakaryocytes. The platelet antibody test is positive in a majority of the patients. Idiopathic thrombocytopenic purpura (ITP) is a diagnosis of exclusion. Some patients with ITP eventually develop SLE; this is more likely to occur in patients with associated autoimmune hemolytic anemia (Evans' syndrome). It is important to obtain a history of drug ingestion in any patient with thrombocytopenia. Drugs may cause either bone marrow suppression directly, or may act as antigens and stimulate antibody formation. In a thrombocytopenic patient, all unnecessary medication should be stopped. Drug-related immune thrombocytopenia usually resolves quickly after discontinuation of the drug. Spontaneous remissions are common in ITP in children with acute infections. Adults with ITP or children who do not have spontaneous remission are treated with corticosteroids. A high dose of prednisone (2 mg/kg/day) is prescribed initially. If the thrombocytopenia resolves, the prednisone dose should be slowly decreased and eventually stopped. Patients not responding to steroids or requiring large doses (more than 10 mg/day of prednisone) for maintenance should be treated by splenectomy. A remission can be induced in about 70% of patients with splenectomy. Patients who have previously responded to prednisone are more likely to improve with splenectomy. Splenectomy failures are treated with immunosuppressive agents such as vincristine, cyclophosphamide, or azathioprine. Patients with secondary thrombocytopenia are treated in the same way as in the idiopathic variety; they may require additional treatment for the primary disorder.

Table 12. Causes of Immune Thrombocytopenia

Idiopathic
Acute
Chronic
Secondary
Lymphoproliferative disorders
Systemic lupus erythematosus
Drug related

Thrombocytosis

Platelets can be increased (above 440,000/mm^3) as a reactive phenomenon referred to as thrombocytosis. A sustained autonomous elevation of the platelet count is called thrombocythemia. Physiologic thrombocytosis occurs after exercise or stimulation of the sympathetic nervous system. Elevation of the platelets may occur in association with severe hemorrhage, surgery, hemolytic anemias, and iron deficiency anemia; following splenectomy, mild thrombocytosis may persist in some of the patients. Transient rebound thrombocytosis occurs during recovery from marrow suppression of any etiology. Various infections, generalized tuberculosis, ulcerative colitis, regional enteritis, rheumatoid arthritis, acute rheumatic fever, solid tumors, and Hodgkin's disease are associated with thrombocytosis; the platelet count seldom exceeds 1 million/mm^3 in these conditions and the platelet function is normal. By contrast, in thrombocythemia there is a progressive autonomous increase in platelets frequently associated with functional abnormalities; the platelet counts may be in excess of 1 million/mm^3. Thrombocythemia may be primary or occur as a part of other myeloproliferative disorders such as CGL, P. vera, and agnogenic myelofibrosis and myeloid metaplasia. Patients with a marked increase in platelets are prone to develop hemorrhagic and thrombotic complications; venous thrombosis is more frequent than arterial thrombosis. These patients can present with iron deficiency anemia. Treatment of the primary disease usually corrects thrombocytosis. Management of thrombocythemia involves bringing the platelet count close to normal with alkylating agents like melphalan, busulfan, or uracil mustard. Plateletpheresis may be employed for temporary removal of platelets in urgent situations. In patients with hemorrhagic complications, normal functioning platelets may have to be transfused to control the acute bleeding episode.

Thrombopathies

Thrombopathies are hemorrhagic disorders caused by functional abnormalities of the platelets and should be considered in bleeding patients with a normal coagulation profile and a normal platelet count with a prolonged bleeding time. Platelet function may be abnormal in congenital or acquired disorders. Congenital thrombopathies are quite rare and may be associated with defective adhesion, aggregation, or release reaction of the platelets; classic examples of the corresponding defects are von Willebrand's disease, thrombasthenia, and storage pool disease. Drugs, uremia, and dysproteinemias are the most frequent causes of acquired platelet dysfunction. Among drugs, aspirin is the most important; but other analgesics and anti-inflammatory drugs, antidepressants, antihistaminics, and some antibiotics can also cause defective platelet function. Fibrin degradation products have some inhibitory effect on platelet function as well. Management consists of treatment of the primary condition in the acquired disorders; in patients with primary platelet dysfunction, transfusion of normal platelets temporarily corrects the bleeding diathesis.

DISORDERS OF COAGULATION

Coagulation of blood at the site of vascular injury is an important component of the hemostatic mechanism. Clot formation provides an effective mechanical barrier to the leakage of blood from the injured vessel; thrombin, which is formed during the coagulation process, enhances hemostasis through stabilization of the platelet plug. The process of blood coagulation consists of a series of enhancing enzymatic reactions culminating in the formation of fibrin. Several intravascular factors and some extravascular tissue factors participate in this complex reaction. By international agreement, coagulation factors have been identified by Roman numerals according to order of discovery (Table 13). For factors I to IV, descriptive terms are more commonly used. With the exception of factor VIII and calcium, all the coagulant factors in the plasma are produced exclusively in the liver. Synthesis of factors II, VII, IX, and X is dependent on the availability of vitamin K. According to the present concept, the formation of fibrin involves the generation of thromboplastin by the intrinsic or the extrinsic pathway. Thromboplastin (activated factor X complex) is involved in the conversion of prothrombin to thrombin, which acts on fibrinogen to form fibrin (common pathway). Stabilization of fibrin is brought about subsequently through the action of factor XIII. Platelets, fibrinogen, and factors II, V, and VIII are consumed during the clotting process.

Most of the coagulation factors are measured by bioassays; the coagulation activity of any given factor in normal pooled plasma is taken to be 100% activity. Primary screening tests of coagulation permit assessment of the integrity of the intrinsic, the extrinsic, and the common pathways (Fig. 1). The sensitivity of these tests is limited to a reduction of individual clotting factor below 20% activity. Specific factor assays permit a sensitive determination of the individual coagulant factor activity. At least 25% activity of all coagulation factors is necessary for normal hemostasis. A decrease in the coagulant factor activity from underproduction or excessive consumption leads to a bleeding diathesis. Coagulation disorders can be caused by congenital deficiency or increased consumption of the clotting factors. In general, congenital coagulation disorders are associated with single-factor deficiencies, whereas acquired coagulopathies involve multiple factor deficiencies. The half-life of individual coagulation factors varies from 5 hours for factor VII to about 5 days for factor XIII (Table 13). The frequency of coagulant factor administration for temporary correction of inherited coagulopathies is determined by the half-life of the deficient factor.

Hereditary Coagulopathies

Hemophilia and Related Disorders

Hemophilia and related disorders include a group of inherited coagulation disorders characterized by an abnormal production of individual clotting factors. There may be either a true deficiency of the factor, such as in von Willebrand's disease, or a qualitative defect in the production of a factor as seen in hemophilia A (factor VIII deficiency). Hemophilia A and hemophilia B (factor IX deficiency) are the most frequent hereditary coagulation disorders and have sex-linked inheritance. In classic hemophilia (A), which is the prototype of the group, there is a defective production of procoagulant factor VIII with normal antigenic activity. Since platelets are normal

Table 13. Coagulation Factors and Their Kinetics

Coagulation Factors		*Biologic Half-Life (hours)*
I:	Fibrinogen	90
II:	Prothrombin	72
III:	Tissue Thromboplastin	-
IV:	Calcium	-
V:	Labile factor	16
VII:	Stable	5
VIII:	Antihemophilic A (AHF)	12
IX:	Antihemophilic B (AHB) (Christmas factor)	24
X:	Stuart-Prower factor	48
XI:	Plasma thromboplastin antecedent (PTA)	60
XII:	Hageman factor	60
XIII:	Fibrin stabilizing factor	120

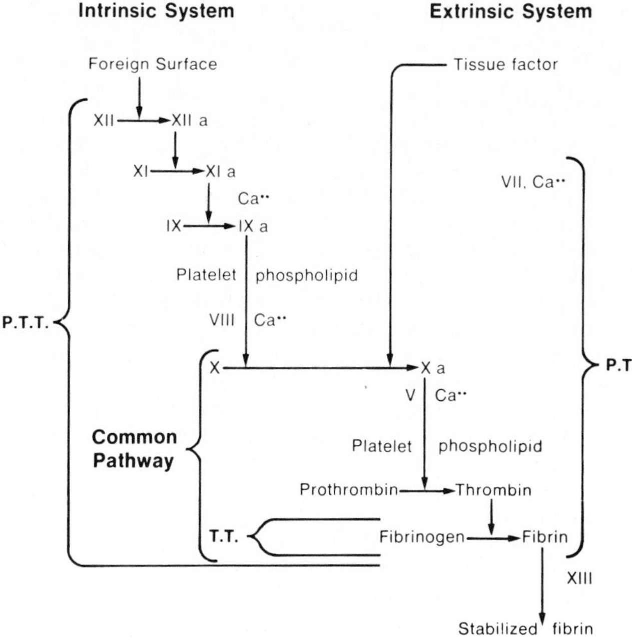

Figure 1. Simplified schema of blood coagulation.

in these patients, the initial hemostatic response to a vascular injury is normal; but bleeding is delayed and may be persistent. Hemophiliacs can be divided into three groups according to the level of coagulant factor and clinical severity of the disease (Table 14). The child with severe hemophilia may present with excessive bleeding after circumcision or minor accidental injuries from learning to walk. Patients with mild hemophilia may not be diagnosed until they are exposed to the major hemostatic stress of surgery. Deep dissecting hematomas and recurrent hemarthroses are common manifestations. History of a bleeding disorder affecting the male members on the maternal side of the family, if present, is characteristic; but a negative family history does not exclude hemophilia. Diagnosis is suggested by an isolated laboratory abnormality of prolonged PTT and is confirmed by the demonstration of decreased factor VIII or factor IX activity. Individual coagulation factor assays are used to distinguish other inherited coagulation disorders. Management consists of making the family aware of the hereditary nature of the problem, instructing them about prevention of bleeding problems, and the treatment of acute bleeding episodes. Long-term control of the bleeding diathesis is not possible at present. However, the hemostatic defect can be eliminated for short periods by the transfusion of the appropriate coagulation factor. The affected boy must be trained to avoid trauma as much as possible without adversely affecting emotional and intellectual development. Prompt and energetic treatment of the individual bleeding episodes with the proper coagulation factor is important in reducing morbidity from the disease. Surgical and dental procedures can be safely carried out with the infusions of coagulation factors. For hemophilia A, the most frequently used replacement products are factor VIII concentrate and cryoprecipitate, which contain factor VIII and fibrinogen. Concentrates of factors II, VII, IX, and X are used in the treatment of hemophilia B and other factor deficiency states. Fresh frozen plasma, which contains all the coagulation factors, can also be used in the treatment of individual bleeding episodes. The introduction of home transfusion programs has further improved the prospects for the hemophilic patient. With modern therapy, most patients can have a self-supporting, productive life. Factor XII deficiency is associated with a marked prolongation of the PTT without clinical bleeding problems; no treatment is necessary. Congenital afibrinogenemia and dysfibrinogenemia are rare. Clinical bleeding episodes are managed with cryoprecipitate or plasma infusions. Factor XIII deficiency is characterized by delayed bleeding after injury, impaired wound healing, and spontaneous abortions. Bleeding episodes are easily controlled by plasma infusions.

Table 14. Clinical Bleeding in Relation to Coagulant Factor Levels in Hemophilia

Severity	*Coagulant Factor Activity*	*Type of Bleeding*
Severe	<1%	Spontaneous bleeding
Moderate	1-5%	Severe bleeding after minor injury, occasional spontaneous bleeding
Mild	5-20%	Severe bleeding after major hemostatic stress, no spontaneous bleeding

Von Willebrand's Disease

Von Willebrand's disease is a hereditary coagulation disorder transmitted in an autosomal-dominant fashion in most cases. It is characterized by a prolonged bleeding time and PTT along with a proportional decrease in the coagulant and antigenic levels of factor VIII. Clinical severity of the bleeding varies considerably. Patients may present with hemorrhage from mucous membranes, (e.g., epistaxis, gastrointestinal bleeding, menorrhagia, and postpartum bleeding); hemarthroses and deep hematomas are rarely seen. Diagnosis is based on family history, abnormal clinical bleeding, prolonged PTT and bleeding time, a low level of factor VIII on bioassay and immunologic assay, synthesis of factor VIII after infusion of factor VIII-deficient plasma, diminished platelet adhesion, and impaired ristocetin-induced platelet aggregation. There is a considerable variability in the laboratory findings in individual patients with von Willebrand's disease. Management of bleeding episodes consists of local measures and transfusion of cryoprecipitate or normal plasma, which also corrects the platelet dysfunction.

Acquired Coagulation Disorders

In clinical practice, acquired coagulation disorders are much more common than the congenital coagulopathies. Bleeding diathesis resulting from inadequate synthesis of multiple factors is seen in association with liver disease, malabsorption

Table 15. Common Causes of Disseminated Intravascular Coagulation

1. Obstetric conditions
   A. Abruptio placentae
   B. Amniotic fluid embolism
   C. Missed abortion
2. Infections
   A. Bacterial
   B. Viral
   C. Rickettsial
   D. Mycotic
   E. Protozoal
3. Disseminated malignant diseases
4. Hematologic disorders
   A. Acute leukemias
   B. Mismatched blood transfusion
5. Vascular disorders
   A. Hemangiomas
   B. Collagen-vascular diseases
   C. Shock
6. Massive tissue injury

syndrome, and the administration of vitamin K antagonist drugs. Rarely, inhibitors of specific coagulant factors (e.g., factor VIII) may lead to hemorrhagic diathesis. Development of the factor VIII inhibitor has been found in association with severe hemophilia, certain drugs, and collagen diseases.

A large number of conditions (Table 15) may cause disseminated intravascular coagulation (DIC) and consumption of fibrinogen, platelets, factor II, factor VIII, and factor V. The fibrinolytic system is activated at the sites of thrombosis and brings about lysis of the clot with a release of fibrin degradation products. Clinically, this results in the paradoxical findings of thrombosis in the microvasculature with organ dysfunction and a hemorrhagic tendency from depletion of platelets, multiple clotting factors, and platelet dysfunction from fibrin degradation products (FDP).

Diagnosis of acquired coagulation disorders is made on the basis of a relatively short history of bleeding, presence of associated disease, nonspecific findings such as petechiae or ecchymoses, and abnormalities in the tests of coagulation indicating characteristic patterns of multiple factor deficiencies. Patients with DIC may have microangiopathic hemolysis, fragmented cells, and raised FDP in the blood. Coagulation tests using mixtures of the patient's plasma and normal plasma are useful in the diagnosis of inhibitors of clotting factors.

Treatment of these disorders is directed at the primary cause of the bleeding diathesis. Infusions of fresh frozen plasma and platelets are useful in the control of episodes of bleeding. In patients with DIC and evidence of organ dysfunction from thrombosis, heparin therapy is useful in improving the hemostatic abnormalities. Heparin therapy does not improve the overall prognosis of patients with DIC. Bleeding episodes in the few hemophiliacs with inhibitors can be treated with factor IX concentrates.

VASCULAR DISORDERS

Vascular purpuras are a group of disorders characterized by a defective vascular contribution to the hemostatic mechanism; the coagulation factors and the platelets are usually normal. Vascular hemorrhagic disorders can be either congenital or acquired (Table 16). Hereditary hemorrhagic telangiectasia is an autosomal dominant disorder characterized by recurrent bleeding with iron deficiency anemia, telangiectasia in the skin and mucous membranes, and visceral vascular malformations. Approximately 20% of the patients have pulmonary arteriovenous fistulae. Vascular purpura may also be seen in hereditary connective tissue disorders such as Ehlers-Danlos syndrome, osteogenesis imperfecta, and pseudoxanthoma elasticum. Except for therapy for the complicating iron deficiency, no treatment is available.

Many bacterial, viral, protozoal, and rickettsial infections are associated with a vasculitis and a hemorrhagic rash. Certain drugs are frequently associated with vascular purpura. A defective intercellular substance of the capillaries leads to the bleeding tendency in scurvy. In Cushing's syndrome and patients receiving steroid therapy, the purpuric skin lesions are thought to be due to a defect in the connective tissue. Skin lesions in senile purpura are characteristically seen on the extensor surface of the arms and hands. Henoch-Schönlein purpura, seen frequently in children, is characterized by polyarthralgia and arthritis, abdominal manifestations, hematuria, and purpuric rash following a streptococcal infection. Paraproteinemias with or without cryoglobulinemia are frequently associated with vascular purpura. Treatment of the acquired vascular purpuras is directed at the primary cause of the disorder.

CLINICAL USES OF BLOOD COMPONENTS

Transfusion of blood components is an important aspect of the practice of medicine and involves sound judgment on the indications for their usage. Specific blood component therapy is preferred over the routine use of whole blood because of the associated morbidity and even occasional mortality with the latter. On rare occasions, fresh whole blood may be indicated in a profusely bleeding patient with hypovolemic shock.

Table 16. Vascular Disorders

Congenital	*Acquired*
Hereditary hemorrhagic telengiectasia	Infections and drugs
Hereditary connective tissue disorders	Senile purpura
	Scurvy
	Cushing's syndrome
	Henoch-Schönlein purpura
	Paraproteinemias

RED BLOOD CELLS

Red blood cell transfusions are used to correct anemia. They are indicated in patients with acute blood loss and severe chronic anemia with cardiac decompensation. Periodic red blood cell transfusions are also required for anemias related to marrow failure in aplactic anemia, malignancies, or uremia. Red blood cells are given usually in the form of packed cells that have a hematocrit of 70%. One unit of packed red blood cells raises the hemoglobin by 1 g/100 ml. Patients who have received multiple transfusions may develop febrile transfusion reactions related to leukocyte and platelet antigens. In these situations, leukocyte-poor packed red blood cells (washed red blood cells) or freeze-preserved red blood cells can be given to avoid febrile reactions. Mild reactions can be treated symptomatically with diphenhydramine (Benadryl).

The patient with acute blood loss of 20% or more of the total blood volume needs intravenous administration of both crystalloid and colloid solutions, starting with a 5% albumin and saline solution. Under exceptional circumstances when the patient is in shock, Group O rhesus-negative packed red blood cells can be given until type-specific blood becomes available. For patients requiring massive red blood cell transfusions, 2 units of fresh-frozen plasma, 4 units of platelets, and 1 g of calcium gluconate should be given for every 4 units of packed red blood cells to prevent hemostatic abnormalities. Elderly patients with cardiovascular disease requiring red blood cells should be transfused slowly; administration of a potent diuretic before starting the transfusion reduces the risk of pulmonary edema in these patients.

GRANULOCYTES

With the advent of cell separators, granulocytes have been made available in a number of major hospitals. In severely neutropenic patients with documented bacterial or fungal infections and poor response to antibiotics, granulocyte transfusions have been effective in reducing the morbidity and mortality from infection.

PLATELETS

Platelet concentrates are prepared from platelet-rich plasma. Each platelet pack raises the platelet count by about 10,000/mm^3 in a person with 1 sq m of body surface area in the absence of bleeding, fever, or infection. Platelet concentrates are indicated in any bleeding patient with thrombocytopenia. Patients with immune thrombocytopenia usually do not benefit from platelet transfusions because of rapid consumption of the transfused platelets; the only indication for platelet transfusion in these patients would be an urgent life-threatening situation like CNS bleeding. Patients with acute leukemia and platelet counts below 20,000/mm^3 should be given prophylactic platelet transfusions to maintain the counts above 20,000/mm^3. Thrombocytopenic patients going for surgery should be transfused to platelet counts of around 100,000/mm^3. In a bleeding patient with a platelet count above 50,000/mm^3, either platelet dysfunction or other additional cause for bleeding should be sought. Bleeding related to a primary platelet dysfunction improves from platelet transfusion. After repeated platelet transfusions, the development of platelet antibodies may lead to a loss of platelet survival and hemostatic effectiveness. Hence, judicious use of platelets is particularly important in patients with prolonged thrombocytopenia. In sensitized individuals, platelets from HLA-compatible donors are more effective than those from random donors.

PLASMA AND ITS FRACTIONS

Fresh frozen plasma contains all the coagulation factors. The main indications for the use of plasma include patients with hypovolemic shock due to loss of plasma as in burns, and in patients with a generalized bleeding diathesis such as disseminated intravascular coagulation, overdosage of oral anticoagulants, and liver disease. It can also be used to restore the circulating blood volume in hemorrhagic shock until red cells become available. Most of the plasma fractions are obtained from pooled plasma. Cryoprecipitate, prothrombin complex concentrate, and albumin are the plasma fractions used in clinical practice. Cryoprecipitate, which contains factor VIII and fibrinogen, is widely used in the control of bleeding episodes in patients with classic hemophilia; dosage and duration of transfusions depend upon the type and severity of the injury. Cryoprecipitate can also be used as a source of fibrinogen in patients with disseminated intravascular coagulation and dysfibrinogenemia. Prothrombin complex concentrates are marketed under different trade names. All of them contain vitamin K-dependent factors, namely, II, VII, IX, and X. In addition to their use in specific factor-deficient patients, they can be used for bleeding complications in patients on oral anticoagulants. They have also been used in patients with classic hemophilia with antibiodies to factor VIII. Administration of the prothrombin complex concentrates may result in thromboembolic complications, particularly in patients with liver disease. Albumn is available as a 5% buffered saline solution and a 25% salt-free solution. These products can be used in patients with hypovolemic shock because of burns or hemmorrhage and for temporary expansion of plasma volume in patients with severe hypoproteinimia. Other available plasma products include immune serum globulins and specific immunoglobulins against a number of infectious agents. RH_0 (D) immune human globulin is used in the prevention of hemolytic diseases of the newborn.

COMPLICATIONS OF TRANSFUSION THERAPY

Immediate Complications

Allergic reactions occur in about 1% of the patients receiving transfusion products; they may develop urticaria, pruritus, and bronchial spasm with wheezing. These should be treated symptomatically with antihistaminics. When transfused with products containing IgA, patients with IgA deficiency may develop an anaphylactoid reaction requiring prompt parenteral administration of epinephrine and steroids.

Febrile reactions related to a transfusion usually start within 4 hours, may last up to 36 hours, and are related to antigen-antibody reactions. Antihistamines and steroids do not usually help.

Circulatory overload in elderly patients with cardiovascular disease and infants make them prone to pulmonary edema. The rate of transfusion should not exceed 2 ml/min in adults with cardiac problems. Administration of furosemide prior to the transfusion decreases the risk of circulatory overload in these patients.

Mismatched blood transfusion may result in rapid intravascular hemolysis or delayed extravascular hemolysis. The most frequent cause of the intravascular hemolysis is an inadvertent administration of ABO-incompatible blood. Depending on the quantity of transfused incompatible blood, there may be restlessness, tachycardia, chest pain, back pain, hemoglobinuria, disseminiated intravascular coagulation or oliguric renal failure that may occasionally result in the death of the patient. Therapy consists of prompt cessation of further incompatible blood transfusion, maintenance of fluid and electrolyte balance, and the treatment of disseminated intravascular coagulation and renal failure, if present.

Delayed hemolytic transfusion reactions are caused by incompatibility of the Rh and other erythrocyte antigens. Coombs' test is positive in most cases. These reactions markedly reduce the efficacy of the transfused blood and can be avoided by the transfusion of erythrocytes devoid of the particular antigen to which the patient is sensitized.

Patients receiving massive transfusion with only red blood cells may develop a bleeding diathesis related to a deficiency of platelets and plasma coagulation factors. This complication can be prevented by the administration of platelets and fresh frozen plasma. Banked blood temporarily depleted of 2,3-diphosphoglycerate may lead to metabolic abnormalities because of impaired oxygen delivery to the tissues. Transfusion of fresh blood (less than 5 days old) will circumvent the problem. Occasionally, microaggregates in the banked blood may cause pulmonary impairment. The risk of this complication can be reduced by the use of appropriate filters.

Delayed Reactions

Viral hepatitis, malaria, syphilis, cytomegalovirus, brucellosis, and toxoplasmosis may be transmitted by transfusion of blood products. Because of improved and strict screening, viral hepatitis remains the main offender. The risk of viral hepatitis and cytomegalovirus infection is high in repeatedly transfused patients especially with plasma and pooled plasma products.

QUESTIONS

1. The normal life span of the red blood cell is approximately:
   A. 90 days
   B. 120 days
   C. 8 hours
   D. 7 days
2. The commonest cause of iron deficiency anemia is:
   A. Chronic blood loss
   B. Inadequate dietary intake
   C. Inadequate absorption
   D. Chronic hemosiderinuria
3. Which statement is true regarding megaloblastic anemia?
   A. Only red blood cell precursors are affected
   B. Morphologic changes caused by vitamin B_{12} and folic acid deficiency are easy to distinguish
   C. Basic defect is impaired RNA and protein synthesis
   D. May present with pancytopenia
4. Find the false statement regarding the anemia of chronic disease:
   A. The anemia is usually normocytic normochromic with a low production index
   B. There is no abnormality of iron metabolism
   C. Iron therapy is not indicated
   D. Treatment is aimed at the underlying disease
5. Regarding aplastic anemia, which is the true statement?
   A. Pancytopenia is always present
   B. Bone marrow is hypocellular
   C. Androgens are always helpful
   D. Bone marrow transplantation is the treatment of choice in all cases of aplastic anemia
6. Hemolytic anemia can be caused by:
   A. Pyruvate kinase deficiency
   B. Valvular heart disease
   C. Thrombotic thrombocytopenic purpura
   D. All of the above
   E. None of the above
7. Regarding chronic myeloproliferative disorders, which of the following is true?
   A. Elevated hematocrit is always associated with elevated red cell mass
   B. Presence of Philadelphia chromosome is essential for the diagnosis of chronic myelocytic leukemia
   C. Therapy has definitely prolonged survival in polycythemia vera
   D. Therapy has definitely prolonged survival in chronic myelocytic leukemia
8. Regarding acute nonlymphoblastic leukemia, all of the following are true except:
   A. Auer bodies are pathognomonic
   B. Disseminated intravascular coagulation may be seen
   C. There is complete normalization of marrow morphology with therapy

D. Survival has not been altered by chemotherapy

9. All of the following are true regarding chronic lymphocytic leukemia except:
   A. It is predominantly a B-cell disorder
   B. Diagnosis is usually based on persistently elevated lymphocytes in the peripheral blood
   C. Immunologic abnormalities are frequently seen
   D. Chemotherapy produces complete remission in a majority of patients
10. Poor prognostic factors for acute lymphoblastic leukemia include all of the following except:
    A. Black race
    B. Ages between 1-10 years
    C. CNS involvement
    D. Mediastinal adenopathy

FOR EACH OF THE FOLLOWING, INDICATE WHETHER THEY ARE:

A. True

B. False

11. Family history is always positive in hemophilia.
12. Patients with factor XIII deficiency have delayed wound healing.
13. Platelet count and bleeding time are useful screening tests for platelet-related problems.
14. Significant hemostatic abnormality is associated with a platelet count of about $100{,}000/mm^3$ even in the absence of thrombopathy.
15. In the treatment of thrombocytopenice purpura, splenectomy should be considered before immunosuppressive therapy with cyclophosphamide.
16. There may be a persistent mild thrombocytosis following splenectomy.
17. Patients with a normal platelet count always have a normal bleeding time.
18. Prolonged PTT related to intrinsic factor deficiencies is always associated with clinical bleeding problems.
19. Platelets and coagulation factors are normal in patients with vascular purpura.
20. Elderly patients receiving red blood cell transfusions may develop pulmonary edema.
21. Any febrile patient with severe neutropenia should receive granulocyte transfusions.
22. Bleeding related to primary platelet dysfunction does not improve with platelet transfusion.
23. Fresh frozen plasma is the treatment of choice for hemophiliacs.
24. Prothrombin complex concentrates may result in thromboembolic complications in patients with liver disease.
25. Patients receiving massive red blood cell transfusions may develop a bleeding diathesis.

ANSWERS

1. B	14. B
2. A	15. A
3. D	16. A
4. B	17. B
5. B	18. B
6. D	19. A
7. C	20. A
8. D	21. B
9. D	22. B
10. B	23. B
11. B	24. A
12. A	25. A
13. A	

BIBLIOGRAPHY

TEXTBOOKS

Beck WS (ed): *Hematology*. Cambridge, Mass, The MIT Press, 1977.

Begemann H, Rastetter J: *Atlas of Clinical Hematology*, ed. 3. New York, Springer-Verlag, New York Inc, 1979.

Williams WJ, Beutler E, Ersley AJ, Rundles RW (eds): *Hematology*, ed. 2. New York, McGraw-Hill Book Co, 1977.

MONOGRAPHS AND ARTICLES

Disorders of Erythrocytes

Bentley DP: Anemia and chronic disease. *Clinics Haemat* 11:465-479, 1982.

Callendar ST: Treatment of iron deficiency. *Clinics Hematology* 11:327-338, 1982.

Gale RP: Aplastic Anemia: Biology & Treatment. *Ann Int Med* 95: 477-494, 1981.

Hillman RS, Finch GA: Red cell manual, ed. 4. Philadelphia, FA Davis Co, 1974.

Hoffman R, Wasserman LR: Natural history and management of Polycythemia vera. *Adv Int Med* 24:225-285, 1979.

Kirshner JP, Cartwright GE: Sideroblastic anemia. *Adv Int Med* 22: 229-249, 1977.

Orkin SH, Nathan DG: The thalassemia. *N Engl J Med* 295 (13):710-714, 1976.

Pirofsky B: Clinical aspects of autoimmune hemolytic anemia. *Sem Hematol* 13: (4):251-265, 1976.

Disorders of Leukocytes

Berard CW, Gallo RC, Jaffe ES, et al: Current concepts of Leukemia and lymphoma: Etiology, Pathogenesis, and therapy. *Ann Intern Med* 83 (3):351-366, 1976.

Beutler E, McMillan R, Spruce W: Brief Review: The role of bone marrow transplantation of acute leukemia in remission. *Blood* 59: 1115-1117, 1982.

Bloomfield CD, Hurd DD: Management of acute myelocytic leukemia in adults. *Curr Concepts Oncol* 2 (4):17-23, 1980.

Boggs DR, Winkelstein A: *White cell manual*, ed. 3. Philadelphia, FA Davis Co, 1975.

Cline MJ, Lehrer RI, Territo MC, et al: Monocytes and macrophages: Functions and diseases. *Ann Intern Med* 88 (1):78-88, 1978.

Silber R: Chronic lymphocytic leukemia in the elderly. *Hospital Practice* 17:131-141, 1982.

Disorders of Hemostasis

Antithrombin, Editorial. *Lancet 1* (7973), 1333-1334, 1976.

Majerus PW, Miletich JP: Relationships between platelets and coagulation factors in hemostasis. *Annu Rev Med* 29:41-49, 1978.

Clinical Pharmacolocy of antithrombotic drugs. *Clinics Haemat* 10: 443-520, 1981.

Clinical Use of Blood Components

Higby DJ, Burnett D: Granulocyte transfusions: Current status. *Blood* 55 (1):2-8, 1980.

Schmidt PJ: Transfusion reactions-status in 1982. *Clinics Lab Med* 2:221-231, 1982.

Valleri CR: Current concepts of blood transfusion. *J Oral Surg* 35 (9): 707-712, 1977.

CHAPTER 9
INFECTIOUS DISEASES

Philip W. Smith

GENERAL CONSIDERATIONS

MICROBIOLOGY

Organisms that cause infectious diseases in humans form a large spectrum in terms of size and complexity (Table 1).

Viruses

Viruses are the smallest infectious agents. The basic structure of a virus is a central core of nucleic acid (DNA or RNA)

Table 1. Characteristics of Organisms

Organism	*Mean Size (μ)*	*Grows Outside of Host Cell*	*Generates Metabolic Energy*
Virus	0.10	No	No
Mycoplasma	0.25	Yes	Yes
Chlamydia	0.30	No	No
Rickettsia	0.45	No	Yes
Bacteria	1	Yes	Yes
Actinomycetes	1	Yes	Yes
Fungus (yeast phase)	4	Yes	Yes
Protozoa	40	Yes	Yes
Helminth	1 cm (length)	Yes	Yes

wrapped in a protective protein coat (capsid). Some viruses also have an outer envelope.

Replication requires the host cell. Early steps in replication are attachment to the host cell, penetration, and uncoating. The virus uses the host's enzymatic machinery to manufacture viral nucleic acid and protein. The nucleic acid is then surrounded by protein and the host cell lyses, releasing mature infectious viruses (virions).

Host defenses against viral infection involve interferon (a protein produced by infected cells), cell-mediated immunity, and antibodies. The antiviral activity of interferon is nonspecific, whereas immunity related to delayed hypersensitivity or antibody formation is specific for the infecting virus.

Intermediate Organisms

Mycoplasmas are the smallest organisms capable of growing in cell-free culture medium. They multiply by binary fission and appear pleomorphic because they lack a rigid cell wall. Antibiotics are active against these organisms.

Chlamydiae were once considered viruses because of their obligate intracellular parasitism. Unlike viruses, chlamydiae possess both DNA and RNA, have a cell wall, multiply by binary fission, and are susceptible to antibiotics.

Rickettsiae are also obligate intracellular parasites, but resemble bacteria with respect to structure, reproduction, and antibiotic susceptibility. Arthropods are the natural vectors for spread of most rickettsiae.

Bacteria

Bacteria possess DNA and ribosomes but no distinct nucleus. Energy is produced anaerobically (fermentation) or aerobically (respiration). A rigid cell wall surrounds the cell membrane and protects the cell from mechanical damage.

Bacteria multiply by binary fission. Some bacteria form endospores that are resistant to adverse environmental conditions. The Gram-positive *Clostridium* and *Bacillus* species are the most important spore-formers.

Bacteria are classified on the basis of shape (cocci, bacilli), staining characteristics (Gram-positive, Gram-negative, acid-fast), oxygen tolerance, motility, encapsulation, and spore formation (Table 2).

Immunity to bacterial infection involves white blood cells (staphylococci), antibodies (pneumococci), or delayed hypersensitivity (tuberculosis).

Actinomycetes

Actinomyces and nocardiae are branching, filamentous organisms that originally were mistakenly classified as fungi. They are actually bacteria, as evidenced by their cell organization (prokaryotic), cell wall structure, and sensitivity to antibiotics.

Fungi

Unlike bacteria, fungi reproduce by sexual and asexual cycles. They occur as single cells (yeasts) or as multicellular organisms (mycelia). Yeasts reproduce by budding or fission, whereas mycelia reproduce by fragmentation of the multicellular filaments (hyphae) or formation of spores. Most fungal pathogens of humans appear in tissue as the yeast phase and in vitro as the mycelial phase.

Fungi also differ structurally from bacteria. The principal material in the fungal cell wall is chitin. Fungi are eukaryotic cells because they possess a nuclear membrane, mitochondria, and several different chromosomes.

Immunity to fungal diseases involves primarily delayed hypersensitivity.

Protozoa and Helminths

Protozoa are unicellular organisms with complex intracellular organization. Protozoa that are pathogenic for humans include flagellates (*Giardia lamblia*), amebae (*Entamoeba histolytica*) and sporozoa (*Plasmodium sp.*).

Helminths are sexually differentiated and reproduce by production of larvae or ova. The pathogenic helminths of man vary in size from 1 mm (*Heterophyes heterophyes*) to 10 m or more (*Diphyllobothrium latum*).

EPIDEMIOLOGY OF INFECTIOUS DISEASES

An infectious disease can be characterized by the number of existing cases in a population (prevalence), the number of new cases in a population (incidence), and the risk of transmission (contagiousness). Diseases may persist at a constant level in the community (endemic) or increase above the baseline level (epidemic).

Importance of Infectious Diseases

On a global level, infectious diseases are responsible for more deaths than cancer or heart disease. Hookworm infection, whipworm infection, ascariasis, filariasis, and schistosomiasis each affect more than 200 million people. The leading infectious cause of death in the United States is bacterial pneumonia.

The field of infectious diseases in one of the most rapidly advancing areas of medicine. Recent years have seen an explosion of new antibiotics, the global eradication of small pox and new or improved immunizations for rabies, pneumococcal

Table 2. Bacterial Classification

Aerobic			*Anaerobic*	
Cocci		Gram-positive	Cocci:	Peptococcus
Staphylococcus				Peptostreptococcus
Streptococcus				
Bacilli			Bacilli:	Clostridia
Lactobacillus				
Corynebacterium				
Listeria				
Cocci		Gram-negative	Cocci:	Veillonella
Neisseria				
Bacilli			Bacilli:	Bacteroides
Escherichia	Brucella			Fusobacterium
Klebsiella	Hemophilus			
Proteus	Salmonella			
Serratia	Shigella			
Pseudomonas	Yersinia			
Franciscella	Vibrio			
Mycobacterium		Acid-fast		
Nocardia		Gram-positive Filaments	Actinomyces	
		Spirochetes		
		Treponema		
		Leptospira		
		Borrelia		

pneumonia and hepatitis B Legionnaries' disease, *Chlamydia* urethritis, toxic shock syndrome and *Clostridium difficile* pseudomembranous enterocolitis have only recently been delineated.

Disease Transmission

The spread of infectious diseases involves the following general sequence: reservoir → vector → host. The reservoir may be humans (influenza), animals (tularemia), or the environment (sporotrichosis). A variety of vectors may be implicated, including insects (malaria), water (cholera), and fomites (staphylococci).

The most contagious diseases of humans are chickenpox, measles, smallpox, influenza, rubella, mumps, and pneumonic plague. The risk of acquisition of disease by a nonimmune host after exposure is over 50% for these diseases. By contrast, a number of diseases that are widely feared are not highly contagious, including leprosy, meningococcal meningitis, diphtheria, and tuberculosis.

PATHOGENESIS OF INFECTION

Microorganisms are beneficial to humans in many ways. Normal bacterial flora inhibit the growth of potential pathogens. Fungi, actinomycetes, and bacteria make antibiotics that are therapeutically useful.

Colonization is the coexistence of microorganisms and host without injury to or reaction by the host. Whether infection develops depends upon the virulence of the organism as well as host defenses.

The virulence, or pathogenicity, of microorganisms relates to two basic mechanisms. First, bacteria may cause disease by invasion of tissues. Invasiveness is enhanced by antiphagocytic capsules (pneumococci) or enzymes that promote spread of the organisms through connective tissue (staphylococci). Second, noninvasive bacteria can injure the host by producing diffusable exotoxins. Botulism, tetanus, diphtheria, and cholera are examples of toxin-related diseases.

Alternatively, tissue damage may be caused by the response of the host to the organism. This mechanism is typified by the delayed hypersensitivity response of the host to infection with *Mycobacterium tuberculosis*, in which mononuclear cell inflammation occurs.

HOST DEFENSES

Man lives in a world of pathogenic organisms. The efficiency of host defenses is fully appreciated when considering the severe infections that affect an immunodeficient host.

Local Defenses

The skin and mucous membranes are the first barrier against potential invaders. Intact skin, urinary flow, and the mucociliary system of the lungs provide mechanical protection.

Chemical factors include gastric acidity and lysozyme, a protein found in all secretions that lyses bacteria. The normal bacterial flora of the skin, mouth, gut, and vagina also exerts a protective effect by virtue of competition with pathogens for nutrients and excretion of toxic substances.

Phagocytosis

The phagocytic system includes polymorphonuclear leukocytes (neutrophils), monocytes, and tissue macrophages. The neutrophil is the most efficient phagocytic cell, but its life span in tissues is only 1 to 3 days.

The phagocytic sequence begins with chemotaxis, the migration of the cell to the site of inflammation. Complement is the primary stimulus for chemotaxis. Following chemotaxis, the phagocyte ingests the organism and kills it in a complicated process involving hydrogen peroxide.

The most common and most severe phagocytic deficiency is neutropenia, which can be detected by white blood cell and differential counts. A neutrophil count of less than 1000/cc is associated with a markedly increased risk of serious bacterial infection. More elaborate in vitro tests of neutrophil function (chemotaxis, ingestion, and killing) are available, but at present serve mainly as research tools.

Humoral Immunity

Humoral immunity involves antibodies produced by the plasma cell. IgG comprises about 70% of serum immunoglobulin. IgM is the earliest antibody produced in response to infection but is short-lived. IgA is the local antibody of respiratory and gastrointestinal tract secretions.

Antibodies function to coat bacteria and facilitate their phagocytosis (opsonization). Other functions include agglutination of organisms, lysis of bacteria, and virus neutralization.

Antibody deficiencies are detected by a quantitative immunoglobulin assay. IgA deficiency is associated with severe and recurrent respiratory and gastrointestinal tract infections. The severe infections with *Streptococcus pneumoniae* and *Hemophilus influenzae* encountered in IgG deficiency reflect deficient opsonization. Multiple myeloma is an example of this deficiency.

Cellular Immunity

Cellular immune reactions are mediated by thymus-dependent lymphocytes. Whereas the end result of humoral immunity is an antibody against a specific microorganism, the end result of cellular immunity is a lymphocyte that recognizes a specific microorganism. The immune lymphocyte produces factors that injure the organism directly or attract macrophages to the site.

Cellular immunity is most easily detected by skin tests for delayed hypersensitivity. Almost all adult patients will react to mumps, *Candida*, trichophytin, streptokinase-streptodornase, or purified protein derivative (PPD). More elaborate testing can be carried out with dinitrochlorobenzene sensitization or in vitro testing of lymphocyte function. Corticosteroid therapy, lymphoma, and renal failure are commonly associated with impaired cell-mediated immunity, which predisposes the host especially to viral and fungal infections.

Other Aspects of Immunity

The complement pathway is a series of proteins that reacts in sequence when triggered by antigen-antibody complexes. The complement system mediates enhancement of vascular permeability, attraction of neutrophils, stimulation of phagocytosis, and cell lysis. Several assays for serum complement activity are available.

Interferon is a glycoprotein produced by lymphocytes in response to viral infection. Interferon inhibits viral multiplication and is an important component of host defenses.

MANIFESTATIONS OF INFECTION

Fever

Normal bod*r* temperature has a diurnal rhythm, with the highest levels occurring in the early evening. Fever is clinically defined as ar. oral temperature above 99°F or 37.2°C. Rectal temperatures are 0.5°C higher. There are many causes of fever including infections, neoplasms, autoimmune diseases, endocrine disturbances, vascular accidents, drugs, and neurologic disorders.

Endogenous pyrogen is a substance produced by phagocytes in response to phagocytosis or bacterial endotoxin. Endogenous pyrogen, released into the bloodstream, stimulates the hypothalamus to mediate cutaneous vasoconstriction, decreased sweating, and rigors. This leads to an elevation in body temperature.

The effects of fever include increased metabolic requirements, heart rate, cardiac output, catabolism, and fluid losses. Fever may also be beneficial. In animals with certain infections, fever significantly improves survival.

Salicylates, acetaminophen, corticosteroids, indomethacin, estrogens, and phenothiazines have antipyretic effects. A fever of 40°C or less is rarely acutely harmful in adults. Patients may be more uncomfortable with antipyretic therapy (especially intermittent therapy) than with the fever, itself.

Hematologic Manifestations

Infections produce anemia by a variety of mechanisms, including iron loss (hookworm infection), vitamin B_{12} deficiency (fish tapeworm infection), decreased blood production (chronic infections), and hemolysis. Hemolysis in malaria is due to the parasite, whereas the hemolysis that occurs in *Mycoplasma* infection is due to cold agglutinins.

Bacterial infections are classically associated with an increase in the neutrophil count and a shift to more immature forms. Parasitic diseases are often manifested by an increased eosinophil count, and viral infections by a lymphocytosis. Mononucleosis is suggested by atypical lymphocytes in the peripheral blood smear.

DIAGNOSTIC ASPECTS

Isolation and Identification of Organisms

Viruses and chlamydiae grow only in tissue culture, embryonated eggs, or suckling mice. Most viruses grow slowly in tissue culture; herpesviruses are an exception, and may be identified in several days. Identification of viruses depends on observation of the viral cytopathic effect on various tissue cultures.

Bacteria can usually be isolated from clinical specimens in 1-2 days. However, anaerobic bacteria may be killed by exposure to oxygen if specimens are not properly collected and transported. Also, *Neisseria gonorrhoeae*, *Brucella sp.*, *Corynebacterium diphtheriae*, *Francisella tularensis*, *Vibrio sp.*, and *Bordetella pertussis* require special media for isolation.

Bacteria are identified by colony morphology, Gram-stained appearance, and biochemical tests. Gas chromatography of fatty acid byproducts is useful in the identification of anaerobic bacteria.

Mycobacteria and fungi grow slowly, final identification often requiring 2 to 8 weeks, and special media are required. Both are identified by colony characteristics and biochemical tests. The microscopic appearance of fungi is helpful in identification.

Protozoa and helminths are identified by direct visualization of the organism. Any stage in the life cycle may be observed.

Specimen Collection

Meticulous specimen collection is critical. The microbiology laboratory cannot compensate for a poorly collected sample.

Spinal fluid and blood are normally sterile. It is essential that cultures be collected aseptically, which is usually accomplished by cleansing the skin with alcohol and iodine solution prior to specimen collection. Three separate 10 ml blood cultures obtained within a 24-hour period will detect 99% of bacteremias. False-positive blood culture results occur most frequently with *Staphylococcus epidermidis* and *Propionibacterium acnes*, which reflects the role of these bacteria as predominant skin flora.

All sputum specimens are contaminated by oral bacteria to some extent. *S. pneumoniae* and *H. influenzae* may be respiratory pathogens or normal pharyngeal flora. A percutaneous transtracheal aspirate bypasses oral flora and is mandatory if anaerobic bacteria are sought. It has the disadvantage of patient discomfort and possible hemorrhage.

Throat culture is not a substitute for sputum culture in the diagnosis of pneumonia. Only group A streptococci, *C. diphtheriae*, and *N. gonorrhoeae* are of diagnostic interest when present in a throat culture.

Urine cultures are contaminated with perineal bacteria, but quantitative midstream cultures distinguish contamination from infection. Lactobacilli and *S. epidermidis* are frequently contaminants. An improperly collected specimen is suggested by the presence of contaminants, of less than 10^4 bacteria per ml of urine, or of multiple bacterial isolates.

In Vitro Antibiotic Tests

The laboratory can perform a number of in vitro tests that may be of assistance to the clinician in directing antibiotic therapy:

1. Antibiotic sensitivity testing for bacteria is most commonly performed by the Bauer-Kirby method. This involves measurement of the zone of inhibition of bacterial growth around an antibiotic-impregnated disk. The size of the zone determines sensitivity or resistance (Fig. 1).

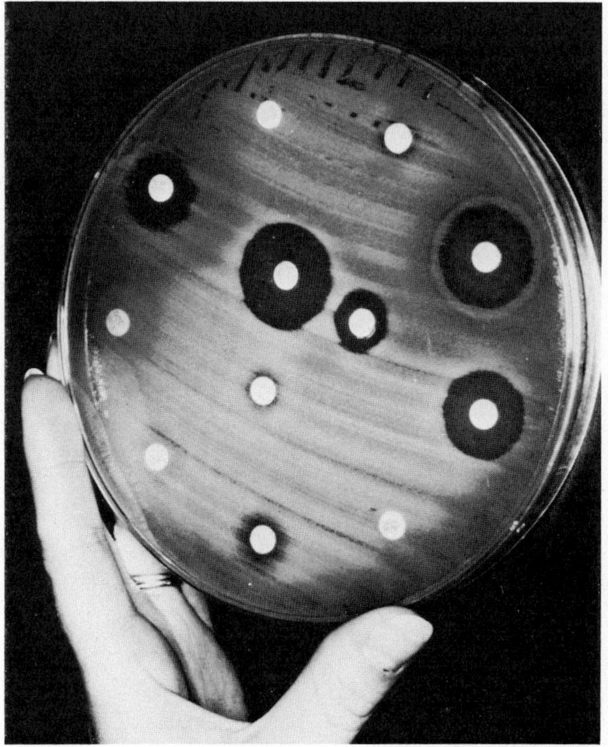

Figure 1. Antibiotic disk sensitivity testing.

2. Broth or agar dilution methods enable the laboratory to quantitatively determine the minimal concentration of an antibiotic that is inhibitory (MIC) or bactericidal (MBC) for an organism.
3. The inhibitory or killing effect of serum on the infecting organism can also be measured by the broth dilution method. This correlates best with antibiotic levels in the serum and is usually measured before (trough) or after (peak) a dose of antibiotic. This assay is helpful in the treatment of bacterial endocarditis.
4. The actual concentration of an antibiotic in the serum can be measured by a variety of techniques. The microbioassay is the standard method, but more accurate and rapid methods are being developed, such as the radioenzymatic assay for gentamicin.

Staining

Information about an infectious process can be obtained rapidly from a properly performed stain of a clinical specimen. Bacteria are best observed by Gram stain, which stains bacteria purple (Gram-positive), or red (Gram-negative). Gram stain provides clues to the adequacy of a sputum specimen by permitting visualization of neutrophils and epithelial cells.

Mycobacteria can be visualized by the acid-fast or auramine-fluorescent stain, actinomycetes by the Gram stain, and fungi by silver or para-aminosalicylic acid (PAS) stains. India ink is used to highlight cryptococci on direct examination of cere-

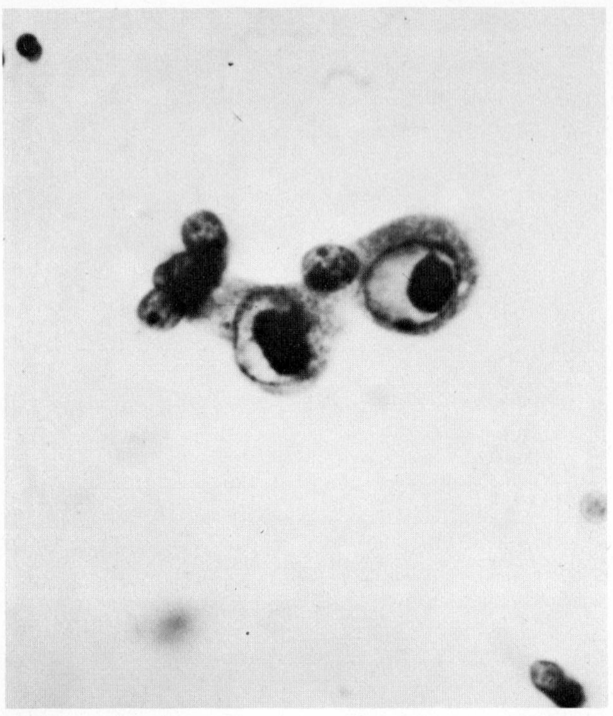

Figure 2. CMV intranuclear inclusion body.

brospinal fluid (CSF). Viral inclusion bodies may be seen by direct examination (Fig. 2).

Counterimmunoelectrophoresis

Counterimmunoelectrophoresis (CIE) is a rapid test for bacterial antigen. An electrical current speeds the standard immunodiffusion reaction; results are available in 1-2 hours. CIE is used primarily for detection of the capsular antigen of *H. influenzae*, *S. pneumoniae*, *N. meningitidis*, and group B streptococci in CSF.

Antibody Titers

Measurement of titers of antibody against organisms by a variety of techniques (complement fixation, immunodiffusion, hemagglutination inhibition) provides helpful diagnostic information. Since a single antibody titer is rarely diagnostic, the clinician should make every effort to obtain paired sera. The first should be obtained early in the course of the disease and the second at least 2 weeks later. A fourfold or greater rise in titer is generally of diagnostic significance.

Diseases that may be diagnosed serologically include viral illnesses (measles, influenza), bacterial diseases (brucellosis, Legionnaires' disease), mycoplasmal and rickettsial infections, fungal diseases (histoplasmosis, coccidioidomycosis), and even parasitic diseases (amebiasis, toxoplasmosis).

Diagnostic Approach

The microbiology laboratory, then, can assist the clinician in several areas:

1. Proper specimen collection
2. Rapid diagnostic aids (e.g., Gram stain, India ink examination, stool examination for parasites, CIE)
3. Isolation and identification of the responsible pathogen (bacteria, mycobacteria, fungi)
4. In vitro testing of antibiotic sensitivity and effectiveness (e.g., disk sensitivity, MIC, serum killing level)
5. Serologic studies (e.g., VDRL, antibody titers, cryptococcal antigen)

VIRUSES AND RELATED ORGANISMS

HERPESVIRUSES

Herpesviruses are DNA viruses that tend to persist in the host and produce recurrent infections. The two most important viruses in this group are herpes simplex virus and varicella-zoster virus.

Epidemiology

Herpesviruses are spread by direct contact. Herpes simplex type 1 involves primarily the mouth and lips and is generally acquired during the first decade of life. Herpes simplex type 2 involves genital sites and is transmitted by sexual contact.

The peak age for chickenpox, which is caused by the varicella-zoster virus, is about 6 years. The virus survives in dorsal root ganglia and may reactivate years later to produce herpes zoster (shingles).

Manifestations: Herpes Simplex

Herpes simplex causes a number of clinical syndromes. Type 1 virus is responsible for ulcerative gingivostomatitis (cold sores). Stress is associated with reactivation of lesions. Primary infections are more severe than recrudescent infections; fever and lymphadenopathy are often seen. Herpetic vesicles or ulcers occur most frequently on the lips but may occur anywhere on the skin. The type 2 virus causes similar lesions on the cervix or labia in women and the penis in men. Herpetic skin lesions are characteristically painful and recurrent.

In the newborn, herpes simplex acquired in the birth canal frequently disseminates. Immunosuppressed adults may also develop widespread disease. The mortality from disseminated herpes simplex infection is high.

Extensive skin lesions may result from cutaneous herpes in patients with atopy or eczema. Herpetic keratitis is a serious ocular problem that may lead to visual impairment. Herpes simplex encephalitis is a devastating infection with a mortality of over 50% and many survivors have permanent neurologic sequelae. Herpes encephalitis is distinguished from other types of encephalitis by the presence of focal signs and focal lesions on brain scan.

Manifestations: Varicella Zoster

Chickenpox is a highly contagious disease with an incubation period of about 14 days. The characteristic skin lesions evolve from macules to papules to vesicles to crusts within 24 hours. The lesions appear in successive crops. Children have no prodrome but may have fever with the rash. The disease is usually mild and has an excellent prognosis. Interstitial pneumonia is the major complication in adults. Chickenpox has a high mortality in the immunodeficient patient.

Herpes zoster peaks at age 50-80. The vesicles resemble chickenpox but occur in a dermatomal distribution. The rash is unilateral and most commonly affects the thoracic dermatomes. Local paresthesias or pain may precede the rash. Severe long-lasting pain (postherpetic neuralgia) is seen particularly in the elderly. The disease may disseminate in the compromised host.

Diagnosis

The diagnosis of cold sores, venereal herpes, chickenpox, and herpes zoster is clinical. The herpes virus can be cultivated in tissue culture, but this procedure is not routinely available. Viral inclusion bodies in clinical specimens may provide a clue to herpes infection. Antibodies are present in a large percentage of the population; hence, antibody studies are not useful diagnostically. The diagnosis of herpes simplex encephalitis is best made by culturing the virus from a brain biopsy specimen.

Therapy and Prevention

There is no cure for mucocutaneous herpes infection. Topical acyclovir hastens resolution of genital type 2 herpes simplex lesions but does not prevent recurrences. Adenine arabinoside is useful for herpes simplex encephalitis and disseminated herpes simplex infection in neonates. Corticosteroids should be avoided, especially in herpetic keratitis.

Cesarean section will prevent neonatal herpes simplex infection and should be seriously considered if the mother has genital herpes. Prevention of herpes zoster infection is feasible only in limited circumstances: zoster immune globulin is available for severely immunosuppressed children who have not previously had chickenpox and who have recently been exposed to the disease.

Cytomegalovirus

Cytomegalovirus (CMV) is a herpes virus that causes mononucleosis in adults and congenital disease in the newborn with jaundice, chorioretinitis and neurologic sequelae. In the renal transplant recipient, CMV causes severe disease including fever, hepatitis, and interstitial pneumonitis.

The diagnosis is suggested by observation of large, inclusion-bearing cells in urine or tissues, but is confirmed only by viral culture of urine, blood, or tissue. Serology is occasionally helpful in diagnosis.

MONONUCLEOSIS

Infectious mononucleosis is a disease with peak incidence in young adults. It is most commonly caused by the Epstein-Barr (EB) virus, although a variety of infectious agents are known to cause a similar clinical picture. The EB virus is found in saliva and presumably spread by oral contact.

Manifestations

Following a prodromal period of several days, fever and sore throat develop. The physical exam discloses enlarged, tender cervical lymph nodes and a whitish exudate on the pharynx or tonsils. About 50% of patients have detectable splenomegaly. Symptoms are frequently of greater severity in elderly patients.

Almost all patients recover without complications, although malaise and lymphadenopathy may persist for several months. Complications, seen in less than 5% of patients, include splenic rupture (the leading cause of death), airway obstruction secondary to severe pharyngeal inflammation, hemolytic anemia, hepatitis, and meningoencephalitis. A generalized skin rash consistently develops with ampicillin administration.

Diagnosis

Mildly abnormal liver function tests are seen, and the blood count shows a lymphocytosis with atypical lymphocytes (large cells with indented nuclei).

Heterophil antibodies are agglutinating antibodies for sheep red blood cells that develop during the first 1-2 weeks. The monospot test is a rapid agglutination test that measures similar antibodies using horse red blood cells. This assay is more sensitive than the heterophil test but is less specific.

A positive monospot test is presumptive evidence of mononucleosis. Titers may persist for a year or more. A few reference laboratories are able to measure EB viral capsid antibodies. A throat culture is advisable since streptococcal pharyngitis may coexist with mononucleosis.

Therapy

No specific therapy is available but bed rest is recommended during the acute illness. Steroids are useful if severe airway obstruction, hemolysis, or thrombocytopenia develop. Relapses may occur.

Non-EB Virus Mononucleosis

Heterophil-negative mononucleosis may be caused by cytomegalovirus (CMV) or toxoplasmosis. Antibody tests are useful in diagnosis, and CMV can be cultured from blood (buffy coat) or urine.

INFLUENZA

Influenza is an enveloped RNA virus that causes cyclic epidemics of respiratory disease. There are three distinct antigenic types: A, B, and C.

Epidemiology

The disease occurs primarily in winter, and preschool children have the highest incidence of disease. Influenza-related deaths occur predominantly among the elderly and the chronically ill. Influenza is spread from person to person by respiratory droplets.

Types A and B cause epidemics every 2 to 4 and 4 to 6 years, respectively; only type A causes pandemics. The virus is notorious for antigenic shifts that make previously acquired immunity obsolete. Type A antigenic subtypes are based on the hemagglutinin (H) and neuraminidase (N) antigens. For instance, in 1968 the predominant A virus changed from H_2N_2 to H_3N_2, and a pandemic (Hong Kong influenza) resulted.

A distinct influenza A viral subtype, swine influenza, is found in pigs. This strain may have been responsible for the influenza pandemic of 1918-1919 and was isolated from several cases in 1976.

There appears to be a finite number of antigenic mutations for the influenza virus. Children have the highest attack rate during an epidemic because they lack the immunologic experience that provides protection to older people.

Manifestations

The incubation period is 1-3 days. The illness begins abruptly with fever, chills, headache, malaise, myalgias, and dry cough. Substernal chest pain and prostration may be seen, but coryza is unusual. Influenza A is more severe than influenza B or C, and symptoms are most severe in elderly or debilitated patients and pregnant women.

In uncomplicated cases the disease resolves in 3 to 6 days. The most common complication is pneumonia, which is usually bacterial but may be due to the influenza virus. *S. pneumoniae*, *H. influenzae* and *S. aureus* are most likely to cause bacterial superinfection of the lungs. A biphasic fever pattern suggests a secondary bacterial infection.

Diagnosis

The diagnosis is obvious during an epidemic but may be difficult in sporadic cases. It is usually made on clinical grounds. The virus can be isolated from throat washings during the first 3 days, but this is a slow procedure. Paired antibody titers by hemagglutination inhibition or complement fixation techniques may demonstrate a diagnostic fourfold rise.

Therapy and Prevention

Antibiotics have no place in the treatment of uncomplicated influenza; treatment of this disorder is symptomatic only. Bacterial superinfections must be diagnosed and treated appropriately.

A killed virus vaccine is available and recommended for pregnant women, the elderly, and patients with chronic diseases such as cardiac disease, diabetes, renal failure, and chronic obstructive lung disease. The vaccine is only about 70% effective, and protection lasts 3 to 6 months. Therefore, an annual vaccination is required. The vaccine consists of the currently prevalent strains; the 1982-1983 vaccine contained influenza A (H_1N_1), A (H_3N_2), and B. Persons over 26 years of age require one dose, while those 26 and under require two doses for an adequate response. Toxicity is minimal and consists of local reactions and a rare case of Guillain-Barré syndrome (10 cases per million vaccinations). Persons allergic to eggs or egg products may develop an anaphylactic reaction.

MUMPS, MEASLES, AND RUBELLA

These three viral illnesses are seen primarily in children but are not uncommon in young adults.

Mumps

Most cases of mumps occur between the ages of 5 and 10. Disease incidence peaks in winter and spring. The incubation period averages 18 days and the disease is spread by respiratory droplets. The most common manifestation is parotitis, which is usually bilateral. Complications include aseptic meningitis, pancreatitis, nerve deafness, arthritis, and epididymo-orchitis. Orchitis is more common in postpubertal men (20%) and is most often unilateral. Sterility occasionally results.

Measurement of antibody titer rises will confirm the diagnosis. The serum amylase is elevated in both parotitis and pancreatitis.

Measles and Rubella

Measles and rubella (German measles) are contagious exanthematous diseases. Both are spread by respiratory droplets, are seen most often in children, and are contagious before the onset of the characteristic rash. Rubella outbreaks have occurred on college campuses and military bases.

Measles is the more severe illness. After an incubation period of 10-14 days, the prodromal symptoms appear: coryza, fever, conjunctivitis, and photophobia. The rash appears 3 to 5 days later, usually spreading downward from the head. Lesions coalesce, turn brown, and desquamate. Physical exam reveals conjunctivitis, rash, lymphadenopathy, splenomegaly, and the pathognomonic Koplik's spots (small red spots with bluish white centers on the buccal mucosa). Complications include interstitial pneumonia, bronchitis, otitis media, encephalitis, and myocarditis.

Atypical measles is seen in patients who were previously vaccinated with the inactivated viral vaccine and have partial immunity. The prodrome consists of fever, cough, headache, myalgias, nausea, and vomiting. The rash is atypical, beginning peripherally and progressing centrally. Severe pneumonia develops.

The incubation period for rubella is 15-24 days. During a mild prodrome, fever and enlarged, tender posterior cervical lymph nodes are found. The pink rash begins on the face and spreads rapidly downward. Complications, except for arthritis, are rare. The most serious consequences of rubella infection occur when women contract the disease during the first trimester of pregnancy. Congenital rubella often causes infant cataracts, deafness, cardiac abnormalities, and other defects.

Both measles and rubella result in a rise in specific hemagglutination-inhibition antibody titers. Measles virus may be cultured from throat washings or conjunctival secretions, but the diagnosis is usually made on clinical grounds.

Therapy and Prevention

Therapy for mumps, measles, and rubella is symptomatic. Theoretically, they can be prevented by vaccination, and natural immunity is lifelong. Live attenuated mumps, measles, and rubella vaccines are very effective and should be given after 15 months of age. The vaccines are generally well-tolerated, although women may develop arthritis or peripheral neuritis following rubella vaccination. These complications are self-limited, however.

The rubella vaccine virus may cross the placenta and result in fetal anomalies similar to those produced by the wild virus. Women should receive the vaccine only if they agree not to become pregnant for 3 months. In some states, a premarital antibody titer is required to determine the immunity of the woman.

Immune globulin interferes with measles immunity when given concurrently with the viral vaccine.

RABIES

Rabies is a viral disease transmitted by the saliva of animals. It is virtually 100% fatal.

Epidemiology

Wild animals are the primary reservoir, although infected domestic animals can transmit the disease. In the United States, the greatest risk is from the bites of skunks, bats, badgers, foxes, and raccoons.

Manifestations

The virus travels along the path of the nerve to the central nervous system. The incubation period is 1-3 months. During the prodromal phase, the patient experiences paresthesias in the area of the bite. The more characteristic excitation phase is entered later, where increased muscle tone and autonomic nervous system imbalance predominate. Attempts to swallow liquids lead to spasmodic pharyngeal muscle contractions, which result in hydrophobia. Finally, flaccid paralysis develops.

Diagnosis

The definitive diagnosis depends on viral isolation or finding the virus in human or animal tissue by the fluorescent rabies antibody (FRA) test. Pathologic examination may demonstrate cytoplasmic inclusion bodies in the neurons of the central nervous system (Negri bodies).

Prevention

The bite wound should be cleaned as quickly as possible. Bites of rats, mice, squirrels, or rabbits do not require prophylaxis but other animal bites (particularly bats or carnivores) may. Domestic cats and dogs should be observed for 10 days. Wild, ill, unvaccinated, or stray animals should be killed and have brain tissue examined by the FRA test. If a dog or cat bite is unprovoked, or if the animal exhibits unusual behavior during observation, it should be similarly examined.

Bites by FRA-positive or escaped animals require prophylaxis, which consists of a single injection of rabies immune globulin and a series of five intramuscular injections of human diploid cell rabies vaccine. The latter is associated with some local reactions and mild systemic symptoms.

ENTEROVIRUSES, INCLUDING POLIOMYELITIS

The enteroviruses include poliovirus, coxsackievirus, and echovirus. They are frequent causes of gastroenteritis and are spread by the fecal-oral route.

Enteroviruses cause epidemic gastroenteritis that manifests as diarrhea and vomiting. Coxsackievirus and echovirus are responsible for a number of syndromes, including hand-foot-and-mouth disease (a vesicular disease caused by coxsackievirus A), herpangina (pharyngeal vesicles caused by coxsackievirus A), pleurodynia (epidemic pleurisy caused by coxsackievirus B), myocarditis (coxsackievirus B), and aseptic meningitis.

Poliovirus is best known for paralytic disease, although gastroenteritis and aseptic meningitis are much more common. Paralytic poliomyelitis presents as a rapidly developing, asymmetric motor disease involving cranial and peripheral nerves. Sensory changes are rare. The case fatality rate is 10-15%, but most survivors recover some function.

The diagnosis of paralytic poliomyelitis is suggested by rising antibody titers or isolation of the virus from stool, but is confirmed by isolation of virus from the CSF.

Prevention

The most effective vaccine is the trivalent oral polio vaccine (OPV), which is a live virus vaccine. Three doses are given to infants in the first year; a preschool booster is also administered. The vaccine has the advantage of inducing alimentary immunity. An inactived polio vaccine (IPV) is available when a live virus vaccine is contraindicated such as in an immunosuppressed child, but the IPV is less effective. The vaccine virus (OPV) itself has rarely been associated with paralytic disease. Recent outbreaks of poliomyelitis among certain religious sects that eschew vaccination have reemphasized the potential of the poliovirus to cause serious disease.

VIRAL HEPATITIS

Viral hepatitis is a syndrome that can be caused by a number of viral agents including hepatitis A, hepatitis B, cytomegalovirus, and EB virus. Hepatitis A and B are the classic examples of viral hepatitis.

Epidemiology

Hepatitis A has an incubation period of 2 to 6 weeks and tends to occur in epidemics. Spread is from person to person by the fecal-oral route. Shellfish, contaminated water, and infected food handlers have been responsible for outbreaks. The virus is found in the stool 2 weeks before the onset of symptoms and remains until the SGOT begins to fall. Twenty to 60 percent of the population in the United States have hepatitis A antibodies. The prevalence of the antibody is increased in urban areas and in areas where sanitation is poor.

Hepatitis B has an incubation period of 1-6 months. Transmission of the virus is usually by the parenteral route. Blood transfusion, hemodialysis, and drug abuse are significant risk factors; health care personnel are at increased risk. The virus can be found in body secretions and in blood. The prevalence of hepatitis B serum antibodies in the general population is less than hepatitis A antibodies.

Manifestations

Many cases are asymptomatic, but fever, anorexia, nausea, or right upper quadrant pain may occur. Ten to 20 percent of hepatitis B patients have a prodrome that consists of fever, arthralgias, and rash. On physical exam an enlarged and tender liver is appreciated; jaundice is often noted. Serum transaminases are high and the bilirubin moderately elevated. A liver biopsy demonstrates a panlobular inflammatory response.

Hepatitis A has a very good prognosis. Symptoms usually resolve within several weeks and chronic liver disease does not develop. Hepatitis B, on the other hand, leads to chronic active hepatitis in as many as 10% of cases. Cirrhosis may eventually result.

Diagnosis

The diagnosis of hepatitis A is usually made on clinical grounds. Hepatitis A antibody (IgG) is present for years after infection and is associated with immunity. The presence of IgM antibody suggests recent infection.

A variety of particles that relate to the hepatitis B virus have been identified including hepatitis B surface antigen (HB_sAg), hepatitis B core antigen, and e antigen. These particles, or the antibodies produced against them, have been used to diagnose hepatitis B. The hepatitis B surface antigen, formerly Australia antigen, correlates well with infectiousness. It appears in the blood before the onset of symptoms. Most patients eliminate the HB_sAg from their blood within several months and develop protective anti-HB_sAg, although 5-10% become chronic HB_sAg carriers.

Therapy and Prevention

There is no specific therapy for hepatitis A or B. Steroids are not indicated in acute hepatitis.

Immune serum globulin (ISG) confers significant protection against hepatitis A; when given within 2 weeks of exposure it is 80-90% effective. It is indicated for household contacts of hepatitis A cases, but should not be given more than 2 weeks after exposure or after the onset of symptoms. The dose is 0.02 ml/kg intramuscularly.

Standard ISG does not reliably protect against hepatitis B. Special high-titer hepatitis B immune globulin (HBIG) may offer some protection especially following accidental needlestick. HBIG should be given at a dose of 0.06 ml/kg IM and repeated one months later.

A hepatitis B vaccine is available which consists of surface antigen of the virus. Three injections are recommended: the primary inoculation, and booster doses at one and six months. It is recommended for high risk groups, including health care workers (especially those routinely exposed to blood products, such as dialysis staff, laboratory personnel and surgeons), renal dialysis patients, institutionalized patients, frequently transfused patients, household contacts of HBsAg carriers, neonates born to HBsAg mothers, drug addicts, and male homosexuals.

The incidence of posttransfusion hepatitis B has been decreased by the screening of all blood for HB_sAg. Blood precautions are mandatory for patients who are known to have HB_sAg in serum.

Miscellaneous Viral Hepatitis

Cytomegalovirus and EB virus can cause viral hepatitis. They are diagnosed by antibody titers. A significant number of cases of viral hepatitis are not caused by one of the four viruses described above. The remaining cases, termed non-A, non-B hepatitis, resemble hepatitis B clinically, and may progress to chronic liver disease. Non-A, non-B hepatitis is now the major cause of posttransfusion hepatitis.

CHLAMYDIA, MYCOPLASMA, AND RICKETTSIA

Rocky Mountain Spotted Fever

Rickettsia rickettsii is the most important rickettsial pathogen in the United States. In spite of its name, Rocky Mountain spotted fever (RMSF) is seen most frequently in the southeastern United States. The disease is spread by the saliva of the dog tick and the wood tick. Peak incidence occurs in spring and summer.

A generalized vasculitis develops 2 to 6 days after the tick bite. This is manifested by a maculopapular or petechial rash that begins on the extremities (notably the palms and soles) and spreads centrally. Other symptoms include fever, headache, myalgias, conjunctivitis, abdominal pain, and confusion. Patients are often quite toxic. Disseminated intravascular coagulation may develop. The mortality is 5-10%.

The diagnosis is serologic. Patients often develop a nonspecific antibody against *Proteus* OX-2 and OX-19 antigens (Weil-Felix reaction). A high or rising Weil-Felix reaction is nonspecific but quite suggestive of RMSF. The diagnosis can be confirmed by complement fixation antibody titers. Meningococcemia and measles may be confused with RMSF, but 80% of RMSF patients have a history of tick bite.

Therapy with either chloramphenicol or tetracycline should be instituted promptly. Early removal of ticks is preventive.

Other Rickettsial Diseases

Rickettsialpox, typhus, and Q fever are rickettsial diseases. All rickettsial diseases except for Q fever require an arthropod vector and produce exanthems in humans.

Chlamydiae

Chlamydiae have been implicated in a number of human diseases. *Chlamydia psittaci* causes psittacosis, a disease of birds that may spread to humans. *C. trachomatis* is the agent of trachoma, a keratoconjunctivitis that is an important cause of blindness in underdeveloped countries. Other chlamydial diseases include nongonococcal urethritis, lymphogranuloma venereum (LGV), neonatal pneumonia, and neonatal conjunctivitis.

Chlamydiae must be cultured in cell lines; they do not grow in media. A complement fixation test is available for detection of antibodies. The drugs of choice for chlamydial infections include tetracycline (psittacosis, trachoma, nongonococcal urethritis, LGV), erythromycin (neonatal pneumonia), and sulfonamides.

Mycoplasmal Pneumonia

Mycoplasma pneumoniae causes about 20% of all pneumonia. Spread occurs by respiratory droplets; the peak age of disease is from 5-19 years.

Mycoplasmal pneumonia is a milder disease than bacterial pneumonia and is virtually never fatal. The patient presents with fever, cough, and upper respiratory tract symptoms. Rales are the most common finding on physical examination. The chest x-ray film often looks worse than the patient does with lower lobe segmental bronchopneumonia. The disease is bilateral in one-third of these patients.

The normal white blood cell count helps distinguish mycoplasmal pneumonia from pneumococcal pneumonia. About 50% of patients will develop cold hemagglutinins (nonspecific antibodies that rarely cause actual hemolysis). The specific diagnosis depends on obtaining paired sera to demonstrate a rise in complement fixation antibody titer. The organism can be cultured on special media, but growth will not occur for 2 to 3 weeks.

Therapy consists of tetracycline or erythromycin, 2 g per day for 1-2 weeks. Hospitalization is usually not required, and complications are rare.

BACTERIAL INFECTIONS

PNEUMOCOCCI

Streptococcus pneumoniae (pneumococcus) is a virulent, Gram-positive bacteria that is the leading cause of bacterial pneumonia. This infectious agent is spread by the airborne route. Up to 50% of normal persons, especially children, may carry the pneumococcus in their throats. The organism is encapsulated and nearly 100 serotypes have been identified on the basis of capsular polysaccharide antigens. Immunity is serotype specific.

Pneumonia

Pneumonia, the most common disease caused by the pneumococcus, often follows a viral upper respiratory tract infection. The postsplenectomy state and antibody deficiency disorders are associated with increased frequency and severity of pneumococcal pneumonia.

The disease classically begins with a single shaking chill. Pleuritic chest pain, fever, and a cough productive of brownish sputum follow. Paralytic ileus and jaundice are not uncommon. The chest x-ray film reveals a lobar pneumonia, most often involving the lower lobes (Fig. 3). Twenty-five percent have a pleural effusion.

The diagnosis is made most easily from microscopic examination and culture of a properly collected sputum sample. A positive sputum culture does not necessarily confirm the diagnosis, since the pneumococcus may be part of the normal pharyngeal flora. Also, a negative sputum culture does not rule out the diagnosis. The Gram-stained smear demonstrates many neutrophils and Gram-positive, lancet-shaped cocci in pairs (Fig. 4). A blood culture should be obtained and will yield the organism about one-third of the time. The peripheral white blood cell count is elevated with a shift to more immature forms.

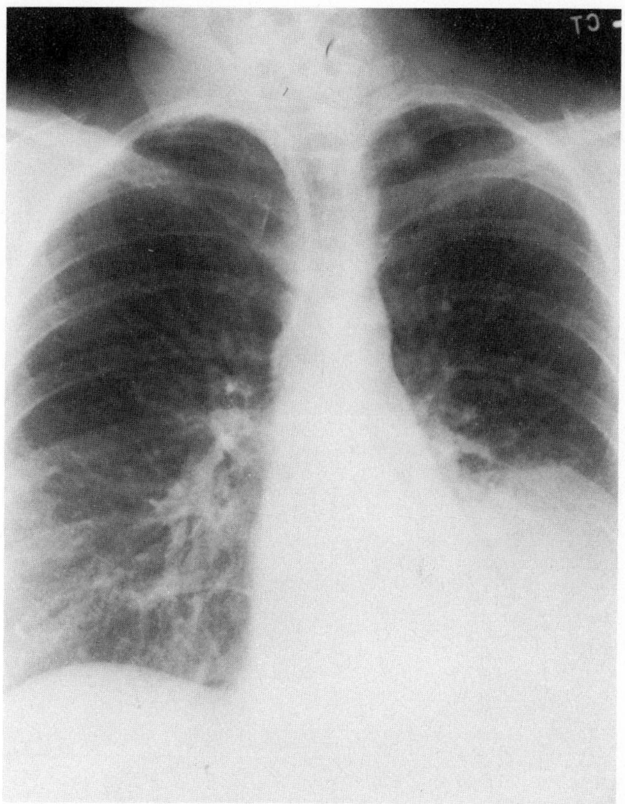

Figure 3. Left lower lobe pneumonia (pneumococcal).

Other Manifestations

The pneumococcus is a leading cause of adult meningitis. The presentation is not different from other bacterial meningitis, and the diagnosis is made on the basis of a positive culture of cerebrospinal fluid or blood. Pneumococcal otitis media is a very common infection of childhood.

Therapy

The most appropriate therapy for pneumococcal pneumonia is 600,000 units of aqueous procaine penicillin G intramuscularly every 12 hours for 7 to 10 days; the organism is generally very sensitive to penicillin. Outpatient therapy with penicillin V 2 g orally per day may be employed if the patient is free of

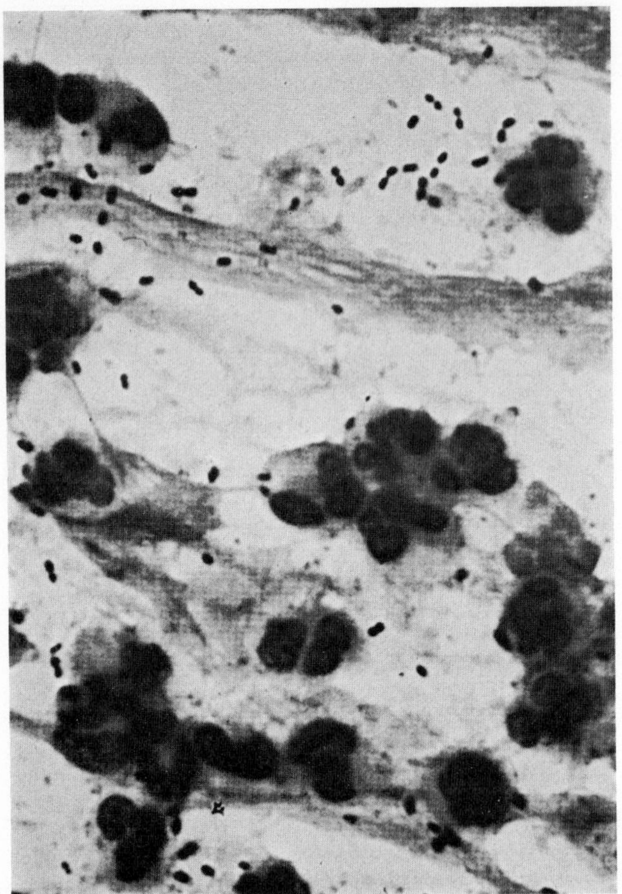

Figure 4. Gram stain of sputum showing white blood cells and diplococci.

complicating medical problems. If penicillin allergy is encountered, the appropriate alternative drugs are erythromycin or cephalosporins.

Dramatic symptomatic improvement usually occurs in 24-48 hours, although the chest x-ray film may not clear completely for several weeks. Lung abscess, empyema, and metastatic infections rarely complicate pneumococcal pneumonia. With proper therapy, the mortality from uncomplicated pneumococcal pneumonia should be less than 5%. The mortality increases with underlying diseases, in the elderly, or if multiple lobes are involved.

Meningitis and endocarditis require high-dose intravenous penicillin therapy, 12-24 million units of aqueous penicillin G per day. Chloramphenicol can be used for meningitis if penicillin allergy is a problem. Pneumococcal meningitis should be treated intravenously for 10-14 days and endocarditis for 3 to 4 weeks.

Prevention

An extract of the capsular polysaccharide of the pneumococcus can induce protective antibodies when injected in humans. In the United States, 14 types account for more than 80% of pneumococcal infections. A vaccine that contains these 14 types of capsular polysaccharides is available and is recommended for patients over 2 years of age with splenic dysfunction (such as sickle cell disease or postsplenectomy) or chronic disease (e.g., diabetes, heart disease, emphysema, lymphoma). The vaccine is not recommended for mass immunization of healthy people, but probably should be given to all patients over the age of 50.

The vaccine is about 80% effective. A single dose is recommended. Side effects are frequent but not severe and consist of local pain and erythema at the site of injection with occasional fever. Periodic revaccination may be necessary every 5 years.

STAPHYLOCOCCI

Staphylococci appear as clusters of Gram-positive cocci when viewed microscopically. *S. epidermidis* is a relatively avirulent species that is present on normal skin. *S. aureus* is a virulent bacteria that produces a variety of extracellular toxins and enzymes that contribute to its pathogenicity. It is spread from person to person by direct contact.

Skin Infections

S. aureus may be carried in the moist areas of the skin (nares, axilla, rectum) without causing disease, but the skin and soft tissues are frequent sites of staphylococcal infection. Staphylococci are the leading cause of furuncles, carbuncles, cellulitis, and wound infections.

Bullous impetigo is a superficial staphylococcal infection, whereas cellulitis is a deeper, spreading infection of the skin and subcutaneous tissues. A furuncle, or boil, is a localized cutaneous infection that begins as an infection of a hair follicle and evolves to a pustule. A carbuncle is a deeper and more destructive abscess that extends into the subcutaneous tissue.

Furuncles generally resolve without therapy. Large boils, carbuncles, and abscesses require surgical drainage. Antibiotic therapy is required for cellulitis and extensive cutaneous infection. Recurrent skin infections should lead to a search for a staphylococcal carrier state.

Bacteremia

S. aureus bacteremia is a serious problem with a 20-40% mortality. This relates to the virulence of the organism, the frequency of coexistent endocarditis (about 20%), and complications such as metastatic abscesses. Approximately one-third of patients will have a definable extravascular source for the bacteremia, one-third will have a definable intravascular source, and one-third will have no definable source.

Bacteremia with *S. aureus* should lead to a search for a primary focus of infection. Soft tissues, intravascular catheters, bones, joints, and lungs are frequent primary sites. Endocarditis must be considered in all cases of bacteremia.

Parenteral antibiotic therapy is mandatory. The optimal duration of therapy is uncertain but ranges from 2 to 3 weeks for bacteremia secondary to a removable focus (e.g., an infected intravenous catheter) to 4 to 8 weeks in a patient with no definable source. Blood cultures should be obtained during antibiotic therapy.

Endocarditis

S. aureus can affect previously normal heart valves. It is the leading cause of acute bacterial endocarditis. Heroin addicts and persons with prosthetic heart valves are at increased risk. Patients present with fever and a heart murmur. Metastatic abscesses of the kidney, spleen, brain, and lung are common. Destruction of valvular tissue may lead to congestive heart failure. The course is typically fulminant and mortality is significant.

The diagnosis is confirmed by blood culture. Therapy with effective intravenous antibiotics should be continued for 6 weeks. The response to therapy as measured by fever and sterilization of blood cultures is often slow. Serum killing levels should be monitored during therapy; a peak serum killing level of 1:8 is desirable.

Bone and Joint Infections

Osteomyelitis is caused most often by *S. aureus*. The most common sites are the vertebrae and the long bones. A history of trauma is often obtained. Parenteral antibiotic therapy for 4 to 8 weeks is frequently required.

Staphylococci are frequently responsible for septic arthritis; the large joints are most commonly involved. Parenteral antibiotics, with daily aspiration or drainage of pus from the joint space, are necessary for successful therapy. Residual functional impairment is common. Parenteral antibiotics are generally administered for 2 to 4 weeks.

Other Manifestations

Staphylococcal pneumonia is a destructive pneumonia that often results in formation of abscesses or empyema. It may develop by inhalation of the organism or showering of the lung with septic emboli. Diagnosis is by sputum culture. The mortality is 30%, even with appropriate therapy.

S. aureus is a leading cause of food poisoning in the United States. Precooked foods, particularly baked goods, may become colonized with staphylococci that produce an enterotoxin. One to 6 hours after ingestion the patient suddenly develops nausea and vomiting but not fever. The disease is self-limited.

Toxic shock syndrome (TSS) is an acute illness which usually occurs in menstruating women. Patients have high fever, vomiting, diarrhea, myalgias, hypotension and, in severe cases, shock. An erythematous, "sunburn-like" rash is present during the acute phase of the illness and is followed by desquamation of the skin, particularly of the palms and soles. The disease has a 5-10% mortality, and up to 30% of patients will have a recurrence.

TSS is associated with menstruation and tampon usage, especially high-absorbency tampons. Most patients with TSS have an increased rate of vaginal colonization with *S. aureus*; a staphylococcal toxin is presumably responsible for the syndrome. TSS occasionally occurs following *S. aureus* wound infections or abscesses.

Therapy is primarily supportive, although antistaphylococcal antibiotics are recommended. Women who recover from TSS should avoid tampon usage in the future.

Therapeutic Approach

The majority of clinically important staphylococci are resistant to penicillin on an enzymatic basis. Some semisynthetic penicillins are not inactivated by penicillinase: methicillin, oxacillin, and nafcillin are the most effective antistaphylococcal drugs available. They have equivalent efficacy and are used intravenously at a daily dosage of 6-12 g per day for serious staphylococcal disease. Dicloxacillin provides the best absorption of the various oral drugs. Penicillin is the drug of choice if the organism is penicillin-sensitive.

Vancomycin, 2-3 g per day, and cephalothin, 6-12 g per day, are effective parenteral antistaphylococcal drugs if the penicillins cannot be used. Rare strains of methicillin-resistant staphylococci have been found; they are usually also cephalosporin-resistant, but vancomycin is effective.

Staphylococci are an important cause of hospital-associated infection. Patients with staphylococcal pneumonia, enterocolitis, and wound or skin infection should be placed in isolation.

STREPTOCOCCI

Streptococci are Gram-positive, chain-forming cocci that produce disease in humans on the basis of invasiveness and toxin production (Table 3).

Microbiology

The identification of streptococci is somewhat complicated. Serologic techniques, hemolytic activity, and biochemical reactions are all used. The Lancefield method is a serologic technique based on the cell-wall polysaccharide: groups A-T can be identified. The hemolytic activity of streptococci on blood agar can be absent (γ), partial (α), or complete (β). Enterococci can be identified by salt tolerance.

Streptococci produce a number of extracellular products, including streptolysins, DNase, DPNase, and an erythrogenic toxin that is responsible for scarlet fever.

Viridans Streptococci

The viridans streptococci are predominantly α hemolytic. These streptococci are organisms of low pathogenicity that are normal flora of the upper respiratory tract and mouth.

Viridans streptococci are the leading cause of subacute bac-

Table 3. Streptococci

Streptococcal Type	*Major Associations*
Group A	Pharyngitis, pyoderma
Group B	Neonatal infections
Viridans	Endocarditis
Group D	Abdominal infections, UTI
Peptostreptococci	Lung abscess
S. mutans	Dental caries

terial endocarditis. The typical patient has a history of organic valvular heart disease. Dental surgery, oral trauma, or periodontal disease provide access for the streptococci to the blood, and the valve is seeded during bacteremia.

A subacute course is the rule, and symptoms may be present for months before the diagnosis is made. The mitral and aortic valves are most often involved. Fever and a heart murmur are almost invariably present; septic complications are rare.

The diagnosis is confirmed by blood culture. Viridans streptococci are generally quite sensitive to penicillin. One approach to therapy is administration of penicillin G 10-20 million units per day intravenously and streptomycin 1-2 g per day intramuscularly for 2 weeks, followed by 2 weeks of oral penicillin. The streptomycin is added to penicillin because of synergy against these organisms.

Group D Streptococci and Enterococci

Group D streptococci, which include enterococci, are found in the human intestine. They are important primarily as causes of urinary tract infections and bacterial endocarditis. Group D streptococcal endocarditis follows urinary tract infection, genitourinary tract surgery, urinary catheterization, or pelvic surgery. The clinical presentation resembles endocarditis due to viridans streptococci. Blood culture confirms the diagnosis.

Therapy is more difficult because enterococci are frequently resistant to penicillin alone. Ampicillin is the drug of choice for urinary tract infections, but endocarditis requires the synergistic combination of penicillin and streptomycin or ampicillin and gentamicin for 6 weeks.

Group B Streptococci

Group B streptococci are well-known as a cause of neonatal sepsis and meningitis. About 30% of healthy women are asymptomatic vaginal carriers of group B streptococci; these organisms may cause pelvic infection in women in association with obstetric procedures.

Group A Streptococci

Group A streptococci are virulent bacteria that are nearly always β hemolytic. Ten percent of children may be asymptomatic pharyngeal carriers.

Streptococcal pharyngitis peaks in winter, and epidemics may occur. It is most common in children. Fever, sore throat, exudative tonsillitis, and tender regional lymphadenitis are usual, but symptoms may be minimal. Suppurative complications are rare, but scarlet fever, rheumatic fever, or glomerulonephritis may follow streptococcal infection. The organism is very sensitive to penicillin, and therapy within 1 week of onset with intramuscular benzathine penicillin or a 10-day course of oral penicillin V (or erythromycin) will prevent late complications.

Streptococcal cellulitis, or erysipelas, is a rapidly progressive cutaneous infection. Fever, warmth, swelling, and redness of the skin are seen, and an associated acute lymphangitis is common. Therapy with penicillin should not be delayed. Erythromycin or a cephalosporin are acceptable alternatives in the face of penicillin allergy.

Streptococcal skin infection can be more indolent. Impetigo is a pustular dermatitis of children with few systemic symptoms. The disease is usually self-limited, but antibiotic therapy with benzathine penicillin is recommended to prevent glomerulonephritis.

Scarlet Fever

An exotoxin produced by the group A streptococcus is responsible for scarlet fever. Initially, there is a punctate rash overlying diffuse erythema. The rash is usually seen first on the neck or upper chest. Erythema of the tongue and lymphadenopathy accompany the rash, which eventually results in desquamation.

Scarlet fever occurs most often between the ages of 2 and 10. It is not associated with an increased incidence of rheumatic fever or glomerulonephritis. The diagnosis is made by the clinical picture and throat culture. Treatment is identical to that for streptococcal pharyngitis.

Rheumatic Fever

Rheumatic fever occurs from 1-5 weeks after group A streptococcal pharyngitis but does not follow skin infection. Up to one-third of rheumatic fever patients give no history of pharyngitis. The proposed mechanism of rheumatic carditis is production of an antibody against the streptococcal cell wall that cross reacts with cardiac tissue.

The diagnosis depends on clinical criteria and evidence of a recent streptococcal infection. The latter is suggested by a positive throat culture, the presence of scarlet fever, or a high or rising antistreptolysin 0 (ASO) titer. An ASO titer of 200 Todd units or greater is elevated.

The five major clinical criteria (Jones' criteria) for the diagnosis are carditis, migratory polyarthritis, chorea, erythema marginatum, and subcutaneous nodules. Fifty percent of the patients have myocarditis or valvulitis, most often mitral regurgitation. Murmurs, cardiomegaly, and pericarditis suggest carditis. Erythema marginatum consists of evanescent, macular pink lesions with central clearing.

The minor criteria include fever, arthralgias, elevated white blood cell count, and elevated erythrocyte sedimentation rate. The diagnosis on the basis of the above criteria requires two major, or one major and two minor, criteria in addition to evidence of prior streptococcal infection.

Therapy consists of rest and salicylates. Steroids may be indicated for carditis. A previous attack of rheumatic fever indicates increased risk for another attack. Consequently, patients with rheumatic fever or rheumatic heart disease should receive antibiotic prophylaxis for group A streptococcal infection for an indefinite period. This is best accomplished with benzathine penicillin 1.2 million units intramuscularly monthly. Oral penicillin G or sulfadiazine are therapeutic alternatives that must be administered daily.

Glomerulonephritis

Poststreptococcal glomerulonephritis may follow skin or throat infection with group A streptococci. The latent period averages 2 weeks and is longer after pyoderma. Edema and hypertension often are present. Laboratory tests reveal low serum complement, elevated streptococcal antibody titer (anti-DNase B, ASO), and an abnormal urinalysis with hematuria, proteinuria, and red blood cell casts. Ninety-five percent of cases resolve, although chronic glomerulonephritis may eventually develop. Treatment is symptomatic.

NEISSERIAE

Neisseriae are Gram-negative, aerobic diplococci. This genus includes *N. Meningitidis*, *N. gonorrhoeae*, and several non-pathogenic species that are normal mouth and pharyngeal flora.

Meningococci

N. meningitidis is found as part of the upper respiratory tract flora in 2-20% of normal persons. A high carrier rate tends to be associated with epidemics of clinical disease, which occur in late winter and particularly in military settings. Several serogroups (A,B,C,D,X,Y,Z) have been identified based on surface polysaccharides. Currently, type B is the most prevalent serogroup. Most meningococcal disease occurs in patients under the age of 20.

The classic clinical picture is that of fulminant bacteremia, meningitis, disseminated intravascular coagulation, and adrenal hemorrhage. The pathologic basis for this picture is a vasculitis. More commonly, the patient presents with a bacterial meningitis with fever, chills, and stiff neck. A petechial rash provides a clue to the diagnosis. The overall mortality is about 20%.

The diagnosis depends on a positive blood or CSF culture. A Gram stain of centrifuged CSF usually reveals intracellular Gram-negative diplococci and many neutrophils. Therapy should be initiated immediately when the diagnosis is suspected. The drug of choice is penicillin in high doses (20-24 million units per day intravenously) to ensure adequate CSF antibiotic levels. In the event of penicillin allergy, chloramphenicol 2-4 g per day intravenously is an excellent alternative. Full-dose therapy is generally continued for 2 weeks intravenously.

The attack rate in household contacts of meningococcal meningitis cases is significantly increased. Consequently, antibiotic prophylaxis is recommended for these persons. Casual contacts do not require prophylaxis. There is no ideal drug for prophylaxis; surprisingly enough, penicillin is ineffective. The current recommendation is 2- to 3-day courses of oral sulfadiazine or rifampin. The former should only be used if the meningococcal strain is known to be sulfonamide sensitive.

Gonorrhea Manifestations

Gonococci are spread by sexual contact; the disease is most common in young adults ages 15-20. Infection does not confer immunity and reucrrent infections are common.

Gonococci penetrate mucosal surfaces. Symptoms appear after a 2- to 7-day incubation period. Men develop a urethritis with purulent urethral discharge, dysuria, or meatal erythema. Asymptomatic infections are more common in women, in whom gonococci may infect the cervix, urethra, or anus. A purulent vaginal discharge is the most frequent complaint. Local complications include endometritis, salpingitis, pelvic abscess, and peritonitis. Salpingitis and endometritis cause abdominal pain; recurrent salpingitis may lead to sterility. In both sexes, the primary site of infection may be the pharynx; patients often complain of a sore throat. Women or homosexual men may develop a painful proctitis.

Usually gonorrhea is a localized infection, but dissemination occurs in about 2% of cases, predominantly in women. Menses are associated with an increased risk for dissemination. Symptoms and signs include fever, tenosynovitis, septic arthritis, and a variety of skin lesions. The arthritis involves especially the wrist, knee, and ankle; gonorrhea is the leading cause of septic arthritis in young adults. Cutaneous manifestations include purpuric lesions, petechiae, pustules, and necrotic ulcers.

Gonorrhea may result in perihepatitis. Typically, a woman with a history of gonococcal pelvic inflammatory disease presents with right upper quadrant tenderness and abdominal pain.

Ophthalmia neonatorum is a purulent conjunctivitis that develops shortly after birth. Blindness may result. The gonococci are acquired in passage through the birth canal. One percent silver nitrate solution is preventive.

Diagnosis

Since gonococci are very sensitive to temperature and dehydration, care should be exercised in obtaining cultures. A successful culture requires prompt inoculation of the specimen on a proper medium (usually Thayer-Martin medium or chocolate agar). Increased atmospheric CO_2 is required for optimal growth.

For a man with symptomatic urethritis, the diagnosis of gonorrhea is strongly suggested by a Gram stain of urethral exudate that demonstrates neutrophils with abundant Gram-negative intracellular diplococci. If gonorrhea is suspected, cultures of the male urethra or female cervix should be done. Culturing the anus and pharynx will increase the diagnostic yield.

Therapy

The recommended drugs of choice for treatment of uncomplicated gonococcal infection are procaine penicillin G, 4.8 million units intramuscularly with 1 g of probenecid orally, tetracycline, 500 mg orally four times per day for 5 days, ampicillin, 3.5 g orally with 1 g of probenecid, and spectinomycin 2 g intramuscularly.

All four regimens are effective over 90% of the time. Only penicillin and tetracycline are recommended for pharyngeal gonorrhea. All the regimens except spectinomycin cure incubating syphilis reliably.

Acute pelvic inflammatory disease should be treated with oral tetracycline, 2 g per day for 10 days, or the above recommended doses of procaine penicillin G or ampicillin, followed by ampicillin 2 g per day for 10 days. If hospitalization is required, penicillin G intravenously is the drug of choice. Similar treatment programs for 7 days are suggested for disseminated gonococcal infection.

The therapy of gonorrhea has been complicated by the recent appearance of penicillin-resistant gonococci. These organisms possess penicillin resistance on the basis of penicillinase production. They are most prevalent in the Far East, but several hundred cases have been reported in the United States. Spectinomycin is the drug of choice for penicillin-resistant gonococci.

Urethritis that develops 2 to 3 weeks after penicillin or ampicillin therapy is frequently nongonococcal urethritis due to chlamydiae. However, relapse or reinfection with gonorrhea must be ruled out. Tetracycline is the drug of choice for nongonococcal urethritis.

Prevention

The optimal public health approach to gonorrhea includes obtaining a VDRL on all patients with gonorrhea, adequate therapy of gonorrhea, followup cultures after therapy with special attention to treatment failures, and disease reporting for the purpose of contact tracing. All known sexual contacts of documented cases of gonorrhea should be examined, cultured, and treated.

A condom will decrease the spread of gonorrhea. Antibiotic prophylaxis for gonorrhea or other venereal diseases is not recommended.

BACTERIAL DIARRHEA

Nontyphoid Salmonella

Salmonellae are Gram-negative bacilli that are subdivided into species biochemically and into surface antigen types serologically. *Salmonella enteritidis* and *S. typhimurium* are the organisms that most commonly produce disease in the United States, although dozens of other serotypes are important. *S. choleraesuis* is notably virulent.

Animals, particularly fowl, are the reservoir of nontyphoid *Salmonella*. Poultry, eggs, dried egg products, raw meat, and pets (especially turtles) have been the source of outbreaks. Spread of the organisms to the human host is by ingestion of contaminated food. Occasionally, a human carrier may be the source of disease. Gastrectomy and prior antibiotic use increase the susceptibility of the intestine to salmonellal infection.

Eight to twenty-four hours after ingestion of salmonellae the patient develops fever, abdominal pain, and diarrhea. Abdominal tenderness is present. A stool smear demonstrates many neutrophils, and culture of the stool on special media yields salmonella. Serum agglutinating antibody titers are rarely helpful in the diagnosis; an elevated titer does not necessarily indicate acute disease. The infection usually remains confined to the intestine, but distant spread occasionally occurs to produce abscesses in liver, bone, or other organs.

Chloramphenicol is the drug of choice for bacteremia, extraintestinal disease, and severe gastroenteritis. The majority of cases of gastroenteritis require no antibiotic therapy; in fact, antibiotics prolong the length of time that *Salmonella* is excreted in the stool. Fifty percent of patients excrete *Salmonella* in their stool for up to 1 month after the acute illness. Periodic stool cultures must be obtained until the salmonellae are gone.

Salmonellosis can be a hospital hazard. Outbreaks in this setting have been ascribed to cross infection, inadequately sterilized endoscopes, and hospital staff who are asymptomatic excretors. Recent community outbreaks have been traced to eggnog, cheese, precooked meat, ice cream, and powdered milk. Good handwashing and proper food preparation would prevent many cases.

Typhoid Fever

S. typhi differs from other *Salmonella* species epidemiologically and clinically. Man is the reservoir and spread of the bacteria occurs from human carriers to susceptibles by way of direct contact and contaminated food or water. The disease is seen primarily in the tropics.

The clinical disease produced by *S. typhi* is more severe than that produced by nontyphoid *Salmonella*, with a mortality of 1-2%. Fever, headache, and abdominal pain develop after an incubation period of 7 to 14 days. Constipation is more common than diarrhea. On physical exam, the physician notes abdominal tenderness, splenomegaly, or faint, rose-colored spots on the abdomen. Rales, hepatomegaly, and relative bradycardia may complete the picture.

The diagnosis is best made by blood culture, although urine, bone marrow, and stool cultures may be helpful. The peripheral white blood cell count is low and a stool smear reveals mononuclear leukocytes. Liver function abnormalities are the rule. Agglutinating antibody titers are not helpful diagnostically. A careful travel history may provide a clue to the diagnosis.

Complications include intestinal perforation, intestinal hemorrhage, delirium, and shock. Recovery is slow and relapse occurs 10-20% of the time, even with proper therapy. The drug of choice is chloramphenicol, 2-4 g intravenously for 2 weeks. Cases acquired in Southeast Asia or Mexico may be chloramphenicol-resistant; ampicillin should be used in that case.

Up to 5% of patients who recover will be found to excrete *S. typhi* in their stool 6 months after the acute illness. These carriers should not serve as food handlers. The source of the *Salmonella* is usually the gallbladder. Ampicillin or cholecystectomy may be of value in eradication of the carrier state. The stool should be cultured periodically until negative.

Immunity after recovery from infection is lifelong. A vaccine is available but only partially effective, and boosters must be given every 3 years. Routine typhoid vaccination is no longer recommended; it is less important in disease prevention than the avoidance of uncooked or potentially contaminated foods.

Shigellosis

Shigella are Gram-negative bacteria that cause diarrhea by invasion of intestinal mucosa. *S. sonnei* and *S. flexneri* are the most common species found in the United States. Man is the reservoir and spread is person to person. Disease is seen most frequently in children and travelers.

Fever, cramping abdominal pain, and watery diarrhea are

seen after an incubation period of 36-72 hours. Dysentery is characterized by severe diarrhea with the passage of blood and mucus; dehydration may develop in children. Stool smear reveals neutrophils, and the diagnosis is confirmed by culture of stool on special media.

The disease is usually self-limited but may be severe, especially in children. Complications include hepatitis, rectal prolapse, and nonseptic arthritis. In general, extraintestinal complications are less common than in salmonellosis and chronic carriers are not a problem. Antibiotic therapy is indicated for significant symptoms such as dysentery. Ampicillin is the drug of choice; trimethoprim-sulfamethoxazole is an alternative when ampicillin resistance is encountered. Antidiarrheal medication should be avoided.

Cholera

Vibrio cholerae causes a severe watery diarrhea. The disease is due to an enterotoxin that stimulates water and electrolyte secretion in the small intestine. Most complications result from massive fluid and electrolyte loss. The disease is endemic in India, but pandemics occur. Spread is waterborne. Fluid administration is the key to therapy; tetracycline shortens the clinical illness.

Escherichia Coli

Recently, *E. coli* has been identified as a cause of diarrhea, especially in travelers. Some strains produce disease by means of a toxin, while others are invasive. Pathogenic strains cannot be distinguished from benign strains by means of culture; elaborate toxin assays are required. The diarrhea is almost always self-limited.

Campylobacter Fetus

C. fetus is an important cause of disease in animals. Two subspecies are implicated in human disease: *C. fetus* subspecies *intestinalis* may cause bacteremia in adults, whereas *C. fetus* subspecies *jejuni* usually causes gastroenteritis. Ingestion of unpasteurized milk and contact with animals have been associated with disease. The stool exam reveals blood and leukocytes. Selective media are required for isolation of *Campylobacter* from stool. The diarrhea is generally self-limited, but antibiotic therapy may be useful. Tetracycline and aminoglycosides have been used with success.

ZOONOSES THAT AFFECT MAN

Brucellosis

Brucellosis is a disease of animals that is spread to humans by contact with sick animals or animal products. The disease is seen primarily in farmers, packing plant workers, and veterinarians. *Brucella suis* and *Brucella abortus* are the most prevalent species. The bacteria enter humans through small cuts in the skin.

The clinical presentation varies from an acute disease with fever, chills, headache, and arthralgias to an indolent disease with fatigue and depression. The physical exam reveals splenomegaly 50% of the time; hepatomegaly is less frequent. The symptoms subside in several weeks, but relapses or a chronic course may develop. Fatalities are rare.

The diagnosis is most secure when the organism can be cultured from blood or pus on special media. Most often the diagnosis depends on high (≥1:160) or rising *Brucella* agglutination titers. Tetracycline is the drug of choice: a 3- to 4-week course is suggested. If relapse occurs, a repeat course of tetracycline with streptomycin is indicated. A falling agglutination titer is a useful indicator of successful therapy.

Plague and Tularemia

Yersinia pestis and *Francisella tularensis* are Gram-negative bacilli that are primarily animal pathogens. The reservoir for plague is sylvatic and urban rodents. The disease is usually spread to man by flea bites; most cases in the United States are seen in the southwestern states. Rabbits and rodents are the major reservoir for tularemia. Spread to humans is most often through the skin after direct contact with these animals or by insect vectors. Most cases of tularemia occur in hunters, trappers, and campers.

Both diseases are serious, but plague has a higher mortality (20%). There are several forms of plague. The dominant finding in bubonic plague is the bubo, a very painful, tender, swollen regional lymph node. Patients with septicemic or pneumonic plague are febrile and very toxic. Pneumonic plague is extremely contagious by the respiratory route.

The patient with tularemia classically has fever, an ulcer at the site of entry of the organism, and enlarged, tender regional lymph nodes. Bacteremia or pneumonia are complications that may ensue.

Blood, sputum, and bubo aspirate should be cultured. Special media are required for isolation of *F. tularensis*. Plague bacilli may be seen on a smear of blood or bubo aspirate. Antibody titers are available. The drug of choice for both diseases is streptomycin. Strict isolation must be observed in suspected cases of plague, and all contacts of pneumonic plague cases should be quarantined. There is no effective preventive measure except the avoidance of sick or dead animals.

OTHER IMPORTANT GRAM-NEGATIVE BACILLI

Enterobacteriaceae

Proteus, *Klebsiella*, *Enterobacter*, *E. coli*, and *Citrobacter* are Gram-negative bacilli that are components of the normal intestinal flora. These enterobacteriaceae are responsible for the vast majority of urinary tract infections; *E. coli* causes about 90% of the cases. *E. coli* is also an important cause of diarrhea and neonatal meningitis. *K. pneumoniae*, as its name implies, is a significant pulmonary pathogen; it is responsible for pneumonia primarily in alcoholics and hospitalized patients.

These organisms have become very important pathogens in the hospital setting for several reasons: (1) the impaired ability of the hospitalized patient to defend against bacterial infection, (2) the access of these bacteria to the patient via urinary catheters, tracheostomy tubes, and the like, and (3) the ability of these bacteria to acquire resistance to multiple antibiotics. Hospital-associated pneumonia, urinary tract infection, wound infection, and intravenous catheter-related sepsis are caused frequently by the enterobacteriaceae.

E. coli and *Proteus mirabilis* are often ampicillin-sensitive, and *K. pneumoniae* may be sensitive to the cephalosporins. However, the aminoglycosides are more uniformly effective against the enterobacteriaceae. Empiric therapy with gentamicin or tobramycin is generally used for serious gram-negative infection; a less toxic drug, such as ampicillin or a cephalosporin, may be substituted when antibiotic sensitivities are known.

Acinetobacter, Serratia, and Pseudomonas

Acinetobacter calcoaceticus, *Serratia marcescens*, and *Pseudomonas aeruginosa* are Gram-negative bacilli that are found in water at low concentrations. *Pseudomonas* is a particularly important pathogen in patients with leukemia, cystic fibrosis, or burns. These bacteria, like the enterobacteriaceae, are important causes of hospital-associated infection.

Aminoglycosides are the drugs of choice for these organisms. Carbenicillin, ticarcillin and piperacillin are effective parenterally for severe *Pseudomonas* infection, but should be used in combination with an aminoglycoside.

Hemophilus

Hemophilus species are short, pleomorphic, Gram-negative bacilli. *H. influenzae* is an encapsulated bacteria that is best-known as a cause of childhood otitis media, meningitis, and pneumonia. Occasionally *H. influenzae* causes pneumonia in adults, usually in chronic obstructive pulmonary disease patients. However, its presence in the sputum of the adult more commonly reflects its role as part of the normal upper respiratory tract flora.

Most strains of *H. influenzae* are sensitive to ampicillin. Chloramphenicol is the drug of choice if allergy or resistance is encountered. Because of the problem of ampicillin-resistant *Hemophilus*, both ampicillin and chloramphenicol may be used in *H. influenzae* meningitis until ampicillin-sensitivity can be confirmed.

ANAEROBIC BACTERIA

Recently, with the improvement of anaerobic microbiology, the importance of anaerobic bacteria has been appreciated. Anaerobes are the major bacteria on mucous membranes. In the intestine, they outnumber aerobic bacteria 1,000:1.

Microbiology

Anaerobes are very oxygen-sensitive. Successful isolation of anaerobes from clinical specimens requires that the sample be moist and protected from oxygen. Special transport tubes are available for this purpose. The specimen should be plated on the specially enriched media required by fastidious anaerobes. Plates must be incubated in an anaerobic atmosphere.

Anaerobic cultures of surfaces that are normally inhabited by anaerobes is meaningless. Expectorated sputum, vaginal swabs, or cultures of a rectal fistula are examples. Anaerobes are virtually never found in normal bladder urine or cerebrospinal fluid. Proper samples would include blood cultures, a swab of an abscess, or a percutaneous transtracheal sputum aspirate.

The microbiology laboratory will usually require 2 to 4 days to establish the presence of anaerobic bacteria in a clinical specimen and up to 1 week for complete identification.

Manifestations

Most anaerobic infections are endogenous and result from the patient's own bacterial flora. *Bacteroides fragilis* is the most commonly isolated anaerobic pathogen. It is also the most numerous bacteria in the colon. Peptostreptococci, peptococci, *Bacteroides melaninogenicus*, and *Fusobacterium nucleatum* are anaerobes that are normal mouth flora and common anaerobic pathogens. *Clostridium* species are also clinically important.

B. fragilis is the leading cause of anaerobic bacteremia, which can result in septic shock or metastatic abscesses. The gastrointestinal tract, pelvis, and lungs are the most frequent sources of anaerobic bacteremia.

Anaerobes are involved in abscesses and other infections adjacent to mucous membranes. Periappendiceal abscess, subphrenic abscess, liver abscess, lung abscess, endometritis, pelvic abscess, oral infection, brain abscess, and synergistic necrotizing cellulitis are infections that frequently involve anaerobes. Impaired blood supply, necrotic tissue, and foreign bodies provide the ideal clinical setting for anaerobic infection.

Diagnosis

Diagnosis requires proper specimen collection, transport, and culture techniques. Anaerobes are rarely isolated in pure culture; typically, an abscess culture will grow several anaerobes and several aerobic bacteria.

Clues to an anaerobic infection include a foul-smelling discharge, location of infection in proximity to a mucosal surface, gangrene, gas in the tissues on physical exam or x-ray film, sulfur granules, and the presence of pus with negative aerobic cultures.

Therapy

Penicillin is the drug of choice for most anaerobic bacteria, including *Clostridium* infections. *B. fragilis* and *B. melaninogenicus* are often resistant to penicillin and require clindamycin, chloramphenicol, or metronidazole.

In general, anaerobic infections of the lungs or facial area are best-treated with penicillin. Gastrointestinal and pelvic anaerobic infections are likely to involve *B. fragilis*; thus, clindamycin or chloramphenicol is a better choice. For successful treatment of anaerobic infections, it is imperative to drain abscesses and remove foreign bodies or devitalized tissue.

CLOSTRIDIA

Clostridia are anaerobic Gram-positive bacilli that form spores. *Clostridium* species may occur as part of normal intestinal flora and consequently may be involved in paraenteric infections such as empyema of the gallbladder or subphrenic abscesses. In addition, several distinctive disease syndromes are produced.

Tetanus

Clostridium tetani spores are found in the soil. They are inoculated into a wound and multiply if anaerobic conditions (deep wound, foreign body, necrotic tissue) exist. The local infection caused by *C. tetani* is usually unimpressive, but the neurotoxin produced by the organism has severe effects.

The toxin, tetanospasmin, produces a strychninelike picture. After a 3- to 21-day incubation period, the patient develops local or generalized tetanus. Classically, trismus is the first symptom. Later, generalized muscle spasms, opisthotonos, abdominal rigidity, and signs of increased sympathetic nervous system activity develop. The mortality is 50%, but recovery, when it occurs, is complete.

The diagnosis is clinical. About one-third of patients have *C. tetani* cultured from the initial wound but definite diagnosis requires the serum toxin neutralization test in mice.

Supportive care is the cornerstone of therapy; in addition, penicillin is usually administered. Human hyperimmune globulin should be given intramuscularly.

Tetanus is theoretically preventable. All children should have the childhood series of tetanus toxoid immunizations and adults should have a booster every 10 years. Wounds should be debrided and cleansed. Tetanus virtually never occurs in fully immunized patients. If immunizations are incomplete, or if immunization status is uncertain, tetanus toxoid alone is recommended for clean, minor wounds. Deep or dirty wounds require tetanus toxoid and tetanus immune globulin. If immunizations are complete, a booster is unnecessary.

Botulism

Botulism is a prototypic toxin-mediated disease. *Clostridium botulinum* produces a potent neurotoxin that resists gastric acid. The toxin interferes with neurologic function by inhibiting the release of acetylcholine at neuromuscular synapses.

The organism is found in fruits, vegetables, fish, and soil. Outbreaks of disease are most often associated with failure to cook vegetables under pressure or allowing fish to putrefy at room temperature. This allows the organism to grow and produce toxin. Seventy-five percent of reported botulism outbreaks are traced to home-processed foods. Infants may develop botulism from endogenous clostridia.

Symptoms develop 24 hours after ingestion of the toxin. Nausea, vomiting, dry mouth, dilated pupils, diplopia, and dysphagia are early symptoms. Later, a symmetrical descending paralysis occurs. Sensory changes, confusion, and fever are notably absent. The mortality is 10-20%, but recovery is complete when it occurs.

The clinical picture is quite characteristic, although myasthenia gravis and Guillain-Barré syndrome must be considered. The diagnosis can be confirmed only by a serum toxin neutralization test in mice. Therapy consists of supportive measures and equine antitoxin. Guanidine hydrochloride may increase acetylcholine release at the neuromuscular junction.

Gas Gangrene

Several *Clostridium* species, especially *C. perfringens*, can cause gas gangrene. The organisms are introduced into a wound externally from the soil, or internally from gut or vaginal flora. The organisms produce potent enzymes that cause tissue necrosis.

Involvement ranges from simple wound colonization to fulminant myonecrosis. When gas gangrene develops, the patient is extremely toxic. The wound is painful; soft tissue gas may be seen on x-ray films. If bacteremia occurs, shock, hemolysis, and disseminated intravascular coagulation may be seen. One-third of patients die of these complications.

The diagnosis requires the presence of necrotic tissue, serous exudate, and tissue gas or crepitation. A positive wound or blood culture is also required to confirm the diagnosis. The presence of *Clostridium* species in a wound culture does not necessarily imply that gas gangrene is present or impending, and organisms other than clostridia can produce soft tissue gas.

Penicillin G, in large doses intravenously, is the drug of choice for gas gangrene. Surgery is also critical; aggressive debridement, amputation of an extremity, or hysterectomy (for uterine gas gangrene) can be lifesaving. Hyperbaric oxygen may be helpful.

Food Poisoning

C. perfringens is a leading cause of foodborne illness in the United States. Meat and poultry are the prime vehicles implicated, especially when they are cooked in large quantities. The patient develops diarrhea and cramps about 12 hours after ingestion. The disease is self-limited; no therapy is required.

Pseudomembranous Colitis

Clostridium difficile can cause a pseudomembranous colitis in patients receiving antibiotics. The disease appears to be toxin-mediated; the toxin may be detected in stool by tissue culture assay. Diarrhea usually resolves with cessation of the offending antibiotic, but may require therapy with oral vancomycin. Fluid losses should be treated.

DIPHTHERIA

Corynebacterium diphtheriae is a Gram-positive, aerobic bacillus. Special media is required for culturing the organism. *C. diphtheriae* is not invasive, but causes disease by producing a toxin that kills cells by interfering with protein synthesis.

Manifestations

The disease is most common in children. The organism is spread by respiratory droplets and *C. diphtheriae* multiplies in the pharynx. Two to 4 days later the patient develops fever, sore throat, and dysphagia. Physical exam reveals cervical lymphadenopathy and the characteristic grayish white, adherent membrane.

Complications include obstruction of the airway by the

membrane, myocarditis, and neurologic problems. Cranial nerve deficits are manifested by dysphagia, nasal voice, and nasal regurgitation of fluids. Later, a peripheral neuropathy may develop. The mortality is 5-15%.

Diagnosis

The pharyngeal membrane must be cultured on special media. The diagnosis requires culture of *C. diphtheriae* and confirmation of the ability of the bacteria to produce toxin by the guinea pig toxin test.

Therapy and Prevention

All diphtheria cases should be placed in strict isolation. Treatment of diphtheria includes equine antiserum to neutralize toxin and antibiotic therapy with penicillin or erythromycin. Five to 10 percent of patients become carriers, they should be treated with erythromycin.

A diphtheria toxoid vaccine is available. It is included in the childhood immunization series with tetanus and pertussis vaccines. Adults should have a booster every 10 years.

SPIROCHETES

Spirochetes are motile organisms that can be seen by darkfield microscopy. Three genera of spirochetes are clinically important. *Treponema pallidum* is the agent of syphilis. *Borrelia*, a louse-borne or tick-borne organism, causes relapsing fever. *Leptospira interrogans* causes leptospirosis, a disease of animals (especially rats) that spreads to humans via contact with contaminated water. Patients have a biphasic illness with fever, chills, and abdominal pain in the first phase and meningitis in the second stage.

Syphilis

Manifestations

Syphilis is spread from person to person by sexual contact. A primary lesions, or chancre, develops at the site of inoculation in about 3 weeks. This is typically a firm, painless ulcer with raised borders on the penis or cervix. Regional lymphadenopathy is seen. The chancre heals in 3 to 6 weeks even without therapy. Secondary lesions appear 6 to 8 weeks later. These include pigmented lesions on the palms and soles, flat papules in moist areas (condyloma lata), alopecia, and a variety of mucous membrane and skin lesions. Fever and lymphadenopathy accompany the rashes.

When secondary syphilis resolves, the disease becomes latent. Tertiary complications may appear later on. About one-third of untreated patients eventually develop destructive lesions, cardiovascular syphilis, or neurosyphilis. Gummas are locally destructive lesions of skin, bone, or viscera. Aortitis, the primary cardiovascular complication, can lead to aortic insufficiency or aneurysmal dilatation of the ascending thoracic aorta. Neurosyphilis is manifested as meningitis with focal signs, general paresis, or tabes dorsalis (posterior column disease). The underlying pathology is an obliterative endarteritis.

Syphilis is a disease with a great variety of presentations. It should be considered in any patient presenting with dermatologic, neurologic, or optic disease.

Diagnosis

The diagnosis of syphilis is serologic because the organism cannot be cultured. Nonspecific antibodies, or reagins, are easily assayed (VDRL). Specific antibodies (FTA-fluorescent treponeme antibody) are sought only if the screening serology is positive. False-positive reagin tests are seen in a variety of conditions including old age, systemic lupus erythematosus, hepatitis, and malignancy. False-positive FTAs are rare.

In primary syphilis the antibody tests may not be positive initially, and the diagnosis is often made on the basis of visualization of spirochetes in scrapings from a chancre by darkfield microscopy. The VDRL is virtually always positive in secondary syphilis, and usually positive in late syphilis. The VDRL, but not the FTA, often reverts to negative after successful therapy.

Neurosyphilis is suggested by the clinical picture or spinal fluid with elevated protein and mononuclear pleocytosis. The diagnosis is confirmed by a positive CSF VDRL.

Therapy

The drug of choice for primary, secondary, or early latent syphilis is benzathine penicillin, 2.4 million units intramuscularly. In the presence of penicillin allergy, a 2-week course of oral tetracycline or erythromycin, 2 g per day, is recommended. For syphilis of greater than 1 year's duration or of indeterminate age, three doses of benzathine penicillin 1 week apart or a 30-day course of erythromycin or tetracycline should be given. A spinal tap should be done prior to initiation of therapy to rule out neurosyphilis.

The VDRL should be checked after therapy. A rising antibody titer may indicate failure of therapy or reinfection. All contacts of an active case should be treated or screened for syphilis. There is no immunity to syphilis; reinfection does occur. A VDRL should be performed on every patient with venereal disease.

LEGIONNAIRES' DISEASE

In 1976 an explosive, common-source outbreak of pneumonia affected persons attending the American Legion convention in Philadelphia. A new bacterium was found to be responsible for this and other previously reported outbreaks.

Microbiology

Legionella pneumophila is a bacillus which does not grow on routine culture media, but does grow on charcoal yeast extract and supplemented Mueller-Hinton agar in 2-10 days. Lung tissue and pleural fluid provide the best material for attempted isolation; the organism is rarely isolated from sputum. Several serotypes have been identified.

The organism can be visualized in tissues by the modified Dieterle or direct immunofluorescent stain. Since it is difficult to see or isolate the organism, the diagnosis is usually made by finding a rising indirect immunofluorescent antibody titer in serum.

Epidemiology

Legionnaires' disease is estimated to cause about 1-2% of all pneumonias. The disease is more common in males, smokers and patients with underlying illnesses, the mean age in several outbreaks is 50-60 years.

Hospital outbreaks have been reported, especially in immunosuppressed patients. The disease is not spread from man to man, but acquired from the environment. *Legionella* has been cultured from a number of environmental sources, including cooling towers, showers, and faucets.

Manifestations

The clinical picture of Legionnaires' disease is not diagnostic and usually consists of high fever, recurrent chills, nonproductive cough, and severe pneumonia. Early gastrointestinal symptoms suggest the diagnosis. The chest x-ray film initially demonstrates a patchy bronchopneumonia; later, a consolidating lobar pneumonia develops, frequently involving more than one lobe. Pleural effusions and cavities are rarely seen. Mortality is 15%.

The white blood cell count is moderately elevated, mild liver function abnormalities are seen, and proteinuria may be detected. Sputum examination reveals neutrophils but no bacteria, on Gram stain.

Therapy

Since the diagnostic antibody titer rise may not appear for 2 to 4 weeks, therapy is initiated on clinical grounds. The drug of choice is erythromycin 2-4 g orally or intravenously per day. Patients often respond with a fall in temperature within 48 hours, but 2 to 3 weeks of therapy is recommended. The chest x-ray clears slowly.

MYCOBACTERIA AND ACTINOMYCETES

The order actinomycetales includes *mycobacterium*, *Actinomyces*, and *Nocardia*. Tuberculosis and leprosy are diseases caused by mycobacteria.

TUBERCULOSIS

Mycobacteria are aerobic bacilli that grow slowly on artificial media. *M. tuberculosis* is the most important human pathogen.

Pathology

Tuberculosis is the prototype for diseases that involve host cell-mediated immunity. The organisms are inhaled on droplet nuclei; they multiply in the alveoli and spread to hilar lymph nodes and other distant sites. About 6 weeks after infection the host develops specific cell-mediated immunity against tuberculosis. The organisms are contained within epithelioid granulomas with central Langhans' giant cells. Macrophages are the most important cells involved in ingestion and killing of the organism. Eventually, necrosis with caseation develops; calcification often follows. Alternatively, softening and liquefaction may develop that, with communication to the bronchus, leads to a cavitary lesion.

Manifestations

Most infected patients do not develop evident clinical disease; however, 5-15% of those who become infected will develop clinical tuberculosis within 5 years. Active pulmonary tuberculosis is classically manifested by fever, weight loss, night sweats, cough, and hemoptysis.

Primary, or childhood, tuberculosis is a disease of the lower lobes of the lungs. Pleural effusion and hilar lymphadenopathy are often seen. The infection spreads hematogenously to other sites, although host defenses contain the majority of cases. The preferred secondary sites are those with high oxygen tension, particularly the apex of the lung, renal cortex, and bony epiphyses.

After the primary infection subsides, the presence of mycobacteria in the body may be manifested only by a positive skin test. Later, dormant lesions may reactivate when host defenses are weakened by old age, corticosteroid therapy, cancer, and so forth. With reactivation (or adult) tuberculosis, the upper lobes are preferentially involved. Cavity formation is common, and endobronchial spread of tuberculosis may lead to extensive pulmonary disease (Fig. 5). The majority of clinical tuberculosis is reactivation disease.

Extrapulmonary Tuberculosis

The lung is, of course, the leading site of tuberculous disease. Extrapulmonary tuberculosis develops from lesions that were seeded during the primary pulmonary infection. Those infections of greatest clinical importance are meningitis, renal disease, skeletal disease, and miliary tuberculosis. Most extrapulmonary tuberculosis is accompanied by clinically evident pulmonary disease that provides a clue to the diagnosis.

Tuberculous meningitis is a basilar meningitis that often results in cranial nerve defects and hydrocephalus. The spinal fluid reveals a mononuclear pleocytosis, depressed sugar, and elevated protein. The mortality is high, and many survivors have residual neurologic sequelae.

Renal tuberculosis classically presents as hematuria and pyuria with a negative routine bacterial culture. The intravenous pyelogram reveals a variety of abnormalities, including calyceal distortion, ureteral stenosis, and calcification. Pathologically, the disease is bilateral. The genitourinary tract is the most common site of extrapulmonary tuberculosis.

Tuberculous osteomyelitis most commonly involves the vertebral column. The infection involves the intervertebral disk space and the anterior part of the spinous process. When destruction of bone has been severe, the involved vertebral bodies may collapse anteriorly with resultant gibbus deformity. Roentgenographic examination reveals the osteolytic process.

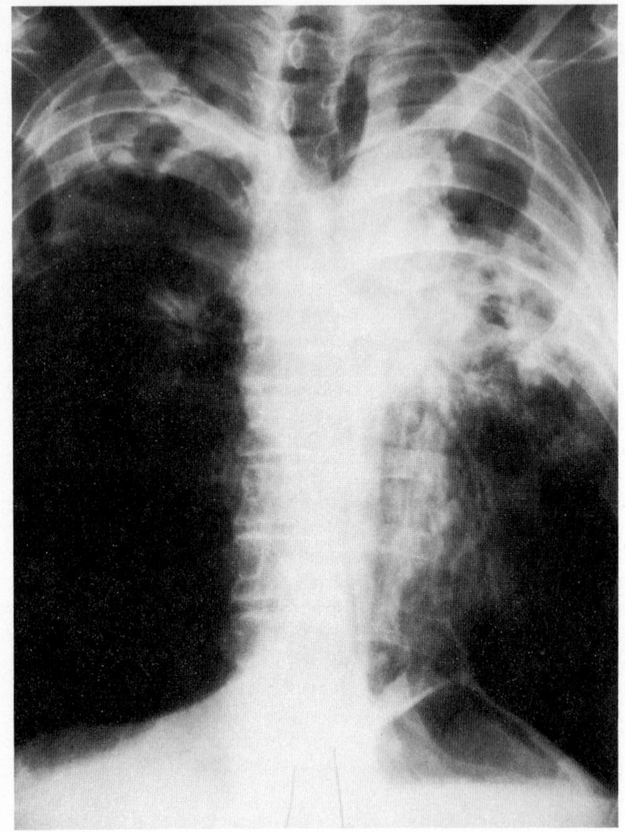

Figure 5. Bilateral, apical cavitary infiltrates (TB).

Miliary tuberculosis may develop in primary or reactivation disease. Many organs are involved and the patient is severely ill. The chest x-ray film reveals the diffuse, fine, nodular densities characteristic of miliary disease.

Diagnosis

Tuberculosis is diagnosed definitively by isolation of *M. tuberculosis* from sputum, tissue, urine, or other sources. Transtracheal aspirate, bronchoscopic washings, expectorated sputum, or early-morning gastric aspirate may confirm pulmonary tuberculosis. Pleural tuberculosis is more likely to be diagnosed by culturing a pleural biopsy specimen than pleural fluid.

M. tuberculosis requires 6 weeks for growth on special media. In general, an early-morning expectorated sputum or clean-catch urine culture is preferred to 24- or 72-hour collections because of the problem of overgrowth by bacteria. The organism may be visualized directly by acid-fast or auramine-fluorescent stain. However, *M. tuberculosis* cannot be distinguished from atypical mycobacteria on smears.

A purified protein derivative (PPD) of *M. tuberculosis* is a reliable skin test for tuberculosis. The skin test is read 48-72 hours after intradermal injection. Ten millimeters or greater induration (erythema is ignored) after an intermediate-strength PPD [5 TU (tuberculin units)] is a positive test. The skin test becomes positive 4 to 8 weeks after infection and remains positive indefinitely. Ninety-five percent of patients with tuberculosis have a positive skin test with 5 TU of PPD. Corticosteroid therapy, acute viral illnesses, immune deficiency states, and overwhelming tuberculosis may result in false-negative results.

Therapy

Therapy for minimal or noncavitary tuberculosis is most commonly isoniazid (INH) and ethambutol for 2 years. For severe pulmonary disease, cavitary disease, miliary disease, meningitis, or renal disease a third drug should be added, usually streptomycin or rifampin. Relapse, which is uncommon, is almost always due to failure of the patient to follow the drug program. Therapy should be guided by antimicrobial susceptibility tests.

Selected patients with uncomplicated pulmonary tuberculosis may be successfully treated with short-course INH and rifampin therapy for 9 months.

Prevention

The incidence of tuberculosis has been rapidly decreasing in the United States. About 5-7% of the U.S. population has a positive PPD, mostly those over 50 years of age. The risk of tuberculous infection still exists, particularly in hospitals, jails, and households exposed to an active case. Consequently, PPDs should be checked routinely on hospital employees and close contacts of active cases. Patients with definite or suspected pulmonary tuberculosis should be placed in respiratory isolation until therapy has been given for 1 to 2 weeks.

Within 5 years of infection, as manifested by conversion of the PPD from negative to positive, 5-15% of patients will develop clinical tuberculosis; the greatest risk is in the first 2 years. INH prophylaxis will significantly decrease that risk. Three hundred mg of INH is given orally per day for 1 year. The indications for prophylaxis include recent conversion of PPD, pediatric contacts of an active case, a postiive PPD in an immunosuppressed patient, and a positive PPD of unknown duration in a patient age 35 or under. The risks of INH hepatotoxicity probably outweigh the risks of developing clinical tuberculosis in those over 35 unless the PPD has recently converted.

Tuberculosis therapy is now largely an outpatient process. Long stays in a sanatorium are unnecessary. The patient who is under treatment poses little risk to the community.

Patients who have converted their PPDs should have periodic chest x-ray examinations. INH alone is not appropriate for a recent convertor who has an abnormal chest x-ray film or evidence of clinically active tuberculosis; multiple drug therapy is indicated in that situation. Case reporting and contact tracing are important aspects of tuberculosis prevention.

Bacille Calmette-Guérin (BCG) is an attenuated mycobacterial strain that is used as a vaccine in some areas of the world.

It results in a false-positive PPD. BCG is not appropriate in an area with a low prevalence of tuberculosis such as the United States.

Atypical Mycobacteria

Nontuberculous mycobacteria are organisms found in the environment that occasionally infect man. Human-to-human spread does not occur, as it does with *M. tuberculosis.*

M. kansasii and *M. intracellulare* produce pulmonary disease that is indistinguishable clinically from pulmonary tuberculosis. *M. scrofulaceum* is an important cause of cervical lymphadenitis in children. *M. marinum* is best known for producing cutaneous nodules in fish tank owners. Other species cause a variety of pulmonary and extrapulmonary diseases.

Atypical mycobacteria can be distinguished from *M. tuberculosis* biochemically. The PPD in atypical disease is usually from 0-9 mm in induration. In general, atypical mycobacteria are more resistant than *M. tuberculosis* to antimicrobial agents.

ACTINOMYCOSIS AND NOCARDIA

Actinomycosis

Actinomyces israelii is an anaerobic actinomycete. It is part of the normal flora of the oropharynx and tonsils. Human disease often follows dental procedures or facial trauma.

The classical presentation is lumpy jaw, with fever, pain, swelling, and fistulas in the cervicofacial area. Physical exam reveals a mass of granulation tissue and cutaneous sinuses. Aspiration of the organism leads to pneumonia, empyema, and chest-wall sinuses. Another primary site of disease is the intestine, particularly the appendix and ileocecal region. Pain, a tender mass, and abdominal wall fistulas are typical. Occasionally, the infection will spread to skin, bone, or brain.

A biopsy of suspicious tissue reveals necrosis and sulfur granules (a mass of organisms). The Gram stain demonstrates branching, Gram-positive filaments. Diagnosis requires culture with proper anaerobic techniques since the organism is a strict anaerobe. Actinomycosis is an indolent infection; the prognosis is good with appropriate therapy. The drug of choice is penicillin.

Nocardia

Nocardia is an aerobic actinomycete that is commonly found in the soil. Infection usually occurs by inhalation. Compromised hosts, especially patients receiving corticosteroid therapy or those with a hematologic malignancy, are at increased risk for nocardiosis. About 50% of patients with nocardiosis have an identifiable immunologic deficit.

Seventy to ninety percent of patients with *Nocardia* infection present with pneumonia. Fever and productive cough are common symptoms. The chest x-ray film is variable: localized infiltrates are most common, but cavities or nodules may be seen (Fig. 6). About half of the cases of pulmonary disease eventually disseminate. The brain is the most common secondary site; a brain abscess is characteristic. The skin is next most frequently involved, as manifested by subcutaneous nodules or abscesses.

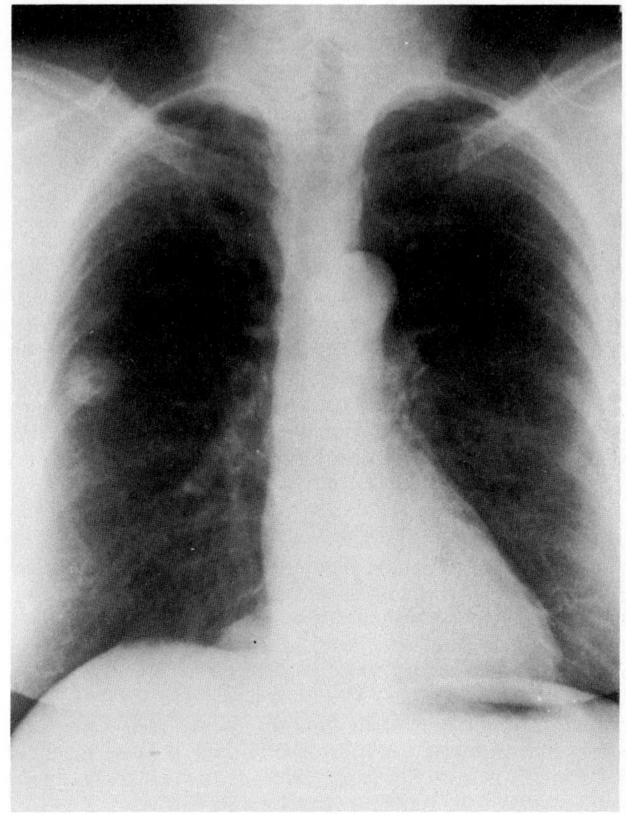

Figure 6. Nocular lesion, right lung (Nocardia).

Pathologically, *Nocardia* produces abscesses. A Gram stain reveals branching, Gram-positive organisms that cannot be distinguished from *Actinomyces*. The diagnosis requires culture and *Nocardia* grows in 3 to 7 days on bacterial or fungal media. *Nocardia asteroides* is the most common species isolated. The drugs of choice for therapy are the sulfonamides and trimethoprim-sulfamethoxazole.

FUNGAL AND PARASITIC DISEASES

ASPERGILLOSIS

Aspergillus is a ubiquitous fungus that is a saprophyte and a frequent laboratory contaminant. Occasionally, the fungus causes disease.

Manifestations

By far the most common site of involvement is the lung, where three distinct presentations can be seen. A mass of hyphae may occur as a fungus ball in a preexisting cavity such as that seen in tuberculosis. Although the fungus is not invasive in this setting, severe hemoptysis can occur.

In immunosuppressed patients, particularly those with hematologic malignancies, *Aspergillus* may cause a hemorrhagic, necrotizing lobar pneumonia. Vascular invasion is common and *Aspergillus* pneumonia may mimic a pulmonary embolus. Fever and a pulmonary infiltrate unresponsive to antibiotics are present. The mortality is at least 80%, which reflects the serious underlying diseases.

The third pulmonary presentation, allergic bronchopulmonary aspergillosis, is due to an allergic response to the fungus rather than direct tissue invasion. Asthma, fleeting pulmonary infiltrates, and eosinophilia are part of the syndrome. Eventually, bronchiectasis may develop.

Extrapulmonary disease is seen only in association with invasive aspergillosis. Disseminated aspergillosis occurs almost exclusively in immunocompromised hosts and is nearly always a fatal infection.

Diagnosis

Patients with allergic bronchopulmonary aspergillosis classically expectorate brown mucous plugs that reveal the fungus microscopically. Additional clues to the diagnosis include a positive immediate skin test, precipitins to *Aspergillus* in serum, and elevated IgE levels.

Aspergillus is a common contaminant, and its presence in sputum does not necessarily indicate disease. In invasive aspergillosis the diagnosis depends on obtaining a tissue specimen. The fungus is seen in tissue sections as branching hyphae readily cultured on standard fungal media (Fig. 7).

Therapy

Medical therapy will not affect a fungus ball; surgery should be considered for severe hemoptysis. Amphotericin B is the drug of choice for invasive or disseminated disease, but therapy is usually unsuccessful. The prognosis for allergic bronchopulmonary aspergillosis is good with steroid therapy.

CANDIDA

Candida is seen microscopically as yeast cells and elongated forms that look like hyphae. *Candida albicans* is the most important species. The organisms are normal flora of the mouth, gut, and vagina. *Candida*, like *Aspergillus*, usually causes serious disease only when host defenses are impaired.

Manifestations

A number of clinical syndromes are seen; mucocutaneous disease is most common. Creamy white patches overlying a red base in the pharynx suggest pharyngeal candidiasis or thrush. Similar lesions in the vagina are seen in *Candida* vaginitis where pruritus is the primary symptom. Antibiotics predispose to both conditions by altering normal bacterial flora of the mucous membranes. Pregnancy and diabetes may also predispose to superficial candidiasis.

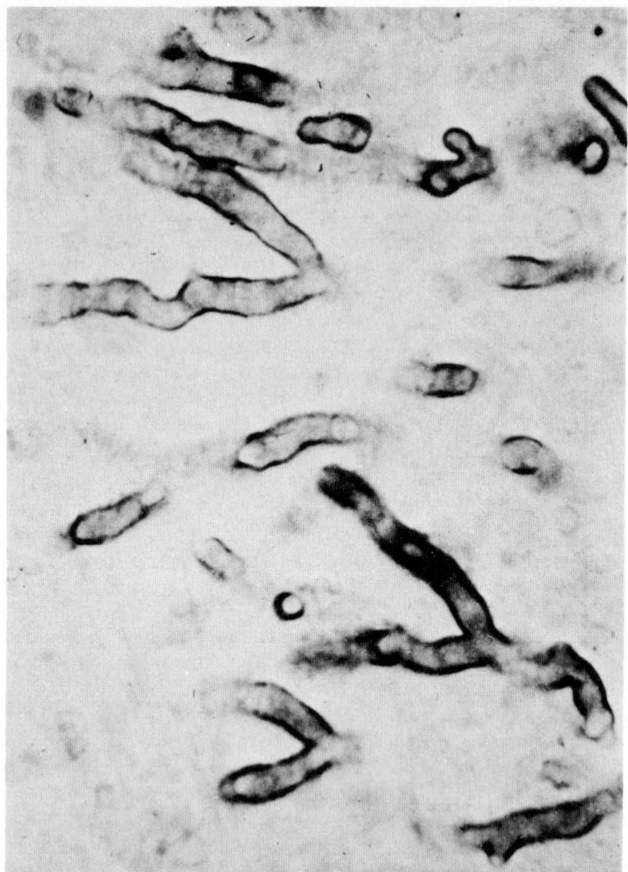

Figure 7. Aspergillosis–hyphae in tissue.

Candida intertrigo is characterized by an area of cutaneous erythema with a palpable margin that occurs in moist skin areas such as the axilla and groin. *Candida* may also cause paronychia and infant diaper rash.

Chronic and severe mucocutaneous candidiasis, particularly in children, is associated with various endocrinopathies and deficiencies in cell-mediated immunity.

Candida may cause cystitis or pyelonephritis, typically in a patient with a urinary catheter who is receiving antibiotics. *Candida* esophagitis results in painful swallowing or chest discomfort. Endoscopy reveals a white pseudomembrane adherent to the esophagus; occasionally, this pseudomembrane can be outlined by barium. Candidemia is an uncommon problem that is seen in the compromised host and in association with hyperalimentation; metastatic infection may develop.

Diagnosis

Candida grows readily on fungal media and blood agar. Growth of this fungus in sputum cultures, urine cultures, vaginal swabs, or stool cultures usually reflects colonization rather than infection. Systemic candidiasis is suggested by the presence of *Candida* in blood cultures or multiple body sites. The presence of a white, raised retinal lesion on fundoscopic exam provides a valuable clue to systemic candidiasis.

Therapy

Superficial disease (intertrigo, thrush, vaginitis) responds readily to topical nystatin or clotrimazole. Oral nystatin is generally adequate therapy for gastrointestinal *Candida* infection. Urinary tract infections usually resolve with discontinuation of antibiotics and urinary catheterization.

Candidemia may resolve without therapy if a primary focus, such as an infected intravenous catheter, can be identified and removed. Secondary lesions (e.g., endophthalmitis or pyelonephritis) require therapy with amphotericin B. *Candida* species are quite sensitive to amphotericin B and low-dose therapy may be successful. *Candida* are also frequently sensitive to 5-fluorocytosine, but resistance develops when this drug is used singly. Ketoconazole is an oral drug useful for some superficial *Candida* infections.

CRYPTOCOCCOSIS

Cryptococcus neoformans is a yeast that is found in high concentration in pigeon droppings. It spreads to humans by inhalation. Most patients with cryptococcosis have an underlying factor that impairs cellular immunity such as lymphoma or corticosteroid therapy.

Manifestations

Although the lung is the portal of entry for the fungus, pulmonary disease is usually mild; an infiltrate or solitary nodule may be seen. The most important manifestation is meningitis, which is more indolent than bacterial meningitis. Headache, confusion, and other neurologic signs develop gradually.

Diagnosis

The cerebrospinal fluid in cryptococcal meningitis is under increased pressure with elevated protein, low glucose, and 50-500 mononuclear leukocytes per cc of CSF. About 50% of the time the yeast cells can be seen on India ink examination of the spinal fluid (Fig. 8). The definitive diagnosis requires a positive culture of CSF.

Stool, sputum, urine, and blood are all potential sources to culture the fungus. Most patients with cryptococcal meningitis have cryptococcal antigen in blood or CSF that can be detected by the latex agglutination method.

Therapy

The mortality from cryptococcal meningitis is 100% without therapy and 50% with appropriate therapy. Amphotericin B intravenously is the drug of choice. If relapse occurs, the drug may have to be administered intrathecally. Amphotericin B and 5-fluorocytosine are often used in combination; synergy against the organism permits therapy with lower doses of amphotericin B. The cryptococcal antigen titer in blood and spinal fluid should be monitored during therapy.

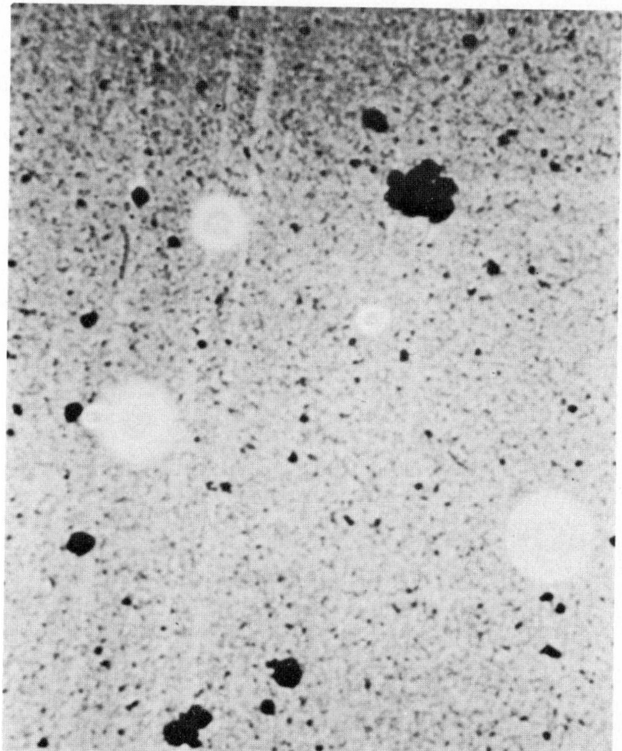

Figure 8. Cryptococcal meningitis–yeast in cerebrospinal fluid with India ink examination.

HISTOPLASMOSIS

The Ohio and Mississippi River valleys are the endemic areas for *Histoplasma capsulatum*. This fungus is found in soil and in bird droppings. Epidemics have been associated with clearing bird roosts and cleaning chicken coops. The organism is acquired by inhalation.

Manifestations

Pulmonary histoplasmosis resembles pulmonary tuberculosis: the primary infection is benign, hematogenous dissemination occurs in many primary cases, and with healing the primary pulmonary lesion and mediastinal lymph nodes calcify. Occasionally primary pulmonary histoplasmosis will progress to chronic cavitary disease.

Disseminated histoplasmosis is an uncommon but serious disease. Interstitial pulmonary disease, mucocutaneous ulcers, and adrenal involvement are seen in disseminated disease. Adrenal insufficiency may eventually develop.

Diagnosis

Pulmonary disease is best diagnosed by culturing the fungus from sputum or lung biopsy specimen. In disseminated disease oral lesions, bone marrow, liver, sputum, blood, or urine may yield the organism. In tissue sections the fungi appear as small, oval yeasts that are often seen inside macrophages.

The diagnosis may be suggested by detection of antibodies in serum by complement fixation or immunodiffusion methods. The histoplasmin skin test should not be used because it is positive in 70-90% of the population in endemic areas and may cause elevations of antibody titers.

Therapy

Primary pulmonary disease almost always resolves without therapy. However, chronic pulmonary disease and disseminated disease are serious problems. The prognosis for both is dramatically improved by therapy with amphotericin B.

OTHER FUNGAL INFECTIONS

Coccidioidomycosis

Coccidioidomycosis is endemic in parts of the southwestern United States. The fungal spores survive for long periods in the soil and are acquired by inhalation. Excavations have triggered epidemics.

The primary pulmonary infection is often asymptomatic. Patients may present with an influenza-like illness; an infiltrate or pleural effusion may appear on chest x-ray examination. Erythema nodosum or arthralgia may also be seen. Primary disease is usually self-limited, but dissemination to bones and meninges may occur.

The diagnosis is by culture, antibody titers, or visualization of *Coccidioides immitis* in tissue. A skin test is available. Therapy is rarely necessary for primary pulmonary disease, but disseminated disease requires amphotericin B.

Blastomycosis

Man acquires the yeast *Blastomyces dermatitidis* by inhalation; spores have been isolated from the soil. Clinical disease is seen especially in the southeastern United States and is much more common in men.

Pulmonary disease and cutaneous disease are each seen in about 75% of cases of blastomycosis. Pulmonary disease varies from an influenza-like syndrome to a chronic pulmonary infiltrate. The skin lesions are the most characteristic, evolving from papules to verrucous, crusted lesions on the hands or face. Other sites of secondary infection are the male genitals, bone, and joints.

Tissue obtained by biopsy often reveals the typical thick-walled yeast with a broad-based bud. Culture of tissue or sputum is diagnostic. Blastomycosis responds well to amphotericin B.

Sporotrichosis

Sporotrichosis is an occupational disease of gardeners and outdoor workers, reflecting the presence of *Sporothrix schenckii* in soil and plants. Spread almost always occurs by traumatic implantation of spores through skin.

The arms are the usual site of involvement. An indolent ulcer or nodule occurs at the site of implantation and multiple subcutaneous nodules appear proximally along the course of the draining lymphatics. Local pain and systemic symptoms are usually absent. Rarely, a disseminated form of the disease is seen.

Biopsy of the lesions will reveal microabscesses and granulomas, but the yeast may be difficult to find. Diagnosis is by tissue culture. The lymphocutaneous form of the disease responds well to potassium iodide, but amphotericin B is required for disseminated disease.

PARASITIC DISEASES

Malaria

Malaria is a mosquito-borne disease seen predominantly in the tropics. Fever, chills, headache, and myalgias in a traveler should raise the question of malaria. *Plasmodium vivax* is the species that most frequently causes disease, but *P. falciparum* infections have the highest mortality. The diagnosis is made by visualizing the parasite in red blood cells on a blood smear.

Travelers to high-risk areas should take malaria prophylaxis, which consists of chloroquine phosphate one tablet (500 mg) weekly, from 1 week before leaving until 6 weeks after return. Chloroquine-resistant malaria is a problem in many areas of the world; different prophylaxis is recommended for these areas.

Amebiasis

Entamoeba histolytica exists as a motile trophozoite or cyst. The cysts are spread from person to person, particularly in areas of poor sanitation. The trophozoite invades the intestinal mucosa to cause disease, and is most common in the tropics.

Infected patients are often asymptomatic cyst-passers. Clinical disease states range from mild diarrhea to invasive colitis with fever and bloody diarrhea. Complications include hemorrhage, intestinal perforation, dysentery, and liver abscess. Diiodohydroxyquin and metronidazole are effective against amebae.

Giardiasis

Giardia lamblia is a flagellate that causes a mild diarrheal disease in man. Outbreaks have been associated with contaminated water in Colorado and other areas. The diagnosis is made by finding the organism in the stool or in a duodenal aspirate. Metronidazole and quinacrine hydrochloride are the drugs of choice for therapy.

Trichomonas Vaginalis

Trichomonas vaginalis is a sexually transmitted cause of vulvovaginitis. This motile flagellate can be seen directly on a wet mount of vaginal secretions. Metronidazole is the drug of choice.

Pneumocystis Carinii

Pneumocystis carinii is a common cause of interstitial pneumonia in immunosuppressed patients; it rarely affects patients with normal host defenses. The diagnosis is made by histologic examination of lung biopsy specimens. Pentamidine and trimethoprim-sulfamethoxazole are effective therapy, but the infection has a high mortality rate.

Toxoplasmosis

Toxoplasma gondii is a parasite that causes several distinct syndromes. Many infected patients have no symptoms. An acute mononucleosis syndrome, congenital infection, chorioretinitis, or severe systemic disease in the immunosuppressed patient may be seen.

Toxoplasma are widespread in nature. Humans acquire the organism by oral ingestion of cysts or by transplacental infection. The two most common sources of cysts are ingestion of undercooked meat and exposure to cat excreta.

The diagnosis is made by demonstrating a rising antibody titer. Most cases do not require therapy, but a sulfonamide with pyrimethamine may be used for severe disease.

Helminths

Trichinella spiralis is the agent of trichinosis. The disease is a zoonosis that humans acquire usually by eating undercooked pork products. Symptoms are due to the larvae encysting in muscle. Fever, periorbital edema, and myalgias are the leading symptoms. Eosinophilia provides a significant clue to the diagnosis, which is confirmed by finding larvae in a muscle biopsy or noting a rising antibody titer.

Trichuris trichiura (whipworm), *Ascaris lumbricoides*, and *Enterobius vermicularis* (pinworm) are the most common helminthic pathogens in the United States. They are diagnosed when characteristic eggs are found in the stool. Effective antihelminthic drugs are available.

INFECTIONS OF MAJOR ORGAN SYSTEMS

PNEUMONIA

Pulmonary Host Defenses

Inhalation of particles occurs with each breath. Large particles are trapped in the upper airway, and small particles remain suspended in air. Particles between 0.1 μm and 10 μm settle in the lower airway. They are cleared largely by the mucociliary system. Alveolar macrophages ingest and kill inhaled bacteria. Some bacteria, such as *M. tuberculosis,* are readily ingested but killed with difficulty unless macrophages are sensitized. Normal IgA activity is also required for defense against respiratory infections.

Epidemiology

Pneumonia is greatly increased in incidence in patients with defective pulmonary host defenses. Tracheostomy and endotracheal tubes bypass upper airway defenses. Chronic obstructive airway disease, dehydration, pulmonary edema, viral upper respiratory infection, and cigarette smoking interfere with mucociliary clearance. Hypoxia and acidosis impair phagocytosis. IgA deficiency is frequently manifested by recurrent and severe pneumonia.

Pneumonia is the leading infectious cause of death in the United States and is reported as the primary cause of death in over 50,000 patients per year. Pneumonia is responsible for about 10% of admissions to acute medical wards.

Etiology

The bacterial pathogens responsible for pneumonia vary with the clinical setting. Ninety percent of adult bacterial pneumonia that develops in the community is caused by *S. pneumoniae*. *M. pneumoniae* occurs most commonly in young adults. Community-acquired *Klebsiella* and *S. aureus* pneumonia may be seen in alcoholics or debilitated hosts. Viral pneumonia is relatively uncommon.

Pneumonia that develops in the hospitalized patient is quite different. Gram-negative bacilli (*K. pneumoniae*, *Pseudomonas*), fungi (*Aspergillus*), and *S. aureus* are the leading pathogens. Patients receiving assisted ventilation are particularly susceptible to hospital-acquired pneumonia.

A special type of hospital-associated pneumonia is aspiration pneumonia. States of altered consciousness (coma, anesthesia, seizures), intestinal obstruction, and disorders of swallowing predispose to vomiting and aspiration of stomach contents. The aspirated fluid results in a chemical pneumonitis if the fluid has a pH less than 2.5. The dependent segments of the lung (right lower lobe and posterior segment of the right upper lobe) are most often involved. A bacterial pneumonia may follow the chemical pneumonitis. Gram-negative bacilli and anaerobic bacteria are likely to be the responsible pathogens.

Manifestations

Patients with bacterial pneumonia appear to be more toxic than those with *Mycoplasma* pneumonia (Table 4). Fever and cough are universal symptoms, and pleuritic chest pain is common. Pneumococcal pneumonia is classically heralded by a single shaking chill; brown, purulent sputum is typical. Rales and signs of consolidation precede radiologic abnormalities by several hours.

In bacterial pneumonia, the white blood cell count is elevated, and hypoxia may be severe. A bacterial pneumonia most often appears as a sharply defined, lobar density on chest

Table 4. Features of Common Pneumonias

	Mycoplasma	*Pneumococcal*
Etiology	Mycoplasma	Bacterial
Peak incidence	Adolescence	Adulthood
Severity	Symptoms often mild	Patient appears quite ill
X-ray	Bronchopneumonia	Lobar pneumonia
White blood cell count	<10,000/cc	>10,000/cc
Cold agglutinins	Present	Absent
Diagnosis	Serology	Culture
Prevention	None	Pneumococcal vaccine

x-ray. *Mycoplasma* and viral pneumonia appear diffuse or interstitial in nature on the chest x-ray and do not usually elevate the white blood cell count.

Mycoplasma pneumonia virtually never results in serious complications. The mortality of bacterial pneumonia varies from 5% with pneumococcal pneumonia to over 70% with Gram-negative pneumonia. Gram-negative, anaerobic, and *S. aureus* pneumonia frequently result in empyema or lung abscesses, complications rarely seen with the pneumococcus (Fig. 9).

Diagnostic Approach

Blood cultures should be obtained from all hospitalized patients with pneumonia; about one-third will yield the causative organism. Bacteria are usually isolated from a good sputum sample. All sputum specimens are contaminated to some degree by the normal bacterial flora of the mouth. A poorly collected sputum specimen that contains saliva rather than purulent sputum will be misleading. Throat cultures have no place in the evaluation of pneumonia. If anaerobic pneumonia is suspected, a transtracheal aspiration or percutaneous lung aspiration is required to bypass oral anaerobes.

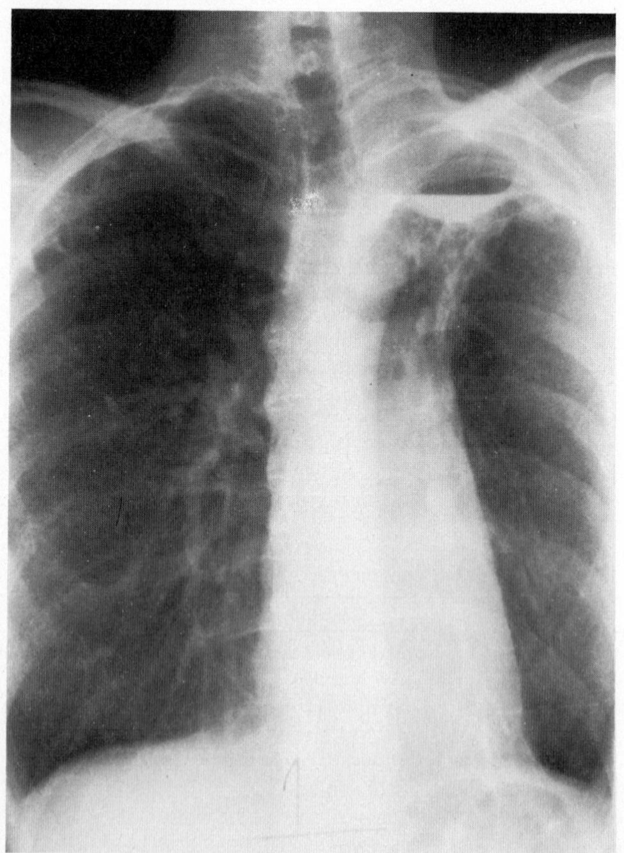

Figure 9. Left upper lobe abscess (anaerobic).

The presence of cold agglutinins is suggestive of *Mycoplasma* pneumonia, but an exact diagnosis depends on demonstration of a rising antibody titer.

Sputum and blood cultures will be positive in 1-3 days. However, useful information can be obtained rapidly from a Gram-stained sputum sample. A bacterial etiology is suggested by the presence of less than 10 epithelial cells and more than 25 white blood cells per high-power field (Fig. 4). Purulent sputum that does not yield a pathogen on routine culture suggests partially treated bacterial pneumonia, anaerobic infection, or Legionnaires' disease.

Therapeutic Approach

Mycoplasma pneumonia is largely an outpatient disease. Uncomplicated pneumococcal pneumonia in a young patient may be treated on an outpatient basis with oral or intramuscular penicillin. Erythromycin is appropriate oral therapy for *Mycoplasma* pneumonia and pneumococcal pneumonia in the penicillin-allergic patient.

Community-acquired pneumonia is usually pneumococcal; penicillin is the most appropriate therapy. Procaine penicillin, 600,000 units intramuscularly twice daily, is adequate therapy. Hospital-acquired pneumonia of uncertain etiology is best-treated with an aminoglycoside and an effective antistaphylococcal agent (a semisynthetic penicillin or cephalosporin) until results of cultures are available. Whenever possible, specific therapy should be based on sputum Gram stain, culture results, and antimicrobial sensitivity testing.

The response of pneumococcal pneumonia to therapy is dramatic. Typically, the temperature falls and the patient feels subjectively better in 24-48 hours. However, the chest x-ray film may not show complete clearing for several weeks. Staphylococcal and Gram-negative pneumonia respond more slowly to appropriate therapy. In addition to antibiotics, attention must be given to oxygenation, fluids, and cardiac status.

Lung Abscess and Empyema

A primary lung abscess is most frequently caused by anaerobic bacteria. Lung abscess and empyema may also follow necrotizing pneumonia due to anaerobic bacteria, *S. aureus*, or Gram-negative bacilli. Fever, pleuritic chest pain, and cough are seen. Anaerobic infections are considerably more indolent than those caused by *S. aureus* and Gram-negative aerobes.

Foul-smelling sputum suggests an anaerobic process. A microbiologic diagnosis requires culture of sputum or pleural fluid. If anaerobes are suspected, a transtracheal aspiration or percutaneous lung aspiration is necessary for culture of a lung abscess.

Chest-tube or surgical drainage of an empyema is necessary in addition to appropriate antibiotics. Lung abscesses often drain endobronchially, a process that may be facilitated by postural drainage. Penicillin, clindamycin, and chloramphenicol have been used with success for anaerobic lung abscesses. Parenteral therapy may be initiated with 6-12 million units of penicillin G per day; oral antibiotics complete a 2- to 4-month course. *S. aureus* and Gram-negative bacteria require specific therapy. Chest x-ray examination and sputum quantitation are useful parameters to follow during therapy (Fig. 10).

RESPIRATORY TRACT INFECTIONS

Upper Respiratory Tract Infection

Upper respiratory tract infection (URI, the common cold) is the most common infectious disease of man. The illness is quite contagious and peak incidence occurs in the winter. Nasal congestion, rhinorrhea, headache, and low-grade fever are the symptoms. URIs are caused by many viruses, especially rhinoviruses. Antibiotics have no place in the therapy of this self-limited viral illness.

Pharyngitis

Pharyngitis is caused by the same viruses that cause URIs. Fever, exudative pharyngitis, and cervical lymphadenopathy suggest group A streptococcal pharyngitis, which is most often seen in children. A throat culture is indicated to rule out streptococcal infection in suspicious cases. Antibiotic therapy, preferably penicillin, is indicated for streptococcal pharyngitis but not for viral pharyngitis.

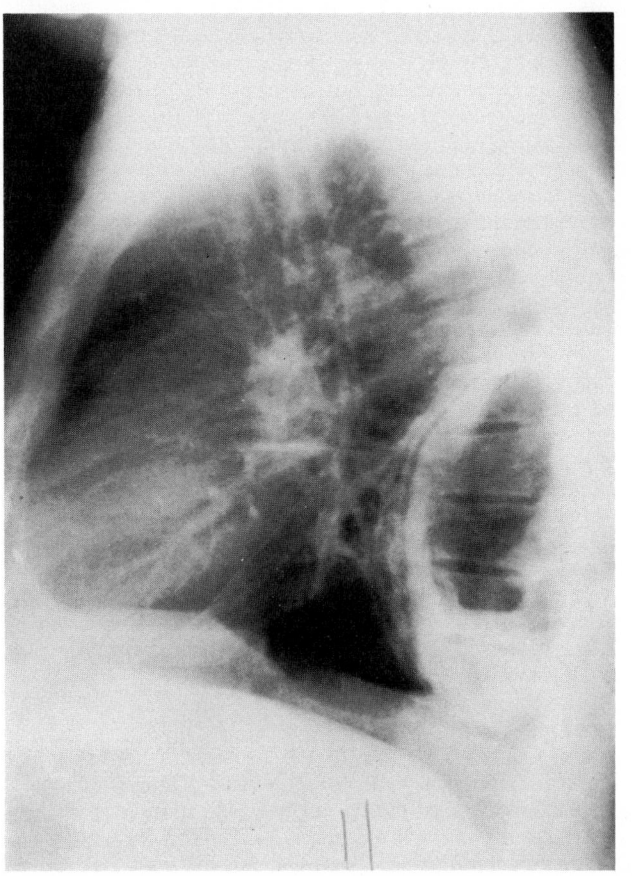

Figure 10. Loculated posterior empyema (*S. aureus*).

Bronchitis

Acute bronchitis most often occurs as part of a viral URI syndrome or in association with a specific viral infection (influenza, measles). Acute bronchitis in a patient without underlying pulmonary disease is rarely bacterial in origin.

Chronic bronchitis occurs in the spectrum of chronic obstructive lung disease. Viral and bacterial infections frequently result in deterioration of pulmonary function in chronic bronchitis. *S. pneumoniae* and *H. influenzae* are the bacteria most often responsible; therapy with ampicillin or tetracycline is frequently helpful.

Sinusitis

Acute sinusitis may follow a viral URI or dental procedure. Manifestations include fever, sinus pain, and cloudy sinuses on head x-ray film. Acute sinusitis in adults is most frequently caused by *S. pneumoniae*. When chronic sinusitis has developed, cultures of sinuses reveal a mixture of anaerobes. Penicillin is the drug of choice for sinusitis. Surgical drainage may be required if sinusitis does not respond to antibiotics or if an air-fluid level is seen on sinus x-ray examination.

URINARY TRACT INFECTIONS

The term urinary tract infection (UTI) refers to urethritis, cystitis, and pyelonephritis. Bacterial cystitis and urethritis are the most common urinary tract infections.

Pathogenesis

The bacteria most often responsible for UTI are the Gram-negative bacilli: *E. coli*, *Klebsiella*, *Proteus*, *Enterobacter*, and *Pseudomonas*. *E. coli* accounts for 90% of UTIs. Enterococcal streptococci, *S. aureus*, *S. epidermidis*, and *Candida albicans* are occasional pathogens.

The external urethra is colonized by perineal bacteria, but normal urine flow usually prevents bacterial access upstream. UTI is much more common in women, which reflects the shorter female urethra and the corresponding greater chance of bacterial ascent.

In women from 15-35 years of age UTI is relatively common, reflecting the effect of sexual activity and pregnancy on local urinary tract defenses. Prostatitis is the leading antecedent to UTI in elderly men. Neurogenic bladder, prostatic hypertrophy, urethrocele, strictures, urinary catheterization, and cystoscopy predispose to UTI by interfering with normal urinary flow.

Most lower tract infections do not develop into pyelonephritis. When pyelonephritis does occur it usually involves the renal medulla, which receives less blood flow than the renal cortex. In addition, the high osmolality and ammonium concentration in the medulla may interfere with the function of neutrophils or complement. Upper tract obstruction, renal calculi, pregnancy, and diabetes mellitus predispose to pyelonephritis.

Manifestations

Dysuria, urgency, and frequency signal a UTI but the patient may be asymptomatic. Fever, flank pain, and costovertebral angle tenderness are classically associated with pyelonephritis. However, symptoms may mislead the physician about localization of a UTI. The urinalysis reveals pyuria and hematuria; white blood cell casts indicate pyelonephritis.

Diagnostic Approach

The urine culture is the cornerstone of the diagnosis. The periurethral area must be cleansed prior to collection of the specimen because the terminal urethra and the periurethral skin are colonized with bacteria, particularly in women and the uncircumcised male. Even clean-catch, midstream urine cultures are contaminated by some bacteria. As a result, quantitative urine cultures are employed, with a level of 10^5 bacteria/ml of urine separating infection from contamination.

Less than 10^4 bacteria/ml, multiple bacterial isolates, and the presence of common contaminants (e.g., lactobacilli) suggest an improperly collected specimen. Occasionally, a suprapubic bladder aspiration for culture will be needed to confirm an infection.

An assay for antibody-coated bacteria in the urine may help differentiate upper from lower tract infection. The presence of antibody-coated bacteria correlates fairly well with renal infection because urinary tract antibodies are produced mainly in the kidney.

Any urinary tract infection in children or adult men should lead to a consideration of correctable anatomic or functional urologic disease. The same consideration applies to women with frequent (more than three) UTIs. An intravenous pyelogram is part of the standard evaluation, as is measurement of renal function (creatinine clearance). The role of cystoscopy is unclear; while correctable genitourinary lesions may be identified, there is a danger of introducing other bacteria into the urinary tract.

Complications

The majority of UTIs resolve even without antibiotic therapy. A perinephric abscess is a rare but serious sequela to pyelonephritis. Bacteremia is not common unless urinary tract instrumentation has taken place.

It is most unusual for even recurrent UTIs to result in chronic renal failure. Most cases of chronic pyelonephritis are associated with obvious structural defects of the urinary tract.

Therapeutic Approach

Patients with acute, uncomplicated lower urinary tract infection are almost always infected with *E. coli.* Because of the sensitivity of most *E. coli* to antibiotics and because of the high urinary levels of many antibiotics, eradication of infection is usually easily achieved. A sulfonamide is the initial agent of choice: sulfisoxazole and sulfamethoxazole are inexpensive and effective. Nalidixic acid, nitrofurantoin, ampicillin, thrimethoprim, trimethoprim/sulfamethoxazole and oral cephalosporins are alternatives. A 5- to 10-day course of therapy is recommended, although some success has been reported with a single large dose of amoxicillin or kanamycin. Liberal fluid intake is advisable; in addition to bacterial washout, it may decrease renal medullary hypertonicity.

Patients who are suspected of having acute pyelonephritis, or who have anatomic or functional abnormalities of the urinary tract, should receive oral ampicillin or a cephalosporin for 10-14 days. If parenteral therapy is desired, either of these agents or an aminoglycoside is indicated. Ultimately, therapy should be guided by urinary culture and antimicrobial sensitivity testing.

The urine should be recultured after therapy is completed. If infection with the same organism recurs within a short period of time after discontinuation of therapy (relapse), a 6-week course of antibiotics may eradicate the infection. Reinfection with another strain of bacteria is common and must be approached differently.

Prevention

Prophylactic antibiotics should be avoided if possible, but if UTIs recur frequently a trial of prophylaxis may be indicated. One tablet of nitrofurantoin (100 mg) or sulfamethoxazole (500 mg) daily may be effective. Trimethoprim-sulfamethoxazole, one-half tablet every other day, has also been useful.

There is a well-known association between sexual intercourse and acute UTIs in women (honeymoon cystitis). Postcoital voiding is recommended but of unproven benefit. In women with severe recurrent cystitis, a single oral dose of various antibiotics (nitrofurantoin, nalidixic acid, sulfonamide) after intercourse may decrease the incidence of UTI.

Mandelamine, a urinary antiseptic, is converted to formaldehyde when the urine pH is less than 5.5. This agent should be administered along with a urine-acidifying agent (such as ascorbic acid) for bacterial suppression. GI upset and acidosis may occur and mandelamine should be avoided with renal insufficiency.

Urinary Tract Catheterization

The risk of UTI after catherization varies from 1-3%, after a single straight catheterization in an outpatient setting, to 95% after a catheter has been in place for 4 days with an open drainage system. A closed drainage system will delay the onset of infection significantly.

The best way to decrease UTIs in a catheterized patient is to remove the catheter as soon as possible, use a closed drainage system, and insert the catheter with good, aseptic technique. Neomycin irrigation and prophylactic antibiotics are ineffective in preventing infection and encourage the emergence of antibiotic-resistant bacteria.

Asymptomatic Bacteriuria

Asymptomatic bacteriuria ($\geqslant 10^5$ bacteria/ml of urine in the absence of pyuria or symptoms) is most often seen in women. Pregnant women with this disorder are at increased risk for pyelonephritis and should receive antibiotic therapy. Asymptomatic bacteriuria in nonpregnant patients is generally benign. Most cases will resolve spontaneously and therapy is usually unnecessary.

Prostatitis

E. coli is responsible for about 80% of the cases of acute bacterial prostatitis, which presents with fever, dysuria, and perineal pain. Chronic prostatitis results in frequency, urgency, and recurrent UTIs. The bacteriologic diagnosis is made by culture of urine or fluid obtained by prostatic massage; the latter procedure may result in bacteremia. Ampicillin and trimethoprim-sulfamethoxazole are the drugs of choice.

VENEREAL DISEASES

The most common sexually transmitted diseases in the United States are gonorrhea and nongonococcal urethritis. Trichomonas vaginitis, nongonococcal cervicitis, and genital herpes are also widely seen. Other venereal diseases that may be encountered include condyloma accuminata (venereal warts), syphilis, pediculosis pubis, chancroid, lymphogranuloma venereum, and granuloma inguinale.

Urethritis

Urethritis presents as dysuria and urethral discharge. Nongonococcal urethritis (NGU) and gonorrhea are the leading causes of urethritis in men. Gonorrhea can be diagnosed by Gram stain and culture of urethral discharge.

NGU is caused by several organisms including *Chlamydia* and *Mycoplasma* (*Ureaplasma urealyticum*). These organisms cannot be readily cultured; hence, the diagnosis depends upon excluding other causes of urethritis (gonorrhea, *Trichomonas*, *Candida*).

A 2- to 3-week course of tetracycline (1-2 g per day orally), sulfisoxazole, or erythromycin is recommended for patients with NGU and their sexual partners. Penicillin and ampicillin are ineffective. Patients may have coexistent gonorrhea and NGU.

Vaginitis and Cervicitis

Vaginal or cervical infection manifests as vaginal discharge, pruritus, and dyspareunia. The gonococcus must be ruled out as a cause of cervicitis by appropriate culture; a purulent discharge is usual with gonorrhea. Nongonococcal cervicitis is most often caused by *Chlamydia*; the diagnosis is by exclusion and therapy is identical to that for NGU.

Candida albicans is not usually transmitted by sexual contact. Pregnancy, antibiotics, oral contraceptives, and diabetes predispose to *Candida* vaginitis. A white, curdlike exudate is noted. The yeast can be seen if a drop of fluid is mixed with 10% KOH or if a smear of vaginal discharge is Gram stained (the yeast is large, Gram-positive). Treatment is best accomplished with nystatin vaginal suppositories.

Trichomonas vaginitis results in a profuse, greenish discharge. Motile organisms are seen microscopically when a drop of fluid is mixed with a drop of saline. Oral metronidazole is the drug of choice. Sexual partners should also be treated to prevent reinfection.

Herpes simplex type 2 is an increasingly important venereal disease for several reasons. This herpes virus causes painful vesicles and ulcers involving the vaginal area and penis. Herpes genital infection in the female is associated with cervical carcinoma and disseminated herpes simplex infection in the neonate. Finally, there is no therapy available to prevent recurrence; however, acyclovir may hasten healing of individual lesions.

Other Venereal Diseases

Calymmatobacterium granulomatis is the cause of granuloma inguinale, a mildly contagious venereal disease. A painless, genital ulcer is seen. Later, inguinal pseudobuboes appear. The diagnosis is made by demonstrating bacteria in mononuclear cells from ulcer scrapings.

Chancroid is caused by *H. ducreyi*. The characteristic lesion is a soft, necrotic, painful genital ulcer with unilateral lymphadenopathy. The organism can be cultured on special media.

Lymphogranuloma venereum, like chancroid and granuloma inguinale, is much more common in Asia and Africa than in the United States. *Chlamydia trachomatis* is the responsible organism. A small, painless primary lesion is followed by painful inguinal lymphadenopathy. Rectal stricture is a late complication. The diagnosis is made by a high or rising complement fixation titer. The drugs of choice for all three of these diseases are tetracycline and the sulfonamides.

All patients with venereal disease should have a serologic test for syphilis. A condom will decrease transmission of most venereal diseases.

Pelvic Inflammatory Disease

Pelvic inflammatory disease (PID) is a disease of young women. The gonococcus is the single most common organism responsible for acute PID, although a variety of anaerobic (vaginal) bacteria may be involved when the process is recurrent or chronic.

PID occurs when the gonococcus spreads from the cervix to the endometrium or fallopian tubes. This event is facilitated by menses or the presence of an intrauterine device.

Cervicitis is often asymptomatic, but when endometritis develops the patient complains of fever and pelvic pain. The patient is often quite uncomfortable. Abdominal pain and tenderness with manipulation of the cervix are noted on physical examination. Complications include pelvic abscess and peritonitis. Recurrent attacks may damage the fallopian tubes, resulting in sterility.

The differential diagnosis includes acute appendicitis, ruptured ectopic pregnancy, and ruptured ovarian cyst. A pregnancy test should be done. Cultures of the cervix on Thayer-Martin medium will usually grow the gonococcus.

Antibiotic therapy with procaine penicillin, 4.8 million units intramuscularly, and 1 g of probenecid orally should be followed by a 10-day course of oral ampicillin, 2 g per day. Another effective regimen is tetracycline 2 g orally per day for 10 days. Hospitalization and parenteral antibiotics are occasionally required; intravenous penicillin G is the drug of choice in the hospitalized patient.

INFECTIOUS DIARRHEA

Intestinal Immunity

Large numbers of organisms enter the upper gastrointestinal tract, but most are killed by the low gastric pH. The normal bacterial flora of the intestine is protective; it competes with potential invaders for space and nutrients. IgA is the predominant antibody in intestinal secretions. Once an infection develops, diarrhea serves as a protective mechanism by increasing clearance of pathogens or toxins.

Achlorhydria, gastric surgery, and antacids raise gastric pH and predispose to bacterial and parasitic infections of the gut. Disturbance of normal gut flora by antibiotics lowers the infective dose of *Salmonella*. Patients with IgA deficiency have severe and recurrent infectious gastroenteritis. Opiates and anticholinergics decrease intestinal motility and may increase the severity of infectious gastroenteritis.

Viral Gastroenteritis

Viral gastroenteritis is a common, self-limited infectious disease that occurs most often in winter. Fever and systemic symptoms are absent. Examination of the stool fails to reveal neutrophils. Rotavirus, Norwalk-virus, and enteroviruses are the usual causes of viral gastroenteritis. Antibiotics are not indicated.

Invasive Pathogens

Salmonella, *Shigella*, *Yersinia*, *Campylobacter fetus*, and *Entamoeba histolytica* produce gastroenteritis by mucosal invasion. The extent of involvement varies from superficial mucosal invasion with *Salmonella* to deep invasion and ulceration with *Shigella*. The incubation period for these diseases is 1-3 days. Patients with invasive gastroenteritis have fever and frequent, small stools with mucus and blood. Examination of the stool reveals may neutrophils. Amebae may be seen directly and stool culture will detect the bacterial pathogens.

All the above pathogens have been involved in foodborne or waterborne outbreaks of diarrhea; hence, any outbreak requires investigation. Human reservoirs are implicated for *S. typhi*, *Shigella*, and amebae, while animals are important in the spread of *C. fetus*, *Yersinia*, and nontyphoid *Salmonella*.

Toxin-Mediated Disease

Cholera is the classic example of toxin-related disease. Toxigenic *E. coli*, *C. perfringens*, *C. botulinum*, and *S. aureus* produce acute, toxin-mediated gastroenteritis (food poisoning). Mucosal invasion is not seen, fever is absent, and examination of the stool does not reveal neutrophils. Nausea, vomiting, and diarrhea develop after an incubation period of 1-24 hours.

S. aureus and *C. perfringens* are the leading causes of foodborne outbreaks in this group. Staphylococcal enterotoxin is acid-stable. Nausea and vomiting begin 1-6 hours after ingestion of precooked food (often custard products). *C. perfringens* has an incubation period of 10-24 hours, and is often associated with ingestion of gravy. Botulism usually follows ingestion of home-canned foods.

Stool cultures are of no value in the diagnosis of toxin-related diarrhea. The diagnosis depends on history, culture of the suspected food, and a serum toxin assay (botulism). Antibiotic therapy is not helpful. Toxin-mediated gastroenteritis due to *E. coli*, *C. perfringens*, or *S. aureus* is self-limited.

Traveler's Diarrhea

Many foreign travelers develop diarrhea while abroad. The disease is unpleasant but rarely serious; the diarrhea is self-limited and systemic symptoms are rare. Toxigenic *E. coli* seems to be the leading cause of traveler's diarrhea but a variety of pathogens may be found. If the diarrhea continues for an unusually long period, a search should be undertaken for manageable causes (*Salmonella*, *Shigella*, amebiasis, *G. lamblia*).

Prophylactic antibiotics are of unproven benefit and have the potential disadvantages of cost, encouragement of antibiotic resistance, and disturbance of normal bowel flora. Consumption of raw foods (especially vegetables) and tap water should be avoided, if possible.

Pseudomembranous Enterocolitis

Pseudomembranous enterocolitis is a serious disease that most commonly follows antibiotic administration or surgery. Many antibiotics have been implicated, including clindamycin, ampicillin, and tetracycline. Fever, diarrhea, and abdominal distention develop rapidly. The stool examination reveals sheets of neutrophils; a pseudomembrane can be seen on proctoscopy.

A toxin-producing organism, *C. difficile*, has been shown to be the major cause of antibiotic-associated colitis. The toxin may be detected in stool by tissue culture assay.

Discontinuation of the offending antibiotic is mandatory. Fluids and bowel rest are also indicated; therapy with oral vancomycin is often beneficial.

ABDOMINAL INFECTIONS

Liver Abscess

Liver abscess is manifested by fever, chills, and right upper quadrant tenderness. An elevated white blood count is usual and the alkaline phosphatase is almost always abnormal. The diagnosis is suggested by radionuclide liver spleen scan, computed tomography, or ultrasound examination. Liver abscesses are usually multiple and are more common in the right lobe of the liver than in the left lobe.

A liver abscess can follow almost any abdominal infection; cholangitis is a common antecedent. Microbiologically, the abscess reflects bowel bacteria with anaerobic bacteria and *E. coli* predominating. Blood cultures may yield the pathogens. Surgical drainage of a large abscess is mandatory and should be supplemented with a 4- to 8-week course of antibiotics.

Biliary Tract Disease

Fever and right upper quadrant colic are the manifestations of cholecystitis. The disease is usually secondary to cholelithiasis. The primary treatment is surgical and the presence of common duct stones should be ruled out by an operative cholangiogram. The mortality is 5%.

Ascending cholangitis is signaled by fever, chills, right upper quadrant pain, and jaundice. Bacteremia is frequent, and mortality is about 60%. Sepsis or hepatic microabscesses may develop. Therapy includes surgery to relieve any obstruction to biliary flow and parenteral antibiotics effective against *E. coli*, enterococci, *Klebsiella*, and anerobes (especially *Clostridia*). Ampicillin and gentamicin provide adequate antibiotic coverage.

Appendicitis and Diverticulitis

The well-known symptoms of appendicitis include nausea, vomiting, fever, and abdominal pain, usually in a young patient. The pain is epigastric at first but later localizes to the right lower quadrant. Rebound tenderness is the rule. Perforation results in an abscess or local peritonitis. Acute appendicitis is a surgical emergency.

Diverticulitis, on the other hand, is a disease of the elderly. Obstruction of the diverticulum may lead to abscess formation, perforation, or a fistula. Manifestations include constipation, abdominal pain, nausea, vomiting, and fever. The physical exam may disclose abdominal tenderness or a tender left lower quadrant mass on rectal exam. Initial therapy for diverticulitis is bowel rest and fluids. Surgery is required for perforation, obstruction, fistula, or an abscess.

Appropriate antibiotic therapy for diverticulitis or appendicitis should provide coverage for anaerobic bacteria (especially *Bacteroides fragilis*) and enteric Gram-negative bacilli. The combination of clindamycin or chloramphenicol with gentamicin is effective.

Peritonitis and Intra-Abdominal Abscess

Peritonitis is usually secondary to an intra-abdominal infection. A microbiologic diagnosis can be made by culturing peritoneal fluid obtained by needle aspiration. Systemic antibiotics are indicated.

Intra-abdominal abscesses follow surgery, trauma, or local infection in the abdomen. Surgery is generally required in addition to antibiotics. The approach to antibiotic selection is similar to that for appendicitis or diverticulitis.

BACTERIAL MENINGITIS

Acute bacterial meningitis is a medical emergency. There is always some degree of encephalitis associated with meningitis. The meninges are usually seeded by blood-borne bacteria.

Etiology

The etiology of meningitis depends on the age of the patient and the clinical setting. Childhood meningitis is most often caused by *Hemophilus influenzae*, whereas *Streptococcus pneumoniae* and *Neisseria meningitidis* are the leading causes of adult meningitis. Meningococci predominates between the ages of 5 and 40 years, and pneumococci predominates above the age 40 (Table 5).

Table 5. Bacterial Meningitis

Age under 2 months	*E. coli*, group B streptococci
Age 2 months to 6 years	*H. influenzae*
Age over 6 years	*S. pneumoniae*, *N. meningitidis*
Sickle cell anemia/splenectomy	*S. pneumoniae*
Immunosuppressed patients	Cryptococcus, Listeria, Gram-negative bacilli
Otitis/mastoiditis/sinusitis	*S. pneumoniae*

Pneumococci are most often found in posttraumatic meningitis (with presumed CSF leak), in recurrent meningitis and in meningitis that follows otitis, mastoiditis, or sinusitis. Immunosuppressed patients tend to be infected with unusual organisms, such as cryptococci or *Listeria monocytogenes*.

Manifestations

Fever, chills, headache, and stiff neck are the classic symptoms of meningitis. The mental status of the patient varies from alert to comatose. Physical exam reveals a stiff neck that resists flexion. Focal signs, except for a sixth cranial nerve paralysis due to increased intracranial pressure, are not common and should raise the question of an abscess. Papilledema is unusual. The presence of petechiae or purpura suggests meningococcal disease.

The overall mortality is 4-10% depending on the pathogen, the promptness of diagnosis, and the therapy selected. The most common residual problem is partial hearing loss, which can be detected by audiograms in up to 25% of survivors. Residual hydrocephalus, blindness, seizures, and cranial nerve deficits are not rare. Sequelae are more prominent after childhood meningitis.

Diagnostic Approach

In the absence of papilledema or focal neurologic signs, a spinal tap should be performed promptly. If these findings are present, it is wise to obtain an emergency brain scan or computed tomography to rule out a mass lesion such as a brain abscess or subdural empyema. A spinal tap in the presence of a mass lesion may result in brain-stem herniation.

The cerebrospinal fluid (CSF) is typically cloudy, with a cell count of 500-5,000 WBC/cc (including at least 95% neutrophils). The pressure is increased, the protein is elevated, and the glucose is depressed (less than 30 mg%, or less than 40% of a simultaneous blood glucose). The Gram stain is positive 50-70% of the time, and the CSF culture is definitive. Blood cultures are positive in about 50% of cases and should be routine.

The patient who has received antibiotics prior to spinal tap and culture poses a difficult problem for the clinician. The culture is often falsely negative in partially treated meningitis. The CSF cell count and glucose are less often affected, and may provide useful information. In addition, some laboratories are able to perform a rapid assay for bacterial antigen in the spinal fluid (counterimmunoelectrophoresis), which is less affected by prior antibiotic therapy.

Therapeutic Approach

Because of the blood-brain barrier, high doses of parenteral antibiotics are required to ensure adequate CSF levels. The drug of choice for both meningococcal and pneumococcal meningitis is penicillin G, 20-24 million units per day intravenously. If penicillin allergy is a problem, chloramphenicol 2-4 g per day intravenously is indicated. Ampicillin is recommended for *H. influenzae* meningitis if the organism is ampicillin-sensitive; chloramphenicol is the alternative drug. Penicillin is the drug of choice for empiric therapy of meningitis in adults.

Therapy should be continued intravenously at full dosage for at least 2 weeks in all cases of bacterial meningitis. It is recommended that adult patients with bacterial meningitis be placed initially in respiratory isolation unless meningococcal meningitis can be excluded with reasonable certainty.

OTHER NEUROLOGIC INFECTIONS

Aseptic Meningitis

Patients with aseptic meningitis present with fever, headache, and stiff neck. They are less toxic than patients with bacterial meningitis.

The spinal tap reveals 0-500 WBC/cc, mostly mononuclear cells. The protein is elevated but the glucose is normal. If the patient has acute meningitis, and the spinal tap does not clearly differentiate aseptic from bacterial meningitis, a repeat spinal tap should be done in 6 hours.

A number of chronic diseases may have spinal fluid findings identical to aseptic meningitis including tuberculosis, neurosyphilis, systemic lupus erythematosus, and leptomeningeal neoplasm. Partially treated bacterial meningitis may also mimic aseptic meningitis.

The enteroviruses (coxsackievirus, echovirus) are the leading pathogens responsible for aseptic meningitis. St. Lous encephalitis, mumps, herpes simplex, and other viruses are less common causes. Epidemics of aseptic meningitis occur, especially in summer.

A specific viral diagnosis is difficult to make and depends on isolation of the virus from spinal fluid or antibody titer rises in serum. In practice, this is usually unnecessary since the disease resolves without therapy.

Encephalitis

Fever and headache are the most frequent manifestations of mild encephalitis. More severe cases are characterized by disturbances of consciousness. Focal signs are not common except in herpes encephalitis.

Arboviruses, most notably St. Louis encephalitis and California encephalitis viruses, are the leading causes of encephalitis. Arboviruses are zoonoses that involve humans as an accidental host. Animal hosts include horses, birds (St. Louis encephalitis), and small mammals (California encephalitis). The viruses are spread to humans by mosquitoes, and the peak incidence is in summer. Most arboviral encephalitis is mild and resolves without sequelae.

Herpes simplex encephalitis is a severe infection that is responsible for only a small percentage of encephalitis cases. Focal findings, especially frontotemporal in location, are commonly noted on physical exam, brain scan, and EEG. The mortality is 70%, and sequelae are common. Mumps, measles, and chickenpox are other agents to be considered in encephalitis.

A specific diagnosis is difficult to make. The CSF may be normal or may resemble that seen in aseptic meningitis. Arboviral infections are diagnosed by a rise in antibody titer; isolation of the virus from CSF is unusual. The diagnosis of encephalitis following childhood diseases is also primarily serologic.

Herpes encephalitis is diagnosed by the isolation of herpes simplex from a brain biopsy specimen; brain biopsy should be considered only for encephalitis with definite focal signs. Adenine arabinoside is an antiviral drug that has some efficacy in herpes simplex encephalitis.

Brain Abscess

A brain abscess may develop by metastatic spread from a distant infection or by direct extension from sinusitis, mastoiditis, or otitis media. Patients present with fever, headache, drowsiness, confusion, seizures, or focal neurologic signs. The diagnosis is confirmed by computed tomography or Tc^{99m} brain scan. A spinal tap may be hazardous.

In the absence of a culture, antibiotic therapy should be directed toward streptococci and anaerobes; penicillin G and chloramphenicol penetrate the central nervous system adequately. Surgery is required when the abscess has become localized. The mortality is 25-30% and residual neurologic sequelae in survivors are not uncommon.

BACTERIAL ENDOCARDITIS

Epidemiology

Bacterial endocarditis may involve damaged or normal valves. α-Hemolytic (viridans) streptococci, the most common cause of endocarditis, involve only valves that were previously damaged (usually by rheumatic fever), while *S. aureus* may involve healthy valves.

Endocarditis follows bacteremia. The leading risk factors are dental procedures (viridans streptococci), drug addiction (staphylococci), and genitourinary tract disease (enterococcal streptococci). Prosthetic heart valves are at increased risk of infection. Right-sided endocarditis is more common in intravenous drug abusers.

Manifestations

Fever is almost invariable. The patient often complains of chills, malaise, myalgias, and arthralgias. Ninety-five percent of cases have a heart murmur, classically a new or changing murmur. The most common murmurs are mitral and aortic insufficiency.

The physical exam may reveal splinter hemorrhages, clubbing, or splenomegaly. Evidence of vasculitis or emboli may be seen in the optic fundus (exudates, hemorrhage) or extremities (nodules, petechiae).

Laboratory results that suggest the diagnosis include elevated ESR, anemia, high WBC count, hematuria, and positive rheumatoid factor assay. The serum complement may be low.

Pathologically, the classic lesion of endocarditis is the vegetation, an amorphous, necrotic mass that contains bacteria. The vegetation may distort valve motion or shower emboli to a variety of organs. The order of frequency of valvular involvement in endocarditis is mitral > aortic > tricuspid > pulmonic.

Complications

Endocarditis has a 15-40% mortality. The leading cause of death is congestive heart failure, which usually follows aortic valve destruction or perforation.

The second most frequent complication is arterial embolization. Emboli vary in size and may involve the central nervous system (cerebrovascular accident syndrome), the lungs, the coronary arteries (myocardial infarction), the spleen, and other organs. Emboli are usually sterile, although *S. aureus* endocarditis may shower septic emboli that cause metastatic infections.

Renal disease may be caused by arterial emboli or immune complex glomerulonephritis. A myocardial abscess may be indicated by the onset of cardiac conduction defects on electrocardiogram (ECG).

Diagnosis

The cornerstone of the diagnosis is the blood culture. Three to six blood cultures should be obtained before antibiotic therapy is begun. The diagnosis is tenuous and therapy extremely difficult if blood cultures are negative. Prior antibiotics often interfere with blood cultures.

A single positive blood culture must be interpreted with caution even if bacterial endocarditis is suspected. At least two positive blood cultures with the same organism, drawn at different times, are preferred before the diagnosis of bacterial endocarditis is entertained. Furthermore, multiple positive blood cultures with the same organisms are seen in many other conditions (e.g., infected intravenous catheter, abscess).

The urinary sediment should be examined for hematuria. An echocardiogram may demonstrate a vegetation, especially on the mitral or aortic valve.

Therapy

Viridans streptococci are generally quite penicillin-sensitive, but therapy is usually initiated with penicillin and streptomycin because the combination is synergistic against streptococci. One approach is to treat with intravenous penicillin, 10-20 million units per day, and streptomycin, 1-2 g per day intramuscularly, for 2 weeks followed by 2 weeks of oral penicillin. Enterococcal endocarditis should be treated with a combination of ampicillin and gentamicin for 4 to 6 weeks. *S. aureus* endocarditis requires at least 6 weeks of a semisynthetic penicillin (e.g., nafcillin). Penicillin should be used if the organism is sensitive.

It is essential to monitor therapy with serum killing levels, which reflect the effectiveness of antibiotics against the causative organism. A peak killing level of ≥1:8 (eight times more than the minimal required level) has been correlated with successful therapy.

The temperature may not return to normal for several days, even with optimal therapy. Blood cultures should be repeated during therapy. Prolonged fever, positive blood cultures on treatment, or large vegetations may signal the need for longer antibiotic therapy.

Surgical intervention is indicated for intractable congestive heart failure, recurrent embolization, or infection that is refractory to medical therapy. Valve replacement is the indicated procedure.

Prevention

Patients with rheumatic or congenital valvular heart disease or prosthetic heart valves are at increased risk of developing endocarditis subsequent to a procedure-related bacteremia. Hence, it is standard practice to administer brief antibiotic prophylaxis directed against the bacteria that are likely to be encountered.

For dental procedures and upper respiratory tract surgical procedures, penicillin or erythromycin is recommended. Streptomycin may be added if the patient has a prosthetic valve. For genitourinary tract and gastrointestinal tract surgery or instrumentation, penicillin or ampicillin with streptomycin or gentamicin is suggested. Vancomycin may be used when penicillin allergy is a problem. Prophylaxis should begin 30-60 minutes prior to the procedure and last only 12-48 hours. The doses of antibiotics recommended for rheumatic fever prophylaxis are inadequate for bacterial endocarditis prophylaxis.

BACTEREMIA AND SEPTIC SHOCK

Bacteremia

Asymptomatic bacteremia often follows tooth extraction and occurs about 10% of the time after sigmoidoscopy, nasotracheal suctioning, barium enema, and other procedures. Usually the bacteria involved are avirulent and host defenses are adequate to eliminate the organisms rapidly from the bloodstream.

Bacteremia in a hospitalized patient is a serious problem, reflecting both pathogenic organisms and impaired host defenses. The leading isolates from blood cultures are the Gram-negative bacilli (*E. coli*, *Klebsiella*, *Enterobacter*, and *Pseudomonas*) and *S. aureus*.

The manifestations of bacteremia are diverse. Fever is almost invariable; tachycardia, hypotension, and tachypnea are common. The elderly patient may present with confusion.

The diagnosis requires a positive blood culture. A diligent search for a primary source should be made with particular attention to the urinary tract, abdomen, lungs, and skin. If empiric antibiotic therapy is required, an aminoglycoside should be included in the treatment regimen.

Septic Shock

Approximately 40% of patients with Gram-negative bacteremia will develop septic shock. Many organisms may cause septic shock, but the majority of cases are due to Gram-negative bacilli. Endotoxin, a component of the Gram-negative cell wall, causes hypotension, fever, disseminated intravascular coagulation, and complement activation. Inadequate perfusion of tissues leads to tissue anoxia, which may become irreversible.

Septic shock is heralded by fever, hypotension, and oliguria. Peripheral vascular resistance is usually decreased, and the extremities are warm. Mental obtundation is the rule. A respiratory alkalosis develops early, but is replaced by lactic acidosis. Disseminated intravascular coagulation or pulmonary edema may complicate the clinical picture.

Cultures of blood, urine, and other potentially infected sites should be obtained at once. The antibiotics of choice for initial therapy are gentamicin or tobramycin, 5 mg/kg/day intravenously in three doses. Supportive therapy is critical and must address fluid balance, acid-base balance, blood pressure maintenance, oxygenation, coagulation status, and myocardial function.

Physiologic salt or plasma protein solutions are useful oncotic agents. Ideally, fluid administration should be monitored by measurement of pulmonary artery wedge or central venous pressure. After intravascular volume has been replaced, vasoactive drugs (dopamine, isoproterenol) may be used to increase arterial pressure. Pharmacologic doses of corticosteroids may be beneficial. Even with appropriate therapy the mortality for septic shock is over 50%.

BONE, JOINT, AND SOFT TISSUE INFECTIONS

Osteomyelitis

Osteomyelitis may occur by hematogenous spread, traumatic inoculation, or direct extension of organisms from a soft-tissue focus. Acute osteomyelitis, which is usually hematogenous in origin, most often involves the long bones of the lower extremities and the vertebrae. It is primarily a disease of children; a history of prior trauma is commonly obtained. Fever, local pain, and inflammation of the surrounding soft tissues are the manifestations.

Chronic osteomyelitis is a more indolent process. Bony necrosis leads to a retained sequestrum, and a fistula to the skin may develop. *S. aureus* is the leading cause of both acute and chronic osteomyelitis, but *Mycobacterium tuberculosis* and a variety of other bacteria have been implicated.

The diagnosis requires a needle or surgical biopsy of involved bone for culture; a swab of skin or draining fistula is not adequate. Blood cultures are positive 50% of the time in acute osteomyelitis. X-ray changes of osteomyelitis are not seen for 2 to 3 weeks after the onset of infection, but a Tc^{99m} bone scan becomes abnormal earlier.

Antibiotic therapy for 4 to 6 weeks is suggested for acute osteomyelitis. Chronic osteomyelitis is extremely difficult to cure and may require long-term antibiotics. Bed rest and immobilization of the involved area are recommended for an acute process. Surgery is required for drainage of abscesses and removal of sequestra or foreign bodies. Closure of a sinus during therapy is a good prognostic sign.

Septic Arthritis

Between the ages of 15 and 45 years, gonococcus is the leading cause of septic arthritis. Below 15 and above 45 years, *S. aureus* is the leading cause. Septic arthritis due to staphylococci or Gram-negative bacilli usually occurs with preexisting joint disease, especially rheumatoid arthritis. Bacteria typically spread to the joint hematogenously.

The manifestations of septic arthritis are fever, joint pain, and swelling. Most cases are monarthric; the large joints, especially the knee and hip, are predominantly involved. Skin lesions suggest gonococcal infection.

The diagnosis is made by arthrocentesis; the synovial fluid is thick and purulent. Protein is elevated, glucose is low, and the cell count reveals over 10,000 white blood cells/cc (mostly neutrophils). Gram stain of joint fluid is positive about half of the time and the culture provides definitive information. Blood cultures should be obtained and are positive in up to 50% of cases.

High-dose parenteral antibiotics should be given for 2 to 4 weeks. Removal of pus by daily joint aspiration or open drainage is necessary to prevent cartilage destruction.

Soft Tissue Infection

Erysipelas is a rapidly-spreading superficial infection caused by group A streptococci. The patient is usually febrile; physical exam reveals lymphangitis and a painful, advancing, red, raised area of dermal inflammation. Prompt therapy is important, especially for facial cellulitis. Penicillin is the drug of choice; oral penicillin V or IV penicillin G may be used, depending on the extent of the infection. Erythromycin should be used in the penicillin allergic patient.

Impetigo is a superficial infection of the skin in children, usually due to group A streptococci. Vesicles appear initially, and evolve into golden-yellow, crusted lesions. Even though the infection is mild, therapy with penicillin is indicated to prevent post-streptococcal glomerulonephritis.

Cellulitis, infection of the skin which extends deeper than erysipelas to invovle subcutaneous tissues, is almost always caused by group A streptococci or *Staphylococcus aureus.* Local heat, swelling and tenderness are seen. IV or PO therapy, usually with an antistaphylococcal penicillin, is appropriate.

S. aureus causes most cutaneous abscesses, ranging from furuncles (pyogenic infections of hair follicles) to more extensive carbuncles. Hidradenitis suppurativa is a deep-seated infection of axillary sweat glands which is difficult to eradicate.

A swab of skin seldom provides useful information; the correct diagnostic approach involves aspiration of fluid or pus for culture. A blood culture may also yield the pathogen.

Staphyloccal skin infections should be treated with a penicillinase-resistant penicillin or cephalosporin. Drainage of abscesses is of critical therapeutic importance. Carbuncles and hidradenitis suppurativa may require more extensive surgery. Most minor cutaneous abscesses will resolve without antibiotics if incision and drainage are performed.

Wound Infections

Overall, 3-10% of all surgical wounds become infected. *S. aureus*, group A streptococci, and Gram-negative bacilli are the leading causes. A percutaneous aspirate for culture is the diagnostic procedure of choice. Therapy involves drainage of pus and appropriate parenteral antibiotics.

Factors that are associated with wound infection include bacterial contamination of the wound, trauma, host factors (diabetes, steroids, obesity, age), poor operative techniques, and local problems (necrotic tissue, hematomas, drains, foreign bodies).

ANTIBIOTICS

OVERVIEW AND MECHANISMS OF ACTION

In 1929, Fleming described an antibacterial substance that was made by the fungus *Penicillium*. Penicillin was first used clinically in the 1940s. Since that time, there has been an explosion of antibiotics that continues to the present.

On a global level, infectious diseases are the leading cause of death. In nations with more primitive socioeconomic conditions and health care systems, antibiotics are unlikely to improve health conditions until nutrition, hygiene, and sanitation are first improved.

Even in the United States, antibiotics have not eliminated the morbidity and mortality from infectious diseases. The reasons for this are that safe, effective antiviral drugs are not available; bacteria have been able to develop some degree of resistance to virtually all new antibacterial drugs; most drugs used for treatment of fungal and parasitic diseases are quite toxic; and antibiotics often fail to eradicate bacterial infections when host defenses are impaired.

Antiviral Drugs

Viruses are intracellular organisms that use host enzymes to reproduce. It is difficult to inhibit viral replication without damaging the host cell.

Adenine arabinoside is a moderately effective systemic agent for some serious herpes simplex infections, and acyclovir can be used topically for herpes genitalis. Amantidine hydrochloride has limited application as prophylaxis against influenza A infection during epidemics.

Antibacterial Drugs

The sulfonamides, trimethoprim, and pyrimethamine are antimetabolic drugs that interfere with bacterial folic acid metabolism; folic acid is required by bacteria for DNA synthesis. Penicillin is the prototype of drugs that interfere with bacterial cell wall synthesis; it interferes with crosslinkage of the mucopeptide structural subunits. Penicillins, cephalosporins, and vancomycin are cell-wall inhibitory agents. The polymyxins cause disruption of the bacterial cell membrane by detergent-like activity.

Many antibiotics inhibit bacterial protein synthesis. Chloramphenicol, erythromycin, clindamycin, tetracyclines, and aminoglycosides inhibit protein synthesis by binding to the bacterial ribosome. Rifampin affects the reading of DNA and nalidixic acid interferes with DNA synthesis.

Bactericidal antibiotics have similar minimal inhibitory (MIC) and bactericidal (MBC) concentrations, whereas with static antibiotics the difference between MIC and MBC is large. Penicillins, cephalosporins, vancomycin, and aminoglycosides are widely used bactericidal antibiotics.

Antifungal Drugs

Amphotericin B is the most reliable drug which is effective in systemic fungal infections. It acts on the fungal membrane, as does ketoconazole, an oral drug most useful for superficial fungal infections. 5-Fluorocytosine interferes with fungal protein synthesis. It is active against several fungi, including *Candida* and *Cryptococci.*

Pharmacokinetics

The pharmacokinetic of an antibiotic depend on absorption, distribution, metabolism, storage, and elimination of the drug. The elimination of a drug is expressed as the half-life ($t^{1/2}$), the time it takes a drug level to decrease by 50% (Table 6). Protein binding decreases the amount of free drug available.

Chloramphenicol, erythromycin, clindamycin, rifampin, isoniazid, nafcillin, and doxycycline are excreted primarily by the liver. The kidney excretes aminoglycosides, penicillins, cephalosporins, vancomycin, tetracyclines, nitrofurantoin, nalidixic acid, trimethoprim, and most sulfonamides. Hence, these drugs should be used with caution in the presence of renal insufficiency.

Patients not requiring hospitalization are usually treated with oral antibiotics. Food, antacids, and malabsorptive disorders often interfere with drug absorption. Intramuscular administration should be avoided in the presence of shock and bleeding disorders. Intravenous administration assures reliable blood levels. The peak antibiotic level occurs immediately after an intravenous infusion and about 1 h after intramuscular or oral administration. The trough (minimal) level occurs prior to the next dose.

Antibiotic Disadvantages

The potential disadvantages of any antibiotic include hypersensitivity, toxicity, encouragement of antibiotic resistance, disturbance of normal flora, and cost. The risk for an adverse reaction to antibiotics in the hospital is about 5% per antibiotic course. The reactions are frequently serious enough to prolong hospitalization (Table 6).

Table 6. Antibiotics

Drug	*Half-Life*	*Primary Route of Elimination*	*Major Side Effects*
Penicillins	30-60 min	Renal	Hypersensitivity
Cephalosporins	40-120 min	Renal	Hypersensitivity
Aminoglycosides	2-3 h	Renal	Nephrotoxicity, ototoxicity
Tetracyclines	6-20 h	Renal, hepatic	Dental staining, rash, gastrointestinal intolerance
Erythromycin	1.5 h	Hepatic	Cholestatic hepatitis, gastrointestinal intolerance
Clindamycin	4 h	Hepatic	Diarrhea, colitis
Chloramphenicol	2-3 h	Hepatic	Bone marrow suppression
Sulfonamides	6-18 h	Renal, hepatic	Hypersensitivity, crystalluria
Trimethoprim	11 h	Renal	Anemia, rash
Vancomycin	6 h	Renal	Nephrotoxicity, phlebitis
Polymyxin	6 h	Renal	Nephrotoxicity
Metronidazole	7 h	Renal	Gastrointestinal intolerance

PENICILLINS

All penicillins have the basic β-lactam ring structure. Addition of side chains may result in altered enzyme resistance, acid stability, or antibacterial spectrum.

Penicillin G

Penicillin G is a narrow-spectrum drug effective against pneumococci, streptococci, meningococci, gonococci, treponemas, and most anaerobes. It can be given intravenously (penicillin G), orally (penicillin V), or intramuscularly (benzathine penicillin, procaine penicillin). Benzathine penicillin provides low levels of penicillin for up to 30 days, while procaine penicillin provides therapeutic levels for 12-24 hours.

Penicillin G doses are measured in units or grams (250 mg equivalent to 400,000 units). The highest doses of penicillin G are 20-24 million units intravenously per day in bacterial meningitis. The doses of procaine penicillin and benzathine penicillin are 600,000-1.2 million units intramuscularly. Penicillin V is given as 1-2 g per day orally in four divided doses.

Penicillin is the drug of choice for infections caused by pneumococci, streptococci (excluding enterococci), anaerobic bacteria (excluding *B. fragilis*), penicillin-sensitive staphylococci, and meningococci. Benzathine penicillin G is the drug of choice for syphilis, group A streptococcal pharyngitis, and rheumatic fever prophylaxis. Procaine penicillin G is recommended for gonorrhea and pneumococcal pneumonia. Penicillin is also optimal therapy for a number of less common infections including anthrax, actinomycosis, and *Listeria* infection.

Anti-staphylococcal Penicillins

Most strains of staphylococci have developed resistance to penicillin on the basis of an enzyme that inactivates the penicillin molecule. Methicillin, oxacillin, nafcillin, cloxacillin, and dicloxacillin are antistaphylococcal penicillins of equal efficacy that are resistant to this enzyme. Methicillin, oxacillin, and nafcillin are for intravenous use, while dicloxacillin gives the best levels after oral administration. The intravenous dosage of methicillin, nafcillin, and oxacillin is 6-12 g per day for serious staphylococcal infections. They are the most effective antistaphylococcal drugs available.

Broad-Spectrum Penicillins

Ampicillin and amoxicillin are equivalent drugs that are effective against Gram-positive bacteria (including enterococci), as well as *H. influenzae*, *Salmonella*, *Shigella*, *E. coli*, and *Proteus mirabilis*. Both drugs can be given orally; amoxicillin is better absorbed but more expensive. The oral doses range from 1-4 g per day. Ampicillin is the intravenous preparation of choice and is administered at a dosage of 6-12 g per day for serious infections.

Ampicillin is the drug of choice for *H. influenzae*; nontyphoid *Salmonella*, *Shigella*, and enterococci. It is widely used against ampicillin-sensitive, Gram-negative enteric bacilli (*E. coli, Proteus mirabilis*) and as a single-dose, oral therapy for gonorrhea.

Several broad spectrum penicillins are notable for their activity against *Pseudomonas aeruginosa*. Carbenicillin, ticarcillin, mezlocillin, and piperacillin are used intravenously at doses of 12-24 grams per day for serious *Pseudomonas* infections, especially in the neutropenic patient. They are generally combined with an aminoglycoside.

General Properties

The penicillins are excreted in the urine and achieve high urinary levels. They penetrate most tissues well and cross the blood-brain barrier in the presence of meningeal inflammation. Probenecid will increase blood levels of all penicillins by decreasing renal excretion of these drugs.

The major side effect of all the penicillins is hypersensitivity; they cross react. A rash is the most common manifestation of allergy, and a great variety of skin manifestations can be seen. Immediate hypersensitivity is the most serious type of allergy. Urticaria, asthma, and anaphylactic shock develop 10-30 minutes after penicillin administration. Serum sickness and vasculitis are late allergic complications.

In all of the above instances, the offending drug should be stopped at once. Penicillin derivatives should be avoided if a history of any type of allergic reaction is obtained. Unfortunately, there is no single skin test that predicts penicillin sensitivity with great accuracy.

Other side effects include hemolytic anemia, seizures (high doses of penicillin), diarrhea (ampicillin), sodium overload and potassium depletion (carbenicillin), platelet dysfunction (carbenicillin), and interstitial nephritis. Methicillin and penicillin have been associated with interstitial nephritis, which presents with fever, eosinophilia, hematuria, proteinuria, and renal functional impairment. Most patients recover completely when the drug is stopped.

CEPHALOSPORINS

Cephalosporins, like penicillins, have a β-lactam ring. Successive generations of cephalosporins have broadening antibacterial spectra.

First Generation Cephalosporins

First generation cephalosporins are quite active against most Gram-positive cocci (except enterococci), and resist enzymatic degradation by staphylococci. They are effective against certain Gram-negative bacilli, notably *E. coli, Klebsiella* and *Proteus mirabilis.*

Cephalothin, cephradine and cephapirin are roughly equivelant drugs given IV at doses of 6-12 grams per day; their half-lives are 30-60 minutes. Cefazolin has a longer half-life of 100 minutes. It is the intramuscular cephalosporin of choice, and can be given IV at doses up to 8 grams per day.

Cephalexin and cephradine are widely used oral cephalosporins. Cefaclor is the most active of the oral preparations against *H. infuenzae,* whereas cefadroxil is notable for its long half-live (90 minutes).

Broad Spectrum Cephalosporins

Cefoxitin and cefamandole, the second generation drugs, have a somewhat expanded spectrum that includes *Enterobacter, Proteus, Hemophilus* and some anaerobes. Cefoxitin, but not cefamandole, is active against most strains of *Bacteroides fragilis.* These drugs, like the first generation cephalosporins, do not penetrate the blood-brain barrier reliably. Both are administered parenterally at doses of 4-12 grams per day.

Third generation cephalospirins have both broader spectra and greater activity against common Gram-negative bacilli. Cefotaxime is very effective against *E. coli, Enterobacter, Klebsiella, Proteus, Serratia* and *Hemophilus.* It has a half-life of 60 minutes, and is given IV at doses of 3-12 grams per day. Moxalactam is somewhat less active; its half-life is longer, about two hours. Both drugs achieve excellent CSF levels. Cefoperazone also has a half-life of two hours, and may be the most active against *Pseudomonas.*

Third generations drugs are less active than first generation cephalosporins against *S. aureus,* and are not reliable against enterococci, *Acinetobacter* or *Pseudomonas.*

Adverse Effects

Any of the allergic reactions described for the penicillins can occur with the cephalosporins. Patients who are allergic to the penicillins have approximately a 10% change of having an allergic reaction to the cephalosporins. Cephalosprins should be avoided when there is a history of immediate hypersensitivtiy to the penicillins.

Other toxicity includes neutropenia, diarrhea, pseudomembranous enterocolitis (moxalactam), and antabuse-like reaction (moxalactam), bleeding due to prolonged prothrombin time (moxalactam) and positive Coombs' test. The drugs are excreted by the kidney; dosage should be decreased in renal failure.

Indications

First generation cephalosporins are of greatest importance in treatment of Gram-positive infections in patients who are allergic to penicillins. They are appropriate in certain Gram-negative infections (*E. coli, Klebsiella*) and as prophylaxis in selected surgical procedures.

Second generation cephalosporins have fewer therapeutic uses. Cefoxitin may be useful prophylactically in certain abdominal or pelvic surgical procedures.

Third generation cephalosporins are expensive and should not be used when a less costly or narrow spectrum drug would suffice, nor should they be used prophylactically. Cefotaxime and others are most valuable in the treatment of certain mixed infections especially when sensitivity is confirmed, and in meingitis caused by entrobacteriaceae.

AMINOGLYCOSIDES

Spectrum and Administration

The aminoglycosides are active primarily against Gram-negative bacilli, but are inactive against anaerobes. They are removed by glomerular filtration and achieve high urinary levels. Protein binding is minimal. None of the aminoglycosides penetrate the blood-brain barrier adequately.

Gentamicin, tobramycin, and amikacin are active against many aerobic Gram-negative bacilli. Many Gram-negative bacilli have acquired resistance to streptomycin, neomycin, and kanamycin.

Gentamicin and tobramycin are equivalent drugs that are administered at a dosage of 3-5 mg/kg/day intramuscularly or intravenously at 8-hour intervals. Recently, there has been an increase in enzyme-mediated gentamicin resistance. Gentamicin-resistant Gram-negative bacilli are generally also resistant to tobramycin, but they are usually amikacin-sensitive. Amikacin is given at a dosage of 15 mg/kg/day in two to three doses.

Toxicity

Unlike the penicillins and cephalosporins, the aminoglycosides have a narrow toxic-therapeutic ratio. Nephrotoxicity is the most important side effect, occurring in about 8-10% of patients; these drugs are highly concentrated in the renal cortex. Nephrotoxicity is more common in the elderly and in patients with preexisting renal disease. The earliest sign is an increase in aminoglycoside half-life; later, renal functional deterioration is noted. The renal impairment is usually reversible. Ototoxicity can present as high-tone hearing loss or vestibular problems; it is often irreversible. Neuromuscular blockade is seen periodically, but allergic complications are rare.

Aminoglycoside therapy requires attention to toxicity, especially renal toxicity. It has been shown that the pharmacokinetics of these drugs are quite variable. Therapy should be monitored with serum aminoglycoside levels and serum creatinine determinations. Ideal gentamicin and tobramycin levels are a peak of 4-8 μg/ml and a trough of <2 μg/ml. Elevated trough levels have been correlated with nephrotoxicity.

The doses of all aminoglycosides must be greatly reduced in renal insufficiency. The half-life of gentamicin increases from 2 hours in normals to 48 hours in renal failure. Several useful methods for dose adjustment are available, notably increasing the interval between doses or decreasing the dosage without changing the interval. In any case, aminoglycoside blood levels should be monitored.

Indications

Streptomycin is used in combination with penicillin in the treatment of streptococcal endocarditis. It is a very useful drug for tuberculosis, tularemia, brucellosis, and plague, usually in combination with other drugs. Neomycin is not used parenterally.

Gentamicin is the drug of choice for a wide variety of Gram-negative infections. It is the preferred drug in septic shock, when culture data are pending. Aminoglycosides must be administered intrathecally if they are used for a central nervous system infection. Amikacin is indicated primarily for gentamicin-resistant, Gram-negative infections.

TETRACYCLINE, ERYTHROMYCIN, CLINDAMYCIN, AND CHLORAMPHENICOL

These antibiotics are bacteriostatic drugs that inhibit bacterial protein synthesis.

Tetracycline

Tetracycline has a half-life of about 10 hours and is excreted by the kidney and liver. Doxycycline, a derivative, has a longer half-life (20 h) and is also excreted by the liver. Tetracyclines are used almost exclusively as oral drugs. Food and antacids will markedly reduce absorption. The standard adult dose of tetracycline is 1-2 g orally per day in four divided doses. The tetracyclines are broad-spectrum drugs with activity against many organisms. They are important drugs in the treatment of *Chlamydia* infections, brucellosis, tularemia, rickettsial diseases, *Mycoplasma* infections, and gonorrhea.

Tetracyclines should be avoided in pregnant women and children under the age of 8 because of tooth enamel discoloration in the fetus and interference with bone development in children. Other side effects include gastrointestinal complaints and diarrhea, *Candida* superinfection, photosensitivity (especially demeclocycline), renal tubular acidosis (outdated tetracycline), vestibular toxicity (minocycline), acute hepatic necrosis (especially in pregnant women), diabetes insipidus (dimeclocycline), elevation of the blood urea nitrogen (related to the catabolic effect), rash, and increased intracranial pressure in infants. The toxicity of minocycline precludes its general use. *Candida* pharyngitis and vaginitis are quite common and reflect the disturbance of normal bacterial flora by these broad-spectrum agents. Tetracyclines other than doxycycline should be avoided in renal failure.

Erythromycin and Clindamycin

Erythromycin and clindamycin are active primarily against Gram-positive bacteria. Erythromycin is the drug of choice for *Mycoplasma* infections, diphtheria, and Legionnaire's disease. Clindamycin is most useful for anaerobic infections and is the drug of choice for *Bacteroides fragilis*. Both drugs can be given orally or intravenously. The dosage of erythromycin is 2 g per day intravenously or orally, while clindamycin is administered in doses of 150-600 mg q 6 h orally or intravenously.

Erythromycin estolate produces cholestatic hepatitis. Other side effects include gastrointestinal upset and phlebitis. The major toxicities of clindamycin are diarrhea and rash. A small percentage of cases of clindamycin-related diarrhea evolve to a pseudomembranous colitis; the drug should be stopped as soon as diarrhea develops.

Chloramphenicol

Chloramphenicol is a broad-spectrum drug that is very useful in rickettsial diseases, anaerobic infections (including *Bacteroides fragilis*), brain abscess, meningitis, *H. influenzae* infections, and *Salmonella* infections. It is well tolerated orally and intravenously at a dosage of 2-4 g per day in four divided doses. Hematologic toxicity and circulatory collapse in infants have prevented its widespread use. The hematologic effect may be either a dose-related, reversible bone marrow suppression or an uncommon bone marrow aplasia (incidence about one in 40,000).

SULFONAMIDES

Sulfonamides are broad-spectrum antibiotics for oral administration. They were first employed in the 1930s and remain useful therapeutic agents. Toxic effects include hypersensitivity (fever, rash, vasculitis), agranulocytosis, serum sickness, hepatitis, crystalluria, hemolytic anemia, methemoglobinemia, gastrointestinal symptoms, and kernicterus in infants. Sulfonamides should be avoided in pregnancy, infancy, and renal failure. Sulfamethoxazole and sulfisoxazole are useful in the treatment of urinary tract infections at total daily doses of 2-4 and 4-8 g, respectively. Sulfadiazine and triple sulfonamides are useful in *Nocardia* infections and silver sulfadiazine is used topically in burn patients.

The combination of a sulfonamide with either pyrimethamine or trimethoprim exerts a synergistic effect against folate metabolism in microorganisms. The former combination is employed in toxoplasmosis. The fixed combination of sulfamethoxazole (400 mg) and trimethoprim (80 mg) is used orally for urinary tract infection, prostatitis, *Pneumocystis* infection, and nocardiosis.

Trimethoprim alone may be used to treat uncomplicated urinary tract infections. Its side effects include rash and anemia.

ANTITUBERCULOSIS DRUGS

Isoniazid (INH) is a key oral antituberculous drug. The standard adult dose is 300 mg per day. Toxic reactions include gastrointestinal complaints, rash, peripheral neuritis, and hepatitis. Allergic hepatitis develops in about 1% of patients, the risk increasing with age. INH hepatitis mimics viral hepatitis in terms of symptoms, liver function abnormalities, and liver histology. Two- to fourfold elevations of SGOT are an indication for discontinuation of INH.

Rifampin is an oral drug that is active against *Mycobacteria* and a number of other bacteria. Resistance to this drug develops quickly when it is used alone. Rash, cholestatic hepatitis, and thrombocytopenia may be seen. Saliva, tears, and urine may also turn orange. Rifampin should be avoided in pregnancy and severe liver disease.

Ethambutol, unlike INH and rifampin, is excreted primarily by the kidney. It is included in many tuberculosis therapeutic programs as a well-tolerated oral agent. The main side effect is a retrobulbar neuritis that is first manifested by decreased red-green vision. This side effect is reversible if the drug is stopped early. Rash and hyperuricemia may also be seen.

p-Aminosalicylate is an oral antituberculous drug. The limiting toxicity is usually gastrointestinal (nausea, vomiting, diarrhea).

OTHER ANTIBIOTICS

Vancomycin is an intravenous drug that is useful against Gram-positive cocci, especially *S. aureus*. Toxicity, which is significant, includes ototoxicity, nephrotoxicity, fever, rash, and phlebitis. The dosage must be greatly reduced in renal failure. Polymyxin is a parenteral drug that is occasionally used against Gram-negative bacilli, especially *Pseudomonas aeruginosa*. It is nephrotoxic.

Nitrofurantoin and nalidixic acid are used as oral therapy for urinary tract infections. Both have limited application because of toxicity or bacterial resistance. Major side effects of nitrofurantoin are allergic pneumonitis, pulmonary fibrosis, peripheral neuropathy, gastrointestinal intolerance, and anemia. Nalidixic acid often causes nausea, vomiting, diarrhea, or rash.

Spectinomycin is used as single-dose therapy for gonorrhea. The dose is 2 g intramuscularly and allergic reaction is uncommon.

Metronidazole is approved for trichomoniasis, giardiasis, amebiasis, and anaerobic infections (including *Bacteroides fragilis*). Gastrointestinal side effects, neutropenia, and an antabuse-like reaction with alcohol may be seen.

Amphotericin B is given intravenously for systemic fungal infections. It is effective but toxic; nephrotoxicity, fever, phlebitis, hypokalemia, and anemia are common side effects. 5-Fluorocytosine is an oral drug useful against several fungi including *Candida* and *Cryptococci*. Gastrointestinal side effects, hepatic dysfunction, and pancytopenia may develop. Its most important application is in combination with amphotericin B in cryptococcal meningitis when synergy is demonstrated. Another oral drug, ketoconazole, is effective in chronic mucocutaneous candidiasis and dermatophyte infections. It may cause nausea, vomiting and rash.

ANTIBIOTIC RESISTANCE

It seems that every new antibiotic is touted as the ultimate weapon against bacteria. However, the history of antibiotics demonstrates bacterial adaptability: bacteria have developed some degree of resistance to virtually all antibiotics that have been formulated.

Mechanisms of Resistance

A number of mechanisms are operative. The genetic information for resistance may be contained on chromosomes or on small pieces of extrachromosomal DNA in the cytoplasm (plasmids). Plasmid exchange among bacteria provides a means for rapid transfer of resistance among Gram-negative bacteria. Resistance is most commonly effected by enzymatic inactivation of the antibiotic (penicillin, aminoglycosides), but may be due to decreased uptake or decreased binding of the antibiotic to the target site in the bacterial cell.

Clinical Problems

Many clinically important examples of antibiotic resistance can be found. Most staphylococci are now penicillin-resistant, and methicillin-resistant strains of *S. aureus* have been found. A β-lactamase is responsible for penicillin resistance in gonococci and ampicillin resistance in *H. influenzae*. Sulfonamide-resistant meningococci are not uncommon. Ampicillin-resistant *Shigella* and chloramphenicol-resistant *Salmonella typhi* are common in tropical countries. Multiply-resistant Gram-negative bacilli have caused large outbreaks of hospital-associated infections. Resistance problems are not confined to bacteria, as is demonstrated by dapsone-resistant leprosy, INH-resistant tuberculosis, 5-fluorocytosine-resistant *Cryptococci* and chloroquin-resistant malaria. Herpes simplex strains resistant to acyclovir lack the thymidine kinase necessary for drug activity.

Causes and Solutions

There is no doubt that antibiotic usage is the cause of the problem. Antibiotics apply selective pressure for antibiotic resistance by eliminating sensitive strains. Hospitals provide an ideal environment for selection and spread of antibiotic resistance.

Multiple studies have consistently revealed extensive overutilization and inappropriate usage of antibiotics. The key to any effort to control antibiotic resistance is to decrease antibiotic abuse. Solutions ranging from physician education to antibiotic restriction have been proposed. In addition, hospital spread of resistant strains should be minimized by an active infection control program.

ANTIBIOTIC PROPHYLAXIS

Generally accepted indications for antibiotic prophylaxis include the prevention of tuberculosis (INH), meningococcal meningitis (sulfonamides or rifampin), rheumatic fever (penicillin), bacterial endocarditis, malaria (chloroquine), and gonococcal ophthalmia neonatorum (silver nitrate). Antibiotics are often used for prevention of infection with CSF rhinorrhea (penicillin) and burns (silver sulfadiazine).

Surgical antibiotic prophylaxis is an area of controversy. In general, prophylaxis is indicated if the consequences of infection are severe (as in prosthetic heart valve surgery or total hip replacement) or if the risk of infection is high (e.g., colon surgery, open fracture reduction). Antibiotic selection depends on the bacteria likely to cause infection, as well as antibiotic safety and cost. Antibiotics should be administered prior to surgery; continuation of antibiotic prophylaxis longer than 24-48 hours postoperatively is of no benefit in the prevention of infection.

APPROACH TO ANTIBIOTIC USAGE

The physician must first decide if an infection is present. A noninfectious process, such as neoplasm or pulmonary embolus, may mimic an infection by producing fever or pulmonary infiltrates.

The presence of a potential pathogen in a culture does not necessarily imply that the organism is responsible for the disease process. For example, *S. pneumoniae* in sputum and *Proteus* on a wound surface may be mere colonizers.

If an infection is documented, it must be amenable to therapy. Therapy for many infectious diseases is either unavailable or unnecessary (e.g., viral pneumonia, URI).

Cultures must be obtained prior to institution of antibiotic therapy, since a single dose of an antibiotic may be enough to inhibit the growth of bacteria in cultures.

Antibiotic Selection

Initial, or empiric, antibiotic therapy may be indicated before identification of the responsible pathogen is possible. The physician selects an antibiotic in this situation on the basis of the pathogen(s) most likely to be found, the probable antibiotic sensitivities of the pathogen(s), and other factors (Fig. 11). Another oral drug, ketoconazole, is effective in chronic mucocutaneous candidiasis and dermatophyte infections. It may cause nausea, vomiting and rash.

Clues to the microbiologic etiology are obtained from the clinical setting (including patient age and immune status) and the site of infection. A Gram stain may provide valuable information. Cumulative antibiotic sensitivity trends for bacteria are available from many microbiology laboratories.

Empiric therapy is then modified when culture results become available: the most effective, safest, and least expensive antibiotic is chosen. In order to minimize toxicity and disturbance of normal flora, a narrow-spectrum drug should be used and a single drug is preferable to multiple drug therapy.

General guidelines for length of antibiotic therapy are available. Examples include treatment of uncomplicated pneumococcal pneumonia for 7-10 days and treatment of staphylococcal endocarditis for 6 weeks. Therapy should be individualized on the basis of clinical response and the results of cultures obtained during therapy.

Approach to Antibiotic Failure

Prolonged fever may not reflect lack of drug efficacy but rather the natural history of the infection, an incorrect diagnosis, or drug-related fever.

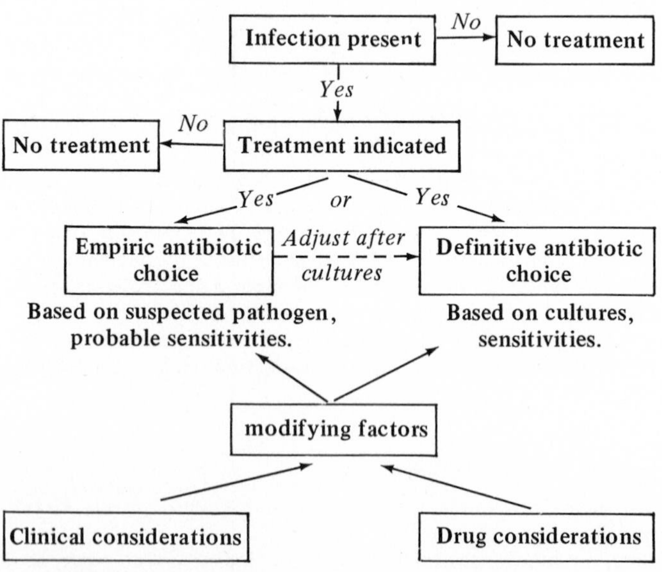

Figure 11. Approach to antibiotics.

Drug-related causes of antibiotic failure include errors in administration, incorrect drug selection, inadequate dosage, adverse drug interactions, and poor tissue levels of antibiotics. Microbiologic causes for antibiotic failure are bacterial drug resistance and superinfection. Host factors to be considered include host defense problems (e.g., neutropenia) and problems that require surgery (abscess, foreign body).

SPECIAL CONSIDERATIONS

HOSPITAL-ASSOCIATED INFECTIONS

Five percent of all patients admitted to acute care hospitals in the United States develop a hospital-associated (nosocomial) infection. One-third of all infections in hospitalized patients are nosocomial.

Pathogenesis

Hospitalized patients are more vulnerable to infectious diseases than outpatients or healthy persons. Normal anatomic and physiologic barriers to pathogens are altered. Intravenous catheters, endotracheal tubes, surgical wounds, and burns may interfere with the integrity of anatomic barriers. Antibiotics may eliminate the protective value of normal bacterial flora of mouth, gut, vagina, or skin. At the same time, the ability of the body to combat potential pathogens that have bypassed local barriers is compromised by certain disease states and therapeutic modalities.

Etiology

The vast majority of nosocomial infections are bacterial in origin. Gram-negative bacilli are now the major cause, particularly *E. coli* (urinary tract infection) and *Klebsiella* (pneumonia). *S. aureus* is still an important cause of wound infection, pneumonia, and other nosocomial infections.

The most common nosocomial infections are urinary tract infection (usually associated with a urinary catheter), pneumonia (often associated with ventilatory equipment), postoperative wound infection, and bacteremia. Sepsis related to intravenous catheters is an uncommon but serious nosocomial infection.

There are two important sources of hospital-associated infections. Many are caused by bacteria that comprise the patient's own microbial flora. Urinary catheters and other factors enable normally harmless bacteria to become pathogens.

Alternatively, bacteria may be acquired in the hospital environment. Nosocomial outbreaks of Gram-negative infections are often traced to equipment that comes into contact with the patient, such as inhalation therapy equipment or hemodialysis machines. Group A streptococcus and *S. aureus* are acquired from human reservoirs, either patients or hospital personnel.

Prevention

Hospital-associated infections cannot be completely eliminated, but they can be minimized by an active infection control program. The major elements of an infection control program are (1) documentation and recording of infections, (2) determination of the nosocomial infection rate for the hospital, (3) detection and investigation of outbreaks of infection, (4) education of hospital staff in infection control procedures, (5) review of antibiotic usage and resistance trends, and (6) review of hospital policies, including isolation.

Compulsive handwashing by physicians and other hospital staff is the most important infection control measure. Handwashing with soap and water removes most transiently acquired organisms and should be done before and after significant patient contacts.

Iodine-containing compounds, 70% alcohol, hexachlorphene, and chlorhexidine are reliable antiseptics that facilitate cleansing of skin. Handwashing with these agents is recommended before surgery and other high-risk invasive procedures.

Infection control programs are designed to eliminate reservoirs of infection (e.g., by disinfection) or to prevent transmission (e.g., by isolation). The infection control committee is responsible for a hospital-wide infection control program. On a state level, public health efforts require input from physicians and hospitals through reporting of communicable diseases such as hepatitis, tuberculosis, and salmonellosis.

INFECTIONS IN THE COMPROMISED HOST

Infection is the leading cause of death in cancer patients. The mortality from infectious complications varies from 40% with solid tumors to 75% in acute leukemia (Table 7).

Immune Deficiencies

Local immunity is frequently impaired in cancer patients. Examples include lung cancer obstructing a bronchus, urinary catheterization, intravenous catheters, and mucous membrane ulcers from chemotherapeutic agents.

Neutropenia, defined as less than 1,000 circulating neutrophils/cc, is clearly associated with a high risk of infection. Bacteremia and pneumonia frequently develop; Gram-negative bacilli are the usual cause. Neutropenia is most often caused by cytotoxic chemotherapy, radiation, or marrow replacement by tumor.

Pneumococci and *H. influenzae* cause severe infections in antibody-deficiency states (multiple myeloma, chronic lymphocytic leukemia) and postsplenectomy. The risk of

Table 7. The Compromised Host

Host Defense Defect	*Type of Infection Associated*
↓ IgG	*S. pneumoniae, H. influenzae*
↓ IgA	Respiratory tract infection, gastroenteritis
Depressed cell-mediated immunity	Fungal, viral, TB infection
Neutropenia	Gram-negative bacteremia
Lung cancer	Bacterial pneumonia
Renal transplant	CMV disease
Hemodialysis	*S. aureus* infection

serious infection after splenectomy is greatest in the first 3 years after surgery. The spleen is an important source of antibody production.

Lymphoma and corticosteroid therapy are common causes of impaired cellular immunity. The organisms that cause infections in this setting are viruses, fungi, *Mycobacteria*, *Pneumocystis*, and Nocardia.

Therapy and Prevention

An aggressive diagnostic approach is mandatory in the compromised host. Therapy, even if appropriate, may fail because of the lack of assistance from the host immune system. Suspected bacterial infection in the neutropenic patient should be treated empirically with broad-spectrum antibiotics without waiting for culture results because of the rapidly fatal nature of such infections.

Pneumonia in the compromised host is a serious problem. The mortality from pneumonia in acute leukemia is 65%. A pneumonia that does not respond to antibiotic therapy requires a transbronchoscopic or open lung biopsy because of the great variety of possible infectious and noninfectious etiologies.

Pneumococcal and influenza vaccines should be given to immunodeficient patients. Pooled gamma globulin injections may be indicated for severe hypogammaglobulinemia associated with recurrent infections. Granulocyte transfusions provide short-lived but occasionally valuable assistance against bacterial infections in selected neutropenic patients.

FEVER OF UNKNOWN ORIGIN

Prolonged fever of undetermined cause is a problem that commonly falls within the realm of infectious diseases. Fever of unknown origin (FUO) is defined as an illness with temperature over 38.3°C with no diagnosis after 1 week of hospital investigation. This definition excludes most viral and self-limited illnesses.

Etiology

The most common diseases that are found to be responsible for FUO are infection (tuberculosis, bacterial endocarditis, abscess), neoplasm (lymphoma), and collagen-vascular disease (systemic lupus erythematosus, temporal arteritis, rheumatoid arthritis). A myriad of causes can be seen occasionally including sarcoidosis, pulmonary emboli, hemolytic anemia, inflammatory bowel disease, atrial myxoma, thyrotoxicosis, and factitious fever.

Evaluation

The fever pattern is seldom diagnostic. Factitious fever can be ruled out by observation temperatures or urinary temperatures. The history should focus on travel and drug usage. The physical exam may reveal splenomegaly, lymphadenopathy, or a heart murmur. The routine evaluation often includes cultures, serologic studies, antinuclear antibody, thyroid function studies, skin tests, and x-ray films of the chest, kidneys, and gastrointestinal tract. Biopsy of clinically involved tissue is often most helpful. Localization of an abscess is often facilitated by ultrasound evaluation, computed tomography, or gallium scan, which is concentrated in inflammatory and neoplastic processes.

An extensive evaluation may not reveal the underlying cause, in which case outpatient followup with repeat examinations is indicated. Blind trials of antibiotics, INH, or steroids are not useful.

IMMUNIZATIONS AND VACCINATIONS

Passive Immunization

The injection of antibody from an immune donor is passive immunization and provides temporary immunity. Passive immunity (i.e., the injection of pooled globulins) is useful for prophylaxis of hepatitis A, hepatitis B, measles, and rabies. Diphtheria and botulism (horse antitoxin) and tetanus (human antitoxin) are also indications for passive immunization.

Active Immunization

The standard vaccination schedule calls for diphtheria-pertussis-tetanus vaccine and oral polio vaccine to be given beginning at 2 months of age. (Table 8). Measles, mumps, and rubella vaccines are given at 15 months of age. Tetanus and diphtheria boosters should be given every 5-10 years throughout adulthood.

Active immunity is preferable to passive immunity because it is generally long lasting. Mumps, measles, rubella, smallpox, and oral polio vaccines are live, attenuated viruses. They should not be given to an immunodeficient host. Rabies, pertussis, and influenza vaccines are inactivated agents. The pneumococcal vaccine consists of cell-wall polysaccharide extract, and hepatitis B vaccine is composed of surface antigen components of the virus.

Smallpox immunization has resulted in elimination of smallpox on a global level. The vaccine is no longer routinely recommended.

Some vaccination preparations contain egg products (yellow fever, influenza, rabies) and should be avoided in patients with egg allergy. Active immunizations should be avoided during a febrile illness or within 3 months of passive immunization since they are less likely to be effective.

Table 8. Standard Vaccination Schedule

Age	*Vaccine*
2 months	DPT, OPV
4 months	DPT, OPV
6 months	DPT, OPV
15 months	MMR
18 months	DPT, OPV
6 years	DPT, OPV
q 5-10 years	Td

Travel Precautions

Malaria prophylaxis is recommended in many areas of the world. Smallpox and yellow fever vaccines are seldom required; typhoid and cholera vaccines are of limited efficacy. Gamma globulin for hepatitis A prevention is recommended in some underdeveloped areas. The current recommendations should be checked with the local or state health departments prior to foreign travel.

QUESTIONS

1. The most contagious disease of the following is:
   A. Diphtheria
   B. Malaria
   C. Measles
   D. Tuberculosis
2. A 48-year-old man presents with a lung abscess; anaerobic bacteria are suspected. A proper specimen for diagnosis would be:
   A. Throat culture
   B. Expectorated sputum Gram stain
   C. Expectorated sputum culture
   D. Transtracheal aspiration culture
3. Which of the following diseases has the highest mortality rate:
   A. Neonatal herpes simplex infection
   B. Influenza A infection
   C. EB virus mononucleosis
   D. Herpes zoster
4. A live virus vaccine is recommended for prevention of all of the following diseases *except*:
   A. Mumps
   B. Poliomyelitis
   C. Measles
   D. Influenza
   E. All of the above
5. Viral hepatitis may be caused by:
   A. Hepatitis A virus
   B. Hepatitis B virus
   C. Cytomegalovirus
   D. EB virus
   E. All of the above
6. The drug of choice for pneumococcal meningitis in a penicillin-allergic patient is:
   A. Ampicillin
   B. Erythromycin
   C. Chloramphenicol
   D. Tetracycline
7. *Staphylococcus aureus* is a frequent cause of all of the following *except*:
   A. Urinary tract infection
   B. Cellulitis
   C. Osteomyelitis
   D. Endocarditis
   E. Furuncles
8. Infection with group A *Streptococcus* is often associated with all of the following *except*:
   A. Scarlet fever
   B. Endocarditis
   C. Rheumatic fever
   D. Glomerulonephritis
9. An animal reservoir is most often associated with:
   A. *Salmonella typhi*
   B. *Salmonella enteritidis*
   C. *Shigella sonnei*
   D. *Vibrio cholerae*
10. Which of the following bacteria is *not* an anaerobic bacteria:
    A. *Bacteroides fragilis*
    B. *Clostridium perfringens*
    C. *Corynebacterium diphtheriae*
    D. *Fusobacterium nucleatum*
11. A positive (>10 mm) PPD skin test usually reflects:
    A. Infection with *M. tuberculosis*
    B. Infection with atypical mycobacteria
    C. Recent exposure to a case of tuberculosis
    D. The need for isolation to prevent spread of tuberculosis to others.
12. A leukemic with fungal pneumonia is most likely to have infection with:
    A. *Histoplasma capsulatum*
    B. *Aspergillus flavus*
    C. *Blastomyces dermatitidis*
    D. *Sporothrix schenckii*
13. The most common organism causing pneumonia is:
    A. *Staphyloccus aureus*
    B. *Mycoplasma pneumoniae*
    C. *Streptococcus pneumoniae*
    D. Influenza
14. A 21-year-old woman develops dysuria, fever, and urgency. Which of the following statements is true?
    A. Pyelonephritis is more likely than cystitis.
    B. A clean-catch, midstream urine culture will probably grow >100,000 *E. coli*/ml on culture.
    C. With recurrent infections, she will probably develop chronic pyelonephritis.

D. Parenteral antibiotic therapy is preferred in this situation to prevent complications.

15. Gonorrhea is a common cause of urethritis and cervicitis. An even more common venereal disease, however, in this country is:
    A. Chancroid
    B. Nongonococcal urethritis
    C. Syphilis
    D. Lymphogranuloma venereum
16. A 37-year-old man presents with meningitis and a petechial rash. The most likely etiology is:
    A. *Streptococcus pneumoniae*
    B. *Neisseria meningitidis*
    C. *Hemophilus influenzae*
    D. *Staphylococcus aureus*
17. Therapy of septic shock should include fluids, oxygen, vasoactive drugs and:
    A. Penicillin
    B. Erythromycin
    C. An aminoglycoside
    D. A cephalosporin
18. Penicillin is the drug of choice for all the following *except*:
    A. Hospital-acquired staphylococcal infection
    B. Pneumococcal pneumonia
    C. Streptococcal pharyngitis
    D. Meningococcal meningitis
19. The most serious side-effect commonly seen with the aminoglycoside antibiotics is:
    A. Rash
    B. Nephrotoxicity
    C. Ototoxicity
    D. Serum sickness
20. Which of the following antibiotics should *never* be used in children under the age of 8:
    A. Gentamicin
    B. Tetracycline
    C. Sulfonamides
    D. Chloramphenicol
21. Common infectious causes of fever of unknown origin include all of the following *except*:
    A. Tuberculosis
    B. Bacterial endocarditis
    C. Occult abscess
    D. Pyelonephritis

ANSWERS

1. C
2. D
3. A
4. D
5. E
6. C
7. A
8. B
9. B
10. C
11. A
12. B
13. C
14. B
15. B
16. B
17. C
18. A
19. B
20. B
21. D

BIBLIOGRAPHY

TEXTBOOKS

Hoeprich PD (ed): *Infectious Diseases: A Modern Treatise of Infectious Processes*, ed. 2. Hagerstown, Md., Harper & Row Publishers Inc, 1977.

Mandell GL, Douglas RG, Bennett JE (eds): *Principles and Practice of Infectious Diseases*. New York, John Wiley & Sons Inc, 1979.

Wehrle PF, Top FH: *Communicable and Infectious Diseases*, ed. 9. St. Louis, C V Mosby, Co 1981.

ARTICLES AND MONOGRAPHS

Microbiology and Epidemiology

Davis BD, Dulbecco R, Eisen HN, Ginsberg HS: *Microbiology*, ed. 3. Hagerstown, Md., Harper & Row Publishers Inc, 1980.

Mausner JS, Bahn AK: *Epidemiology: An Introductory Text*. Philadelphia, W B Saunders Co, 1974.

Viral Infections

Evans AS (ed): *Viral Infections of Humans: Epidemiology and Control*. New York, Plenum Publishing Corp, 1978.

Nahmias AJ, Hall CB: Diagnosis of viral diseases: Today and tomorrow. *Hosp Pract* 16(4):49-61, 1981.

Nahmias AJ, Roizman B: Infection with Herpes simplex viruses 1 and 2. *N Engl J Med* 289:667-74, 719-25, 781-9, 1973.

Bacterial Infections

Musher DM, McKenzie SO: Infections due to *Staphylococcus aureus*. *Medicine* 56:383-409, 1977.

Peter G, Smith AL: Group A streptococcal infections of the skin and pharynx. *N Engl J Med* 297:311-7, 365-70, 1977.

Finegold SM, Bartlett JG, Chow AW: Management of anaerobic infections. *Ann Intern Med* 83:375-89, 1975.

Young LS, Martin WJ, Meyer RD, Weinstein RJ, Anderson ET: Gram-negative rod bacteremia: Microbiologic, immunologic, and therapeutic considerations. *Ann Intern Med* 86:456-71, 1977.

Mycobacterial Infections

Stead WW, Dutt AK (eds): Tuberculosis. *Clin Chest Med* (May)1:165-285, 1980.

Fungal Infections

Medoff G, Kobayaski GS: Strategies in the treatment of systemic fungal infections. *N Engl J Med* 302:145-55, 1980.

Infections of Organ Systems

Kunin CM: *Detection, Prevention and Management of Urinary Tract Infections*, ed. 3. Philadelphia, Lea & Febiger, 1979.

Lerner PI: Bacterial infections of the nervous system: Etiologic and therapeutic aspects. *Cleve Clin Q* 42:83-99, 1975.

Antibiotics

Hermans PE: General principles of antimicrobial therapy. *Mayo Clin Proc* 52:603-10, 1977.

Kucers A, Bennett NM: The Use of Antibiotics, ed. 3. London, Heinemann Medical Books, 1979.

Special Problems

Bennett JV, Brachman PS (eds): *Hospital Infections*. Boston, Little, Brown & Co, 1979.

Bodey GP: Infections in cancer patients. *Cancer Treat Rev* 2:89-128, 1975.

CHAPTER 10
NEPHROLOGY

Mahendr S. Kochar

DISEASES OF THE KIDNEYS AND URINARY TRACT

ROLE OF THE KIDNEYS

The kidneys have three major functions: excretion of the products of metabolism, maintenance of fluid and electrolyte balance, and endocrine functions.

Excretion

The prime function of the kidney is to excrete nonmetabolized solute in the diet and the nonvolatile end products of metabolism through the processes of glomerular filtration and selective tubular absorption. Although several hundred substances can be identified in the urine, the major constituents in addition to water are urea, sodium, chloride, potassium, phosphate, sulfate, and creatinine. Depending on requirement for water conservation and the osmotic load of solutes, the normal urine volume varies from 500 ml to several liters a day. In chronic renal disease symptoms of uremia appear only after 90% of the renal function is lost. It is not known which of the waste products of metabolism are responsible for the various uremic symptoms. Blood urea and serum creatinine, which are monitored to evaluate the renal function, probably play an insignificant role in causing the clinical manifestations of uremia. Guanidines, phenols, amines, and sulfates have been blamed for some of the symptoms. Middle molecule substances with a molecular weight of 300-1,500 have been thought to be responsible for some of the neuromuscular manifestations of chronic renal disease.

Maintenance of Fluid and Electrolyte Balance

The next major function of the kidney is to excrete or conserve water so as to maintain the tonicity of body fluids, to regulate the amount and concentration of major electrolytes, and to assist in maintaining the acid-base balance. Water excretion is controlled primarily by the antidiuretic hormone that affects the water permeability of the distal tubule and the collecting duct. Osmotic load also influences water excretion, particularly when fluid intake is low. Rates of glomerular filtration, particularly when decreased, and the state of distal nephron transport functions also play important roles in certain clinical situations. Sodium excretion is determined by the glomerular filtration rate, aldosterone, and poorly understood mechanisms of adaptaion that include the Starling forces expressed across the tubule membranes, renal ultrastructure, and the peritubular capillary walls. Under normal circumstances, less than 0.5% of the filtered sodium is actually excreted in the urine. Due to certain adaptive mechanisms in renal failure, up to 20% or more may be excreted in order to compensate for the decrease in glomerular filtration rate (GFR). Potassium is continually and slowly absorbed in the distal tubule. Aldosterone increases potassium excretion in the distal tubule and promotes sodium absorption. If a greater sodium load is present in the distal tubule, more potassium is excreted along with hydrogen ions in exchange for the sodium.

The kidney participates in the maintenance of acid-base balance in a number of important ways. First, it retains or excretes bicarbonate and generates new bicarbonate to replace that already used to buffer nonvolatile acids. Bicarbonate is reabsorbed in both the proximal and distal tubules. In addition, in acidosis the kidney eliminates large amounts of hydrogen ions by titrating them with urinary buffers and producing ammonium that combines with the hydrogen ions to produce ammonia. In prolonged acidosis, the ammonium production may increase tenfold or more so that more acid can be excreted as ammonia.

Endocrine Functions

The kidney performs at least four endocrine functions: secretion of renin, production of erythropoietin, conversion of vitamin D into its active metabolite, and secretion of prostaglandins. Renin is an enzyme with a molecular weight of about 40,000. It is produced in the juxtaglomerular apparatus that consists of a series of microscopic structures intimately associated with the afferent arteriole of the glomerulus and the macula densa of the distal convoluted tubule. Renin acts on a substrate in plasma to produce the decapeptide angiotensin I that is further split by a converting enzyme, Kininase II, in the lung capillaries to form the active octapeptide angiotensin II. Angiotensin II stimulates the adrenal to produce aldosterone and is the most potent known vasoconstrictor. Renin secretion is increased by sodium depletion, hypovolemia, stimulation of sympathetic nerves, secretion of catecholamines, adoption of the upright posture, and several drugs such as diuretics and antihypertensives. Secretion is decreased by the administration of mineralcorticoids or β blockers.

Renal erythropoietic factor (REF) secreted by the kidney acts on a plasma substrate of hepatic origin to produce a glycoprotein called erythropoietin. Erythropoietin stimulates committed stem cells in the marrow to differentiate into pronormoblasts, the earliest recognizable red cell blood precursors. The exact site of origin of REF in the kidney is doubtful since it can be extracted from both the medulla and the cortex. Its output is increased by hypoxemia, which may occur at high altitudes, in cyanotic heart disease, and in chronic lung disease. Androgens increase its output and estrogens block its action.

Vitamin D is first converted into vitamin D_3 (cholecalciferol) by untraviolet irradiation of the skin. Vitamin D_3 is then converted into 25-hydroxycholecalciferol (25-HCC) in the liver. The next and most important step in vitamin D metabolism occurs in the kidneys, where 25-HCC is converted into 1,25-dihydroxycholecalciferol (1,25-DHCC), the most active form of the vitamin. This substance acts like a hormone. 1,25-DHCC stimulates calcium and phosphate absorption from the gut and mobilizes calcium from the bone.

Prostaglandins are ubiquitous 22-carbon fatty acids. The renal medullary prostaglandins play an important role in the regulation of renal circulation and maintenance of blood pressure.

EVALUATION OF RENAL DISEASE

For evaluating the diagnosis and prognosis of a patient with kidney disease the physician depends on the history, the physical findings, results of certain laboratory investigations, and x-ray findings.

Clinical Manifestations of Urinary Dysfunction

A patient with renal or urinary tract disease may present with one or more of the following clinical findings.

Nocturia and Polyuria

Very often nocturia is one of the first symptoms of renal insufficiency. Normally, a much larger volume of urine is excreted during the waking period. The diurnal rhythm is frequently reversed in patients with renal insufficiency and accumulation of fluid. As the extracellular fluid accumulates during the day with activity and upright posture, the patient may notice edema towards the end of the day. At night when the patient is supine, the excessive interstitial fluid is mobilized into the vascular compartment, increasing the plasma volume. This leads to increased urine formation and thus nocturia. In addition, patients with renal insufficiency very often excrete urine of a fixed osmol close to serum and therefore have polyuria. This may be on the basis of a constant osmotic diuresis per nephron. During the day the patient may be unaware of passing excessive urine, but when it interrupts sleep, polyuria is noted. Patients with prostatic hypertrophy causing partial obstruction of the bladder often complain of nocturia.

Dysuria and Incontinence

Dysuria denotes difficulty or pain during voiding. Symptoms such as frequency, hesitancy, burning, urgency, and strangury (slow and painful urination) are often included under the general term dysuria. Urgency results from tirgonal or posterior urethral irritation by inflammation, stones, or tumor. Frequency of urination results from either a decreased capacity or pain on distention of the bladder. It is a common symptom of cystitis. Tuberculosis produces frequency as a result of diminished bladder capacity from scarring. It may be an early presenting symptom of bladder malignancy. Diseases of other pelvic organs by invading, compressing, or distorting the lower urinary tract may also produce dysuria. Prostatic hypertrophy commonly causes hesitancy and slowing of the stream.

True incontinence must be distinguished from overflow incontinence. In the latter condition the bladder is distended because of a mechanical or functional obstruction and the incontinence is characterized by small, frequent, involuntary (overflow) voidings. True incontinence may occur as a result of certain congenital malformations of the bladder neck, urethra, spinal cord, and cauda equina. True incontinence may also result from diseases or injury of the spinal cord as seen in tabes dorsalis, multiple sclerosis, tumor of the spinal cord, or following fractures of the spine. Stress incontinence may result from stretching or disruption of the structures of the pelvic floor and perineum during a difficult labor. Overflow incontinence occurs as a combination of neurologic and obstructive causes such as in elderly atherosclerotic patients with prostatic hypertrophy and in cases of diabetic neuropathy, resulting in a flaccid, overdistended bladder. The accumulation of residual urine in the bladder may lead to infection and pyelonephritis.

Enuresis, or bed-wetting, without gross urologic abnormality may occur in up to 15% of boys and 10% of girls up to the age of 5. By the age of 9 only 5% of all children remain bed wetters. It is important early in the management of these patients to distinguish incontinence due to organic urologic disease from functional enuresis. In cases of functional enuresis management of the child's general health, physical environment, and emotional state are necessary. Imipramine (Tofranil), a mood-elevating drug or similar agents, administered at bedtime, may be helpful in certain patients.

Hematuria

Microscopic or gross bleeding from the urinary tract may occur both in renal parenchymal diseases or disorders of the urinary tract. Total hematuria or bleeding throughout the urinary stream may suggest its origin in either the kidney or the ureter. Initial hematuria is associated with urethral disease and terminal hematuria is a sign of a lesion in the area of the bladder trigone. Severe hemorrhage from the bladder, however, will always present as total hematuria. Red or dark urine may occur in the absence of hematuria. A positive dipstick test for blood in the absence of red blood cells on microscopic examination of urine may indicate hemoglobinuria or myoglobinuria. Certain dyes and pigments may be excreted in the urine, causing it to become dark. Rifampicin (Rifampin), an antibiotic used primarily in the treatment of tuberculosis, may stain the urine dark yellow or pink. After the presence of blood has been established in the urine it is important to determine if the urine contains red blood cell (RBC) casts. Presence of RBC casts indicates glomerular disease, usually glomerulonephritis. Other renal parenchymal diseases such as polycytstic kidneys, medullary sponge kidney, polyarteritis nodosa, systemic lupus erythematosus (SLE), renal arterial infarction, and renal vein thrombosis often lead to hematuria. Hematuria may also result from a disorder of blood clotting or due to the administration of anticoagulant drugs. However, an increased tendency to bleed in anticoagulant-treated patients may often bring to light an unsuspected urinary tract disease. Sickle cell disease may cause microinfarcts in the renal medulla, causing hematuria. Tumors, calculi, and infections of the urinary tract account for hematuria in about 75% of patients. Chronic infections such as tuberculosis of the urinary tract or infection with *Schistosoma haematobium* may cause hematuria as the only presenting symptom. The latter is the most common cause of hematuria in the Middle East and Africa, where it is endemic.

Trauma to the kidney may cause painless hematuria persisting for several days. The majority of these cases may be treated conservatively with bed rest and careful observation. The appearance of hematuria following vigorous exercise or febrile diseases is termed pseudonephritis and is of no significance.

Arteriovenous malformations of the urinary tract may be responsible for hematuria in a small number of patients. A few cases may remain undiagnosed and require follow-up despite all the investigations, including a renal biopsy.

Anuria or Oliguria

Urine volume of less than 50 ml per day is termed anuria and a volume of less than 500 ml per day is termed oliguria. In addition to acute and chronic renal failure, oliguria may signify dehydration and reduced effective plasma volume. Abrupt oliguria also occurs in acute glomerulonephritis and acute tubular necrosis. Renal cortical necrosis and bilateral renal artery occlusion may result in anuria. Oliguria due to renal parenchymal disease is usually accompanied by both diminished GFR and impaired tubular reabsorption of salt and water. Obstruction of the lower urinary tract or bilateral ureteral obstruction may result in oliguria or anuria. It is essential, therefore, that urinary tract obstruction be ruled out in every patient with these symptoms.

Hypertension

Hypertension is a frequent manifestation and can occur in almost all renal diseases. In addition, it can occur in patients with urinary tract obstruction causing hydronephrosis. Although it is not necessary to investigate the urinary tract in every patient with hypertension, urinalysis and serum creatinine measurement should always be performed in the evaluation of hypertension. Hypertension in patients with chronic renal insufficiency probably results from fluid retention and expanded plasma volume. In patients with renal disease without significant renal insufficiency, hypertension is probably mediated through the renin-angiotensin-aldosterone system.

Laboratory Investigations

Certain laboratory investigations are essential to the evaluation of renal diseases. These include examination of the urine, measurement of serum creatinine, and other biochemical and serologic tests depending on the suspected diagnosis.

Urinalysis

Urine specific gravity has been used traditionally as the criterion of urinary concentration. The ability to concentrate urine is impaired as the population of nephrons decreases with progressive renal disease. If one or more of several early morning urine specimens have a specific gravity of 1.020, a defect in urinary concentration can almost always be excluded. Measurement of osmolality is a more sensitive and accurate indication of urine concentration than the specific gravity. A specific gravity of 1.020 corresponds roughly to an osmolality of 700. The presence of protein, glucose, or x-ray contrast medium in the urine increases the urinary specific gravity without altering the osmolality.

Proteinuria is an important manifestation of renal disease. Urine should be tested with both dipstick and sulfosalicylic acid for proteinuria. The dipstick, impregnated with bromphenol blue and a buffer (Albustix, Labstix, etc.) turns green in the presence of albumin. Upon addition of eight drops of sulfosalicylic acid to 5 ml of urine, the urine turns turbid when protein (albumin or globulin) is present. Whenever protein is noted in the urine a 24-hour specimen should be collected for quantitation of the protein. Protein excretion in excess of 150 mg/day or 20 mg/100 ml is considered abnormal. Heavy proteinuria in excess of 4 g/day usually signifies generalized glomerular disease. Proteinuria may also be observed in patients with malignant hypertension, severe congestive heart failure, renal vein thrombosis, or constrictive pericarditis. A high molecular weight mucoprotein (Tamm-Horsfall protein) orginating in the cellular lining of the ascending limb of the loop of Henle and the distal convoluted tubule usually forms the matrix of hyaline casts that may be seen in the normal urine. Proteinuria can be induced in certain normal adolescents and young adults by prolonged standing in the erect position and strenuous excercise. In these individuals there is usually no protein in the morning urine sample, 24-hour excretion of protein is less than 1 g, serum creatinine is normal, and there are no abnormal findings on careful examination of the urinary sediment. The orthostatic proteinuria under these circumstances is almost always benign and often disappears spontaneously in a few years.

The dipstick test for protein detects only albumin. When proteinuria is composed primarily of globulins without albumin, as may happen in multiple myeloma, dysgammaglobulinemias, and amyloidosis, the dipstick test is negative. The sulfosalicylic acid test for protein, however, detects both globulins and albumin in the urine. Urine protein electrophoresis and immunoelectrophoresis are helpful in determining the exact nature of proteins in the urine and should be performed in all patients above the age of 50 years with proteinuria.

Urinary Sediment. Examination of urinary sediment by the physician is important to the diagnosis of renal disease. A 15-ml sample of a freshly voided morning midstream urine specimen is centrifuged for 5 minutes at 3,000 rpm. The supernatant is discarded and the sediment resuspended immediately and efficiently in two to three drops of the remaining urine. It is covered with a coverslip and first examined under low power for the presence of various formed elements. The individual formed elements are then identified under high power of the microscope. A normal urine contains no more than one or two red blood cells, white blood cells, and epithelial cells per high power field. An occasional hyaline cast may also be seen.

Hyaline casts are clear and colorless. They result from the precipitation of the renal tubular protein, Tamm-Horsfall protein, whose solubility decreases in the presence of albumin and highly concentrated urine. Small numbers may be normal or indicate dehydration. Red blood cell casts are usually orange or rusty brown in color, with red blood cells incorporated in the matrix. They are best identified by focusing up and down through the cast under medium or high power. They are usually surrounded by RBCs and have greater diagnostic significance than other casts. They indicate glomerular bleeding that may occur in poststreptococcal glomerulonephritis, membranoproliferative nephritis, focal glomerulonephritis, and malignant hypertension. Hemoglobin casts have the same significance as red blood cell casts. Granular casts consist of immunoglobulin aggregates in a matrix of Tamm-Horsfall protein. They may also represent a further stage in the degeneration of cellular casts. Except for an occasional granular cast, they almost always indicate renal disease but do not point to any particular pathology. Dense granular casts may appear black under the microscope and may be confused with red cell casts. Leukocyte casts surrounded by white blood cells (WBCs) suggest acute pyelonephritis or interstitial nephritis. Broad casts, also referred to as renal failure casts, represent advanced and chronic renal disease. The broadness is explained on the basis of hypertrophy of the remaining renal tubules and slow progression of urine through the collecting duct system. Oval fat bodies and Maltese crosses are fat-laden renal tubular cells that appear birefringent in polarized light. They, as well as fatty casts, are found in the urine of patients with heavy proteinuria typically seen in the nephrotic syndrome. Muddy brown casts representing shredded renal tubular epithelium are typically seen in acute tubular necrosis.

Uric acid and calcium oxalate crystals may be present in the normal urine; however, large amounts may indicate precipitation of these substances in the urinary tract resulting in stone formation.

Serum Creatinine and Creatinine Clearance

Creatinine is an end product of muscle metabolism. Raised serum creatinine indicates depression in GFR, but normal serum creatinine concentration does not exclude renal disease. The clearance of endogenously produced creatinine approximates more rigorous measurements such as inulin clearance; thus, for clinical purposes creatinine clearance is an accurate measurement of glomerular filtration rate. Creatinine is excreted independently of urine flow and its plasma level is relatively stable except when the GFR is rapidly changing. The clearance of creatinine is calculated based on the following formula:

$$C_{Cr}{}^{a} = \frac{\text{Urine creatine concentration} \times \text{volume of urine}}{\text{Plasma or serum creatinine concentration}} \text{ or } \frac{U \times V}{P}$$

$$= \frac{\text{mg creatinine/ml urine} \times \text{ml urine/24 h}}{\text{mg creatinine/ml plasma or serum}^{b}}$$

$$= \frac{\text{mg creatinine/24-h urine specimen}}{\text{mg creatinine/ml plasma or serum}^{b}}$$

The 24-h creatinine clearance can also be readily calculated by the following formula:

$$C_{Cr}\,(\text{L/day}) = \frac{\text{mg creatine/24-h urine specimen}}{\text{serum creatinine mg/100 ml} \times 10}$$

[a] For expressing C_{Cr} in L/day the above value has to be divided by 1,000.

[b] Most laboratories provide the level as serum creatinine/100 ml. To obtain serum creatinine/ml, the laboratory value has to be divided by 100.

When renal function is stable, creatinine clearance can thus be determined by collecting a 24-hour urine specimen and drawing a sample of blood for measurement of serum creatinine during this period. Normal creatinine clearance for men is 140-200 L/day (98-140 ml/min). For women it is 120-180 L/day (85-125 ml/min).

Although creatinine clearance is of value in the initial determination of renal function, serum creatinine concentration alone can be used to follow a patient's renal function. The relationship of creatinine clearance to serum creatinine concentration is hyperbolic (Fig. 1). A large change in creatinine clearance produces a small change in serum creatinine close to the normal range, whereas a small change in creatinine clearance causes a large change in plasma creatinine in late renal failure. At near-normal serum levels, the usual laboratory methods for creatinine measurement are not sufficiently accurate; however, when the creatinine levels are higher, the measurement is quite reliable for monitoring abnormal kidney function.

Plotting reciprocal serum creatinine (1/Scr), which roughly indicates the remaining renal function, on the ordinate and months of observation on the abscissa gives useful information on the progression of renal failure in chronic kidney diseases. Extending the regression or trendline obtained from such a plot can predict with reasonable accuracy when an individual patient would reach a level of renal failure requiring dialysis or transplantation. It can also be used to monitor improvement in renal function. (Fig. 2).

Blood urea nitrogen (BUN) level is affected by factors other than renal function and is therefore not always a reflection of kidney function. It rises with a high protein diet and falls with a low protein diet. Fluid depletion, gastrointestinal bleeding, and administration of antianabolic drugs such as tetracycline and corticosteroids raise the BUN level without affecting renal function.

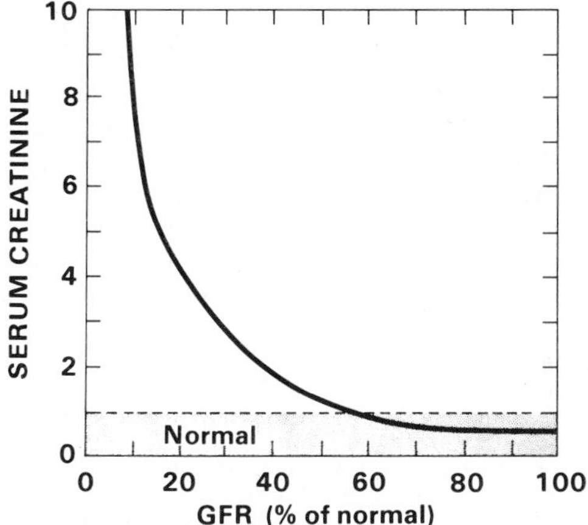

Figure 1. Relation between serum creatinine and glomerular filtration rate (GFR). The serum creatinine levels change very little until the GFR falls below 50% of normal.

Other Laboratory Tests

The kidney may be involved in systemic diseases such as systemic lupus erythematosus (SLE) and metabolic diseases such as diabetes. Appropriate investigations should be undertaken to evaluate the patient for the presence of a suspected systemic disease involving the kidney. Serum complement measurement is a useful serologic test. The serum complement levels are persistently low in patients with membranoproliferative glomerulonephritis. Certain lymphomas, such as Hodgkin's disease and other malignancies, may present as proteinuria. Proteinuria may also occur in patients with hepatitis, malaria, and certain systemic bacterial and viral infections. Thus, if a certain cause for renal disease is suspected or needs to be excluded, proper investigations should be undertaken.

Radiologic Investigations

The radiologic investigations of the kidney and urinary tract include (1) a plain x-ray film of the abdomen (kidney, ureter, and bladder-KUB), (2) excretory urogram (intravenous pyelogram or IVP), (3) retrograde pyelography, (4) retrograde urethrocystography, (5) radiosotopic visualization of the kidney and renogram, (6) ultrasonic examination, (7) computed tomography, and (8) angiography.

KUB

A plain film of the abdomen is particularly useful when there is minimal gas that does not obscure the kidneys. The examination can provide useful information on the presence, size,

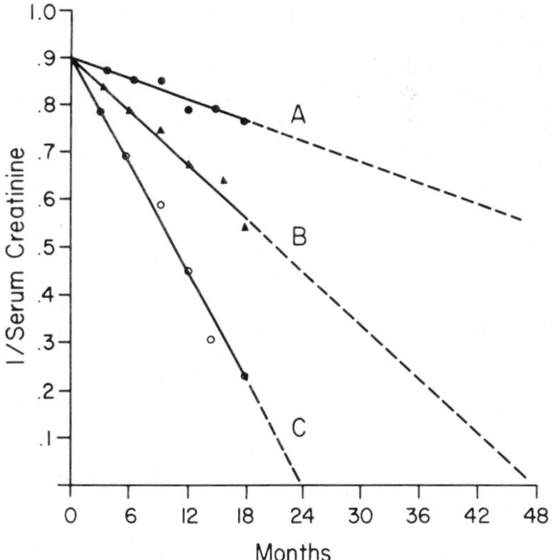

Figure 2. Plotting 1/serum creatinine against time can help predict the time of occurrence of end-stage renal disease (ESRD) (creatinine clearance less than 10 L/day). Follow-up of three patients (A, B, and C) over an 18-month period is shown (solid lines). By extending the lines (dashed lines) one can say with reasonable confidence that in the case of patient A it would be several years before ESRD occurs. Patient B will need dialysis in another 2 years and patient C within the next 6 months.

and location of the kidneys. A radio-opaque stone in the renal pelvis or urinary tract can be readily identified and its presence later confirmed within the urinary tract by excretory urography. Normally, the right kidney is generally situated lower than the left because of displacement by the liver.

Urography
The kidneys and the urinary tract are visualized by intravenous injection or infusion of iodine containing radiocontrast medium. The contrast agent is concentrated in the renal tubule providing a nephrogram and is later excreted into the collecting system outlining the renal pelvis, ureters, and the bladder. Adequate renal function is necessary for proper visualization of the kidneys and urinary tract. By using a larger dose of the contrast medium, the kidneys and urinary tract can be visualized even in the presence of renal insufficiency; however, this can cause deterioration in renal function especially in patients with diabetes and multiple myeloma. A film obtained during voiding can provide useful information about the male urethra and a postvoid film is helpful in gauging the residual urine in patients with prostatic or bladder neck obstruction.

The retrograde pyelogram requires introduction of the dye directly into the urinary tract following cystoscopy and catheterization of the ureter. It is a useful test in evaluating the urinary tract when the excretory urogram has failed to provide the necessary information to rule out urinary tract disease. It can also be carried out in patients allergic to intravenous radio-opaque dyes. Retrograde cystogram is helpful in diagnosis of vesicoureteral reflux, neurogenic bladder and rectovesical fistulas.

Antegrade pyelography performed by direct injection of radiocontrast material into a distended upper urinary tract or cyst under fluoroscopy or ultrasonography is useful in distinguishing cysts from hydronephrosis. Percutaneous placement of a catheter in the renal pelvis, calyces or perirenal space permits drainage and irrigation of pyonephrosis, abscesses and obstructions.

Ultrasound Evaluation of the Kidneys and the Urinary Tract
This technique does not depend on renal function and can be utilized in anatomic evaluation of the urinary system even in patients with profound renal insufficiency. It should be the initial method for evaluation of the urinary tract in patients with renal failure of unknown etiology. Ultrasound is extremely accurate in differentiating solid from cystic masses. Since ultrasound is a noninvasive and innocuous procedure, it is used for the follow-up of cystic lesions and after treatment for hydronephrosis. When the IVP does not visualize the kidneys, ultrasound may be used to locate the lower pole of the kidney for the purposes of renal biopsy.

Radionuclide Scintillation Imaging
^{99m}Tc-glucoheptonate is used for static imaging which provides information on the location, size and contour of functional renal tissue. Dynamic imaging is obtained after intravenous injection of ^{99m}Tc-diethylenetriamine pentacetic acid (DTPA) and recording its course through the vascular, renal parenchymal and urinary collecting system by external monitoring of regional activity with a scintillation camera placed over the renal area on the back.

Computed Tomography
Computed tomography, performed with or without contrast material, permits visualization of the kidneys and the urinary tract and is useful as a tertiary test if ultransonograph and IVP prove insufficient in evaluating a mass lesion or obstruction.

Angiography
By injection of the contrast medium into the aorta and selectively into the renal arteries, both the extrarenal and the intrarenal arteries can be studied. This test is useful in the definitive anatomic diagnosis of renovascular stenosis. Displacement of intrarenal vessels by a vascular mass is highly suggestive of a neoplasm. On the other hand, an avascular mass would be more compatible with a diagnosis of an intrarenal cyst.

Renal Biopsy

Renal biopsy is helpful in establishing a histologic diagnosis, gauging the prognosis of renal disease, and monitoring the value of therapy. It should never be undertaken in the presence of a bleeding disorder. A needle biopsy should also be avoided when there is only one functioning kidney. The biopsy is extremely useful in establishing the exact renal pathology in patients with proteinuria. Visualization of the kidney by x-ray or ultrasonic techniques during the kidney, biopsy has increased its safety. The kidney biopsy specimen must be studied by light and electron microscopy and immunofluorescence examination in order to obtain the maximal and most accurate information on the histology of the renal disease.

NEPHROTIC SYNDROME

The nephrotic syndrome is defined as a clinical syndrome consisting of heavy proteinuria, hypoalbuminemia, and generalized edema. Proteinuria is the cornerstone of the syndrome, other manifestations being its consequences. In general, these criteria are met when 5 g of protein a day (or 4 g/day/1.73 m^2 body surface) are lost in the urine and the plasma albumin falls below 3 g/dl. Renal failure, hypertension, and hypercholesterolemia are frequently present.

Pathogenesis
Heavy proteinuria leads to reduced plasma albumin concentration, decreased plasma oncotic pressure, and a redistribution of body fluid between the interstitial and intravascular spaces. As a consequence of diminished intravascular volume, the renin-angiotensin system is activated and the kidney begins to retain salt and water. Numerous other factors such as salt intake and mineralocorticoid activity play significant roles in the development of edema.

Clinical Manifestations
Proteinuria is the hallmark of the nephrotic syndrome.

Normally the glomerular capillary wall is impermeable to proteins; the low molecular weight protein filtered through the glomeruli is either reabsorbed or metabolized by the renal tubule. The exact reason for proteinuria in patients with the nephrotic syndrome is not well understood. Under normal conditions, there is evidence that portions of the glomerular capillary wall are negatively charged and repel the positively charged albumin molecules. Damage to the glomerular capillaries may abolish this electrical barrier and allow filtration of albumin. Certain patients with severe nephrotic syndrome may have massive proteinuria, often in excess of 15 g/day. Even in the absence of therapy the proteinuria may diminish. The magnitude of the proteinuria is not a good index of prognosis. Diminishing proteinuria is usually interpreted as improvement in a patient with the nephrotic syndrome, but may actually be a consequence of decreasing GFR. Albumin/creatinine clearance ratio ($C_{ALB}/C_{CR} \times 100$) is a useful way to monitor the severity of albuminuria in the presence of changing renal function. Hypoalbuminemia is not present in all patients with heavy proteinuria. Serum albumin level is determined by the rate of albumin synthesis, its catabolism, and, in renal disease, its rate of excretion in the urine. In the nephrotic syndrome urinary losses of albumin and its catabolism are increased. Hyperlipidemia (increased serum cholesterol, triglycerides, and phospholipids) and lipiduria are frequently present in patients with the nephrotic syndrome. Increased synthesis and decreased metabolism of lipids seem to contribute to this abnormality. Casts containing lipid are often present in the urinary sediment. Oval fat bodies, as stated before, are epithelial cells containing cholesterol esters. They appear birefringent in polarized light and are called Maltese crosses. The fat accumulates in the renal tubular cells; hyperlipidemia causes its increased excretion in the urine. Edema, often accompanied by ascites and pleural effusion, is the sine qua non of the nephrotic syndrome.

Causes

Causes of the nephrotic syndrome are numerous. A few selected causes include

1. Intrinisic Renal Diseases
   - A. Various forms of glomerulonephritis
   - B. Homograft rejection
   - C. Heavy metal-induced renal damage (eg., Hg, Bi, and Au compounds)
   - D. Allergen-induced renal damage (e.g., bee stings, pollen, poison ivy, insects, vaccines, and serum sickness)
   - E. Drug-induced renal damage (e.g., penicillamine, anticonvulsants, probenecid, and sulfonamides)
2. Systemic Diseases Affecting the Kidneys
   - A. Various connective tissue disorders
   - B. Metabolic diseases, such as diabetes, amyloidosis, and myxedema
   - C. Infectious diseases, such as syphilis, malaria, hepatitis B, bacterial endocarditis, schistosomiasis, and cytomegalic inclusion disease
   - D. Malignancies, such as Hodgkin's disease, multiple myeloma, carcinomas, and lymphatic leukemia
   - E. Accelerated hypertension and toxemia of pregnancy
3. Diseases Altering Renal Hemodynamics by Increasing Renal Venous Pressure
   - A. Renal vein and inferior vena cava thrombosis
   - B. Constrictive pericarditis
   - C. Tricuspid insufficiency
   - D. Severe congestive heart failure

Complications

Although edema is the prominent clinical manifestation of the nephrotic syndrome other serious, even life-threatening, complications may occur.

Hypovolemia and shock. The reduction of plasma volume, cardiac output, and blood pressure may result from loss of fluid into the interstitium and predispose to syncopal episodes and shock. Injudicious use of diuretics, paracentesis, thoracentesis, and antihypertensive medications may contribute to this complication. Hypotension and impaired renal perfusion may produce a degree of prerenal azotemia that may be falsely interpreted as progression of renal insufficiency. Treatment with infusions of hyperoncotic albumin or other plasma volume expanders may be urgently indicated in these situations.

Protein malnutrition. Massive proteinuria may lead to negative nitrogen balance and malnutrition that may manifest as parallel transverse white bands in the fingernails and toenails and puckering of the muscles on percussion (myoedema). The plasma protein deficiency may also have an effect on various protein-binding functions; severe hypotransferrinemia may contribute to anemia and loss of thyroxine-binding globulin may produce low T4 and raise T3 resin uptake.

Accelerated atherosclerosis. Many patients with a nephrotic syndrome manifest acceleration of vascular and coronary artery disease. Prolonged and severe hyperlipidemia and uncontrolled hypertension may predispose patients with nephrotic syndrome to these diseases.

Increased susceptibility to infections. This is not an uncommon complication, especially among children. Not only bacterial infections but also fungal infections and parasitic infestations may occur. Peritonitis and severe enterocolitis may be manifested by fever, leukocytosis, abdominal pain, vomiting, constipation, and coma. Prior to the introducton of antibiotics, pneumococcal peritonitis and erysipelas were the major cause of death in these patients. Acquired IgG deficiency may be partly responsible for this susceptibility to infections.

Renal failure. Depending on underlying disease, renal insufficiency may progress and ultimately lead to end-stage renal disease. Hypertension and its consequences are often early signs of such progression and make the renal failure worse.

Thromboembolism. The incidence of renal vein thrombosis, pulmonary arterial embolism, and peripheral venous thrombophlebitis is increased. The precise mechanism is not clear although several abnormalities of clotting tests suggest a hypercoaguable state. Renal vein thrombosis is of particular interest because it may be the cause as well as a consequence of the nephrotic syndrome. Membranous nephropathy is especially likely to be associated with this complication.

Pulmonary Edema. The profound fall in plasma oncotic pressure due to severe hypoalbuminemia may cause accumulation of fluid in the low pressure pulmonary vasculature. Even minor increases in the left atrial pressure may induce pulmonary edema in these patients. Judicious use of diuretics, vasodilators, and infusion of salt-poor hyperoncotic albumin may alleviate the situation.

Treatment

Treatment of the underlying cause of the glomerular disease is the best approach to reversal of the nephrotic syndrome. This may be readily achieved in patients with elevated renal venous pressure due to one of the mechanical causes or in whom a drug, heavy metal, or an allergen can be identified as the causative agent.

Diet. As long as glomerular filtration rate is not severely impaired, a high-protein diet should be encouraged. Salt intake should be low (20 mEq/day) in order to avoid edema formation.

Diuretics. Proper use of diuretics is important in patients with severe edema that is limiting activity and impairing respiration. Thiazide diuretics cause a slow decrease in edema without producing hypovolemia. Use of loop diuretics such as furosemide (Lasix) and ethacrynic acid (Edecrin) should be reserved for selected patients. If potassium deficiency occurs, potassium-sparing diuretics should be used cautiously, carefully avoiding hyperkalemia.

Thoracentesis and paracentesis. These should be carried out only in extreme cases after an adequate trial of diuretic therapy has proved ineffective.

Corticosteroids. Nephrotic syndrome due to lipoid nephrosis and SLE is usually amenable to treatment with corticosteroids. Prednisone, 40-60 mg daily for 4-6 weeks, and then 80-120 mg on alternate days for another 4-6 weeks limits the syndrome in most patients. Treatment of the nephrotic syndrome due to membranous nephropathy with 120 mg prednisone on alternate days for 12 weeks has been demonstrated to be beneficial with minimal side effects.

Immunosuppressive agents. Azathioprine (Imuran) or cyclophsphamide (Cytoxan) may be used in patients who have not responded to steriod therapy; however, there is a lack of well-controlled studies to fully support their valure. Patients with azotemia and chronic proliferative or sclerosing glomerulonephritis are not likely to respond to steroid or immunosupressive therapy. Older patients do not usually respond to therapy and suffer adverse effects more often.

GLOMERULAR DISEASES

The terms glomerulopathy and glomerulonephritis, usually used synonymously, include a group of diverse conditions in which the disease appears to affect primarily the glomeruli.

Clinical Spectrum

The clinical presentation of glomerulopathies can be grouped into the following categories: acute onset, persistent symptomless urinary abnormalities, nephrotic syndrome, and chronic renal failure.

Acute Onset

The acute onset is usually characterized by gross hematuria or smoky urine. The hematuria may be microscopic and the patient may present with periorbital edema and edema of the distal extremities. Hypertension and circulatory overload also may dominate the clinical presentation. It is almost impossible to correlate the clinical presentation with the histologic renal disease and prognosis.

Persistent Urinary Abnormalities

These patients are generally symptom free and diagnosis of glomerulopathy is suspected upon urinalysis that reveals red blood cells, red blood cell casts, and proteinuria. The renal function, as measured by creatinine clearance, is usually normal or only moderately impaired. The long-term prognosis for asymptomatic patients with normal serum creatinine and either proteinuria or hematuria appears to be better than if both abnormalities persist.

Nephrotic Syndrome

With severe proteinuria, edema and other manifestations of the nephrotic syndrome may be the dominant clinical features. As with acute onset glomerulopathy, the renal pathology and natural history may be considerably different in patients presenting with the same clinical features. In general, the longer the duration of the nephrotic syndrome, the poorer is the prognosis.

Chronic Renal Failure

The manifestations of end-stage renal disease (ESRD), such as hypertension, circulatory fluid overload, and symptoms of uremia, may be already present when the patient with glomerular disease first seeks care.

Pathogenesis and Morphologic Classification of Glomerular Diseases

Much has been learned in recent years about the immune mechanisms in the pathogenesis of glomerular diseases. In immune complex glomerular diseases antigen-antibody complexes form in the blood stream and are trapped in the glomeruli during the process of ultrafiltration of plasma. These immune complexes initiate an inflammatory reaction in the glomerulus. Activation of the complement system by the antibody or the complexes is of prime importance in initiating this inflammatory reaction. The activation of the complement system also leads to triggering of the clotting mechanisms and deposition of fibrin in the glomeruli. The organization of fibrin eventually results in fibrosis and obliteration of the glomeruli. The complement system can also be activated by properdin, which is normal serum β globulin, without the participation of antibody or antigen-antibody complexes. This is called the alternate pathway of activation of the complement system. In these conditions the C3 (β1C globulin) component of the complement is low while the other components of the complement are normal in the blood. Some glomerular diseases do not involve the antigen-antibody complexes or the complement system but seem to result from direct activation of the coagulation system. In certain glomerular diseases antibodies may form against the glomerular basement membrane (GBM). They are classified as anti-GBM diseases. Glomerulopathy may also result from dysfunction of the glomerular mesangium. The mesangial cells normally serve as reticuloendothelial cells and remove foreign particles, preventing their sequestration in the glomerular capillaries. Dysfunction of these cells may lead to trapping of immune complexes in the glomeruli. Glomerular disease may also result from abnormalities of metabolism. Glomerular involvement also occurs in certain hereditary diseases.

Due to the limited number of ways that a glomerulus can respond to various injuries, it is not always possible to define the etiology of renal disease from histopathology. The glomerulus consists of cells and extracellular material. The cells may increase in number (proliferation) or there may be infiltration by neutrophils (exudation). The glomerular capillary basement membrane may be thickened due to antigen-antibody complex deposition. As the disease progresses there may be destruction of the cells and the glomerulus may be sclerosed or scarred. The disease may affect all the glomeruli (diffuse change), a few glomeruli (focal change), or only parts of a few glomeruli (segmental change). The glomerular damage is almost always associated with increased glomerular capillary permeability manifesting as proteinuria, hematuria, and RBC casts in the urine.

No classification of the glomerular diseases is perfect because of the lack of complete knowledge and the involvement of multiple mechanisms in pathogenesis of many glomerular diseases. A morphologic classification based on the light, electron, and immunfluorescence microscopy incorporating the known pathogenic mechanisms of the glomerular diseases is presented here.

Minimal Change Glomerulopathy

Munk, in 1939, termed this condition lipoid nephrosis, referring to the presence of fat bodies in the urine that are now known to result from a glomerular leak. Hamburger has called the condition minimal change glomerulopathy. The other synonyms for this condition include nil disease, glomerular epithelial cell disease, and foot process disease. The peak incidence occurs between ages 3 and 4 years, but no age is exempt. It accounts for 10 to 20 percent of adult patients with nephrotic syndrome; males are affected more often than females, in a ratio of 3 to 1. The etiology and pathogenesis remain unknown. In adults it may occur in association with Hodgkin's disease and other lymphomas.

Light microscopy usually shows no abnormalities except for occasional small areas of glomerular proliferation or adhesions to Bowman's capsule. The tubules usually show presence of protein and doubly refractile lipid vacuoles in the proximal tubular cells. The blood vessels appear normal. Vascular changes, when present, usually are related to the age of the patient and unrelated to hypertension, if present. There may be edema of the interstitium. Electron microscopy reveals characteristic glomerular changes consisting of swelling and fusion (smudging) of the epithelial foot processes. The basement membrane usually has a normal appearance but may show small vacuoles or irregular thickening. Immunofluourescent findings are noteworthy for the lack of deposition of IgG and complement in the glomeruli.

The disease characteristically presents as florid nephrotic syndrome. The urine sediment contains hyaline, granular, and fatty casts and occasional red cells. Red cell casts are usually absent. Azotemia may occur in the early stages of the disease, perhaps due to hypovolemia or obstruction of tubules by the protein casts. In most instances, the BUN and creatinine remain normal. Hypertension is uncommon. C3, C4, and properdin levels are usually within normal limits. IgG levels may be profoundly depressed, accounting for the notorious susceptibility to infection with pneumococci.

Oral diuretic therapy for edema and appropriate antimicrobial drugs for infections constitute appropriate supportive therapy. Steroids exert a beneficial influence on proteinuria and facilitate the natural tendency for spontaneous remission. More than 90% of the patients respond to prednisone therapy. The recommended dose is 60 mg/m^2/day for children and 1 mg/kg/day for adults for 4 weeks, followed by alternate-day therapy at this dose for 4-8 weeks, to reduce side effects and supression of the pituitary-adrenal axis. Although the proteinuria usually subsides in 4 weeks, occasionally it may take up to 8 weeks. Steroid therapy is tapered after the urine is protein free for 4 weeks. Relapses may be treated by temporarily resuming or increasing the dosage.

Patients who develop multiple relapses or steroid-induced complications are probably best treated with alkylating agents such as cyclophosphamide (Cytoxan) and chlorambucil (Leukeran). Azathioprine (Imuran) is not as effective. Cyclophosphamide at a dosage of 2-2.5 mg/kg/day for 8 weeks is generally considered effective. Genitourinary toxicity, consisting of azoospermia, amenorrhea, and cystitis, limits its applicability. Bone marrow suppression and alopecia are also common. The mechanism of action of the salutary effects of steroids and alkylating agents in lipoid nephrosis is unknown.

Most cases follow a benign course with respect to development of renal failure. Relapses may continue to occur for many years after the initial occurrence. Approximately two-third of patients who receive treatment with cyclophosphamide (Cytoxan) remain in remission for 5 years or more after therapy.

Focal Glomerulosclerosis

This condition is also known as segmental hyalinosis and focal sclerosis. It may be clinically indistinguishable from lipoid nephrosis and early cases of membranous nephropathy. Some pathologists consider it part of the pathologic spectrum of lipoid nephrosis. The lesion is encountered in 10-20% of adults with idiopathic nephrotic syndrome but is less common in children. The etiology and pathogenesis of the disorder is unknown. Some regard it as an immune complex disease, but the antigen is not known. Several cases of rapid recurrence of this lesion in the transplanted kidney have been noted.

Light microscopy characteristically shows segmental glomerulosclerosis and hyalinosis affecting a variable minority of the glomeruli, especially those in the deeper juxtamedullary cortex. There is no associated proliferation or necrosis. The extent of segmental lesions vary from glomerulus to glomerulus and, as the disorder progresses, a picture of global sclerosis may develop. Tubular changes consisting of focal thickening of the basement membrane and atrophy are common. The blood vessels and the interstitium are usually normal. Serial biopsies show progression at a highly variable rate. Electron microscopy shows diffuse or segmental fusion of the foot processes. Areas of the glomeruli that are abnormal on light microscopy reveal subendothelial and mesangial deposits and areas of sclerosis and capillary collapse. On immunofluorescence the affected glomeruli show granular and nodular deposits of IgM and C3 in a segmental distribution.

Patients may be initially discovered with asymptomatic proteinuria. A few may present with frank nephrotic syndrome. The majority of patients demonstrate persistent proteinuria, hypertension, and a progressive decline in GFR. Hematuria and abnormalities of tubular function such as glycosuria, aminoaciduria, and phosphaturia may be also found. Serum C3 concentration is usually normal.

Resistance to steroids is the rule although some patients, predominently children, may show an initial steroid response. Cytotoxic agents have no proven value.

Progression to renal failure, although not uncommon, usually takes many years.

Membranous Glomerulopathy

The disorder is also known as membranous glomerulonephritis and epimembranous nephropathy. It accounts for more than 50% of instances of adult idiopathic nephrotic syndrome. The condition is uncommon in children. A similar or identical histopathologic lesion occurs in SLE, upon exposure to heavy metals such as mercury and gold, treatment with penicillamine (Cuprimine), and infections such as congenital and secondary syphilis, malaria, leprosy, filariasis, schitosomiasis, and hepatitis B. Diabetes, sarcoidosis, Sjögren's syndrome, and chronic allograft rejection can also cause histopathologic changes similar to membranous nephropathy. An underlying carcinoma may be ultimately detected in 6 to 10% of the patients with idiopathic membranous nephropathy. The term glomerulonephritis is inappropriate for the condition since there is usually no histologic evidence of glomerular inflammation.

Light microscopy reveals a diffuse and uniform thickening of the capillary wall; however, the capillary lumina are widely patent in the early stages. With progression of the disease the capillary wall becomes increasingly thickened, encroaching on the lumen. Tubular alterations are minimal initially; however, with progression of the glomerular disease tubular atrophy becomes pronounced. Vascular changes are usually absent in the early stages but are common in advanced disease. Renal vein thrombosis, generally regarded as a complication rather than a cause of membranous nephropathy, is associated with significant edema and fibrotic changes in the interstitium. Under the electron microscope, the basement membrane shows thickening, vacuolation, irregularity, and subepithelial electron-dense deposits. Immunofluorescence reveals heavy granular IgG and C3 deposits.

The usual presentation is a florid nephrotic syndrome. Asymptomatic proteinuria, renal hypertension, or chronic renal failure are uncommon presentations. The condition may be distinguished from lipoid nephrosis by a higher average age of patients, hypertension, renal failure, nonselective proteinuria, and a rarity of clinical remission. Serum C3 concentration is typically normal. Renal vein thrombosis is not uncommonly present and may precipitate episodes of acute renal failure or pulmonary embolization.

Recent data from a multicenter prospective study conducted in the United States reveal a role for alternate-day steroid therapy. The adult dose is 120 mg prednisone every other day for 6-8 weeks followed by tapering over the next 4-6 weeks. Those not responding to steroids or showing reccurrence despite steroid therapy should be given a trial of cyclophosphamide (Cytoxan). The dosage is 2-2.5 mg/kg/day for 8-12 weeks. White blood cell count should be monitored on a weekly basis when administering cyclophosphamide to detect bone marrow suppression and the dose modified accordingly.

Spontaneous remission of proteinuria occurs in approximately 33% of patients without treatment. In the remainder, the course is one of slow progression with renal failure occurring in 5-10 years after the onset of the disease. In patients who respond to treatment the prognosis is improved.

Proliferative Glomerulonephritis

This term is used to describe glomerular diseases with cellular proliferation in the absence of systemic disorders such as SLE and other collagen vascular diseases. Until quite recently, it was widely believed that most cases were poststreptococcal in origin. This now is clearly recognized as incorrect. The group is heterogenous but immunecomplex renal injury seems to play a part in almost all cases.

Acute Poststreptococcal Glomerulonephritis. The condition in also known as postinfectious glomerulonephritis. This may occur after streptococcal pharyngitis or pyodermal skin infection. The pharyngitis-associated glomerulonephritis occurs most frequently in the winter and spring months and is twice as common in men. The pyoderma-associated nephritis occurs more frequently in the summer and early fall, has an equal sex incidence, and is more common in the southern parts of the United States. The streptococcal serotypes associated with nephritis are generally not associated with rheumatic fever and it is not clear if penicillin treatment prevents the occurrence of glomerulonephritis. The latent period between the throat infection and glomerulonephritis averages 10-14 days; between the skin infection and nephritis it averages 3 weeks. Staphylococcal infection of subarachnoid-jugular shunts used in the treatment of hydrocephalus and subacute bacterial endocarditis may be also associated with glomerulonephritis.

On light microscopy, the glomeruli appear swollen and hypercellular. The cellularity is contributed by proliferation of the epithelial and the endothelial capillary wall cells and infiltration with polymorphonuclear leukocytes. Electron microscopy reveals prominent electron-dense deposits known as humps on the epithelial side of the basement membrane. These deposits generally correspond to discrete nodular deposits of IgG and C3 observed by immunofluorescence.

Most patients give a history of preceding severe throat infection, otitis media, leg ulcer, or a surgical wound. Bacteriologic cultures in untreated patients often reveal the nature of the infection. Sometimes the only evidence of a preceding streptococcal infection may be raised antistreptolysin-O (ASLO) titer. One to 3 weeks following the infection the patient develops edema and hematuria. Edema is most pronounced in the face on first arising. The urine is described as smoky brown in color but may be occasionally frankly blood stained. Reduced urine output, bilateral flank pain, vague malaise, nausea, and headache are other common symptoms. Fever is, however, unusual. Mild to moderate hypertension is present in more than 50% of patients. Occasionally, the patient may manifest features of malignant hypertension. Fluid retention, if marked, may lead to clinical manifestations of fluid overload. Urine output is usually reduced. A rare patient may manifest anuria. Persistent renal failure leads to symptoms of uremia.

Urinanalysis characteristically reveals proteinuria and RBC casts. In addition granular casts, hemoglobin casts, RBCs, and leukocytes may be observed. The serum creatinine is generally elevated in 1.5-4 mg/dl range. Appropriate cultures may reveal a nephrogenic strain of streptococcus or other organisms responsible for initiating the neprhitis. Early treatment of the infection may abort the rise in ASO titer. The serum titer of type-specific antibody to streptococcal M antigen persists considerably longer but is difficult to measure. A marked drop in serum complement characteristically occurs. The sedimentation rate is moderately raised. Cryoglobulinemia may be present.

The condition may need to be differentiated from nephritis associated with Henoch-Schönlein purpura, SLE, and other collagen vascular diseases. It can be confused occasionally with maligant hypertension, various forms of hematuria, and acute tubular necrosis, particularly when the latter occurs in a setting of septicemia.

In the acute stages, penicillin is given to eradicate any remaining streptococcal infection. Fluid retention during the oliguric phase is treated by sodium restriction to 20-60 mEq/day, and fluid restriction to about 500 ml/day. Furosemide (Lasix) in doses of 40-1,000 mg/day may be used in patients with severe edema. Digitalis is ineffective. In rare cases life-threatening fluid overload requires dialysis. Severe hypertension may require intravenous infusion of diazoxide (Hyperstat) at a rate of 15 mg/Min until 300-600 mg is infused. Diazoxide infusion should be preceded by intravenous furosemide to overcome fluid retention and propranolul to prevent tachycardia and angina. Concomitant oral antihypertensive therapy should be started with a diuretic and a sympathetic blocker. Bed rest is advised during the acute phase of the disease but normal activity may be undertaken during convalescence. Neither corticosteroids nor immunosupressive drugs are of value. Follow-up requires frequent determination of blood pressure, urinalysis, and plasma creatinine measurements. Acute urinary tract infections that occur occasionally should be treated at the first opportunity.

The proteinuria may persist for several months and hematuria may outlast proteinuria. Complete recovery, however, has been reported as long as one year after the acute attack. Prognosis for complete recovery is better in children than in adults. As many as 50% of the adults either deteriorate rapidly or develop chronic glomerulonephritis. Complete recovery is less likely after repeated attacks of glomerulonephritis in both children and adults.

Membranoproliferative Glomerulonephritis. This condition is also known as mesangiocapillary or mesangioproliferative glomerulonephritis. The condition is found most commonly between the ages of 5 and 30 years, with a slight predominance of females over males. On the basis of electron microscopy the conditon can be divided into two types (I and II). The term persistent hypocomplemententemic glomerulonephritis is used because of frequent occurence of prolonged depression of serum complements, and because of the frequent finding of centralobular nodules in renal biopsy specimens the term lobular glomerulonephritis is also applied to the entity. The disease, especially type II, has been noted to recur in renal allotransplants.

The principle feature on light microscopy is proliferation of mesangial cells with a variable tendency for expansion of the mesangial matrix. The capillaries are narrowed by the expanding lobular mass, causing the glomerulus to look enlarged. Silver methanamine stains the glomular basement membrane and basement membranelike material. With the extension of the mesangial material into the basement membrane the peripheral capillary loops may show apparent reduplication of the basement membrane. Polymorphonuclear leukocyte exudation may be extensive in some cases. The tubules may show atrophy and fibrosis in patients with decreased GFR and the interstitium may show focal mononuclear infiltration and foam cells in some patients. Electron microscopy reveals extension of mesangial cell cytoplasm and matrix into the peripheral capillary wall, causing mesangialization of the peripheral capillary loops. On the basis of electron microscopy, two variants can be recognized. Type I demonstrates electron-dense subendothelial deposits and type II shows electron-dense deposits within the substance of the glomerular basement membrane, causing it to split in two layers (dense deposit disease). On immunfluorescence, deposition of IgG, and C3, and occasionally IgM and IgA is usually found variably distributed in the capillary walls and certain mesangial regions.

Heavy proteinuria usually associated with manifestations of

the nephrotic syndrome and hematuria are the initial symptoms in almost 75% of the patients. The remainder commonly present with asymptomatic proteinuria. Occasionally a patient may present with features of acute nephritis. In most patients the course is slowly downhill with episodes of hematuria and nephrotic syndrome gradually leading to renal failure. The urine sediment shows RBC casts, RBCs, and oval fat bodies if proteinuria is heavy. The most characteristic laboratory feature is the decreased serum level of complement. The earliest serum complement components, C1, C2, and C4 are usually normal. In a patient with depressed levels of C3 a circulating factor capable of cleaving native C3 may be demonstrated. This is known as C3 nephritic factor (C3NeF).

Since the etiology of the disease is unknown and the pathogenesis uncertain, no specific therapy has been devised. Recent studies suggest that treatment with alternate-day steroids as outlined for treatment of membranous glomerulopathy may result in better preservation of renal structure and function. Therapy with immunosuppresive agents does not seem to alter the clinical course.

Generally the disease progresses to end-stage renal disease in a period of 5-10 years.

Focal Glomerulonephritis. This condition is also termed focal nephritis, essential or benign recurrent hematuria, and Berger's disease. The disorder is characterized by repeated attacks of profuse hematuria following nonspecific respiratory infection, systemic infections, or strenuous physical exercise. The symptoms occur several hours to 1-2 days after the infection as compared to acute poststreptococcal nephritis where hematuria occurs after 1-3 weeks of infection.

By light microscopy, there is a focal increase in the mesangial matrix and mesangial cells. Only portions of some glomeruli are involved. Characteristically there is no scarring or tubular atrophy. Electron microscopy reveals only local proliferation of mesangial cells and an increase in the matrix material. Immunofluorescence characteristically reveals IgA deposition although IgG and C3 may also be present.

As indicated above, the syndrome is characterized by recurrent hematuria occurring in children and young adults following respiratory and systemic infections. It is more common in males. Hypertension is usually present. Proteinuria occurs in less than 50% of patients and is generally less than 1 g/24 h. Bacteriologic and serologic tests for streptococcal infection are characteristically negative. The passage of blood clots may cause ureteral colic.

Corticosteroids and immunosuppressives are not indicated and there is no evidence that they alter the natural history of the disease. Penicillin prophylaxis to reduce bacterial respiratory infection is usually disappointing.

The course is not always benign as some of the long-term complications such as hypertension and renal failure occur not infrequently.

Latent Glomerulonephritis. This term refers to that period of time following an attack of acute glomerulonephritis when evidence of nonhealing persists. Latent glomerulonephritis either results in complete healing or progression to chronic glomerulonephritis. On light microscopy there is usually residual hypercellularity. On electron microscopy granular subepithelial deposits are present. On immunofluorescence the diffuse nodular IgG and C3 deposits of acute nephritis subside and immunoglobulins are discernible only in the central stalk area.

Chronic Glomerulonephritis

This is the outcome of several different types of glomerular diseases. At the time the diagnosis is made, in most patients there is no prior history of renal disease. Approximately 50-70% of all patients requiring dialysis or transplantation carry the diagnosis of chronic glomerulonephritis.

By light microscopy most of the glomeruli are distorted with loss of glomerular architecture. Partial or complete hyalinization and sclerosis are common. Occasionally mesangial hypercellularity may be present. There is usually conspicuous interstitial fibrosis, tubular atrophy, and hyaline arteriosclerosis. Electron microscopy reveals mesangial sclerosis. Immunofluorescence shows nonspecific changes and is not helpful in the diagnosis.

Initial manifestations include persistent, asymptomatic proteinuria, and nephrotic syndrome with or without symptoms of renal failure. As the GFR deteriorates, complications of uremia appear. There is no definable sytemic disorder present. Hypertension is common. Radiologic investigations reveal bilaterally small, fibrosed kidneys. Urine sediment may reveal RBC casts.

Protein and salt restriction, antihypertensive therapy, sodium bicarbonate to combat uremic acidosis, and phosphate binders, such as aluminium hydroxide-containing antacids, constitute the conservative medical therapy. Steroids and immunosuppressives are not helpful. Chronic hemodialysis and kidney transplantation are usually not necessary until the GFR falls below 5 ml/min.

After the appearance of uremic symptoms, most patients require chronic hemodialysis or transplantation within 1 year.

Antiglomerular Basement Membrane Disease

This entity is also known as anti-GBM disease. The renal lesion classically occurs in the clinical condition called Goodpasture's syndrome. The other entity included in this category of glomerular diseases is rapidly progressive glomerulonephritis (RPGN).

Goodpasture's Syndrome. Goodpasture, in 1919, described a syndrome characterized by life-threatening pulmonary hemorrhage, hemoptysis, hemosiderin-laden macrophages in the sputum, and necrotizing glomerulitis. The disease is more frequent in men and has a high mortality. Although the etiology remains uncertain, hydrocarbon exposure, influenza, and other infectious processes are believed to damage alveolar basement membrane that releases certain antigens, causing formation of antibodies. Since there is cross reactivity between alveolar and glomerular basement membranes the antibodies also act against the glomerular basement membrane.

On light microscopy, the glomerular lesions are characterized by extensive crescent formation. Occasionally, there may be only minimal changes or focal proliferation and necrosis. Electron microscopy reveals subendothelial fibrin deposition. Immunofluorescence reveals linear deposition of IgG and/or

IgM and C3 along the peripheral capillary wall. This classic linear deposition of antibodies indicates that they are directed against the basement membrane. Linear deposition of immune globulins that are not anti-GBM antibodies may also be seen in cases of mild lupus nephritis, diabetic nephropathy, focal glomerulosclerosis associated with heroin abuse, and, rarely, in poststreptococcal glomerulonephritis.

The extent of pulmonary hemorrhage varies, but it frequently develops about the same time as the renal manifestations. Chest x-ray film reveals characteristic infiltrates and the sputum contains iron-laden macrophages. Severe or malignant hypertension is uncommon. Massive proteinuria may be seen occasionally. Levels of C3 are most often within normal range. Circulating anti-GBM antibody is often detectable. Abnormal circulating levels and increased urinary excretion of fibrin split products may also be found. The onset of renal disease is characterized by oliguria and anuria. Rapidly advancing azotemia, proteinuria with RBC casts in the urine, and hypertension are common. The renal function usually declines rapidly; however, in some patients the kidney function stabilizes. Goodpasture's syndrome may have to be differentiated from pulmonary hemorrhage and renal failure in patients with polyarteritis nodosa, Wegener's granulomatosis, bacterial endocarditis, and fluid overload with pulmonary edema in a uremic patient.

Plasmapheresis to remove the cirulating anti-GBM antibodies along with administration of glucocorticoids and immunosupressive drugs to prevent further synthesis of these antibodies has been successful in some patients with Goodpasture's syndrome. Bilateral nephrectomy has also been reported to be of value in aborting life-threatening pulmonary hemorrhage in certain patients. This approach, however, has not been uniformly successful. Since spontaneous remissions of pulmonary hemorrhage may occur and also pulmonary hemorrhage may be life threatening in certain patients with adequately functioning kidneys, bilateral nephrectomy is not an ideal treatment. Anticoagulant therapy has been recommended by some investigators, but it requires further evaluation.

The prognosis is generally poor. Recurrence of original renal disease in transplants has been noted.

Rapidly Progressive Glomerulonephritis. This condition is characterized by progressive and often irreversible loss of renal function accompanied by urinary findings of glomerular disease. The histopathologic findings on kidney biopsy are similar to those seen in Goodpasture's syndrome. Clinically there is no involvement of the lungs. Anti-GBM antibodies can be detected in the circulation. The treatment is the same as for Goodpasture's syndrome, except that there is no need to worry about pulmonary hemorrhage. If the patient does not respond to conservative management and develops severe renal failure, dialysis may be necessary. Transplantation should be delayed until anti-GBM antibodies can no longer be detected in the circulation.

Glomerular Diseases Associated with Systemic Diseases

Many connective tissue disorders, disorders of coagulation, metabolic diseases, and malignancies may be associated with glomerulonephritis, which is not always clearly distinguishable from other forms of glomerulonephritis. A discussion of glomerulonephritis in various systemic diseases follows.

Connective Tissue Disorders. Several connective tissue disorders such as SLE, polyarteritis nodosa, Wegener's granulomatosis, and scleroderma may be associated with renal disease involving the glomeruli and the blood vessels. A discussion of the renal involvement in these disorders follows.

Glomerular involvement in *systemic lupus erythematosus* (SLE) is extremely common; some 50-75% of patients with this condition develop renal disease at some time. Extensive glomerular disease may be present with minimal clinical findings. The renal lesion is an example of immune complex glomerular injury; the complexes consist of DNA antigen, IgG, and complement. Although a viral etiology for SLE has been proposed, a specific virus has not been isolated from patients with SLE. The disease is more frequent in women. When the lupus syndrome occurs secondary to drugs such as procainamide (Pronestyl), hydralazine (Apresoline), and so on, the kidneys are usually spared.

On light microscopy, the glomerular involvement takes several forms: the kidneys may appear normal on light microscopy but show evidence of diffuse mesangial deposits of immunoglobulins and complement by immunofluorescence, focal proliferative glomerulonephritis with hypercellularity and thickening of the basement membrane, membranous nephritis without cellular proliferation, and diffuse proliferative glomerulonephritis with areas of necrosis and subepithelial crescent formation. Another characteristic histologic finding is the presence of hematoxylin bodies consisting of depolymerized ribonucleic acid. On electron microscopy, electron-dense deposits representing the antigen-antibody complexes are seen in the subendothelial areas. They may contain a fingerprint pattern. Deposits of microtubular structures resembling viral particles are often present. In patients with membranous changes on light microscopy, electron microscopy reveals epimembranous deposits and irregular thickening of the capillary basement membrane. Immunofluorescence studies show deposits of IgG, IgA, and C3.

The disease is characterized by exacerbations and remissions with a typical butterfly rash over the malar eminences, fever, leukopenia, joint involvement, proteinuria, and hematuria. Renal involvement may be manifested as a symptomless proteinuria that may remain unchanged for a long period, nephrotic syndrome, and a severe and progressive acute glomerulonephritis with the urine sediment showing telescopic changes composed of white and red blood cells, red blood cell casts, broad granular casts, and proteinuria. Renal tubular acidosis and Fanconi's syndrome also may occur when the renal involvement is severe.

Serum levels of C1q, C4, and C3 tend to be diminished during active renal and connective tissue disease. High titers of anti-DNA antibody is often present when the renal disease is active. Serum titers of antinuclear antibody (ANA) is not useful in predicting the presence or severity of renal disease. Serum complement levels fall before acute exacerbation of SLE and their measurement is probably a useful way to monitor the activity of the disease.

Steroids are indicated to control the extrarenal manifestations. Diffuse proliferative glomerulonephritis may respond favorably to the addition of an aklylating agent such as cyclophosphamide (Cytoxan) or chlorambucil (Leukeran). Azathioprine (Imuran) is not as useful. The cytotoxic agents should be used with great caution as they cause increased susceptibility to serious fungal, bacterial, and viral infections. The role of cytotoxic agents in the management of mild and focal proliferative or membranous lesions has not been established. Hypertension, when present, should be vigorously treated.

Attempts have been made to gauge prognosis on the basis of histopathology. It is generally believed that minimal or focal glomerulonephritis is associated with a good prognosis. Membranous nephropathy has a prognosis similar to the idiopathic disorder. Diffuse proliferative involvement of the glomeruli is associated with a poor prognosis. Some cases of proliferative glomerulonephritis, upon treatment with steroids and immunosupressive agents, have resulted in membranous transformation.

Renal involvement occurs in 75-85% of the patients with *polyarteritis nodosa* (periarteritis nodosa). Drug sensitivity such as to amphetamines, sulfonamides, or penicillin, and hepatitis B infection have been implicated in the production of the vasculitis characteristic of this disease.

On light microscopy, there are two varieties of changes. Fibrinoid necrosis of the walls of medium-sized arteries within the kidneys associated with microaneurysms is a more common pattern. In the second variety, fibrinoid changes involving all or part of a glomerular tuft with adhesions to Bowman's capsule, along with proliferation and occasional crescent formation, may be present. Hemorrhage into the capsular tufts may be present; however, the glomerular capillaries appear bloodless. Although an immunecomplex mechanism is suspected, electron-dense material is not conspicuous on electron microscopy. On immunofluorescence no immunoglobulins are usually found, although fibrin deposition is often seen.

Unexplained fever, leukocytosis, eosinophilia, abnormal liver function tests, and bronchospasm are usually present. Skin involvement is particularly common in those with renal disease. Small tender areas, 2-4 mm in diameter, representing infarcts may be present in the pulp of the fingers and toes. The renal manifestations may vary. Gross hematuria due to renal infarction and flank pain may be the presenting complaint in some patients. Certain patients may present with manifestations of acute oliguric nephritis with microscopic hematuria, red blood cell casts, and proteinuria. Chronic glomerulonephritis with proteinuria and progressive reduction in renal function may be the third manifestation. Hypertension is quite common and may be severe.

A renal arteriogram may demonstrate microaneurysms. If they are present, kidney biopsy should not be performed because of danger of hemorrhage.

Control of hypertension is of primary importance to prevent further renal damage. Corticosteroids usually control the systemic manifestations and may cause partial or complete remission of the renal manifestations. They seem most helpful when the renal lesion is not far advanced.

The usual course is progressive deterioration, particularly in patients with proliferative glomerulonephritis. Rarely the disease may spontaneously become stationary or even remit temporarily. Polyarteritis may recur in the transplanted kidney.

Wegener's Granulomatosis is closely related to polyarteritis nodosa. The clinical manifestations are prominent in the respiratory tract. The lung lesions appear nodular on chest x-ray and upper respiratory symptoms of severe sinusitis and perforation of the nasal septum are prominent. Pathologically these lesions consist of necrotizing and granulomatous inflammatory changes.

Light microscopy usually reveals focal proliferative glomerulonephritis. Electron microscopy and immunofluorescence generally fail to reveal the presence of immune complexes.

The renal manifestations may vary from normal kidney function to severe renal failure. Urine sediment contains red and white blood cells, red cell casts, and proteinuria.

Cyclophosphamide (Cytoxan) or azathioprine (Imuran) with or without corticosteriods is generally very effective. Early diagnosis and treatment is important.

The untreated disease usually progresses relentlessly; however, with treatment, dramatic and prolonged remissions are common.

Scleroderma or systemic sclerosis involves the kidney in almost two-thirds of the patients.

On light microscopy, renal biopsy shows changes indistinguishable from malignant hypertension. Fibrinoid necrosis, intimal thickening, and patchy necrosis of arterioles and interlobular arteries is present. Electron microscopy does not reveal any specific changes. Immunofluorescence reveals fibrin, IgM, $C1_a$, C4 and C3 deposits in the glomerular capillaries and arterioles.

Proteinuria and hypertension usually occur at the onset of renal disease. As renal insufficiency progresses, hypertension becomes severe. Other typical manifestations of scleroderma such as sclerodactyly, telangiectasia, Raynaud's phenomonon, and esophageal involvement are usually present.

Treatment of hypertension is of paramount importance to retard the progression of renal disease. Captopril has proved especially useful in controlling hypertension in this condition. Treatment of scleroderma with penicillamine may be helpful in further slowing the renal disease. Hemodialysis is necessary once the GFR falls below 5 ml/min.

Because of multisystem involvement and despite hemodialysis, the prognosis is generally poor. With continued control of hypertension and treatment with penicillamine, on rare occasions there may be reversal of the renal disease allowing discontinuation of hemodialysis.

Disorders of Coagulation. In several varieties of glomerulopathies, enhanced coagulation seems to play a primary pathogenic role. These include toxemia of pregnancy, postpartum renal failure, hemolytic-uremic syndrome, Henoch-Schönlein purpura, and thrombotic thrombocytopenic purpura. Other pathogenic mechanisms operate in varying degrees.

Toxemia of pregnancy, or preeclampsia, characteristically occurs late in pregnancy and is characterized by hypertension, edema, and proteinuria. It is called eclampsia when associated with convulsions. It is more common in patients with pre existing renal disease, hypertension, diabetes, with twin pregnancies, and in blacks. The etiology of the disease is unknown, and the pathogenesis is poorly understood.

On light microscopy, the glomeruli appear swollen and the capillaries occluded by the swollen epithelial cells. Electron microscopy may reveal focal basement membrane thickening and immunofluorescence may show fibrin deposits.

Hypertension usually appears first. This is followed by proteinuria. Since blood pressure normally falls in the second trimester of pregnancy, a blood pressure of 130/80 mm Hg during this period should be considered elevated. Edema is present in the periorbital region, the hands, and ankles. Headache, blurred vision, and midabdominal pain may frequently be present. The fundi may show changes of hypertensive retinopathy. Proteinuria may range from trace to 10 g/24 h. Urine sediment may show granular or hyaline casts. Although reduction in the GFR occurs, azotemia is seldom present because of the increase in GFR accompanying normal pregnancy. Hyperuricemia is often present because of a disproportionate reduction in urate clearance.

Bed rest and mild sedation constitute the initial therapy. Magnesium sulfate is widely used because of a depressant effect on the central nervous system (CNS) and a mild antihypertensive action. If hypertension is severe, hydralazine or methyldopa may be used in addition to a small dose of a diuretic. The definitive therapy is termination of pregnancy.

Maternal death is now rare. Blood pressure usually returns to normal within 2-4 weeks after delivery; however, proteinuria may persist longer. There is to date no evidence that infants born of toxemic pregnancies are predisposed to the development of hypertension. Multiparous women developing toxemia seem to have a higher incidence of hypertension in later life.

Postpartum renal failure, also known as postpartum nephrosclerosis, is a rare disorder that occurs in multiparous women within days or weeks after an apparently normal delivery. It is not related to toxemia of pregnancy. Intravascular hemolysis, retained fragments of placenta, or certain undefined factors may trigger release of thromboplastin and intravascular coagulation causing consumptive coagulopathy.

On light microscopy, there is evidence of advanced nephrosclerosis and cortical necrosis. Fibrin microthrombi may be present in the glomerular capillaries. Electron microscopy and immunofluorescence do not reveal any specific changes.

Nausea, vomiting, lethargy, and fever may precede the onset of the syndrome. Vaginal bleeding, epistaxis, purpura, and other evidence of bleeding may be present. Severe uncontrollable hypertension appears at the onset of renal involvement, resulting in hypertensive encephalopathy and pulmonary edema. The heart may be involved independent of hypertension. Laboratory examination reveals evidence of consumptive coagulopathy and microangiopathic hemolytic anemia.

Heparin has been recommended but may cause increased hemorrhage. Plasmapheresis is probably worth a try. Emergency bilateral nephrectomy has been reported to correct the consumptive coagulopathy in some patients. Despite support of renal function with hemodialysis, the patient may die of cardiovascular complications.

The prognosis is generally very poor. Renal failure is almost always irreversible.

Hemolytic uremic syndrome is a disorder of unknown etiology that usually occurs in children, although it has been reported in adults.

Light microscopy of the kidney reveals fibrin thrombi in the glomerular capillaries and evidence of cortical necrosis. In addition, fibrinoid necrosis of the arterioles may be present. Electron microscopy and immunofluorescence show nonspecific changes.

After nonspecific prodromal symptoms of respiratory and gastrointestinal infection, hemolysis and renal failure appear. The patient rapidly becomes anemic and thrombocytopenic. The blood smear demonstrates evidence of microangiopathic hemolytic anemia in the form of burr cells and fragmented erythrocytes. Hypertension and neurologic signs appear as the patient's condition deteriorates.

Heparin has been recommended but has not always proved valuable.

Almost 50% of the patients succumb to this disease. The remainder recover in 2-4 weeks. Some children may continue to have hypertension and evidence of renal failure.

Henoch-schönlein purpura is also known as anaphylactoid purpura. The kidneys are involved in almost 50% of patients with this syndrome. It generally occurs in children but is also seen in adults, regardless of age.

On light microscopy, focal or diffuse glomerulitis is present. Crescent formation may be extensive. Electron microscopy reveals dense deposits in the mesangium and subendothelial region of the glomerular basement membrane, sometimes splitting the membrane. Immunofluorescence reveals the presence of IgA, IgG, and properdin.

Purpuric lesions are usually confined to the lower extremities. In addition there may be colicky pain, gastrointestinal bleeding, and joint pains. Heavy porteinuria is often present. Hematuria varies from microscopic to severe gross hematuria. Urine sediment reveals RBC casts.

No satisfactory treatment is known. Corticosteroids and cytotoxic agents may be tried in severe cases.

Prognosis is good in children; 90% improve spontaneously. Mortality is higher in adults.

Thrombotic Thrombocytopenic Purpura. Thrombotic thrombocytopenic purpura is also known as Moschowitz's disease. It usually occurs between the ages of 10 and 39 with females being affected more commonly. Although the etiology of the disease has not been well established, certain viral and bacterial infections are believed to trigger the disorder. The disease closely resembles adult hemolytic-uremic syndrome, the major differences being a more generalized thrombotic involvement of small arteries, less severe renal involvement, and the severity of neurologic symptoms in thrombotic thrombocytopenic purpura.

On light microscopy, some glomeruli may be totally involved while others may show focal areas of fibrinoid necrosis. Interstitial edema and focal tubular necrosis eventually lead to tubular atrophy and interstitial fibrosis. The most characteristic changes are in the afferent arterioles and small arteries where there is intimal hyperplasia, subintimal deposition of fibrin, and fibrin thrombi. On electron microscopy there is loss of glomerular epithelial cell foot processes and thickening of the basement membrane. On immunofluorescence, fibrin deposition is typically seen in the capillary loops of the glomeruli.

The onset is characterized by a prodromal phase of nonspecific gastrointestinal or upper respiratory tract symptoms. Neurologic manifestations consisting of headaches, mental changes, altered states of consciousness, and seizures are commonly present. Fever is present in almost all patients. Renal involvement consisting of proteinuria, hematuria, pyuria, casts, and azotemia is noted in 50% of the patients.

The blood smear shows evidence of microangiopathic hemolytic anemia. Reticulocytosis, thrombocytopenia, and decreased platelet survival are common. Coagulation disturbances are usually absent.

The most widely accepted form of treatment for these diseases used to be the combination of steroids and splenectomy. Plasmaphereis and plasma infusion are now the treatment of choice. With employment of plasmapheresis some patients have obtained complete remissions of long duration, whereas others have required continued plasma infusions.

Metabolic Disorders. Metabolic disorders such as diabetes and amyloidosis not uncommonly involve the kidney.

The term *diabetic nephropathy* includes glomerulosclerosis, arteriolar nephrosclerosis, and pyelonephritis. Diabetic glomerulosclerosis is believed to be a manifestation of the generalized microangiopathy that may occur in diabetics independent of glucose intolerance. The majority of patients with juvenile diabetes of 20 years duration develop nephropathy. It is frequently associated with diabetic retinopathy and neuropathy.

The nodular glomerulosclerosis (Kimmelstiel-Wilson syndrome) is present in 10-15% of patients with diabetic nephropathy and is specific for diabetes. Diffuse glomerulosclerosis with thickening of the glomerular basement membrane and increase in the mesangial matrix is a nonspecific change that may be present in other renal diseases. On electron microscopy, there is marked basement membrane thickening in generalized glomerulosclerosis. Diabetic glomerulosclerosis is considered to be nonimmunologic in origin, however in many cases linear staining of the glomerular basement membrane (GBM) with IgG and IgM is not uncommon.

Proteinuria is usually the first evidence of kidney involvement in diabetic nephropathy. As the disease progresses, nephrotic syndrome often results. Uremic symptoms may, however, develop in the absence of nephrotic syndrome. Hypertension is common. Renal and urinary tract infection, pyelonephritis, and occasionarlly papillary necrosis are not uncommon. These causes for rapid deterioration in renal function should always be kept in mind for every diabetic patient. Congestive heart failure and compromised renal plasma flow may contribute to prerenal azotemia and bladder distention due to autonomic neuropathy may cause postrenal azotemia. As indicated above, retinopathy and peripheral neuropathy are common accompaniments.

Meticulous control of diabetes with multiple daily doses of insulin seems to not only retard progression but may even reverse renal insufficiency in many patients. Avoidance, and early detection and treatment, of urinary tract infections are of great help in slowing the progression of renal insufficiency. Hypertension should be controlled whenever present. Steroids and immunosuppressives are of no help and may even be contraindicated.

Once end-stage renal disease results, chronic dialysis may be necessary. Due to difficulty with vascular access, chronic ambulatory peritoneal dialysis (CAPD) is the treatment of choice in many patients with end-stage renal disease. It was long believed that diabetics would not make good transplant candidates because the large doses of steroids in the posttransplant state cause difficulty in controlling diabetes and immunosuppressives make these patients very susceptible to infections. Despite these difficulties, renal transplantation in selected patients is successful in rehabilitating them.

After the appearance of a nephrotic syndrome, end-stage renal disease usually results within 3 years. Most patients with diabetic end-stage renal disease treated with hemodialysis succumb to cardiovascular complications. Even renal transplantation does not retard the relentless progression of vascular disease and many successfully transplanted patients develop severe peripheral vascular disease causing gangrene and requiring amputations. Eventually these patients also succumb to cardiovascular disease.

The kidney is involved with great frequency in the secondary forms of *amyloidosis.* The underlying conditions include: osteomyelitis, regional enteritis, rheumatoid arthritis, multiple myeloma, tuberculosis, familial Mediterranean fever, and certain malignancies. The kidney may also be involved without any apparent predisposing condition.

On light microscopy amyloid is best visualized with special stains containing iodine, metachromatic dyes, or Congo red. It appears as an amorphous homogeneous extracellular deposit. The glomeruli are primarily affected, although extensive vascular and interstitial deposition of amyloid may also occur. In the glomerulus it is generally found deposited along the mesangium and the glomerular capillaries. Tubular loss and dilatation with casts associated with interstitial deposition of amyloid and papillary necrosis may also occur. On electron microscopy, amyloid has a beaded nonbranching fibrillar appearance. Immunofluorescence is usually positive for IgG because of the prescence of light chains in the amyloid deposits.

Heavy proteinuria and nephrotic syndrome are the clinical hallmarks of the disease. Hypertension is uncommon. Upon radiographic examination, the kidneys are either normal or slightly enlarged. The only other conditions with end-stage renal disease and enlarged kidneys are rapidly progressive glomerulonephritis, diabetes, scleroderma, and renal vein thrombosis. Renal vein thrombosis complicates renal amyloidosis in a small percentage of patients. Azotemia and urinary complications appear with progression of the disease. Involvement of the tubules may cause bicarbonaturia, renal tubular acidosis, and nephrogenic diabetes insipidus. Urinary sediment reveals typical findings seen in the nephrotic syndrome.

Treatment of the underlying disorder may rarely be associated with the improvement or even disappearance of renal amyloidosis. Steroids and immunosuppressives are not helpful. Peniciliamine, colchicine and dimethyl sulfoxide (DMS) have been reported useful in isolated cases.

The disease generally progresses slowly over a number of years to end-stage renal failure.

Glomerulopathy Associated With Malignancies. Nephrotic syndrome can occur in association with Hodgkin's disease and lymphoproliferative disorders. Renal biopsy is compatible usually with a diagnosis of lipoid nephrosis; however, some patients may show membranous nephropathy. Proteinuria can precede the discovery of malignancy by several months. Nephrotic syndrome has been also described in association with several solid tumors. Immune complexes composed of tumor-associated antigen and antibody have been implicated in the pathogenesis of glomerular lesions in many patients.

Glomerulopathies in Hereditary Diseases

Hereditary Nephritis. This condition is also known as Alport's syndrome. The disease is inherited as an autosomal dominant, affects men more severly than women, and is often transmitted by the mother. Nerve deafness is frequently present.

When renal function is normal the biopsy may show RBC casts in the tubules on light microscopy. The glomeruli may be normal. In advanced cases chronic glomerulonephritis or interstitial nephritis may be seen. Fat-laden cells called foam cells are often seen in the interstitium. They are, however, not specific for this disease. On electron microscopy, splitting of the glomerular basement membrane may be present. Immunofluorescence is usually negative.

Hematuria preceded by a systemic infection is frequently the presenting symptom. Proteinuria is usually mild. With progressive renal insufficiency, hypertension is common. History of nerve deafness and renal disease in immediate relatives is helpful in the diagnosis.

In addition to proteinuria, the urine frequently reveals RBCs and RBC casts.

There is no definitive treatment known for this disease. Control of hypertension and treatment of urinary tract infections can forestall renal failure. Symptomatic treatment of renal failure in the early stages, and dialysis and transplatation when end-stage renal disease develops are indicated.

Most male patients develop end-stage renal failure by age 40. Women only rarely get to this stage.

Fabry's Disease (Glycosphingolipidosis). This is also known as an angiokeratoma corporis diffusum. It is a familial disorder characterized by deposition of an abnormal glycolipid, galactosylgalactosylglucosyl ceramide in vascular smooth muscle, the myocardium, sympathetic ganglia, the central nervous system, and the renal glomeruli. This disorder of metabolism is due to deficiency of the enzyme α-galactosidase.

On light microscopy the epithelial cells of the glomerular capillaries have a honeycomb appearnace. The arteries also show deposition of the glycolipid. Electron microscopy reveals presence of round, laminated, electron-dense bodies called myelin figures in the epithelial cells. Immunofluorescence is negative.

Punctate, red-purple papules on the skin of the lower trunk, thighs, and scrotum are typically present. In addition, the patients also complain of acroparesthesias, leg edema, heat intolerance, unexplained attacks of fever, and pain. Proteinuria usually develops in the second decade of life; uremia and hypertension appear in the fourth or fifth decade. Urine sediment shows lipid globules containing foam cells. These are called mulberry bodies. Serum, urine and tissue levels of the specific α-galactosidase are depressed.

It has been reported that renal transplantation may provide a source of the deficient enzyme and reverse the disease; however, this therapy has not proved as effective as originally claimed. Symptomatic treatment of uremia, followed by dialysis and transplanatation, are required for renal failure. Phenytoid combined with carbamazepine and low dose corticosteroid therapy provides symptomatic relief from pain.

Most male patients develop end-stage renal disease by the fifth decade of life. Women, however, seldom develop end-stage renal disease due to Fabry's disease.

The information on histopathologic lesions and serum complement levels is summarized in Table 1.

TUBULOINTERSTITIAL DISEASES

Acute Pyelonephritis

The term implies the immediate effects of bacterial infections of the kidney. The most common infecting organisms are *Eschericia coli, Proteus marabilis,* and *Pseudomonas aeruginosa.* Infection when present without urinary obstruction can usually be traced to instrumentation of the urinary tract. Most cases of acute pyelonephritis result from infection ascending the urinary column from the bladder. Hematogenous pyelonephritis occurs most often in immunosuppressed and terminal patients. Diabetes, urinary tract obstruction, and vesicoureteral reflux predispose to acute and chronic pyelonephritis.

The kidneys are usually swollen and small abscesses may be seen on the surface throughout the kidney but occur mainly in the cortex. In mild infections, the inflammation may involve only the pelvis of the kidney. The microscopic changes are usually patchy. Polymorphonuclear leukocyte infiltration and microabscesses may be present in the inner part of the medulla. Glomeruli and blood vessels are usually spared. Lymphocytes and plasma cells may also be present.

The symptoms generally develop rapidly, within a few hours. Aching pain in the flank with high fever (103-105°F) and shaking chills are the characteristic symptoms. Nonspecific

Table 1. Histopathologic Lesions and Serum Complement in Various Glomerulopathies

Glomerulopathy	*Light Microscopy*	*Electron Microscopy*	*Immunofluorescence*	*Serum Complement*
I. Lipoid nephrosis	Normal	Swelling and fusion of the foot processes	Negative	Normal
II. Focal glomerulosclerosis	Focal and segmental mesangial sclerosis of the juxtamedullary glomeruli	Foot process fusion, mesangial deposits, and sclerosis	Granular deposits of IgM and C3 in a segmental distribution	Normal
III. Membranous glomerulopathy	Diffuse uniform capillary wall thickening	Thickening, vacuolation, and irregularity of the basement membrane along with electron dense deposits	Heavy granular IgG and C3 deposits	Normal
IV. Proliferative glomerulonephritis				
A. Acute poststreptococcal glomerulonephritis	Capillary wall cell proliferation and exudation	Subepithelial "humps"	Nodular deposits of IgG and C3	Low C3 initially
B. Membranoproliferative glomerulonephritis	Lobular accentuation with mesangial proliferation, "tram-tracking" of the basement membrane, and exudation	Electron dense deposits; intramembranous deposits splitting the basement membrane	Lumpy, bumpy IgG, C3, IgM, IgA, and fibrin	Persistently low C3 and properdin
C. Focal glomerulonephritis (Berger's disease)	Focal and segmental increase in mesangial matrix	Mesangial hypercellularity	Mesangial IgA deposits; sometimes IgG, C3, and fibrin.	Normal
D. Latent glomerulonephritis	Residual hypercellularity	Granular subepithelial deposits	IgG, IgA, and C3 in the central stalk area	Normal
V. Chronic glomerulonephritis	Glomerular hyalinization, interstitial scarring, and tubular atrophy	Mesangial sclerosis, occasionally mesangial deposits.	No consistent pattern	Normal
VI. Anti-GBM disease				
Goodpasture's syndrome and rapidly progressive glomerulonephritis	Crescent formation, focal proliferation, and necrosis	Subendothelial fibrin deposits	Linear IgG, IgM, and C3	Normal
VII. Glomerulonephritis associated with systemic disorders				
A. Connective tissue disorders				
1. Systemic lupus erythematosus	Minimal focal and segmental proliferation; diffuse membranous thickening; generalized or focal, segmental or diffuse proliferation, necrosis, and crescent formation	Minimal focal sclerosis Epimembranous deposits and irregular thickening of the basement membrane; microtubular deposits. Subendothelial, mesangial, and subepithelial deposits; microtubular deposits	No pattern Confluent capillary lumpy, bumpy IgG, IgM, and IgA Capillary and mesangial lumpy, bumpy IgG, IgM, IgA, C3, and C1q	Usually normal Low C1-C9 Low C1-C9
2. Polyarteritis nodosa, Wegener's granulomotosis	Generalized or focal fibrinoid necrosis of glomeruli, adhesions, proliferation, and occasional crescent formation.	Fibrin deposition with mesangial proliferation; no deposits	Mesangial and subendothelial fibrin	Normal
3. Scleroderma	Fibrinoid necrosis, intimal thickening, and patchy necrosis of the arterioles	No specific changes	Fibrin, IgM, $C1_a$, C4 and C3 deposition in the arterioles and glomeruler capillaries	Normal
B. Disorders of coagulation				
1. Toxemia of pregnancy	Capillaries occluded by swollen epithelial cells	Focal basement membrane thickening	Fibrin deposits	Normal

Table 1. Histopathologic Lesions and Serum Complement in Various Glomerulopathies (Cont.)

Glomerulopathy	*Light Microscopy*	*Electron Microscopy*	*Immunofluorescence*	*Serum Complement*
2. Postpartum renal failure	Advanced nephrosclerosis, cortical necrosis; fibrin microthrombi in the glomeruli	Noncontributory	Noncontributory	Normal
3. Hemolytic-uremic syndrome	Fibrin thrombi in the glomerular capillaries; cortical necrosis	Noncontributory	Noncontributory	Normal
4. Henoch-Schönlein purpura	Focal or diffuse proliferation with segmental necrosis; crescent formation	Dense deposits in the subendothelial and mesangial regions; splitting of the basement membrane	IgA, IgG and properdin deposits	Normal
5. Thrombotic thrombocytopenic purpura	Focal or diffuse fibrinoid necrosis	Basement membrane thickening	Fibrin deposits in the glomerular capillary loops	Normal
C. Metabolic disorders				
1. Diabetes	Nodular or diffuse glomerulosclerosis	Basement membrane thickening	In certain patients linear IgG and IgM deposits	Normal
2. Amyloidosis	Amorphous, homogenous extracellular deposit	Accumulation of 75-80 Å fibrils	IgG because of light chains	Normal
VIII. Heredofamilial diseases				
A. Alport's syndrome	Proliferative changes; foam cells	Splitting of the basement membrane	Negative	Normal
B. Fabry's disease	Honeycomb appearance of the glomerular capillaries	Myelin figures in the epithelial cells	Negative	Normal

gastrointestinal and urinary tract symptoms are often present. Frequently, there is tenderness on pressure in one or both subcostal areas. In mild infections the symptoms subside spontaneously. In severe infections they persist despite appropriate antibiotic treatment for 4-7 days.

Polymorphonuclear leukocytosis is often present. The urine sediment reveals clumps of leukocytes and WBC casts with occasional red blood cells. When there is severe cystitis, gross hematuria may be present. Typically, examination of uncentrifuged urine under the microscope reveals bacteria. For confirmation of the diagnosis, 100,000 colonies/ml is essential. Less than 10,000 colonies/ml usually indicates contamination. Carefully performed intravenous pyelogram may show hypotony of the calicyes, pelvis, and ureters. Stones, tumor, or scarring from tuberculosis, which may predispose an individual to acute pyelonephritis, can usually be diagnosed on IVP. Kidney biopsy is of limited value.

Prompt treatment with an appropriate antibiotic is the hallmark of therapy. After appropriate cultures are obtained ampicillin or amoxicillin, administered orally or parenterally 1-1-4 g daily, depending upon the severity of infection, is the treatment of choice. When the urine culture report becomes available, if the organism is insensitive to the already administered antibiotic, the appropriate antibiotic should be initiated immediately. Encouragement of oral fluids or adminstration of intravenous fluids, depending upon the patient's condition, is necessary to avoid dehydration due to high fever and to maintain adequate urine output. The antibiotic treatment should be contiued for at least 10 days even though symptoms disappear. A repeat culture should be obtained in 2 months to assure a complete cure. In patients with recurrent acute pyelonephritis, suppression of infection can be achieved by daily administration of 0.5-1 g of a soluable short-acting sulfonamide such as sulfisoxazole (Gantrisin). Recurrent acute pyelonephritis is best treated with a combination of trimethoprim and sulfamethoxazole available as co-trimoxazole (Bactrim, Septra).

Except in patients with papillary necrosis such as may occur in sickle cell disease, diabetes, analgesic abuse, and urinary tract occlusions, the symptoms of acute pyelonephritis readily subside with treatment. It is not always possible to gauge which patients will go on to develop renal insufficiency following recurrent episodes of acute pyelonephritis.

Renal and Perinephric Abscess

Renal abscess may result from hematogenous spread of a distant infection usually from staphylococci or as a complication of acute pyelonephritis with one of the Gram-negative organisms such as *E. coli*, *Proteus sp.*, and *Klebsiella-Enterobacter*. Perinephric abscess results from rupture of a renal abscess into surrounding tissues.

A distinct abscess cavity in the interstitium of the renal

medulla is usually present. With antibiotic therapy the abscess may partially heal with a thick wall around it, causing a chronic renal carbuncle. On microscopic examination, collections of polymorphonuclear leukocytes can be seen in and around the tubules. The glomeruli are usually normal. The perinephric abscess is usually confined to the area around the kidney, but may rupture into the abdominal cavity or through the diaphragm into the pleural space.

The diagnosis is frequently missed since it is not suspected. The onset is usually abrupt with fever and chills accompanied by dysuria and costovertebral pain. Tenderness and spasm in the flank area and a palpable mass may be present. Elevation of the diaphragm on the side of the abscess may lead to an erroneous diagnosis of subphrenic infection. Psoas muscle involvement may cause the patient to keep the thigh on the involved side in flexion.

Urinary sediment often contains red blood cells and pus. Urine culture usually reveals the infecting organism.

A roentgenogram may reveal a mass in the renal area. The kidney margins are blurred and the psoas indistinct. The kidney may be displaced with scoliosis on the side of the lesion. There may be gas in the perinephric area that should not be confused with gas in the colon. Chest x-ray may show basal infiltrates and pleural effusion.

Administration of appropriate antibiotics, hydration, analgesics, and, most importantly, surgical drainage constitute appropriate treatment for this condition.

Many patients with perinephric abscess carry the diagnosis of fever of unknown origin (FUO) for varying lengths of time and the condition goes undiagnosed. The overall prognosis is, therefore, poor. If a diagnosis is made early and appropriate treatment rendered, the prognosis is good. Concomitant diabetes mellitus, uremia, septicemia, and urinary tract obstruction make the prognosis worse. Surgical treatment of obstruction, when present, is of paramount importance.

Chronic Interstitial Nephritis

Chronic interstitial nephritis is the preferred term for what used to be called chronic pyelonephritis. There is a great deal of uncertainty regarding the true prevalence of chronic nonobstructive pyelonephritis. Since the realization that not every chronic interstitial nephritis is bacterial in origin, the diagnosis of chronic pyelonephritis is not as commonly made as before. As obstruction is found only infrequently, it is believed that certain factors may make the kidney susceptible to infection leading to chronic bacterial pyelonephritis.

The kidneys appear shrunken and irregular in outline due to underlying scars. Light microscopy reveals a chronic inflammatory reaction with foci of lymphocytes and plasma cells in the interstitium. Eventually there is extensive scar tissue formation. The glomeruli initially appear normal. With progression of the disease they appear shrunken and surrounded by a cuff of fibrosis. The tubules appear distorted, some small and some dilated, containing large amounts of homogenous amorphous material giving the appearance of thyroid tissue (thyroidization of the kidneys). Vascular involvement varies. With the appearance of hypertension there is afferent arteriolar sclerosis. Papillary sclerosis and deformity along with dilated calyces is considered characteristic of chronic interstitial nephritis.

A patient with chronic interstitial nephritis may present with varying manifestations. Even though the patient may be entirely asymptomatic, urinalysis reveals WBCs, WBC casts, slight protein, and bacteria. In the second group of patients, the BUN on a screening test may be found to be elevated with minimal abnormality on urinalysis. A third group of patients may present with florid symptoms and signs of uremia without any previous history of renal disease.

Mechanical obstruction must always be excluded. Enlarged prostate, congenital malformations of the urinary tract, kidney stones, neurogenic bladder, and vesicoureteral reflux may predispose to chronic interstitial nephritis. In most patients with chronic interstitial nephritis there is no evidence of obstruction. Other causes of chronic interstitial nephritis such as analgesic abuse, heavy metal poisoning, urate nephropathy, chronic potassium depletion, nephrocalcinosis, and tuberculosis should be considered in the differential diagnosis. Hypertension is frequently present. Unexplained splenomegaly is not uncommon finding. Nephrotic syndrome is seldom seen.

Urine sediment may reveal leukocytes and leukocyte casts. Presence of immunoglobulins on the surface of WBCs is believed to indicate pyelonephritis rather than cystitis. The urine culture may be positive. Twenty-four-hour urine protein is usually less than 1.5 g. Due to renal tubular function abnormality the patient may have polyuria, decreased concentration, sodium wasting, and hyperchloremic acidosis due to inadequate secretion of acid by the kidney. With progression of the disease, BUN and creatinine rise and other biochemical abnormalities of uremia appear.

Renal biopsy is of little help as the histologic changes are patchy and the biopsy needle may not hit the abnormal tissue.

If a remediable obstructing lesion or other reversible abnormality is present, it should be corrected promptly. Appropriate antimicrobial therapy on the basis of urine culture findings is usually undertaken. Hypertension when present is treated, which may help prevent further renal damage. Appropriate treatment to delay the symptoms of uremia and correct the biochemical abnormalities is also indicated. With development of end-stage renal disease, dialysis is initiated and the patient considered for renal transplantation.

Radiation Nephritis

When in a period of 5 weeks or less a dose of 2300 rads is administered to the kidneys, radiation nephritis may result. The kidneys are probably the most radiosensitive major organ in the body. With appropriate shielding the condition can be avoided in most instances.

The most remarkable finding occurs in the blood vessels where fibrinoid necrosis and fibrosis of the intima and hyalinization of the media is a common finding. As the disease progresses other components of the renal tissue become involved. The glomeruli show focal necrosis, proliferation, and hyalinization. The tubules are atrophic and there is extensive interstitial fibrosis.

The clinical presentation may be acute when the clinical

manifestations appear within 6 months of radiation, or chronic when manifestations appear insidiously 1 year or later after radiation. The clinical manifestations include: proteinuria, hypertension, edema, and renal insufficiency. Hypertension may be mild or severe.

Antihypertensive therapy to control hypertension is indicated. If malignant hypertension is due to unilateral radiation nephritis, removal of the affected kidney may relieve the condition. Treatment of the uremic manifestations by appropriate medical therapy and hemodialysis is indicated. Since radiation may also involve the ureters, the bladder, and may cause abdominal adhesions, renal transplantation may not be feasible.

In acute cases mortality may be 50%; the remaining patients gradually improve.

Hypersensitivity Nephritis

Acute tubulointerstitial nephritis due to hypersensitivity may occur in certain patients treated with sulfonamides, methicillin, or large doses of other penicillins, diuretics such as furosemide, thiazides, and other drugs. The condition is reversible when the triggering agent is discontinued.

Patchy interstitial accumulation of lymphocytes, plasma cells, and eosinophils is the characteristic histologic picture on light microscopy. On immunofluorescence there is usually no vasculitis. Allergic manifestions such as fever, eosinophilia, and a pruritic rash may be present. Mild to moderate proteinuria and varying degrees of hematuria are usually observed. Oliguria may be a prominent manifestation, causing the condition to be confused with acute tubular necrosis or acute glomerulonephritis.

Withdrawal of the inciting agent and treatment with prednisone are indicated.

If the condition is diagnosed early and appropriately treated, the prognosis is excellent.

Disorders Associated with Metabolic Derangements

Hypercalcemic Nephropathy

Renal tubular injury may result with persistent hypercalcemia. The disease is insidious in onset and progresses slowly. Regardless of the cause for hypercalcemia, changes in the structure and function of the kidney are usually the same. Nephrocalcinosis is not always associated with stones or with radiographic evidence of calcification in the kidneys.

The epithelium of the distal tubule and collecting ducts shows necrosis and calcification. The tubules may be blocked by calcified casts and atrophy. In late stages, calcification may involve the blood vessels, interstitium, and the glomeruli. As hypertension develops, nephrosclerosis occurs.

Polyuria and polydypsia are usually the early signs of impaired urinary concentration. Renal tubular injury may occur. Fanconi's syndrome comprising glucosuria, aminoaciduria, and phosphaturia may be manifest. Hypertension is common when nephroacalcinosis is established but may occur with acute hypercalcemia. Urine sediment may contain red blood cells and leukocytes. Proteinuria is uncommon. Polyuria, salt depletion, and dehydration may occur, causing azotemia that may progress as a consequence of tubular obstruction. Hypercalciuria may lead to nephrolithiasis complicated by pyelonephritis. KUB may demonstrate nephrocalcinosis chiefly in the region of the renal pyramids.

The cause for hypercalcemia should be promptly detected and specific treatment, if any, rendered. Hypercalcemia, if severe, may have to be treated promptly with hydration and furosemide (Lasix) administration. Mithramycin (Mithracin) and phosphate infusion are only necessary when hypercalcemia does not respond to hydration and diuretic therapy. Hemodialysis against a calcium-free dialysate may have to be undertaken in rare circumstances.

The prognosis depends on the severity and chronicity. Renal failure of recent onset due to hypercalcemia is completely reversible. The prognosis is poor if nephrosclerosis and pyelonephritis are present.

Hyperuricemic Nephropathy

Urate calculi may develop in approximately 15% of patients with gout. Acute hyperuricemia during treatment of leukemia, polycythemia vera, lymphoma, or other malignançies may pre cipitate acute renal failure. Regardless of the treatment, destruction of malignant cells releases large amounts of nuclear protein that are metabolized to uric acid.

Urate crystals are deposited in the interstitium and the medulla of the kidney. Obstruction of the renal tubules and urinary tract with urate calculi may lead to pyelonephritis. Hypertension leads to nephrosclerosis.

Reduction in concentrating ability, mild proteinuria, and slowly progressive azotemia are the usual clinical manifestations. Hypertension is common. Urine sediment is usually nonrevealing.

Hydration and allopurinol (Zyloprim) therapy constitute the cornerstones of treatment. Uricosuric agents are contraindicated. Attempts to alkalinize the urine with sodium bicarbonate without adequate hydration may cause percipitation of sodium urate crystals that are less soluble than uric acid.

Hypokalemic Nephropathy

It is not certain how long a potassium deficiency must persist before renal damage results. In most instances, hypokalemia is of several years duration. The usual causes of hypokalemia are primary aldosteronism, diuretic therapy, Cushing's syndrome, Fanconi's syndrome, and gastrointestinal loses such as chronic diarrhea and vomiting.

The renal tubular epithelial cells, particularly those of the distal convoluted tubule and cortical collecting ducts, show multiple vacuoles. The glomeruli and blood vessels are usually normal.

Most patients are asymptomatic; however, nocturia, polyuria, and polydypsia may be prominent. Urinalysis may reveal slight proteinuria and cylindruria but is very often normal. Azotemia results only with dehydration and onset of pyelonephritis. Renal potassium wasting is usually a manifestation of the underlying disorder of adrenal or renal origin.

Treatment of the underlying disease causing hypokalemia

is important. Correction of hypokalemia with potassium replacement or potassium-sparing diuretics prevents further renal damage and leads to improvement.

Prognosis is good when the disease is treated early. In the late stages, irreversible damage to urinary concentrating ability may result.

Renal Tubular Acidosis

Two main types of renal tubular acidosis (RTA) are recognized; distal (classic or type I) and proximal (type II). A hybrid of RTA with both distal and proximal acidification defects is termed Type III RTA. Type IV RTA is hyporenenimic hypoaldosteromism present in some patients with diabetes and mild chronic renal insufficiency. The primary defect in the distal RTA lies in the kidney's ability to produce a H^+ gradient between urine and blood at the distal tubule. In the proximal RTA the bicarbonate absorption in the proximal tubule is defective. Both forms can occur either as a primary disease or secondary to other causes.

Distal Renal Tubular Acidosis (Type I RTA). The usual manifestation of RTA is hyperchloremic metabolic acidosis of varying severity with an inappropriately high urine pH, usually >6.0. When the disease appears as a primary disorder, it manifests early in life. It is more common in women. Osteomalacia, hyperphosphaturia, hypophosphatemia, bone pains, and gait disturbances are common. Hypercalciuria is another common feature of the disease, frequently causing nephrocalcinosis and renal calculi. As potassium is exchanged for sodium in the distal tubule due to the latter's inability to secrete hydrogen ion, hypokalemia results. It leads to muscle weakness and, in long-standing cases, to hypokalemic nephropathy. Renal insufficiency appears in the late stages due to urinary tract obstruction from renal calculi and pyelonephritis.

Secondary distal RTA may occue in hyperglobulinemic states such as Sjögren's syndrome and cryoglobulinemia. It may occur as a result of amphotericin B (Fungizone) toxicity or toluene toxicity (glue sniffing). It has also been observed in patients with Fabry's disease

Sodium bicarbonate in a dose of 1-1.5 mEq/kg/day in three divided doses will help correct acidosis, hypercalciuria, and potassium wasting. Alkali replacement is usually better tolerated as Shohl's solution (140 g citric acid + 98 g sodium citrate/L), administered 50-100 ml/day in divided doses. Supplementary potassium, calcium, and vitamin D may be temporarily required.

Proximal Renal Tubular Acidosis (Type II RTA). Primary proximal RTA is more common in male infants and is primarily manifested by growth retardation. Hyperchloremic acidosis is also usual in this type of RTA; however, the urine pH is only inappropriately high at levels of serum HCO_3 between 15 and 20 mEq/L. If acidosis is severe enough a maximally acid urine with a pH below 5.5 can be produced. Osteomalacia and nephrocalcinosis are uncommon. Alkali therapy leads to marked improvement. The defect in bicarbonate reabsorption usually disappears spontaneously in a few years.

Secondary proximal RTA is observed in association with cystinuria, Wilson's disease, administration of outdated tetracyclines, heavy metal toxicity, multiple myeloma and other dysproteinemias, nephrotic syndrome, or transplant rejection. A mild form may occur with primary or secondary hyperparathyroidism.

As mentioned previously, acidosis occurs because of a bicarbonate leak. Potassium wasting results from flooding of the distal tubules with sodium ions. Thus, sodium bicarbonate therapy may exacerbate hypokalemia. Potassium supplementation is therefore often necessary. Large amounts of sodium bicarbonate or citrate are required due to urinary bicarbonate wastage. For severe bone disease Vitamin D may be indicated. Thiazides may be used to cause modest volume depletion and enhance proximal bicarbonate absorption.

Toxic Nephropathy

Toxic nephropathy may be defined as a functional or structural alteration in the kidney caused by a chemical or biologic product. There are several reasons for vulnerability of the kidney to toxins. Some of the more important ones are large blood supply, high oxygen consumption, large vascular endothelial surface, high solute concentrations achieved in the medulla because of the countercurrent mechanism, high intratubular concentration, uncoupling of protein-toxin binding by the renal tubule, and effects of the toxins on the enzymatic activity in the renal epithelial cells. There are several mechanisms by which various nephrotoxic agents can cause kidney disease. They may have a direct effect on the nephron, induce an immune reaction causing nephrotic syndrome, produce angitis or vasculitis, cause a chronic interstitial nephritis, or predispose to secondary renal disease such as pyelonephritis. Although many substances are found to be nephrotoxic there are three main classes of nephrotoxic agents; heavy metals, solvents, and drugs including antibiotics.

Heavy Metals

Mercury toxicity is the prototype of heavy metal-induced kidney damage. Other heavy metals that may produce kidney damage include arsenic, bismuth, cadmium, gold, iron, lead, silver, and uranium.

Mercury Poisoning. Acute inorganic mercury poisoning causes tubular necrosis and renal failure. Organic mercury and prolonged exposure to inorganic mercury can cause nephrotic syndrome and chronic renal damage. Inorganic mercury poisoning can occur by accident or in suicide attempts. Mercury exposure may occur during the manufacturing of paint, alloys, and scientific instruments. Exposure to disinfectants and pesticides may occur in farming. Medicinal sources of organic mercury include mercurial diuretics, merbromin (Mercurochrome), and ammoniated mercury ointments used in the treatment of psoriasis. Urinary concentration of inorganic mercury does not normally exceed 1 μg/L.

Granular or vascular degeneration of the epithelium of the proximal tubular usually occurs quite early. This change is followed by calcification at the site of necrosis. By combining with sulfhydryl groups in the mitochondria of the mucous membranes, heavy metal poisoning leads to disintegration of mitochondria, necrosis of nuclei, and loss in enzyme activity of the gastrointestinal tract cells. Mercury deposition also involves the liver, spleen, myocardium, and cerebral cortex causing cellular degeneration in those organs.

Acute severe mercury poisoning is manifested by symptoms of gastroenteritis, circulatory collapse, and acute renal failure. The urinalysis shows albuminuria, glucosuria, aminoaciduria (Fanconi's syndrome due to proximal tubular damage), epithelial cell casts, and erythrocytes. Urinary concentration of mercury is very high, usually in excess of 100 μg/L.

Prevention is extremely important. Acute ingestion is a medical emergency. Attempts should be made to remove mercury from the stomach by inducing vomiting or lavage. Activated charcoal is then administered for adsorption of the remaining mercury in organic mercurial salts. Dimercaprol (BAL) is an effective antidote. Intramuscular injections of 2.5-3 mg/kg are administered every 4 hours. Depending upon the severity of mercury poisoning up to six injections may be needed. Dialysis can be used in severe cases to remove the mercury-BAL complexes.

Prognosis is good if the overdose is treated early.

Solvent and Glycol-Induced Nephropathy

Carbon tetrachloride is the prototype of solvent-induced nephropathy and ethylene glycol (antifreeze) is a typical example of an agent causing glycol-induced nephropathy.

Carbon Tetrachloride Poisoning. Carbon tetrachloride is used as a cleaning agent, grease solvent, vermifuge, and a fire-extinguishing material. Both inhalation and ingestion can cause nephrotoxicity. The toxicity is aggravated by simultaneous alcohol ingestion.

The primary damage occurs in the renal tubule. The proximal tubules are dilated and the epithelial cells swollen. Bile-stained cellular and hyaline casts can be identified in the distal tubules.

Gastrointestinal symptoms are usually the first to appear. Oliguria and anuria usually occur a week later. Neurologic symptoms and manifestations of liver damage are also common. Urinary findings include proteinuria, hematuria, cylindruria, and uric acid crystaluria. Due to hepatic damage and impairment of the hepatic urea synthesis, the creatinine/BUN ratio is usually considerably higher than 11%; this is also generally observed in other causes of acute renal failure.

Removal of the patient from the area of exposure, adequate ventilation and removal of carbon tetrachloride by gastric lavage, catharsis, or cleaning of the skin are important therapeutic measures. Appropriate treatment for liver failure, renal failure, and hemorrhagic complications should then be undertaken. Avoidance of alcohol during exposure is of paramount importance to prevent carbon tetrachloride toxicity.

If carbon tetrachloride poisoning is detected early and alcohol avoided, the prognosis is good.

Ethylene Glycol Poisoning. Ethylene glycol is a colorless, odorless liquid commonly used as antifreeze in automobile radiators. Approximately 10% is metabolized rapidly to oxalic acid that crystalizes in the kidneys and meninges. Approximately 100 ml of ethylene glycol can prove fatal.

The light microscopy shows tubular dilatation and necrosis along with intraluminal calcium oxalate crystallization. Interstitial reaction consisting of edema and mononuclear cell infiltration is common. In addition to the kidneys and brain, the lung and heart are also involved.

After ingestion of ethylene glycol, central nervous system manifestations resembling ethanol intoxication occur within 30 minutes. In the next 12 to 24 hours signs of severe cardiopulmonary distress develop. After the first day, flank pain, tenderness, proteinuria, and oxalate crystaluria develop. Anuria and metabolic acidosis due to oxalic acid and uremia lead to death.

Ethylene glycol poisoning is a medical emergency. Infusion of sodium bicarbonate and removal of circulating ethylene glycol and oxalic acid by hemodialysis are indicated. Subsequent management of acute renal failure may be necessary if anuria develops.

Drug-Induced Renal Damage

Both diagnostic agents, such as contrast media, and therapeutic agents, such as sulfonamides and antibiotics, can cause renal damage.

Contrast Media-Induced Renal Damage. Contrast media used for intravenous pyelography, angiography, and cholecystography can cause renal damage. The incidence rises as the dose delivered to the kidney is increased. Possible mechanisms of nephrotoxicity include direct cellular toxicity, reduction in renal blood flow and GFR, intrarenal osmotic effects, obstructuve crystaluria due to uric acid crystals and idiosyncrasy to the contrast medium. Although all contrast media contain iodine, it is not clear if iodine plays a role in nephrotoxicity.

Contrast media-induced nephrotoxicity is particularly common in patients with multiple myeloma and diabetes who are dehydrated before administration of the dye. Proliferative changes in the glomeruli and vacuolar degeneration of the proximal tubules has been described. Medullary necrosis has been reported following angiography in children. Interstitial hemorrhage and uric acid depositon in the tubules also contribute to nephrotoxicity.

Oliguria is usually the first manifestation of nephrotoxicity following administration of the contrast media. Anuria and azotemia may follow. Urinalysis reveals proteinuria, hemauria, cylindruria, and pyuria.

Contrast media should be avoided in patients with multiple myeloma, other dysgammaglobulinemias, and diabetes. If it is essential to perform such a radiographic study, the patient should be well hydrated and only the minimal necessary amount of contrast medium should be administered. Once nephrotoxicity occurs hydration of the patient and, if necessary, dialysis to overcome the acute renal failure phase constitute appropriate treatment.

Antimicrobial-Induced Renal Damage. Nephrotoxicity due to drugs has been described in association with sulfonamides, aminoglycoside antibiotics such as gentamicin (Garamycin), kanamycin (Kantrex), tobramycin (Nebcin), and other antibiotics such as neomycin (Mycifradin, Myciguent), cephalosporins, and amphotericin B (Fungizone). Polymyxin B (Aerosporin) and colistin (Coly-Mycin) were previously used in the treatment of pseudomonal infections but are no longer in common use because of nephrotoxicity. Underlying impairment of renal function increases this complication of antibiotic therapy. The incidence of nephrotoxicity increases with age. In most cases nephrotoxicity is dose related. Administration of more than one nephrotoxic antibiotic increases the incidence and severity of nephrotoxicity.

Gentamicin toxicity is the prototype of aminoglycoside-induced renal damage. Slight proteinuria and progressive azotemia are the usual clinical manifestations. Histopathology reveals dilated tubules, flattened epithelium, and interstitial edema. The condition is usually reversible upon discontinuing the drug. It is best avoided by altering the dose based on serum creatinine and monitoring gentamicin levels.

Intrarenal crystallization with degeneration and necrosis of the tubular epithelium used to be a common complication with sulfonamide therapy. Hypersensitivity reaction may be characterized by interstitial inflammation. The usual clinical manifestations are flank pain, occasional renal colic or anuria, hematuria, crystaluria, leukocyturia, cylindruria, and azotemia. The use of soluble sulfonamides has made sulfonamide toxicity due to crystallization a rare event. If crystallization occurs, hydration and alkali therapy should be undertaken immediately.

Cephaloridine (Loridine), the most toxic of all cephalosporins, is no longer used. The presently available cephlosporins have minimal nephrotoxicity. However, when used in combination with gentamicin (Garamycin) or in patients with compromised renal function, nephrotoxicity may be seen. It is manifested by proteinuria, cylindruria, hematuria, and azotemia. It is usually reversible on discontinuing the drug.

Despite its nephrotoxicity, the beneficial antifungal effect of amphotericin B (Fungizone) calls for its continued judicious use. The development of azotemia requires reduction in dosage or cessation of therapy. The predominant findings are tubular dilatation and necrosis. The renal damage is usually reversible.

Acute Tubular Necrosis

Often the term acute renal failure is used to indicate acute tubular necrosis (ATN), previously known as lower nephron nephrosis. Acute renal failure can occur due to many causes other than acute tubular necrosis. Acute renal failure is discussed in a later section of this chapter. The term acute tubular necrosis is used to indicate the clinical and pathologic syndrome that results from tubular dysfunction and/or degeneration usually caused by renal ischemia. Certain toxic agents as described above can also cause renal tubular damage.

Acute tubular necrosis occurs typically in a setting of hypotension, shock, and intense vasoconstriction. Common causes are extensive burns, rapid hemorrhage, hypotension on the operating table, septicemic shock, crush injuries, mismatched blood transfusion, and distilled water infusion, such as may occur during transurethral prostatectomy. Renal ischemia during cardiac, aortic, or renovascular surgery may also cause varying degrees of acute tubular necrosis. Placenta previa, septic abortion, postpartum hemorrhage, or eclampsia may also cause acute tubular necrosis. Dehydration and renal ischemia predispose to kidney damage caused by nephrotoxic agents.

Renal injury caused by ischemia affects parts of the nephron at random. Complete destruction of the tubular lining occurs in a scattered fashion along the course of an otherwise well-preserved nephron. The basement membrane may also be disrupted. The glomeruli are generally intact unless renal cortical necrosis has occurred. Epithelial and hemoglobin casts can be seen in the tubules of the medulla. In renal tubular damage caused by toxins the basement membrane is spared. There is frequently a poor correlation between the degree of tubular damage and the degree of impairment in renal function. Thus it has been suggested that as yet poorly understood pathophysiologic mechanisms have important roles in the development of acute renal failure.

Oliguria lasting 2-8 weeks is the most characteristic feature of ATN. This is succeeded by a diuretic phase lasting 1-4 weeks. During the second week of ATN, symptoms of azotemia may be quite marked. Due to fluid overload, pulmonary congestion and cardiac failure may appear during the oliguric phase. Diastolic hypertension occurs in approximately 25% of patients during the second week of oliguria. Arrhythmias and pericarditis are not uncommon. Pulmonary and blood stream infections with hospital organisms frequently occur and are a common cause of death. Coma and convulsion are not uncommon in these patients.

Urinalysis reveals mild to moderate proteinuria, slight hematuria, and glucosuria. The urine osmolality is usually low or normal; however, the specific gravity may be high owing to the presence of red blood cells and protein. Serum amylase and lipase concentrations may be elevated due to their low renal clearance. BUN, serum creatinine, and phosphate are elevated and continue to rise until either the renal failure reverses or dialysis is instituted. Metabolic acidosis and hyperkalemia occur due to inability to excrete H^+ and K^+ and enhanced catabolism of the body tissues. Anemia usually occurs in the second week probably due to subclinical bleeding, increased hemolysis, and relative bone marrow suppression. Coagulation deficiencies in the form of thrombocytopenia and abnormal prothrombin consumption time are not uncommon.

Prevention of ATN is of paramount importance. Avoidance of dehydration and rapid correction of hemorrhagic or septic shock will help to achieve this. After fluid volume is restored, diuresis with mannitol or furosemide (Lasix) is also helpful.

Correction of the circulatory failure that may have initiated ATN is usually the first priority. However, overhydration must be avoided by careful monitoring of the pulmonary artery pressure or at least the central venous pressure. As oliguria progresses, fluid restriction becomes necessary. Under the average environmental and body temperature conditions, 600 ml plus the measured daily fluid loses in the urine, diarrheal stools, and gastric suction should be adminstered on a daily basis. Ideally the patient should lose ¼ to ½ lb daily as a result of consuming intrinsic fat calories. Intake of 100-150 g of carbohydrate is essential to avoid rapid breakdown of body tissues. Juices should be avoided because of their high potassium content. Oral feedings should not be attempted in the presence of nausea or vomiting because of fear of aspiration. Hyperalimentation has been demonstrated to increase survival and possibly reduce the duration of renal failure. Potassium intoxication is treated by administration of a potassium-exchange resin such as sodium polystyrene sulfonate (Kayexalate). Dialysis may be necessary if hyperkalemia is not controlled or reversed by Kayexalate. Heart failure is treated with digoxin in half the usual dosage. Monitoring the digoxin blood level is quite helpful in this situation. Treatment of infections with appropriate antibiotics in reduced doses, taking into account the patient's renal failure status, is extremely important. However, prophylactic antibiotics should be avoided. Correction of acidosis with sodium bicarbonate may be necessary. The major indications for dialysis are uncontrollable hyperkalemia, fluid overload causing pulmonary edema, and severe uremic symptoms. Close attention should be paid to the nutritional status of these patients utilizing hyperalimentation if oral intake is not possible.

Although ATN is theoretically reversible, the mortality remains high in spite of careful medical management and dialysis, due primarily to the nature and severity of the patient's underlying problem. Rapid reversal of the underlying cause and precipitating event is helpful. If renal ischemia is prolonged, acute cortical necrosis with destruction of the glomeruli may occur which is not reversible.

VASCULAR DISEASES OF THE KIDNEY

In this section, those diseases of the kidney that involve primarily the vascular system or have vascular involvement as the intitating event will be discussed.

Nephrosclerosis

Structural alterations occur in the small arteries and arterioles of almost all patients with essential hypertension. Similar but less marked changes are found in about 10% of nomotensive patients on postmortem examination. The severity increases with age. Nephrosclerosis probably is responsible for the mild renal insufficiency often observed in elderly patients.

Medium-sized and small arteries and arterioles show intimal thickening. As the disease progresses, ischemic damage to the glomeruli results causing hyalinization, atrophy, and scarring. Patients dying of malignant hypertension have severe intimal and medial proliferation (onion-scale thickening) and patches of necrosis of the preglomerular arterioles. Hemorrhage into Bowman's capsule and crescent formation occasionally may be seen.

Elevated blood pressure is the hallmark of this condition. The retina shows arteriolar spasm narrowing and arteriovenous (AV) nicking. Patients with severe accelerated hypertension may in addition show flame-shaped hemorrhages and cotton wool exudates. The term malignant hypertension is used if papilledema is also present. Proteinuria is usually minimal; however, it may be heavy ($\geqslant$4g/dl) if severe hypertension persists for a long time causing ischemic damage to the glomerular capillaries. Microscopic hematuria is not uncommon. Occasionally gross hematuria may occur with accelerated hypertension. As renal insufficiency progress, normocytic normochromic anemia appears. Malignant hypertension is usually associated with signs of heart failure, hypertensive encephalopathy, and uremia.

Early detection and treatment of hypertension are important in preventing renal insufficiency due to nephrosclerosis. If nephrosclerosis is already present, treatment of hypertension may cause a slight deterioration of renal function. This, however, reverses with continued treatment. Patients with malignant hypertension should be treated aggressively with blood pressure reduced to a safe level. Patients who have already developed extensive renal damage may require artificial kidney support. Even if hypertension is not readily controlled with antihypertensive therapy, bilateral nephrectomy should be avoided since there are reports of return of renal function after several months of total renal failure requiring dialysis.

If hypertension is treated early, the prognosis is excellent. In patients with severe renal insufficiency and malignant hypertension, despite aggressive antihypertensive therapy, the prognosis of recovery of renal function is not good. Although these patients can be kept alive with dialysis, cardiovascular and cerebrovascular complications are common and often fatal.

Renal Arterial Occlusion

The most common cause of renal arterial occusion is embolism. This leads to partial or complete infarction of the kidney. The most common presenting features are sudden, sharp, remitting flank pain and hematuria. The BUN and creatinine are usually normal; IVP shows a nonfunctioning kidney that is normal in size. The treatment consists of anticoagulation with intravenous heparin followed by oral anticoagulants if recurrent embolism is expected. Hypertension, if present, should be agressively treated. Fever and moderate leukocytosis are common. Usually kidney function is regained, albeit slowly.

Partial renal occlusion due to atherosclerotic narrowing, and fibromuscular hyperplasia is discussed in the chapter on hypertension.

Bartter's Syndrome

Since the histopathologic lesion is in the afferent arterioles, it is classified here under vascular diseases of the kidney.

Renal biopsy shows hyperplasia of the cells of the juxtaglomerular apparatus. Although the exact pathogenesis of the syndrome remains to be understood, it is now believed that decreased absorption of chloride ions in the ascending limb of the loop of Henle is the primary abnormality. Increased secretion of prostaglandins stimulates juxtaglomerular apparatus cells causing their hyperplasia. Large amounts of renin are secreted from these cells that leads to severe hyperaldosteronism and hypokalemia.

Weakness, tiredness, lethargy, and nocturia are the predominant symptoms primarily caused by severe hypokalemia. Blood pressure is either normal or low and edema is absent. Moderate alkalosis is usually present.

Potassium repletion and spironolactone (Aldactone) is the traditional therapy for this condition. Indomethacin (indocin), a prostaglandin synthetase inhibitor, has been demonstrated to be effective in reversing hypokalemia. The combination of indomethacin 25 mg-50 mg t.i.d. and spironolactone 50-100 mg daily is now the treatment of choice.

In many patients who have the clinical and laboratory picture of Bartter's syndrome, a specific cause of chronic volume depletion such as diuretic or cathartic abuse is present. These patients are designated as having pseudo-Bartter's syndrome.

DISEASES OF THE RENAL MEDULLA

Cystic Diseases of the Kidney

Polycystic Kidneys

There are two types of polycystic kidney diseases: infantile and adult. Infantile polycystic kidney disease usually results in death in infancy or early childhood. The adut variety is an autosomal dominant condition. The disorder is bilateral although one kidney may be more involved than the other.

The kidneys enlarge with age and by the time renal failure occurs they may be five to ten times the normal size. Grapelike clusters of cysts containing clear or hemorrhagic fluid are the characteristic gross finding. The cysts perform the usual function of the nephron and communicate with the renal pelvis. In some patients there may be cysts in the liver, pancreas, and spleen; however, these are usually asymptomatic. Twenty percent of these patients have an intracranial aneurysm in the circle of Willis that may rupture, causing subarachnoid hemorrhage.

The diagnosis is often made in the course of routine physical examination or as part of an evaluation of hypertension or hematuria. The condition usually manifests between the ages of 40 and 60. However, an IVP performed at an earlier age usually reveals enlarged kidneys with elongation of the pelvis and flattening and indentation of the calyces due to the cysts. Both kidneys are usually palpable. The patients complain frequently of lumbar and abdominal ache that is often increased by exertion. Passage of clots during episodes of hematuria may cause renal colic. Symptoms of uremia usually develop after the fifth decade of life. Most patients have polyuria rather than oliguria.

Urinalysis reveals low specific gravity due to reduced concentrating ability, hematuria, and mild to moderate proteinuria. The urine sediment reveals hyaline and granular casts. Superimposed pyelonephritis, which occurs frequently, may be manifested by WBCs and WBC casts. Sonography reveals well-defined sonolucent systs and is probably the most useful test for early diagnosis of the condition. IVP reveals the findings stated above. Biochemical abnormalities of uremia are present in the later stages.

Treatment of hypertension to prevent further renal damage is of paramount importance. Hematuria usually responds to bed rest. If urine culture reveals infection, it must be treated aggressively with appropriate antibiotics. Invasive procedures such as cystoscopy and retrograde pyelography must be avoided to prevent infection. Sometimes one or more cysts may become infected and lead to abscess formation that may require surgical drainage. Surgery is otherwise of no benefit. When end-stage renal disease develops chronic dialysis and transplantation therapy help to prolong life and rehabilitate these patients.

Medullary Cystic Disease

This is a rare disorder that also seems to have a familial tendency.

Cysts varying in size from a few microns to a centimeter are present at the corticomedullary junction. The cortex is thinned and the glomeruli hyalinized. Evidence of chronic interstitial inflammation and fibrosis is often present.

The disease usually manifests during adolescence or early adulthood. As renal insufficiency progresses, hypertension is common. Most patients develop end-stage renal disease by the age of 30.

Treatment of hypertension and uremia are indicated before the development of end-stage renal disease, at which time chronic dialysis and transplantation are necessary.

Unless hemodialyzed or transplanted, patients with medullary cystic disease usually succumb to renal disease in the fourth decade of life.

Medullary Sponge Kidney

This is benign condition as compared to medullary cystic disease.

Ectasia of the collecting ducts causes formation of small cysts in the medulla. The lesions may be localized to one pyramid or be diffuse and bilateral.

These patients are usually asymptomatic. The condition is often first suspected on a KUB that reveals oval calcifications in the region of the papilla. The IVP reveals spongelike patterns in the papilla due to the collection of dye in the dilated collecting tubules. Occasionally small calculi may form, causing renal colic and hematuria. Disorders of distal tubular function such as renal tubular acidosis may occur. Because of calcification the condition may be mistaken for renal tuberculosis or diffuse nephrocalcinosis.

No treatment is usually necessary. Instrumentation of the urinary tract must be avoided; if urinary tract infection develops, it should be treated aggressively.

The condition of medullary sponge kidney is compatible with a normal life span.

Nephrolithiasis

The majority of urinary tract stones originate in the kidney. They affect almost one of every 1,000 persons. Eighty percent of the stones contain calcium, 10% contain uric acid, and 2% contain cystine.

Caclium Stones

These are the most common type of stone. Most calcium stones are a mixture of calcium oxalate and phosphate; a significant number have a core of uric acid. Formation of these stones is favored by increased amounts of calcium or oxalate in the urine.

Caclium oxalate stones frequently occur in conditions associated with hypercalcemia such as hyperparathyroidism, sarcoidosis, and immobilization. They also occur in conditions that produce hypercalciuria without hypercalcemia such as renal tubular acidosis, Cushing's syndrome, and hypoparathyroidism treated with calcium and vitamin D. However, the most common cause of calcium oxalate stones is idiopathic hypercalciuria. Idiopathic hypercalciuria may occur because of augmented intestinal absorption, increased calcium mobilization from the bones, or reduced renal tubular reabsorption of calcium. Calcium oxalate stones are common in patients with malabsorption syndromes or after intestinal bypass surgery due to increased absorption of oxalate. A family history of kidney stones is often present in patients with idiopathic hypercalciuria.

Colicky pain in the flank radiating to the lower part of the abdomen, genitals, and inner thigh is often the first manifestation. The attack may last from several minutes to several hours. Urinary tract symptoms such as dysuria, frequency, and hematuia are common. Fever may indicate presence of an associated urinary tract infection. Urinalysis reveals mild proteinuria, red cells, and, if there is an associated infection, white cells and white cell casts. A 24-hour urine specimen usually contains more than 300 mg of calcium. The absorptive type of idiopathic hypercalciuria is characterized by normal serum calcium, normal fasting urinary calcium excretion, and high calcium excretion after an oral calcium load. Measurement of urinary 3',5'-adenosine monophosphate (cyclic AMP) can help differentiate idiopathic hypercalciuria from primary hyperparathyroidism. A high oral calcium load generally fails to reduce the increased urinary cyclic AMP in primary hyperparathyroidism.

Treatment of the primary disorder responsible for hypercalciuria helps prevent recurrence of renal stones. In idiopathic hypercalciuria, thiazide diuretics along with modest salt restriction reduce calcium excretion. Fluid intake should be increased to maintain a daily urine volume of at least 2500 ml. Urinary calcium can also be reduced by increasing the phosphate intake. Many calcium oxalate stones are found to have a uric acid nidus. Allopurinol can help prevent formation of this nidus.

The above therapeutic measures can substantially reduce the incidence of renal stones in patients predisposed to the condition.

Uric Acid Stones

Eighty-five percent of uric acid stones occur in a pure form.

Hyperuricemia and hyperuricosuria such as may occur in gout or in a variety of hematologic diseases such as polycythemia or leukemia are often associated with uric acid stones. Almost 50% of uric acid calculi occur without hyperuricemia and increased uric acid excretion. These patients tend to excrete highly acid urine with a pH below 5.5, probably due to a defect in ammonia excretion.

Renal colic is often the presenting manifestation. The urinalysis reveals uric acid crystals in large numbers. On KUB the uric acid stones are radiolucent. They appear as filling defects on IVP.

Hydration and alkalinization of the urine help dissolve and prevent formation of uric acid stones. Allopurinol therapy is very effective in the treatment and prevention of these stones.

Cystine Stones

Cystine stones occur in association with cystinuria, a congenital disorder characterized by decreased tubular reabsorption of cystine, arginine, ornithine, and lysine. Cystine is a relatively insoluble amino acid and therefore precipitates in the urine to form stones. The crystals appear hexagonal upon microscopic examination of the urine. Due to their sulfur content, the cystine stones are partially radiopaque. Treatment consists of hydration and alkalinization of the urine. When these measures prove inadequate, treatment with penicillamine is helpful.

Struvite Stones

Struvite or magnesium ammonium phosphate stones occur in the face of recurrent urinary tract infection with urea-splitting organisms such as *E. coli* proteus and klebsiella. Staghorn calculi are usually of this variety. They often cause no symptoms but should always be suspected in patients with recurrent urinary tract infections. If they cause obstruction, surgical removal may be necessary.

Papillary Necrosis

This condition is often associated with diabetes, sickle cell disease, acute bacterial infection, gout, and analgesic (phenacetin) abuse.

The pathology may be indistinguishable from that of pyelonephritis. Ischemia of the renal tubules seems to play an important role in the pathogenesis of this condition.

Hematuria, pain in the flank or abdomen, fever, and chills are often the presenting symptoms. Acute renal failure with oliguria or anuria may sometimes occur. Dysuria and urinary frequency are often present. Straining of the urine will often reveal presence of tissue fragments that on microscopic examination are confirmed to have papillary tissue. IVP typically reveals a ring shadow.

Analgesics may be necessary for the symptomatic treatment of pain. Hydration, treatment of infection with appropriate antibiotics, and treatment of the underlying disorder is often helpful in preventing the progression of the disease.

Analgesic-induced papillary necrosis can progress slowly and lead to end-stage renal disease. Despite intensive counseling, many of these patients continue to abuse analgesics. Avoidance and early treatment of infection are of paramount importance.

Nephrogenic Diabetes Insipidus

This disorder is distinguished from pituitary diabetes insipidus by its inability to respond to vasopressin. The acquired form of the disease can occur in patients with pyelonephritis, mutiple myeloma, amyloidosis, obstructive neuropathy, polycystic disease, sarcoidosis, hypercalcemic nephropathy, hypokalemic nephropathy, Sjögren's syndrome, sickle cell anemia, and those taking such drugs as lithium, methoxyflurane (Penthrane), and demeclocycline (Declomycin). Congenital nephrogenic diabetes insipidus is a rare entity and believed to have an x-linked recessive transmission.

The pathogenesis seems to be a defect in the activation of adenyl cyclase by vasopressin in patients with congenital diabetes insipidus.

The condition is characterized by excretion of large volumes of dilute urine with osmolality well below that of plasma. Polyuria and polydipsia are apparently an early occurrence in the lives of water babies suffering from congenital diabetes insipidus. Hydronephrosis and atonic bladder often result from high rates of urine flow. A relatively high incidence of mental retardation has been reported, which may be related to repeated episodes of dehydration.

Management of the primary disorder or discontinuation of the drug causing diabetes insipidus is helpful in reversing the condition in many patients.

An early diagnosis of congenital diabetes insipidus is essential to prevent brain damage. Adequate water intake must be maintained. Thiazide diuretics are helpful in reducing the urinary volume by producing mild salt depletion and allowing increased fluid absorption in the proximal segment of the nephron.

Drug-induced diabetes insipidus is completely reversible on discontinuation of the drug. Congenital diabetes insipidus, if diagnosed early and treated, usually does not reduce life expectancy.

DISEASES OF THE URINARY TRACT

The diseases of the urinary tract include infections, tumors, obstructive lesions, and malformations. Only the relatively common disorders are discussed here.

Infections

Most urinary tract infections are due to invasion of the urinary tract by bacteria that constitute normal colonic flora. *Mycobacterium tuberculosis*, although uncommon, still causes urinary tract and kidney infections. There is no convincing evidence that viruses cause urinary tract infection and anaerobic bacteria seldom involve the urinary tract. Urinary tract obstruction, stones, and instrumentation may lead to infections with uncommon organisms such as *Proteus*, *Enterobacter*, and *E. coli* resistant to the commonly used antibiotics. Staphylococcus, when isolated from the urine, is usually a contaminant.

Cystitis is more common in sexually active women and usually presents with dysuria and frequency of urination. Severe cystitis may lead to hematuria. Systemic signs of infection such as fever, chills, and malaise are usually absent. Urinalysis reveals WBCs. Bacteria may be seen in an unspun specimen of urine when examined under high power of a microscope. Urine culture usually reveals more than 100,000 colonies/ml. White blood cell casts are rarely present. The treatment consists of sulfonomide therapy. Antibiotics, such as ampicillin or tetracycline, are rarely necessary for the first or second episodes of cystitis. In patients with repeated infections either due to relapse (indicating a chronic focus of infection) or reinfection, co-trimoxazole (Bactrim, Septra) is the therapy of choice.

Renal Tuberculosis

Next to pulmonary tuberculosis, the kidney is the most common site for the late appearance of localized tuberculosis. Implantation of infection takes place by hematogenous spread early in the course of the disease, the pathogen remaining dormant for many years.

As infection spreads from the cortex into the medulla where the environment is more favorable, the renal lesions undergo necrosis and excavate. Local obstruction may cause segmental renal destruction. Infected papillary tissue traveling down the ureter and bladder causes spreading of the infection along the urinary tract. Ureteral obstruction may lead to hydronephrosis. As the infection spreads along the bladder wall, it may cause scarring and contracture of the bladder as well as infection of the epididymis and testes.

Tuberculous infection of the kidney and urinary tract remains asymptomatic for a long period of time. When the symptoms occur, they are usually insidious. Cystitis or epididymitis may be the first manifestation. Microscopic hematuria and pyuria with a sterile urine should always raise the possibility of tuberculosis. A positive tuberculin skin test is present and culture of urine for acid-fast bacillus (AFB) is positive in almost all patients. Intravenous pyelography demonstrates calcification in one or both kidneys and in addition may reveal a cortical cavity communicating with the caliceal system.

Antituberculous therapy with a two-drug regimen should be undertaken for at least 18-24 months. Surgical resection is seldom necessary.

With early diagnosis and appropriate treatment, the prognosis for full recovery from renal tuberculosis is excellent.

Prostatitis and Nongonococcal Urethritis

This term is loosely applied to various conditions in men presenting with lower urinary tract symptoms when no specific organisms can be isolated.

The patient may present with dysuria, frequency, mucous discharge from the urethra, low back pain, and perineal or testicular discomfort. Acute bacterial prostatitis causes fever, chills, and dysuria; the prostate on rectal examination feels very tender and boggy. There may be no tenderness upon examination in chronic prostatitis; however, upon massaging, prostatic secretions exude from the urethra. A Gram stain may show polymorphonuclear leukocytes and lymphocytes. Urine culture is almost always negative.

Treatment with sulfonomides may be helpful. Chronic prostatitis may require tetracycline therapy. Co-trimoxazole (Bactrim, Septra) has been employed with considerable success in some of these infections.

Despite adequate treatment, many patients with chronic prostatitis continue to have recurrent symptoms and may require repeated therapy.

Tumors

Many types of benign and malignant tumors occur in the urinary tract. Benign tumors such as fibroma, lipoma, and adenomas are small and usually of no clinical importance. Malignant tumors of the kidney occur chiefly in childhood and after the age of 40. The most common malignant tumor of the kidney in adults is renal cell carcinoma; in children it is Wilms' tumor. Other types of renal cancer are extremely rare.

Renal Cell Carcinoma (Hypernephroma)
It represents 65% to 90% of all malignant tumors of the kidney in adults and 3% of all visceral malignancies. The patients are most often in the fifth to seventh decade of life and the tumor is twice as common in men than in women.

The tumor is usually large, 3-15 cm in diameter at the time of discovery. Most often it is located in the upper pole of the kidney, is yellowish orange, and has large areas of cystic softening and hemorrhages. Although the margins are usually well defined, localized invasion of the renal veins and pelvis frequently occurs. Upon microscopic examination the tumor consists predominately of vacuolated clear cells. The vacuoles contain lipid and and glycogen material. Also seen are tubular epithelial cells exhibiting marked anaplasia.

Renal cell carcinoma has been called the internist's tumor because of systemic manifestations such as fever, polycythemia, leukocytosis including leukemoid reaction, gastrointestinal symptoms, polyneuritis, myopathy, disturbances in liver function, hypercalcemia with low serum phosphorus, and hypertension. Hematuria is often the first manifestation. Flank pain and a mass are present in over 50% of cases.

Calcification of the tumor mass is occasionally seen on plain x-ray films of the abdomen. IVP may show distortion of the calyceal system. Ultrasound examination reveals a solid lesion. Arteriography reveals characteristic neovascularity and pooling of the contrast material in the venous sinusoids as a result of small arteriovenous communications in the tumor mass. Epinephrine injection into the renal artery during the procedure may accentuate visualization of tumor vessels by causing contraction of the normal blood vessels.

Nephrectomy is usually the treatment of choice. There have been a few case reports of regression of the metastases following nephrectomy. However, in most instances metastases are not affected by resection of the primary tumor. The tumors are relatively resistant to radiotherapy. Chemotherapy with vinblastine (Velban) has produced significant regression of metastatic lesions.

Although the prognosis in renal cell carcinoma varies considerably, overall 5-year survival is about 35% and 10-year survival is 25%.

Wilms' Tumor (Nephroblastoma)
This is the third most common malignant tumor in children after leukemia and tumors of the nervous tissue. Ninety percent of cases occur before the age of 7.

The tumor arises from the embryonic nephrogenic tissue and contains both epithelial and connective tissue elements. The gross appearance varies depending on the predominant tissue component. Histologically, the characteristic features are primitive glomeruli and abortive tubules within a spindle-cell stroma. In addition striated muscle fibers, smooth muscle, cartilage, bone, and fat cells may be present.

The most common presenting symptom is a palpable abdominal mass, which may be enormous. Hypertension is commonly present. The tumor may need to be differentiated from an enlarged kidney due to multicystic disease, hydronephrosis, a renal cyst, or a neuroblastoma.

A combination of surgery and chemotherapy in combination with radiotherapy is the treatment of choice. After nephrectomy, chemotherapy with actinomycin D (Cosmegen) and vincristine (Oncovin) during the first week postoperatively, and subsequently at regular intervals during the next year, is very helpful. Radiotherapy is given when there is invasion of surrounding tissues and regional lymph nodes. When the tumor is very large, preoperative irradiation may help by causing it to shrink.

The most favorable prognosis is in those children in whom the diagnosis is made before the age of 2. With the above therapy, the 2-year survival rate is 90%. Cure is now possible in the majority of patients.

Tumors of the Urinary Collecting System (Renal Pelvis, Ureter, Bladder, and Urethra)
Since the entire urinary collecting system is lined with transitional epithelium, tumors arising in these areas have similar cellular patterns. They range from small benign papillomas to large invasive carcinoma. Bladder tumors are 50 times more frequent in people exposed to intermediate products in the manufacture of aniline dyes. Chronic cystitis and schistosomiasis also predispose to bladder cancer. A small lesion in the ureter may cause urinary obstruction and has more serious clinical implications than a large benign tumor in the bladder. Painless hematuria is often the first clinical manifestation regardless of the site of origin and the degree of anaplasia.

Nodular Hyperplasia of the Prostate (Benign Prostatic Hypertrophy)
Beginning with the fifth decade of life there occurs a progressive increase in the incidence of nodular hyperplasia of the prostate. About 50% of men have symptoms of prostatic hypertophy; however, only 10% require surgical relief.

The prostate gland becomes enlarged and nodular. The nodules usually occur in the median and lateral lobes, in contrast to prostatic carcinoma, which usually involves the posterior lobe. The median lobe projects into the prostatic urethra that can also be compressed from the sides by the hypertrophic lateral lobes. Histologically, hyperplasia of the glands and fibromuscular hyperplasia are the predominant features.

Nocturia is usually the first symptom. Frequency and hesitancy are also common. Obstruction with overflow incontinence or complete obstruction of the urethra are not uncommon in severe cases. If the obstruction is not relieved, renal failure and uremia occur.

Estimation of residual urine by straight catherization of the bladder soon after voiding gives an indication of the degree of obstruction. If the residual urine volume is more than 50 ml, cystoscopy should be performed for evaluation of the obstruction.

If the symptoms are prominent or the obstruction is compromising renal function, transurethral resection (TUR) of the prostate is advisable.

The prognosis for nodular hyperplasia of the prostate is good. There is no known association with the development of prostatic cancer.

Carcinoma of the Prostate

This is the most common malignancy in men but accounts for only 10% of deaths from malignant disease. The incidence rises rapidly with advancing age. Microscopic lesions in autopsy studies have been found to be present in as many as 60% in the eighth decade of life.

Seventy-five percent of prostatic cancers arise in the posterior lobe. Histologically, the tumor blends imperceptibly into the prostatic tissue. Most tumors are adenocarcinomas with varying degrees of differentiation. The tumor cells are usually uniform and cuboidal.

Carcinoma of the prostate is usually asymptomatic because it arises in the posterior lobe, away from the urethra. The aggressive variety invades the bladder and produces clinical manifestations such as frequency, dysuria, and hematuria. Upon rectal examination the prostate may feel hard, irregular, and nodular. One-fifth of the patients present with symptoms due to distant metastases, usually to the vertebrae via the paravertebral veins. The serum alkaline phosphatase is frequently elevated in prostatic carcinoma but is a nonspecific test. The prostatic fraction of the serum acid phosphatase is a more sensitive estimation and is elevated in a high proportion of cases when local or distant dissemination has occured. The bony metastases are usually osteoblastic. Radioactive technetium scanning of the skeleton is a very sensitive test for detection of metastases in the absence of radiographic changes. Needle biopsy is a useful method of obtaining a histologic diagnosis.

Radical prostatectomy remains the treatment of choice when tumor is confined to the gland. Orchiectomy and estrogen therapy are useful palliative measures as adjuncts to surgery. Estrogen therapy may, however, increase the mortality from cardiovascular disease. Transurethral resection of the prostate is often used to relieve the obstruction. Supervoltage irradiation and direct injection of radioactive substances may be used for treatment of tumors confined to the pelvis. Local irradiation of skeletal metastases may effectively relieve pain.

Only 5-10% of patients with carcinoma of the prostate live 5 years without treatment. If dissemination is not present, with treatment 44% survive more than 5 years, but in the presence of metastatic disease, only 20% survive that long.

Malformations of the Urinary Tract

Horseshoe Kidney

This condition occurs twice as commonly in men. The two kidneys are fused at the lower pole. They have an increased risk of infection and are subject to stone formation largely because of urethral distortion. It may be possible to see the soft tissue outline of the isthmus across the vertebral column. IVP shows malrotation of the renal pelvis and nephrogram shows fusion of the two kidneys. Instrumentation of the urinary tract should be avoided and infection treated at the first sign of occurrence. Separation of the two kidneys is seldom necessary.

Renal Dysplasia

This may be unilateral or bilateral. The dysplastic process may involve the entire renal mass or a segment of it. Microscopically, cysts lined by cuboidal or columnar epithelium are surrounded by mesenchymal tissue including cartilage. Other congenital anomalies such as ureteral malformations, ventricular septal defects, and bronchoesophageal fistulae may be present. Segmental hypoplasia (Ask-Upmark kidney) is limited to the upper pole of one kidney and is demarcated by a transverse groove on the kidney surface. The condition is found in young women and is associated with hypertension.

Congenital Anomalies of the Ureter and Bladder

The most common congenital anomalies of the ureter are double and bifed ureters and ureteral strictures at the ureteropelvic junction. All these patients are more susceptible to urinary tract infections. Extrophy of the urinary bladder is one of the most common anomalies of the urinary bladder. The anterior wall of the bladder and overlying abdominal wall are absent.

ACUTE RENAL FAILURE

Acute renal failure is characterized by a sudden reduction in renal function causing rapid (in a matter of days) elevation of BUN and creatinine, oliguria, and uremic symptoms. Instead of oliguria, in rare circumstances, there may be anuria or polyuria.

Acute renal failure must be distinguished from oliguria and azotemia due to prerenal causes and urinary tract obstruction (postrenal failure). Acute prerenal failure occurs due to decreased renal perfusion and glomerular filtration. This may occur due to decreased intravascular volume from hemorrhage or extracellular fluid losses (gastrointestinal, burns, or third-spacing as in bowel obstruction), severe congestive heart failure, or septicemic shock. Acute postrenal failure occurs due to obstruction of the urinary passage. The ureteral obstruction has to be bilateral and may occur in retroperitoneal fibrosis or due to stones, clots, or tumors. The most common cause of obstructive uropathy is prostatic hypertrophy or obstruction of the urethra. The renal causes of acute renal failure include vascular complications such as renal arterial obstruction or vasculitis, the glomerular diseases mentioned earlier, tubular damage due to either prolonged ischemia or nephrotoxins, interstitial diseases, and papillary necrosis.

The pathology and pathogenesis of acute tubular necrosis have already been discussed. The pathology of acute renal failure due to other causes is discussed under each respective disease.

Manifestations of fluid overload comprising congestive heart failure and hypertension are often present due to inability of the kidneys to excrete salt and water. Electrolyte imbalance causing hyperkalemia and acidosis are also common. As uremia occurs, nausea, vomiting, neuromuscular irritability, asterixis, somnolence, and coma may be present. The oliguric phase usually lasts approximately 2 weeks although it may last as long as 12 weeks. It is usually followed by a diuretic phase when polyuria occurs due to impaired tubular renal reabsorption of salt and water. The patient can become dehydrated during this phase unless extracellular fluid volume is maintained by adequate replacement.

The appropriate laboratory studies consist of urinalysis and measurements of BUN, serum creatinine, serum electrolytes, urine sodium concentration, plasma and urine osmolality, urine creatinine concentration, and, if indicated, serum CPK levels and urine examination for myoglobin in patients suspected to have rhabdomyolysis, antistreptolysin-O titer in patients suspected to have poststreptococcal glomerulonephritis, and blood levels for methanol, ethelene glycol, or other nephrotoxic agents in those suspected to have ingested one of these agents.

Radiographic studies to delineate the anatomy of the urinary tract and detect obstruction may need to be performed. Renal biopsy is usually not necessary.

Table 2 summarizes the laboratory features of prerenal, renal, and postrenal causes of kidney failure.

Removal or treatment of the remedial causes is of paramount importance. This may comprise removal of nephrotoxic agents, relief of urinary tract obstruction, replenishing the extracellular fluid volume, or treatment of severe heart failure. To minimize the effects of loss of renal excretory function, restriction of daily fluid intake to no more than 500 ml plus the visible losses is necessary. Restriction of salt intake to avoid thirst is also necessary. Potassium intake should be kept to a minimum. Administration of potassium-exchange resin (Kayexalate) along with sorbitol, which prevents constipation produced by the resin, is often necessary to remove potassium from the body through the gastrointestinal tract.

Intravenous hyperalimentation with essential amino acids and hypertonic dextrose infusion (Nephramine/$D_{70}W$) administered through the central venous catheter with careful aseptic precautions has been shown to reduce the duration of renal failure and decrease morbidity and mortality.

Dialysis (peritoneal or hemodialysis) may be necessary for removal of fluid, potassium, or reversal of the uremic symptoms. Frequent dialysis (to keep serum creatinine below 10 mg/dl) also has been demonstrated to improve prognosis.

Early detection and appropriate treatment of infection of the urinary tract, pneumonia, or septicemia constitute an integral part of the management of acute renal failure.

Once the diuretic phase sets in, in addition to the above management appropriate fluid replacement is necessary.

Prognosis is generally related to severity of the underlying condition that predisposes to acute renal failure and the duration of renal failure before appropriate management is instituted. Despite the aggressive therapy outlined above, almost 50% of patients with acute renal failure succumb, mostly due to underlying disease.

CHRONIC RENAL FAILURE

Many renal diseases lead to chronic renal failure (end-stage renal disease or ESRD). Approximately 100 people per million population can be expected to develop ESRD per year. Common causes of chronic renal failure include: glomerulonephritis, diabetes, nephrosclerosis, polycystic disease, and interstitial nephritis, in approximately that order.

Pathophysiology

The pathophysiology of uremia has a great deal of bearing on its clinical manifestations. Uremia is a complex clinical syndrome resulting from multiple metabolic derangements arising from renal failure. Some of the biochemical impairments are as follows.

Due to impaired concentrating ability and solute diuresis, polyuria and polydipsia are among the first signs of renal insufficiency. Nocturia may be the first manifestation of polyuria. Dehydration can be readily produced by relatively brief abstention from fluids. Although the restriction of fluid intake

Table 2. Differential Diagnosis of Acute Renal Failure

Test	*Prerenal*	*Renal*	*Postrenal*
Urinalysis			
Specific gravity	>1.015	⩽1.010	⩽1.010
Osmolality (U_{osm}/P_{osm})	>1.5	⩽1.0	⩽1.0
Proteinuria	Absent	Usually present	Absent or minimal
Urine sediment	Unremarkable	RBC casts in acute glomerulonephritis, muddy-brown (renal failure) casts in ATN	Unremarkable
Urine Na^+ (mEq/L)	<10	>20	Usually >20
U_{creat}/P_{creat}	>40	Usually <40	Usually <40
BUN/creatinine	>10	⩽10	⩽10

is seldom indicated, excessive fluid ingestion is unnecessary. Maximal urea excretion occurs at a daily urine volume of approximately 3,000 ml. Excessive water administration can lead to hyponatremia with its attendant symptoms of nausea, muscle cramps, and mental disturbances.

Patients with renal insufficiency are unable to diminish renal sodium loss when salt is restricted. Initially water and sodium are lost proportionately; however, with progression of renal insufficiency water is no longer lost as much as sodium and therefore hyponatremia develops. Salt wasting is particularly common in patients with chronic pyelonephritis, interstitial nephritis, polycystic disease, medullary cystic disease, and urinary tract obstruction when salt intake is low; however, with high salt intake, there might be retention. In chronic glomerulonephritis salt loss is not prominent. In salt-losing conditions as much as 200 mEq daily sodium intake may be necessary. In addition to urinary losses, vomiting and diarrhea may produce salt depletion in uremic patients. Since hyponatremia commonly causes nausea, a vicious circle may ensue. Depletion of extracellular volume may further reduce GFR and cause progression of uremia. Repletion of salt and water may partially reverse uremia. In azotemic patients without fluid overload as manifested by edema, hypertension, or congestive heart failure, restriction of salt is unnecessary. However, in patients who develop hypertension and signs of heart failure that are not controlled with digitalis, salt restriction may be necessary.

Hyperkalemia usually complicates renal insufficiency only when the daily urine output falls below 500-1,000 ml. The distal tubule has an enormous capacity to secrete potassium in the urine. Increased secretion of aldosterone and increased flow of anions such as sulfates and phosphates through the distal tuble further enhance potassium excretion. Salt restriction, acidosis, adrenal insufficiency, or selective hyporeninemic hypoaldosteronism may be responsible for hyperkalemia in some patients even when the urine output is adequate. Hypokalemia and potassium wasting may be prominent in renal tubular acidosis, nephrocalcinosis, and during the diuretic phase of recovery from acute tubular necrosis. Hypokalemia results in further renal damage and should be corrected without delay.

Approximately 40-60 mEq of acid in the form of hydrogen ion (H^+) is excreted daily by the kidneys of a healthy person ingesting a 70 g protein diet per day. Almost half the load of H^+ is excreted as ammonium (NH_4^+). In renal insufficiency there is reduced excretion of ammonia (NH_3) in the distal tubule; therefore, the excretion of NH^+_4 is also reduced. Inability to reabsorb the filtered bicarbonate from the proximal tubule also contributes to acidosis. Accumulation of sulfuric and phosphoric acids generated by oxidation of sulfur-containing amino acids also contributes to uremic acidosis.

Systemic acidosis causes nausea, lethargy, malaise, and dyspnea. Sodium bicarbonate administration of 40-60 mEq/day (each 600-mg tablet of sodium bicarbonate provides 12 mEq HCO_3) maintains serum bicarbonate at 18-20 mEq/L. Excessive sodium administration can lead to congestive heart failure and should therefore be avoided.

Phosphate is excreted in the glomerular filtrate but 80% of the filtered phosphate is reabsorbed, chiefly in the proximal tubule. As the GFR falls, phosphate is retained and deposited as calcium phosphate salts in various soft tissues. This causes serum calcium to fall, which in turn stimulates the parathyroids to secrete more parathormone. Parathormone diminishes phosphate reabsorption from the renal tubule, mobilizes calcium from the bone, and increases renal calcium absorption, thus restoring both serum phosphorus and calcium levels. When the GFR decreases to approximately 20% of normal, serum phosphorus begins to rise despite excessive parathormone since the kidney cannot excrete phosphate into the urine in excess of the amount filtered. The secretion of parathormone rises further, causing secondary hyperparathyroidism. Although more calcium is mobilized from the bone, calcium phosphate deposition in the soft tissue continues causing serum calcium to remain low. Since half the serum calcium is bound to albumin in low serum albumin states, a portion of the decrement in calcium may be due to hypoalbuminemia. A third reason for low serum calcium is inability of the kidney to convert vitamin D into its active form 1,25-$(OH)_2$ cholecalciferol (1,25-DHCC). As indicated before, 1,25-DHCC is a hormone synthesized in the kidney from 25-(OH)cholecalciferol and is responsible for facilitating the calcium absorption from the gastrointestinal tract. As less of this hormone becomes available, calcium absorption from the gastrointestinal tract is reduced.

Bone disease in renal failure may manifest as renal rickets characterized by widening of the osteoid seams at the growing end of bones, and osteomalacia characterized by ribbonlike radiolucent zones perpendicular to the free bone surfaces (Looser's transformation zones, Milkman's syndrome) most commonly seen in the upper third of the femur; subperiosteal reabsorption of bone in the phalanges and long bones, eventually leading to cystic changes of osteitis fibrosa; and osteosclerosis seen characteristically in the spine (rugger jersy spine). Aseptic necrosis of the hip is also common in patients kept alive on dialysis for long periods.

The treatment involves vigorous control of serum phosphorus by use of aluminum hydroxide-containing antacids, calcium supplementation either orally or by use of increased dialysate calcium concentration and by the judicious use of vitamin D (calcitriol or one of the less-active forms).

Urea has a molecular weight of 68 and is a product of protein metabolism. Although there is a buildup of urea in renal failure and the symptom complex is called uremia, not all uremic symptoms are due to urea. Anorexia, nausea, and vomiting are best correlated with blood urea levels. The formation of ammonia by urea-splitting organisms in the gut is probably responsible for the uremic odor and gastrointestinal irritation.

The serum magnesium level may rise in uremia particularly upon ingestion of magnesium-containing antacids and laxatives. Due to a breakdown of tissues and compromised excretion of uric acid, uremic patients may also develop hyperuricemia and gout. However, joint swelling caused by deposition of calcium phosphate crystals is more common than that due to uric acid crystals. Due to insulin resistance mild carbohydrate intolerance is present in more than 50% of patients with chronic uremia; however, it disappears after several weeks of adequate dialysis. Hyperlipidemia including hypercholesterolemia is quite common in uremic patients, particularly those on prolonged hemodialysis. This biochemical abnormality is probably partly responsible for the increased cardiovascular deaths observed in uremic patients. Besides the abnormality mentioned above, there is accumulation of indoles, certain amino acids, various organic acids, sulfates, and guanidinosuccinic acid, the latter being probably responsible for the defect in platelet aggregation observed in uremia.

Clinical Manifestations

The onset of chronic uremia is usually insidious. Weakness, easy fatiguability, loss of appetite, and breathlessness are the usual presenting features. Polyuria and nocturia are common and usually precede any other manifestation of uremia. The patient appears pale and has a uriniferous odor on the breath. Bleeding into the skin, mucous membrane, and gastrointestinal tract is usually a late manisfestation. The patient appears somnolent and may have signs of congestive heart failure. Uremia affects almost all the major organ systems. Manifestations pertaining to various organ systems are as follows.

Neuromuscular Manifestations

Disturbances of mentation such as mental clouding, inability to concentrate, drowsiness, and psychosis are common in advanced uremia. Hyponatremia, acidosis, or dehydration may cause coma that can be corrected by appropriate therapy. Peripheral neuropathy, which is usually sensory and affects the distal lower extremities appears late but may progress rather rapidly. Nerve conduction time is prolonged. Vitamins are not helpful; however, intensive hemodialysis may slow progression of the disease. Successful kidney transplantation can be curative.

Cardiovascular Manifestations

Hypertension is commonly present in patients with end-stage renal disease. Very often it is due to fluid overload and can be controlled by ultrafiltration with hemodialysis. In a minority of patients hypertension is very severe and requires intensive medical therapy. Intermittent cardiac failure is common in uremic patients on hemodialysis. Fluid overload, hypertension, and anemia frequently contribute toward this complication. Uremic pneumonia is a misnomer for pulmonary edema occuring in patients with ESRD and is characterized by agitation, restlessness, dysnea, and a loud S_2 heart sound. The treatment consists of digitalis, diuretics, and ultrafiltration with dialysis. Almost 50% of deaths in chronic dialysis occur from myocardial infarction and other cardiovascular complications. Arteriosclerosis is accelerated in dialysis patients, probably from risk factors such as hypertension, hyperlipidemia, and vascular calcification due to secondary hyperparathyroidism. Pericarditis is common in uremics, particularly those in whom dialysis has been postponed. It also occurs in patients inadequately dialyzed and is often complicated by a hemorrhagic tamponade. Indomethacin, intensive dialysis, and steroids are the usual treatment. Pericardial tap or pericardiectomy may be necessary.

Gastrointestinal Manifestations

Ammonia produced from breakdown of the urea along with mouth breathing, acidosis, and dehydration lead to mouth ulcers and parotitis. Gastrointestinal symptoms such as anorexia, hiccups, nausea, and vomiting are common. Bleeding from gastrointestinal ulcers is a distressing complication. Pancreatitis may occur and cause abdominal pain. The diagnosis of pancreatitis is difficult to make since patients with renal insufficiency have hyperamylasemia without pancreatitis due to reduced amylase clearance. Phenothiazines and small frequent feedings combined with dialysis usually alleviate the gastrointestinal symptoms.

Hematologic Manifestations

Normocytic normochronic anemia occurs regularly and is often proportional to the degree of azotemia. It results from hemolysis in a uremic environment, suppression of erythropoiesis due to decreased production of erythropoietin, and a direct toxic effect of urea on the bone marrow. Additional contributory factors may be suppression of erythropoiesis due to transfusions, gastrointestinal bleeding, blood loss during dialysis, iron deficiency due to impaired absorption or inefficient utilization, folic acid deficiency due to dialytic losses, and hypersplenism.

Hematocrit as low as 20% is tolerated quite well by most patients. Replacement iron and folic acid along with androgen injections are helpful in increasing the hematocrit in many patients. Transfusion of packed red cells may be necessary particularly if the patient develops cardiac failure due to anemia or is unable to function because of weakness and shortness of breath. Complications of repeated transfusions include hepatitis, transfusion reaction, and hemosiderosis.

Coagulation defects include prolonged bleeding time, abnormal prothrombin consumption, thrombocytopenia, abnormal platelet adhesiveness, and decreased platelet factor III activity. Regular dialysis restores the platelet function. Leukopenia is common and is corrected only by renal transplantation.

Skin manifestations

A sallow, yellow color and generalized pruritus are the typical skin manifestations of uremia. Both anemia and deposition of carotenelike uremic pigments impart the typical color to the skin. Severe itching is sometimes due to calcium deposition in the skin from secondary hyperparathyroidism and may be relieved by parathyroidectomy. The medical treatment of itching consists of daily baths, bland lubricating ointments, use of antipruritic agents such as diphenhydramine (Benadryl), hydroxyzine (Atarax), and ultraviolet light treatment.

Infections

Depressed cellular immunity, poor nutrition, pulmonary congestion, coma, vascular insufficiency, and indwelling tubes predispose uremic patients to sepsis. Next to cardiovascular complications, infections are the most common cause of death in the uremic patients on dialysis.

Endocrine Manifestations

Secondary hyperparathyroidism, impaired sexual function and fertility, hyperreninemia, and in rare instances hypergastrinemia are the endocrine manifestations of renal failure. Although many uremic patients appear to have features of myxedema, thyroid functions are usually normal. Prolonged hemodialysis may lead to adrenal insufficiency due to certain unknown mechanisms; these patients may require replacement steroid therapy.

Nutrition and Growth

Children with uremia requiring hemodialysis suffer from retarded growth. Therefore, every attempt should be made to maintain proper nutrition. Renal transplantation, if performed early and successfully, can help these patients grow normally.

Evaluation of a Patient with Chronic Renal Disease

The evaluation of a patient with chronic renal disease should answer the following four questions:

1. What is the nature of the renal disease?
2. What is the extent of renal failure?
3. Are there any aggravating factors present?
4. What other associated medical and social problems are present?

Diagnosis of Renal Disease

For an accurate diagnosis of the underlying renal disease it is important that the patient be evaluated early in the course of renal failure. Once end-stage renal disease appears the kidneys usually do not visualize on IVP, and renal biopsy reveals hyalinization of the glomeruli and fibrosis of the renal tissue. Every effort should be made to recognize reversible and treatable diseases so that appropriate measures can be taken. Past history of renal disease or urinary symptoms and exposure to or ingestion of phenacetin-containing or other nephrotoxic agents should be elicited. Family history should include inquiries about renal disease, hypertension, gout, collagen diseases, and deafness. Laboratory tests should include urinalysis including microscopic examination, urine culture, measurement of serum creatinine, electrolytes, calcium, phosphate, alkaline phosphatase, proteins, and serum protein electrophoresis. Twenty-four-hour urine collection is carried out for measurement of protein and creatinine clearance. A chest x-ray film and electrocardiogram are necessary for adequate evaluation of the heart. If the kidneys are not visualized on a KUB or IVP, high-dose infusion pyelography with renal tomograms and films taken up to 24 hours later often provide information on kidney size and calyceal pattern. Evaluation of the cardiovascular, gastrointestinal, and skeletal systems should be carried out and, if affected, appropriate measures undertaken.

Degree of Renal Failure

Measurement of creatinine clearance is the most practical and accurate measurement of GFR. Progression of the disease can be monitored by repeated measurement of serum creatitine over several months and plotting 1/creatinine against time as explained before.

Aggravating Factors

Every effort should be made to identify reversible aggravating factors. Hypovolemia, systemic infections, hemorrhage, urinary infection, rapid rise or fall in blood pressure, and administration of nephrotoxic drugs can aggravate previously existing renal failure. Deterioration in renal function should not be blamed on the primary disease unless the above-mentioned contributory factors have been excluded.

Associated Medical and Social Problems

Dialysis and transplantation may place heavy demands on a patient's physical and social resources. Services of a social worker should be sought whenever possible to evaluate the patient's housing, social, economic, and family needs.

Treatment of End-Stage Renal Disease

The treatment of end-stage renal disease usually starts with dietary and medical management. As renal failure progresses and dietary and medical measures prove inadequate, dialysis is initiated. Once the patient's condition is stabilized and there are no contraindications, kidney transplantation is performed. The kidney may come from a live donor or from a cadaver, whichever is available first and can be appropriately matched.

Dietary and Medical Management

A low-protein diet is extremely effective in reducing the BUN. When the protein intake consists of high biologic value (eggs and milk) and the intake of carbohydrate and calories is sufficient to prevent catabolism of endogenous proteins, weight loss is minimal. When the GFR falls to 10 ml/min and symptoms of uremia develop, a 40 g protein diet is indicated. The Giordano-Giovannetti diet has a high essential amino acid content mostly derived from eggs and milk. Calories are provided in the form of bread and pasta made from protein-free flour with modifications to suit the patient's taste. Once the GFR falls below 10 ml/min, further protein restriction may be necessary. The diet becomes rather unattractive when simultaneous sodium, potassium, and water restriction become necessary. Fruits high in potassium should be avoided. Patients should be allowed as much salt as they can tolerate. Some salt restriction is necessary in most patients with chronic renal failure except in the presence of sodium-losing nephropathies such as chronic pyelonephritis and polycystic kidney disease.

Water restriction to a point where the patient stops gaining weight without becoming dehydrated is often necessary. In addition to the above restrictions, phosphate restriction may also be necessary. Food items such as bread and cheese contain high inorganic phosphates.

Diuretics may be necessary for treatment of hypertension and congestive heart failure associated with chronic renal disease. Furosemide (Lasix) and metolazone (Zaroxolyn) are more efficacious than thiazides in patients with renal failure. Antihypertensive therapy is often necessary in these patients. If hypertension does not respond to diuretic therapy alone, one of the step 2 drugs should be added. If there is no contraindication to its use, propranolol (Inderal) is a good drug since high renin levels are often present in these patients. If a combination of the diuretic and propranolol proves inadequate, addition of prazosin (Minipress) constitutes a good step 3 drug. In patients with intractable hypertension, minoxidil (Loniten) has proved to be a superior vasodilator to hydralazine. Captopril (Capoten) in reduced doses is also useful in many patients. Bilateral nephrectomy should be carried out only in rare instances for management of severe intractable hypertension that has not responded to maximal medical therapy despite good compliance on the part of the patient. For correction of acidosis, adminstration of sodium bicarbonate may be necessary. Phosphate binders such as aluminum hydroxide (e.g., Amphogel, Basalgel, Dialume) are almost always necessary for treatment and prevention of hyperphosphatemia. For treatment of hypocalcemia adminstration of calcium carbonate or vitamin D may be necessary in certain patients. Early treatment of infections with appropriate antibiotics is necessary. Aminoglycosides such as gentamicin (Garamycin), tobramycin (Nebcin) and amikacin (Amikin) should be adminstered in appropriately lowered doses as they are excreted mainly by the kidneys. Penicillin G, cephalosporins, co-trimoxazole (Bactrim, Septra), ethambutol (Myambutol), clindamycin and rifampin (Rifadin) require moderate reduction in doses since they are predominantly excreted through the kidney; however, in renal failure, they are excreted through the liver. Methicillin, dicloxacillin, ampicillin, amoxicillin, erythromycin, and carbenicillin are excreted primarily by the liver and require only slight reductions in dosage. Tetracyclines, except doxycycline (Vibramycin), are contraindicated in renal failure. For the treatment of heart failure, adminstration of digitalis may be necessary. Digoxin should be adminstered in half the normal dose. Digitoxin is excreted primarily through the liver and can be adminstered in normal doses.

Dialysis

Dialysis involves separation of two fluid compartments by a semipermeable membrane, through which low-molecular-weight substances such as electrolytes, BUN, and creatinine can cross from high to lower concentration compartments. Larger particles such as protein molecules and RBCs do not cross the membrane. In the case of peritoneal dialysis, the peritoneum acts as the semipermeable membrane. For hemodialysis, the semipermeable membrane is a synthetic material such as cellophane or cuprophan.

The major criterion for the initiation of chronic dialysis in chronic renal failure is the patient's inability to maintain a useful and comfortable life. Patients in need of chronic dialysis are no longer turned down because of underlying cardiovascular or other systemic diseases, with the exception of inoperable cancer. Age is no longer considered a limiting factor for selection of patients unless they are disabled or debilitated. Diabetes is no longer considered a contraindication to chronic dialysis, and diabetic nephropathy is rapidly becoming a common cause of renal failure in dialysis patients.

There are now almost 70,000 patients on long-term dialysis in the United States. The cost of outpatient chronic dialysis is staggering. The cost of home dialysis is considerably less. The other advantages of home dialysis include psychologic independence, flexibility of scheduling, and reduced risk of hepatitis.

Hemodialysis

For vascular access a subcutaneous A-V fistula is made by surgically creating a window between a peripheral artery and vein, usually in the forearm. As the blood flows continuously from the artery into the vein the proximal veins become prominent and, after a few weeks, they can be easily used for venipuncture. If the patient's blood vessels don't lend themselves to creation of a junctional A-V fistula, a graft made of synthetic material such as polytetrafluoroethylene (PTFE, Gore-Tex) is placed as a large bore arteriovenous connection thay may be "venipunctured" for dialysis. Single-needle dialysis is now commonly used. With the assistance of a pump, the blood is intermittently sucked and pushed though the same needle, or the two steps are carried out simultaneously through a double-lumen needle. As compared to previously used A-V shunts, fistula has the advantage of reduced infection and more freedom for the patient as no prosthetic material sticks out of the skin. A hemodilaysis system consists of a dialyzer where the mass transfer occurs and a second portion that delivers fresh dialysate of suitable composition to the dialyzer. Three basic types are in common clinical use today: coil, parallel-flow, and capillary (or hollow-fiber) dialyzers. A coil dialyzer consists of two cellophane or cuprophan tubings spirally wound and supported by a screen. Blood passes through the tubes and the dialysate is pumped through the supporting structures over the outside of the blood conduits. The parallel flow dialyzers consist of dialysing membrane layers stretched over the supporting structure. The capillary dialyzer consists of 10,000-15,000 capillaries with an internal diameter of 200-250μ, through which blood is passed. The dialysate is circulated outside the capillary. All three types of dialyzers are available in disposable form. All are efficient and the choice depends on the experience and preference of the nephrologist in charge of dialysis. Extracorporeal hemodialysis is usually conducted with the patient anticoagulated with heparin. When systemic heparinization is contraindicated, regional heparinization may be used with protamine sulfate introduced into the efferent blood line at a rate sufficient to precisely neutralize the heparin being infused into the afferent limb.

The patient should begin on dialysis early on rather than later to prevent complications of renal failure such as bone disease and peripheral neuropathy. Severe protein restriction is usually unnecessary after dialysis is initiated; however, water and sodium restriction is necessary in most cases. Peripheral neuropathy may be prevented and in some cases reversed by adequate dialysis. For prevention of anemia from blood loss, iron supplementation is necessary. Intravenous iron dextran complex (Imferon) is convenient to administer after a hemodialysis run and assures prevention of iron deficiency. Since folic acid and some of the water-soluble vitamins are removed during dialysis, supplemental vitamin therapy is necessary in these patients.

Chronic Peritoneal Dialysis
The indwelling plastic prosthesis first introduced by Tenckhoff has made it possible for patients to receive chronic intermittent peritoneal dialysis. When access to circulation through a shunt or fistula is difficult or impossible, chronic peritoneal dialysis is undertaken. The dialysis fluid is cycled in and out of the peritoneal cavity with appropriate dwell-time, using automated equipment. Difficulty with protein loss has not been a problem and infection around the site is not common. If peritonitis occurs, continuing peritoneal dialysis and antibiotic therapy usually controls the infection. Chronic ambulatory peritoneal dialysis (CAPD) uses the continuous presence of peritoneal dialysis solution in the peritoneal cavity except for periods of drainage and installation of fresh solution five times per day. After each drainage and fresh installation the patient is disconnected from all tubing, the chronic indwelling peritoneal catheter is capped and the patient is free to participate in his usual daily activities. The risk of peritonitis is the greatest stumbling block but can be usually treated on an outpatient basis with oral antibodies.

Renal Transplantation
Renal transplantation has become an established therapy for end-stage renal disease. The problems include unavailability of a sufficient number of transplantable kidneys, the rejection process, and complications of immunosuppressive therapy. The factors that need to be taken into consideration before a kidney transplantation include: availability of a living related donor, histocompatibility, nature of the renal disease and its likelihood of recurrence in the transplant, the age, general health, and emotional status of the recipient, and experience of the transplant team in the area. An identical twin makes an ideal living donor. A first-degree relative, especially a sibling, is the next best donor. Immunologic prerequisites include ABO compatibility, a negative cross match, and HLA compatibility. The histocompatibility antigens were first identified on leukocytes and thus names HLA (human leukocyte antigens). A combination of five genetic lock within the short arm of the sixth human chronosome is known as the major histocompatibility locus (MHL). It encompasses the HLA antigens, A, B, C and D. There may be other still undefined histocompatibility gene sites on other chromosomes. On the basis of HLA antigens prospective donors and recipients can be matched from grade A, when the donor and recipient are identical, to grade E, when there are more than two antigens in the donor not present in the recipient. Mixed-lymphocyte culture reaction (MLR) is another histocompatibility test performed by mixing lymphocytes of the potential donor and recipient in tissue culture and grading their transformation into blast cells. This is particularly useful for selecting the best donor from among several potential donors. The test is possible only for liver related donors. Cytotoxic antibodies and a cross-match test is performed with the recipient's serum and complement and the potential donor's hymphocytes to detect free preformed cytotoxic antibodies in the recipient to antigens of the donor. Serologic testing for and subsequent marching by D-related (DR) antigens or other recently described antigens may prove to be more predictive of cadaver transplant success in the future.

The cadaveric donor should have no malignancy (except of brain) or infection and normal or near normal renal function. ABO compatibility is necessary. HLA testing for cadaveric transplantation is usually a secondary consideration in the selection of recipients in the United States but is shown to be of significance in Europe.

The majority of cadaveric donors are those with head trauma. The kidneys can be preserved up to 24 hours in cold storage or up to 36 hours by continuously perfusing the organ with hypothermic intracellular-type fluid. The kidney is placed in the recipient extraperitoneally in the iliac fossa with the donor's renal artery anastomosed to the recipient's hypogastric artery, the donor's renal vein to the recipient's iliac vein, and the donor's ureter to the recipient's bladder. Prednisone or methyl prednisone (Medrol) and azathioprine (Imuran) are the mainstays of antirejection therapy. Other immunosuppressive techniques include irradiation of the transplant, used particularly when rejection is first detected. The results of transplantation are better with live donor transplants. At the end of 1 year, approximately 75% of these kidneys continue to function. With cadaveric transplant, only 50% of the kidneys continue to function at the end of 1 year. Causes of death after transplantation include infection, rejection, cardiovascular and cerebrovascular diseases, gastrointestinal hemorrhage, and other causes.

The advantages of a successful uncomplicated transplantation include improved health, a better quality of life, and rehabilitation. The disadvantages of transplantation include: major surgery, serious complications like infection, and an increased incidence of malignancy, particularly lymphomas.

DISORDERS OF FLUID, ELECTROLYTE, AND ACID-BASE BALANCE

SODIUM AND WATER METABOLISM

Normal Sodium and Water Metabolism

Sodium and water metabolism are closely interrelated. In health, renal sodium excretion is closely regulated to match the intake; the extrarenal losses of sodium are negligible. Approximately two-thirds of the filtered sodium load is reabsorbed isotonically in the proximal convoluted tubule. Twenty to thirty percent of the filtered sodium is reabsorbed in the ascending limb of Henle's loop, where active chloride transport has been demonstrated. Approximately 9% is absorbed in the distal tubule and the collecting duct, and less than 1% is excreted in the urine. All but 2-5% of the sodium in the body is located in the extracellular fluids; the plasma composition can be considered representative of the entire extracellular compartment. The normal plasma sodium concentration is 140 mEq/L (range, 135-145 mEq/L). The intracellular sodium concentration is less than 5 mEq/L. The total extracellular sodium content is approximately 2,000 mEq; the total intracellular sodium content is only about 150 mEq. Besides sodium, the other principal electrolytes in the extracellular fluid are chloride and bicarbonate. The major electrolytes of the intracellular compartment are potassium, magnesium, calcium, phosphorus, and organic ions, including proteins.

Distribution of Body Water
Water constitutes 50% of the body weight of an average adult woman and 60% of that of a man. Fatty tissue contains very little water. Of the total body water, 55% is intracellular and the remaining 45% is extracellular (7.5% plasma, 20% interstitial fluid, 15% in bone and dense connective tissue, and 2.5% secretions). Water moves freely across both cell and capillary membranes. Hydrostatic, osmotic, and oncotic forces are important determinants of water and electrolyte distribution.

Osmolality (Osmotic Pressure)
Osmotic pressure is often misunderstood. Osmolarity denotes the concentration of osmotically active particles in a solution. Osmolality is the property of a solution that depends on the concentration of the solute per unit of solvent. The effect of solute concentration on the freezing point of water is the basis for the clinical measurement of osmolality in body fluids. If a solute is added to pure water, the solute molecules interfere with the movement of water molecules, making it more difficult for the water to crystallize and freeze. One osmole is theoretically defined as the number of molecules necessary to lower the freezing point of water from 0°C to −1.86°C. A milliosmole (mOsm) equals .001 of an osmole. The osmolality of solutions can also be calculated if the solute content is known. Each millimole (mM) of an undissociated molecule equals 1 mOsm; for example, 1mM of glucose equals 1 mOsm. For a dissociated molecular species, each mM times the number of molecules released into solution equals the number of mOsm. For example,

$$1 \text{ mM NaCl} = 1 \text{ Na} + 1 \text{ Cl} = 2 \text{ mOsm};$$

$$1 \text{ mM CaCl}_2 = 1 \text{ Ca} + 2 \text{ Cl} = 3 \text{ mOsm}$$

The osmolality of normal extracellular fluid (ECF) is determined almost entirely by sodium (2 × 140 mOsm/L). There is also a small contribution from other nonelectrolyte solutions such as glucose (5 mOsm/L) and urea (5 mOsm/L), which amounts to about 10 mOsm/L. Normal plasma osmolality is thus 290 mOsm/L. In the presence of mild hyperglycemia or azotemia, glucose or urea contribute more to the osmolality. The contribution of glucose to the osmolality is calculated by dividing glucose concentration in mg/100 ml by 18, and urea concentration in mg/100 ml by 2.8. In complicated situations such as hyperglycemia, azotemia, or hyperlipemia, it is usually easiest to measure osmolality directly by freezing point depression in a laboratory rather than attempting to calculate the osmolality. Alcohol, another small molecule, increases osmolality when large amounts of liquor are consumed. In the presence of mild hyperlipemia or hyperproteinemia, plasma water is displaced by the lipid or protein; thus, the measured amount of sodium per ml of plasma will appear to be abnormally low. However, since the concentration of sodium in plasma water is normal, plasma osmolality is unaffected. The normal concentration of various electrolytes in the plasma are shown in Table 3.

Table 3. Ionic Composition of Plasma

Cations (mEq/L)		*Anions (mEq/L)*	
Na^+	142	Cl^-	103
K^+	4	HCO_3^-	27
Ca	5	PO_4^-	2
Mg	2	SO_4^-	1
		Organic acids	5
		Proteins	15
Totals	153		153

Oncotic Pressure (Colloid Osmotic Pressure)
The plasma oncotic pressure is a function of plasma proteins. The oncotic pressure is expressed in mm Hg. Because of the large molecular weight of plasma proteins (the molecular weight of albumin is 68,000), there are many fewer molecules of proteins in the plasma than there are of electrolytes. Therefore, the contribution of plasma proteins to osmotic pressure is negligible. Although the oncotic forces are small relative to osmotic forces, they are very important in maintaining the homeostatic balance. Since the plasma proteins are confined to the intravascular space, they pull the water from the interstitial space into the vascular space. The interaction of oncotic and hydrostatic forces at the capillary level is responsible for the water exchange that occurs between the capillaries and the interstitial space. The normal plasma oncotic pressure is 25 mm Hg. Since the hydrostatic pressure at the arterial end of the capillaries is 35 mm Hg, there is a net outflux of fluid at the arterial end. As the hydrostatic pressure falls to 15 mm Hg at the venous end of the capillary, there is a net influx of fluid at the venous end. In health, the rate of fluid outflow from the arterial end of the capillary equals the rate of uptake at the venous end of the capillary.

Clinical Assessment of Sodium and Water Balance
Serum electrolyte concentration reflects the ECF electrolyte composition. The next step is to determine the volume status of the patient, the critical volume being the intravascular volume that determines the cardiac output of the patient. The following clinical and laboratory parameters are used to evaluate the volume status of the patient.

Tissue Turgor. If the tissue becomes depleted of interstitial fluid, it loses its elasticity. Skin turgor is best judged on the forehead and anterior chest. In older individuals, the elasticity is normally decreased, making the skin turgor unreliable in interpreting the state of interstitial volume.

Edema, Ascites, and Pleural Effusion. In general, the effective intravascular volume is increased in the presence of edema, pleural effusion, and ascites. However, this assumption is not correct in the presence of hypoalbuminemia, venous obstruction, or third spacing (loss of intravascular volume into the interstitial compartment).

Blood Pressure. Orthostatic hypotension (a drop in systolic blood pressure greater than 10 mm Hg upon sitting or standing from a supine position) in the absence of antihypertensive therapy or autonomic neuropathy is a reliable indication of sodium and water depletion.

Renal Function. Measurements of BUN, serum creatinine, and urine output along with urine and plasma osmolality are also used for evaluating the volume status of a patient. Normal BUN to serum creatinine ratio is 10:1. Elevation of BUN out of proportion to serum creatinine suggests dehydration. Reduced urine output ($<$30 ml/hr), concentrated urine (Uosm/Posm $>$ 1.5), along with sodium concentration (UNa $<$ 10 mEq/L) are usually present in volume or sodium depletion without kidney damage.

Central Venous Pressure. The normal central venous pressure (CVP) is between 4 to 8 cm H_2O. The CVP is an index of the filling pressure of the right atrium and, therefore, the right ventricle. In uncomplicated circumstances, expansion of the intravascular volume results in an increased CVP and vice versa. In the presence of left ventricular failure, CVP becomes an unreliable measurement.

Pulmonary Capillary Wedge Pressure. Measurement of the pulmonary wedge pressure (PWP) is the most reliable aid to assess the status of intravascular volume. Pulmonary capillary wedge pressure provides a direct measurement of the filling pressure of the left ventricle. It can be measured at the bedside by using a Swan-Ganz balloon-tip catheter. A normal PWP is less than 12 mm Hg. A high PWP indicates left ventricular failure. A low PWP along with a low CVP is a reliable indication of volume contraction. In patients being ventilated with high levels of positive end-expiratory pressure, PWP becomes an unreliable index of left ventricular filling pressure.

Measurement of Intravascular Volume. Measurement of intravascular volume using indicator-dilution techniques or radioactive iodinated serum albumin (RISA) does not necessarily reflect the effective intravascular volume and is seldom used in the assessment of volume status.

Disorders of Sodium and Water Balance

Volume Depletion

The most common disorder of fluid and electrolyte equilibrium is a combined deficit of sodium and water. Although the term dehydration is often used synonymously with volume depletion, dehydration implies water depletion without the concomitant sodium loss leading to hypernatremia. The causes of volume depletion are listed in Table 4.

Table 4. Causes of Volume Depletion

Gastrointestinal losses
Vomiting
Gastric or small bowel drainage
Diarrhea
Bowel fistulas (colostomy, ileostomy, etc.)
Renal losses
Chronic renal failure
Diuretic phase of acute tubular necrosis
Postobstructive nephropathy
Adrenal insufficiency
Osmotic diuresis (diabetic glycosuria)
Diuretics
Skin losses
Sweating
Burns
Paracentesis

Clinical Features and Diagnosis. The symptoms of volume depletion are nonspecific and include nausea, lightheadedness, and weakness, particularly upon standing. History of inadequate salt and water intake together with vomiting, diarrhea, excessive sweating, poorly controlled diabetes mellitus, and renal or adrenal disease may be elicited. Physical findings include decreased skin turgor, orthostatic hypotension, and, in extreme cases, shock. The hematocrit and plasma protein concentration are increased. Plasma sodium may be decreased, normal, or increased, depending upon the proportion of deficits between sodium and water. Plasma creatinine and BUN are often increased (prerenal azotemia); urinary sodium is less than 10 mEq/L.

Treatment. Modest deficits of sodium and water can often be corrected by increased oral intake in the absence of gastrointestinal disorders. Serious depletion requires intravenous infusion of isotonic saline. Patients with moderate volume contraction usually require 2-3 liters of saline in addition to their continuing losses and daily requirements, while patients with serious depletion may require much larger volumes. In patients with metabolic acidosis, infusion of sodium bicarbonate and, in the presence of potassium depletion, addition of potassium to the intravenous fluids is necessary. Patients should be carefully monitored to avoid fluid overload and congestive heart failure.

Hyponatremia

Loss of sodium without a proportional loss of water, increased intake of water without sodium, and retention of water may all induce hyponatremia. The serum sodium concentration yields no direct information concerning the state of total sodium stores; rather, it indicates only a disturbance in the ratio of sodium to water.

Clinical Manifestations. The severity of symptoms is related to the degree of hyponatremia and the rapidity with which it develops. Neurologic dysfunction in the form of lethargy, confusion, stupor, or coma are the principal clinical features of hyponatremia. If hyponatremia develops rapidly, signs of neuromuscular hyperexcitability may occur. Clinical manifestations of hyponatremia are believed to be due to movement of fluid from the extracellular space into the relatively more hypertonic cells. Hyponatremia rarely causes clinical symptoms when serum sodium is above 125 mEq/L.

Pathogenesis and Diagnosis. Table 5 lists the clinical circumstances in which hyponatremia is encountered. Pseudohyponatremia is the spurious reduction in serum sodium concentration resulting from a displacement of plasma water by an abnormal accumulation of lipid or protein. In severe hyperlipemia, a part of any unit of volume of plasma taken for analysis will be lipid, which is sodium free. In patients with extreme hyperproteinemia, proteins occupy more than the normal 7% of plasma volume, again reducing the proportion of aqueous sodium-containing fluid. Although the laboratory would report hyponatremia, sodium concentration per liter of plasma water and plasma osmolality are normal; therefore, this type of hyponatremia is artifactual and without any clinical implications.

In the syndrome of inappropriate secretion of antidiuretic hormone (SIADH), hypotonicity of the plasma fails to suppress the release of ADH, with the result that renal excretion of water is impaired. The consequent expansion of ECF not only causes dilution of body fluids, but also induces a sodium diuresis by virtue of an increase in the rate of glomerular filtration and other as yet unknown factors. The combination of water retention and salt wasting produces a decrease in serum sodium concentration to as low as 110 or even 100 mEq/L. The syndrome has been noted in association with bronchogenic carcinoma of the oat cell type, carcinoma of the pancreas, and other malignant tumors that appear to produce a vasopressorlike polypeptide. The syndrome is also seen in association with CNS disturbances such as head injuries, brain tumors, encephalitis, and lung diseases such as cavitating tuberculosis or pneumonia. Although in most cases with SIADH the urinary sodium is high (>20 mEq/L), when the serum sodium concentration falls to less than 110 mEq/L, a new steady state of sodium concentration is achieved and the urine may become virtually sodium free if the sodium intake is extremely low. The salt wasting can, however, be readily unmasked by the administration of salt, either orally or intravenously.

A variety of drugs, including chlorpropamide, vincristine, cyclophosphamide, carbamazepine, tolbutamide, clofibrate, morphine, barbiturates, and acetaminophen interfere with the excretion of water load by the kidneys and can produce enough retention of water to cause volume expansion and hyponatremia. These agents are believed to stimulate the release of ADH and, at least in the case of chlorpropamide, augment the action of ADH on the renal tubule. The resulting syndrome is indistinguishable from the classic SIADH.

Treatment. The treatment of hyponatremia depends on the cause. In the presence of volume depletion, hyponatremia is best treated with isotonic saline. Severe hyponatremia can be treated by the intravenous administration of hypertonic (3%) sodium chloride. Elevation of serum sodium to 125-130 mEq/L ordinarily suffices to eliminate central nervous system

Table 5. Hyponatremia

State of ECF volume	Decreased (volume depletion)	Normal or modestly increased (no edema)	Increased (edema)
Sodium and water balance	↓Water, ↓↓sodium	↑Water, N sodium	↑Water, ↑↑sodium
Causes	Renal losses Diuretics Mineralocorticoid deficiency Salt-losing nephritis Proximal renal tubular acidosis	Glucocorticoid deficiency Hypothyroidism Pain Psychogenic polydipsia Drugs SIADH	Nephrotic syndrome Cirrhosis CHF Acute and chronic renal failure
	Extrarenal losses Vomiting Diarrhea "Third spacing" Pancreatitis Traumatized muscle		
Urinary sodium concentration (mEq/L)	Renal losses >20 Extrarenal losses <10	>20	Nephrotic syndrome Cirrhosis CHF <10 Renal failure >20
Treatment	Isotonic saline	Water restriction	Sodium/water restriction

ECF = Extracellular fluid volume

SIADH = Syndrome of inappropriate antidiuretic hormone

dysfunction. Mild SIADH symptoms are best treated simply by restricting fluid intake without the restriction of salt. Fluid restriction has to be stringent enough to produce a loss of at least one pound of weight every day. An intake of 400-500 ml of fluid per day will usually accomplish this goal. When the serum sodium concentration is very low and signs of severe water intoxication such as coma and convulsions are present, hypertonic sodium chloride solution along with intravenous furosemide should be administered to correct hyponatremia and overhydration. Demeclocycline and lithium interfere with the action of vasopressin on the renal tubule and are useful agents for long-term use. Demeclocycline is the safer of the two agents and is administered in a 600-1200 mg per day oral dose to correct the syndrome of inappropriate ADH release. Demeclocycline is metabolized by the liver and should be avoided in patients with liver dysfunction because of the risk for nephrotoxicity and azotemia.

Hypernatremia

Hypernatremia is much less common than hyponatremia and may occur in the presence of low, normal, or excess total body sodium. An intact thirst mechanism normally stimulates intake of sufficient water to prevent hypernatremia. The presence of hypernatremia, therefore, may indicate a hypothalamic lesion causing adipsia or an inability to take water, as may happen in unconscious states, vomiting, and unavailability of water. Causes and diagnostic features of hypernatremia are listed in Table 6.

Clinical Features. The principal symptoms and signs of hypernatremia are related to central nervous system functions. Hypernatremia causes cellular dehydration and therefore brain shrinkage. Acute hypernatremia is more dangerous than slowly developing chronic hypernatremia.

Treatment. It is best to correct hypernatremia at a rate commensurate with its rate of development. Rapid correction of hypernatremia may lead to cerebral edema and convulsions. The nature of intravenous fluid needed to correct the various types of hypernatremia is listed in Table 6. Lysine vasopressin (lypressin, Diapid) and desmopressin acetate (DDAVP) are synthetic analogs of Vasopressin with longer antidiuretic and little pressor effects. They are adminstered by nasal insufflation and are the preferred drugs for central diabetes insipidus.

POTASSIUM METABOLISM

Normal Potassium Balance

Potassium is the principal intracellular cation. It plays a significant role in control of intracellular osmotic pressure and a number of enzymatic reactions. In addition, it is responsible for the excitability of both skeletal and cardiac muscle and functions of the kidneys. The normal serum potassium concentration is 3.5-5.5 mEq/L in extracellular fluid and approximately 150 mEq/L in intracellular fluid. Thus, only a small fraction of the 2,500-3,000 mEq of potassium within the body is contained in the extracellular space. The ratio of intracellular potassium concentration is the principal determinant of membrane potential in excitable tissues. The relationship between plasma and cellular potassium is influenced by a number of factors; prominent among them is acid-base balance. Acidosis tends to shift potassium out of cells, and alkalosis favors movement of potassium into the cells. During potassium depletion, plasma potassium initially decreases about 1 mEq/L for each 100-200 mEq potassium. Upon administration of potassium, renal excretion of the ion increases promptly; therefore, sustained hyperkalemia is rarely caused by excess

Table 6. Hypernatremia

Mechanism	Sodium and water losses	Water losses	Sodium addition
Total body sodium	Low	Normal	Increased
Causes	Renal losses Osmotic diuresis (mannitol, glucose, urea)	Renal losses Diabetes insipidus (central, nephrogenic partial) Hypodipsia	Primary hyperaldosteronism Cushing's syndrome Hypertonic dialysis Hypertonic saline sodium bicarbonate
	Extrarenal losses Excessive sweating Diarrhea in children	Extrarenal losses Respiratory and dermal insensible losses	Sodium chloride tablets
Urinary concentration (urine Na^+ in mEq/L)	Renal losses Iso- or hypotonic (>20)	Renal losses Hypo-, iso-, or hypertonic urine (variable)	Iso- or hypertonic urine (>20)
	Extrarenal losses Hypertonic (<10)	Extrarenal losses Hypertonic urine (variable)	
Treatment	Hypotonic saline	Water replacement	Diuretics and water replacement

potassium intake in the presence of normal renal function. Of the usual potassium intake of 50-150 mEq/L, most is excreted in the urine. Although the excess potassium is excreted promptly, the renal response to potassium depletion is more sluggish. The bulk of filtered potassium is reabsorbed by the proximal tubule and the loop of Henle, so that only 10% of the filtered load reaches the distal tubule. Urinary potassium is derived mostly from potassium secreted by distal portions of the nephron. Potassium secretion along the distal tubules is modulated by urinary flow rate, the sodium concentration in the distal tubule, the acid-base status, potassium intake, aldosterone secretion, and integrity of the distal tubule cells. Net excretion is the result of secretion and concurrent reabsorption in the distal segments. Alkalosis enhances, whereas acidosis depresses, renal potassium secretion.

Disorders of Potassium Balance

Hypokalemia

The causes of hypokalemia fall into three major categories: inadequate intake, excessive gastrointestinal or renal losses, and shifts of potassium from the extracellular to the intracellular compartment (Table 7). More than one mechanism may be simultaneously active. Typically, serum potassium concentration is reduced to 2.5-3.5 mEq/L; but, with severe potassium depletion, it may fall below 2 mEq/L. The serum potassium may be normal despite low body potassium by the concomitant presence of acidosis that shifts the intracellular potassium into the extracellular compartment.

Clinical Features and Diagnosis. The most prominent features of hypokalemia are those affecting the neuromuscular system. Depending on the degree and rapidity with which hypokalemia develops, the symptoms may vary from slight muscle weakness to total paralysis and rhabdomyolysis. The electrocardiographic manifestations of hypokalemia include flattening and inversion of the T wave, increased prominence of the U wave, and sagging of the S-T segment. In digitalized patients, the sudden development of hypokalemia may precipitate serious arrhythmias. Long-standing potassium depletion may affect the renal tubular function. So-called hypokalemic nephropathy is manifested by decreased concentration ability, polyuria, and polydipsia. Potassium deficiency can also cause dysfunction of the smooth muscle of the gastrointestinal tract leading to paralytic ileus. The cause of hypokalemia and potassium depletion is usually evident from the history. However, a history of chronic abuse of laxatives and self-induced vomiting are rarely volunteered by the patient. Hypokalemia and hypocalcemia may occur together in patients with malabsorption syndrome. The neuromuscular effects of each electrolyte abnormality is masked by the other, and treatment of one may bring out manifestations of the other.

Treatment. When possible, potassium depletion should be corrected by increased dietary intake or supplementation with potassium salts. Potassium chloride is preferred, especially in alkalotic patients. Organic salts such as gluconate or citrate are adequate in patients who are not severely alkalotic. Potassium salts are best administered after meals to avoid gastrointestinal discomfort.

Intravenous treatment is required when the potassium deficiency is severe or in the presence of gastrointestinal disorders. Concentrations in intravenous infusion should not exceed 40 or, at the most, 60 mEq/L. Potassium is best administered at a rate of no more than 20 mEq/h or approximately 200-250 mEq/day. If more rapid administration is required, the patient's heart beat should be monitored for changes due to hyperkalemia.

Table 7. Causes of Hypokalemia

Causes
Inadequate dietary intake
Gastrointestinal losses (vomiting, diarrhea, villous adenoma, fistulas, ureterosigmoidostomy, chronic laxative abuse)
Renal losses
Diuretics and osmotic diuresis (glycosuria)
Excessive mineralocorticoid effects
Primary aldosteronism (adenoma, bilateral hyperplasia)
Secondary aldosteronism (including accelerated hypertension, renovascular hypertension, renin-producing tumor)
Glucocorticoid excess (adrenal steroid therapy, Cushing's syndrome, ectopic ACTH production)
Licorice ingestion
Renal tubular disorders (renal tubular acidosis, Liddle's syndrome, antibiotic-induced renal damage, metabolic acidosis)
Recovery phase of acute tubular necrosis
Cellular shift (alkalosis, periodic paralysis, insulin administration)

Hyperkalemia

The causes of hyperkalemia are listed in Table 8.

Clinical Features and Diagnosis. The clinical manifestations of potassium intoxication are related primarily to the heart and the neuromuscular system. Electrocardiographic abnormalities are the earliest and most frequent sign of potassium

Table 8. Causes of Hyperkalemia

Causes
Pseudohyperkalemia (improper venipuncture technique, thrombocytosis, leukocytosis, in vitro hemolysis)
Exogenous potassium load (oral or intravenous KCl, K^+-containing drugs and salt substitutes, transfusion, geophagia)
Inadequate excretion
Renal failure (acute, chronic with marked acidosis or oliguria)
Mineralocorticoid deficiency
Addison's disease
Bilateral adrenalectomy
Hypoaldosteronism (hyporeninemic hypoaldosteronism, heparin, specific enzymatic defect, tubular unresponsiveness)
Potassium-sparing diuretics (spironolactone, triamterene, amiloride)
Shift or release of potassium from tissues
Tissue damage (trauma, burns, rhabdomyolysis, hemolysis, tumor necrosis)
Drugs (succinylcholine, digitalis, poisoning, arginine infusion)
Metabolic acidosis
Hyperkalemic periodic paralysis

intoxication occurring when the serum potassium concentration reaches 7-8 mEq/L. The earliest manifestations are the development of high, peaked T waves, especially prominent in precordial leads. It is usually followed by a prolongation of the P-R interval, widening of the QRS complex, complete heart block, and atrial asystole. The QRS becomes progressively prolonged and finally tends to merge with the T waves in a sine-wave configuration. Cardiac standstill is likely to occur at a serum potassium concentration of 9-10 mEq/L. Skeletal muscle weakness and paralysis occur occasionally with moderate or severe hyperkalemia.

Treatment. The cause of hyperkalemia should be eliminated whenever possible. Minimal hyperkalemia (serum potassium 5.5-6.5 mEq/L and electrocardiographic changes limited to peaking of T waves) can usually be treated with elimination of the cause or by treatment of accompanying acidosis. More severe or progressive hyperkalemia requires aggressive therapy. Cardiac toxicity responds best to infusion of calcium, which counteracts the adverse effects of potassium on neuromuscular membranes. Ten to 30 milliliters of 10% calcium gluconate should be infused intravenously within 1-5 minutes. The effect of calcium infusion, while almost immediate, is relatively transient. In moderately severe hyperkalemia (serum potassium 6.5-8 mEq/L, T-wave peaking on the electrocardiogram), infusion of hypertonic glucose solution along with intravenous insulin decreases potassium toxicity by shifting the ion into cells. One liter of a 10% glucose solution with 30-40 units of insulin is generally employed for this purpose and may reduce serum potassium by 1-2 mEq/L, the effect persisting for a number of hours. Intravenous sodium bicarbonate, 44-132 mEq, helps lower serum potassium rapidly by causing potassium shift into the cells. Although sodium bicarbonate is most valuable in acidotic patients, it also is effective when the acid-base balance is normal. The effect occurs within 1 hour and persists for 6-12 hours. None of the above measures removes potassium from the body. A cation-exchange resin in the sodium cycle, such as sodium polystyrene sulfonate (Kayexalate), removes the potassium from the body when administered by mouth at a dosage of 20-30 g every 6 hours along with 20 ml of a 70% solution of sorbital, the latter to prevent constipation. The resin can also be given as a retention enema of 100 g in several hundred milliliters of water. A single enema can reduce potassium by 0.5-2 mEq/L within 1 hour. Hemodialysis and peritoneal dialysis are efficient alternative measures that are used in the presence of renal failure.

ACID-BASE METABOLISM

Normal Acid-Base Balance

Physiologic Considerations

Normal metabolism continuously produces acids. These acids are produced intracellularly and diffuse or are transported into the extracellular fluid. The volatile acids are excreted by the lung, whereas nonvolatile acids are excreted only by the kidneys. The single, important volatile acid significant to health is carbon dioxide. Carbon dioxide reacts with water to form H_2CO_3 at the sites of metabolic production and is transferred to the lungs. At the alveolar membranes, the reaction is reversed and the carbon dioxide (CO_2) gas is liberated and expelled in the expired air. Some 20,000 mM of CO_2 are produced each day in the adult. The alveolar ventiation maintains the P_{CO_2} of arterial blood at approximately 40 mm Hg; that is, 1.2 mM of dissolved carbon dioxide per liter of plasma.

As the food is oxidized, both carbon dioxide and nonvolatile acids such as sulfuric and phosphoric acids are added to the extracellular fluid. Immediate buffering within the interstitial fluid, plasma, and red blood cells minimizes the changes in pH and permits a large quantity of acid to be transferred to the lungs and kidneys for excretion.

Nonvolatile acids are excreted solely by the kidney. Virtually all hydrogen ion (50-100 mEq/day) is excreted as either titratable acid or ammonium. Hydrogen ion is excreted by the distal renal tubule where it binds with phosphates ($HPO_4 + H \rightarrow H_2PO_4$). In the process sodium is absorbed back into the renal tubular cell. The secreted hydrogen ions also combine with the ammonia that diffuses from the tubular cells into the lumen to form ammonium ions. The term metabolic describes an acid-base disturbance initiated by a change in bicarbonate concentration; the term respiratory denotes a disturbance initiated by a change in P_{CO_2}. Each initiating event, whether metabolic or respiratory, sets in motion secondary physiologic responses. The metabolic disturbances induce a ventilatory response that alters the P_{CO_2}, and the respiratory disturbances result in an immediate titration of tissue buffers that abruptly alter the level of bicarbonate. If the respiratory disturbance lasts a few days, a change in renal acid excretion and bicarbonate absorption occurs, which results in further adjustments in acid-base equilibrium. Respiratory disturbances are, therefore, classified as acute or chronic. A simple acid-base disturbance denotes the presence of one primary process and its appropriate physiologic response. A mixed acid-base disturbance refers to the coexistence of two or more primary processes. The two primary events may alter the body's hydro-

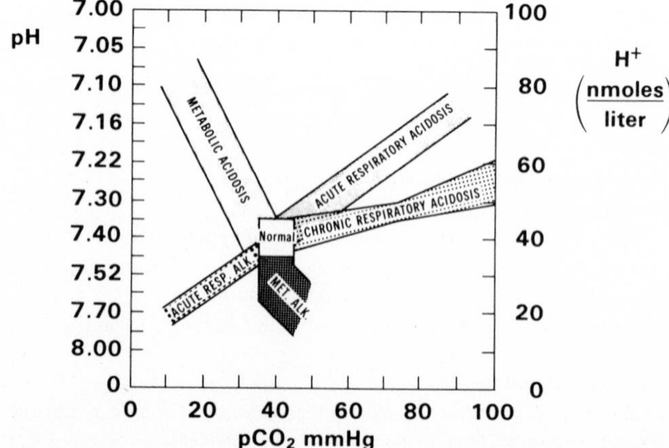

Figure 3. A simplified way to diagnose various acid-base disorders based on P_{CO_2} and pH (H^+).

gen ion concentration (or pH) in the same or opposite direction. Figure 3 illustrates how to reasonably diagnose the acid-base disorder based on arterial P_{CO_2} and pH (or H^+).

Bicarbonate generated in tubular cells moves into peritubular blood and replenishes the bicarbonate stores for buffering of more acid. Derangements of pulmonary or renal function and stresses that may overwhelm the normal regulatory mechanisms can produce disturbances of acid-base equilibrium.

Evaluation of Acid-Base Balance

The bicarbonate-carbonic acid system, the principal buffer of extracellular fluid, is functionally linked with the intracellular buffers and provides a meaningful and convenient expression of the acid-base status of the organism. The relationship among the elements of the acid-base system is best expressed by the following equation:

$$[H^+]\ (nEq/L) = 24\ \frac{P_{CO_2}\ (mm\ Hg)}{[HCO_3^-]\ (mEq/L)}$$

(Henderson equation)

or by the logarithmic form:

$$pH = 6.1 + \log \frac{[HCO_3^-]}{0.03\ P_{CO_2}}$$

(Henderson-Hasselbalch equation).

In practice, the value for the total carbon dioxide concentration is substituted for bicarbonate in both of the above equations without introducing any signficant error. Ideally, arterial blood samples should be used for acquiring acid-base data; venous blood sample analysis without stasis can provide sufficiently reliable information.

Definitions and Terminology

Acidemia and alkalemia are terms used to denote increases and decreases in hydrogen ion concentration, respectively (or, conversely, decreases and increases in pH). The terms acidosis and alkalosis are used to describe primarily pathophysiologic processes that tend to alter the hydrogen ion concentration or pH.

Clinical Disorders of Acid-Base Balance

Metabolic Acidosis

Pathophysiology. Metabolic acidosis is caused by increased production of nonvolatile acids, decreased acid excretion by the kidney, and loss of alkali. In each case, the reduction in bicarbonate concentration is accompanied by a rise in hydrogen ion concentration, that is, a decrease in pH. Body buffers provide the large reservoir of hydrogen ion acceptors distributed throughout the extracellular and intracellular compartments. In the extracellular space, bicarbonate is the principal buffer; hemoglobin and plasma proteins contribute only to the buffering ability of blood. Intracellular buffers consisting largely of protein and organic anions sequester acid load, providing indirect protection against lethal reductions in extracellular pH. To maintain electroneutrality, as hydrogen ions accumulate, both potassium and sodium are forced out of cells. In the presence of normal renal function, the displaced potassium is excreted in the urine. In the presence of renal dysfunction and dehydration, potassium is retained and potentially dangerous hyperkalemia may occur. Respiratory compensation takes place by an increase in both depth and rate of respiration, lowering alveolar and arterial P_{CO_2}; but respiratory defense is never sufficient to restore pH to normal. Even with the most severe metabolic acidosis, P_{CO_2} does not fall below 10 mm Hg. In the patients with plasma bicarbonate of 10 mEq/L, for example, normal respiratory compensation reduces the P_{CO_2} to 25 mm Hg, keeping the pH in the 7.20-7.25 range, whereas without the reduction in P_{CO_2}, the pH would be 7.00. Renal compensation is a final step in the defense against metabolic acidosis, but it takes place slowly and does not contribute to the immediate protection of pH. In the presence of renal dysfunction or renal tubular disease, an even longer period may be required for compensation.

Pathogenesis and Diagnosis. The diagnostic approach to the metabolic acidosis is based on the presence or absence of an increase in unmeasured anions (anion gap):

$$\text{Unmeasured anion} = [Na^+](mEq/L) - [Cl^- + HCO_3^-](mEq/L);$$

$$\text{Normal unmeasured anion} = 8\text{-}12\ mEq/L.$$

In health, the unmeasured anions are mostly protein anions along with small quantities of sulfate, phosphate, and organic acids. The causes of metabolic acidosis based on unmeasured anions are listed in Table 9.

Lactic acidosis is a frequent cause of life-threatening metabolic acidosis. The production of lactic acidosis results most often from an interference with oxidative metabolism. Liver can regenerate bicarbonate ions from lactic acid; but, in the presence of liver dysfunction, lactic acidosis can be severe. The most common lactic acidosis is secondary to circulatory failure, as in shock, low cardiac output states, severe anemia, and sepsis. In these situations, tissue hypoxia accelerates glycolysis and lactic acid is formed more rapidly than it can be metabolized. Lactic acidosis is also observed with phenformin

Table 9. Causes of Metabolic Acidosis

With increase in unmeasured anions
Diabetic ketoacidosis
Lactic acidosis
Azotemic renal failure
Ingestions (salicylates, methyl alcohol, ethylene glycol, paraldehyde, chronic alcoholism)
Normal unmeasured anions
Excessive HCO_3^- loss (diarrhea, drainage of pancreatic juice, ureterosigmoidostomy, proximal renal tubular acidosis, carbonic anhydrase inhibitors, hypoaldosteronism, hyperparathyroidism)
Decreased renal HCO_3^- regeneration (distal renal tubular acidosis)
Excessive HCl production (ammonium chloride, arginine hydrochloride administration; intravenous hyperalimentation solution containing cationic amino acids)
Combinations of the above

therapy, alcoholism, diabetes mellitus (with or without ketoacidosis), and certain types of leukemia. Spontaneous lactic acidosis may develop without a recognized cause, especially in chronically ill, debilitated patients. Firm diagnosis can be made only if the serum lactate level is found to be elevated (normal venous lactate in 0.5-2.2 mM/L). In the absence of lactate determination, a strong presumptive diagnosis can be entertained if the anion gap is elevated in the absence of any obvious cause.

Treatment. Correction of the cause of metabolic acidosis is the first step in treatment of the disorder. Moderate metabolic acidosis (plasma $HCO_3^- > 18$ mEq/L) is usually well tolerated and does not require treatment. Acute and moderately severe to severe metabolic acidosis (plasma $HCO_3^- < 10$ mEq/L) requires intravenous infusion of sodium bicarbonate to correct the acidosis. Effective space of distribution of bicarbonate is approximately equal to body water. Thus, a 60-kg woman with approximately 30kg of body water would require 120 mEq of sodium bicarbonate to increase plans bicarbonate by 4 mEq/L. Sodium bicarbonate should be infused slowly, and serum HCO_3^- should not be raised to levels greater than 15-18 mEq/L. The restoration of serum HCO_3 to normal may produce alkalosis because of persistence of a low P_{CO_2} and can cause cardiac arrhythmias, tetany, and seizures.

Dichloroacetate is undergoing clinical trials and may be used for the treatment of lactic acidosis. The drug reduces lactate concentration by increasing the affinity of the enzyme pyruvate dehydrogenase.

Metabolic Alkalosis

Metabolic alkalosis results from either an abnormal loss of acid or an excessive retention of alkali. In each case, a rise in bicarbonate concentration induces a fall in hydrogen ion concentration, that is, an increase in pH.

Pathophysiology. As in metabolic acidosis, tissue buffers defend the pH to a significant extent. In response to alkalinization of the extracellular fluid, hydrogen ions migrate out of cells in exchange for sodium and potassium, mitigating the severity of the acid-base disturbance. Respiratory compensation may serve as an additional mitigating factor. Diminished ventilation and the resulting rise in P_{CO_2} tends to restore the ratio between carbonic acid and bicarbonate. Each mEq/L increment in bicarbonate, on the average, evokes only 0.5-0.7 mm Hg increment in P_{CO_2}. Even with severe metabolic acidosis, P_{CO_2} does not usually rise above 50 mm Hg. Respiratory compensation usually becomes significant only when plasma bicarbonate concentration rises to 35 or 40 mEq/L. Renal excretion of excess alkali is ultimately responsible for the correction of metabolic alkalosis. Despite elevation of plasma bicarbonate, the urine pH is usually less than 7 in patients with sustained metabolic alkalosis, indicating relatively high reabsorption of bicarbonate by the kidney probably due to an associated volume-concentrated state.

Pathogenesis and Diagnosis. The causes of metabolic alkalosis are outlined in Table 10. Loss of body chloride out of proportion to the loss of sodium is the most frequent cause of sustained metabolic alkalosis. Due to a reduction in the effect of extracellular fluid volume, the kidney attempts to conserve sodium. Since filtered sodium is no longer accompanied by a normal complement of chloride, the rate of sodium-hydrogen exchange is accelerated, thus sustaining the alkalosis. The diagnostic hallmark of conditions characterized by volume and chloride depletion is virtual absence of urinary chloride.

Table 10. Causes of Metabolic Alkalosis

Volume and chloride depletion
Vomiting and gastric drainage
Diuretic therapy
Abrupt relief of hypercapnia
Congenital chloride diarrhea
Hypercalcemia
Potassium depletion
Cushing's syndrome
Primary aldosteronism
Bartter's syndrome
Licorice ingestion
Chronic diarrhea
Excessive alkali intake
Bicarbonate infusion
Milk-alkali syndrome

Severe potassium depletion probably causes intracellular acidosis that, at the renal tubular cell level, results in increased renal acid excretion (renal bicarbonate production) and an increased renal threshold for bicarbonate, so that the high filtered loads of bicarbonate can be retained by the kidneys. These forms of metabolic alkalosis are associated with abundant urinary chloride.

There are no specific clinical signs or symptoms. Severe alkalosis may cause apathy, confusion, and stupor. Serum calcium is borderline or low; rapid development of alkalosis may lead to tetany. Diagnosis of metabolic alkalosis depends on recognition of the clinical setting and appropriate laboratory studies. Plasma potassium concentration is often reduced, and ECG may reveal changes in T and U waves typical of hypokalemia.

Treatment. Treatment of the underlying cause to prevent further progression of metabolic alkalosis is important. In patients with volume and chloride depletion (Urine $Cl^- < 10$ mEq/L), infusion of saline solutions is usually sufficient to enhance renal bicarbonate excretion and to correct alkalosis. Consequently, these forms of metabolic alkalosis are termed chloride responsive. Moderate potassium deficits can be repaired readily with potassium chloride administration. Metabolic alkalosis with potassium depletion is not correctable by sodium chloride infusion and is thus termed chloride resistant. Potassium chloride administration, however, corrects the situation. In patients with prolonged gastric losses where metabolic alkalosis is not correctable by sodium and potassium chloride infusion, intravenous administration of ammonium chloride or arginine hydrochloride may be necessary. However, in most patients, the use of these potentially toxic acidifying agents can be avoided by appropriate early treatment with saline and potassium chloride.

Milk-alkali syndrome occurs as a result of alkali ingestion in the presence of renal dysfunction. Nephropathy limits bicarbonate excretion, thus maintaining the alkalosis.

Respiratory Acidosis

Pathophysiology. Respiratory acidosis results from decreased alveolar ventilation and an increase in P_{CO_2}. In acute respiratory acidosis, immediate tissue buffering is insufficient because of rapid production of carbon dioxide and rise in carbonic acid. This leads to an increased plasma hydrogen ion concentration; however, after 24 hours of hypercapnia, there is a significant increase in renal acid excretion and bicarbonate production, which results in a rise of plasma bicarbonate concentration and a fall in plasma hydrogen ion. This usually reaches a steady state by 3-7 days so that plasma bicarbonate rises approximately 3 mEq/L for each increase of 10 mm Hg in P_{CO_2}.

Pathogenesis and Causes. The causes of respiratory acidosis are listed in Table 11. Acute respiratory acidosis occurs whenever there is a sudden failure of ventilation as in patients with airway obstruction, narcotic or sedative overdosage, severe pulmonary edema, and cardiopulmonary arrest. Acute and chronic diseases characterized principally by interference with alveolar gas exchange, such as chronic pulmonary fibrosis, pneumonia, and pulmonary edema, usually cause hypocapnia as hypoxia stimulates increased ventilation.

Clinical Features and Diagnosis. When P_{CO_2} exceeds 70 mm Hg, patients manifest confusion and obtundation. Asterexis, papilledema, and congestion of the conjunctiva and face may be noted. Respiration is depressed and shallow. Arterial blood gas measurements reveal elevated P_{CO_2} and acidemia. Acidosis in acute cardiopulmonary arrest is usually a combination of lactic metabolic acidosis and acute respiratory acidosis. Plasma bicarbonate is normal in acute respiratory acidosis but is elevated in chronic respiratory acidosis.

Table 11. Causes of Respiratory Acidosis

Acute respiratory acidosis
Sudden airway obstruction (foreign body in the trachea, trauma, hemorrhage in a tumor compressing or obstructing the trachea)
Depression of respiratory center (sedatives and narcotics, CNS diseases, respiratory arrest)
Neuromuscular disorders
Chest-wall disorders (fractured ribs)
Decreased alveolar ventilation (pulmonary edema, pneumonia, aspiration pneumonitis)
Chronic respiratory acidosis
Obstructive pulmonary disease (chronic bronchitis, emphysema, asthma)
Alveolar hypoventilation (Pickwickian syndrome)
Chronic respiratory muscle weakness

Treatment. The treatment of acute respiratory acidosis is directed toward the underlying cause of impaired ventilation. Treatment of chronic respiratory acidosis is to increase alveolar ventilation by such means as an endotracheal tube, mechanical ventilators, or bronchodilators. In severe hypercapnia, the sensitivity of the respiratory center to carbon dioxide may be diminished and hypoxemia may be the major stimulus to respiratory activity. If hypoxemia is suddenly corrected, ventilation may be further depressed, causing hypercapnia to become severe. Thus, during oxygen therapy, the patient must be watched closely and blood gases monitored to ensure that improvement in hypoxemia does not depress ventilation. In patients with chronic respiratory acidosis, posthypercapnic alkalosis develops if P_{CO_2} is rapidly restored to normal. This can be corrected by administration of NaCl and KCl, which leads to bicarbonate diuresis and correction of metabolic alkalosis. Administration of alkali has no role in management of respiratory acidosis.

Respiratory Alkalosis

Pathophysiology. Respiratory alkalosis results from an increase in alveolar ventilation causing a decrease in P_{CO_2}. Acute reduction in carbon dioxide concentration releases hydrogen ions from tissue buffers, which minimizes alkalemia by reducing plasma bicarbonate. An abrupt reduction in P_{CO_2} to 20-25 mm Hg is associated with a 3-4 mEq/L fall in plasma bicarbonate concentration. On the other hand, prolonged reductions in P_{CO_2} (chronic respiratory alkalosis) reduces renal acid excretion and bicarbonate reabsorption, causing plasma bicarbonate concentration to fall further. Each millimeter of mercury decrement of P_{CO_2} causes 0.4-0.5 mEq/L reduction of plasma bicarbonate concentration.

Pathogenesis and Causes. The causes of respiratory alkalosis are listed in Table 12. The most common cause of respiratory alkalosis is hyperventilation resulting from extreme anxiety. Ventilation perfusion defects in certain pulmonary diseases produce hypoxemia and hyperventilation, leading to hypocap-

Table 12. Causes of Respiratory Alkalosis

Acute respiratory alkalosis
Hyperventilation due to anxiety
Fever
Exercise
Acute hypoxia (asthma, pneumonia, acute pulmonary edema)
Salicylate intoxication
Overzealous mechanical ventilation
Gram-negative septicemia
Chronic respiratory alkalosis
CNS diseases (tumor, encephalitis)
Chronic hepatic insufficiency
Pregnancy
Chronic hypoxia (lung disease, cyanotic heart disease, adaptation to high altitude)

nia. Persistence of respiratory compensation after the correction of metabolic acidosis produces changes that are chemically indistinguishable from primary respiratory alkalosis.

Clinical Features and Diagnosis. Patients with acute respiratory alkalosis complain of paresthesias, numbness, tingling, and lightheadedness and may demonstrate tetany due to enhanced neuromuscular excitability. Diagnosis is suspected from the clinical setting and confirmed by analysis of blood gases that demonstrate hypocapnia together with a variable degree of alkalemia. Usually, plasma bicarbonate is decreased but is rarely below 15 mEq/L.

Treatment. The treatment of respiratory alkalosis is directed toward correction of the underlying causes. In the acute hyperventilation syndrome, sedation, reassurance, and, if symptoms are sufficiently severe, rebreathing into a bag usually terminates the attack. In patients with salicylate intoxication, the goal is removal of the offending drug. Renal excretion of salicylates is augmented by urinary alkalinization along with adminstration of osmotic diuretics or by hemodialysis.

Mixed Acid-Base Disturbances

The coexistence of two or more simple acid-base disturbances is not an uncommon finding in hospitalized patients. When the magnitude of the secondary change in P_{CO_2} or bicarbonate concentration (in the metabolic and respiratory disorders, respectively) is inappropriate with respect to the magnitude of the initiating process, the presence of a mixed disturbance should be suspected. Clues to the presence of complicating disturbances should be sought from the patient's history and a close examination of the laboratory data. The following are frequently encountered examples of mixed acid-base disturbances.

Metabolic Acidosis Plus Respiratory Acidosis. This combination is most frequently encountered following acute cardiopulmonary arrest and acute pulmonary edema. It results from accumulation of carbon dioxide and lactic acidosis triggered by poor tissue perfusion. The treatment consists of artificial ventilation and sodium bicarbonate administration. Frequent monitoring of blood gases is essential to ensure optimal treatment.

Chronic Respiratory Acidosis Plus Metabolic Alkalosis. This is a frequent occurrence in patiens with pulmonary insufficiency and cor pulmonale who are treated with diuretics and a low-salt diet. The metabolic alkalosis can become pronounced when long-standing hypercapnia is partially corrected by mechanical ventilation. The treatment is slow correction of respiratory acidosis and enhanced bicarbonate excretion by acetazolamide.

Chronic Respiratory Acidosis Plus Acute Respiratory Acidosis. Sudden worsening of pulmonary function due to sedative administration, oxygen therapy, or acute pneumonitis in patients with moderately severe carbon dioxide retention due to chronic obstructive disease can develop the above mixed acid-base disorder. The treatment is slow correction of hypercapnia, usually with the assistance of mechanical ventilation.

Respiratory Alkalosis Plus Metabolic Acidosis. This disorder is typical of salicylate intoxication that independently affects the ventilation and cellular metabolism. Gram-negative septicemia can also lead to this combination by producing lactic acidosis and hyperventilation. The treatment is correction of the underlying disorders and infusion of sodium bicarbonate.

HYPERTENSION

Blood pressure (BP) is a physiologic measurement similar to body temperature, heart rate, respiration rate, height, and weight. Elevated blood pressure often leads to complications and therefore needs to be lowered. For all practical purposes in adults under the age of 50 years, a blood pressure ⩾140/90 mm Hg and in persons 50 years or older, a blood pressure ⩾160/95 mm Hg is considered elevated and the condition is termed hypertension.

EPIDEMIOLOGY OF HYPERTENSION

Hypertension is the most common cardiovascular disease and probably the greatest public health problem of our time. The estimates of the number of hypertensive patients in the United States range from a low of 23 million (BP ⩾160/95 mm Hg) to a high of 60 million (BP ⩾140/90 mm Hg). Hypertension contributes to the deaths of at least 250,000 Americans each year.

The major complications of hypertension include stroke, coronary artery disease, and chronic renal failure. Most strokes that occur between the ages of 35 and 65 result from hypertension. Stroke is responsible for as many as 175,000 deaths and 250,000 disabilities per year in the United States. Stroke deaths have been declining in recent years, probably because of early detection and better control of hypertension. Hypertension is the major risk factor for coronary artery disease, which occurs 3-5 times more frequently in people with hypertension than in those with normal arterial pressure. Although the incidence of kidney failure due to hypertension has been declining markedly in recent years, hypertension remains an important cause of kidney failure among the black population. The above complications of hypertension are estimated to cost the nation more than 30 billion dollars per year in direct medical expenditures and lost income through illness, disability, premature loss of productivity, and death, in addition to an incalculable toll of social disruption and agony.

It is obvious, from the body build and blood pressure study of the Society of Actuaries first reported in 1959, that the higher the arterial blood pressure, the higher the mortality over the years. This is true from the lowest to the highest arterial pressure, the relationship being quantitative. Elevated blood pressure of 150/100 mm Hg at age 35 reduces the life expectancy by 16-½ years in men and 13 years in women. The same blood pressure at age 45 reduces the life expectancy by 11½ years in men and 8½ years in women.

Intensive antihypertensive therapy reduces both morbidity

and mortality from complications of hypertension. Only recently has attention been directed toward preventing hypertension. Although the role of excessive sodium intake in causing hypertension remains somewhat controversial, since daily sodium intake is 10-20 times the physiologic need, a lower sodium intake is clearly indicated for most people. Obesity has been known for many years to be a contributing factor to the development of hypertension. Every effort should be made to avoid childhood obesity as obese children develop into obese adults. Obese patients with hypertension should be encouraged to make a concerted effort to lose weight.

Severe hypertension among children (diastolic blood pressure $\geqslant$115 mm Hg) is usually due to secondary hypertension. However, mild to moderate hypertension is usually due to essential hypertension. Children 3 years of age and older should have their blood pressure measured annually as part of their continuing health care.

PATHOPHYSIOLOGY OF HYPERTENSION

Normal Regulation of Blood Pressure

Under normal circumstances, blood pressure is maintained by interplay of various mechanisms. Blood pressure is primarily a function of cardiac output and peripheral resistance. This relationship is summarized by the formula:

$$\text{Blood pressure} = \text{cardiac output} \times \text{peripheral resistance}$$

Cardiac output is the volume of blood ejected by the left ventricle into the aorta per minute. It is the major determinant of systolic blood pressure. Diastolic blood pressure is primarily determined by the resistance in the arterioles. Cardiac output and peripheral resistance are directly and indirectly and indirectly affected by such factors as blood volume, blood viscosity, sympathetic nervous system activity, the renin-angiotensin-aldosterone system, and autacoids (vasoactive substances) such as prostaglandins and bradykinin.

Essential Hypertension

More than 95% of patients with elevated blood pressure have essential (idiopathic, primary) hypertension. These patients do not have an identifiable cause for their hypertension, but have a disease of blood pressure regulation. In earlier stages in mild hypertension, the cardiac output is elevated. As the pressure rises further, cardiac output falls and the elevated blood pressure becomes a reflection of increased peripheral resistance. The state of vasoconstriction is maintained by excess sodium content of the arteriolar smooth muscle cells, increased sympathetic nervous system activity, imbalance between angiotensin (a vasoconstrictor) and prostaglandins and kinins (vasodilators), and other unknown mechanisms. Other factors associated with hypertension include obesity, increased heart rate, heredity, physical activity, and increasing age.

Secondary Hypertension

A specific cause of high blood pressure can be identified in less than 5% of people with hypertension. This type of hypertension, with an identifiable cause, is called secondary hypertension. It is discussed in greater length later in this chapter.

EVALUATION OF THE HYPERTENSIVE PATIENT

Purpose of the Evaluation

The purpose of the elevation is to answer the following questions:

1. *Does the patient have hypertension?* Before a patient is labeled hypertensive, at least three readings of blood pressure should be recorded. Two of the three readings and the average of the three should be elevated.
2. *Is it secondary hypertension?* During initial evaluation, in most patients with secondary hypertension, it should be possible to suspect the presence of secondary hypertension requiring further laboratory and radiologic investigations to prove the diagnosis.
3. *Is there target organ damage?* Presence of target organ damage usually signifies long-standing or severe hypertension. Patients with target organ damage have a worse prognosis.
4. *Are other cardiovascular risk factors present?* Presence of other risk factors such as obesity, smoking, diabetes mellitus, and elevated blood cholesterol should be documented and treated along with control of hypertension.
5. *Are certain antihypertensives contraindicated?* Obesity, peptic ulcer disease, depression, and allergic rhinitis are considered contraindications to reserpine. Asthma, congestive heart failure, and heart block are contraindications to β blockers. Detection of contraindications to certain antihypertensive agents is part of the hypertensive patient's evaluation.
6. *How much does the patient know about hypertension?* Since hypertension is a chronic disorder requiring lifelong treatment, it is imperative that the patient understand this and participate in medical care as much as possible.

History

After the patient identification information is obtained, the first question asked is on the duration of hypertension and previous treatment. Although most patients with mild to moderate hypertension are symptomatic and are surprised to find that their blood pressure is elevated, the severely hypertensive may be quite symptomatic. The symptoms of hypertension include

Headache that is typically located in the occipital region and is worse on rising in the morning

Epistaxis or nose bleed

Cardiovascular symptoms of angina, dyspnea, and ankle edema indicate coronary artery disease and congestive heart failure; claudication or leg pains with walking is indicative of arteriosclerosis in the lower extremities

Cerebrovascular symptoms of dizziness, blackouts, numbness, tingling, or weakness in one side of the body

Review of systems may reveal symptoms suggestive of secondary hypertension. Family history in regard to hypertension, heart disease, diabetes, stroke, and kidney disease must be recorded. The personal history is an extremely important part of the evaluation and includes information on diet, smoking, alcohol consumption, drug abuse, exercise, and sleep.

All medications including oral contraceptives and over-the-counter preparations are recorded. Allergies should not be overlooked.

Physical Examination

The patient's general appearance is noted, particularly in relation to gait, coordination, and speech. Hirsutism and truncal obesity are indications of Cushing's syndrome. Weight, height, and body frame are recorded and compared with standard charts to see if the patient is overweight or obese. The body frame is judged by having the patient hold his left wrist between the right thumb and index finger. If the tips of the fingers touch, the patient has a medium frame; if they do not, a large frame; and if they overlap, a small frame. Pulse rate and regularity should then be noted. Peripheral pulses, that is, the radial, carotid, and femoral pulses, are palpated. A weak pulse or a bruit indicates the presence of arteriosclerosis.

At the time of the first visit, the blood pressure should be recorded in both arms and a note made as to which side is higher. A discrepancy of up to 5 mm Hg is not unusual. However, a larger difference may indicate the narrowing of an artery in the side in which blood pressure is lower. On follow-up visits the blood pressure is always recorded on the side with the higher blood pressure.

A larger cuff should be used for obese people. The rubber bladder of the blood pressure cuff should have a width equal to one-third to one-half the length of the upper arm and a length equal to at least two-thirds of its circumference. The arm with the cuff wrapped around it is placed at the level of the heart so that hydrostatic pressure does not alter the blood pressure reading. Leg blood pressure is recorded by wrapping a leg cuff around the thigh and auscultating over the popliteal artery, with the patient preferably lying prone. Leg blood pressure should be recorded routinely in children and adolescents with hypertension and in adults who have a delayed or weak femoral pulsation.

The fundi are examined in a dark room with the patient looking straight at a distant point. The hypertensive retinopathy is graded from I to IV in increasing severity. Grade I signifies arterial narrowing or spasm; grade II, arteriovenous nicking; grade III, hemorrhages and exudates; and grade IV, papilledema. Grades III and IV are considered indicative of accelerated and malignant hypertension, respectively.

The neck is examined for a goiter or any other swelling. A note is made if the jugular veins are prominent and distended.

The cardiac examination consists of palpating the point of maximal impulse (PMI, or apex beat), which is shifted downward and laterally as the heart enlarges. Auscultation is then performed for rhythm, heart sounds, and the presence of murmurs. As indicated earlier, an S_4 sound indicates a rigid left ventricle due to left ventricular hypertrophy and an S_3 sound is an early sign of congestive heart failure.

The lungs are then auscultated for rales or wheezing. Basal rales are present in congestive heart failure. Wheezing may indicate heart failure, chronic bronchitis, or asthma.

The abdomen is inspected and palpated to determine whether the kidneys are enlarged. Polycystic kidneys and grossly enlarged, hydronephrotic kidneys usually are easily palpable. Careful auscultation over the epigastrium usually reveals a continuous bruit in patients with renal artery stenosis. It is not uncommon to hear a systolic bruit in the epigastrium, particularly in older patients. This is produced by the flow of blood through the celiac artery and is of no significance.

The legs are then examined for the presence of edema and signs of peripheral vascular disease such as discoloration of the skin, loss of temperature, or absence of dorsalis pedis pulsations. The skin should be closely inspected for neurofibromatosis and café-au-lait spots, which are often seen in patients with pheochromocytoma.

A neurologic examination for muscle strength and deep-tendon reflexes is performed to detect the presence of stroke, of which the patient may or may not be aware.

The prostate is examined in older men. Enlarged prostate and urinary retention may cause kidney damage, which can lead to or contribute to hypertension.

Laboratory Investigations

Certain laboratory investigations are routinely performed as part of the evaluation of a hypertensive patient.

Urinalysis is necessary, since proteinuria usually indicates renal disease and hypertension may be secondary to the renal parenchymal disease. However, long-standing hypertension can cause nephrosclerosis, ischemic glomerulopathy, and mild to moderate proteinuria.

Glycosuria can be easily diagnosed with dipstick urinalysis. Almost 10% of hypertensives have diabetes. The presence of occult blood may indicate a renal or urinary tract disorder. A microscopic examination of the urine must always be undertaken if the dipstick urinalysis is abnormal (presence of protein or blood). This helps determine the nature of renal disease. Red blood cell casts are pathognomonic for glomerulonephritis. However, granular casts simply indicate the presence of a renal disease.

It is a good practice to routinely record the patient's hematocrit before undertaking treatment of hypertension. Many hypertensives tend to have a somewhat higher hematocrit. If the patient is anemic, he may be dizzy from anemia rather than hypertension.

Fasting blood glucose or a 2-hour postprandial blood sugar measurement should be done for the diagnosis of diabetes. BUN or creatinine elevation indicates renal insufficiency, which may be either the cause or the result of hypertension. A slight rise in BUN can be expected to occur after diuretic therapy. If BUN is normal, it is usually not necessary to measure creatinine. However, if BUN is elevated, serum creatinine should always be measured because it is a more accurate indicator of renal dysfunction.

Serum potassium measurement is an excellent screening measure for primary aldosteronism. A normal serum potassium (3.5-5 mEq) on a normal diet excludes primary aldosteronism for all practical purposes.

Serum cholesterol and triglyceride measurements are done to determine the presence of other risk factors such as hypercholesterolemia. After prolonged diuretic therapy, serum lipids may show slight elevation.

Uric acid measurement is not essential for evaluation or to determine the presence of a risk factor; however, the uric acid level may rise with diuretic therapy, and some patients may develop clinical gout.

Serum calcium measurement is useful in determining the presence of hyperparathyroidism, which can cause hypertension. Also, the serum calcium level may rise with thiazide therapy.

Electrocardiogram should be done routinely in patients 40 years of age or older and in younger patients with severe hypertension (diastolic BP $\geqslant$115 mm Hg), cardiac symptoms, arrhythmias, or a strong family history of heart disease. Evidence of left ventricular hypertrophy or myocardial ischemia are signs of hypertensive cardiovascular disease.

Chest x-ray examination is done primarily to determine the heart size and presence of congestive heart failure.

Special Investigations

After the initial evaluation, if a patient is suspected to have secondary hypertension, appropriate laboratory and radiologic investigation are undertaken to prove or disprove the suspected diagnosis. It is fruitless to investigate a patient for all possible causes of secondary hypertension. Only those investigations need be carried out that would help in the diagnosis of a certain suspected cause of secondary hypertension. These are indicated later in this chapter in the section on secondary hypertension.

Table 13. Classification of Antihypertensive Drugs

Diuretics
Thiazides and related diuretics
Loop diuretics: furosemide and ethacrynic acid
Potassium sparing diuretics: spironolactone, triamterene, and amiloride
Sympathetic Inhibitors
Centrally acting: reserpine, methyldopa, and clonidine
Baroreceptor action: veratrum alkaloids (protoveratrine A & B and veratridine)
Ganglion blockers: trimethaphan camsylate
Adrenergic nerve ending blockers: reserpine, guanethidine, bethanidine, and debrisoquin
Receptor blockers:
α blockers: phentolamine, phenoxybenzamine and prazosin
β blockers:
nonselective: alprenolol, nadolol, oxprenolol, pindolol, propranolol, sotalol, and timolol
selective: acebutolol, atenolol, metoprolol, and practolol
α and β blockers: labetolol
Monoamine oxidase inhibitors: pargyline
Blockers of the Renin-Angiotensin System
Renin inhibitors
Converting enzyme inhibitors: taprotide, captopril and enalapril
Angiotensin II blockers: saralasin
Vasodilators
Hydralazine
Minoxidil
Diazoxide
Sodium nitroprusside
Calcium Channel Blockers
Nifedipine
Verapamil
Diltiazem

CLINICAL PHARMACOLOGY OF ANTIHYPERTENSIVE DRUGS

The antihypertensive drugs can be classified in various ways. Table 13 lists a classification based on site of action and Fig. 4 illustrates this.

Diuretics

Most experts consider diuretics first for the treatment of essential hypertension. Table 14 lists various diuretics available for clinical use.

Thiazide Diuretics

Chlorothiazide was the first of these agents. Many analogs are now available that differ only in potency (the dose required to attain the desired effect) and duration of action. In terms of antihypertensive efficacy (maximal beneficial effect), there is little advantage in choosing one over another. Hydrochlorothiazide is probably the most commonly used thiazide diuretic. The thiazides cross the placental barrier and are found in human milk; therefore, they should be avoided in the nursing mother. The early predominant action of thiazides is to enhance sodium and water excretion, producing a mild to moderate volume contraction. In addition, the mobilized sodium and chloride ions from the arteriolar smooth muscle decrease vascular reactivity, blunting the effects of sympathetic reflexes. This results in a blood pressure drop by an average of 10-15 mm Hg. Adverse reactions of clinical importance are hypokalemia, hyperuricemia, hyperglycemia, hypercalcemia, and hyperlipidemia. Hypokalemia is more common with long-acting diuretics such as chlorthalidone and metolazone and may require potassium supplementation or the simultaneous use of potassium-sparing diuretics. Although hyperuricemia is not uncommon. Approximately 10% of patients develop hyperglycemia with chronic diuretic usage. Hyperglycemia and

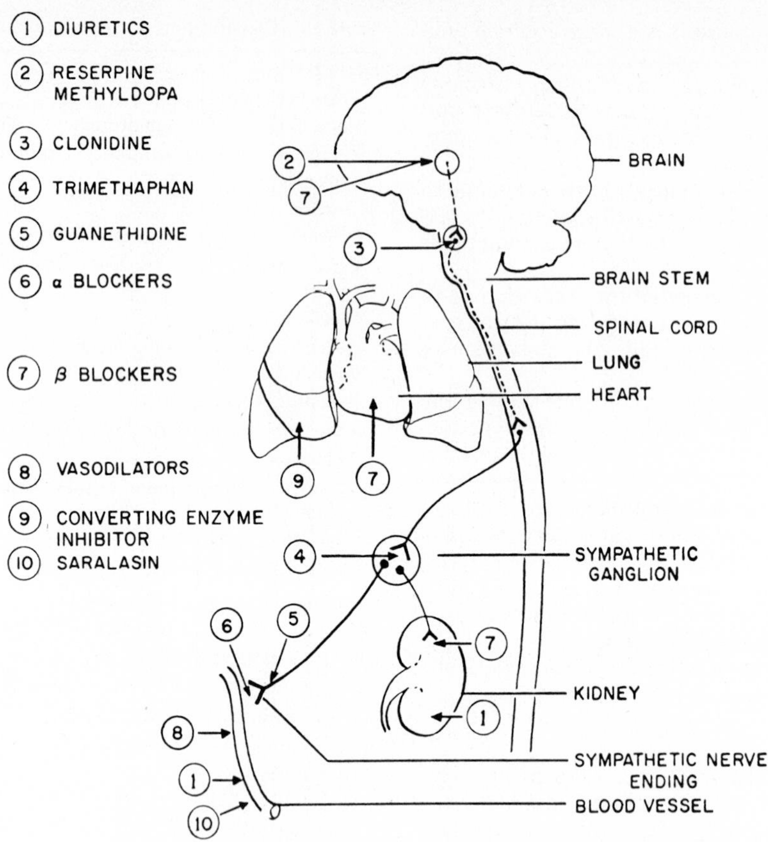

Figure 4. Site of action of various antihypertensive drugs.

diabetes are not contraindications to the use of diuretics for treatment of hypertension. Hypercalcemia after thiazides is seldom of clinical importance. The clinical implications of hyperlipidemia remain to be defined. In pregnancy, fetal jaundice and thrombocytopenia have been reported after thiazides.

Loop Diuretics

The loop diuretics constitute a pharmacologic rather than a chemical class. They produce diuresis far greater than thiazides and act at the loop of Henle. Their antihypertensive mode of action is similar to that of the thiazide diuretics. Their major use in treatment of hypertension is in patients with renal insufficiency and fluid retention. Patients who develop hypercalcemia secondary to thiazides are also candidates for furosemide since the latter increases calcium excretion. Furosemide does not interfere with the excretion of lithium but thiazides do so. Furosemide is therefore preferable to thiazides in patients receiving lithium for treatment of manic depressive illness. The side effects of loop diuretics are essentially similar to thiazides.

Potassium-Sparing Diuretics

These include spironolactone (Aldactone), triamterene (Dyrenium), and amiloride (Midamor).

Spironolactone is a steroid compound with a structural formula similar to aldosterone; it is an antagonist of aldosterone. It increases sodium and water excretion and diminishes potassium excretion. Gynecomastia in the male and menstrual irregularity in the female are important side effects. It should be avoided in pregnancy and during nursing. Aldactazide is a combination of hydrochlorothiazide (25 mg) and spironolactone (25 mg) in a single tablet.

Triamterene is used primarily to conserve potassium and prevent hypokalemia in patients treated with thiazide or loop diuretics. It is contraindicated in patients with renal insufficiency, in whom it can cause fatal hyperkalemia. Dyazide is a combination of hydrochlorothiazide (25 mg) and triamterene (50 mg) in a single capsule.

Amiloride is similar to triamterene as a potassium-retaining diuretic. Moduretic is a combination of hydrochlorothiazide (50 mg) and amiloride (5 mg).

The commonly used antihypertensives other than diuretics are listed in Table 15.

Inhibitors of the Sympathetic Nervous System

This group includes drugs that interfere with sympathetic nerve impulses at different sites from the brain to target organs. The decreased arterial and venous constriction causes a

Table 14. Diuretics for Treatment of Hypertension

Generic Name	*Trade Name*	*Size of Tablets (mg)*	*Dose Range (mg/24 h)*
Thiazides and related diuretics			
Short acting (6-12 h)			
Chlorothiazide	Diuril	250 and 500	250-1,000
Flumethiazide		500	500-1,000
Hydrochlorothiazide	Esidrix Hydrodiuril, Oretic	25 and 50	25-100
Medium acting (12-24 h)			
Bendroflumethiazide	Naturetin	2.5 and 5	2.5-5.0
Benzthiazide	Exna	50	50-100
Cyclothiazide	Anhydron	2	1.0-2.0
Hydroflumethiazide	Saluron	50	50-100
Long acting (24-36 h)			
Methylclothiazide	Enduron	2.5 and 5	2.5-5.0
Metolazone	Diulo, Zaroxolyn	2.5, 5, and 10	2.5-10
Polythiazide	Renese	1, 2, and 4	2.0-4.0
Quinethazone	Hydromox	50	50-100
Trichlormethiazide	Naqua, Metahydrin	2 and 4	2.0-4.0
Ultralong acting (36-72 h)			
Chlorthalidone	Hygroton	25, 50, and 100	25-100
Uricosuric diuretics			
Ticrynafen	Selacryn	250	250-500
Loop diuretics			
Ethacrynic Acid	Edecrin	25 and 50	25-200
Furosemide	Lasix	20 and 40	20-160
Potassium-sparing diuretics			
Spironolactone	Aldactone	25	25-200
Triamterene	Dyrenium	50 and 100	50-300

fall in blood pressure. The adverse effects depend on the site of action and include orthostatic hypotension, nasal congestion, increased gastrointestinal motility, impotence, delayed ejaculation, and bradycardia.

Centrally Acting Sympathetic Inhibitors
These include reserpine, methyldopa, and clonidine. The β-adrenergic blocking agents may also have central action.

Reserpine. Reserpine is the most commonly used rauwolphia alkaloid, although a number of other natural and semisynthetic alkaloids are also available. Effects are cumulative and may require up to 3 weeks for the maximal reduction of blood pressure with usual oral doses. After discontinuance of reserpine, its autonomic action persists for 7-10 days; a month may pass before the drug effects completely disappear from the body. It need be given only in a single daily dose because of its long duration of action. Reserpine has both central and peripheral nervous actions. It depletes stores of catecholamines and serotonin and prevents their reuptake into nerve endings. It is contraindicated in mental depression, peptic ulcer, and ulcerative colitis. It is also not recommended in obese patients as it stimulates the appetite. Adverse reactions include mental depression, nasal stuffiness, weight gain, activation of peptic ulcer, parkinsonism, and sexual dysfunction. A carcinogenic potential has been described in laboratory animals. Numerous preparations are available for oral use.

Methyldopa (Aldomet). The mechanism of antihypertensive action of methyldopa is presently thought to be a consequence of its conversion to methyl norepinephrine in the brain, causing central α-adrenergic stimulation. This reduces peripheral adrenergic activity and causes a reduction in blood pressure within 1-2 hours of administration. It is useful in the treatment of hypertension when a thiazide diuretic alone proves inadequate. It is contraindicated in the presence of liver disease, hemolytic anemia or if previous methyldopa therapy has been associated with hypersensitivity reactions such as liver dysfunction, fever, and skin rash. Sedation, malaise, orthostatic hypotension, and dizziness can occur as side effects.

Clonidine. Clonidine (Catapres) acts by central α-adrenergic stimulation that causes a decrease in sympathetic outflow from the brain. Blood pressure declines within 30-60 minutes after an oral dose. The maximal effect occurs within 2-4 hours, and the antihypertensive response lasts approximately 6-8

Table 15. Commonly Used Antihypertensives

Generic Name	Trade Name	Size of Tablets (mg)	Usual Dose Range (mg/24 h)	Contraindications
Sympathetic inhibitors				
Reserpine and analogues	Many	0.1, 0.25, 0.5, 1, 2, and 5	0.1-1	Mental depression peptic ulcer, obesity, epistaxis, sinusitis
Methyldopa	Aldomet	125, 250, and 500	250-2,000	Liver disease, hemolytic anemia
Clonidine	Catapres	0.1, 0.2, and 0.3	0.1-2	None
Trimethaphan	Arfonad	IV infusion only 500 mg/10 ml ampule	500 mg in 500 ml of 5% dextrose in water Start 3-4 mg/min, increase to titrate BP	Uncorrected anemia, hypovolemia, asphyxia, uncorrected respiratory insufficiency, glaucoma
Guanethidine	Ismelin	10 and 25	10-100	Sexual dysfunction, pheochromocytoma, congestive heart failure
Prazosin	Minipress	1, 2, and 5	3-20	Syncope
Propranolol	Inderal	10, 20, 40, and 80	40-480	Congestive heart failure, asthma, brittle diabetes, bradycardia
Metoprolol	Lopressor	50 and 100	50-400	Same as above
Nadolol	Corgard	40, 80, and 120	40-320	Same as above
Atenolol	Tenormin	50 and 100	50-100	Same as above
Timolol	Blocadren	10	20-40	Same as above
Vasodilators				
Hydralazine	Apresoline	10, 25, 50, and 100	20-200	Angina, mitral valve disease, SLE, syncopal episodes
Minoxidil	Loniten	2.5 and 10	5-40	Pheochromocytoma
Diazoxide	Hyperstat	IV infusion; 15-30 mg/min; 300 mg/20 ml ampule	75-600 mg	Angina, uncontrolled diabetes, heart failure
Sodium nitroprusside	Nipride	IV infusion only; 50 mg/5 ml ampule	50 mg in 500 ml of 5% dextrose in water Start 200 μg/min, increase to titrate BP	Absence of facilities for continuous BP monitoring
Converting Enzyme Inhibitors				
Captopril	Capoten	25, 50, 100	50-300	Neutropenia

hours. The orthostatic effects are mild and infrequent. In combination with a diuretic, it is useful for the treatment of most patients with hypertension. Its hypotensive effect may be reduced by simultaneous administration of a β-blocking agent. Dry mouth, drowsiness, and sedation are the most common side effects. Constipation, dizziness, headache, and fatigue may also occur. On abrupt cessation of therapy, rapid reversal of the antihypertensive effect has been reported. Clonidine is particularly useful in control of hypertension in patients with renal insufficiency and end-stage renal disease.

Ganglion Blockers

Trimethaphan camsylate (Arfonad) is available for intravenous use in treatment of hypertensive emergencies and dissecting aneurysm of the aorta. It blocks both the sympathetic and parasympathetic ganglia. Blockade of the parasympathetic system causes such unacceptable side effects as paralytic ileus, urinary retention, dryness of mouth, and cycloplegia. In addition, angina pectoris or syncope may occur without warning if hypotension is excessive. Trimethaphan is administered by adding 500 mg to 500 ml of 5% dextrose. It is infused initially at the rate of 0.5-1.0 mg/min and the rate gradually altered until the blood pressure is lowered to the desired level. Oral antihypertensive drug therapy is initiated simultaneously to wean the patient from trimethaphan at the first opportunity.

Adrenergic Nerve-Ending Blockers
These drugs are taken up by and displace norepinephrine from the nerve endings. Guanethidine is the prototype of these drugs.

Guanethidine. The pharmacologic effect of guanethidine (Ismelin) develops slowly as it is taken up by the sympathetic nerve endings, displacing norepinephrine. The norepinephrine depletion persists for several days after the drug has been discontinued. Tricyclic antidepressants, amphetamines, and tyramine displace guanethidine at the nerve endings and reduce its antihypertensive effect. The blood pressure response to guanethidine is most intense in the upright posture. The drug is reserved for treatment of unresponsive and uncontrolled hypertension after diuretics and other sympathetic inhibitors and vasodilators have been tried. It is contraindicated in pheochromocytoma. Side effects include postural hypotension, reduction in cardiac output, fluid retention, and sexual dysfunction.

Receptor Blockers
Antihypertensive agents are available which block α and β receptors selectively.

Alpha Blockers. The α-adrenergic blocking agents include phentolamine, phenoxybenzamine, and prazosin. Phentolamine and phenoxybenzamine are potent agents but are seldom used because of severe reflex tachycardia.

Prazosin was initially thought to be a direct vasodilator but has now been shown to be a postsynaptic α-adrenergic blocking agent. It diminishes vascular constriction without affecting the α-adrenergic presynaptic negative-feedback mechanism that inhibits norepinephrine release. It is used with a diuretic agent, with or without additional sympathetic agents, for treatment of hypertension of all grades of severity. It is also useful for treatment of hypertension in patients with renal insufficiency since cardiac output and renal blood flow are preserved. Prazosin can cause postural syncope after the first dose in a small percentage of patients. The therapy is initiated with 1 mg of prazosin, usually given at bedtime, and the patient instructed not to stand up for several hours. It has also proved useful in the treatment of congestive heart failure because of its ability to reduce both preload and afterload. Postural dizziness and drowsiness, lethargy, palpitations, and nausea are infrequent adverse effects.

Beta Blockers. β-adrenergic receptors are classified into two main groups: β-1 in the heart, and β-2 receptors in the bronchi and blood vessels. The chemical structures of β-blocking agents have several features in common with the β agonist isoproterenol. Most β blockers are completely metabolized and excreted by the liver. However, nadolol is poorly metabolized and excreted unchanged by the kidney. All the β-blocking drugs are competitive antagonists of catecholamines at β-adrenergic receptor sites. They are classified as selective or nonselective according to their relative ability to antagonize the different classes of β receptors. The selective β-1 receptor blockers, when employed in low doses, do not affect the bronchial and vascular β-2 receptors; however, in higher doses, both β-1 and β-2 receptors are blocked. Nonselective β blockers that have both β-1 and β-2 inhibitory properties include alprenolol, nadolol, oxprenolol, pindolol, propranolol, sotalol, and timolol. Those with β-1 cardioselectivity are acebutalol, atenolol, metoprolol, and practolol. Labetol is a non-selective β blocker which is also an α blocker and a vasodilator.

The β blockers are contraindicated in patients with bronchial asthma, allergic rhinitis during the pollen season, sinus bradycardia, heart block, cardiogenic shock, right ventricular failure secondary to pulmonary hypertension, congestive heart failure, and brittle diabetes. The major adverse reactions include the precipitation of congestive heart failure in the presence of heart disease, dizziness, tiredness, depression, nightmares, gastrointestinal disturbances, paresthesias, asthma, and impotence. Nadolol and atenolol are long-acting β blockers that require only once-a-day adminstration.

Blockers of the Renin-Angiotensin System

Since the renin-angiotensin system often has an important role in maintenance of hypertension, agents that inhibit the production or action of the pressor hormone angiotensin II are potentially useful hypotensive drugs. Three classes of compounds are available as inhibitors of renin release, angiotensin I-converting enzyme blockers, and angiotensin II receptor antagonists. They are particularly useful in renin-dependent forms of hypertension such as renovascular hypertension, malignant hypertension, and other conditions associated with elevated plasma renin levels. The β-receptor antagonists, already in wide use for treatment of hypertension, partially block the release of renin. Other sympatholytic agents such as clonidine and methyldopa also inhibit renin release.

Converting Enzyme Inhibitors
Angiotensin I converting enzyme (ACE) blockers have been found to be useful in many patients with essential and renal hypertension. These are competitive inhibitors of the enzyme dipeptidylcarboxypeptidase, which converts angiotensin I to angiotensin II. In addition, they inhibit the kininase enzyme responsible for the breakdown of bradykinin. Thus, these drugs can lower blood pressure by preventing the formation of the endogenous vasoconstrictor angiotensin II, or decreasing the metabolism of the endogenous vasodilator bradykinin. *Teprotide* is a converting enzyme inhibitor that can only be used intravenously and has a half-life of approximately 3 hours after a single injection. *Captopril (Capoten)* is a synthetic proline derivative that is active orally. It can control blood pressure in patients in whom other antihypertensive drugs have failed. The side effects include rash, fever, proteinuria, and, rarely, agranulocytosis. *Enalapril* is another oral ACE inhibitor which is very similar to captopril.

The angiotensin II blocker saralasin (Sarenin) is available only in intravenous form.

Vasodilators

These agents cause direct relaxation of vascular smooth muscle. They may act predominantly on arteriolar smooth muscles (precapillary or resistance vessels) or venules (postcapillary or capacitance bed). Examples of the first type include hydralazine, minoxidil, and diazoxide. The second type of agents include sodium nitroprusside and the nitrates. Due to a reflex increase in sympathetic activity, heart rate, cardiac contractility, and cardiac output may increase, partially blunting the blood pressure reduction produced by vasodilatation. Angina pectoris, headache, and orthostatic hypotension may occur as adverse effects.

Hydralazine (Apresoline)
Hydralazine is well absorbed from the gastrointestinal tract and metabolized in the liver. It is generally used as a step 3 drug for treatment of essential hypertension after a combination of diuretic and a sympathetic inhibitor has proven insufficient. Coronary artery disease causing angina is a relative contraindication to the use of hydralazine as reflex tachycardia and increased cardiac work increase susceptibility to myocardial infarction.

Minoxidil (Loniten)
Minoxidil is also well absorbed after oral ingestion; it is metabolized by the liver and only 10% is excreted unchanged in the urine. It is rapidly taken up by the arteriolar smooth muscle cells and only slowly released from these sites. It markedly reduces peripheral resistance, causes a pronounced reflex tachycardia, and increases cardiac output. Vasodilatation resulting from minoxidil is more pronounced than that from hydralazine. Sodium retention and weight gain are common with minoxidil therapy. Combined with β blockers, reflex sympathetic activity is attenuated and there is less fluid retention. Another relatively common side effect includes hypertrichosis of the face, chest, and brow. Minoxidil is usually administered in a once-daily dosage; however, if the blood pressure fall is precipitous after a single large dose, a divided daily dose is recommended.

Diazoxide (Hyperstat)
Diazoxide is chemically related to the thiazide diuretic agents but, instead of causing diuresis, it causes fluid retention. It used to be adminstered rapidly as an intravenous bolus, but due to precipitous fall in blood pressure causing angina and even myocardian infarction, it is recommended that it be administered as an intravenous infusion at a rate of 15 to 30 mg per minute until the blood pressure falls to a desired level. It dilates arterioles directly and has little effect on the veins. The vasodilatation is accompanied by increased reflex sympathetic activity resulting in tachycardia and increased cardiac output. In common with other thiazides, it inhibits tubular secretion of uric acid and produces glucose tolerance. It is indicated for reduction of blood pressure in hypertensive emergencies when prompt treatment is required. In order to avoid the side effects stated above, diazoxide infusion should be preceded by intravenous injections of furosemide and propranolol.

Sodium Nitroprusside (Nipride)
Sodium nitroprusside is a potent vascular smooth muscle relaxant, causing vasodilatation of the arterial and venous vascular beds. The hypotensive effect of the drug is immediate and short-lived, ending when the intravenous infusion is stopped. The aqueous solution is degraded by light. The drug is indicated for the immediate reduction of blood pressure in hypertensive crises. With prolonged therapy (2-3 weeks) cyanide and thiocyanate may accumulate, which raises the possibility of toxic reaction to the compounds.

Calcium Channel Blockers

Nifedipine and *verapamil* are coronary and peripheral vasodilators that act by interfering with the excitation-contraction coupling of smooth muscle by blocking the entrance of calcium into the cell. The drugs are presently undergoing clinical trials in the United States for treatment of hypertension but are available for treatment of angina and arrhythmias.

DRUG THERAPY FOR ESSENTIAL HYPERTENSION

For treatment of essential hypertension, a stepped-care approach is recommended. It consists of the following steps:

1. Nonpharmacologic measures such as caloric and salt restriction
2. Diuretics
3. Add clonidine, methyldopa, metoprolol, nadolol, prazosin, propanolol, or reserpine
4. Add hydralazine (prazosin if not used after diuretics); substitute minoxidil for hydralazine if blood pressure is still elevated
5. Substitute captopril for sympathetic inhibitor and vasodilator

The approach is based on the long-term experience of most practitioners, the Veterans Administration Cooperative Group, and the experiences of the Hypertension Detection and Follow-Up Program. Approximately 10% of hypertensive patients can be controlled without drug therapy. An additional 40% or more patients with essential hypertension can be controlled with diuretic therapy. Continuation of diuretic therapy prevents pseudotolerance to the effect of other antihypertensive agents. Most patients respond well to a thiazide diuretic dose equivalent to 50 mg hydrochlorothiazide. The antihypertensive efficacy of the step 2 drugs are similar, although there are differences in the types and frequency of side effects. Postural hypotension with clonidine and propranolol is minimal, and these drugs are useful when this problem must be avoided. Prazosin is a useful agent in treatment of congestive heart failure and may be preferable in hypertensive patients with heart disease. β blockers are helpful in patients with angina or migraine and may be the choice agents for patients with these problems. Reserpine is especially long-acting and cheap and has a beneficial tranquilizing effect on anxious patients.

The drugs are first administered in small doses and increased gradually until the desired therapeutic effect is achieved, side effects develop, or the maximal recommended dose is attained, whereupon the next-step agent is added to the regimen. For the convenience of patients and to help compliance, several combination preparations of antihypertensive drugs are available.

SECONDARY HYPERTENSION

Although the majority of hypertensive patients have essential hypertension, a significant number (approximately 5%) have secondary hypertension. In children, severe hypertension is almost always secondary in nature. In evaluation of recent onset hypertension in adults above the age of 50, one should seriously entertain the possibility of secondary hypertension. Table 16 lists the important causes of secondary hypertension. Following is a discussion of the major forms of secondary hypertension.

Renal Hypertension

Kidney disease of almost any nature can cause hypertension; the more important causes are listed in Table 16. The exact mechanism of hypertension in these renal disorders is not always clear. Fluid retention may be responsible in patients with end-stage kidney disease. This is called renoprival hypertension. In many patients with severe renal disease, plasma renin is elevated and the renin-angiotensin-aldosterone system may be responsible for hypertension. In patients with normal plasma renin activity, hypertension is presumed to be due to accumulation of certain vasopressor substances that may be normally metabolized and excreted by the kidney, or a result of the inability of the diseased kidney to generate certain vasodilator substances such as prostaglandins and kinins.

Laboratory investigations usually reveal proteinuria with or without hematuria and an elevated serum creatinine. Sonography is undertaken for detecting kidney size followed by intravenous pyelography if better delineation of individual kidney function is desired. If one kidney is smaller (≥2 cm) than the other, split renal vein renin studies along with renal angiography may be undertaken to confirm unilateral renal disease as the cause of secondary hypertension. The renal vein renin on the abnormal side is usually 1.5-2 times the opposite kidney. If parenchymal renal disease is suspected, kidney biopsy may have to be performed to make an accurate diagnosis.

When hypertension is a result of bilateral kidney disease, medical therapy, as prescribed for control of essential hypertension, is indicated. When hypertension is due to unilateral kidney disease such as a dysplastic or severely traumatized kidney, removal of the diseased kidney can often cure hypertension. Removal of a kidney should never be considered lightly, and a prior trial of medical therapy is always indicated. Renoprival hypertension usually responds to dialysis and removal of excess fluid. Minoxidil, when used in combination with furosemide and a β blocker, has proved particularly useful in controlling blood pressure in patients with severe intractable hypertension. If despite adequate antihypertensive therapy hypertension remains uncontrolled and the kidneys have been damaged irreversibly, removal of nonfunctioning kidneys either cures the hypertension or makes it relatively simple to manage with medical therapy.

Table 16. Causes of Secondary Hypertension

Renal diseases
Acute glomerulonephritis
Chronic glomerulonephritis
Polycystic kidney disease
Dysplastic kidney
Diabetic nephropathy
Hydronephrosis
Connective tissue diseases
Renin-producing tumors
Renal trauma
Analgesic nephropathy
Renal artery stenosis
Fibromuscular hyperplasia
Atherosclerosis
Adrenal disorders
Cortical
Primary aldosteronism
Cushing's syndrome
Congenital adrenal hyperplasia
Medullary
Pheochromocytoma
Medications
Estrogens
Corticosteroids
Sympathetic stimulators
MAO inhibitors and tyramine-containing foods
Coarctation of the aorta
Toxemia of pregnancy
CNS disorders

Renal Artery Stenosis

Constriction of one or both renal arteries, as may happen in congenital fibromuscular hyperplasia or atherosclerotic narrowing of the renal arteries, often results in hypertension. Fibromuscular hyperplasia, also called fibrous dysplasia, is more commonly encountered in white women under the age of 50 years. Various varieties of pathologic lesions have been described but they have little clinical relevance. Renal ischemia leading to excessive renin secretion and activation of the renin-angiotensin-aldosterone mechanism leads to elevated blood pressure. A continuous upper abdominal bruit that radiates to the side of the lesion is often present. Rapid-sequence (hypertensive) IVP, split renal vein renin studies and renal angiography are utilized for confirmation of the diagnosis. Captopril is particularly useful in controlling blood pressure in many patients. If blood pressure is not readily controllable with medical therapy, surgical treatment should be considered. Dilatation of the narrowed segment by an inflatable balloon catheter has proved successful in selected cases. Surgical treatment consists of resection of the stenotic lesion, bypass of the lesions using either a Dancron graft or saphenous vein graft, and an endarterectomy with path plasty. Nephrectomy is considered only if a revascularization procedure is technically impossible or has failed. Surgical treatment cures hypertension in most of these patients. In certain patients, the disease is progressive and can recur after surgery.

Renal artery stenosis due to atherosclerosis usually occurs in patients over the age of 50. The atherosclerotic narrowing is most frequently present at the origin of the renal artery. In almost all cases, there is evidence of extensive atherosclerosis elsewhere. Most of these patients have a history of long-standing untreated essential hypertension. In most patients blood pressure can be controlled with medical therapy utilizing captopril. Selected patients can be treated with percutaneous transluminal angioplasty using the balloon catheter. Surgical therapy should be undertaken only in patients with severe uncontrolled hypertension or in those with inevitable risk of losing kidneys due to ischemia. Unilateral nephrectomy of an unsalvagable kidney combined with contralateral revascularization is sometimes lifesaving in properly selected patients.

Adrenal Disorders

Adrenal, cortical, and medullary disorders can cause hypertension.

Primary Aldosteronism

Primary aldosteronism is usually caused by an aldosterone-secreting adenoma (Conn's syndrome) but can also be caused by adrenal hyperplasia. Primary aldosteronism is more common in white females. Excessive aldosterone leads to sodium retention, expansion of extracellular volume, and elevation of blood pressure. In addition, potassium loss occurs in the urine leading to hypokalemia that causes muscular weakness, fatigue, areflexia, tetany, paresthesias, electrocardiographic abnormalities, and impaired concentration of the urine by the kidney leading to polyuria and nocturia. Edema is seldom seen as progressive expansion of extracellular volume is avoided by certain physiologic adjustments; this is termed the escape phenomenon. The serum potassium is almost always less than 3 mEq/L in untreated patients. Metabolic alkalosis is frequently present and the urinary potassium excretion exceeds 40 mEq for 24 hours despite hypokalemia. Peripheral plasma renin activity even after stimulation with 2-3 days of a low-salt diet (sodium, 10 mEq per 24 hours), furosemide (40 mg daily for 2-3 days) and 3-4 hours of ambulation is either low or undetectable. Increased 24-hour urinary aldosterone and elevated plasma aldosterone help confirm the diagnosis. Aldosteronomas can be localized by CAT scanning, adrenal venography, and measurement of adrenal venous aldosterone levels. Resection of the adrenal gland containing the adenoma is the treatment of choice. Patients with primary aldosteronism due to bilateral adrenal hyperplasia are treated by bilateral adrenalectomy. A trial of spironolactone (300-400 mg daily) prior to surgery may be carried out. Patients who respond to spironolactone therapy respond well to surgery; those who do not respond to surgery may be treated with the usual antihypertensive drugs.

Cushing's Syndrome

Cushing's syndrome results from a chronic excess of cortisol (hydrocortisone). The well-established causes of Cushing's syndrome are adrenocortical tumors, ACTH production by the pituitary gland usually due to a basophil or a chromophobe adenoma, ectopic ACTH syndrome due to a nonpituitary malignant neoplasm, and the extrinsic administration of glucocorticoids in pharmacologic doses. Cortisol promotes potassium excretion and sodium retention similar to aldosterone, causing hypertension and hypokalemia. Clinically, Cushing's syndrome is characterized by hypertension, truncal obesity, deposition of fat on the nape of the neck, pigmentated striae on the abdomen, proximal weakness of muscles, and hypoglycemia. The diagnosis is confirmed by measurement of plasma cortisol and by the dexamethasone suppression test. The latter is carried out by administration of 1 mg dexamethasone at 11 PM and measurement of plasma cortisol the next morning. Patients with Cushing's syndrome maintain increased secretion of cortisol despite dexamethasone.

The treatment of Cushing's syndrome depends on its cause. Removal of the tumor-bearing gland is often curative.

Congenital Adrenal Hyperplasia

Two distinct enzymatic defects may induce hypertension and congenital adrenal hyperplasia. The first is 11-hydroxylase deficiency, in which hypertension is accompanied by virilization from excessive androgens. The second is 17-hydroxylase deficiency, in which there is a failure of secondary sexual development because sex hormones are also deficient. In both situations hypertension is from excessive synthesis of deoxycorticosterone. The treatment consists of lifelong cortisone acetate administration that suppresses excessive ACTH production and restores the patient's condition to nearly normal.

Pheochromocytoma

Pheochromocytoma is a catecholamine-producing tumor usually located in the adrenal gland; it can also occur in the paravertebral sympathetic ganglia. Most patients have a single benign pheochromocytoma but 10% may have a malignant tumor. Hypertension is due to excessive production of catecholamines and is classically paroxysmal in nature. It is often associated with palpitation, tachycardia, feeling of malaise, apprehension, and excessive sweating. Some patients have persistent hypertension with superimposed paroxysmal rises in blood pressure. Orthostatic hypotension, polycythemia, impaired glucose tolerance, and constipation are also often present. The diagnosis is confirmed by a 24-hour urinary assay for total catecholamines, metanephrines, and vanillylmandelic acid; the tumor is best-localized by CAT scanning. Treatment of choice is excision of the tumor-bearing gland. α-Receptor blockade with prazosin and β-receptor blockade with β-blocker therapy has been used for control of hypertension before surgery. Tyrosine hydroxylase inhibitor, α-methyl-L-tyrosine (metyrosine, Demser) can be used for control of hypertension in patients with pheochromocytoma who are not surgical candidates.

Medication-Induced Hypertension

Oral contraceptive ingestion is the most common cause of secondary hypertension among women. Between 5 and 7 percent of women receiving oral contraceptives develop hypertension, requiring discontinuation of medication. Although the exact mechanism of hypertension in this situation is not well-understood, oral contraceptives stimulate production of angiotensin and aldosterone, causing hypertension. Discontinuation of hormone therapy usually leads to lowering of blood pressure within 6 months.

Therapy with corticosteroids (hydrocortisone, prednisone, fludrocortisone, and analogs) is not an uncommon cause of iatrogenic hypertension. Upon discontinuation of therapy, hypertension is usually reversible.

Sympathetic drugs such as amphetamines and analogs used for appetite suppression, and ephedrine and analogs used for asthma and nasal congestion, produce vasoconstriction and therefore hypertension. Amphetamine has been described to produce vasculitis in the kidney and can cause hypertension through renal mechanisms as well.

Mono amine oxidase (MAO) inhibitors such as tranylcypromine (Parnate) and phenelzine (Nardil), sometimes indicated in the treatment of depression, when used in combination with tyramine-containing foods such as cheese and pickles can lead to excessive plasma catecholamine levels and hypertension.

Licorice, present in black candy, contains glycerrhizic acid that has a mineralocorticoid effect causing salt and water retention and can lead to hypertension.

Coarctation of the Aorta

Coarctation of the aorta is a narrowing of the aortic lumen due to a localized deformity of the vascular media and a curtain-like infolding. It is characteristically located distal to the origin of the left subclavian artery but can occasionally occur proximal to the orifice of that vessel. Patients may complain of headache, spontaneous epistaxis, and leg fatigue. There can be an associated bicuspid aortic valve and an aneurysm of the circle of Willis. Hypertension in the upper extremities are the hallmarks of the condition. The femoral pulses are feeble and delayed. Collateral arteries may be seen and felt on the patient's back. Chest x-ray films may show rib notching due to collateral arteries and a poststenotic dilatation of the aorta but an aortogram is usually necessary for confirmation and exact localization of the coarctation. Section of the narrowed segment with end-to-end anastomosis or bypass with a Dacron graft are the surgical procedures of choice. Postoperative hypertension requiring medical therapy is not uncommon.

Toxemia of Pregnancy

Toxemia usually occurs late in pregnancy and is characterized by hypertension, edema, and proteinuria. It is more common with preexisting renal disease, hypertension, diabetes, with twin pregnancies, and in black women. Although the exact mechanism of hypertension in toxemia is unclear, salt retention caused by reduction in the glomerular filtration rate, excessive renin production by the placenta because of ischemia, and increased sensitivity to angiotensin have been implicated. The role of prostaglandins in the pathogenesis of toxemia has been much speculated but is still unsettled. Most obstetricians still prefer to treat this condition with intravenous magnesium sulfate injection and early evacuation of the uterus either by induction of labor or cesarean section. Antihypertensive therapy with diuretics and other pharmacologic agents may help in reversing the hypertension but does not necessarily improve the prognosis for the fetus and mother.

CNS Disorders

Disorders causing increased intracranial pressure such as may occur in respiratory acidosis, encephalitis, brain tumor, and hemmorrhagic stroke can cause increased sympathetic outflow from the brain and hypertension that can be very severe and often labile. Reduction of intracranial pressure by reversal of the underlying cause usually leads to normalization of blood pressure.

HYPERTENSIVE EMERGENCIES

A hypertensive emergency or hypertensive crisis is a clinical situation in which the blood pressure is so elevated as to constitute a threat to life or certain organ systems. Some conditions such as acute left ventricular failure and acute dissecting aneurysm of the aorta qualify as hypertensive emergencies, not so much because of the severity of hypertension but as a result of coexisting life-threatening complications. The clinical situations that constitute hypertensive emergencies can be classified as follows according to the rapidity with which reduction in blood pressure is required:

1. Life-threatening situations requiring immediate reduction in blood pressure
   A. Hypertensive encephalopathy
   B. Acute dissecting aneurysm of the aorta
   C. Acute pulmonary edema (hypertension with acute left ventricular failure)
2. Situations requiring urgent reduction in blood pressure
   A. Malignant or accelerated hypertension
   B. Intracerebral or subarachnoid hemorrhage
   C. Severe hypertension in a patient with acute coronary insufficiency or myocardial infarction
3. Situations requiring relatively rapid reduction in blood pressure
   A. Diastolic blood pressure above 130 mm Hg
   B. Hypertension association with acute glomerulonephritis
4. Curable conditions that may require prompt reduction in blood pressure
   A. Pheochromocytoma
   B. Toxemia of pregnancy
   C. Oral contraceptive-induced severe hypertension

D. Renovascular hypertension

Management of hypertensive emergencies usually requires intravenous administration of antihypertensive drugs. The medications presently used include furosemide (Lasix), sodium nitroprusside (Nipride), diazoxide (Hyperstat), and trimethaphan (Arfonad). The clinical pharmacology of these drugs has already been described.

During administration of these potent antihypertensive agents, close monitoring of arterial blood pressure, preferably using an intra-arterial line, is essential; these patients are therefore best treated in an intensive care setting.

QUESTIONS

(For each question one or more answers may be correct)

1. Usually the first symptom of renal insufficiency is
   A. Oliguria
   B. Dizziness
   C. Dysuria
   D. Nocturia
   E. Fluid retention and weight gain
2. Serum creatinine measurement is a useful test of renal function for the following reason(s):
   A. Normal serum creatinine excludes renal disease.
   B. The measurement is quite reliable for monitoring abnormal kidney function.
   C. Except when the GFR is rapidly changing, creatinine is excreted independently of the urine flow and its plasma level is relatively stable.
   D. A large change in creatinine clearance produces a corresponding change in serum creatinine even when close to the normal range.
3. A 70 kg man has a serum creatinine of 2 mg/dl. His 24-hour urine volume is reported to be 2500 ml and contained 3000 mg of creatinine. His creatinine clearance is
   A. 150 L/day
   B. 15 L/day
   C. 100 L/day
   D. None of the above
   E. Probably 75 L/day
4. In a patient with serum creatinine of 10 mg/dl, the best method for evaluation of the renal size is
   A. Renal scan
   B. Intravenous pyelography
   C. Angiography
   D. Ultrasonography
   E. Retrograde pyelography
5. The nephrotic syndrome consists of
   A. Proteinuria
   B. Hypertension
   C. Hypercholesterolemia
   D. Hypoalbuminemia and generalized edema
6. Which of the following glomerulopathies respond to steroid therapy?
   A. Minimal change glomerulopathy
   B. Focal glomerulosclerosis
   C. Proliferative glomerulonephritis
   D. Membranoproliferative glomerulonephritis
   E. Membranous glomerulopathy
7. Minimal change glomerulopathy is characterized by
   A. Normal histology on light microscopy
   B. Normal electron microscopic appearance
   C. Negative immunofluorescence
   D. Normal serum complement
   E. Poor prognosis
8. Examples of immune complex mediated glomerulonephritis include
   A. Poststreptococcal glomerulonephritis
   B. Goodpasture's syndrome
   C. Systemic lupus erythematosus
   D. Diabetes mellitus
   E. Hereditary nephritis
9. Acute poststreptococcal glomerulonephritis
   A. Can follow streptococcal skin and throat infections
   B. Can occur at any age
   C. Is an immune-complex-mediated disorder
   D. Is frequently associated with hypocomplementemia
   E. Has a poor prognosis
10. Renal biopsy and serum complement findings in SLE include
    A. Focal and segmental proliferation
    B. Diffuse membranous thickening
    C. Subepithelial and microtubular deposits
    D. Linear IgG, IgM, and C_3
    E. Usually normal serum complement
11. Goodpasture's syndrome is characterized by
    A. Most patients are older females
    B. Linear glomerular basement membrane fluorescence
    C. Crescent formation and focal proliferation on light microscopy
    D. Intensive therapy with steroids, cyclophosphamide, and plasmapheresis may help some patients
    E. Associated Legionnaire's disease is responsible for hemoptysis in many patients
12. Which of the following statements regarding Alport's syndrome are true?
    A. It is an autosomal dominant trait.

B. It is phenotypically more severe in men than in women.
C. Foam cells may be present in the interstitium.
D. There is deafness for high frequency sounds.
E. It is reversible.

13. Which of the following clinical situations require intravenous urography?
A. Symptomatic bacteriuria in a 5-year-old girl
B. Asymptomatic bacteriuria in a 15-year-old boy
C. Asymptomatic bacteriuria in a 65-year-old man
D. Asymptomatic bacteriuria in a married 25-year-old woman
E. Asymptomatic microscopic hematuria without proteinuria in a 50-year-old man

14. The diagnosis of chronic interstitial nephritis is suggested by the following findings:
A. Heavy proteinuria
B. RBC casts in the urine
C. Small, scarred kidney on ultrasonography
D. Hypertension
E. Hyperchloremic acidosis

15. Which of the following findings are incompatible with the diagnosis of distal renal tubular acidosis?
A. Serum sodium 138 mEq/L
B. Serum potassium 3.4 mEq/L
C. Serum chloride 98 mEq/L
D. Serum bicarbonate 20 mEq/L
E. Urine pH 5.5

16. The following statement(s) regarding ethylene glycol poisoning is/are true.
A. It damages kidneys by deposition of calcium oxalate crystals in the tubules.
B. As little as 100 ml of ethylene glycol can prove fatal.
C. Hemodialysis is the treatment of choice.
D. Most patients recover spontaneously.

17. The following statement(s) regarding contrast media-induced renal damage is/are true.
A. The renal toxicity is dose dependent.
B. It is particularly common in patients with multiple myeloma and diabetes who are dehydrated before administration of the dye.
C. It can be prevented by intravenous furosemide.
D. It is often irreversible.

18. Which of the following statement(s) regarding acute tubular necrosis is/are true?
A. Renal ischemia plays a central role in most cases.
B. Oliguria or anuria is always present.
C. The urine osmolality is usually high.
D. Dialysis expedites recovery.
E. The condition has an excellent prognosis.

19. Bartter's syndrome is characterized by
A. Hyperplasia of the cells of the juxtaglomerular apparatus and hyperreninemia
B. Symptomatic hypokalemia and alkalosis
C. Hypertension and edema
D. Indomethacin has proved useful in treatment
E. Decreased chloride absorption seems to be the primary abnormality

20. True statements regarding adult polycystic disease include
A. Hypertension and hematuria are common clinical features.
B. Most patients experience anemia, oliguria, and proteinuria early in the course of the disease.
C. Retrograde pyelography is recommended for confirmation of the diagnosis.
D. Cyst puncture is best avoided.
E. Early treatment of urinary infections constitutes important therapy.

21. Which of the following statements pertaining to kidney stones are true?
A. Most kidney stones are a mixture of calcium oxalate and phosphate.
B. The most common cause of calcium stones is idiopathic hypercalciuria.
C. Thiazide diuretics and modest salt restriction reduce calcium excretion.
D. Eighty-five percent of uric acid calculi occur without hyperuricemia and increased uric acid excretion.
E. Cystine stones are radiolucent.

22. Papillary necrosis caused by phenacetin abuse is characterized by
A. Presence of tissue fragments detected on straining of the urine
B. IVP typically reveals a ring shadow
C. Surgical removal of the broken pupilla is the treatment of choice
D. Discontinuation of phenacetin-containing analgesics can stabilize the condition
E. History of analgesic abuse is readily obtained in almost all patients

23. Which of the following is/are the most reliable indicator(s) of acute renal failure?
A. Increase in BUN
B. Decrease in urine output
C. Urine sodium greater than 20 mEq/L
D. Hyperkalemia
E. Elevated serum creatinine

24. Prerenal azotemia is usually characterized by
A. Urine specific gravity >1.015

B. Proteinuria
C. Urine Na^{+} <10 mEq/L
D. U_{creat}/P_{creat} >40
E. Uosm/Posm >1.5

25. The diuretic phase of acute renal failure may be related to
A. Increased GFR
B. Impaired tubular reabsorption
C. Expansion of extracellular fluid volume during the oliguric phase
D. Increased cardiac output
E. Diuretic therapy administered during oliguria

26. Chronic renal insufficiency is usually associated with
A. Low serum thyroxine
B. Hyperlipoproteinemia
C. Peripheral neuropathy
D. Increased receptor sensitivity to insulin
E. Increased skeletal responsiveness to parathormone

27. Which of the following is/are presently used in the treatment of patients with end-stage renal disease?
A. Antihypertensive drugs
B. Phosphate binders
C. Calcitriol
D. Calcitonin

28. Which of the following statements regarding hemodialysis are true?
A. A-V fistula is preferable to A-V shunt for vascular access.
B. Coil dialyzers are better than capillary dialyzers.
C. Dialysis should be delayed as long as possible.
D. Some patients have used hemodialysis for more than 20 years.
E. Hemodialysis is superior to renal transplantation.

29. The following conditions constitute contraindications to using kidneys from a cadaver donor.
A. Septicemia
B. Primary intracranial malignancy
C. Hepatorenal syndrome
D. A positive test for hepatitis B surface antigen
E. Flat EEG without sedation

30. The following statements regarding normal sodium and water balance are true.
A. All but 2-5% of the sodium in the body is located in the extracellular fluids.
B. The normal serum sodium concentration is 135-145 mEq/L.
C. Dissociated molecules contribute more to osmolality than the undissociated molecules.
D. The plasma oncotic pressure is primarily a function of plasma proteins.
E. A normal serum sodium concentration indicates normal total body sodium as most of the body sodium is located extracellularly.

31. A decrease in the ability to excrete sodium chloride frequently occurs in patients with
A. Primary aldosteronism
B. Syndrome of inappropriate ADH
C. Chronic hypokalemia
D. A normally functioning renal transplant
E. Essential hypertension

32. The causes of hyponatremia include
A. Diuretics
B. Primary aldosteronism
C. Diabetes insipidus
D. Congestive heart failure
E. Syndrome of inappropriate ADH

33. Acquired diabetes insipidus may occur as a result of
A. Hypokalemia
B. Chlorpropamide therapy
C. Doxycycline therapy
D. Lithium carbonate therapy
E. Hypercalcemia

34. Potassium replacement therapy is usually necessary in patients with
A. Diuretic-induced alkalosis
B. Laxative abuse
C. Uremic acidosis
D. Diabetic ketoacidosis
E. Hyporeninemic hypoaldosteronism

35. High urinary potassium excretion (> 20 mEq/L) despite hypokalemia (<2.5 mEq/L) may occur in
A. Bartter's syndrome
B. Nasogastric suction
C. Renin-producing tumor of the kidney
D. Magnesium depletion
E. Persistent diarrhea for more than 3 weeks

36. Electrocardiographic signs of hyperkalemia include
A. Peaked T waves
B. Prominent U waves
C. Widened QRS complex
D. Prolonged P-R interval
E. ST elevation

37. Causes of metabolic acidosis include
A. Ingestion of ethylene glycol
B. Bartter's syndrome
C. Hyporeninemic hypoaldosteronism
D. Obstructed ileal loop bladder
E. Amphotericin B-induced nephrotoxicity

38. Which of the following causes of metabolic alkalosis may be expected to result in a urine chloride concentration of

less than 10 mEq/L?

A. Diuretic therapy
B. Primary aldosteronism
C. Cushing's syndrome
D. Bartter's syndrome
E. Protracted vomiting

39. Respiratory alkalosis may occur as a result of

A. Renal insufficiency
B. Pulmonary embolism
C. Hepatic insufficiency
D. Gram-negative sepsis
E. Pulmonary edema

40. Which of the following statement(s) concerning the incidence and severity of hypertensive disease in the United States is/are true?

A. The incidence of hypertension increases with age regardless of race.
B. The incidence of hypertension is higher in white men than in white women.
C. The incidence of systolic hypertension is higher in young blacks than whites.
D. The incidence of diastolic hypertension is twice as high in blacks as in whites.
E. Blacks suffer more severe complications of hypertension.

41. Substances that increase vascular resistance include

A. Bradykinin
B. Catecholamines
C. Ionized serum calcium
D. Angiotensin II
E. Histamine

42. A complete history and physical examination are necessary in the evaluation of hypertension for the following reason(s):

A. Establish baseline data
B. Define the possibility of a secondary form of hypertension
C. Detect evidence of damage to target organs
D. Identify other risk factors in atherosclerotic cardiovascular disease
E. Evaluate the patient's understanding about hypertension

43. Laboratory investigations that should be routinely performed in the evaluation of hypertension include

A. Urinalysis
B. Blood glucose
C. Serum potassium
D. Plasma renin
E. IVP

44. Which of the following statements regarding diuretics is/are correct?

A. Longer-acting diuretics produce hypokalemia less often than short-acting diuretics.
B. Loop diuretics are better antihypertensives than thiazides.
C. Diuretic-induced hyperuricemia causes renal damage.
D. Diuretics increase plasma renin activity.
E. Diuretics can cause hyperglycemia, hypercalcemia, and hyperlipidemia.

45. Contraindications to β-blocker therapy include

A. Hepatic insufficiency
B. Asthma
C. Bradycardia
D. Congestive heart failure
E. Renal insufficiency

46. Which of the following drug(s) cause(s) both arteriolar and venous dilatation?

A. Diazoxide
B. Guanethidine
C. Hydralazine
D. Sodium nitroprusside
E. Methyldopa

47. When hypertension remains uncontrolled despite the combination of a diuretic and a sympathetic inhibitor, which of the following can be added to the drug regimen as a step 3 agent?

A. Prazosin
B. Hydralazine
C. Minoxidil
D. Guanethidine
E. Diazoxide

48. Which of the following are appropriate in the followup examination of a well-controlled hypertensive patient?

A. Monthly serum potassium
B. Annual general examination and laboratory tests of blood surgar, serum potassium, creatinine, uric acid, and lipids
C. Annual rapid-sequence IVP
D. Annual plasma renin
E. Annual chest x-ray

49. Drugs known to elevate arterial blood pressure include

A. Oral contraceptives
B. Corticosteroids
C. Appetite suppressants
D. Phenylephrine nose drops
E. Indomethacin

50. Symptoms of pheochromocytoma include

A. Weight gain
B. Palpitations

C. Headache
D. Sweating
E. Nocturia

51. The IVP findings of renovascular hypertension include the following on the affected side:
    A. Delay in the appearance of the contrast material
    B. Decrease in the concentration of the contrast medium
    C. Notching of the ureter
    D. Small kidney
    E. Slow excretion (delayed clearance)
52. The features of primary aldosteronism include
    A. Weakness, polyuria, and paresthesias
    B. Hypokalemia
    C. High plasma renin
    D. High plasma cortisol
    E. High urinary aldosterone

ANSWERS

1. D
2. B, C
3. D, E. Men excrete 15-20 mg creatinine per kg of body weight per day. Presence of 3000 mg of creatinine in the urine indicates a 48-hour collection rather than 24-hour.
4. D
5. A, D
6. A, E
7. A, C, D
8. A, C
9. A, B, C, D
10. A, B, C
11. B, C, D
12. A, B, C, D
13. A, B, C, E
14. C, D, E
15. C, E
16. A, B, C
17. A, B, D
18. A
19. A, B, D, E
20. A, D, E
21. A, B, C
22. A, B, D
23. E
24. A, C, D, E
25. A, B, C
26. A, B, C
27. A, B, C
28. A, D
29. A, D
30. A, B, C, D
31. C
32. A, D, E
33. A, C, D, E
34. A, B, D
35. A, B, C, D
36. A, C, D
37. A, C, D, E
38. E
39. B, C, D, E
40. A, B, D, E
41. B, C, D
42. All
43. A, B, C
44. D, E
45. B, C, D
46. D
47. A, B, C
48. B
49. All
50. B, C, D
51. A, C, D, E
52. A, B, E

BIBLIOGRAPHY

TEXTBOOKS

Diseases of the Kidney

Brenner BM, Rector FC (eds): *The Kidney*, ed. 2. Philadelphia, WB Saunders Co, 1981.

Earley LE, Gottschalk CW (eds): *Strauss & Welt's Diseases of the Kidney*, ed. 3. Boston, Little, Brown & Co, 1979.

Hamburger J, Crosnier J, Grunfield P (eds): *Nephrology*. New York, John Wiley & Sons, Inc., 1979.

Heptinstall RH: *Pathology of the Kidney*, ed. 3. Boston, Little Brown & Co, 1974.

Fluid and Electrolytes

Maxwell MM, Kleeman CR (eds): *Clinical Disorders of Fluid and Electrolyte Metabolism*, ed. 3. New York, McGraw-Hill Book Co., 1980.

Hypertension

Kaplan NM: Clinical Hypertension, ed. 3. Baltimore, Williams and Wilkins Co, 1982.

Kochar MS, Daniels LM: *Hypertension Control*. St. Louis, The CV Mosby Co, 1978.

ARTICLES

Role of the Kidney

Haussler MR, McCain TA: Basic and clinical concepts related to vitamin D metabolism and actions. *N Engl J Med* 297:974-83, 1041-50, 1977.

Glomerular Diseases and the Nephrotic Syndrome

Appel GB, Silva FG, Pirani CL, et al: Renal involvement in SLE: A study of 56 patients emphasizing histologic classification. *Medicine* 57:371-410, 1978.

Coggins CH et al: A controlled study of short-term prednisone treatment in adults with membranous nephropathy: Collaboration study of the adult idiopathic nephrotic syndrome. *N Engl J Med* 301: 1301-6, 1979.

Glassock RJ: The nephrotic syndrome. *Hosp Pract* 14:105-109, 115-118, 123-124, passim, 1979.

Hayslett JP, Siegel NJ, Kashgarian M: Glomerulopathy. *Adv Intern Med* 20:215-248, 1975.

Tubulointerstitial Diseases

Heptinstall RH: Interstitial nephritis. A brief review. *Am J Pathol* 83: 214-236, 1976.

Vascular Diseases of the Kidney

Fauci AS, Haynes BF, Katz P: The spectrum of vasculitis: Clinical, pathologic, immunologic, and therapeutic considerations. *Ann Intern Med* 89:660-676, 1978.

Nephrolithiasis

Pak CYC, Finlayson B, Fleisch H: Symposium on urolithiasis. *Kidney Int* 13:341-426, 1978.

Dialysis

Popovich RB, Moncrief JW, Nolph KD, et al: Continuous ambulatory peritoneal dialysis. *Ann Intern Med* 88:449-456, 1978.

Renal Transplantation

Guttman RD: Renal transplantation. *N Engl J Med* 301:975-982; 1038-1048, 1979.

Fluid, Electrolyte, and Acid-Base Balance

Dirks JH, Seely J, Levy M: Control of extracellular fluid volume and the pathophysiology of edema formation. In Brenner BM, Rector FC (eds): *The Kidney*. Philadelphia, WB Saunders Co, 1976, pp. 495-552.

Felig P: Combating diabetic ketoacidosis and other hyperglycemic-keto-acidotic syndromes. *Postgrad Med* 59:150-153, 1976.

Gennari FJ, Cohen JJ: Renal tubular acidosis. *Annu Rev Med* 29:521-541, 1978.

Kreisberg RA: Lactate homeostasis and lactic acidosis. *Ann Intern Med* 92:227-237, 1980.

Szylman P, Better OS, Chaimowitz C, et al: Role of hyperkalemia in the metabolic acidosis of isolated hypoaldosteronism. *N Engl J Med* 294:361-365, 1976.

Hypertension

Report of the Joint National Committee on Detection, Evaluation, and Treatment of High Blood Pressure. *Arch Intern Med* 140:1280-1285, 1980.

CHAPTER 11
DISEASES OF THE NERVOUS SYSTEM

Anthony A. Da Costa

Assa Mayersdorf

INTRODUCTION

During the last half century neurology has taken a giant leap forward. The accumulated knowledge of the basic mechanisms and functions of the central nervous system has expanded understanding and improved diagnostic and therapeutic approaches. The availability of better methods of investigation, coupled with new kinds of treatment, has converted the art into a science. Various entities considered untreatable or even unknown 50 years ago are now recognized, correctly diagnosed and, in many instances, successfully treated. The space-age technology of the 1960s and 1970s has benefitted the medical sciences in general and the neurosciences in particular. Following the introduction of x-rays around the turn of the century, other techniques followed rapidly—to name a few, pneumoencephalography in the 1920s, electroencephalography and angiography in the 1930s, isotope scanning in the 1950s, and computed tomography (CT) in the 1970s. New scanning devices are being developed and the 1980s should prove even more exciting. The accumulated information and knowledge in the basic neurosciences, especially the development of neurophysiology and neuroanatomy, coupled with newer horizons in biochemistry, pharmacology, virology, and immunology, have made the modern neurologist more capable of tackling what was previously thought of as unknown. Although neurology has become more and more scientific, the art has not been discarded. No substitutes have yet been found for a thorough history and examination that, together with knowledge, experience, and appropriate investigations, lead to a correct diagnosis.

This chapter is not intended to make the reader a qualified neurologist. The authors wish to stimulate the student to refer to more comprehensive textbooks and medical journals on neurology.

APPROACH TO A NEUROLOGIC PATIENT

HISTORY

A complete and accurate history is the crux of a neurologic evaluation. In most instances the patient is able to give a detailed account of the symptoms and their evolution. In some instances a good history cannot be obtained. These conditions might be disorders of communication, dementia, an altered state of awareness, or language problems. It might also be as simple as an infant who cannot communicate and the parents are the main source of information, or as complicated as in patients following a seizure or head injury who have retrograde amnesia. Therefore, it is important to interview a close relative who is aware of the patient's problem. In a pediatric practice, the parents or relatives should always be called upon to give an account of the patient's complaint(s). Inquiries should be made using simple words, avoiding the use of confusing medical terminology and jargon. When possible, past medical records and other data should be utilized to collaborate the patient's account of symptoms and progression. It is frequently stated that if a good history is obtained, it is easy to elicit the appropriate physical signs and reach a presumptive diagnosis with a greater degree of certainty.

In establishing a neurologic diagnosis, the physician should address the following questions:

Where is the lesion (anatomic localization)?

What is the nature of the disturbance (physiologic disturbance)?

What could be the cause of the illness (pathologic factors)?

Are there any accompanying or complicating features?

A review of systems with special reference to cardiovascular and musculoskeletal assessment should always precede a neurologic examination. It is also important to assess bodily functions and observe the skin closely for cutaneous lesions.

THE NEURLOGIC EXAMINATION

The neurologic examination need not be a lengthy or compulsive ritual but is aimed at elucidating certain points brought out by the history. The patient's cooperation should be always sought. The intent of this chapter is not to explain the details of a neurologic examination; the reader should refer to other textbooks for these. The student should be familiar with the primary components of the neurologic examination and try to be methodic and systematic in the assessment. It is not essential to have a full kit of instruments to examine a neurology patient. To reach a presumptive neurologic diagnosis, the only equipment necessary, in addition to a stethoscope, is an ophthalmoscope, reflex hammer, tuning fork, cotton wool, and a few safety pins. Some of the more detailed techniques are called upon for further localization.

Particular emphasis must be given to asymmetrical signs and focal or lateralized abnormalities. These findings should be correlated with other abnormalities found during systemic examination. Subtle signs of neurlogic dysfunction are frequently revealed by close observation. It is of paramount importance to observe the patient, particularly children and infants, for a considerable length of time.

Mentation and higher cortical functions are usually checked by evaluating the state of alertness, recall, and orientation to time, place, and person. The presence of delusions, illusions, or hallucinations, the ability to perform simple arithmetic, understanding the meaning of simple phrases, and speech are also assessed.

An attempt to check gait should be made on almost all patients. If the patient cannot stand or walk, or this assessment is contraindicated (e.g., acute cord lesions), this fact should be noted as a positive finding. The manner in which a patient stands, the nature of the gait, movements of the legs, and arm swing should be closely observed. There are certain types of abnormal gaits that are usually obvious, such as hemiplegic, ataxic, spastic, festinating (parkinsonian), apraxic, and hysterical (astasia-abasia) gaits. Difficulties arise when there is more than one lesion or when other systemic and skeletal disorders also exist.

It is essential to examine all 12 cranial nerves. Particular attention should be given to the ocular movements, pupillary function, optic fundi, facial movements and sensation, and the oropharynx.

It is important to assess the motor power, presence or absence of atrophy or hypertrophy, muscle tone, abnormal muscular twitches (e.g., fasciculations), and the existence of abnormal movement (e.g., tremor, focal seizures, chorea, athetosis, ballismus). Examination of the reflexes is an integral part of the neurologic examination. The superficial (cutaneous) and deep tendon reflexes should be compared on both sides. The presence or absence of clonus and of pathologic reflexes (e.g., Babinski's sign) should be carefully documented.

Posterior columns sensations (light touch, vibration, and joint position), in addition to spinothalamic tracts dysfunction (pain and temperature), should be routinely checked. Tactile localization, two-point discrimination, and stereognosis should be tested, too, but are less vital in patients where cortical or thalamic problems are not suspected.

Cerebellar functions are assessed by testing coordination and equilibrium. The battery of tests includes checking the patient's stance and gait, the absence or presence of intention tremor, pastpointing, diadochokinesis, nystagmus, and other subtle signs and symptoms. Much attention has been focused on the Romberg test. However, the results of this test should be interpreted carefully as other conditions like neuropathy can also cause the results to be abnormal.

In patients with retention, dribbling, or incontinence of urine and feces, the sphincters should be evaluated. They should also be examined in all cases involving the spinal cord, the cauda equina, and in most cases of spinal roots involvement as well as in some cases of upper motor neuron disorders.

In a comatose patient, it is important to elicit responses to painful stimuli and to determine if any localized abnormalities are present. In addition, techniques such as introducing ice-cold water into the ears (calorics) and doll's eye phenomenon are used to determine if the brain stem is intact.

INVESTIGATIONS

Routine laboratory evaluation of the patient with a neurologic illness is essential. The general laboratory workup helps evaluate the patient's overall state of health and aids in the clarification of the differential diagnosis of the particular neurologic problem at hand.

Lumbar Puncture (Spinal Tap, LP)

Examination of the cerebrospinal fluid (CSF), when carefully performed, is of value in numerous neurologic disorders including meningitis, cerebrovascular accidents, brain tumor, multiple sclerosis, and so forth. The test should be avoided in cases with increased intracranial pressure and, on many occasions, should be delayed until fully assured of its absence. In certain cases, spinal fluid should be examined at the time of neuroradiologic procedures such as intrathecal radioisotope scanning, pneumoencephalography, or myelography. Spinal fluid is usually obtained from the lumbosacral subarachnoid space, but special techniques can be utilized for cisterna magna or ventricular puncture if a localized lesion is suspected. It is essential to utilize aseptic techniques and combine lumbar puncture with manometry and Queckenstedt's test comprising of compression of neck veins to elicit a rapid rise in the CSF pressure. Normally 5-10 ml of spinal fluid is sufficient for most purposes, but more fluid can be obtained when special cultures and immunologic tests are planned. Post-lumbar puncture headache is occasionally encountered and is usually relieved by forcing oral fluids, bed rest, and simple analgesics. In patients with persistent headache, intravenous saline or glucose may be helpful. The cerebrospinal fluid is routinely examined for gross appearance, number and types of cells, microorganisms, protein, sugar, and serology. Special tests are performed when indicated.

X-Ray Examination

The introduction of the CT scan diminished the importance of the radiographic examination of the skull, but the test remains very helpful in certain instances. Plain skull films may be of benefit in patients with head injuries. Mass lesions may cause a shift in the pineal gland that might be visualized on plain skull films. In patients with paranasal problems and in developmental defects of the skull, an x-ray film may reveal asymmetry of the skull or cranial nerve foramina, fractures, and areas of bone lucency or increased density. Intracranial calcifications, leading the examiner to an accurate diagnosis, can be identified through this procedure. Orbital views are useful in patients with anosmia or visual disturbance. Special views of the petrous temporal bone and base of the skull are indicated in patients with auditory or vestibular abnormalities. Although CT scanning can demonstrate abnormalities in the spinal cord, there is no replacement as of yet for the routine radiographic examination of the spine. Traumatic lesions, primary and metastatic neoplasm, congenital birth defects, and other entities identified by the test supply the clinician with valuable information. In patients with suspected herniation of the intervertebral disk, narrowing of the intervertebral space might point toward the diagnosis. The same is true when the spinal roots are compressed, which is indicated by visualization of a narrowed intervertebral foramen.

Electroencephalogram

The electroencephalogram (EEG) is of paramount importance in the assessment of epilepsy and related disorders. Although its value in other structural cerebral disorders has been largely superseded by neuroradiologic techniques, such as radioisotope scanning and computed tomography, the EEG is very helpful in certain situations, such as encephalitis, encephalopathies, and some cerebral degenerative disorders. The radiographic and isotopes techniques test mostly the anatomic structure and outlay of the diseased brain; the EEG checks the electrophysiologic properties of the brain, similar to the electromyogram (EMG) in the neuromuscular system. Thus the EEG reflects dynamic changes that make it harder to interpret, and therefore somewhat less acceptable to the novice as a clinical tool. However, its importance in evaluating neurologic patients is unsurpassed and indicated in most conditions affecting the brain.

Electromyogram and Nerve Conduction

In disorders affecting the lower motor neuron and in muscular and neuromuscular diseases, it is important to have expert electromyographic assessment. Nerve damage, nerve entrapment, neuropathies, various kinds of myopathies, and disorders affecting the neuromuscular function like myasthenia gravis are best assessed by EMG. In addition to assessment of spinal reflex changes, nerve conduction consists of motor and sensory stimulation and measurements of the conduction velocities through the nerve trunk. Needle electromyography should be assessed at rest and during limited and maximal muscular contraction. It provides valuable information by identifying the characteristic EMG findings, which are in many cases pathognomonic.

Radioisotope Brain Scanning

Radioisotope brain scanning is beneficial in assessing conditions in which the blood-brain barrier has been broken, such as infarction, abscesses, and cerebral tumors. These areas concentrate radioisotope and appear as zones of increased density. Intrathecal radioisotope scans are most useful in patients with normal-pressure hydrocephalus. They are performed by injecting radioactive iodinated serum albumin (RISA) into the subarachnoid space and observing its concentration in the ventricles, over the convexities, in the basilar systems, and in areas around the superior sagittal sinus. Dynamic radionuclide brain scanning is employed to evaluate cerebral blood flow and patency of the venous sinuses.

Computed Tomography

This technique has revolutionized neurodiagnosis and is based on the principle that structures inside the calvarium have varying densities. It yields greater detail of anatomy without resorting to invasive techniques and, in some instances, has replaced angiography and pneumoencephalography. CT examines the brain by taking serial transverse or sagittal sections that, when coupled with computer-assisted techniques, display the anatomic picture on a screen or film. When this system of scanning is combined with enhancement techniques such as injection of iodinated radiocontrast material, the degree of definition is greatly improved. This is especially important in the differential diagnosis of cerebral tumors, infarcts, subdural and intracerebral bleeds, brain atrophy, and hydrocephalus.

Angiography and Pneumoencephalography

Cerebral angiography is of great value in ascertaining the exact structure of the cerebrovascular circulation (both arterial and venous), in localizing cerebral aneurysms and arteriovenous malformations, site of bleeding, planning neurosurgical approaches, delineating vascular tumors, and studying normal and abnormal cerebral vascular patterns. Angiography can be undertaken by direct carotid puncture coupled with cross compression to fill the whole carotid tree or by examination of the carotid and vertebral arteries (four-vessel angiography) via an aortic arch catheter introduced through the femoral artery.

Until recently, pneumoencephalography was a useful technique for assessment of the ventricular system and the study of basal cisterns. Cortical atrophy, space-occupying lesions (by shifting the ventricular system), hydrocephalus, and other structural lesions were originally identified and diagnosed via this test. This procedure has considerable morbidity and is now replaced by CT scanning.

Noninvasive Techniques for the Study of Extracranial Vascular Disorders

These procedures are detailed under the chapter on cerebrovascular disorders.

Myelography

Although CT scanning techniques have invaded this field, myelography is still considered the crucial test to identify many of the structural lesions around the cord and in the spinal canal. Extradural lesions like primary or metastatic tumors will cause a block in the flow of contrast material introduced via a spinal tap to the subarachnoid space. Arteriovenous malformations leave typical fingerprints and a herniated disk will show an indentation around the root sleeves. Intra-axial lesions like tumors, syrinx, hematoma, and others will expand the cord again blocking the normal flow.

Evoked Responses (Evoked Potentials)

Each sensory stimulus (visual, auditory, or somatosensory), when reaching the brain will create a neuronal response in the appropriate representative area. These responses, too minute to be seen by regular recording devices, can be seen when multiplied by repetition, averaged by computing devices, and separated from normal background activity (noise). The visual evoked response (VER) involves the presentation of a light stimulus to the retina and recording the response at the occipital cortex by scalp electrodes (Figs. 1, 2). The test helps detect subclinical involvement of the visual pathways as seen in multiple sclerosis, optic neuritis, and other conditions. Auditory evoked responses are currently utilized in testing infants for patency of the auditory pathways in the brain stem. The tests, although used as research tools, have significant clinical use and are being utilized more often in daily clinical practice.

Other Techniques

These tests include biochemical techniques utilized in the study of metabolic and hereditary cerebral disorders. Immunologic testing for demyelinating and autoimmune disorders are called upon in a large number of patients. The identification of increased gamma globulin and its IgG fraction in the CSF of patients with multiple sclerosis has become part of the routine workup in that disorder.

Cerebral biopsy is largely used in cases when a storage disease is suspected and, more recently, has been used in the study of slow viruses affecting the brain. This is usually undertaken after appropriate burr holes have been made and a block piece of grey and white matter removed from a silent area of the brain for histologic and histochemical examination and for inoculation into a laboratory animal.

DEVELOPMENTAL ANOMALIES

A variety of developmental abnormalities can affect the central nervous system (CNS). Most can be traced to genetic faults, infection, and metabolic diseases acquired in utero or during early life that manifest in childhood. A few may present later in life or persist through adulthood. Various arteriovenous malformations are in this category and may present as space-occupying lesions or bleeds, causing a catastrophic cerebral insult.

Structural defects in the region of the foramen magnum can result in a variety of neurologic syndromes. Arnold-Chiari malformation is characterized by caudal displacement of the brain stem, including the pons, medulla, and cerebellum with

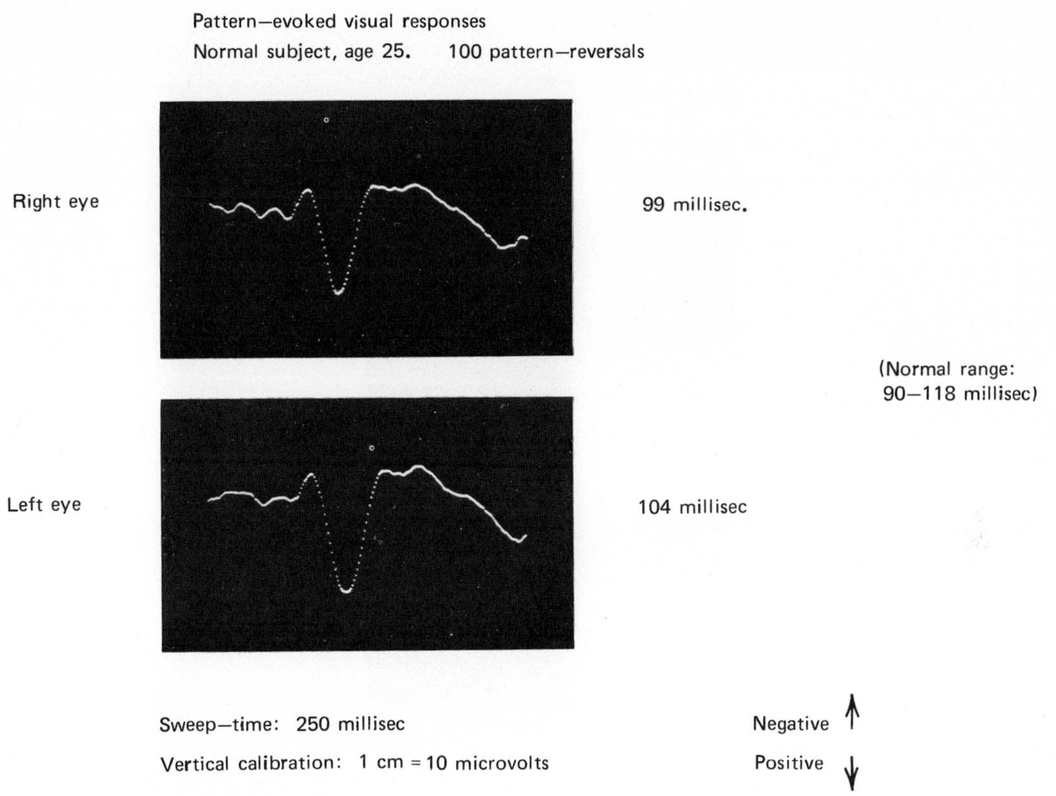

Figure 1. Normal visual evoked responses.

elongation of the fourth ventricle. It is frequently associated with meningomyelocele in the suboccipital region. The spinal cord is tethered caudally; this produces elongation of the brain stem, hydrocephalus, and secondary atrophic changes affecting posterior fossa structures. The clinical picture is that of hydrocephalus, involvement of lower cranial nerves, cerebellar defects, and spasticity affecting primarily the lower limbs. A positive diagnosis can be established by myelography. In order to reduce tension and pressure on the posterior fossa structures, treatment consists of high cervical laminectomy and suboccipital decompression.

Maldevelopment of the vertebrae or part of a vertebral body may produce hemivertebrae, which is noted in the Klippel-Feil syndrome. Fusion of one or more cervical vertebrae may occur or the patient might have a hemivertebra with scoliosis and kyphoscoliosis. A short neck, neck deformity, low hairline, spasticity, and bladder and bowel problems may occur. The diagnosis is established by plain x-ray films and myelography that help demonstrate site and degree of spinal cord and root damage. Other developmental anomalies are spina bifida and related malformations like meningocele, meningomyelocele, and encephalomyelocele. Those are congenital malformations involving closure defects of the spine (spina bifida) or along the cranial sutures (cranium bifidum), with herniation of either meninges alone or in combination with spinal cord or cerebral hemispheres. For other malformations (like anecephaly, prozoncephaly, hydranencephaly, and hydrocephalus) the reader is referred to a more comprehensive textbook on child development and pediatric neurology.

DEMYELINATING DISORDERS

The demyelinating disorders are a group of diseases characterized either by abnormalities of formed myelin (multiple sclerosis) or by production of abnormal myelin (the leukodystrophies). Several demyelinating disorders have been described and can be classified as follows:

1. Conditions associated with breakdown of formed myelin
   - A. Multiple sclerosis
   - B. Neuromyelitis optica (Devic's disease)
   - C. Schilder's disease
   - D. Postvaccinal leukoencephalitis

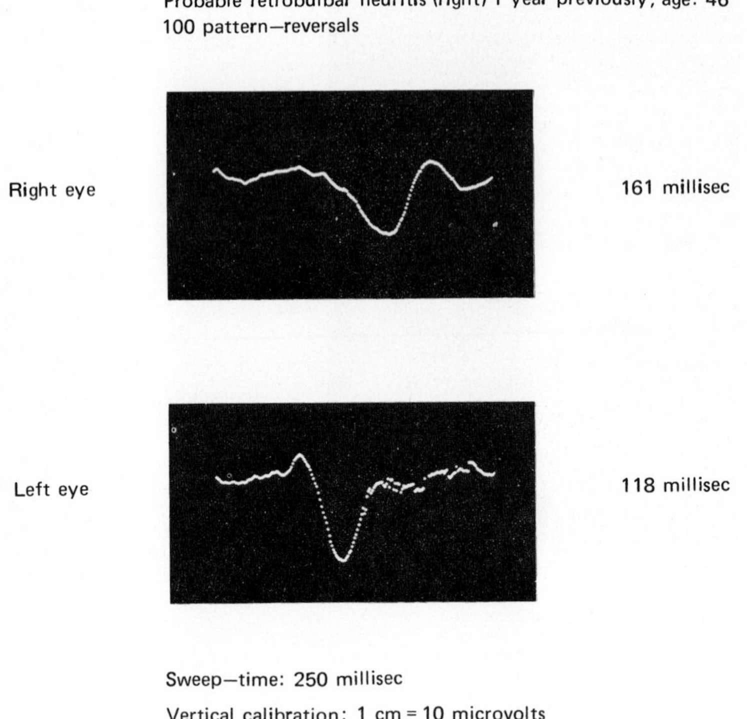

Figure 2. Abnormal visual evoked response from the right eye.

   E. Postinfectious leukoencephalitis (also known as acute disseminated encephalomyelitis)
   F. Acute hemorrhagic encephalitis
   G. Balò's disease
   H. Central pontine myelinolysis
2. The leukodystrophies
   A. Spongy degeneration
   B. Krabbe's leukodystrophy
   C. Sudanophilic leukodystrophy
   D. Pelizaeus-Merzbacher disease
   E. Metachromatic leukodystrophy
3. Viral (slow virus) demyelinative and degenerative CNS disorders
   A. Subacute sclerosing panencephalitis (SSPE)
   B. Progressive multifocal leukoencephalopathy (PML)
4. The lipidoses-these disorders have a combined neuronal-axonal and myelin degeneration. Many of these are familial. The lipidoses include
   A. Gangliosidoses (like Tay-Sachs disease and others)
   B. Sphingomyelin lipidosis also known as Niemann-Pick disease
   C. Gaucher's disease
   D. Fabry's disease
   E. Wolman's disease

MULTIPLE SCLEROSIS

Multiple sclerosis (MS, disseminated sclerosis), progressive and often crippling CNS demyelinating disorder, is characterized by exacerbations and remissions (dissemination in time) and lesions distributed widely in the CNS (dissemination in space). Not all patients follow a progressively downhill course; in some, prolonged quiescent periods are seen.

Epidemiology and Etiology

This disease has been recognized worldwide but is most common in cold or temperate climates. The role of genetic factor(s) is interesting. Studies carried out in Israel have shown that the prevalence of MS is highest in Israeli immigrants from Northern and Eastern Europe, while the incidence of MS in the native-born population of Israel is very low. It appears, therefore, that birthplace and childhood residence are important factors. This is supported by the fact that MS is extremely rare in adult immigrants from East Asia to temperate climates. Although Japan and Korea lie in the temperate zone, for unknown reasons MS is extremely rare in those countries. Another implicating factor is socioeconomic status. It is known that MS is more common in those of higher socioeconomic scale and in Caucasians, as compared to the Afro-Asian and Spanish population of North America. The risk of contracting MS is higher if one sibling is affected and even greater if one or both parents have the disease. Despite these findings, there is no positive evidence that MS is a familial or inherited disease.

The slow virus theory of MS came into vogue when studies of kuru in Eastern New Guinea showed that viral agents could be transmitted from human beings to monkeys with production of progressive dementia, ataxia, and pseudobulbar symptoms resulting in death. Human transmission of kuru has been explained on the basis of cannibalism. Another degenerative disorder affecting sheep, visna, has features similar to MS. Characteristics of a slow virus infection and the immunologic mechanisms are as follows:

1. Although the infection is probably acquired early in life, overt symptoms do not appear until the teens or later years due to a long incubation period.
2. A relapsing and remitting course is in favor of an infective disorder with bouts of hypersensitivity.
3. Elevation of gamma globulin and alteration of the albumin-globulin ratio in the CSF, as seen in patients with MS, is also a feature of chronic infective CNS disorders.
4. Recent studies have shown that measles antibodies are raised in the serum and CSF of patients with MS. Although most children have measles, only a small minority develop MS. Multiple other viruses have been implicated too. Some unknown autoimmune factor is therefore responsible for eventual development of the disease.

A host of other factors, such as trauma, allergy, other CNS infections, and even pregnancy, have been implicated as precipitating factors for MS. Relapse of MS may be associated with rise of body or ambient temperature. A patient with MS may notice that transient disability sometimes appears after a hot bath and/or increase in air temperature.

Pathophysiology

Normal myelin is broken down in MS resulting in the formation of a brownish, gelatinous area of demyelination in the white matter of the brain. The sites of involvement are usually the periventricular areas and the zones with high myelin content such as the medial longitudinal fasciculus, optic nerves, pyramidal tracts, and the lumbosacral region. The pathologic hallmark of MS is plaque. Other features include lymphocytic infiltration, shrinkage of axons and neurons, and perivascular lymphocytic cuffing as well as plasma-cell infiltration. In the later stages there is destruction of axons and proliferation of microglial cells and astrocytes, resulting in the production of glial scars. The intensity of MS varies from an incomplete lesions called shadow plaque to intense demyelination with resultant cyst formation or areas of extreme shrinkage. Physiologically, MS results in delayed conduction of nerve impulses along the axons due to demyelination, plaques, and secondary nerve damage. Raised temperature levels and electrolytic changes adversely affect the nerve conduction.

Clinical Features

The tendency to relapse and remit is a classic feature. The onset of MS is extremely variable, usually beginning in healthy young adults 20-40 years of age. Women are affected somewhat more than men. The onset is frequently characterized by blurred vision, pain on eye movement, vague spots in front of the eyes, and ill-defined discomfort or sometimes pain in ocular or other skeletal muscles. The symptoms are frequently labeled as psychoneurotic or growing pains, are usually multitudinous, and can occur in various permutations and combinations. A description of symptoms according to the organ systems follows.

Visual symptoms include blurred vision, impairment of color vision, pain behind the eye aggravated by eye movement, visual field defects, double vision, and progressive loss of visual acuity. These symptoms, characteristic of retrobulbar neuritis or optic neuritis, occur due to myelin destruction and axonal irritation in the heavily myelinated optic tract. Optic neuritis, with its papillitis or papilledema, can be distinguished from retrobulbar neuritis by fluorescence angiography; this is normal in retrobulbar neuritis but distorted in patients with papillitis or papilledema.

There is marked variation in motor symptoms. The patient may complain of mild weakness or lack of coordination that may remit or progress to severe motor disability, paraparesis, or even total incapacitation. In addition to muscle weakness, signs of pyramidal tract involvement such as increased tone, hyperactive deep tendon reflexes, and extensor plantar responses are evident. The abdominal reflex is frequently absent, even in the earlier stages of MS.

Vague paresthesiae and thermal dysesthesias consisting of a feeling of warmth or burning pain are common complaints. Signs of a spinothalamic tract involvement such as bands of anesthesia, hypoalgesia, or even zones of heightened intensity or soreness to touch or pinprick are also common. Posterior column dysfunction usually produces sensory ataxia and loss of joint position and vibration sense. These symptoms are very crippling in the advanced form. In the upper limbs they may produce a useless hand, while in the lower limbs severe sensory ataxia sometimes mimics the unsteadiness seen in patients with tabes dorsalis and advanced cerebellar disorders. Lhermitte's sign is due to cervical spinal cord involvement and consists of a sudden, shocklike, unpleasant sensation extending down the spine into the back and even lower limbs on sudden flexion or jerking of the head or neck. It is believed to be due to traction on posterior columns of the spinal cord by stretching the spinal roots during movement of the neck.

The heavily myelinated tracts linking the third, fourth, and sixth cranial nerves, the medial longitudinal fasciculus (MLF), other tracks linking the cerebellum to the brain stem, and the cerebellar and brain-stem nuclei are frequently affected. The scattered plaques of demyelination can produce cranial nerve, intranuclear, or cerebellar disconnection syndromes. The most common presentation is diplopia due to MLF involvement. This is manifest by near-normal conjugate eye movement but abnormal lateral eye movement, with nystagmus of the abducting eye and diplopia. Other ocular dysfunctions, such as paralysis of individual cranial nerves, are less common. Sensory changes of the face are common and are due to plaques involving the spinal tract of the trigeminal nerve. There is also a slight increase in incidence of trigeminal neuralgia in patients with MS. Facial palsy and facial hemispasm are less common. Pontine involvement can produce peculiar vestibular problems, but deafness is rare. Bulbar and pseudobulbar signs due to corticobulbar tract involvement and eleventh and twelfth cranial nerve damage are rare. In addition to ataxia, cerebellar involvement produces a scanning or staccato speech. Severe flapping of the arms and sometimes hemiballismus is noted when the tracts to the basal ganglia are affected. In very advanced cases, bulbar and cerebellar involvement can produce a totally noncommunicative and helpless patient with severe dysphagia, dysarthria, and body incoordination.

The degree of spinal cord involvement varies, but bladder and bowel functions are often severely affected. Involvement of the posterior columns may cause ataxic gait with a positive Romberg's sign; this often compounds the deficit associated with cerebellar involvement. Spinothalamic tract involvement may produce disorders of pain and thermal sensations with unpleasant dysesthesia and zones of hyperesthesia. The bladder is frequently affected in patients with MS with varying degrees of incontinence, retention, and retention with overflow. Chronic bladder infection often complicates neurogenic involvement of bladder function. In men, impotence is frequently noted.

Diagnosis

There is no single diagnostic test for MS. The CSF might be normal, a fact that does not exclude the diagnosis. Raised gamma globulins (>45 mg%) in the CSF is of considerable importance. CSF examination may also show a slight mononuclear pleocytosis during active disease.

Visual field examination may show a central or centrocecal scotoma.

Visual evoked response is a useful test in this disorder. Most patients with MS have some involvement of the optic tracts. A delay in latency of visual response is seen in a great number of patients and does not improve, although visual acuity may improve on clinical testing (Fig. 2).

Blink reflex is a useful test to determine whether brain-stem involvement has occurred. Asymmetries of response, especially delay and temporal dispersion of waveforms, are important factors.

The somatosensory responses are occasionally delayed or asymmetrical and might serve as a clue when other disorders have been ruled out.

EEG abnormalities are usually nonspecific. Slow activity and asymmetries are seen in many patients with MS. Epileptiform discharges may occur, and clinical seizures happen in about 5-10% of the patients.

Management

Management during the relapse and remission stages is totally different. During the relapse stage bed rest, passive physiotherapy, steroids (especially adrenocorticotropic hormone-ACTH), and immunosuppressive therapy are used. Plasmapheresis is emerging as a useful mode of therapy in severe cases and is currently under intensive investigation at several major centers. In the remission stage graded physiotherapy, mobilization, and gait training are useful. The value of social workers, physiotherapists, and occupational therapists should not be underestimated. Bladder care, particularly in patients with retention, is of utmost importance. In patients with early urine retention, bethanechol chloride (Urecholine) is often effective. In patients with retention or loss of bladder tone, the long-term use of indwelling catheters is the only alternative. Constipation is frequently a severe problem in MS patients. Mild laxatives and agents to increase roughage, together with periodic enemas, may prove effective.

The use of steroids, especially ACTH, during exacerbations is usually advocated. ACTH is better than oral prednisone and is started in a dosage of 80-100 units intramuscularly or intravenously daily. Recently, daily oral administration of dexamethasone in reducing doses has been introduced as a successful treatment. The side effects of steroids, such as hypertension, edema, peptic ulceration, gastrointestinal bleeding, osteoporosis, susceptibility to infection, and electrolyte disturbances, should be closely monitored. Intrathecal hydrocortisone is sometimes used in acute relapse but does not have widespread application. Immunosuppressive therapy, using methotrexate (Amethopterin), azathioprine (Imuran), and cyclophosphamide (Cytoxan), has been tried with varying results. Some patients show dramatic improvement, especially those who are steroid-resistant, but on the whole response is limited. Other treatments, such as with high polyunsaturated fats, are of doubtful significance. The role of interferon in treatment of MS is also being studied.

The relief of bladder infection by appropriate antibiotics should be instituted at an early stage. In severe cases, relief of spasticity with diazepam (Valium), dantrolene (Dantrium), or baclofen (Lioresal) is useful. In patients with severe contractures and continued flexor spasms, intrathecal phenol has been tried.

Prognosis

The prognosis of MS is variable. Some patients are confined to a wheelchair, while others are minimally affected. Visual symptoms, paraplegia, and ataxia due to cerebellar or spinal involvement may be incapacitating. In some patients contractures, sphincter dysfunction, and secondary bedsores resistant to treatment may be the end result.

TAY-SACHS DISEASE

The pathochemistry of this entity is the accumulation of GM_2 ganglioside in the neurons. Poor development, seizures (mostly myoclonic and generalized), blindness, and the appearance of macular cherry red spots coupled with psychomotor retardation (or regression) are the hallmarks of this disease. Later, nystagmus appears with disconjugate eye movements and long-tract (pyramidal) signs. Very few of these patients live past their fourth birthday. It is transmitted as an autosomal recessive trait and approximately 80% of the patients are of Jewish ancestry. Rarely, a variant can be found in children and young adults (partial or juvenile GM_2 gangliosidosis).

DEGENERATIVE DISORDERS

Degenerative diseases form a group of disorders in which there is gradual but relentlessly progressive degeneration of neurons. The pathologic process may be focal, widespread, or involve anatomically or functionally related neurons. The following disorders are included under this category:

1. The dementias
2. Diseases of the basal ganglia and extrapyramidal syndromes
3. Dystonias
4. The spinocerebellar degenerations
5. Syringomyelia
6. Motor neuron disease

THE DEMENTIAS

The dementias are a heterogenous group of central nervous system disorders wherein progressive deterioration of intellectual capacity is the major factor. The etiology of dementias is varied; in certain types, a slow virus has been implicated, while in others, genetic, metabolic, and systemic factors are responsible. In the vast majority, however, no definitive factor has as yet been established.

The classic division of dementias is into the so-called presenile and senile groups. This is an arbitrary distinction based on age at onset. When dementia is suspected it is essential to establish the patient's capability, intelligence, memory, and functioning levels preceding the illness. Deterioration must be documented with collaborative evidence from the patient's records and relatives and the rapidity of deterioration determined. The neurologic examination should include a battery of simple and more complicated neuropsychologic tests to assess the degree and presence of dementia. A useful mnemonic to remember is TOMMI:

T = thought (intellect)
O = orientation
M = mood
M = memory
I = insight (judgment)

If a patient fails more than three parameters and there is no obvious psychiatric illness, it can safely be concluded that the patient is demented. It is, however, important to exclude diseases such as subdural hematoma, slow-growing neoplasm, and associated cerebrovascular disease. Syphilis, hypothyroidism, pernicious anemia, lead intoxication, and exposure to other heavy metal or industrial toxins should be excluded.

The plain skull x-ray film, radioisotope brain scan, and arteriography are useful to exclude specific disorders. CT scanning demonstrates the nature, location, and degree of cerebral shrinkage and ventricular dilatation and adds to the exclusion of tumors and other lesions. This is well demonstrated in Figure 3.

Radioisotope cisternography by injection of RISA (radioactive iodinated serum albumin) into the lumbar subarachnoid space is useful in determining CSF flow and absorption. Normally there is uptake demonstrated in the subarachnoid cranial and ventricular system within 24 hours with flow into the venous sinuses over the next 48 hours. Depending on levels of obstruction, no CSF would enter the ventricles, as seen in aqueductal stenosis, or flow into the venous sinuses via the arachnoid granulations, such as in low-pressure hydrocephalus.

The EEG may be normal in patients with mild dementia, but when dementia is established, scattered or diffuse slow-wave abnormalities are seen. In Jakob-Creutzfeldt disease, semiperiodic bursts of sharp waves occur over both cerebral hemispheres; this may be associated with brief myoclonic and somatic jerking.

Whenever a slow virus disorder, such as Jakob-Creutzfeldt disease, is suspected, a block of cerebral tissue for histologic, histochemical, and, most important, animal inoculation is taken.

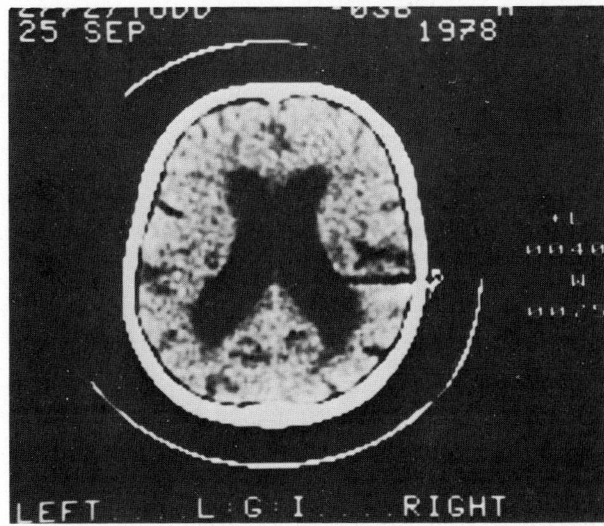

Figure 3. CT scan showing atrophy of the brain and enlarged lateral ventricles.

Salient features of the individual dementias are described below.

Alzheimer's Disease

In 1907, Alzheimer reported the clinical and pathologic findings of this disorder in a 51-year-old woman with progressive memory loss, disorientation, and dementia. The etiology is unknown, but abiotrophy or premature death of neurons has been postulated. The neuropathologic characteristics are diffuse neuronal loss, neurofibrillary tangles within the neuron, especially in Sommer's sector of the hippocampus, and granulovacuolar degeneration within the neurons, together with increases of microcytes and astrocytes. The onset usually occurs in the middle forties or fifties and consists of progressive dementia, a disinhibited state, and deterioration over several months to produce severe intellectual decline. Seizures, particularly myoclonic jerks, are frequent. Brain biopsy is the only means of obtaining a definitive diagnosis. Treatment is conservative and aimed at alleviating aggression, depression, paranoid behavior, and seizures. Medical advice is frequently sought regarding the legal competence of such patients. Since the condition is irreversible and progressive, the prognosis is poor.

Pick's Disease (Lobar Cerebral Atrophy)

This entity is rare in the United States. In contrast with Alzheimer's disease, women are more frequently affected and there is sometimes a familial incidence. The disorder frequently picks out selected areas of the cerebral cortex, particularly in the parietal and frontal lobes, causing significant granulovacuolar degeneration. Personality changes, speech disorders, agnosia, and apraxia frequently occur. In many cases, the clinical picture between Pick's and Alzheimer's disease is indistinguishable.

Jakob-Creutzfeldt Disease

Jakob-Creutzfeldt disease (J-C, spongiform encephalopathy) disease is a degenerative neurologic disease caused by a slow virus. Gajdusck's studies on this disease are the backbone of the slow virus theory of dementias and other CNS degenerative disorders. Recently, some investigators hypothetized that occasionally the transmission of the virus occurs by eating affected raw sheep's brain, especially in endemic areas like North Africa. Light microscopic examination of brain tissue is usually unimpressive, except for atrophy, but electron microscopy reveals viral bodies resembling papovavirus. The disorder affects the entire nervous system. Visual problems and myoclonic jerks often precede progressive dementia. In a few patients, musculoskeletal involvement, reminiscent of motor neuron disease, is prominent, but later there is progressive dementia, ataxia, tremors, dysarthria, mute state, and eventual death. The diagnosis is confirmed by cortical biopsy and slow virus culture. Atrophy of the brain can be demonstrated by CT scanning (Fig. 3). EEG abnormalities are typical in the late stage and consist of a disorganized background with frequent bursts of semiperiodic (every 1-2 seconds), moderate-amplitude sharp discharges at rest and during auditory and photic stimulation, which are associated with myoclonic jerks. Treatment is supportive. Recently antiviral agents such as amantadine hydrochloride have been tried with limited success. The course of this illness is variable, but death usually occurs between 6 months to 3 years.

Occult Hydrocephalus

This is a chronic, progressive dementing illness first described in the 1960s by Hakim and Adams as a normal-pressure hydrocephalus. The main features are dementia, gait disturbances (gait apraxia), and urinary incontinence. Variable spasticity, apraxia, and limitation of upward gaze may be seen. The CSF pressure is normal. CT scan and/or a pneumoencephalogram demonstrate a communicating hydrocephalus with ventricular dilatation; the extraventricular air is limited to the basal cisterns with little or no air overlying the cerebral convexities (Fig. 4). The RISA scan shows prolonged concentration of radioactivity in the ventricles and minimal concentration in the supracallosal cistern even 2 or 3 days after an injection; this is due to defective CSF absorption. Absorption is impaired at the arachnoid granulation level, usually due to previous subarachnoid hemorrhage, cerebral trauma, or chronic meningitis, causing protein deposition over these granulations. Treatment consists of shunting CSF from the dilated ventricles to the superior jugular vein or pleural or peritoneal cavities.

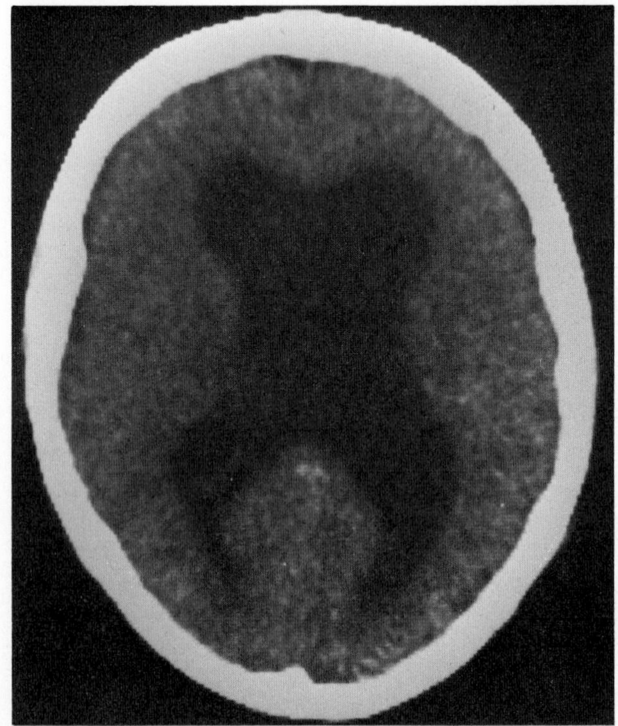

Figure 4. CT scan. Symmetrical dilatation and enlargement of the lateral ventricles with no apparent cortical atrophy.

DISEASES OF THE BASAL GANGLIA AND EXTRAPYRAMIDAL SYNDROMES

This group includes parkinsonism and other extrapyramidal disorders. They affect 0.5-1% of the population over 60 years of age.

Parkinson's Disease (Paralysis Agitans)

The classic syndrome of shaking palsy or paralysis agitans was first described by James Parkinson in 1817.

Pathology

The most well-known feature of Parkinson's disease is a deficiency of dopamine in the striatonigral pathways and caudate nucleus. Whether this is a primary dopamine disorder or is compounded by altered levels of acetylcholine-like substances is as yet undetermined. There seems to be an imbalance between α and γ motor systems. In most cases, atrophy and depigmentation of the substantia nigra can be demonstrated. Detailed histologic examination shows involvement of efferent pathways from the midbrain to the basal ganglia region, as well as damage to more minor pathways between the basal ganglia themselves.

Clinical Features

In the early stages, weakness, fatigue, lethargy, and a general sense of ill-being are the most common complaints, but as the disease progresses the diagnosis is clearly evident.

The three cardinal clinical features of Parkinson's disease are tremor, rigidity, and bradykinesia. Tremor usually begins in the hands and fingers with classic pill-rolling movements. It spreads slowly to affect both hands (often asymmetrically) and then the face and trunk. The tremor is abolished during sleep and is increased by muscular exertion or emotional stress. It is present at rest and diminishes with activity. It is a coarse to-and-fro tremor with three to six cycles per second, the severity bearing an inverse ratio to rigidity. Rigidity affects the neck, trunk, and limbs with classic cogwheeling due to irregular contraction and relaxation of the muscles on stretching. When rigidity affects facial muscles, characteristic masklike facies with immobility, loss of skin creases, and infrequent blinking and smiling are evident; the so-called reptilian stare. Speech may be affected in later stages. Handwriting gets progressively smaller (micrographia). Gait is affected with the patient leaning forward and taking small, fast steps as if chasing the center of gravity (festinating gait). Similarly, retropulsion and lateropulsion are seen and can be clearly demonstrated by the patient tending to fall or stumble if suddenly moved backward or sideways. Mental capabilities are classically not affected in early parkinsonism, but in established cases slowness of intellect is common. This is probably due to associated cerebral degeneration.

In addition to classic paralysis agitans, there are other well-described categories of parkinsonism.

Post-encephalitic parkinsonism was a sequela of encephalitis lethargica, a severe pandemic influenza that occurred between 1916 and 1928. It produced an acute encephalitic illness, followed by slow recovery and residual neurologic dysfunction. Clouding of consciousness, cranial nerve palsies, hyperkinetic syndromes, and somnolent states were associated with bradykinesia tremor and rigidity. In addition to basal ganglia damage, upper brain stem structures and reticular formation were also affected.

More recently, a mild encephalitic illness, followed by some parkinsonian features with or without somnolence, has been reported. The etiologic agent is probably related to the original virus now appearing in a mutant form. The severe autonomic manifestations seen in patients with encephalitis lethargica are less obvious in the postencephalitic parkinsonism reported recently. Another feature that distinguishes paralysis agitans from postencephalitic parkinsonism is the frequent occurrence of oculogyric crises in the latter group.

Arteriosclerotic parkinsonism results from multiple strokes involving the basal ganglia. In addition to features of parkinsonism, dementia, and other features of cerebrovascular disease, the patient presents with signs of pseudobulbar palsy consisting of inappropriate crying, dysphagia, dysarthria, and sometimes frontal lobe signs. These patients have a short steppage gait often referred to as petit pas gait.

Treatment

From a medical standpoint, several groups of drugs are useful; the anticholinergic drugs and levodopa form the mainstay of treatment. The anticholinergic drugs are most useful in controlling rigidity and bradykinesia, and levodopa for reducing tremor. The pharmacologic basis for the use of anticholinergic drugs is to antagonize the relative increase in the levels of acetylcholine-like substances, thus restoring the equilibrium in favor of dopamine.

The most commonly used anticholinergic drugs are trihexyphenidyl (Artane), 4-10 mg/day; benztropine (Cogentin), 2-6 mg day; and biperiden (Akineton), 2-10 mg/day in individual doses. In addition, there are at least 10 other anticholinergic drugs that act on a similar basis to those mentioned above. The clinician should be well versed with one or two of these and have good knowledge regarding dosage, duration or action, and possible toxic effects.

Orally administered levodopa (L-dopa, Dopar) is converted by decarboxylation to dopamine in the brain and replaces deficient dopamine in the brain stem and basal ganglia. High doses are required for a therapeutic effect as only a small portion crosses the blood-brain barrier. Levodopa treatment is commenced with approximately 1 g/day and increased steadily to the level of tolerance, usually 2-4 g/day. The patient usually notices improvement within a week after commencing treatment with increased mobility, a more free feeling, and progressive decrease in tremor. Common side effects to levodopa are nausea, vomiting, orthostatic hypotension, and mild involuntary movements. The side effects are frequently dose related. When the amount of levodopa is increased, grimacing movements or facial dyskinesia combined with restlessness of the limbs (akathisia) may occur. Symptoms are relieved by decreasing the amount of levodopa. Sinemet is a combination of levodopa and a peripheral dopa decarboxylase inhibitor (carbidopa). The carbidopa inhibits the peripheral use of L-dopa, freeing it for its main purpose; thus, less amounts are necessary. This leads to decreased side effects and better patient acceptance. It is available as Sinemet-10/100 (10 mg of carbidopa plus 100 mg of levodopa) or Sinemet-25/250 (25 mg of carbidopa plus 250 mg of levodopa). The starting dose is Sinemet-10/100 four times daily. The dose is increased slowly up to an optimal dose, usually in the range of 50-100 mg carbidopa and 500-1,000 mg of levodopa. A combination of another peripheral dopa decarboxylase inhibitor, benserazide and levodopa, is Madopa.

Amantadine hydrochloride (Symmetrel) is an antiviral compound used in the prevention and treatment of influenza. It was accidently found to be effective in the treatment of parkinsonism and is now used for mild parkinsonism and for cases that are resistant to other forms of therapy. It is postulated that this substance stimulates release of catecholamine stores in the brain, but has no specific action on dopamine metabolism.

Antihistamines and amphetamines are also helpful in treating some patients. The exact mechanism of action is unclear, but these drugs can be used as adjuncts to anticholinergic preparations. Pyridoxine (vitamin B_6) is an antagonist to dopamine and should not be given during levodopa therapy.

A recently introduced antiparkinsonian drug is bromocriptine (Parlodel). Bromocriptine in combination with levodopa often yields significant improvement when additional amounts of levodopa are liable to produce serious side effects.

Surgical treatment consists of a stereotaxic approach to destroy the ventrolateral nucleus of the thalamus and is useful in patients with severe unilateral parkinsonism, especially if the nondominant cerebral hemisphere is affected. Bilateral involvement, bulbar and musculature involvement, and speech problems preclude surgical treatment.

Since the advent of levodopa, the need for stereotactic operations has decreased, although this procedure is of undoubted benefit in selected patients.

Parkinsonism Variants

Parkinsonism-Dementia Complex

Although dementia can be seen in many patients with Parkinson's disease, this syndrome is commonly seen in the Chamaro Indians of Guam where there is a definite familial incidence.

This syndrome is composed of progressive parkinsonism with dementia and spinal cord involvement. Sporadic cases have been described in other parts of the world. Slow virus infection has been postulated as the etiologic agent, but this is not proven. In addition to progressive parkinsonism, a mild form of amyotrophic lateral sclerosis is also present. Levodopa is of limited help; most patients have a progressively downhill course.

Striatronigral Degeneration

These patients have features similar to parkinsonism except that rigidity is more prominent. In some patients, additional signs of cerebellar dysfunction are seen. Response to levodopa is limited.

Progressive Supranuclear Palsy

This condition presents with progressive paralysis of upward gaze, parkinsonism, dysequilibrium, and increasing dementia. The neck muscles become rigid causing retrocollis. Corticospinal tract involvement is seen in some patients.

Essential Tremor

This condition occurs in families and can be rather incapacitating. The onset is between 30 and 50 years of age with progressive tremor of the hands and titubation of the neck. There is little if any rigidity. The tremor is more rapid than in parkinsonism, is present at rest, and is more obvious during intention or action. There is no dysmetria or cerebellar signs. Hypotonia is sometimes noted, but nystagmus is absent. The patients do not respond to levodopa, but benzodiazepines help by reducing anxiety that is frequently a contributory factor. In many patients, propranolol (Inderal) gives dramatic relief.

The Dystonias

These are a group of neurologic diseases with abnormal postures at rest that frequently interfere with voluntary movements. They affect the head, neck, trunk, and extremities. Posture is maintained for a few minutes to hours; in some cases, for more prolonged periods leading to contractures and skeletal deformities. Some of the more commonly encountered forms are discussed below.

Dystonia Musculorum Deformans (DMD)

This occurs as an autosomal recessive disorder as a sporadic form. The symptoms usually begin during the teens with odd posture of the head and neck and slow writhing movements of the limbs. As the disorder progresses there is tonic contraction of axial muscles, contorting movements of the limbs, and prolonged muscle spasm producing strikingly abnormal body postures with ultimate deformities. The dystonic movement largely disappears during sleep. The pathologic basis of this disorder is still unclear. There is severe neuronal loss in the basal ganglia. Diagnosis is established by exclusion of other causative factors or treatable conditions. There is no specific treatment for progressive dystonia, but haloperidol (Haldol), amantidine, and diazepam have been tried with dubious results. In the infantile form, the disorder is slowly progressive with death occurring 5-10 years after onset; in a few cases, there may be eventual arrest of the disease process.

Spasmodic Torticollis (Wryneck)

This is a contracted state of the cervical muscles, producing twisting of the neck and an unnatural position of the head. In a few patients, organic factors such as postencephalitic state, carbon-monoxide exposure, or Wilson's disease may be present. In most cases, the cause is unclear and psychologic factors are frequently blamed. Long-term phenothiazine therapy can cause torticollis and should be avoided in these patients. Torticollis may occur as a heralding sign of generalized extrapyramidal disease or present in isolation. The muscular activity is often provoked by stress and decreases significantly during relaxation and sleep.

Investigations are aimed at excluding organic and treatable causes such as Wilson's disease and phenothiazine intoxication. Treatment with diazepam, amantidine, and haloperidol is of limited value. In a great majority of patients and invariably in those with underlying psychiatric disorders, there is symptomatic relief with psychiatric counseling and behavior therapy. Stereotactic lesions in the thalamus with destruction of pallidothalamic fibers may give relief in patients with fixed and intractable torsion of the neck; however, other surgical procedures such as division of nerve roots is of doubtful significance.

Chorea and Athetosis

Chorea and athetosis cover a spectrum of extrapyramidal disorders where semipurposive, involuntary, and slow writhing movements, or problems in gait and speech may occur. In patients with marked athetosis, distinction from the dystonias is sometimes very difficult.

The most classic form of athetosis is athetotic cerebral palsy or so-called double athetosis. This is due to anoxic brain damage that produces striatopallidal damage together with neuronal loss in the cerebrum, globus pallidus, and demyelination of the long tracts. In addition to signs of cerebral palsy, involuntary slow writhing movements affecting the face and upper and lower limbs frequently appear.

The two most classic forms of chorea are Sydenham's (rheumatic) chorea and Huntington's chorea. There are several other causes of chorea such as anoxic cerebral damage, kernicterus, postencephalitic, in association with Wilson's disease, and with phenothiazine therapy. In a small proportion of cases, chorea and athetosis may occur as a manifestation of systemic illnesses such as hepatic encephalopathy or systemic lupus erythematosus.

Sydenham's Chorea (Acute Chorea, St. Vitus' Dance)

This is due almost invariably to rheumatic fever and presents during adolescence with increased involuntary movements, incoordination, weakness, hypotonia, and brief jerking movements affecting the limbs and face. The patient appears restless, has an explosive dysarthria, facial grimacing, and rapid involuntary movements during rest that are worse with effort but subside during sleep. The patient is often unable to protrude the tongue or keep hands motionless during extension. The deep-tendon reflexes are usually pendular. Coordination is severely affected. In a few patients, unilateral involvement (hemichorea) is noted. Pathologically, there is widespread involvement of the basal ganglia. Evidence of prior rheumatic fever should be investigated and appropriate tests carried out for the diagnosis of rheumatic fever and active carditis.

Bed rest and good nursing care are essential to the treatment of this condition. Mild sedation with phenobarbital and diazepam is recommended. In patients with severe movement disorders, phenothiazine or haloperidol may be used. Any concurrent streptococcal infection should be treated to prevent further episodes of chorea and, more important, carditis and arthritis. These patients have a rather long period of convalescense. Most make a full recovery, but some remain emotionally unstable.

Huntington's Chorea

This is a progressive neurologic disorder inherited as an autosomal-dominant trait. It produces progressive chorea, dementia, cerebral degeneration, and, ultimately, death. The disease is due to severe neurotransmitter failure in the basal ganglia. There is a deficiency of choline acetylase, an enzyme responsible for acetylcholine synthesis, γ-aminobutyric acid and certain other amino acids. Dopamine metabolism is normal. Pathologicaly, there is cerebral atrophy, ventricular dilatation, and atrophy of basal ganglia, particularly the caudate nucleus and putamen. The disorder usually begins in adulthood or middle age with a combination of athetosis and dementia. Dystonic posturing and unsteady gait with peculiar grimacing facial movements are often present. In some, dementia is paramount while in others involuntary movements predominate. The disorder is slowly progressive with continuous deterioration over a period of months and eventual death within a few years. In the terminal phase, the patient is totally demented, movements largely subside, and there is urinary incontinence. Several variants of Huntington's chorea have been described, notably the juvenile form, and another type wherein rigidity is the dominant feature. Diagnosis in the early stage is frequently difficult, but is made easier given a positive family history and observation spaced over a few months. The CT scan often shows significant ventricular dilatation, particularly of the frontal horns and lateral ventricles. Caudate nucleus atrophy is clearly visible. The EEG is often disorganized and of very low voltage. IQ testing shows progressive intellectual deterioration. In relatives of patients with suspected Huntington's chorea, abnormal choreiform movements can be precipitated by administering small doses of levodopa. This test is useful for genetic counselling. Treatment is mainly palliative and consists of administering drugs to decrease abnormal involuntary movements. The phenothiazines, and more recently haloperidol, have been tried. Choline chloride (20 g daily) can ameliorate the choreiform movements in some.

Ballismus

The most common form of ballismus is hemiballismus; this is due to a vascular incident affecting the subthalamic nucleus and its connections to the globus pallidus. It often occurs in combination with stroke, but if it occurs alone it may be particularly distressing and present with severe unilateral flinging movements of the arms and legs with total incapacitation. The movements may be very severe, requiring restraint in bed and the administration of high doses of diazepam. After 2-3 weeks of violent movements the disorder subsides in intensity and may result in severe hemiplegia.

Wilson's Disease (Hepatolenticular Degeneration)

This is inherited as an autosomal recessive disorder. Both males and females are affected equally and there is almost invariably a family history of the disease or a history of consanguinity. It is associated with deranged copper metabolism, resulting in deposition of copper in the liver and other tissues. This produces hepatocellular damage ultimately ending in cirrhosis and liver failure. Renal tubular damage results in aminoaciduria and occasionally glycosuria. In the brain, copper is mainly deposited in the basal ganglia, notably the putamen and caudate nucleus, but is also seen in the cerebellum and cerebral neurons. Wilson's disease frequently begins during the teens and presents as peculiar dystonic movements. Choreoathetotic movements with facial grimacing, flapping tremor, and gait disorders are frequent and are followed by features resembling parkinsonism. In addition to a festinating gait, lack of arm swing, and tremor, there is usually dystonic posturing. As the disease progresses, memory failure, emotional lability, and seizures appear. Death usually occurs in 5-10 years after onset of the disease if the patient remains untreated. Diagnosis is established on the basis of a positive family history, evidence of liver failure, the pathognomonic corneal Kayser-Fleischer ring, and abnormal biochemical tests. These include reduced copper-binding protein, a reduced ceruloplasmin level, raised serum-free copper, and increased urinary excretion of copper. Tissue dignosis can be established by a liver biopsy that shows hepatocellular cirrhosis and copper deposition in the liver. Dimercaprol was the initial breakthrough in the treatment of Wilson's disease, but newer chelating agents, such as penicillamine, have proved more effective and less toxic. Oral penicillamine (Cuprimine), 1-4 g/day, in divided doses prior to a meal helps bind copper ingested in the diet. Asymptomatic siblings of patients with Wilson's disease should be examined to see whether their ceruloplasmin levels are abnormally low; if so, penicillamine will help prevent the disease.

Shy-Drager Syndrome

This condition is characterized by orthostatic hypotension, parkinsonism, and long-tract signs. When neurologic signs are absent, the term idiopathic orthostatic hypotension or idiopathic autonomic insufficiency is used. On autopsy, degenerative changes are detected in the putamen, substantia nigra, cerebellum, brain stem, and intermediolateral column of the spinal cord. The peripheral nerves remain intact. Postmortem biochemical studies have revealed reduced levels of catecholamine biosynthetic enzymes in various areas of the nervous system. The pathogenesis of the disease remains unclear. Early symptoms are related to autonomic failure and include postural hypotension, retention of urine, constipation, impotence, and anhidrosis. Syncope due to postural hypotension is common. The most conspicuous neurologic signs are those of parkinsonism that are often accompanied by signs of long-tract and cerebellar involvement. The disease is steadily progressive, with a fatal outcome in 5-7 years after onset. Levodopa is rarely helpful in ameliorating extrapyramidal symptoms. Orthostatic hypotension is treated by elastic stockings, fludrocortisone (0.1-0.4 mg/day), vasoconstrictors and indomethacin, in that order. Urinary retention may respond to bethanechol, 10 mg three times daily, but catheterization is often necessary.

SPINOCEREBELLAR DEGENERATION

Spinocerebellar degeneration is part of a group of hereditary disorders in which the cerebellum and spinal motor and sensory systems undergo progressive deterioration. In a few instances, toxic or metabolic factors play a role.

Friedreich's Ataxia

This is the most typical form of spinocerebellar degeneration and is probably inherited as an autosomal recessive trait. There is selective degeneration of the spinal cord, cerebellar atrophy, some peripheral nerve involvement, and, in a few cases, myocardial fibrosis. Symptoms usually begin in the early teens with unsteadiness of gait, progressive ataxia, and incoordination. This is followed by cerebellar signs, skeletal deformities, and dementia. Optic atrophy, visual failure, and dysarthria are invariably seen. Although nystagmus and dysarthria are frequent, specific cranial nerve disorders are rare. The gait is spastic and ataxic with involvement of both pyramidal and posterior column functions. Coordination is affected with marked cerebellar signs in both upper and lower limbs. In severe and advanced cases, marked kyphoscoliosis is seen and, in most patients, foot deformity in the form of pes cavus is noted. Diagnosis is confirmed by establishing a positive family history, classic neurologic signs, and the absence of any CSF abnormalities or evidence of immunologic dysfunction. There is no specific treatment, but palliative measures directed toward gait disturbance, skeletal deformities, and cardiorespiratory failure are helpful. Respiratory involvement and cardiac failure are late features with death usually occurring 10-20 years after onset of the disease.

Syringomyelia

This disorder of uncertain origin results in cystic degeneration within the cervical spinal cord and sometimes spreads rostrally to affect the fourth ventricle and aqueduct (syringobulbia). Whether this is a primary degeneration or secondary to proliferation of embryonic cells rests within the developing neural tube; subsequent atrophic changes are unclear. In addition, the role of increased CSF pressure within the spinal canal and altered mechanics of CSF flow due to obstruction at the foramen magnum level or fourth ventricle remain a matter of speculation. The pathologic basis of syringomyelia is the formation of a cystlike structure or syrinx in the cord. Onset is usually in the mid-twenties with neurologic symptoms and signs related to the anterior horn cells and corticospinal and spinothalamic tracts. Spinothalamic-tract involvement produces dissociated anesthesia with no response to pain and thermal sensation, but relative preservation of superficial touch. This results in painless ulcers and accidental burns. Spastic changes develop in the lower limbs. In the upper limbs, a cardinal feature is absent deep-tendon reflexes and arthropathic changes affecting joints, especially the elbows. In the lower limbs, spasticity is invariable and bladder involvement appears when the disorder is well established. Radicular burning pain at the site of involvement is frequent. In patients with brain-stem or cervical cord involvement, Horner's syndrome may be seen. In those with disturbances at the level of the fourth ventricle, progressive hydrocephalus may eventually appear. Additional points, such as spinal deformity, may give a clue, but in all patients the foramen magnum region should be investigated by contrast neuroradiography. If surgical treatment is considered, its purposes are

1. Irradiation of the syrinx in an attempt to decrease the size.
2. Surgical decompression of the spinal cord and syrinx. This is done if the syrinx is very large and is causing bony compression and significant long-tract involvement.
3. The release of adhesions and correction of abnormalities at the base of the brain such as platybasia, Arnold-Chiari malformation, and adhesions at the foramen magnum region.

In most instances, the disorder progresses over several years. Sudden deterioration may occur due to infarction of the spinal cord.

Toxic Cerebellar Degeneration

All patients presenting with ataxia and cerebellar signs should be investigated to determine whether toxic and metabolic factors are responsible. The main offenders are alcohol, underlying carcinoma, myxedema, anticonvulsants, and the post-hyperthermia state. In the United States, alcohol abuse is the major cause of toxic effects on the nervous system. Some of its effects will be summarized below.

Alcohol cerebellar degeneration is associated with marked trunkal ataxia and unsteadiness of gait due to combined cerebellar degeneration and associated peripheral neuropathy.

Long-term anticonvulsant drug therapy, especially with phenytoin (Dilantin) might produce, among other symptoms, macrocytic anemia (due to folic acid deficiency), osteomalacia (due to relative vitamin D_3 deficiency in institutional patients who lack enough exposure to sunshine), and progressive ataxia (due to cerebellar involvement, mainly in the immature brain). Mild peripheral neuropathy might be encountered on rare occasions. CT scanning occasionally reveals cerebellar atrophy and distinct cerebellar folia.

NEUROLOGIC SYNDROMES ASSOCIATED WITH ALCOHOL

These manifestations will be identified by name only; the reader is referred to other chapters of this book and to the extensive work of Maurice Victor in this field. These syndromes are:

1. Acute and chronic alcoholic intoxication (including pathologic intoxication, blackout spells, and coma)
2. Withdrawal syndrome (delirium tremens, rum fits, acute hallucinosis, etc.)
3. The nutritional diseases: cerebellar degeneration, Wernicke's disease, Korsakoff's psychosis, amblyopia, and pellagra
4. Hepatic encephalopathy
5. Other manifestations: neuropathy, myopathy, central pontine myelinolysis, Marchiafava-Bignami disease, fetal alcohol syndrome, and so on

PAROXYSMAL DISORDERS

Episodic and transient loss of consciousness is a common presenting complaint in a neurology practice. Syncope and epilepsy are the two major reasons for loss of consciousness.

SYNCOPE

Fainting or syncopal spells need careful history taking, neurologic assessment, and, most important, general physical review. The patient should be requested to give a detailed account of symptoms in chronologic order. It is essential to ascertain the preceding circumstances, nature of the blackouts, and sequence of events after recovery of consciousness. If possible, this history should be supplemented by collaborative evidence from witnesses. In a young child, information supplied by a parent or a schoolteacher is frequently of crucial significance. It is also important to know whether the patient is receiving any medication and if there is a history of drug or alcohol abuse.

Some of the common causes of syncope are discussed below.

Vasovagal Syncope

This consists of sudden onset of lightheadedness and unsteadiness followed by loss of consciousness and collapse. The precipitating factors include the sight of blood, needle puncture, and severe emotional shock. The episodes are usually brief and are accompanied by marked pallor, sometimes slight cyanosis, and occasionally jerking and shivering of the limbs. In some patients, the jerking may be violent and appear as a convulsive seizure. The attacks are brief, usually lasting a few seconds to a minute. After regaining consciousness, the patient is often dizzy and hyperventilates. Cardiovascular examination usually reveals no abnormality; however, in a few instances, marked sinus arrhythmia or sinoatrial block may be seen on the ECG. Vasovagal syncope is due to vagal overactivity, producing slowing of the heart rate and a sudden fall in blood pressure. During an attack the patient may be pulseless. Reassurance frequently alleviates the attacks.

Orthostatic Hypotension

Dizziness or sudden loss of consciousness upon assuming an erect posture along with a fall in blood pressure of $\geqslant 20$ mm Hg are typical features. Although the mechanism is not always clear, autonomic insufficiency, venous pooling, and reduced cardiac output are the usual underlying factors. The causes of postural hypotension include dehydration, antihypertensive drugs, surgical sympathectomy, Addison's disease, severe cardiac failure, diabetes, amyloidosis, alcoholism, and neurologic illnesses such as Shy-Drager syndrome, parkinsonism, syringomyelia, tabes dorsalis, and familial dysautonomia. Treatment includes reversal of causative factors, whenever possible, hydration, elastic stockings, fludrocortisone, and nonsteroidal anti-inflammatory agents, such as indomethacin.

Carotid Sinus Sensitivity

In normal subjects pressure on the carotid sinus may produce bradycardia and a fall of blood pressure. In patients with arteriosclerotic plaques involving the carotid sinus there may be a great deal of vasomotor change following stimulation due to shaving, pressure from a collar or jewelry, and sometimes even movement of the neck resulting in hypotension, slow pulse, asystole, and unconsciousness. Recovery is often accompanied by palpitation and a feeling of blood surging through the head. The patient should avoid wearing tight or starched collars. A trial with drugs, such as ephedrine, atropine, or dextroamphetamine, may prove beneficial.

Hyperventilation Syndrome

This is a common symptom in patients with underlying anxiety. In tense patients, hyperventilation may be one of the symptoms among a complex group of anxiety and psychoneurotic features. The fact that the patient is hyperventilating may not be obvious and careful psychologic and psychiatric assessment is important in evaluating these complaints. Attacks may be precipitated by requesting the patient to hyperventilate. After 20 to 30 breaths, following a drop in the carbon dioxide (CO_2) contents, the patient may experience a cold feeling, shortness of breath, tightness of the chest, lightheadedness, blackouts, and, in extreme cases, tetany. Treatment consists of reassurance and increasing the CO_2 contents of the breathing air by the use of a plastic or paper bag for breathing. Diamox is of limited value. In patients with a clear-cut psychoneurotic element, long-term psychotherapy may be of benefit.

Stokes-Adams Syndrome

These attacks are due to sudden heart block or cardiac dysrhythmia resulting in asystole or brief periods of ventricular tachycardia with little or no cardiac output. The attacks are observed in patients with established cardiac disease and are confirmed by detecting cardiac abnormalities on examination, ECG, or Holter monitoring.

Drop Attacks

These are sudden onset attacks wherein the patient collapses without warning. They are almost invariably related to vascular problems in the distribution of the vertebrobasilar system. The etiologic factors include vertebrobasilar arteriosclerosis, cervical spondylosis, and other abnormalities involving the craniocervical regions. The patient frequently has brain-stem and long-tract signs. Cardiac disorders and epilepsy must be excluded. A cervical spine x-ray film should be taken, and, if required, vertebral angiography should be carried out. Treatment is generally of little help but anticoagulants, antiplatelet agents, such as aspirin, vasodilators and sympathectomy may be tried.

EPILEPSY

The epilepsies or seizure disorders are characterized by a sudden alteration in the electrical activity of the brain resulting in motor, sensory, autonomic, or psychic features that might (or might not) be associated with loss of consciousness. A detailed history of the preictal symptoms (aura), the onset and characteristics of the seizure (ictal phase), and the immediate period following the seizure (postictal phase), together with a review of past medical history constitute the most important factors in the investigation of patients with epilepsy. Epilepsy is a major public health problem. Approximately 1% of the adult population is affected. It poses difficulties in relation to employment and the patient's life-style.

Classification of the Epilepsies

An international classification has been formulated to group seizure disorders into subdivisions. This classification is based on clinical symptoms and signs with some influence on the EEG findings. It is used in daily management of patients.

The international classification is given below:

1. Partial seizures (seizures beginning locally; formerly known as focal)
   - A. Partial seizures with elementary symptomatology (generally without impairment of consciousness)
     - 1) With motor symptoms (includes jacksonian and adversive seizures)
     - 2) With special sensory or somatosensory symptoms
     - 3) With autonomic symptoms
     - 4) Compound forms
   - B. Partial seizures with complex symptomatology (generally with impairment of consciousness; formerly known as temporal lobe or psychomotor seizures)
     - 1) With impairment of consciouness only
     - 2) With cognitive symptomatology
     - 3) With affective symptomatology
     - 4) With "psychosensory" symptomatology
     - 5) With "psychomotor" symptomatology (automatisms)
     - 6) Compound forms
   - C. Partial seizures secondarily generalized
2. Generalized seizures (bilaterally symmetrical and without local onset)
   - 1) Absences (petit mal)
   - 2) Bilteral massive epileptic myoclonus
   - 3) Infantile spasms
   - 4) Clonic seizures
   - 5) Tonic seizures

6) Tonic-clonic seizures (grand mal)
7) Atonic seizures
8) Akinetic seizures
3. Unilateral seizures (or predominantly)
4. Unclassified epileptic seizures (due to incomplete data)

Childhood epilepsy cannot be easily grouped into these individual sections as it is liable to evolve with time and in many instances is of a mixed type. Status epilepticus is not included in the above classification as it is primarily related to generalized seizures or partial seizures becoming continuous.

The etiologic factors concerning epilepsy are many and include hereditary and familial conditions, developmental defects, birth trauma, anoxia, infections of the brain, neoplastic, nutritional and toxic disorders, as well as vascular disturbances and degenerative conditions of the CNS. It is important to emphasize that a seizure is a symptom of disordered cerebral function and is not a disease in itself. The presence of epilepsy should alert the physician to investigate the problem further as very few cases of epilepsy are truly idiopathic, especially if they occur in adults.

The EEG has made great strides in the understanding of epilepsy, its etiology and classification, and in follow-up of patients with a view to adjusting medication. Certain forms of seizure disorders have a characteristic EEG picture. In patients with photosensitivity, abnormal EEG responses can be demonstrated to variable rates of flash flicker. It is important to emphasize that the EEG reveals spikes or dysrhythmic activity but does not in itself prove that the patient has a seizure disorder. Thus, a normal EEG tracing does not exclude epilepsy and, if abnormal, the patient's symptoms rather than the EEG findings form the mainstay of management.

Some of the common forms of seizure disorders are briefly described below.

Simple Absence Seizures (Petit Mal Epilepsy)

This is associated with classic, generalized three cycles per second spike and wave EEG discharges. A typical absence consists of a brief lapse of awareness during which the patient may twitch the eyelids, roll the eyes upward, be momentarily unaware, drop things, or have a brief loss of body posture.

Generalized Tonic-Clonic Seizures (Grand Mal)

In the classic form, there is sudden loss of consciousness with no aura, accompanied by tonic (stiff) and clonic jerking phases. The so-called idiopathic forms usually have no evidence of structural CNS disease. Genetic factors were described. In patients with such seizures, it is important to fully investigate if there are focal features preceding or following the major attack. If an aura or preictal symptoms appear, or postictal signs are evident like postictal transient paralysis (Todd's paralysis), further investigation is necessary to rule out structural lesions. In these cases, the seizures are not true primary generalized ones but really focal seizures with secondary generalization.

Simple Partial (Focal) Seizures (Including Jacksonian and Adversive Seizures)

These seizures are of the utmost clinical importance, especially if they occur in adults. They almost invariably indicate cerebral damage. Careful observation and assessment of these seizures gives good clinicopathologic correlation. The EEG helps localize and classify the type of seizure disorder. Partial seizures on many occasions may generalize. As stated before, the diagnostic clues to focal origin are the aura and postictal manifestations. Focal or partial seizures can sometimes be aborted, the patient being able to stop the progression of attacks by distraction, forced thinking, or purposeful movements.

Partial Complex Seizures (Temporal Lobe Seizures, Psychomotor Seizures)

This constitutes over 50% of seizures in the adult population. The medial aspect of the temporal lobe is particularly liable to damage by anoxic factors at the time of birth and during the perinatal period. Furthermore, head injuries and other cerebral insults frequently involve the temporal lobes and in time produce epileptogenic areas within the hippocampus, amygdala, and other grey matter islands in the depths of the temporal lobe. The temporal lobe is closely allied to special senses, the gastrointestinal tract, the autonomic system, memory, and behavior. The manifestations of complex partial seizures are therefore numerous and include automatism, psychosensory, and cognitive and affective manifestations, separately or in combination.

Seizures in Childhood

Epilepsy in childhood does not have the same connotation as seizures in adults. Focal seizures, especially in infants and very young children, do not indicate localized cerebral abnormality but may be due to toxic-metabolic factors. Disorders such as hypocalcemia, anoxia, and minor cerebral abnormalities may produce focal seizures. The presence of Todd's palsy should alert the clinician to localized cerebral damage. In children, West's syndrome (infantile spasms) is sometimes seen. This is a potentially serious disorder that occurs due to cerebral anoxic damage, developmental defects, and severe structural cerebral lesions of vascular, atrophic, postinfectious, or traumatic etiology. The EEG characteristics are high-voltage, chaotic, irregular waveforms called hypsarrhythmia. The prognosis in these patients is uniformly poor, although a few eventually improve.

Reflex Epilepsy

These are a heterogenous group of seizure disorders in which attacks are precipitated by certain stimuli such as flashing lights, noises, music, or reading. The source of epileptogenic activity is unclear, but in photosensitive epilepsy abnormal visually evoked responses may be seen. The reflex epilepsies, particularly photosensitive epilepsy, are often related to primary generalized epilepsy.

Hysterical Seizures

This term is a misnomer since hysteria and epilepsy are two different clinical entities. However, in a small proportion of patients with epilepsy, certain types of functional attacks occur in addition to the seizure disorder and present as peculiar behavioral problems. The EEG is of paramount importance in the assessment of these patients as serial studies do not demonstrate any ongoing epileptic activity during a hysterical episode.

Status Epilepticus

Continued epilepsy occurs in three forms: repetitive seizures, absence continua, and major status epilepticus. Repetitive seizures consists of repeated attacks with return of consciousness between the individual spells. Major status epilepticus is a very serious disorder and consists of continuous seizures for more than an arbitrary period of 20 minutes (or repetitive seizures without gaining consciousness in between for over 20 minutes). Absence continua is a peculiar syndrome consisting of variable confusion, motor twitching, and drowsiness accompanied by irregular EEG phenomena consisting of spike and wave discharges and irregular sharp and slow wave discharges. In children, the attacks may constitute prolonged absence states while in older patients, especially women, periods of prolonged confusion may occur. Many of these patients end up in psychiatric institutions and hence the importance of identifying it with EEG recordings. The syndrome of transient global amnesia is believed by some not to be an epileptic phenomena but to be related to vascular disturbances affecting the temporal lobes. However, this subject is still controversial.

Diagnostic Evaluation

In the evaluation of a seizure disorder, the EEG is of great importance. Routine EEG consists of recording with the eyes open and closed, followed by hyperventilation and photic stimulation. An EEG with sleep induction using chloral hydrate or with no medication using sleep depreviation is often tried to induce epileptiform discharges. Sphenoidal and nasopharyngeal leads are other helpful aids in the localization of seizure disorders, especially if they are thought to arise from the temporal lobes (Fig. 5). These are often combined with the use of special activating agents (i.e., combination of Metrazol and photic stimulation, injections of methohexital). Other techniques include the use of telemetry EEG, which adds new dimensions to the study by allowing the subject to continue a normal life routine. Using the many variants of telemetry also enables investigators to study the influence of psychosocial events and the patient's environment on his seizure patterns. Split-screen audio-videotaping allows the physician to compare the clinical signs with the electrical activity by displaying the patient and the EEG tracing on the same monitor and recording for extended periods of time.

Skull x-ray films are of some benefit and might show calcifications and occasionally other abnormalities. The CT scan is of importance in patients in whom localized seizures have been demonstrated on clinical and EEG examinations. A glucose

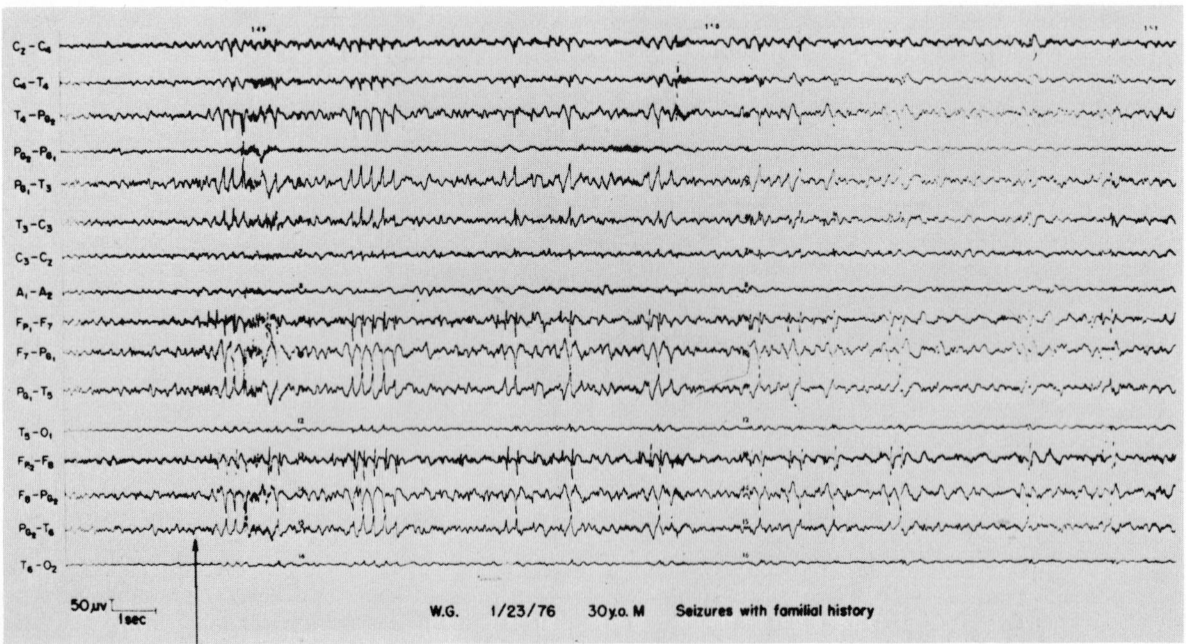

Figure 5. EEG. Bilateral trains of spikes originating from both nasopharyngeal electrodes (P_{G_1} and P_{G_2}). Electrode placement according to the international 10-20 system. 30-year-old man with history of familial seizures.

tolerance test, serum calcium, and electrolytes may be abnormal in some patients. Syphilis should be routinely excluded in patients with epilepsy, but the incidence of epilepsy in syphilis is very low. In young children, amino acid assays, chromosomal studies, a metabolic screen, and perhaps a lumbar puncture are indicated. Cerebrospinal fluid examination is of little help in assessment of epilepsy in adults and is usually performed last in the list of tests.

Management

The objective of treatment is to suppress the seizures by maintaining an effective brain concentration of the administered drugs. Various drugs available for treatment of epilepsy are listed in Table 1.

The approach to drug therapy has changed significantly with knowledge of plasma half-life of drugs and pharmacokinetics. As numerous patients with epilepsy fail to comply with therapy, it is important to prescribe the least number of tablets and make treatment as convenient as possible. The drugs of choice in various seizure disorders are listed below.

Generalized tonic-clonic seizures—Phenytoin, carbamazepine and valproic acid

Absence seizures—Ethosuximide, valproic acid, and clonazepam

Partial complex seizures—Phenytoin, carbamazepine

Epilepsy in childhood—Depends on the type of seizures; phenytoin and valproic acid are most commonly used

Hypsarrhythmia—ACTH and clonazepam.

Status epilepticus—intravenous phenytoin and intravenous diazepam

It is best to begin with one drug and increase the dosage until the seizure is controlled or toxic effects appear. Monitoring plasma drug levels assures compliance. When one drug is not sufficient in controlling seizures, a second drug should be added. Two drugs might be necessary in patients with two types of seizures such as grand mal and petit mal. Frequent and rapid changes of medication produce side effects and can precipitate further seizures. Drug interactions between anticonvulsants and other drugs should be avoided whenever possible.

Status epilepticus is a medical emergency and if not controlled might result in brain damage. Establishing an adequate airway and proper oxygenation is of paramount importance. Most neurologists use the intravenous injection of phenytoin (very slow injection, approximately 50 mg/min in a normal saline solution as phenytoin might crystalize in glucose solution). The dose is 12-18 (average 15) mg/kg body weight. If bradycardia or hypotension develop, the procedure should be discontinued. Intravenous diazepam in slow injections (5-20 mg) is another alternative. This might be repeated every 20-30 minutes.

HEADACHE

Headache is a common complaint. In a large proportion of patients, the cause is unclear but happily is of no serious consequence. In others, headaches can be totally incapacitating or might be related to a primary or progressive cerebral disorder. Headaches can be defined as pain or discomfort in the head including the orbit, paranasal sinuses, and cranium, extending

Table 1. Commonly Used Anticonvulsants

Generic Name	*Trade Name*	*Average Daily Adult Dose (mg)*	*Mean Half-Life (h)*	*Therapeutic Level (μg/ml)*	*Toxic Effects*
Acetazolamide	Diamox	1,000-2,500			Acidosis, drowsiness, numbness of extremities
Carbamazepine	Tegretol	200-800	6-12	6-12	Gastrointestinal symptoms, drowsiness, rash, leukopenia, and thrombocytopenia
Clonazepam	Clonopin	3-12	26		Drowsiness, ataxia, behavioral problems, anorexia, anemia, leukopenia
Diazepam	Valium	10-20	22	0.5	Sedation, habit forming, respiratory depression
Ethosuximide	Zarontin	750-1,500	55	50-100	Pancytopenia
Phenobarbital	Luminal	100-300	96	20-50	Drowsiness, rash, fever, ataxia, nystagmus
Phenytoin	Dilantin	300-500	24	10-20	Rash, fever, gum hypertrophy, gastric distress, diplopia, nystagmus, ataxia, hirsutism, megaloblastic anemia, lymphadenopathy
Primidone	Mysoline	750-1,500	12	5-12	Drowsiness, ataxia, dizziness, rash, nausea
Trimethadione	Tridione	750-2,000	14	20-40	Rash, gastritis, visual symptoms, agranulocytosis, nephrotic syndrome
Valproic acid	Depakene	1,000-2,000	8-12	150	Gastrointestinal symptoms, sedation, ataxia, rash, hair loss, emotional reactions, altered bleeding time, leukopenia, ↑ phenobarbital level, ↑↓ phenytoin level

from the orbital region to suboccipital areas. Facial, dental, and neck pain do not constitute headache, but are frequently related to head pain. The most common types of headaches are tension headache, migraine, cluster headache, and headaches related to specific causes. The neuralgias will be considered separately.

Head pain originates from disturbances involving the meninges, venous and arterial systems, cranial bones, scalp, and cranial nerves, especially the fifth, ninth, and tenth. Pain can result from pressure, stretching, compression, invasion, or inflammation of these structures. The vascular system may be affected by traction, dilatation (aneurysm), vessel spasm, inflammation, direct or indirect pressure, and compression. In addition, emotional disturbances such as anxiety or depression tend to aggravate and modify the nature, distribution, and severity of head discomfort.

VASCULAR HEADACHES

These include migraine and its variants.

Migraine

The common factor is a periodic instability of vasomotor control affecting cranial arteries with episodes of vasconstriction and vasodilatation. The events leading up to and associated with migraine attacks vary and frequently alter with time. Vasoconstriction produces the aura. Headache and discomfort arise from arterial distention and dilatation. The variability of migraine is due to the scope and nature of vessel involvement and peculiar reaction and interaction with various causative and precipitating factors.

Pathophysiology

A positive family history is obtained in more than one-half of migraine sufferers. The incidence of this disorder is greater in higher socioeconomic groups and professional people. Migraine is more common in women, the onset is frequently at puberty, and attacks are often related to menstrual periods. Pregnancy frequently alleviates migraine attacks, and it is considered, therefore, that an endocrine imbalance is a significant factor in precipitation of migrainous episodes. High levels of estrogen are known to alleviate these episodes, the attacks being precipitated by a relative fall in estrogen level. The oral contraceptive pill, probably due to suppression of the body's estrogen synthesis, aggravates migraine, although this is not an invariable occurrence. Stress, frustration, and nervous tension coupled with such factors as fatigue, bright lights, and hypoglycemia often precipitate attacks. Many patients develop migraine after and not during stressful situations; for example, the migraine often occurs on weekends rather than during a busy workweek. Certain foods containing nitrites and monosodium glutamate are known to precipitate migrainous attacks. Avoidance of certain foods and beverages, such as cheese and other dairy products, nuts, chocolate, and intoxicating liquors, usually decrease the incidence and severity of migraine. Drugs, including vasodilators, reserpine, and several psychotropic medications, are often blamed as the precipitating factor. Mild trauma and change in atmospheric pressure and humidity often serve as subsidiary factors. An alteration in sympathetic tone and vasomotor reaction are often incriminated. The plasma level of 5-hydroxytryptamine (serotonin) is known to fall, sometimes precipitously, at the onset of a migraine attack and remain low for the duration of the attack. Another contributory factor is the role of prostaglandins, which may affect adrenergic responses and vessel tone. The relation of migraine and epilepsy is unclear but, in general, the incidence of migraine in patients with generalized epilepsy is higher than in the population at large. The EEG in patients with migraine might also demonstrate paroxysmal events.

Clinical Features

Migraine usually commences during late childhood or early adolescence and tends to decrease in intensity and frequency after menopause. The frequency of attacks is highly variable. The prodromal symptoms are those of restlessness, a sensation of mounting tension, or fluid retention and stuffiness. The classic migraine attack consists of an aura followed by headache with fairly rapid subsidence and return to normal after the attack has passed. The aura consists of blurred vision, hemisensory or motor involvement, dysphasia, and sometimes scintillating streaks of light, photophobia, or visual field loss. The symptoms vary from case to case, but are usually fairly classic and repeated in a given patient. Over the years the severity and duration of these prodromata often change. The headache is variable and is often described as pulsating, throbbing, splitting, or awful. Headache often involves one side of the head (hemicrania), is often accompanied by pupillary alterations, and may end in marked diuresis. Vomiting, in many instances, relieves the pain. After an attack passes the patient may report a feeling of relief and sometimes feels elated. In a significant minority of migraine sufferers, transient hemiplegia, hemianopia, well-defined ophthalmoplegia, or hemisensory disorders are evident usually with no headaches. In children, gastrointestinal disturbances including vomiting, abdominal pain, and pallor (abdominal migraine) are sometimes seen; this is often confused with the entity of so-called abdominal epilepsy. An unusual form of migraine consists of vascular disturbances in the vertebrobasilar system (basilar migraine) during which attacks of vertigo, dysarthria, motor weakness, and ataxia associated with occipital headaches and sometimes loss of consciousness are seen. In other attacks, episodes of dysphasia, confusion, and spatial disorientation occur; these are related to ischemic changes affecting the temporal and temporoparietal regions.

Diagnosis

The diagnosis is based primarily on history and course of events. Although there are no specific diagnostic tests, these are often called upon to exclude more sinister problems. Transient EEG changes often occur during migraine attacks and consist of α-asymmetry, excessive θ activity, and, in a small proportion of cases, clear epileptogenic discharges. In patients with migraine headaches and blackouts, the label of migraine/epilepsy is often used. In a very small number of patients with migraine, an arteriovenous malformation or angioma is found. Therefore, in the workup of patients with migraine, it is important to listen for nuchal and cranial bruits and confirm these suspicions by angiography. Cerebral blood flow studies using radioactive xenon reveal a decrease in blood flow during the ischemic phase with a relative increase during the headache. The CT scan often shows brain edema after the headache is established. These changes are reversible and fully subside during the remission period.

Treatment

This consists of avoiding precipitating factors. Sedatives, antiemetics, and ergotamine are of use during full-blown episodes. Ergotamine preparations such as sublingual tablets of ergotamine tartrate (2-4 mg/day), rectal suppositories of ergotamine, and, in severe cases, subcutaneous or intramuscular ergotamine (0.25-0.5 mg) often help during the early phases of a migraine episode. The most important side effect is severe vasoconstriction (ergotism). Ergotamine is contraindicated in patients with thrombophlebitis, poor circulation angina pectoris, and in pregnancy. Nausea and vomiting are common side effects of ergot preparations.

Analgesics such as aspirin or acetaminophen are beneficial and, in severe cases, codeine (30 mg) may be added. Narcotics and addictive drugs should be avoided if possible. Intramuscular barbiturates may be necessary in severe episodes.

Severe and continued migraine sometimes results in so-called status migrainosus. This is characterized by severe prostration, intermittent vomiting, and continuous splitting headache with or without focal neurologic deficits. Ergotamine is singularly ineffective. Intramuscular barbiturates or chlorpromazine, together with strong analgesics and intravenous fluids, may be necessary. Methysergide maleate (Sansert) prevents vascular headache by serotonin antagonism. It is given orally starting with 2-6 mg/day, the dosage being gradually increased during the course of treatment that lasts for 4-12 weeks. Methysergide treatment should not be repeated until 2-3 weeks have elapsed since the previous course. Side effects, such as drowsiness, ataxia, nausea, and abdominal pain, are common. The most dreaded complication is retroperitoneal fibrosis, which follows injudicious and prolonged therapy. Methysergide should be avoided in patients with peripheral vascular disease or angina pectoris and should be used very cautiously and only as a last resort. Even then, only a very short course is usually advised. In patients with intractable and refractory migraine, a combination of methysergide and oral steroids has been tried; the latter drug is used to negate the fibrotic effects of the former. Clonidine, an antihypertensive agent, is also helpful in the early stages of migraine, the daily dosage being 0.2-0.5 mg. Propranolol and amitryptiline have been employed with some success in the prevention of migraine. Propranolol is currently used in many instances of patients with migraine. Its effects are thought to be related to its antiplatelet-adhesion properties.

Cluster Headaches

These headaches are broadly similar to migraine, except that they occur in clusters or groups and are most common in men. Various labels are given to them, such as migrainous neuralgia, Horton's histaminic cephalagia, sphenopalatine neuralgia, and Sluder's syndrome. They differ from migraine in that vasodilatation is a significant factor, serotonin metabolism is not affected, and there is an increased turnover of histamine and histamine-like substances. Alcohol and stress are common precipitating factors. A typical headache consists of discomfort amounting to pain in the orbital and frontotemporal regions and watering of the corresponding eye lasting for minutes to hours and appearing in groups or clusters over hours or days. The headaches often awaken the patient from sleep and are associated with a flushed facial appearance. Vomiting is rare.

Treatment is similar to that of migraine, but antihistamines tend to relieve headaches better than ergot preparations. In severe and intractable cases, sphenopalatine ganglionectomy is helpful.

TENSION HEADACHES

Headaches related to nervous tension, anxiety, and overt depression are a frequent occurrence. The mechanism of these headaches is unclear. Increased muscular contraction of the neck and shoulder muscles, together with a furrowing or frowning appearance and associated diffuse or vertex headaches, is a common clinical presentation. Pain is variously described as a diffuse ache, unbearable, bursting, crushing, gripping, viselike, and more infrequently throbbing. Treatment consists of using simple analgesics, avoidance of habit-forming drugs, and attention to emotional or personality problems. Firm reassurance and demonstration to the patient that organic factors have been excluded is of great benefit. In some, a short course of phenothiazines or mood elevators like imipramine or amitriptyline may be tried. In intractable cases, psychiatric referral may be necessary.

HEADACHES DUE TO SPECIFIC CAUSES

Headache in Cerebrovascular Disease

Subarachnoid hemorrhage and intracranial aneurysm produce unilateral or focal headache due to meningeal involvement, vessel spasm, or irritation. Hypertensive encephalopathy causes constant and diffuse severe headache. Over one-fifth of patients with cerebral embolism complain of severe headache. The incidence of head discomfort is less obvious in those with carotid or vertebrobasilar insufficiency. Giant-cell or temporal arteritis causes severe and incapacitating headache in the temporal region. The superficial temporal arteries are often dilated and tortuous. The disorder typically occurs in elderly patients and is a giant-cell arteritis. It is associated with raised erythrocyte sedimentation rate and blindness. Giant cells can be demonstrated in biopsy of the superficial temporal artery. Headaches are also noted in patients with polyarteritis nodosa and systemic lupus erythematosus; this is due to cerebral infarction, brain swelling, or arterial involvement.

Headaches due to Meningeal Inflammation

Meningeal irritation due to infection, increased CSF pressure, irritation secondary to trauma, or invasion due to malignant or other processes can produce headache, neck stiffness, and severe backache.

Post-lumbar-Puncture Headache

Following lumbar puncture, patients often complain of severe headache. This is due to leakage of CSF at the site of puncture and changes in CSF pressure. Strict bed rest, oral fluids, analgesics, and maintenance of a supine posture are beneficial. In intractable cases, intravenous saline and inhalation of 5% carbon dioxide with oxygen is helpful. A short course of fludrocortisone acetate (Florinef), 0.1 mg 3-4 times a day is useful, especially in patients who have recently had pneumoencephalograms.

Raised Intracranial Tension

Headache is due to one or more of the following factors: increased CSF production, impedance of flow, or stretching of nerve endings to meninges. Headache is a late symptom of brain tumors and is of very limited localizing value. This is often associated with papilledema, blurred vision, and vomiting.

Posttraumatic Headache

This is due to meningeal involvement or damage to the calvarium or paranasal structures. In some patients its origin is considered to be psychogenic. The clinical features and management depend upon the nature and site of injury.

Toxic-Metabolic Factors

Retention of carbon dioxide, hypoglycemia, cerebral anoxia, heat exhaustion, dehydration, and electrolyte imbalance are often incriminated as causative factors for toxic-metabolic headaches. The patient responds well to reversal of specific causes. Hangover headaches following alcohol abuse (binge) are due to vasodilatation, fluid imbalance, and effects of aromatic compounds in the alcoholic beverage. Certain alcoholic drinks such as rum produce more severe headache. Treatment consists of abstinence, rest, simple analgesics, and plenty of oral fluids.

Ocular Headaches

Headaches due to eye strain are a common complaint. Refractory factors and inflammation of the eye, conjunctiva, and orbital tissues are blamed. Uveitis, iritis, and, in older patients, chronic glaucoma can present with headaches.

Headaches Due to Paranasal Sinus Involvement

Inflammation and other disorders affecting the maxillary, mastoid, and frontal sinuses are commonly incriminated in headaches. In these patients, there is usually clear-cut sinus pathology with tenderness over these regions, bogginess of the skin, and primary disorders affecting the ear, nose, or throat. Chronic sinusitis is an overdiagnosed condition. Headaches in these patients are usually fairly typical and respond to antibiotics and drainage of the sinuses.

Vacuum Headaches

Vacuum related to a sudden decrease of pressure in the nasal passages and eustachian tubes due to a precipitous fall in atmospheric pressure during descent can cause severe pain over the sinuses and ear regions. These headaches are relieved by Valsalva's maneuver and nasal decongestants.

Neuralgias

The classic neuralgia is trigeminal neuralgia also called ticdouloureux. Other neuralgias such as glossopharyngeal, geniculate, and sphenopalatine are less common.

Trigeminal Neuralgia

This is a most distressing disorder with severe lightning pain affecting one side of the face in the distribution of a division of the trigeminal nerve. The pain is thought to be related to an electrical discharge in the trigeminal nerve or its spinal nucleus. In most cases, the etiology is unclear, but in a few patients degenerative changes affecting the ganglion, demyelination, tortuosity of the basilar artery, arteriosclerotic plaques, aneurysm, and sometimes trauma to the nerve or ganglion may be demonstrated. The disorder most commonly affects middle-aged and elderly patients, except when due to multiple sclerosis when it might affect those under 40 years of age. The pain is usually precipitated by chewing, talking, touching the face, or blowing the nose. The patient usually notices a trigger zone and learns to avoid precipitating factors. Neurologic examination is usually negative, although trigger zones can be demonstrated, and, in a small minority of patients, sensory changes in one or more divisions of the trigeminal nerve are found. In these cases organic causes should be excluded (i.e., tumors, arteriovenous (AV) malformation). Diagnosis is established by a classic history, trigger zone, and often a total absence of abnormal physical signs. However, skull x-ray including views of the base of the skull and foramen rotundum for erosion, foramen enlargement, or damage to the petrous temporal bone may reveal a structural cause. Simple analgesics are usually of little help in relieving the acute pain, but are called upon in treating nagging and persistent discomfort.

The specific drugs are carbamazepine and to a lesser effect phenytoin. These drugs are thought to act by diminishing electrical activity in the damaged neurons, the rationale being similar to that in epilepsy. Carbamazepine is the drug of choice and should be administered at a dose of up to 1.2 g daily. Side effects are described in the chapter on epilepsy. In the past, alcohol injection of the trigeminal ganglion was popular. The selective operation for relief of trigeminal neuralgia is retrogasserian neurotomy, in which the sensory root of the trigeminal nerve is permanently severed. Surgical interference is used less today since the introduction of carbamazepine. In patients with clear-cut basilar artery ectasia or intractable pain, or when other organic causes are demonstrated, surgery might prove to be the only solution.

INFECTIONS

Infectious agents can enter the nervous system by at least four routes: direct entrance through penetrating wounds, via the CSF, through the blood, and by retrograde extension along nerve trunks.

MENINGITIS

Inflammation of the dura mater is called pachymeningitis, and of the piarachnoid is called leptomeningitis. The term meningitis is used synonymously with leptomeningitis. Meningitis is divided into three groups: acute bacterial meningitis, aseptic (or viral) meningitis, and subacute or chronic meningitis.

Acute bacterial meningitis and aseptic meningitis are described in the chapter on infectious diseases.

Subacute or Chronic Meningitis

The most common causes of subacute or chronic meningitis are tuberculosis, fungal infections (i.e., cryptococcus), carcinomatous meningitis, and involvement of the meninges in sarcoid. The tuberculous and fungal forms of the disease are infective in origin and will be dealt with under this heading.

Tubercular Meningitis

The natural course of tuberculosis and tubercular meningitis (TBM) has changed dramatically since the introduction of effective antituberculous chemotherapy. In the West, tubercular meningitis is more common in adults, while in Asia it is more common in infants and children. Diagnosis is frequently a problem as the illness may masquerade as other neurologic disorders.

TBM may occur secondary to primary pulmonary tuberculosis, miliary tuberculosis, or spread from other foci such as the spine (Pott's disease), a paravertebral abscess, paranasal sinuses, or cervical lymph glands. The pathology of TBM varies somewhat from other meningitides in that the process is slower and there is an abundance of exudate and fibrinous response. The latter results in adhesions, causing entrapment of arteries and cranial nerves. The onset is frequently insidious, sometimes appearing secondary to a systemic illness but on occasion may be fulminating. The usual features are low-grade fever, headache, neck stiffness, vomiting, malaise, myalgia, and confusion. In some patients, the illness may be heralded by seizures, psychotic behavior, or cranial nerve involvement. In the early stages, TBM is often mistaken for less serious systemic disorders, other CNS infections, or a neoplastic process. Diagnosis is established by lumbar puncture. There is frequently moderate lymphocytic pleocytosis (50-100 cells), but in the acute stage polymorphonuclear cells and mild turbidity may be seen. Biochemical analysis shows a moderate reduction of glucose (approximately 40 mg/dl), significant reduction of chloride, and moderate elevation of protein. A Ziehl-Neelsen stain for acid-fast bacilli and CSF culture confirm the diagnosis. Problems often arise when TBM has to be distinguished from viral meningitis. A positive PPD reaction supports the diagnosis of TBM, but skin tests may be negative in immunocompromised patients even when TBM is present. In established cases of TBM, especially when cranial nerves or focal cerebral signs are seen, it is useful to follow with cerebral angiography to determine whether or not there is encroachment or obstruction to arterial blood flow. Pneumoencephalography is sometimes undertaken to demonstrate adhesions and loculated spaces secondary to chronic arachnoiditis.

Treatment with antitubercular drugs should be commenced when the diagnosis is suspected. Initially, isoniazid, ethambutol, and rifampicin are administered. Rifampicin is discontinued after 3 months, but the other two continued for approximately 12 months. In the acute phase, steroids may be required to overcome fulminating infection and prevent adhesions.

Cryptococcal meningitis and other fungal infections are described below.

BRAIN ABSCESS AND EMPYEMA

Epidural abscess, subdural empyema, brain abscess, and leptomeningitis are included under this heading.

Epidural Abscess

Epidural abscesses are seen in the cranium and spinal cord where they pose distinct diagnostic problems.

Cranial epidural abscesses commonly occur due to direct extension of infection from adjacent sinuses or osteomyelitis of the skull. Neurologic manifestations occur due to expansion of the abscess and compression of adjacent structures. Rupture into the subdural or subarachnoid space produces catastrophic results. Abscesses presenting over the calvarium are fairly obvious. Those near the midline may affect the sagittal sinus, producing severe cerebral venous thrombophlebitis. Diagnosis is established by plain skull x-ray film, which may show paranasal sinus involvement and a variable degree of bony erosion, hyperostosis, or expansion. Treatment consists of surgical drainage of the abscess and appropriate antibiotics. In addition, the source of infection must be eliminated.

Spinal epidural abscesses may be acute or chronic. The chronic form is more common and is frequently related to underlying tuberculosis (Pott's disease) but may result from syphilitic granuloma or fungal infections. An orthopedic deformity producing kyphosis or gibbus is the usual presenting feature. Neurologic involvement due to spinal cord damage, infringement of its arterial blood supply, or collapsed vertebrae may produce transverse myelitis and paraplegia. Thus, the patient may present with a spinal deformity, paraspinal swelling, a history of infection, root pains, or paraplegia. Spine x-ray films may reveal destruction of vertebrae, calcification, and paravertebral abscess. Spinal puncture should be avoided unless combined with myelography and as a prelude to surgical correction as the chances of disseminating infection are high. Treatment consists of appropriate antibiotics, relief of spinal compression, and orthopedic procedures to stabilize the spinal column.

Acute epidural spinal abscess may occur in healthy persons

but is seen more frequently in those suffering from diabetes mellitus or furunculosis. This is an acute process presenting with localized back pain and sudden severe paraparesis. Spine x-rays reveal a zone of erosion. Spinal manometry and myelography should be undertaken to demonstrate the site and extent of block. Treatment consists of laminectomy and drainage of the abscess, followed by appropriate antibiotic therapy.

Subdural Empyema

In some ways, this is similar to cranial epidural abscess in that infection from adjacent bones and paranasal sinuses is frequently the causative factor. Infection may, however, gain access to this space from cranial venous sinuses or by infection of a subdural effusion or hematoma. As the subdural space is not bound into compartments, lateral spread of effusion and empyema may attain considerable size, especially in infants and children. Subdural empyemas occur most frequently over the dorsolateral aspects of the cerebral hemispheres, but are sometimes seen in the falx or undersurface of the brain. Loculations sometimes occur; granulations may follow and there is usually a great deal of adhesion and arachnoiditis. Plain skull x-rays may show bone erosion. The CT scan clearly reveals the area, size, and extension of subdural collection of fluid or pus. Treatment consists of surgical drainage and antibiotics. In children, subdural hygromas are more common than empyema and may occur as a sequela to *Hemophilus influenzae* meningitis or follow mild head injury. The clinical presentations are protean but should be suspected in children with altered levels of alertness. Transillumination of the head usually demonstrates fluid.

Cerebral Abscess

Brain abscesses (cerebral or cerebellar) may arise as the result of direct extension from overlying bone and paranasal sinuses, penetrating wounds of the skull, septic embolization, or secondary to cortical thrombophlebitis. Of these, septic emboli are most common and are frequently related to pulmonary infections or occur secondary to bacterial endocarditis. If the patient's general condition is poor, less pathogenic (opportunistic) bacteria and fungi may embed in the brain and produce chronic abscesses. The type of brain abscess depends on the source, method of spread, and the offending organisms. The most common organism is *Streptococcus hemolyticus* followed by *Staphylococcus aureus*, *Escherichia coli*, and other enteropathic bacteria. Bloodborne cerebral abscesses are usually multiple and most often arise at the junction of white and grey matter or in the temporoparietal regions of the cerebrum. An abscess tends to grow rapidly in white matter (due to its limited blood supply) and responds less actively to antibiotic agents. In patients with a fulminant abscess, purulent meningitis due to superficial spread into the subdural space or deeper spread into the ventricular system may occur. An acute brain abscess is a severe and fulminating illness with systemic and neurologic manifestations. Headaches, neck stiffness, focal neurologic signs, convulsions, papilledema, and obtundation are common. Underlying cardiopulmonary pathology should be sought in every patient. Skull x-ray may demonstrate a paranasal sinus source. The EEG shows severe disorganization of activity with localized or lateralized, polymorphous, high-amplitude δ waves. Spinal puncture should be undertaken with care, especially if papilledema is present. A raised CSF protein, low sugar, leukocytosis, and growth of bacteria on culture is invariably found. Computed tomography demonstrates the size, nature, and extension of cerebral abscess, as well as delineating the acute and more chronic forms of abscess. Treatment consists of appropriate systemic antibiotic therapy and surgical drainage. Prophylactic anticonvulsants are recommended. The mortality is high, especially in the acute situation.

NEUROSYPHILIS

Neurosyphilis can simulate a vast majority of neurologic disorders. Diagnosis is a relatively simple matter and, with the advent of penicillin therapy, tertiary manifestations of syphilis have largely disappeared. Syphilis should, however, always be considered as an etiologic factor in young patients presenting with cerebrovascular episodes or other unusual CNS disorders. In the primary stage no neurologic features are noted. In the secondary stage, perivascular cuffing and, more typically, endarteritis are evident together with endothelial proliferation and lymphocytic infiltration. In the brain this produces vascular accidents, meningoencephalitis, or chronic meningitis. In the tertiary stage, there is organization of syphilitic deposits, production of granulomata, and a great degree of gliosis. This can produce pachymeningitis, degeneration of fibers, or tracts and gummata. In congenital syphilis, the time scale of CNS dysfunction is further compressed. Some of the salient clinical syndromes in neurosyphilis are described below.

Meningeal and Meningovascular Syphilis

In the majority of patients with meningovascular syphilis in the granulomatous form with vascular insufficiency or strokes, chronic basal meningitis, cranial nerve palsies, and brain stem involvement are seen. Some patients with secondary syphilis have psychotic episodes, clouding of consciousness, and mental dulling culminating in pseudodementia. Extrapyramidal involvement with some parkinsonian features may also occur. Diagnosis is established by positive serologic tests for syphilis. In the secondary stage of syphilis, spinal fluid examination reveals mild lymphocytic pleocytosis with a first or midzone colloidal gold (Lange) curve. In the tertiary stage, the CSF gamma globulins are raised and there is a well-developed first zone gold curve together with positive serologic tests for syphilis. Distinction between meningovascular syphilis and other vascular disorders is important as the former can be effectively treated with high doses of penicillin.

Spinal Syphilis

The spinal cord may be affected by diffuse syphilitic meningoencephalitis in a manner similar to the cerebral process of meningovascular syphilis and by chronic basal meningitis. The common factor is syphilitic arteritis, resulting in small infarcts of the spinal cord. There is also thickening of the leptomeninges and mild arachnoiditis. The onset is insidious with fleeting motor and sensory signs culminating in sphincter involvement, zones of analgesia, and hypalgesias. Muscle wasting and fasciculations may be seen; this is due to anterior horn cell involvement. Serologic tests for syphilis are positive. Lumbar puncture reveals high protein, partial block, positive gold curve, and altered globulin levels. Treatment consists of high doses of penicillin.

Pachymeningitis Cervicalis Hypertrophica

In the latter stages of syphilis, the pathologic process consists of severe thickening of the meninges, fibrinous deposits compressing vessels, nerves, and the spinal cord, and severe arachnoiditis. Pachymeningitis frequently occurs in the cervical region and presents with features similar to cervical spondylosis but, in addition, root signs and other features of syphilis predominate. The serologic tests are positive and diagnosis is confirmed by spinal puncture and myelography. On myelography there is partial obstruction to CSF flow with evidence of arachnoiditis and thickened meninges; this shows a classic stippled pattern of multiple blocks and adhesions.

Tabes Dorsalis

This is a late complication of syphilis and is seen 20-25 years after primary infection. In this disorder, the dorsal columns, dorsal nerve roots, and dorsal ganglia show severe atrophy. Proprioception is first affected and results in ataxia, unsteadiness, and incoordination. In addition, there are some peculiarities unique to tabes dorsalis consisting of tabetic lightninglike pains. They may occur in the lower limbs but frequently involve visceral structures and even thoracic and facial nerves. Tic douloureux and anginal pains have been described. Tabetic crises are often present with severe abdominal pain. Urinary retention, abdominal rigidity, and severe colic have been described. In some forms, laryngeal crises may occur with paroxysms of coughing or dyspnea. The main feature of tabes dorsalis is the inability to stand erect with eyes closed (Romberg's sign) and severe paresthesia in the limbs, primarily affecting light touch and joint position. Bladder and bowel dysfunction are common, resulting in a large flaccid and painless urinary bladder. This is frequently the source of infection culminating in cystitis, pyelitis, or pyelonephritis. Constipation is frequent. Due to severe joint position loss and autonomic changes, marked arthropathy is common and usually begins in the lower limbs. Gross deformity of joints, especially the knee, effusion within the joints, and secondary changes result in neuropathic (Charcot's) joints. Brain stem involvement leads to Argyll Robertson pupil. This consists of an irregular small pupil that reacts to accommodation but not to light. Diagnosis of tabes dorsalis is established by positive serologic tests for syphilis. The CSF may show a positive first- or second-zone gold curve and lymphocytic pleocytosis. Treatment is mainly palliative and consists of relief of pain, treating various crises, and adequate support by orthopedic assistance to deformed joints. Lightning pains may respond to phenytoin or carbamazepine. Trophic ulcers should be treated with appropriate footwear and local dressings. Procaine penicillin G, 900,000 units daily intramuscularly for 15-20 days, is an accepted treatment regimen. Patients allergic to penicillin should be treated with oral tetracycline, 2 g per day, for 20 days. In a few patients, paradoxical reactions to penicillin may occur, resulting in crises and increased lightning pains. This is thought to be related to a severe antigen-antibody response from the dead organisms.

General Paralysis of the Insane

General paralysis of the insane (general paresis, GPI) is a form of tertiary or late neurosyphilis with parenchymatous cerebral involvement. Patients with GPI usually do not get tabes dorsalis, and those with tabes dorsalis are protected from GPI. In this disorder, there is diffuse cerebral degeneration and atrophy. Brain biopsy shows spirochetes diffusely distributed in the cerebral substance. The onset is ill defined and consists of altered behavior and progressive loss of intellectual and mental capabilities. At the onset of this disorder, abnormal judgement, poor memory, and altered personality and temperament are frequent. Hallucinations, delusions, and paranoid states follow. Sudden fluctuation in intellectual capability, mood, and seizures are a common occurrence. Hemiplegia and other focal neurologic deficits are sometimes seen but are comparatively rare. Physical examination reveals a demented patient with involuntary movements, slurred speech, dysphasia, and sometimes dysarthria. Cranial nerve paresis is infrequent. Focal neurologic signs are rare. The most common CNS manifestation is Argyll Robertson pupil. Diagnosis is confirmed by positive serologic tests for syphilis, an abnormal first-zone gold curve, and signs of brain atrophy on CT scanning or pneumoencephalography. The EEG is progressively disorganized. In the early stages, penicillin in the doses mentioned under tabes dorsalis is helpful. Once the disorder is well established, most patients need institutional care.

Syphilitic Gumma

This almost exclusively affects the cerebrum and begins as a solitary space-occupying lesion with or without other features of neurosyphilis. The patient usually presents with seizures and signs of an expanding cerebral lesion. The CSF and blood show positive serology. Treatment consists of antibiotic therapy and surgical removal of the lesion.

Primary Optic Atrophy

Primary optic atrophy is commonly seen in patients with tabes dorsalis but is sometimes noted with GPI. It is thought to be related to degeneration of blood vessels, demyelination, and secondary gliosis. The patient complains of constriction of visual fields and progressive visual loss. Fundus examination reveals a chalky white disk with small blood vessels. Penicillin is the treatment of choice.

FUNGAL INFECTIONS

Coccidioidomycosis occurs in the southwestern United States as an endemic infection. Other mycotic infections occur as opportunistic infections in debilitated patients.

Cryptococcal Infection

Cryptococcus neoformans is a yeastlike organism found in droppings of birds that produces a mild respiratory illness in healthy adults. It may cause a systemic illness in immunosuppressed patients or those with debilitating disorders. The neurologic picture is that of meningoencephalitis, papilledema, and cranial nerve dysfunction. The diagnosis is confirmed by CSF examination, where an India ink preparation shows encapsulated budding yeast bodies. Indirect fluorescent antibody and agglutination tests are also positive. Other fungal infections are very rare.

Amphotericin B and flucytosine are used in combination in the treatment of fungal infections. Amphotericin B is given slowly as an intravenous infusion, increasing the daily dose from 5-10 mg to 1 mg/kg. Hydrocortisone is added if a febrile reaction occurs. Intrathecal amphotericin B is given in cases with inadequate clinical response or relapse. Flucytosine is administered orally for 4-6 weeks. The principal toxic effect of amphotericin B is nephrotoxicity. Renal function must be monitored carefully as this drug is a good example of the common saying that the treatment might be more dangerous than the primary disorder.

CEREBROVASCULAR DISORDERS

EPIDEMIOLOGY

Cerebrovascular diseases result in approximately 200,000 deaths annually in the United States. It is estimated that as many as 2 million people suffer from cardiovascular disease of one form or another. During the past decade early detection and control of hypertension has reduced the incidence of strokes. Nevertheless, as many as 500,000 new stroke cases occur annually. For the survivors, disability and dependency are the usual result. As cerebrovascular disorders constitute the most common neurologic illness, these disorders must be considered in the differential diagnosis of most neurologic cases.

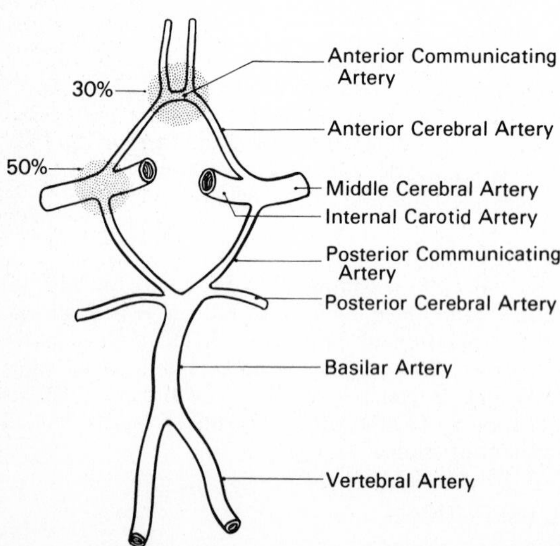

Figure 6. The circle of Willis, showing the common sites and frequency of the aneurysms.

CEREBRAL BLOOD FLOW

The brain is supplied by the carotid and vertebrobasilar systems. The common carotid arteries divide into internal and external branches. The internal carotid branch enters the skull through the carotid canal and cavernous sinus to supply a major portion of the cerebrum, the eye, and deep cerebral structure. The main branches of the carotid and vertebrobasilar system forming the circle of Willis are detailed in Figure 6. The vertebral and basilar arteries have several branches that supply structures in the posterior cranial fossa and upper portion of the spinal cord. The capacity of cerebral neurons to survive ischemia is very limited. The circle of Willis enables collateral circulation from various main branches. In addition to the circle of Willis, there are at least four other systems of collateral circulation. The blood supply to the brain depends on adequacy and adjustments in cerebral blood flow.

Cerebrovascular disorders can be classified as follows:

- Cerebral ischemia
  - Carotid insufficiency
  - Vertebrobasilar insufficiency
  - Subclavian steal syndrome
- Cerebral thrombosis
  - Internal carotid artery occlusion
  - Middle cerebral artery occlusion
  - Anterior choroidal artery occlusion
  - Anterior cerebral artery occlusion
  - Vertebrobasilar artery occlusion
  - Posterior cerebral artery occlusion
  - Lacunar states
- Cerebral embolism
- Intracranial hemorrhage
  - Cerebral hemorrhage
  - Cerebellar hemorrhage
  - Subarachnoid hemorrhage
- Hypertensive encephalopathy
- Inflammatory disorders of cranial arteries

CEREBRAL ISCHEMIA

Cerebral ischemia results from diminished circulation, the most common cause being cerebral arteriosclerosis. Cerebral arteriosclerosis is believed to be a chronic degenerative disorder of the cerebral arteries usually beginning in adult life and manifesting during middle age. The primary risk factors are hypertension, diabetes mellitus, hyperlipidemia, and familial predisposition. Dietary excess, coagulation disorders, obesity, lack of exercise, and smoking have been incriminated. The common denominator of cerebral arteriosclerosis is an arteriosclerotic plaque. Whether the initial lesion is in the vessel wall due to deposition of lipids, including cholesterol, or whether a thrombus is formed in the vessel due to endothelial ulceration or vessel weakness is as yet unclear. A plaque has three effects: narrowing and occlusion of the lumen, ulceration of the vessel wall, and embolization within the arterial tree. The plaque spreads around the vessel wall, resulting in progressive thrombosis and eventual occlusion. Cerebral arteriosclerosis results in transient ischemic attacks, cerebral infarction and so-called arteriosclerotic dementias.

Transient ischemic attacks (TIAs) are brief neurologic disturbances due to carotid and vertebrobasilar insufficiency. TIAs result in transient neurologic disturbances lasting less than 24 hours followed by complete recovery. A precipitating factor may be difficult to ascertain. Factors such as transient fall of blood pressure, movement of the head and neck, and cardiac arrhythmias are known to precipitate attacks. If untreated, one-third of these patients will suffer a complete stroke, one-third will continue to have TIA without infarction, and one-third will have a spontaneous remission. Ischemic attacks occur in the two main vascular territories: carotid and vertebrobasilar. In contrast to the TIAs, reversible ischemic neurologic deficits (RINDs) are completed strokes with reversion and disappearance of the symptoms and signs in less than 72 hours.

When the anterior (carotid) system is involved, stenosis of major vessels in the neck usually occur. These may involve the carotid arteries. An ulcerated arteriosclerotic plaque is often demonstrated in that site, attributed to platelet embolization. Circulatory problems involve the eyes and cerebral hemispheres. Ocular involvement may result in transient blindness (amaurosis fugax), floating figures, or diminished vision. Carotid bruit is usually heard when the stenosis is between 50-80% and the carotid pulse might be decreased. If the dominant cerebral hemisphere is affected, transient dysphasia is common. Other clinical manifestations include transient weakness, numbness, or confusion. Examination of fundi for pulsations, suction ophthalmodynamometry, and ocular plethysmography are helpful in the differential diagnosis. Vascular echoes recorded by sonography (Doppler) can also help locate the lesion. Arteriography provides a definite diagnosis (Figs. 7 and 8).

When the insufficiency occurs in the vertebrobasilar system, the symptoms are vast and are related to the involved vessel, thus causing symptoms and signs originating in the upper spinal cord, hind brain, and posterior half of the cerebrum. Drop attacks, visual difficulties, ataxia, facial paresthesia, and transient auditory symptoms are common. Neurologic examination after an episode is usually normal. Aortic arch arteriography with vertebral artery catheterization to demonstrate involvement of the vertebrobasilar system is the final diagnostic study.

Symptoms of claudication of an exercised arm accompanied by symptoms of vertebrobasilar insufficiency constitute the subclavian steal syndrome. The pathologic lesion is arteriosclerotic occlusion of the subclavian or innominate artery. Reversal of blood flow in the ipsilateral vertebral artery causes stealing of blood from areas of the brain supplied by the vertebrobasilar system. An audible bruit over the stenosed artery, delay in radial pulse, and reduction of systolic blood pressure of over 20 mm Hg on the affected side are pathognomonic signs.

Noninvasive Techniques for the Study of Extracranial Vascular Disease

Over the last few decades it has become increasingly clear that extracranial atherosclerotic disease plays an important role in the pathogenesis of stroke. About 18% of all strokes are in relation to carotid artery disease and about 65% of these patients have TIAs before stroke. In such a group of patients,

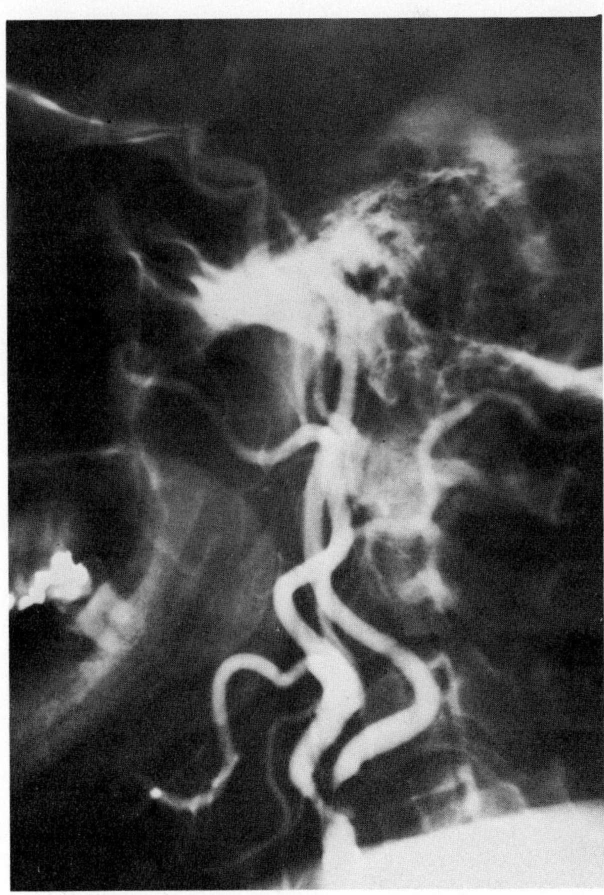

Figure 7. Carotid angiogram. Note the ulcerative atherosclerotic plaque causing severe narrowing of the carotid bifurcation and the origin of the internal carotid artery. Extension to the external carotid artery is also seen. 58-year-old man with TIAs.

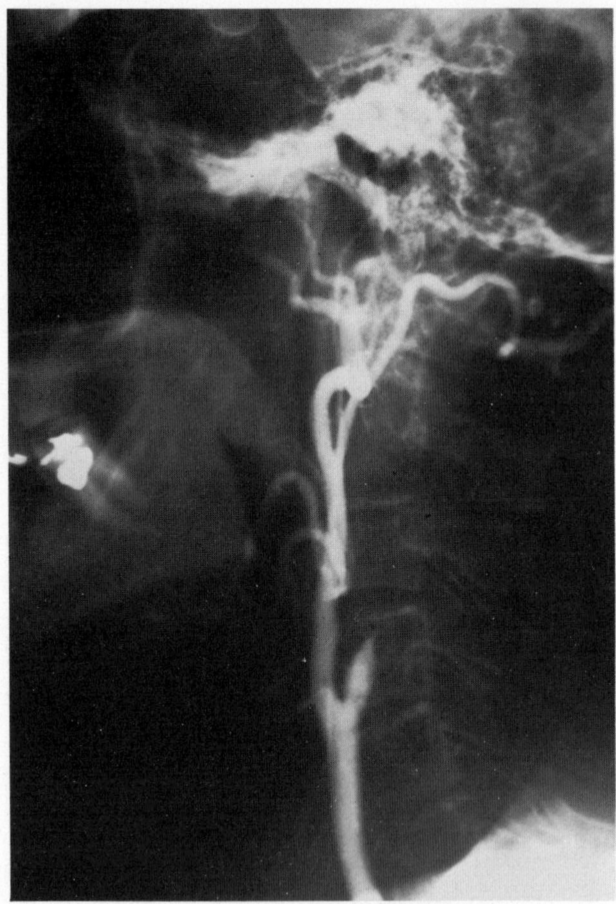

Figure 8. Carotid angiogram. Complete occlusion of the internal carotid artery distal to the bifurcation. 62-year-old man with TIAs.

carotid endarterectomy, in appropriate settings, is considered to have a definite role in management of these patients. Angiography still remains an accepted method of defining the extent and nature of the disease in the carotid system, but it is time-consuming, uncomfortable, and poses some risks to the patients. Recognition of these problems have led to the development of various noninvasive investigative techniques in recent years. The noninvasive techniques are of two types; indirect and direct.

Indirect techniques assess the hemodynamics of the carotid system distal to the bifurcation, and thus indirectly provide information about its morphology. These try to assess stenosis of more than 50%, which is considered hemodynamically significant. Included in this group are techniques like ophthalmodynamometry, ocular plethysmography, ocular pneumoplethysmography, periorbital directional Doppler sonography, and fluid-filled ocular plethysmography.

The direct techniques try to assess the carotid bifurcation directly and provide physiologic and/or morphologic observations about the bifurcation. Carotid phonoangiography provides audio-frequency analysis of cervical bruits, while various ultrasound imaging techniques provide anatomic data with regard to stenosis and ulcerated lesions.

By using various techniques in combination, physiologic and morphologic information about the carotid system can be obtained accurately in up to 90% of the patients.

Treatment

Associated medical conditions such as hypertension, anemia, obesity, and diabetes should be appropriately treated. Further management depends on the area of vessel involvement and nature of the neurologic deficit. In patients with unilateral carotid stenosis of 50-85%, and in those with ulcerated atherosclerotic plaque or subclavian stenosis, surgery might prove to be the most beneficial (Fig. 9). Medical therapy is indicated in patients with normal arteriograms, multiple vascular lesions, in a few cases of asymptomatic carotid bruits, vertebrobasilar insufficiency, in low-risk patients, and when patients refuse surgery. As the pathophysiology often consists of platelet emboli, medical management consists of long-term administration of antiplatelet drugs such as aspirin, dipyridamole (Persantine), and sulfinpyrazone (Anturane), or anticoagulants such as heparin (acute) and warfarin (Coumadin-more chronic).

CEREBRAL THROMBOSIS

Cerebral infarction may result from vessel thrombosis or severe spasm. Secondary cerebral embolism may occur if a thrombus is dislodged. The precipitating factors are similar to those producing cerebral ischemia, but the rate of progression of events is more rapid. A preliminary TIA frequently gives a clue to an impending cerebrovascular accident, which results from a catastrophic reduction of blood flow to a given area of brain and associated failure of collateral circulation. Clinical features depend on area of involvement and rate of progression.

When the occlusion occurs in the middle cerebral artery (Fig. 9), the preliminary symptoms might consist of transient episodes of failure of vision in one eye (amaurosis fugax), diminution of vision in that eye, and transient numbness or weakness in the contralateral upper and lower limbs. Failure of collateral circulation produces hemiplegia with dysphasia if the dominant hemisphere is affected and variable visual involvement in the ipsilateral eye. Secondary changes resulting from brainstem edema due to infarction may further compound the picture.

It is frequently difficult to distinguish between middle cerebral and internal carotid artery occlusion. In the former, visual symptoms are minimal but severe dysphasia and hemiplegia are present. Also, examination of the neck might reveal good carotid pulsation. This is an inaccurate sign as the artery palpated is usually the common carotid artery. The severity of neurologic deficit depends on efficacy of collateral circulation.

The anterior choroidal artery supplies the optic tract, a portion of the cerebral peduncle, the lateral geniculate body, and the internal capsule. Occlusion produces symptoms similar to

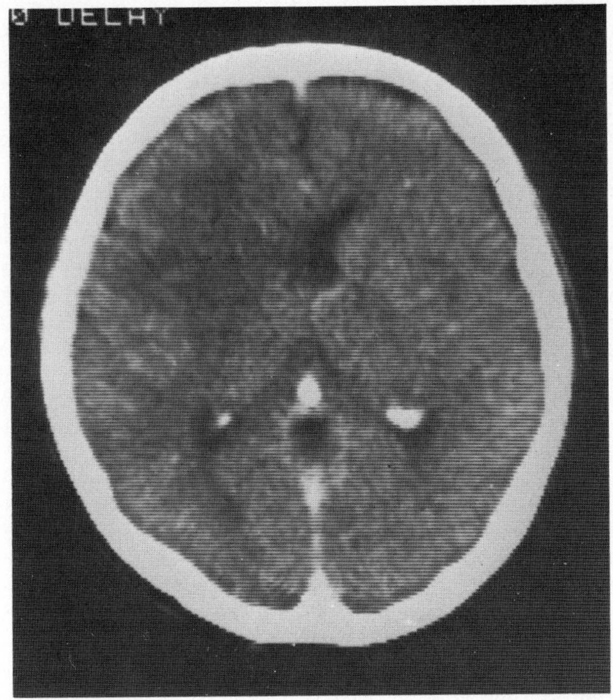

Figure 9. CT scan. Acute infarction of the right middle cerebral artery. Low density lesion in the distribution of the artery in a 58-year-old man.

middle cerebral artery blockage, but visual involvement is severe (contralateral homonymous hemianopia) with other features of internal capsular involvement. Speech is usually spared.

When the anterior cerebral artery is involved, depending on site of involvement, infarction of the frontal lobe, cingulate area, and deep structures occurs. Bilateral occlusion produces a peculiar altered level of consciousness varying from drowsiness to an akinetic mute state. Thrombosis of the artery supplying the anterior limb of the internal capsule produces contralateral monoparesis. More distal obstruction of the callosomarginal and pericallosal arteries leads to ischemia of the frontal lobe and the paracentral lobules. In these cases, the lower limbs are more severely affected.

Ischemic damage of the occipital lobes as well as the upper brain-stem and posterior portion of the basal ganglia are seen when the posterior cerebral artery is involved. In addition to homonymous hemianopia, upper brain-stem signs are noted in most cases. Involuntary movements may occur, the most severe being hemiballismus due to occlusion in the posterior choroidal artery.

Numerous syndromes have been described in occlusions of vessels in the vertebrobasilar system, depending on the site of brain-stem or cerebellar involvement. In addition to selected cranial and other nuclei, the ascending and descending tracts are involved. Crossed motor and sensory disorders, cranial nerve dysfunctions, and problems with balance, respiration, temperature, blood pressure, and consciousness are common.

The lacunar state is due to small areas of infarction in the area of supply of penetrating branches of the major cerebral arteries. The well-recognized lacunar syndromes include pure motor hemiplegia, dysarthric clumsy-hand syndrome, pure sensory stroke involving the face, arm, and leg, and homolateral ataxia and spastic weakness with greatest involvement in the legs.

Prevention and Treatment of Cerebral Thrombosis

The most important preventive measure is the early diagnosis and treatment of hypertension. Hypotension and dehydration must also be prevented during acute illnesses and surgery. Treatment of cerebral infarction has four goals: to preserve life, to limit the amount of brain damage, to minimize disability and deformity, and to prevent recurrence.

In the acute phase, treatment consists of attention to respiration, blood pressure, temperature regulation, and general care of the unconscious patient. Bladder care, frequent change of posture, and feeding together with physiotherapy are necessary. Specific measures consist of managing cerebral edema, improving cerebral blood flow, and preventing recurrence of another catastrophic episode. Cerebral edema occurs in a few hours to days after infarction and is a major cause of death in patients with acute stroke. To relieve edema, agents such as intravenous urea, mannitol, glycerol, and low molecular weight dextran have been used. The corticosteroid preparations, especially dexamethasone (Decadron), given parenterally may be effective in reducing cerebral edema over a short period. Cerebral vasodilators have limited value in the acute situation and are potentially dangerous as they may divert blood flow from the infarcted and ischemic areas. Anticoagulants are useful in the treatment of stroke-in-evolution but may be hazardous in patients with high blood pressure. The use of thrombolytic agents such as urokinase and streptokinase is still experimental. Surgical correction of isolated carotid stenosis in patients with a mild neurologic defect is effective in reducing future morbidity and mortality. Cerebral arterial bypass surgery is presently undergoing clinical trials. Early physiotherapy and mobilization helps lessen deformity and disability.

CEREBRAL EMBOLISM

Emboli may lodge in the carotid or vertebrobasilar vessel tree to produce catastrophic changes. In a small portion of patients, larger vessels may be the source of emboli that lodge more distally in the arterial tree. Cardiac causes for embolism are numerous. In young patients, right-to-left shunts and rheumatic heart disease and, in older patients, cardiac arrhythmias, myocardial infarction, and subacute bacterial endocarditis are common factors. Rare causes include cardiomyopathy, atrial myxoma, and paradoxical embolism. In addition to vascular emboli, other causes of embolism such as fat, air, foreign bodies, and tumor metastases should be considered. The symptoms of cerebral embolism are similar to those of infarction, except that the chain of events is more rapid. The presenting CNS picture depends on the site of cerebral infarction and the state of collateral circulation. Management is similar to that described for patients with thrombotic CVAs, except that if the source of embolism is identified, it should be adequately dealt with. Anticoagulants in patients with proven emboli from the aortic arch or heart are more effective than in patients with cerebral infarction.

INTRACRANIAL HEMORRHAGE

Spontaneous intracranial hemorrhage can be either intra-axial (into the brain) or extra-axial (subarachnoid hemorrhage).

Cerebral hemorrhage may be either primary or secondary due to lysis of a preexisting infarct. The patient with primary intracerebral hemorrhage is invariably hypertensive with evidence of retinal, cardiac, and perhaps renal damage. Onset is rapid with headache, vomiting, severe neurologic deficit, and altered consciousness. Respiration is frequently disordered and irregular. Depending on the site of bleeding and anatomic localization of the hemorrhage, various neurologic syndromes are noted. If blood leaks into the subarachnoid space or ventricles, signs of meningism appear. If the hemorrhage is confined to the cerebral mass, a localized hematoma results and produces effects of an expanding space-occupying lesion.

Cerebellar hemorrhage is less common and presents the patient with severe occipital headaches, vomiting, and signs of brain-stem and cerebellar dysfunction. It is difficult to distinguish cerebellar hemorrhage from a primary vascular brain-stem disturbance, but if there are prominent cerebellar features, occipital headache, and progressive obtundation, the diagnosis of cerebellar hemorrhage is more likely. Prompt angiography and ligation of the bleeder or resection of part of the cerebellum sometimes retrieves a patient who would otherwise almost invariably perish.

Intracranial bleeding frequently occurs in the subarachnoid space and is often related to cerebral aneurysms, vascular malformations, and other arterial or venous anomalies. Bleeding may also occur spontaneously in hypertensive patients. Less frequent causes of bleeding are mycotic infections involving the arterial wall and blood dyscrasias. The blood may be restricted to the subarachnoid space or spread to adjacent intracerebral or subdural structures. In addition, the presence of blood in the subarachnoid space produces severe vessel spasm; this may lead to infarction in the area of supply. A rare occurrence is for an artery to rupture into a venous channel, thus producing an arteriovenous fistula. The clinical presentation of subarachnoid hemorrhage is acute and consists of severe headache, neck stiffness, vomiting, disturbed consciousness, and cranial nerve and brain-stem signs together with cardiorespiratory dysfunction. In patients with congenital and developmental disorders, facial nevi (as in Sturge-Weber syndrome) or other pointers may be seen. Bleeding is commonly related to the circle of Willis. Examination of fundi may show subhyaloid hemorrhage. Pepilledema is seen in over 10% of patients and cranial nerve palsies are frequent in patients with aneurysms involving the posterior part of the circle of Willis. If the aneurysm is large, it may act as a space-occupying lesion, especially if localized to nonstrategic sites. In some patients, a large aneurysm may be confused with a cerebral tumor or metastatic intracranial deposit. Diagnosis of subarachnoid hemorrhage is confirmed by performing a lumbar puncture that shows a grossly bloody tap and xanthochromia of CSF if bleeding has occurred 6 hours to 3 weeks previously. Skull x-ray may show areas of calcification or erosion of bone adjacent to the aneurysm. The EEG is of limited value, but is useful in patients with bilateral aneurysms to assess the side most severely affected by vessel spasm and consequent cerebral ischemia. The isotope brain scan is of limited value. CT scanning is very useful in patients who are extremely ill, it may reveal intracerebral hematomas and other extension from aneurysms. Diagnosis is confirmed by angiography that shows the site of the lesion, feeding and draining blood vessels, and distortion of adjacent cerebral tissue.

Patients with intracranial hemorrhage must be treated with strict bed rest and headache relieved by potent analgesics. Control of hypertension, if present, is essential. If consciousness is impaired and respiration disordered, measures to alleviate this should be undertaken in an intensive care unit where constant nursing care, monitoring facilities, and assessment of neurologic dysfunction can be carried out concurrently. Seizures are frequent and should be treated with anticonvulsants. The use of antifibrinogen agents such as ϵ-aminocaproic acid (Amicar) to inhibit lysis of the clot has recently come into vogue, but its efficacy needs further evaluation. Cerebral edema is treated with intravenous 10% glycerol or intramuscular dexamethasone. Surgical treatment depends on the extent and location of hemorrhage, site of the aneurysm, associated complications, and efficacy of collateral vascular supply.

HYPERTENSIVE ENCEPHALOPATHY

This entity is described under the discussion of hypertensive emergencies.

INFLAMMATORY DISORDERS OF THE CRANIAL ARTERIES

This heterogeneous group includes various connective tissue disorders: systemic lupus erythematosus, polyarteritis nodosa, temporal (giant cell) arteritis, and other vascular disorders of uncertain origin such as Takayasu's arteritis. These conditions are discussed in the chapter on rheumatology.

BRAIN TUMORS AND INCREASED INTRACRANIAL PRESSURE

A detailed discussion of tumors is presented in the chapter on oncology. However, no chapter on neurology can be complete without a brief note on this subject.

Tumors of the nervous system cause two types of symptoms and signs: general, usually due to increased intracranial pressure, and focal, due to their presence in a specific location. The focal symptoms and signs are paresis or paralysis; seizures; ataxia and gait disturbances; language and communication abnormalities like aphasia, apraxia, and agnosia; pituitary and hormonal malfunction like diabetes insipidus and abnormal growth; specific cranial nerve palsies; signs originating in the different lobes of the brain like personality changes in frontal lobe lesions, astereognosis in parietal lobe lesions, and so forth.

The general symptoms and signs, commonly referred to as signs of increased intracranial pressure, are usually caused by one or more of the following reasons: pressure by the tumor mass, pressure by cerebral edema, obstruction of CSF flow and absorption, and obstruction of the venous system. These symptoms and signs consist of one or more of the following: headache; vertigo; vomiting; changes in personality; convulsions; enlargement of the head, especially in infants and children; papilledema; changes in vital signs (bradycardia, increased systolic blood pressure and slowing of the respiratory rate—known as Cushing's triad). The various herniations (temporal lobe or uncal, below the falx, the gyrus rectus, and cerebellar tonsils) and occasional cranial nerve manifestations (like the Foster Kennedy syndrome) are considered false localizing signs and are also due to increased intracranial pressure.

The tumors of the nervous system consist of 10 major groups (WICC classification), which are

1. Tumors of the nerve cells
2. Tumors of neuroepithelial origin (ependymomas)
3. Tumors of the eye and retina
4. Tumors of glial cells (astrocytomas, oligodendrogliomas, glioblastomas, spongioblastomas, and medulloblastomas)
5. Tumors of peripheral and cranial nerves (neurinomas)
6. Tumors of the meninges (meningiomas)
7. Vascular tumors (hemangiomas)
8. Paraganglia tumors (carotid body tumor, chemodectoma)
9. Tumors of the pineal gland (pinealomas)
10. Tumors of the hypophysis (the various adenomas, craniopharyngiomas, etc.)

Figs. 10 through 13 show typical CT scan pictures of primary and metastatic tumors.

DISORDERS OF THE CRANIAL AND PERIPHERAL NERVES

CRANIAL NERVE DISORDERS

This section deals with specific disorders of cranial nerves that are unrelated to other problems such as tumors, infections, and so on.

Optic Atrophy

Primary optic atrophy occurs in cases where the optic nerve tracts and nerves degenerate without evidence of edema, compression, or prior inflammation. On funduscopic examination the disks appear white with sharp edges and the physiologic cup is well developed. Primary optic atrophy is seen in certain hereditary disorders such as Leber's optic atrophy, hereditary ataxias, and spinocerebellar degenerations.

Secondary optic atrophy usually follows optic or retrobulbar neuritis, papilledema, or compression of the optic nerve. In this condition, the disk appears grey or white, the margins are

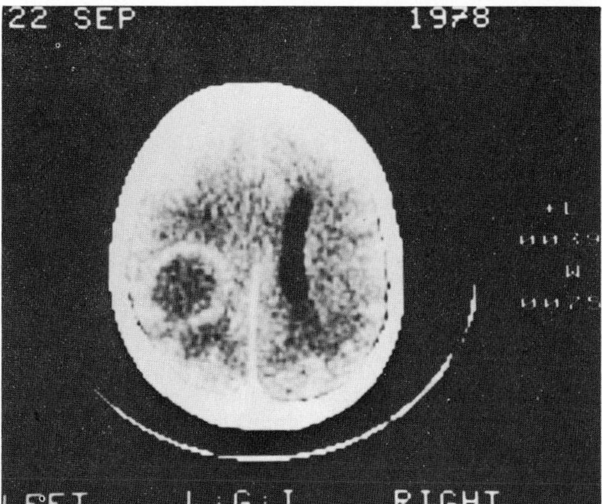

Figure 10. CT scan. Primary brain tumor in the left hemisphere.

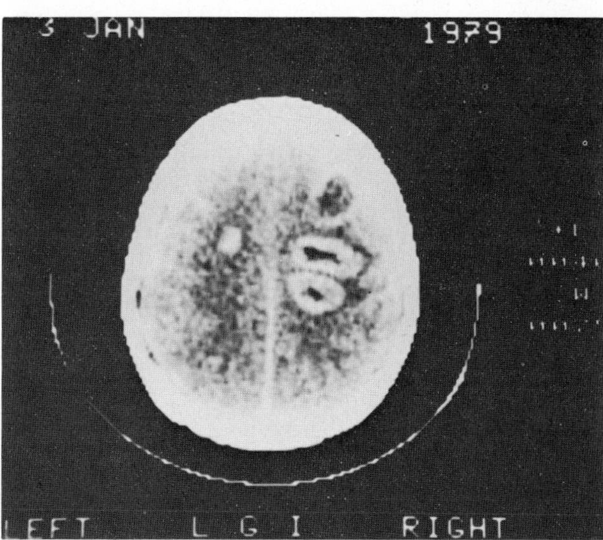

Figure 11. CT scan. Metastatic tumor shadows in the right hemisphere.

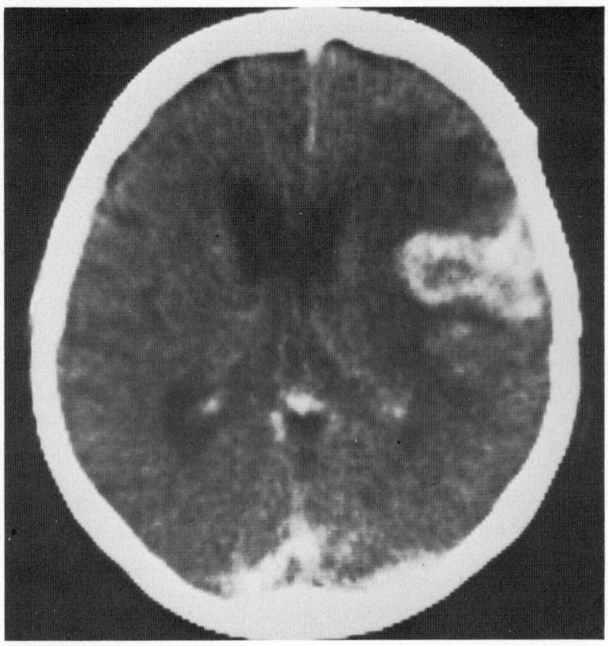

Figure 12. CT scan. Recurrent primary tumor in the left hemisphere (glioblastoma) in a 60-year-old man.

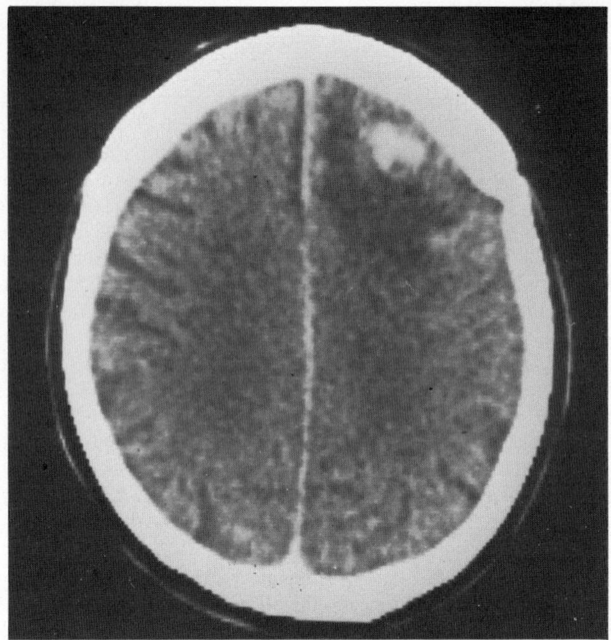

Figure 13. CT scan. Metastatic tumor to the left hemisphere (carcinoma of the lungs) in a 61-year-old man.

indistinct, and the physiologic cup is distorted. Other causes of secondary optic atrophy include rasied intraocular pressure as in glaucoma, or extraocular compression on the optic nerve from mass lesions in the anterior or middle cranial fossa. This is commonly seen in patients with aneurysms or tumors compressing the optic nerve and its subsequent decussation. Toxic and metabolic disorders frequently produce optic atrophy. Skull fractures and trauma to the orbit may damage the optic nerve with resultant secondary optic atrophy. Demyelination (multiple sclerosis) is a common cause of optic atrophy. In this disorder, the temporal sector of the optic disks is initially affected and appears pale. Temporal pallor is due to demyelination of the papulomacular bundle. A chalky-white disk is sometimes seen in patients with methyl alcohol poisoning. Tobacco amblyopia may produce mild optic atrophy but, more significantly, a visual deficit. Diabetes mellitus and underlying carcinomatosis are other causes of optic atrophy.

Patients with optic atrophy should receive a detailed neurologic examination, followed by a thorough visual examination including assessment of visual fields, ocular movements, and measurement of intraocular tension. Conditions such as head injury, congenital syphilis, optic nerve tumors, craniopharyngiomas, and congenital glaucoma should be excluded before diagnosis of primary optic atrophy is established. In some children, no cause may be evident, but careful family history would suggest the diagnosis of so-called Leber's optic atrophy. Electroretinography (ERG) and visual evoked responses (VER) help to better delineate the problem. In patients with primary choroidoretinal involvement, there is slowing and eventual absence of activity on ERG, whereas in patients with conditions such as multiple sclerosis that involve the visual pathways, the ERG is normal but the VER is deformed, delayed, or absent.

Treatment depends on the causative factor. In patients with an uncertain diagnosis or when demyelination is suspected, a course of prednisolone or ACTH may be beneficial. In patients with tobacco amblyopia and in most cases where the diagnosis has not been established, vitamin B_{12b} (hydroxocobalamin) is administered.

Myotonic Pupil (Holmes-Adie Syndrome)

This is a benign disorder of uncertain etiology that is not associated with progressive central nervous system (CNS) dysfunction. It is commonly seen in women complaining of blurred vision, sometimes photophobia, and problems related to accommodation in needlework, reading, and so forth. The pupils are usually unequal, sometimes irregular, and frequently dilated. They respond slowly to light: a bright light may not produce any pupillary reactions or may cause slow constriction over a matter of minutes. Pupillary constriction to convergence is usually more rapid, but the pupil does not dilate fully after the patient has stopped converging. The pupil is very active to small amounts of cholinergic drugs instilled in the conjunctiva. The cause of Holmes-Adie syndrome is unknown but is thought to be related to degenerative changes in the parasympathetic preganglionic fibers to the ciliary ganglion and central connections to pupillary motor centers in the midbrain. Other neurologic findings consist of depressed or absent deep-tendon reflexes, especially at the ankle or knee levels. In addition, patchy facial numbness and reduction of corneal reflexes may be seen. The condition is harmless and the patient should be reassured after other causes of ophthalmic and ocular motor disturbances have been excluded.

Cranial Nerve Paresis

Paresis of the third, fourth, and sixth cranial nerves occurs due to disorders affecting brain-stem nuclei, their connections, or compression of these nerves within the cranium or orbit. Neuromuscular disorders such as myasthenia gravis may also produce unusual cranial nerve disturbances. Due to its long course, the nerve most commonly affected is the sixth (abducent) nerve. The next most vulnerable is the third (oculomotor) nerve, which is often compressed by the uncus of the temporal lobe during cerebral herniation. Transient paresis of these nerves may occur after pneumoencephalography or lumbar puncture. In all patients, detailed neuro-ophthalmologic and neurologic examination, together with a metabolic workup, should be undertaken. Diabetes mellitus sometimes presents with curious cranial nerve disorders.

Trigeminal Neuralgia (Tic Douloureux)

This has been referred to in the section on headaches. Trigeminal neuralgia is a disorder seen in the fifth or sixth decade of life and is frequently related to previous herpes zoster infection. In young patients, multiple sclerosis is a common cause for severe facial pain. In older patients, aneurysms or ectasia of the basilar artery or its branches can cause tic douloureux.

Disorders of the Facial Nerves

Unilateral weakness or paralysis of the facial nerve is due to supranuclear, nuclear, or infranuclear lesions. Supranuclear weakness results from involvement of the corticopontine pathways and is characterized by weakness or paralysis of the lower facial muscles. Due to bilateral innervation, the upper part of the face is spared. The lower facial movements are affected but, in most patients, emotions can produce some movements of both the upper and lower parts of face. Upper motor neuron lesions are frequently associated with monoplegia, hemiplegia, or dysphasia.

Nuclear facial lesions are due to damage in the pons. The facial nucleus is closely related to the abducent nerve nucleus as well as the spinal tract of the ipsilateral trigeminal nerve. The facial nerve exits from the anterolateral aspect of the pons and may be affected at this site or at the level of the cerebellopontine angle, facial canal, or the parotid gland. Cerebellopontine involvement frequently produces concurrent vestibular and cerebellar problems. A lesion in the facial canal can involve the nerve to the stapedius muscle and the nerve from the taste buds. Tumors of the parotid gland can produce paralysis affecting individual branches of the facial nerves.

Bell's palsy occurs due to a host of factors, both local and systemic. Local factors consist of otitis media, mastoid infection, mumps, or exposure to cold. The nerve may be directly infiltrated as in leprosy, leukemia, sarcoidosis, and viral infections such as herpes zoster. Systemic disorders such as diabetes mellitus and Guillain-Barré syndrome should also be considered. In most patients with Bell's palsy, no clear etiology can be identified. Bell's palsy is common in cold weather, occasionally occurs as minor epidemics, and is sometimes noted after patients have exposed their face or temporal region to cold winds or drafts. Some facial discomfort or pain in or around the ear is frequently evident and is followed by severe unilateral facial weakness. The patient is unable to move the mouth fully or close one eye. Food accumulates between the cheek and jaw with dribbling, and there is often watering of the eye on the affected side due to inadequate eyelid movements. In approximately 5-10% of the patients, taste is affected due to involvement of the chorda tympani. In these patients, one side of the tongue sometimes feels numb. In a small proportion of patients, hyperacusis is noted; this is due to involvement of nerve twigs supplying the stapedius muscle.

Full recovery is accomplished in over 90% of patients. In the remainder, recovery is slow and protracted, but in approximately 5% little if any improvement occurs. In some patients with Bell's palsy, facial nerve damage is due to compression from surrounding structures. It is important to detect those with severe compression as the nerve may be irreversibly damaged. Nerve conduction (distal motor latency) and EMG is useful in assessing denervation; this usually begins 2-3 weeks after onset. The prognosis is poor if there is complete denervation and no motor responses traverse the facial nerve when it is stimulated at the stylomastoid foramen. In advanced cases, severe fibrillation activity is noted. Reinnervation may produce excessive watering of the eyes while eating. This is due to misguided migration of nerve fibers from the lacrymal to salivary glands. Early treatment with intramuscular ACTH, 40-100 units a day with gradual tapering after 2 weeks is recommended. Oral steroids can also be used. In all patients, systemic problems such as diabetes, sarcoidosis, and local parotid disease such as mumps should be excluded.

Hemifacial Spasms

This disorder sometimes occurs as a sequela to Bell's palsy but is more frequently related to facial tics or habit spasm. Facial spasm may be due to structural causes such as arteriosclerotic dilatation or aneurysm of the vertebrobasilar arteries or tumors in the cerebellopontine angle pressing on the seventh cranial nerve. In a few patients, facial spasms form part of the torsion dystonia syndrome. The spasm may be minimal or produce startling facial contractions and grimacing. The EMG shows bursts or clusters of high-amplitude discharges with normal motor units and anatomically intact nerves. Treatment consists of correction of the cause. Carbamazepine and phenytoin are helpful. In severe cases with incapacitating symptoms, alcohol injection of one or more branches of the facial nerve may be of benefit.

Geniculate and Glossopharyngeal neuralgia

Glossopharyngeal neuralgia is similar to trigeminal neuralgia.

This discomfort involves the throat and pharynx. These patients have paroxysmal pain precipitated by swallowing or chewing. Bradycardia and hypotension due to vagal inhibition may occur. Geniculate neuralgia due to involvement of the nervus intermedius consists of bouts of pain in the external auditory canal with radiation to the orbit, face, jaw, and throat. The causes are obscure and treatment is unsatisfactory.

PERIPHERAL NEUROPATHIES

The peripheral nerves are susceptible to a great deal of metabolic, endocrine, and toxic disturbances. They react by either axonal or segmental degeneration. Diabetes is the most common cause of neuropathies in the Western Hemisphere, while vitamin deficiencies and leprosy still cause the vast bulk of neuropathies in underdeveloped countries. There are at least 100 known etiologic factors causing various forms of neuropathy (Figs. 14, 15). In patients with neuropathic symptoms and a positive family history it is essential to palpate the nerves as well as conduct a more detailed examination of spine, cerebellum, brain stem, and special senses. Careful hematologic investigation should also be undertaken.

Hereditary Neuropathies

Only the more common forms of hereditary neuropathies are discussed here.

Dejerine-Sottas' Disease (Progressive Hypertrophic Interstitial Neuropathy)

This is a familial neuropathy inherited as an autosomal dominant trait associated with thickening of the nerves due to marked proliferation of endoneurium and Schwann's cells. In time, the nerve appears thickened with progressive degeneration of axons. The disorder runs an indolent course with exacerbations and remissions. It primarily affects lower limbs producing numbness, gait problems, trophic changes, and ataxia. A thickened nerve, very slow nerve conduction, and classic neuropathologic changes (onion-skin nerve) confirm the diagnosis. There is some evidence that thiamine injections are helpful. During exacerbations oral methylprednisolone may be tried. Physiotherapy is essential.

Refsum's Disease

This is an autosomal recessive trait due to accumulation of various forms of phytanic acid within the nervous tissue. Nerves are most commonly affected but, since it is a metabolic disorder, other systems may also be involved. Clinical features include atypical retinitis pigmentosa, cerebellar ataxia, some skeletal deformities, hearing defects, and peculiar ichthyosis-like cutaneous lesions. The nerves show degeneration with concentric hypertrophy of Schwann's cells, hypertrophic nerve sheaths, and degenerated axons. There is progressive sensory and motor neuropathy in the limbs resulting in absent reflexes, skeletal deformities, cutaneous abnormalities, deafness, visual disturbances, and ataxia. Estimation of phytanic acid by gas-liquid chromatography of serum confirms the diagnosis. Treatment consists of reducing chlorophyll in the diet and moderate amounts of oral steroids and physiotherapy.

Familial Amyloid Neuropathy

This is distinct from amyloidosis secondary to chronic infections or myelomatosis. Neuropathy occurs in either lower or

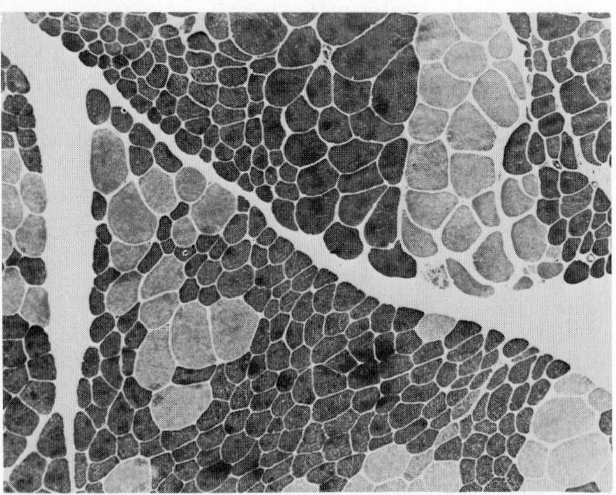

Figure 14. Muscle biopsy specimen. Chronic denervation and renervation in a patient with neuropathy. ATP (adenosine triphosphatase) stain at pH 9.4. Characteristic fiber type grouping is demonstrated. The type I fibers are lighter staining, while the type II fibers are darker staining.

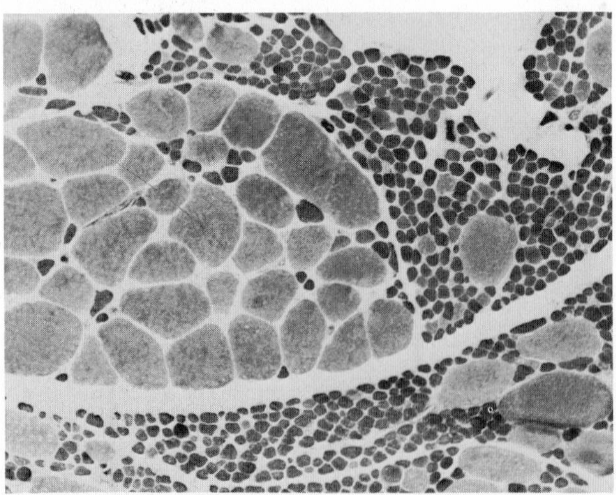

Figure 15. Muscle biopsy specimen. Group atrophy, characteristic of denervation in a patient with spinal muscular atrophy (gastrocnemius muscle). ATP (adenosine triphosphatase) stain at pH 9.4. Atrophy of both fiber types (I & II) and hypertrophy of type I (lighter staining) is demonstrated.

upper limbs with systemic manifestations of amyloidosis such as hepatosplenomegaly, cardiomegaly, and other vascular disorders. The diagnosis is confirmed by a positive family history, slow nerve conduction, signs of denervation, and raised CSF protein levels. Nerve and other tissue biopsies (particularly of the rectum) with special staining confirm the diagnosis. Treatment is symptomatic.

Infectious Neuropathies

Leprosy

This is a primary infectious neuropathy with cutaneous and peripheral nerve changes. Depending on the site of infection, various nerve syndromes and musculoskeletal deformities may occur. Nerve thickening is easily demonstrated in the ulnar, great auricular, and facial nerves. In addition, other cutaneous nerves may be thickened and easily palpable. The cutaneous patch of leprosy is hypoesthetic or anesthetic and the nerves to this patch may be thickened. On occasion, small nodules representing nerve abscesses are palpable along the course of a nerve. Neuritic pains are common and become more acute in patients with so-called lepra reaction. These reactions may present spontaneously but often occur after administration of antileprotic agents (diaminodiphenylsulfone, or dapsone). Diagnosis is established by characteristic cutaneous features, nerve thickening, and isolation of acid-fast bacilli in skin scrapings or nerve biopsy. Treatment consists of general measures, specific antileprotic agents, and physiotherapy. In patients with severe deformity calipers, walking aids, or artificial limbs may be used. Orthopedic procedures and plastic surgery should be undertaken only after the disease has run its course.

Guillain-Barré Syndrome

This is a form of postinfectious allergic polyneuroradiculopathy with some degree of spinal cord involvement. In extreme cases, cerebral tissue may be affected. The essential pathologic disorder is inflammation of the nerve roots; this is secondary to a hypersensitive autoimmune response to unknown viral agents. The posterior horn and nerve roots are severely inflamed.

The striking clinical features consist of ascending symmetrical flaccid paralysis with subjective sensory symptoms but little objective sensory loss. In addition, total areflexia with mild bladder and bowel problems are seen. In approximately 10% of all patients, facial involvement results in facial diplegia and, in a few, cervical and thoracic nerve root involvement produces respiratory insufficiency. Diagnosis is confirmed by demonstrating areflexia, no definite sensory level, raised CSF proteins with few cells (dissociation cytoalbuminique), and very slow to absent nerve-conduction latencies. In established cases, denervation changes may occur. The illness continues for 2-4 weeks and usually results in good recovery. In some patients, a relapsing form is seen with indolent phases and periods of exacerbation and remission.

Treatment consists of general nursing measures with particular attention to prevention of secondary infection and care of bladder and bowel function. In patients with breathing difficulties, tracheostomy and respiratory assistance may be necessary. In the acute phase, parenteral ACTH for several days, followed by oral corticosteroid therapy, is indicated. Physiotherapy and mobilization should be encouraged during remission and as improvement occurs.

Entrapment Neuropathies

The nerve trunks, plexuses, roots, or nerve fibers may be trapped or compressed at various levels due to a host of factors such as fibrous bands, accessory ribs, bony protruberances, thickening of local structures, edema, and trauma. In addition, systemic metabolic and endocrine factors may be responsible. A few of the more common forms of entrapment neuropathy are considered below.

Carpal Tunnel Syndrome

In its course from forearm to palm, the median nerve may be easily compressed by the flexor retinaculum at wrist level. The classic features include pain, numbness, and paresthesia affecting the thumb, index, middle fingers, and the lateral aspect of the ring finger. In addition to pain over the volar aspect of the wrist, some bogginess over the flexor retinaculum is frequently noted. Pain is alleviated by rest and diuretics, but commonly occurs at night or when using the hand. Carpal tunnel syndrome can be caused by local trauma, occupational injury, tenosynovitis, osteoarthritis, rheumatoid arthritis, gout, amyloidosis, and metabolic or endocrine disorders such as myxedema, acromegaly, and diabetes mellitus. Occasionally, a mild carpal tunnel syndrome is noted during pregnancy. An x-ray of the wrist may show underlying bone deformity but the diagnosis is confirmed by electromyography, which reveals delayed sensory and motor latency across the wrist with denervation on needle testing of the thenar muscles. In severe cases, there is marked wasting of the abductor pollicis and opponens pollicis muscles with gross atrophy of the thenar group of muscles producing a striking deformity. Treatment consists of injections of 0.5-2 ml of hydrocortisone acetate through the flexor retinaculum medial and lateral to the median nerve. In established cases of carpal tunnel syndrome, surgical exposure of the nerve and division of the flexor retinaculum affords lasting relief.

Ulnar Nerve Compression

In some patients with carpal tunnel syndrome, the ulnar nerve may be affected in the region of the pisiform bone but more commonly this nerve is involved at the elbow. The nerve has a long course through the arm and is liable to damage in the region of the medial epicondyle or olecranon of the humerus. Certain occupations such as draftsmen and railroad or locomotive engineers, where the arm is actively used or the elbow rested on a hard surface, predispose to stretching of the nerve and fibrotic damage. The clinical features consist of pain or discomfort at the elbow, limitation of extension, pain or numbness in the ring and little fingers, and wasting of intrinsic muscles of the hand. Diagnosis is established by performing nerve conduction studies and finding slow conduction across the elbow. Treatment consists of surgical decompression of bands of fibrous tissue and anterior transposition of the ulnar nerve.

Radial Nerve Palsy

During sleep, especially after large doses of narcotics or alcohol and usually with an impaired nutritional state, compression neuropathy occurs. The most common involvement is that of the radial nerve (Saturday night palsy). This results from sleeping with the arm hanging over the back of a chair or the bedside, or due to the head resting on the arm and compressing the nerve in the spiral groove of the humerus. The most prominent feature is a wrist drop with weakness of the hand extensors. Diabetes and uremia should be ruled out. The outcome is often favorable.

Thoracic Outlet Syndrome

This is due to compression of the neurovascular bundle containing brachial plexus and subclavian vessels in the neck. Compression may result from a cervical rib, postfixed brachial plexus, fibrous bands, or between the two heads of the scalenus anterior muscle and the scalenus medius muscle. Other conditions, such as a mass lesion of the apex of the lung (Pancoast's tumor) or compression between the clavicle and first rib, may also cause a thoracic outlet syndrome. Depending on the area of involvement and compensatory changes, the upper brachial nerve or lower nerve roots may be affected. In addition, vascular supply may be impaired. Symptoms are due to combined nerve and vessel involvement and consist of reduced peripheral pulsations, coldness of the limb, venous engorgement, and sometimes edema. The blood pressure is usually asymmetrical in the arms. Involvement of the cervical sympathetic nerve may produce Horner's syndrome, which is especially common in apical pulmonary neoplastic (Pancoast's) tumors. Nerve damage produces irritative signs in the distribution of the affected segment. The C7, C8, and T1 roots are most commonly affected, and produce burning pain or numbness in the ring and little fingers together with numbness over the medial aspect of the hand and forearm.

Investigation includes x-ray film of the chest and neck together with nerve conduction and EMG studies. Proximal slowing of nerve conduction with distal denervation is frequently observed. Diagnosis is confirmed by subclavian angiography to demonstrate the vascular tree and is useful when surgery is contemplated. In patients with mild compression, relief may be afforded by not using the affected hand in carrying heavy objects, a course of physiotherapy, or a supporting sling. Once the diagnosis has been established and symptoms are progressive, surgical exploration and decompression is the treatment of choice.

Neuropathies Associated with Systemic Diseases

This group includes neuropathies occurring in metabolic disorders, malignancy, collagen vascular diseases, deficiency states, and other systemic illnesses such as sarcoidosis and atherosclerosis. Some of the more common neuropathies are described below.

Diabetes

The incidence of neuropathy increases with age and duration of diabetes. Nerve conduction velocities are diminished and the EMG shows features of denervation. The CSF protein level is elevated (50-240 mg/dl). Five major clinical syndromes have been delineated: diabetic ophthalmoplegia, peripheral polyneuropathy, proximal polyneuropathy (amyotrophy), mononeuropathy or mononeuritis multiplex, and autonomic neuropathy. A combination of neuropathies often occurs, particularly in those with autonomic disturbances.

Treatment is unsatisfactory. Meticulous regulation of diabetes, vitamin B supplements, and analgesics are the mainstay of treatment. Phenytoin and carbamazepine may be tried in severe cases, especially in those with neuritic pains.

Uremia

Distal sensorimotor polyneuropathy that is worse in the lower limbs frequently develops in patients with end-stage renal disease. Pathologically, axonal degeneration and segmental demyelination are detectable. Intensive chronic hemodialysis and peritoneal dialysis slow the progression, but a successful kidney transplantation usually leads to clinical improvement.

Porphyria

Acute intermittent porphyria is inherited as an autosomal dominant trait and is associated with predominant motor polyneuropathy. Accompanying clinical features include psychiatric disturbances and attacks of abdominal pain. Cranial nerves and respiratory muscles may be seriously involved. The diagnosis of porphyria is confirmed by detection of porphobilinogen in the urine. The course of polyneuropathy is extremely variable.

Cancer

Neuropathy may occur as a remote effect of malignant tumors of the lung, ovary, breast, and stomach. Cancer should always be suspected in older patients with polyneuropathy.

Collagen-Vascular Diseases

Some 20% of patients with systemic lupus erythematosus, polyarteritis nodosa, rheumatoid arthritis, and scleroderma have associated peripheral nerve involvement. They can produce mononeuritis multiplex; this is due to vasculitis of the vasa nervorum.

Toxic Polyneuropathies

Many drugs, heavy metals, alcohol, and household or industrial poisons can produce neuropathy.

Drugs

Neuropathy can occur in patients treated with isoniazid, vincristine, nitrofurantoin, hydralazine, phenytoin, disulfiram, ethambutol, chloramphenicol, sodium cyanate, or gold. Pyridoxine and folic acid can correct neuropathies caused by isoniazid and phenytoin, respectively. In most instances, the neuropathy reverses after discontinuing the offending drug.

Heavy Metals
Chronic exposure to or ingestion of practically any heavy metal results in polyneuropathy; common examples are arsenics, lead, mercury, and thallium. Their presence in hair, fingernails, serum, and urine should be determined. Treatment consists of diminution of toxic exposure and removal of heavy metal from the body by penicillamine, 250 mg by mouth four times daily.

Alcohol
Vitamin deficiency (of the B-complex type) is commonly associated with chronic alcoholism and causes polyneuropathy. Both axonal degeneration and segmental demyelination are found on nerve biopsy. The initial symptoms are pain and numbness of the feet, followed by weakness and tenderness of intrinsic muscles of the feet and absent ankle reflexes. The course of polyneuropathy is quite variable. Treatment is aimed at restoration of an adequate diet, abstinence from alcohol, and multivitamin therapy.

Chemicals
Large outbreaks of polyneuropathy can occur from inhalation of toxic substances in factories and from adulteration of food and drinking water. Organophosphorous compounds, DDT, kepone (an ant insecticide), organic solvents, plasticizers, *n*-hexane (used in shoe factories and misused as a euphoriant agent), hexachlorophene, carbon disulfide, and trichloroethylene are examples of chemicals associated with polyneuropathy.

DISEASES OF THE MUSCLE AND NEUROMUSCULAR JUNCTION

Disorders of skeletal muscles are due to a host of inflammatory (Fig. 16), metabolic and hereditary defects. In addition, in a large group of idiopathic muscle disorders, autoimmune mechanisms may be responsible for weakness and wasting. In many cases, muscle disorders produce skeletal deformities and these compound problems with locomotion. The complaints of difficulty in rising from a chair or arranging items on a high shelf distinguish true muscle weakness from fatigue, stiffness of joints, or bradykinesia.

MUSCULAR DYSTROPHIES

This section describes the more common disorders of muscles. These are a group of genetically determined and usually progressive primary muscular disorders resulting in degeneration and wasting of muscles. These are sometimes associated with systemic involvement. There are over a dozen forms of muscular dystrophies. The main types are considered below.

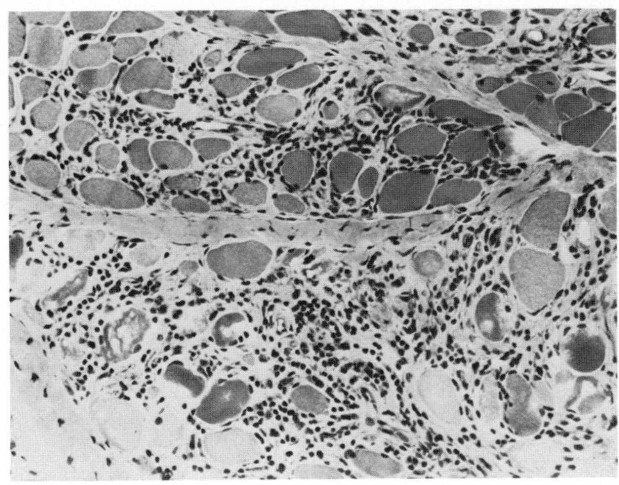

Figure 16. Muscle biopsy specimen. Note diffuse inflammatory cell infiltration, muscle fiber necrosis, myophagia, and focal loss of muscle fibers. Patient with polymyositis.

Duchenne's Muscular Dystrophy

This common form of muscular dystrophy, also called pseudohypertrophic muscular dystrophy, usually occurs in boys and is inherited as a sex-linked recessive trait (Fig. 17). In a small proportion of patients, an autosomal recessive inheritance has been noted, in which instance girls are also affected. In an even smaller proportion of cases, sporadic occurrence has been reported. This disorder is usually detected when the child

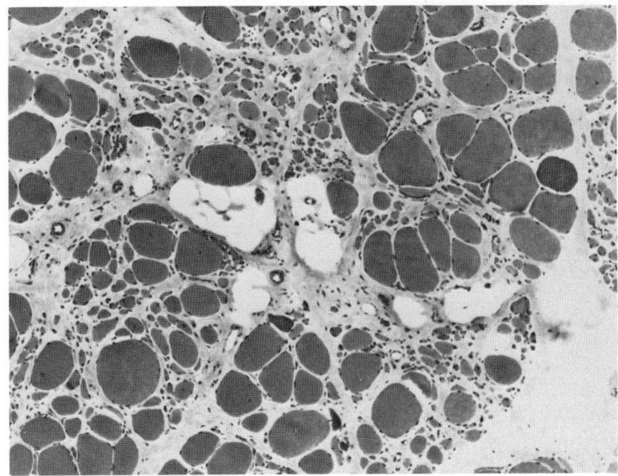

Figure 17. Muscle biopsy specimen. Patient with Duchenne's muscular dystrophy (quadriceps muscle). Note random variation in fiber sizes with presence of atrophic and hypertrophic fibers and connective tissue proliferation. Several fibers have internal nuclei. (H & E stain)

begins to walk. There is progressive proximal muscle weakness with characteristic lordosis, a wide-based waddling gait, and weakness of the shoulder girdle muscles. The child climbs up on himself from the lying position in order to stand up (Gowers' sign). In over 70% of children, pseudohypertrophy of muscles (especially the calves) is seen. Respiratory insufficiency occurs a few years after the onset of disease. Cardiac involvement is common. Central nervous system manifestations are rare, but in a small proportion of cases cerebral involvement results in mild mental retardation. There is no specific treatment and most patients die before adulthood. General supportive measures and management of respiratory and cardiac problems, in addition to minor orthopedic procedures, should be undertaken when necessary. It is important that the parents receive genetic counseling. Approximately 70% of the female carriers have an elevated creatinine phosphokinase (CPK) level.

Becker's Muscular Dystrophy

This is a relatively benign, sex-linked, recessive disorder. It has many features akin to Duchenne's muscular dystrophy, but the striking feature is that the course is nonprogressive and most patients survive.

Facioscapulohumeral Muscular (Landouzy-Dejerine) Dystrophy

This is most probably an autosomal dominant myopathic disorder. The lower part of the face and shoulder girdle muscles are maximally affected. Deglutition is spared.

Limb Girdle (Erb's) Muscular Dystrophy

This is an autosomal recessive trait. The myopathic process begins in the second or third decade of life. Muscle weakness is restricted to the pelvic and shoulder girdles with problems in gait, rising from a sitting position, and peculiar posture.

Distal Muscular Dystrophy (Gowers' Disease)

This is inherited as an autosomal dominant trait. The distal muscles are involved with maximal changes in both feet. It is a rare disorder and has to be distinguished from myotonic dystrophy. In Gowers' myopathy, no myotonia is demonstrable by clinical or electromyographic testing.

Ocular Myopathy

In this disorder, ocular involvement with ptosis, diminished extraocular movements, and characteristic facies occurs. The disease is transmitted as an autosomal dominant trait. Many patients also have pharyngeal involvement (oculopharyngeal myopathy) resulting in difficulty in deglutition and speech. Myasthenic disorders should be excluded in such cases.

Myotonic Dystrophy

Myotonic dystrophy is the most common form of myotonic disorders and is inherited as an autosomal dominant trait. These patients have muscular as well as systemic involvement, the latter frequently limiting life expectancy. The most common age of onset is the middle twenties or thirties. Infrequently, the disorders occurs in neonates. The classic features are frontal baldness, cataracts, and wasting of the masseter and temporal muscles. In addition, mild ptosis and severe wasting of the sternocleidomastoid muscles is seen. A hoarse voice due to involvement of the pharyngeal muscles and weakness of the hands are often present. Invariably, myotonia is found; this is demonstrated by prolonged gripping and inability to release objects. Cardiac abnormalities, conduction defects, poor ventricular contractions, and cardiac failure are sometimes seen. Gonadal atrophy due to testicular or ovarian failure are invariable; this results in impotence and infertility. Endocrine involvement is frequent with impaired glucose tolerance. Smooth-muscle involvement is less frequent, but difficulty in deglutition is often present. Immunologic disturbances are due to reduced immunoglobulins and predispose to chronic infection, bronchitis, and pneumonias. Diagnosis can be invariably established on clinical grounds. EMG reveals features of myotonia. Muscle biopsy demonstrates signs of denervation and atrophy of muscle fibers. There is no specific therapy for myotonia, but physiotherapy is of some benefit. Muscle stiffness may be relieved by procainamide or quinine.

Investigations of Patients with Muscular Dystrophy

The most important investigations are the assessment of muscle enzymes and electromyography. It is sometimes essential to have at least two readings, spaced over time for comparison, to be able to assess the degree of deterioration. Serum aldolase and CPK are invariable raised and are frequently extremely high. Raised muscle enzymes indicate progressive muscle lysis and degeneration. The enzyme levels are markedly elevated during the initial illness but tend to decrease in the later stages of the disorder. The serum glutamic oxaloacetic transaminase (SGOT) and lactate dehydrogenase (LDH) levels are also high but these are nonspecific. The raised enzyme levels help distinguish between neuropathic and myopathic disorders. Electromyographic examination reveals disordered motor units with low amplitude, brief duration motor unit potentials, and abundant recruitment on minimal contractions. Fibrillations are sometimes seen but are less frequent than those noted in a neuropathic disorder. Muscle biopsy reveals variation in size of muscle fibers, loss of cross striation, and migration of sarcolemmal nuclei to the center. In addition, atrophy of fibers, muscle necrosis, or lysis is seen. In some sections regeneration may be noted. Pseudohypertrophy is due to replacement of muscle fibers by fatty tissue. Of the muscular dystrophies, Duchenne's shows maximal cardiac involvement, but heart infiltration may also be seen in patients with limb girdle muscular dystrophy.

TOXIC-METABOLIC MYOPATHIES

Proximal muscle weakness may occur in metabolic disorders, either systemic or confined to the muscles.

Alcoholic Myopathy

Both acute and chronic forms of proximal muscle weakness have been described in alcoholics. Rapid development of muscular weakness, especially in the legs, swelling and tenderness of muscles, and myoglobinuria may follow after very heavy alcohol intake. On the other hand, chronic myopathy with muscle atrophy is a complication of protracted drinking. Alcoholic myopathy is characterized by proximal muscle involvement, elevation of creatinine phosphokinase (CPK), myoglobinuria, and, in acute cases, rapid recovery on abstinence. The latter is the only treatment known.

Drug-Induced Myopathy

Drugs such as colchicine and fluorinated corticosteroids such as triamcinolone, phenytoin, and chloroquine are known to cause reversible myopathy.

Thyroid Disorders

Hyperthyroidism may produce severe muscular involvement in the form of myasthenia gravis, periodic paralysis, thyrotoxic myopathy, and ophthalmoplegias. Thyrotoxic myopathy occurs in moderate to severe hyperthyroidism and manifests as proximal muscle weakness and other features of thyrotoxicosis. Deep tendon reflexes are not affected and serum enzyme levels are normal. Myopathy subsides when the patient is rendered euthyroid. In addition, β-adrenergic blocking agents may be helpful. Ophthalmoplegia is usually seen when the thyroid disorder is fulminant and presents as ptosis and weakness of the ocular muscles. Severe thyrotoxicosis may progress to malignant exophthalmos with conjunctival edema, proptosis, and very weak ocular muscles. These patients are usually acutely ill. High doses of corticosteroids, β-adrenergic blocking agents, and decompression of the orbit in addition to prompt and adequate treatment of thyrotoxicosis is usually necessary.

Hypothyroidism (myxedema) is sometimes associated with myopathy but myotonic disorders are more frequent. The most common symptom is that of apathy and lethargy. Muscle cramps are sometimes seen and the tendon jerks reveal slow relaxation. If a muscle is tapped with a reflex hammer, some dimpling may be noted. The delayed relaxation of muscles in myxedema is also called Hoffmann's syndrome. In children, cretinism may present with myotonia coupled with hypertrophy. EMG shows some myopathic activity and the muscle enzymes are almost invariably raised.

Parathyroid Disorders

In hyperparathyroidism proximal muscle weakness, muscle pains, and tenderness may be noted. Myopathy is, however, more frequent in hypoparathyroidism and is due to insufficient levels of calcium and vitamin D.

Adrenal Disorders

Hyperadrenalism may produce a severe degree of proximal weakness associated with other signs of hypercorticism. Treatment consists of dealing with the primary disease.

Glycogen Storage Diseases

Myopathy results in Types II, III, V, and VII glycogen storage diseases (Table 2).

Myoglobinuria (Rhabdomyolysis)

Certain glycogen and lipid storage diseases are frequently associated with myoglobinuria. More importantly, severe muscle injury as may happen in crushing, convulsions, hyperthermia, ischemia, alcoholism, and drug ingestion may lead to increased muscle membrane permeability causing release of myoglobin and CPK. Myoglobinuria may cause intratubular casts and tubular necrosis leading to acute renal failure. Treatment consists of hydration and diuresis to prevent renal failure. If renal failure develops, the patient should be managed as a patient with acute renal failure.

MYASTHENIC DISORDERS

These include myasthenia gravis, the myasthenic syndrome, and botulism.

Myasthenia Gravis

It is now widely believed that myasthenia gravis results from the presence of circulating antibodies to acetylcholine receptors (AChR) located at the muscle end-plate. There are morphologic changes at the neuromuscular junction, especially simplification of the postjunctional folds, and antibody can be demonstrated on the postjunctional membrane by immunocytochemical methods; consequently, the postjunctional membrane becomes less sensitive to the application of acetylcholine and analogues. It is not known what initiates the formation of the antibodies. There is abnormality of the

Table 2. Glycogen Storage Diseases Involving Muscle

Type	*Eponym*	*Deficient Enzyme*	*Clinical Manifestations*
II	Pompe's disease	α-1,4-Glycosidase (acid maltase)	Infantile form involves CNS, liver, and heart; adult form shows proximal muscle weakness only
III	Forbe's disease	Amylo-1,6-glucosidase (debrancher enzyme)	Hepatomegaly and hypoglycemia
V	McArdle's disease	Myophosphorylase	Onset in late teens, exercise-induced stiffness and paroxysmal myoglobinuria

thymus gland in most patients, either germinal centers or thymoma. There is an increased incidence of other autoimmune disorders in myasthenics.

This disorder is more common in women and occurs in two peaks: between 20 and 30 and between 60 and 70 years of age. When myasthenia gravis occurs in the elderly, it is more common in men. The symptoms vary in severity but are primarily limited to the orofacial region and eyes. The first symptoms are those of diplopia, ptosis, restriction of ocular movements, and difficulty in swallowing or speaking as the day progresses. Temporary aphonia may sometimes occur. In patients with severe involvement, dysphagia and nasal regurgitation of food is noted. Peripheral skeletal musculature is relatively spared until later. When the limbs are affected, the hands are maximally involved. Eye involvement is demonstrated by external ocular muscle weakness, but pupillary function and accommodation are spared. In approximately 30% of patients, the disorder progresses to generalized myasthenia gravis. The dreaded complication is respiratory dysfunction producing the so-called myasthenic crisis. A crisis may occur during severe infections, in pregnancy, in association with thyroid disease, or in patients who are refractory to anticholinesterase drugs.

Diagnosis of myasthenia gravis is established by demonstrating weakness after exertion, and response to intravenous edrophonium (Tensilon). On EMG, repetitive nerve stimulation with supramaximal impulses produce progressive fallout in amplitude of response and is associated with clinical fatigue. Stimulation is begun at one per second and continued to 20 pulses per second. Posttetanic exhaustion can be clearly demonstrated by repetitive nerve stimulation. Intravenous endrophonium, 10 mg injected slowly over a 2-minute period in small boluses, produces dramatic improvement in strength and recovery from diplopia, nasal voice, and ptosis. The test is also useful in assessing whether the patient is over- or undermedicated. Additional investigations such as chest x-ray to reveal a mediastinal (thymic) mass and thyroid function tests should be undertaken in all patients. Detailed tests for antinuclear antibodies and antibodies to thyroid and gastric mucosa, together with a full evaluation for collagen disorders, should also be undertaken in all cases.

Treatment

In mild myasthenia, medical treatment with cholinesterase inhibitors is the mainstay of management. This helps raise the level of acetylcholine at the neuromuscular junction. Oral neostigmine (Prostigmin), 15 mg every 3-4 hours, or pyridostigmine (Mestinon), 60 mg every 4 hours, provides dramatic and continued relief. The dosage should be gradually increased and patients seen periodically to determine if more medication is necessary. It is essential to monitor these patients closely so that effective control is achieved. Other drugs such as ephedrine sulfate and ambenonium (Mytelase) are less helpful but may be used in patients with severe side effects to anticholinesterase drugs. Infections, particularly of the respiratory system, should be treated early with antibiotics. It is important to avoid aminoglycoside antibiotics since they have neuromuscular blocking side effects. Substances containing quinine such as tonic water should be avoided as they increase myasthenic symptoms. Severe myasthenia gravis is a medical emergency necessitating hospitalization. Treatment should commence after performing the Tensilon test to determine whether a patient is appropriately medicated. If the patient is undermedicated, oral neostigmine or, in severe cases, intramuscular neostigmine is administered. Respiratory difficulties should be overcome by artificial ventilation. Corticosteroids help dramatically in many patients by reducing the amount of neostigmine required and also produce significant muscle improvement. Careful assessment of electrolytes, particularly potassium loss, should be monitored. In a myasthenic crisis, artificial respiration is essential to maintain proper oxygenation. If required, tracheotomy is performed. Thymectomy is of value in patients with severe and incapacitating weakness who show minimal improvement on anticholinesterase therapy. It is also effective in those with a thymoma or repeated myasthenic crises. Removal of antibodies by plasma exchange (plasmapheresis) is beneficial in many patients.

Myasthenic (Lambert-Eaton) Syndrome

A syndrome of defective neuromuscular transmission is seen in some patients with oat cell carcinoma of the bronchus. On the surface this condition appears similar to myasthenia gravis but there are certain distinguishing features. Ocular muscles are relatively spared, weakness primarily affects proximal muscle groups, and strength frequently improves after exercise. The response to Tensilon is poor. Other disorders such as hypothyroidism, pernicious anemia, Sjögren's syndrome, hyperthyroidism, and thyroiditis can also cause this syndrome. These patients have little or no response to the anticholinesterase drugs but improve with guanidine hydrochloride (200-1,000 mg/day).

Botulism

This is a rare but potentially fatal disorder due to exotoxin of *Clostridium botulinum*. This anaerobic bacillus produces a powerful exotoxin. Botulism occurs when defective home-prepared canned products are consumed and, in rare instances, when commercially canned food is infected due to defective packaging. Symptoms appear 6-20 hours after ingestion and consist of muscle weakness, dysphagia, dysphonia, and respiratory paralysis. Diarrhea is notably absent. Diagnosis is established by a high index of suspicion. The patient should be admitted to an intensive care unit and maintained on artificial respiration. Botulism antitoxin is beneficial. Guanidine has been tried but its value is dubious.

Tick Paralysis

This is exceedingly rare and is due to tick bites producing partial or complete block of neurotransmission. The wood tick and dog tick are usually responsible. Patients develop variable degrees of muscle weakness, anorexia, and unsteadiness of gait followed by bulbar weakness. If there is any suspicion of respiratory embarrassment, artificial respiration is indicated. The local wound should be incised and drained.

Table 3. Periodic Paralyses

Type	*Age of Onset*	*Precipitating Factors*	*Serum K^+ Concentration during Attack (mEq/L)*	*Diagnostic Features*
Hypokalemic	20-30	Large meal, strenuous exercise, glucose and insulin effusion	<3	ECG changes, hypokalemia
Normokalemic	1-10	Alchol, exercise, stress	3.4-5.5	Attack may last up to 2 weeks
Hyperkalemic	1-10	Exercise, potassium, exposure to cold	>5.5	Myotonia of the tongue and eyelids

PERIODIC PARALYSES

Three types of periodic paralyses are recognized: hypokalemic, normokalemic, and hyperkalemic. The clinical features are summarized in Table 3.

There is believed to be an abnormal flux of potassium between serum and muscle cells, causing alterations in the muscle membrane potential and electrically unexcitable muscle. The muscle biopsy shows vascular changes and dilatation of sarcoplasmic reticulum. Treatment consists of acetazolamide (Diamox), 500-1,000 mg daily by mouth.

Periodic paralysis can also result from hypokalemia due to diuretics, steroids, gastrointestinal losses, licorice, or from thyrotoxicosis. Treatment is directed at the underlying disorder.

Factors known to precipitate attacks include muscular exertion, a high-carbohydrate diet, exposure to cold, and certain drugs such as corticosteroids and thiazides. Licorice ingestion may also induce attacks. The prodromal symptoms consist of muscle aching and severe thirst, followed by weakness and total paralysis. Respiratory muscle involvement is rare. Examination reveals hyporeflexia, sometimes areflexia, and on palpation the muscles are flaccid. Sensations are intact. Muscular strength is very limited during an attack but slowly improves in minutes to hours. Serum potassium during an attack is low and EMG reveals electrical silence of muscles. When the patient improves, diagnosis may be confirmed by the use of intravenous glucose and insulin under close observation. Treatment consists of oral potassium. If diuretic treatment is necessary, only potassium-sparing diuretics should be used.

Thyrotoxic Periodic Paralysis

Thyrotoxicosis, especially in individuals of Japanese descent, sometimes produces severe muscle weakness resembling hypokalemic periodic paralysis. The disorder is mild and improves when thyrotoxicosis is treated.

QUESTIONS

Multiple choice questions: For each question, choose the best answer.

1. A 23-year-old woman collapses at work with a mild right hemiparesis and garbled speech. She had been well except for increasingly troublesome migraine headaches in the prior 6 months. She uses no drugs or medications other than oral contraceptives. The *most* likely etiology is
   A. Ruptured aneurysm
   B. Primary astrocytoma
   C. Cerebral infarction related to ulcerated carotid plaque
   D. Cerebral infarction related to hormone use
   E. Cerebral infarction related to collagen vascular disease

2. The drug of choice for a 4-year-old girl who presents with brief spells of staring and with an EEG that shows a three-per-second spike and slow wave would be
   A. Phenobarbital
   B. Carbamazepine (Tegretol)
   C. Clonazepam (Clonopin)
   D. Ethosuximide (Zarontin)
   E. Phenytoin (Dilantin)

3. A 55-year-old known alcoholic presents to the emergency room confused, unsteady, and combative. On examination, paresis of the extraocular muscles, impaired recent memory, and profound ataxia are demonstrated. The attending physician should
   A. Suspect acute intoxication and send the patient to jail
   B. Send for immediate angiography to rule out a subdural hematoma
   C. Give 50 cc 50% glucose after obtaining serum for glucose determination
   D. Suspect Wernicke's syndrome and give thiamine
   E. Suspect Wernicke's syndrome and give vitamin B_{12}

4. Cerebral embolism or infarction may complicate
   A. Subacute bacterial endocarditis
   B. Sickle cell disease
   C. Subendocardial myocardial infarction
   D. Cardiomyopathy
   E. All of the above

5. The risk of cerebral infarction is *most* closely related to
   A. Obesity
   B. Hypertension
   C. Cigarette smoking
   D. Physical inactivity
   E. Racial origin
6. Agents and neurotransmitters that improve Parkinson's disease include
   A. Dopa agonists such as Sinement
   B. Dopa antagonists such as chlorpromazine (Thorazine)
   C. Acetylcholine agonists such as choline chloride
   D. Benzodiazepines such as diazepam (Valium)
   E. Any one of the above
7. Cardinal signs of Parkinson's disease include
   A. Spasticity
   B. Rigidity
   C. Intention tremor
   D. Bradykinesia
   E. Both B and D
8. The tremor of Parkinsonian patients
   A. Is present at rest
   B. Worsens with anxiety
   C. Responds poorly to treatment
   D. All of the above
   E. Only A and B are correct
9. In multiple sclerosis, the most likely finding in the cerebrospinal fluid (CSF) is
   A. Decreased sugar
   B. Increased mononuclear cells, normal protein
   C. Mildly increased pressure
   D. Normal total protein, increased globulin content
   E. Increased protein, normal globulin content
10. When testing muscle tone, cogwheeling is characteristic of
    A. Senility
    B. Parkinsonism
    C. Stroke
    D. Hypothyroidism
    E. Peripheral neuropathy
11. Treatable causes of dementia include
    A. Vitamin B_{12} deficiency
    B. Myxedema
    C. Normal pressure hydrocephalus
    D. Tuberculous meningitis
    E. All of the above
12. Parkinson-like symptoms can result from each of the following *except*
    A. Manganese intoxication
    B. Carbon monoxide intoxication
    C. Anticonvulsant drugs
    D. Lacunar infarcts
    E. Norma-pressure hydrocephalus
13. Involuntary, irregular, random, rapid jerky movements of the extremities are characteristic of
    A. Parkinson's disease
    B. Huntington's chorea
    C. Congenital athetosis
    D. Essential tremor
    E. Dystonia musculorum deformans
14. The most prominent and frequently the first symptom to occur in dementia is usually disturbance in
    A. Calculation
    B. Comprehension
    C. Memory
    D. Abstract reasoning
    E. Spontaneous speech
15. A 43-year-old man, "found down" in a rooming house, exhibits a dense right hemiplegia, a dilated fixed left pupil, a stiff neck, and fever. Chest x-ray shows hilar adenopathy. *The CT scanner is broken down.* The first diagnostic study to obtain is
    A. Lumbar puncture
    B. Cerebral angiography
    C. Toxic screen on blood and urine
    D. Serum and urine osmolalities
    E. Lung scan
16. A slowly progressive right hemiparesis developed over a period of 8-12 weeks in a 50-year-old woman accompanied by headaches, disturbances in expressing thoughts, and inability to see the right half of the visual field. The most likely diagnosis is
    A. A progressive infarction
    B. A neoplasm
    C. Presenile dementia
    D. Parkinson's disease
    E. Multiple sclerosis
17. Partial complex (psychomotor) seizures are usually best treated with
    A. Carbamazepine (Tegretol)
    B. Phenobarbital
    C. Clonazepam (Clonopin)
    D. Valproic acid (Depakene)
    E. Phenytoin (Dilantin)

ANSWERS

1. D
2. D
3. D
4. E
5. B
6. A
7. E
8. D
9. D
10. B
11. E
12. C
13. B
14. C
15. B
16. B
17. A

BIBLIOGRAPHY

TEXTBOOKS AND MONOGRAPHS

Adams RD, Victor M: *Principles of Neurology*, ed. 2. New York, McGraw-Hill Book Co, 1981.

Baker AB, Baker LH (eds): *Clinical Neurology*. New York, Harper & Row Pubs, Inc, 1981.

Merritt HH: *A Textbook of Neurology*, ed. 6. Philadelphia, Lea & Febiger, 1979.

Plum F, Posner JB: *The Diagnosis of Stupor and Coma*, ed. 3. Philadelphia, FA Davis Co, 1980.

Swaiman KF, Wright FS (eds): *The Practice of Pediatric Neurology*, ed. 2. St. Louis: The CV Mosby Co, 1982.

Walton JN: *Brain's Diseases of the Nervous System*, ed. 8. New York, Oxford University Press, 1977.

Walton JN (ed): *Disorders of Voluntary Muscle*, ed. 4. New York, Churchill Livingstone, Inc, 1981.

ARTICLES

CT Scanning of the Head

David DO: CT in the diagnosis of supratentorial tumors. *Semin Roentgenol* 12:97-108, 1977;

Diaconis JN, Rao KC: CT in head trauma: A review. *CT* 4:261-70, 1980.

Forbes GS, Sheedy PF II, Piepgrass DG, et al: Computed tomography in the evaluation of subdural hematomas. *Radiology* 126:143-8, 1978.

Multiple Sclerosis

Cook SD, Dowling PC: Multiple sclerosis and viruses: An overview. *Neurology* 30(Pt. 2):61-79, 1980.

Ellison GW, Myers LW: Immunosuppressive drugs in multiple sclerosis: Pro and con. *Neurology* (NY) 30(Pt. 2):28-32, 1980.

Kurtzke JF: Epidemiologic contributions to multiple sclerosis: An overview. *Neurology* (NY) 30(Pt. 2);61-79, 1980.

Lisak RP: Multiple sclerosis: Evidence for immunopathogenesis. *Neurology* (NY) 30 (Pt. 2):99-105, 1980.

Poser CM: Multiple sclerosis. *Med Clin North Am* 63:729-43, 1979.

Dementias

Ropper AH: A rational approach to dementia. *Can Med Assoc J* 121: 1175-90, 1979.

Terry RD: Dementia: A brief and selective review. *Arch Neurol* 33:1-4, 1976.

Wells CE: Chronic brain disease: An overview. *Am J Psychiat* 135:1-12, 1978.

Parkinsonism

Calne DB, Kebabian J, Silbergeld E, et al: Advances in the neuropharmacology of parkinsonism. *Ann Intern Med* 90:212-29, 1979.

Rinne UK: Recent advances in research on parkinsonism. *Acta Neurol Scand Suppl* 69:77-113, 1978.

Teravainen H, Calne DB: Developments in understanding the physiology and pharmacology of parkinsonism. *Acta Neurol Scand* 60:1-11, 1979.

Huntington's Disease

Shoulson I, Fahn S: Huntington disease: Clinical care and evaluation (editorial). *Neurology* 29:1-3, 1979.

Alcohol-Induced Neurologic Disorders

Edmondson HA: Pathology of alcoholism. *Am J Clin Pathol* 74:725-42, 1980.

Holt S, Skinner HA, Israel Y: Early identification of alcohol abuse. II. Clinical and laboratory indicators. *Can Med Assoc J* 124:1279-94, 1981.

Schenker S, Henderson GI, Hoyumpa AM Jr, et al: Hepatic and Wernicke's encephalopathies: Current concepts of pathogenesis. *Am J Clin Nutr* 33:2719-26, 1980.

Metabolic Disorders

Raskin NH, Fishman RA: Neurologic disorders in renal failure. *N Engl J Med* 294:143-7, 204-9, 1976.

Epilepsy

Penry JK, Porter RJ: Epilepsy: Mechanisms and therapy. *Med Clin North Am* 63:801-12, 1979.

Headache

Caviness VS Jr, O'Brien P: Current concepts: Headache. *N Engl J Med* 302:446-50, 1980.

Raskin NH: Chemical headaches. *Annu Rev Med* 32:63-71, 1981.

Migraine

Diamond S, Medina JL: Review article: Current thoughts on migraine. *Headache* 20:208-12, 1980.

Scheife RT, Hills JR: Migraine headache: Signs and symptoms, biochemistry, and current therapy. *Am J Hosp Pharm* 37:365-74, 1980.

Cerebrovascular Disease

Hirsh J: Selection and results of antiplatelet therapy in the prevention of stroke and myocardial infarction. *Arch Intern Med* 141:311-5, 1981.

Kartchner MM, McRae LP: Noninvasive evaluation and management of the "asymptomatic" carotid bruit. *Surgery* 82:840-7, 1977.

Ostfeld AM: A review of stroke epidemiology. *Epidemiol Rev* 2:136-52, 1980.

Robertson JT, Watridge CB: The surgical management of extracranial and intracranial occlusive disease. *Med Clin North Am* 63:681-93, 1979.

Brain Tumors

Lieberman A, Ransohoff J: Treatment of primary brain tumors. *Med Clin North Am* 63:835-48, 1979.

Naidich TP, Moran CJ, Pudlowski RM, et al: Advances in diagnosis: Cranial and spinal computed tomography. *Med Clin North Am* 63: 849-95, 1979.

Wikstrand CJ, Bigner DD: Immunobiologic aspects of the brain and human gliomas. A review. *Am J Pathol* 98:517-68, 1980.

Wilson CB: Current concepts in cancer: Brain tumors. *N Engl J Med* 65: 145-7, 149-50, 1979.

Neuropathies

Hilsted J, Madsbad S, Krarup T, et al: Hormonal, metabolic, and cardiovascular responses to hypoglycemia in diabetic autonomic neuropathy. *Diabetes* 30:626-33, 1981.

Noronha JL, Bhandarkar SD, Shenoy PN, et al: Autonomic neuropathy in diabetes mellitus. *J Postgrad Med* 27:1-6, 1981.

Myasthenia Gravis

Argov Z, Mastaglia FL: Drug therapy: Disorders of neuromuscular transmission caused by drugs. *N Engl J Med* 301:409-13, 1979.

Drachman DB: Myasthenia gravis. *N Engl J Med* 298:136-42, 186-93, 1978.

Elias SB, Appel SH: Current concepts of pathogenesis and treatment of myasthenia gravis. *Med Clin North Am* 63:745-57, 1979.

Whitaker JN: Myasthenia gravis and autoimmunity. *Adv Intern Med* 26: 489-510, 1980.

CHAPTER 12
ONCOLOGY

James C. Arseneau

Susan N. Rosenthal

INTRODUCTION

Incidence

Malignant neoplasms, a varied group of over 100 disease entities, are collectively referred to as cancer. As a group, malignant lesions are second only to cardiovascular diseases as a cause of morbidity and mortality in the United States. Malignant disease may arise in any tissue and may occur at any age, but malignancies of certain organs such as the lung, breast, and colon constitute the greatest proportion of clinically important cancers. The frequency of cancers in men and women is listed in Table 1. As the incidence of malignant disease increases with age, and as the mean age of the population in this country increases, cancer is expected to become an even greater medical problem in future years.

Etiology and Epidemiology

The etiology of malignant neoplasms is not known, but many predisposing factors have been identified. It is noteworthy that the organs that seem most susceptible to developing cancers are those in which there is a rapid cell turnover. If there is, as many authorities speculate, a small inherent risk of neoplastic transformation in any cell division, this increased frequency of neoplasms in organs that have a rapid cell turnover may be simply a consequence of statistics. More likely, populations of cells that are rapidly dividing, in addition to whatever inherent risks are applicable, are also more exposed to exogenous factors that almost certainly have a major role in the etiology of cancer.

Physical influences, mainly in the form of ionizing radiation, have long been known to increase the incidence of malignant neoplasia in exposed individuals. The earliest data were observed in uranium miners (high incidence of lung cancer) and fluoroscopists (high incidence of skin cancer). More recently, population studies of the survivors of the atomic bombing of Hiroshima have shown an increased incidence of malignant disease, chiefly leukemia, that correlates both with the dose of radiation and the time since exposure.

Table 1. Frequency of Cancer by Origin and Sex

	Male (%)	*Female (%)*
Skin	2	2
Head and neck	5	2
Lung	22	8
Breast	–	27
Colon and rectum	14	15
Other digestive	10	8
Prostate	17	–
Uterine	–	13
Ovary	–	4
Urinary	10	4
Leukemia and lymphoma	8	7
All other	12	10

Environmental factors, chiefly chemicals and toxins, are being increasingly recognized as contributory etiologic factors. Examples include the association of asbestos exposure with mesotheliomas and lung cancers, of vinyl chloride with hepatic malignancies, of inhaled tobacco tars with lung cancers and oropharyngeal cancers, and the controversial possible association of iatrogenic estrogen exposure with endometrial malignancy in postmenopausal women. Population studies have recorded a low incidence of colorectal cancer in Africans, who eat a diet low in meat and fat and high in roughage. These data have led to the suggestion that American and Western European diets may account in part for their high incidence of colorectal carcinoma.

Viral agents have long been suggested as an etiology of human malignant disease. Perhaps the best evidence for a viral cause of human cancer is found in Burkitt's lymphoma. Consistently high titers of serum antibody to the Epstein-Barr (EB) virus are found in patients with this disease. Whether the virus is a cause or simply an associated factor is not yet known. Because viruses are known to cause a variety of malignant tumors in animals, great interest remains in their potential role in human malignant tumors, but no conclusive evidence for a viral cause of human cancer has yet been demonstrated.

The association of many congenital immunodeficiency states with an increased incidence of malignancy and observations of an increased incidence of malignancy in iatrogenically immunosuppressed renal transplant patients have emphasized the importance of the intact immune system in prevention of malignant neoplasia. The etiology of most human malignancies is probably multifactorial and may represent interactions of inherent susceptibilities, environmental predisposing factors, and defects in host defense mechanisms.

Development of Medical Oncology

Great changes have occurred over the past 20 years in the ability of medicine to deal with malignant tumors. These changes have resulted from a better understanding of the behavior of malignant neoplasms and the development of effective systemic therapy for widespread cancers. Historically, the effective therapy for cancer was largely dependent on the ability to identify localized disease and either resect it surgically or destroy the malignant tissue with ionizing radiation. As a consequence, until the mid-1960s, treatment of cancer patients was largely the province of surgeons and radiation therapists. Successes in the cure of cancer resulted from the development of surgical and/or radiation therapy techniques to eliminate localized malignant tumors. The limitation of these techniques, however, was dramatized by the failure of ever more radical surgical procedures or radiation therapy techniques to control some tumors that, although apparently localized, all too often recurred locally or at distant sites (metastases). These failures led to a modification in clinical theories of tumor development and growth to include the concepts that malignant tumors may have an extended period in their natural history when disease is subclinical and that certain tumors may have the capacity to spread widely and

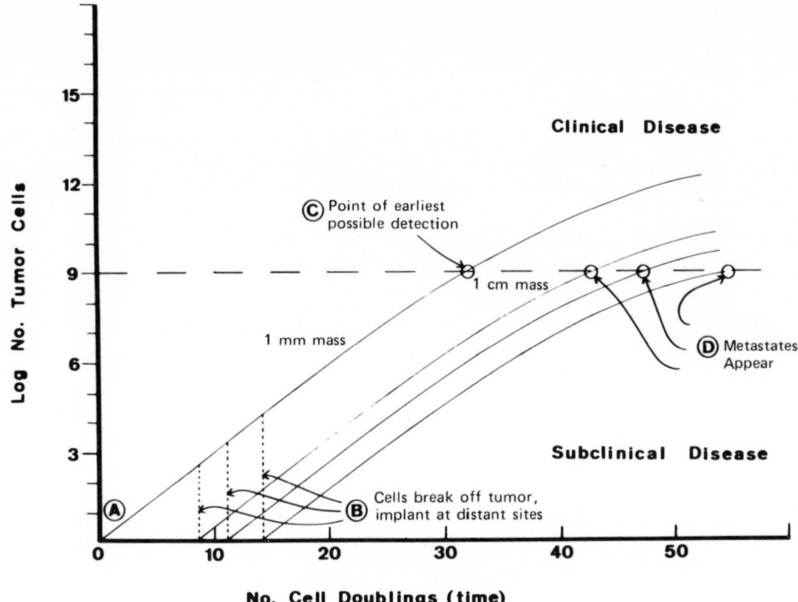

Figure 1. A single or small group of neoplastic cells begins to proliferate (A) and reaches a clinically detectable size (C). However, while the tumor was subclinical metastasis occurred (B). Even if the original tumor (C) is eradicated, disease will recur (D) unless some sort of systemic treatment can eliminate the subclinical metastatic disease.

metastasize during the subclinical period (Fig. 1) and therefore are not amenable to cure by local measures.

Recognition of the systemic nature of many seemingly localized malignant tumors took place in the context of developing systemic therapies for widespread cancers. The first effective use of systemic therapy for widespread malignancy was hormonal ablation for advanced prostatic carcinoma (orchiectomy) and breast carcinoma (oophorectomy and adrenalectomy) pioneered by Huggins. Almost at the same time, in the 1940s, the first efforts at systemic therapy for advanced cancer with cytotoxic drugs (chemotherapy) took place when Farber demonstrated the ability of the antifolate compounds aminopterin and methotrexate to produce temporary remissions in childhood acute leukemia. A milestone was reached in the early 1950s when choriocarcinoma, previously a universally and rapidly fatal disease, was shown to be curable with methotrexate even in advanced stages. Over the ensuing years a great variety of natural and synthetic compounds with cytotoxic properties have been identified. Table 2 lists many of these drugs that are in clinical use. Their mechanisms of action are outlined in Table 3.

Principles of Therapy

The development of chemotherapy with cytotoxic agents has proceeded from a knowledge of their effects on normal and neoplastic cells. These drugs mainly affect cells, normal as well as malignant, that are dividing. Some drugs affect dividing cells in a particular phase of cell division, or the cell cycle (Fig. 2). It has become evident that combinations of cytotoxic drugs are more effective than single-agent therapy in almost every instance in which cytotoxic drug therapy is effective. Optimal combinations use active agents with differing dose-limiting toxicities. This strategy allows employment of the component drugs at doses very near their optimal dose when used individually, greatly strengthening the therapeutic effect of the combination as a whole. As an example, a combination that has resulted in great improvement in the therapy of testicular malignancies employs vinblastine (dose-limiting toxicity—myelosuppression), bleomycin (dose-limiting toxicity—pulmonary) and *cis*-diamminedichloroplatinum (dose-limiting toxicity—renal). Each drug is individually active and used at full single-agent dosage, which is possible because the dose-limiting toxicities do not overlap. It has also been learned that cytotoxic drugs given on intermittent schedules have better antitumor effect and far less toxicity to normal tissues, which can recover during the intervals between cycles of chemotherapy. Use of intermittent schedules allows cytotoxic chemotherapy to be carried out over much longer periods than if given continuously. In some cases, knowledge of drug action in the cell cycle can be used to plan scheduling of the drug so that its killing effect on malignant cells will be maximized (e.g., scheduling of cytosine arabinoside, a phase-specific drug that interferes with DNA polymerase, as therapy for acute myelocytic leukemia).

Table 2. Major Cytotoxic Drugs

Drug	*Clinical Indications*	*Toxicity*
Alkylating agents		
Cyclophosphamide (Cytoxan)	Leukemias, lymphomas, sarcomas, breast, ovary, prostate, bladder, lung, many combintions	ST[a], hematuria
L-phenylalanine mustard (Melphalan, Alkeran)	Leukemia, breast, ovary, many combinations	ST
Nitrogen mustard (Mustargen)	Hodgkin's disease, malignant effusions	ST
Chlorambucil (Leukeran)	Leukemias, lymphomas, some combinations	ST
Thiotepa	Ovary, malignant effusions	ST
Mitomycin C (Mutamycin)	Gastric, colorectal, esophagus, many combinations	ST, severe soft tissue necrosis if extravasated
Antimetabolites		
Methotrexate	Leukemias choriocarcinoma, breast, lung, many combinations, intrathecal use	ST, mucositis, dermatitis
6-mercaptopurine (Purinethol)	Leukemias	ST
6-thioguanine	Leukemias	ST
5-fluorouracil	Colorectal, breast, prostate, lung, gastric, bladder, many combinations	ST, mucositis, neurotoxicity (rare)
Cytosine arabinoside (Cytosar)	Leukemias, lymphomas, intrathecal use	ST
Vinca alkaloids		
Vincristine (Oncovin)	Leukemias, lymphomas, breast, lung, many combinations	Neurotoxicity, soft tissue necrosis if extravasated
Vinblastine (Velban)	Leukemias, lymphomas, testicular, some combinations	ST, severe soft tissue necrosis if extravasated
Antibiotics		
Doxorubicin (Adriamycin)	Myeloma, testicular, gastric, prostate, leukemias, lymphomas, breast, lung, ovary, uterine, bladder, sarcomas, many combinations	ST, cardiotoxicity, severe soft tissue necrosis if extravasated
Bleomycin (Blenoxane)	Lymphomas, testicular, head and neck, squamous cell tumors, some combinations	Pulmonary, dermatitis fever, and chills
Actinomycin D (Cosmegen)	Testicular, ovary, choriocarcinoma, sarcomas	ST, severe soft tissue necrosis if extravasated
Mithramycin (Mithracin)	Testicular, hypercalcemia	ST, hepatotoxicity, severe soft tissue necrosis if extravasated
Daunomycin	Leukemias	ST, cardiotoxicity, severe soft tissue necrosis
Miscellaneous		
Cis-diamminedichloroplatinum (Platinol)	Testicular, ovary, cervix, head and neck, esophagus, some combinations	Nephrotoxicity, neurotoxicity
Procarbazine (Matulane)	Hodgkin's disease, lymphomas, lung	ST, dermatitis
BCNU	Colorectal, gastric, lymphomas, brain	ST
CCNU (CeeNU)	Colorectal, gastric, lymphomas, brain	ST
MethylCCNU	Colorectal, melanoma	ST
Dimethyltriazino imidazole carboxamide (DTIC)	Melanomas, lymphomas, sarcomas	ST, flushing
Hydroxyurea (Hydrea)	Leukemias, lymphomas	ST
Streptozotocin	Islet cell carcinomas, carcinoid	Nephrotoxicity, nausea
Hexamethylmelamine	Ovarian, breast, lymphomas, lung	ST, neurotoxicity
Hormones and Antagonists		
Prednisone	Leukemias, lymphomas, breast	Fluid retention, diabetes, catabolism, psychosis
Diethylstilbesterol	Breast, prostate	Fluid retention, nausea, feminization

Table 2. Major Cytotoxic Drugs (Cont.)

Drug	*Clinical Indications*	*Toxicity*
Fluoxymesterone (Halotestin)	Breast	Fluid retention, masculinization, polycythemia
Progesterone (Megace)	Uterine, breast, prostate, renal cell	Fluid retention, impotence
Tamoxifen (Nolvadex)	Breast	Nausea, thrombocytopenia

[a]ST (standard toxicity) common to most cytotoxic drugs includes GI upset (nausea, vomiting, diarrhea), myelosuppression (leukopenia, thrombocytopenia), and often alopecia.

The toxicity of cytotoxic drugs can be formidable and is related to the susceptibility of proliferating normal cells to these agents. Normal tissues with rapid cell turnover include the skin and appendages, mucous membranes, GI (gastrointestinal) epithelium, bone marrow, and germinal epithelium of the testes. As a consequence, most cytotoxic agents will cause GI distress, alopecia, mucositis (and sometimes dermatitis), and myelosuppression with resultant leukopenia, thrombocytopenia, and the attendant risks for severe infection and/or bleeding. In addition, many cytotoxic drugs have unique toxic effects that are outlined in Table 2. Obviously, cytotoxic chemotherapy is a potentially hazardous undertaking; it should be performed by specialists experienced in the selection and use of these drugs and the management of complications of chemotherapy.

With the recognition that many seemingly localized tumors have already metastasized widely at the time of diagnosis and that large tumor masses often contain populations of cells that are viable but divide slowly or not at all and are thus relatively impervious to killing by cytotoxic drugs, great interest has

Table 3. Mechanisms of Action of Cytotoxic Drugs

Drug	*Mechanism of Cytotoxic Action*
Alkylating Agents	Cross links DNA
Antimetabolites	
Methotrexate	Inhibits dihydrofolate reductase, interferes with purine synthesis
6-mercaptopurine	Blocks purine synthesis, inhibits purine interconversions
6-thioguanine	Blocks purine synthesis, inhibits purine interconversions
5-fluorouracil	Blocks thymidylate synthetase, interferes with pyrimidine synthesis
Cytosine arabinoside	Blocks reduction of cytidylic to deoxycytidylic acid, inhibits DNA polymerase
Vinca Alkaloids	Bind to mitotic apparatus, produce metaphase arrest
Antibiotics	Bind to DNA, block RNA production
Bleomycin	causes DNA strand breakage
Miscellaneous	
Cis-dimminedichloroplatinum	Cross links DNA, ? other action
Procarbazine	Depolymerizes DNA
Nitrosoureas (BCNU, CCNU, MeCCNU)	Cross links DNA, ? Other action
DTIC	Cross links DNA, ? other action
Hydroxyurea	Blocks ribonucleotide reductase, inhibits DNA synthesis
Streptozotocin	? cross links DNA, ? other action
Hormones and Antagonists	
Prednisone Diethylstilbesterol Fluoxymesterone Progesterone	Influence RNA-directed protein synthesis, act on hormonally responsive cells, alter production of pituitary hormones
Tamoxifen	Blocks action of estrogen at cellular level, ? direct cytotoxic action

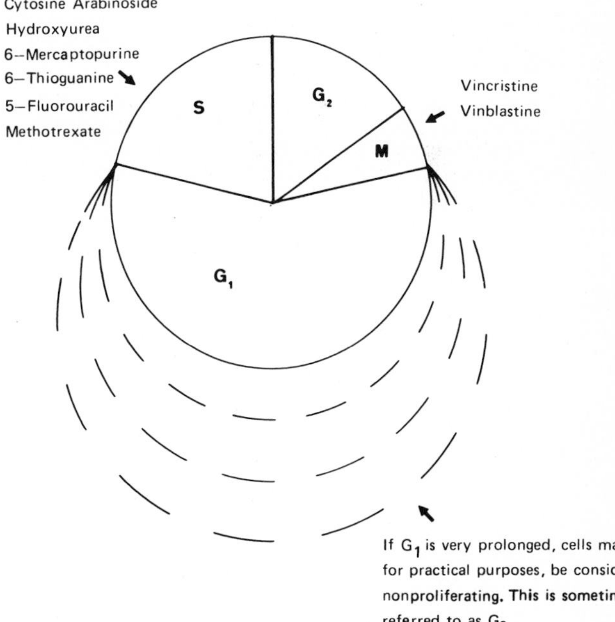

Figure 2. G_1 = Resting phase. DNA-directed RNA synthesis, protein synthesis. Time highly variable. S = DNA synthesis and replication. Time varies from 8-60 hours. G_2 = Premitotic phase. DNA synthesis stops, RNA and protein synthesis continue. M = Mitosis. Time fairly constant 30-90 minutes. G_0 = Hypothetical phase, either for totally nonproliferating cell or for cell with very long G_1. Cell is viable but relatively resistant to cytotoxic drug killing in this state.

developed in combining different anticancer therapeutic modalities to make the best use of the particular strengths of each and to use one modality to cover the weakness of another.

The strength of surgery and radiotherapy is the ability to eliminate large masses of tumor, but neither is capable of dealing with subclinical areas of distant dissemination (occult metastases). The strength of cytotoxic chemotherapy is its ability to deliver antitumor effects throughout the body. Its weakness is its frequent inability to eliminate large masses of tumor. Combined-modality therapy is an obvious answer and has been employed with early success in small-cell lung cancer, breast cancer in premenopausal women, and possibly in osteosarcoma. The use of adjuvant chemotherapy to treat patients at high risk for metastatic disease following elimination of the primary tumor by surgery or radiation therapy is being explored in many other malignant diseases and may lead to improved management, but until benefits of such an approach are clearly demonstrated, this treatment is best carried out in an investigational setting.

Clinical observations have demonstrated the importance of the intact immune system in the etiology of cancer. Laboratory investigations in animals have shown that techniques that stimulate the immune system can cause regression or prevent the development of both carcinogen-induced and transplantable tumors. These observations have prompted clinical trials of both nonspecific immune stimulation (with BCG C-parvum, transfer factor) and specific immune stimulation using killed tumor cells mixed with nonspecific stimulators. Early results of these trails are mixed as yet, and, other than the ability of some nonspecific agents such as BCG to cause regression of cutaneous malignant tumors when directly injected into them, there has been no consistent data to support widespread use of these techniques. A great deal of laboratory and clinical research is in progress and may result in another effective means of systemic therapy through manipulation of the immune system.

Cancer Staging

Recognizing the variety of treatments available for malignant disease and dependence of the selection of therapy on the location, extent, and apparent or inapparent spread of the disease, it is clear that the initial evaluation of a cancer patient is critical to an intelligent selection of initial and subsequent therapy. Various criteria have been advanced for the initial evaluation or staging of the cancer patient; these criteria will be dealt with in detail in subsequent sections. Efforts have been made to standardize tumor staging for the purpose of simplifying reporting and allowing published data to be compared. The most widely used standard staging system is the TNM classification that is summarized in Table 4. As an example of the use of this classification, if a 2-cm breast tumor were confined totally within the breast, and two mobile lymph nodes were found to contain tumor at surgery and other studies did not reveal additional sites of disease the tumor would be stage $T_2N_1M_0$. The advantage of this classification is

Table 4. TNM Classification of Tumors[a]

Primary tumor		T_1	T_2	T_3	T_4
Size		<2 cm	2-5 cm	>5 cm	>10 cm
Depth of invasion					
Solid organs		Confined within organ	Involves capsule or muscle	Involves surrounding bone or cartilage	Involves adjacent viscera
Hollow organs		Confined within submucosa	Involves muscularis	Involves serosa	Extends beyond serosa
Neighboring structures		Uninvolved	Adjacent involved	Surrounding but unattached involved	Viscera involved
Lymph nodes	N_0	N_1	N_2	N_3	N_4
Location	–	Ipsilateral	Ipsilateral, contralateral, or bilateral	Ipsilateral, contralateral, or bilateral	Contralateral or distant
Number	0	Solitary	Multiple	Multiple	Multiple
Size	–	<2-3 cm	>3 cm	>5 cm	>10 cm
Mobility	–	Mobile	Muscle invasion	Fixed	Fixed and destructive
Metastases	M_0	M_1	M_2	M_3	M_4
Number	0	1	>1	Multiple	Multiple
Number of organs	–	1	1	Multiple	Multiple
Impairment	–	0	Minimal	Moderate	Severe

[a]T refers to characteristics of the primary tumor; N refers to involvement of lymph nodes; M refers to metastases.

its wide acceptance and utility for surgeons and radiotherapists because of the detailed description of the main tumor mass and its spread to adjacent organs and/or lymph nodes. The disadvantage is the rather vague description of widespread disease, which limits the usefulness of such a staging system in systemic malignancies such as the lymphomas.

When the initial evaluation of a cancer patient is complete and an accurate evaluation of the clinical stage has been made, initial therapy can be selected. Selection obviously will depend a great deal on the size and location of the tumor and on the presence or absence of obvious metastases; it also depends on a knowledge of the natural history of the disease, the condition of the patient, the presence or absence of other medical problems, the personal wishes of the patient and the patient's family and, to no small extent, the therapeutic philosophy of the attending physician.

Therapeutic Goals

Therapy for any disease, but particularly of cancer, can be classified into therapy with intent to cure, therapy with intent to prolong life, therapy directed against the disease process to alleviate symptoms, or symptomatic therapy only without any attempt to influence the disease process. The choice of therapeutic philosophy is often straightforward, as in the case of a young person with a localized malignant tumor (curative therapy with surgery or radiotherapy); or a responsive but widespread malignant lymphoma (curative or life-prolonging treatment with cytotoxic chemotherapy); or in the case of an elderly patient with advanced metastatic disease refractory to known treatment modalities (symptomatic therapy only). Many cases, however, will fall between these extreme examples, and therapeutic philosophy then depends on weighing the potential gains from antitumor treatment against the potential side effects or toxicities of therapy. Such decisions are best made in consultation with oncologic specialists, whose particular treatments may be applicable, and with the patient and family. In Table 5, malignant tumors are classified according to responsiveness to cytotoxic and hormonal therapy for purposes of quick reference.

Good medical care of the cancer patient frequently requires more than treatment of the specific disease process. Perhaps more than any other disease, cancer is surrounded by misinformation that often has profound psychologic and social effects on both the patient and family. Support from and communication with the family physician and oncologic specialists are essential for both physical and psychologic recovery. A general policy of honesty and open, compassionate communication with the patient and family will result in better cooperation and serve to lessen the anxiety derived from rumors or popular misconceptions about the disease or the proposed therapy. Attempts to conceal the diagnosis are not only dishonest, but risk a breach of trust between physician and patient that is essential for effective therapy, whether it be curative or simply palliative. A great variety of supportive services for cancer patients exists in most communities. The wise physician will be familiar with local services and will use them to benefit these patients.

Table 5. Responsiveness of Various Malignant Tumors to Cytotoxic or Hormonal Therapy

Tumors in which cure is possible with systemic therapy	
Acute lymphocytic leukemia	Embryonal rhabdomyosarcoma
Hodgkin's disease	Ewing's sarcoma
Histiocytic lymphoma	Wilm's tumor
Testicular carcinoma	Retinoblastoma
Choriocarcinoma	Burkitt's lymphoma
Responsive tumors in which survival can be prolonged with systemic therapy	
Ovarian carcinoma	Diffuse lymphomas
Breast carcinoma	Neuroblastoma
Acute myelocytic leukemia	Malignant islet cell carcinoma
Multiple myeloma	Endometrial carcinoma
Small-cell carcinoma of lung	
Responsive tumors in which clinically useful prolongation of survival has not yet been demonstrated	
Head and neck carcinomas	Osteogenic sarcoma
Gastrointestinal carcinomas	Soft tissue sarcomas
Malignant brain tumors	Bladder carcinoma
Malignant carcinoid	Prostate carcinoma
Tumors which at present are marginally responsive or unresponsive to systemic therapy	
Renal cell carcinoma	Hepatocellular carcinoma
Malignant melanoma	Thyroid carcinoma
Carcinoma of pancreas	Carcinoma of esophagus
Carcinoma of lung (non-small-cell)	

Development of the field of medical oncology and increasing coordination of systemic anticancer therapy with surgery and radiation therapy has led to major advances in cancer treatment. Efforts to improve management are constantly in progress. These efforts involve the introduction and screening of new drugs, the development of new surgical and radiation therapy techniques, the integration of different modalities of anticancer therapy, and the testing of new treatments in cancer patient populations. Basic research into tumor cell growth and host defense mechanisms offers the possibility that completely new means to affect malignant disease may be available in the future. Such basic and clinical cancer research is carried out in cancer centers and by national clinical research cooperative groups. These clinical research efforts are worthy of the support and participation of the medical profession so that further improvements in cancer management will continue.

HODGKIN'S DISEASE

Hodgkin's disease is a malignant lymphoproliferative disorder usually arising in lymph nodes or other lymphoid tissue. The cause is unknown, but reports of Hodgkin's disease occurring in space-time clusters have suggested the possibility of an unidentified infectious agent, although no direct evidence for an infectious cause has been discovered.

Hodgkin's disease may be encountered in all age groups. In the United States a bimodal incidence curve is seen. The first peak occurs in young adults, and the second after age 50. Childhood Hodgkin's disease occurs predominantly in males; the female incidence rises sharply in adolescence. Overall, the male/female ratio is 1.4:1.

Pathology

The diagnosis of Hodgkin's disease and its distinction from other lymphomas, infectious disorders, or immunologic conditions depend on the histopathologic examination of an involved lymph node under light microscopy. To make a diagnosis of Hodgkin's disease, Reed-Sternberg cells (characteristic binucleate giant cells) in an appropriate histologic milieu must be recognized. Reed-Sternberg cells alone, however, are not sufficient for diagnosis; they may be seen in other lymphomas, carcinomas, and viral diseases such as infectious mononucleosis.

Hodgkin's disease has been classified by Lukes and Butler into four main histologic types. These include, in order of decreasingly favorable prognosis: lymphocyte predominant, nodular sclerosis, mixed cellularity, and lymphocyte depletion. The first three types tend to present with more limited disease, whereas lymphocyte depletion Hodgkin's disease is often widespread at the time of diagnosis. Nodular sclerosing Hodgkin's disease has a predilection for the mediastinum, especially in young women. With modern treatment regimens the prognostic importance of the histologic subtype has tended to recede.

Clinical Features

Most patients with Hodgkin's disease present to their physician with the complaint of a painless mass, most commonly in the neck, but occasionally in the axilla or groin. On examination, rubbery nontender lymphadenopathy is noted. Occasionally, an abdominal mass, representing enlarged retroperitoneal nodes, or splenomegaly, is the initial finding. Some patients are totally asymptomatic, and the physician may discover lymphadenopathy during the course of a routine physical examination or may detect mediastinal adenopathy on a chest x-ray obtained for other indications. On careful questioning, however, most patients presenting with mediastinal adenopathy will be aware of subtle changes in exercise tolerance, cough, shortness of breath, or alcohol-induced chest pain.

Occasionally, extensive lymphadenopathy may cause symptoms by compression of adjacent organs. Venous obstruction in an extremity, hydronephrosis (with renal failure if bilateral ureteral compression occurs), superior vena cava syndrome, tracheal compression, dysphagia due to extrinsic compression of the esophagus, and spinal cord compression are all unusual presenting features in patients with Hodgkin's disease. These problems may also occur late in the course of the disease if progressive adenopathy cannot be controlled by therapeutic interventions. Compression of the superior vena cava, trachea, ureters, and spinal cord are medical emergencies that, if recognized early and treated promptly, are reversible; if overlooked or neglected, however, they can result in either permanent disability or death.

A minority of patients with Hodgkin's disease present with systemic symptoms. Unexplained fever, anorexia and weight loss, and night sweats, when present in a patient with Hodgkin's disease, are designated by the addition of the letter B to the clinical stage. The presence of B symptoms implies a less favorable prognosis in any given stage. Pruritus may also occur in patients with Hodgkin's disease and may precede the diagnosis by months or even years. Localized pain in areas containing enlarged lymph nodes following consumption of alcohol is an unusual symptom that should alert the physician to the possibility of underlying Hodgkin's disease.

Evaluation and Staging

After a pathologic diagnosis of Hodgkin's disease is established (usually by lymph node biopsy), further clinical, radiologic, and laboratory evaluation is directed toward defining the extent of disease or clinical stage. Such staging is essential for the selection of the most appropriate therapy. The initial evaluation includes a careful history and physical examination with particular attention to lymph node-bearing areas, screening blood chemistries, and chest x-ray. If the chest x-ray is suspicious for mediastinal or hilar adenopathy, tomograms may be useful. Retroperitoneal node involvement is assessed with bipedal lymphangiography or computed tomography (CT) of the abdomen. A needle or open biopsy of bone marrow should be obtained. Any finding that directs attention to any other organ system should be evaluated by appropriate diagnostic studies.

During the past decade, exploratory laparotomy has been employed frequently in Hodgkin's patients to improve diagnostic accuracy in assessing disease stage. Provided the patient is an acceptable surgical risk, a staging laparotomy is indicated if results of the laparotomy would alter the choice of treatment. If, however, the selection of therapy is already determined by the clinical findings (e.g., a patient who has both nodal and extranodal involvement and would receive combination chemotherapy regardless of laparotomy findings) or would not be altered by the results of a laparotomy, then it can be omitted.

The stage of disease at the time of diagnosis is the most important prognostic factor. The staging of Hodgkin's disease (and the non-Hodgkin's lymphomas) is shown in Table 6.

Treatment

The treatment of Hodgkin's disease has improved dramatically in the past two decades. With modern therapeutic techniques most patients with limited Hodgkin's disease at diagnosis (stages I and II) will be cured. A majority of patients with advanced disease will achieve prolonged disease-free remission and cure in some cases.

Radiation therapy is the preferred treatment modality for stages I and II Hodgkin's disease. Radiation fields are designed to encompass areas of known disease as well as adjacent nodal areas that may contain occult disease. Modern radiotherapy equipment allows treatment of the most common presenta-

Table 6. The Staging of Hodgkin's Disease[a]

Stage	*Definition*
I	Involvement of a single node or node group, or of a single extranodal site (I_E)
II	Involvement of two or more node groups on the same side of the diaphragm
III	Involvement of nodes on both sides of the diaphragm, with or without splenic involvement
IV	Diffuse or disseminated involvement of one or more extranodal sites

[a]The presence or absence of systemic symptoms (see text) is denoted by B or A, respectively.

tions in two or three large fields including the mantle, the upper para-aortic chain, and the inverted Y. Radiation therapy to all lymph node-bearing areas (total nodal treatment) may also be curative in stage III Hodgkin's disease, but treatment with chemotherapy may be equally successful.

Chemotherapy is the treatment of choice for advanced (stages IIIB and IV) Hodgkin's disease. It is also effective in the salvage treatment of patients whose disease has relapsed following radiation therapy. Combination chemotherapy has been unequivocally demonstrated to be far superior to single-agent treatment. Single-agent chemotherapy has no role in the initial management of Hodgkin's disease.

The most widely used regimen, MOPP, includes nitrogen mustard, vincristine (Oncovin), procarbazine, and prednisone. Many other effective combinations have been devised and employ a variety of agents including adriamycin, bleomycin, vinblastine, and the nitrosoureas. Some of these combinations are useful in treating patients who have relapsed after an initial response to MOPP. Single-agent therapy may be used for palliation in patients wtih advanced disease who have failed the standard regimens.

Testicular and ovarian failure, carcinogenesis, and immunosuppression are all long-term complications of the treatment of Hodgkin's disease. In patients treated with both intensive radiation and chemotherapy, the incidence of second malignancies, predominantly leukemia, approaches 5%. There should be no hesitation, however, to treat a patient with one modality following relapse after initial therapy with another, since the risk of progressive Hodgkin's disease far exceeds the potential long-term risks of combined-modality therapy.

NON-HODGKIN'S LYMPHOMAS

The non-Hodgkin's lymphomas (NHL) are a group of diseases that vary widely in natural history, prognosis, and specific histopathologic features; nevertheless, they all represent neoplastic proliferations of lymphoid cells. The lymphomas usually arise in lymph nodes or other sites of lymphoid tissue including the spleen, Waldeyer's ring, gastrointestinal tract, and bone marrow. In some cases the disease may remain localized to one node, a group of nodes, or to a single extranodal site for prolonged periods. In other instances multiple lymph nodes are involved at the outset and widespread dissemination to the liver, lungs, bone marrow, and other organs may be present as well. As a group, the NHL differ from Hodgkin's disease in their greater tendency to involve extranodal sites and their lesser frequency of attaining long-term remissions or cures.

Incidence and Etiology

The etiology of the NHL is unknown. In the case of Burkitt's lymphoma, an infectious cause has been implicated. This is an undifferentiated lymphoma endemic to children of Central Africa, with a particular tendency to involve the jaw and facial bones. Epidemiologic studies have suggested that a mosquito-borne virus may be involved, and electron microscopy and serologic studies have incriminated the Ebstein-Barr virus, the causative agent of infectious mononucleosis. However, it is not yet clear whether the association of EB virus with Burkitt's lymphoma is etiologic, secondary, or merely fortuitous.

An increased incidence of malignant lymphomas occurs in a variety of immunologic deficiency states and in immunosuppressed patients, suggesting that defects in immune surveillance may permit an oncogenic stimulus (possibly viral) to cause the lymphoma to arise in susceptible hosts. The association of lymphomas with Sjögren's syndrome and with prolonged use of the antiepileptic agent phenytoin is unexplained.

The NHL comprise approximately 5% of human malignancies. They occur in all age groups, but the incidence rises with age and peaks in the 65-74 year age group. The male/female ratio is about 1:1.

While several different classification schemes for the NHL are in current use, the Rappaport classification shown in Table 7 is by far the most useful clinically. In terms of prognosis, the presence of nodularity is the most important histologic feature of the NHL and has major therapeutic implications.

Clinical Features

Like Hodgkin's disease, NHL commonly presents with painless lymphadenopathy. Massively enlarged nodes may cause symptoms by compression of adjacent organs: superior vena cava syndrome, hydronephrosis, venous obstruction of an extremity, spinal cord compression, back pain, and bowel obstruction. Occasionally, enlarged nodes in the porta hepatis may compress the common bile duct and cause obstructive jaundice. Superior vena cava syndrome, spinal cord compression, and bilateral hydronephrosis represent medical emergencies that, as in Hodgkin's disease, require prompt treatment, usually with radiation therapy.

The NHL, especially the diffuse histiocytic variety, may present with extranodal involvement. Lytic bone lesions may produce pain and pathologic fracture. Gastrointestinal lymphoma can cause obstruction, ulceration, or malabsorption. Extensive bone marrow replacement, especially with the lymphocytic varieties, may produce pancytopenia and consequent hemorrhage or infection, or may lead to overt circulation of malignant cells termed lymphosarcoma-cell leukemia

Table 7. Classification and Relative Frequency of Non-Hodgkin's Lymphomas

	Nodular		*Diffuse*	
	Frequency (%)	*Median Survival (years)*	*Frequency (%)*	*Median Survival (years)*
Lymphocytic				
Well differentiated	1	>5	6	>5
Poorly differentiated	27	7-8	15	1-2
Histiocytic	5	2-3	23	0.5-1.5
Mixed lymphocytic-histiocytic	13	7-8	8	1-2
Undifferentiated	–		2	0.3-1.0

in the case of poorly differentiated lymphocytic lymphomas and chronic lymphocytic leukemia (CLL) in the case of well-differentiated lymphocytic lymphomas. Confusion may arise as to whether such patients have leukemia or malignant lymphoma in a leukemic phase; the distinction is probably not of great importance since these conditions merely represent two ends of the spectrum of the same lymphoproliferative disorder.

In advanced cases, or late in the course of the disease, progressive lymphoma may involve almost any organ system. Central nervous system involvement with diffuse meningeal infiltration may cause headache, coma, cranial nerve palsies, or nerve root symptoms. Lumbar puncture with spinal fluid cytology reveals malignant lymphoid cells in the cerebrospinal fluid (CSF). Lumbar myelography may demonstrate the characteristic plaquelike involvement of the meninges. Pleural or pulmonary involvement produces respiratory symptoms with pleural effusions and/or pulmonary infiltrates on chest x-ray. Extensive hepatic involvement can ultimately lead to hepatic failure. Bone marrow failure as a consequence of lymphomatous replacement or extensive myelosuppressive chemotherapy and radiotherapy may lead to thrombocytopenic hemorrhage or marked granulocytopenia and infection. Severe infection with bacteria, viruses, parasites, or fungi represent the most common cause of death in advanced lymphomas.

Diagnosis and Staging

The diagnosis and clinical evaluation of patients with NHL are similar to the evaluation of Hodgkin's patients. Biopsy and histologic examination of an involved node are essential for diagnosis and classification. Careful physical examination, chest x-ray examination, bone marrow biopsy, and lymphangiogram or abdominal CT scan are performed routinely. Additional investigations may be performed as indicated by clinical findings. Staging laparotomy is of limited utility in the NHL since in the majority of patients therapeutic decisions can be made without input from the laparotomy findings. The staging system for the NHL is the same as that used for Hodgkin's disease.

Treatment

Radiation therapy and cytotoxic chemotherapy are both effective in the NHL. The remissions obtained, however, are generally not as durable as those achieved in Hodgkin's disease. Because of the variable natural histories and responsiveness to treatment among the malignant lymphomas, the selection of initial therapy depends as much on the particular histologic type as it does on the clinical stage. Discussion of therapy is best carried out using the concept of favorable and unfavorable histologies. Favorable histologies include all the nodular lymphomas (although some evidence indicates that nodular histiocytic and nodular mixed may not be as favorable as initially thought) and diffuse well-differentiated lymphocytic lymphoma. All the other diffuse lymphomas are unfavorable histologies.

Favorable Histologies

Intensive therapy of the favorable lymphomas has not been shown to prolong survival, except perhaps in patients with nodular mixed lymphomas. Therefore, treatment is directed at palliation. In asymptomatic patients it may be appropriate to withhold treatment, simply observing the patient for the development of progressive disease and consequent symptoms. Local radiation therapy may be used to treat enlarged nodes that are producing local symptoms, or for cosmetic or psychologic reasons. Widespread adenopathy, especially if B symptoms are present, is best treated with chemotherapy. In these situations a single-agent alkylator or simple combination therapy is as effective and less toxic than more aggressive combination regimens. In patients with widespread disease and extensive parenchymal organ involvement intensive combination chemotherapy is appropriate. The duration of treatment depends on the particular clinical circumstances but, in general, is limited to what is necessary to cause disease regression. Treatment is usually stopped after all clinical evidence of disease regresses, but may be reintroduced when symptoms recur.

Unfavorable Histologies

The unfavorable NHL, mainly diffuse histiocytic lymphoma, frequently present with widespread disease and systemic symptoms; they tend to progress rapidly. Aggressive therapy that succeeds in producing a complete remission (i.e., complete disappearance of lymphoma in all areas in which it had previously been present, as documented by clinical, radiologic, and pathologic examinations) results in prolonged survival, unlike the situation in the favorable histologies. In diffuse histiocytic lymphoma 30-40% of patients treated with intensive combination chemotherapy will achieve a complete remission; the majority of these patients remain in complete remission for over 5 years. Such patients are considered cured. Those patients who do not achieve a complete remission undergo a rapid deterioration caused by progressive lymphoma and usually die within a year of diagnosis.

Radiation therapy is the treatment of choice for localized nodal or extranodal disease (stage I or I_E). Patients with apparent stage I NHL after a complete staging evaluation should undergo laparotomy to confirm the absence of more widespread disease and hence the potential ability of local treatment to cure the patient. Clearly, if occult intra-abdominal lymphoma is discovered, local radiation therapy would be inappropriate, and combination chemotherapy would become the treatment of choice.

Burkitt's Lymphoma

Burkitt's lymphoma, a subtype of diffuse undifferentiated lymphoma, deserves special mention because of its remarkable responsiveness to chemotherapy. Burkitt's lymphoma is one of the few malignancies in which single-agent chemotherapy (usually cyclophosphamide) may produce a cure, even in patients with advanced disease. Rapid tumor destruction following initiation of treatment may result in hyperkalemia, hyperuricemia, hyperphosphatemia, and hypocalcemia with the consequent risks of severe cardiac arrhythmias and acute renal failure. This tumor lysis syndrome occasionally follows treatment of other very sensitive lymphomas and leukemias and must be recognized so that life-threatening consequences may be avoided.

Angioimmunoblastic Lymphadenopathy

Angioimmunoblastic lymphadenopathy appears to be a nonneoplastic immunoproliferative condition with similarities to lymphomas and a tendency to evolve into frank lymphoma in some cases. The disorder presents in older patients as generalized adenopathy, hepatosplenomegaly, skin rash, fever, weight loss, anemia, and polyclonal hyperglobulinemia. Node biopsy specimens reveal infiltration with a mixed population of plasma cells, lymphocytes, eosinophils, and immunoblasts. PAS-positive intercellular deposits and a poliferation of capillary vessels are also characteristic. In most cases, these patients undergo a progressive deterioration regardless of treatment and succumb to the disease within a year or two.

Mycosis Fungoides

Mycosis fungoides is a chronic lymphoproliferative disorder of T lymphocytes. It begins generally as a chronic dermatitis and progresses over a period of years to produce extensive skin infiltration with plaques and nodules of tumor. Eventually, local or generalized adenopathy and widespread visceral involvement, the so-called tumor phase, occurs, and death follows in 1-3 years.

Sézary's syndrome is a variant of mycosis fungoides consisting of a generalized exfoliative erythroderma and circulation of abnormal monocytoid (Sézary's) cells in the peripheral blood. Sézary's syndrome can be thought of as the leukemic phase of mycosis fungoides.

Treatment of early stage mycosis fungoides employs electron-beam irradiation or topical applications of nitrogen mustard. Advanced disease has been treated with various cytotoxic drugs, with brief partial responses in most cases. No controlled trial of combination chemotherapy has been reported.

PLASMA CELL TUMORS

The plasma cell dyscrasias are a group of related disorders each characterized by the excessive proliferation of a single clone of immunoglobulin-producing cells; in most cases, this results in the presence in the serum of a monoclonal immunoglobulin, detected as an M spike on serum-protein electrophoresis. This proliferation may be benign, as in the case of benign monoclonal gammopathy, or clearly malignant, as in multiple myeloma or Waldenström's macroglobulinemia; or it may be somewhere in between, as in heavy-chain disease or amyloidosis. In this section, discussion will be limited to the malignant plasma-cell disorders.

MULTIPLE MYELOMA

The etiology of multiple myeloma is not understood, but observations made on plasma cell tumors in laboratory animals suggest that protracted antigenic stimulation, oncogenic viruses, and genetic factors may all play an etiologic role.

The incidence of multiple myeloma appears to be rising; it occurs at a rate of two to three per 100,000 population, about as frequently as Hodgkin's disease. The disease is now as common in women as in men, although in the past there was a male predominance. The reason for this apparent change in sex distribution is not known. The disease may arise at any age from young adulthood to elderly; peak incidence occurs in the middle fifties.

Clinical Features

At present, multiple myeloma is detected in many patients in an asymptomatic stage. This may occur when routine blood work or urinalysis reveals an M protein on serum electrophoresis, increased blood sedimentation rate, mild anemia, or unexplained proteinuria. Investigation of these abnormalities leads to a diagnosis of early myeloma, which may persist for years before the classic picture of symptomatic myeloma supervenes.

Bone pain is the most frequent presenting symptom of overt myeloma. This pain is often of sudden onset and extremely severe, especially if it is due to a pathologic fracture. X-ray films usually reveal multiple osteolytic or punched-out lesions throughout the skeleton. On occasion, diffuse osteoporosis rather than lytic lesions is seen. As the disease progresses, the lytic lesions enlarge and increase in number, vertebral compression fractures occur, and marked skeletal deformities result. The patient may actually lose several inches in height.

Table 8. Factors Contributing to Renal Impairment in Patients with Multiple Myeloma

Myeloma kidney
Amyloidosis
Hyperuricemia
Recurrent pyelonephritis
Ureteral stone
Dehydration
Invasion of kidney with abnormal plasma cells
Hyperviscosity (possibly)

Patients with multiple myeloma have increased susceptibility to bacterial infections, particularly pneumococcal, and recurrent infections frequently complicate the course and management of these patients. Decreased antibody synthesis is the major cause of this susceptibility and is reflected in the low levels of normal immunoglobulins in most myeloma patients. Deficiencies in cellular immunity and neutropenia may also play a role.

Renal impairment in myeloma occurs in over 80% of patients and may be the presenting complaint. Renal disease in myeloma has multiple causes (Table 8), but the most common is the so-called myeloma kidney, which results from tubular damage related to the reabsorption of large amounts of Bence Jones proteins (monoclonal light chains). In the past it was thought that proteinaceous casts obstructing the tubules caused the renal damage, but recent evidence makes this seem less likely, and the nephrotoxicity of Bence Jones proteinuria is not well understood.

Neurologic problems develop in many myeloma patients and involve all levels of the nervous system. Peripheral neuropathies can result from amyloid infiltration and nerve root symptoms may follow vertebral compression fractures. Spinal cord compression from adjacent vertebral involvement may be seen and represents a medical emergency. Confusion and stupor may accompany many metabolic abnormalities, most prominently azotemia and hypercalcemia.

Laboratory Manifestations

The presence of a monoclonal immunoglobulin composed of a single heavy-chain type and a single light-chain class (κ or λ) is characteristic of myeloma. An M protein and/or Bence Jones protein can be detected by serum and urine electrophoresis in over 99% of myeloma patients. IgG is the most frequent M-protein type, followed by IgA and IgD. Very rarely a patient may have two different M proteins. In about 25% of cases, Bence Jones proteinuria alone is encountered, without an M protein in the serum.

Bone marrow examination in multiple myeloma generally reveals increased numbers of abnormal plasma cells, usually greater than 10%. In advanced cases normal marrow elements may be replaced entirely by sheets of malignant plasma cells. Peripheral blood findings almost invariably include anemia and rouleau formation. The erythrocyte sedimentation rate is markedly elevated in most cases. White blood cell and platelet counts are normal in most patients, but in about one-third the counts are low before myelotoxic treatment. Circulating plasma cells are rarely a prominent finding, although they may be detected on careful buffy coat examination in up to 70% of cases.

Hypercalcemia, azotemia, and hyperuricemia are frequent chemical findings in myeloma patients and may cause difficult problems in management.

Diagnosis

The diagnosis of overt multiple myeloma is usually not difficult and depends on the following: increased numbers of abnormal plasma cells in the bone marrow, the presence of a monoclonal protein in the serum or urine, and osteolytic bone lesions. Early cases, presenting only with an M protein, must be distinguished from benign monoclonal gammopathy, which rarely evolves into overt myeloma. Similarly, increased numbers of immature plasma cells may be seen in the bone marrows of patients with chronic inflammatory diseases, such as rheumatoid arthritis, and, without other findings, should not lead to a diagnosis of myeloma.

Treatment

Treatment with chemotherapy is clearly indicated for patients with overt symptomatic myeloma, but for those with early disease manifested only by laboratory abnormalities, a policy of observation with frequent clinical and laboratory reevaluations is preferable. The disease may remain stable and asymptomatic for years before treatment is required.

Chemotherapy with an alkylating agent (melphalan or cyclophosphamide) and prednisone, given intermittently, is the standard therapy for myeloma and produces significant subjective and objective improvement in 70-80% of patients. Responses can be recognized by a rise in hemoglobin level, improvement in renal function, decline in M-protein level and in Bence Jones proteinuria, and diminution of pain with eventual radiologic improvement in skeletal lesions. Remissions may last from several months to many years; the median survival of treated patients is about 4 years in most series. Patients who respond to treatment survive longer than those who do not. The likelihood of response to chemotherapy is greatest among patients with a serum creatinine of less than 2 mg/dl and a normal serum calcium.

In addition to chemotherapy, general supportive measures play an important role in the management of myeloma patients. Careful attention to proper hydration, caloric intake, regular ambulation, and adequate analgesia will be rewarded by increased patient comfort and avoidance of hypercalcemia and renal failure. Palliative radiation therapy to painful bony lesions may be helpful but should be used sparingly to avoid compromise of marrow reserve. Pneumococcal vaccine (Pneumovax) is recommended in an attempt to prevent pneumococcal pneumonia. Prophylactic gamma globulin injections have been advocated for the purpose of reducing the risk of bacterial infections; however, such injections were not shown to offer any benefit in a randomized trial. Sodium fluoride has been given to myeloma patients in an attempt to increase bone density and remineralize lytic and osteoporotic areas. Fluoride treatment, however, does not seem to produce any subjective or objective improvement in the clinical course of the skeletal disease, nor does it prolong survival.

In a patient who fails to respond to the standard melphalan-prednisone regimen or in one who relapses after an initial remission, several other chemotherapeutic agents may be useful. Adriamycin, vincristine, and carmustine (BCNU) each are active against myeloma; occasionally, a patient who is resistant to melphalan will respond to cyclophosphamide and vice versa. Second remissions in this disease are usually brief. The most common causes of death in myeloma are infections and renal failure. In recent years, an increased incidence of acute myelomonocytic leukemia, possibly as a result of treatment with cytotoxic agents or due to the natural history of myeloma itself, has been recognized in myeloma patients.

MACROGLOBULINEMIA

Macroglobulinemia, first described by Waldenström in 1944, is a malignant plasma cell dyscrasia involving IgM-producing cells and is, therefore, characterized by the presence of large amounts of monoclonal IgM in the serum. Macroglobulinemia differs from multiple myeloma in that the proliferating cells in macroglobulinemia include malignant lymphocytes, plasma cells, and intermediate forms. In advanced stages, macroglobulinemia resembles the lymphomas with lymphadenopathy, hepatosplenomegaly, and bone marrow invasion as prominent findings. Lytic bone lesions of the type seen in myeloma are rare, and renal impairment is uncommon.

Most patients with macroglobulinemia present with symptoms related to anemia or to the presence of the abnormal protein. These problems include cryoglobulinemia (Raynaud's phenomenon, cold sensitivity, cold urticaria), hyperviscosity (visual, circulatory, auditory, and neurologic complaints), and protein-protein interactions (interference with platelet function and coagulation proteins leading to a bleeding diathesis). There is an increased susceptibility to bacterial infections in macroglobulinemia, but this is not as severe as in myeloma.

The diagnosis of macroglobulinemia requires the demonstration of a monoclonal IgM in the serum and the characteristic plasmacytoid lymphocytes in marrow, peripheral blood, and lymph nodes. Treatment with chlorambucil generally controls the disease for several years. Plasmapheresis to relieve severe manifestations of hyperviscosity may be necessary on an emergency basis and for several weeks until chemotherapy can take effect.

MALIGNANT NEOPLASMS OF BREAST

Pathology

Malignant neoplasms of the breast are most often carcinomas that arise from the epithelial lining of the ducts or from the glandular tissue of the breast itself. Histologic subvarieties are listed in Table 9. The great majority of breast carcinomas are of the infiltrating ductal variety. Lobular carcinomas, the second most common subtype, may be localized or in situ, but this tumor is so frequently multicentric and so often associated with infiltrating disease that limited surgical excisions may not eradicate local disease. Medullary carcinomas may appear cytologically undifferentiated and may present as very large masses. Nevertheless, they are said to have a somewhat better prognosis, perhaps because of the tendency of this variety to remain localized to breast tissue longer than the more common ductal carconomas. It is not uncommon to see several histologic subtypes of carcinoma within a single mastectomy specimen. Sarcomas and malignant lymphomas comprise most of the rare (<1%) noncarcinomatous breast malignancies.

Table 9. Histologic Varieties of Breast Cancer

Type	*Frequency (%)*
Infiltrating duct carcinoma	70-80
Infiltrating lobular carcinoma	8-10
Medullary carcinoma	4-5
Colloid carcinoma	2-3
Comedo carcinoma	4-5
Papillary carcinoma	1-2

Paget's disease of the breast refers to carcinomatous infiltration of skin around the nipple. An underlying infiltrating duct carcinoma is almost always present. Inflammatory carcinoma of the breast is a clinical entity consisting of a malignant breast tumor (usually infiltrating duct carcinoma) presenting with associated skin changes of redness, warmth, edema, and dimpling of the skin (peau d'orange). Tumor emboli in dermal lymphatic channels are noted pathologically. This clinicopathologic variant of breast cancer has the worst prognosis of all breast malignancies. Inflammatory breast carcinoma should not be confused with neglected breast tumors, present for many months or years, in which skin changes are simply a consequence of locally advanced disease.

The biologic behavior of breast cancer is variable. This variability may account for much of the confusion regarding the ability of local therapies (surgery, radiation therapy) to cure this disease. The traditional concept of the natural history of breast cancer, consisting of the development of the tumor within the breast, followed after a period of time by spread to regional lymph nodes, followed after a further interval by metastases to distant organs, has undergone revision in the light of clinical studies that show that more aggressive surgical procedures and/or radiation therapy do not improve survival. Recent pathologic evidence shows that metastatic involvement of axillary lymph nodes predicts systemic spread of the disease. Apparently, breast cancers that are capable of metastasizing to regional lymph nodes are also capable of metastasizing to distant organs via the bloodstream, and frequently do so before the primary tumor is clinically detectable. The poor prognosis of inflammatory breast cancer is due to the tendency of this variant to metastasize widely and very early in its natural history.

Incidence and Etiology

Breast cancer is the most common malignant disease of women and the leading cause of death in those aged 35-55. The incidence of breast cancer in women becomes substantial at age 30 and increases with age. Breast cancer rarely occurs in men.

The etiology of breast cancer is not known, but a variety of environmental and familial risk factors have been identified. Low risk is correlated with early pregnancy, multiple pregnancies, and castration at a young age, emphasizing the important role of hormonal factors. A history of breast cancer in close female relatives defines a high-risk population. Exposure to ionizing radiation is now widely accepted as a risk factor. Iatrogenic estrogen exposure has not been demonstrated to increase the risk of breast cancer. Demographic studies have shown a low incidence of breast cancer in Oriental women, yet studies of women of Japanese ancestry born in the United States show an incidence of breast cancer similar to that found in white American women. These studies tend to implicate other, as yet unidentified, environmental factors. Carcinoma of the breast is clearly caused by a virus in certain inbred mouse strains and is transmissible from generation to generation. Efforts to demonstrate a viral etiology of human breast cancer have not been successful to date.

Presenting Signs and Symptoms

Breast cancer almost always presents as a painless lump or mass in the breast. It is discovered by the patient in about one-half of cases, and in the other half it is found by the physician in the course of a routine physical examination. Lymph node enlargement in the ipsilateral axilla should be sought and is occasionally a presenting complaint. Many breast masses are, of course, not malignant. Characteristics that should raise suspicion of malignancy include hardness, immobility, ill-defined margins, dimpling of skin, or peau d'orange, and the presence of enlarged regional lymph nodes. An enlarged, painful, inflamed breast probably represents acute mastitis rather than malignancy, especially in a younger woman. However, it may be a presenting complaint of breast cancer, particularly of the highly malignant inflammatory variety. Any case of suspected mastitis that does not resolve completely and promptly with antibiotic therapy warrants suspicion of underlying carcinoma and further investigation. Discharge from a nipple, particularly when bloody, is a fairly frequent presenting complaint. An underlying mass is usually found on physical examination. Despite extensive efforts at public education, it is not rare for women to ignore breast masses. The physician may occasionally be confronted with a very large breast mass, often with ulceration of the skin, and sometimes with total destruction of the breast or automastectomy. A brief history will reveal that disease has been present for many months or even years.

Breast carcinoma may present occasionally with signs or symptoms of metastatic disease. The particular complaint will depend on which organ or organs are involved. Pain from metastatic bone disease is sometimes a presenting symptom, as is painless lymphadenopathy, usually in the axilla. When breast masses are not palpable in such patients, mammograms will sometimes reveal the primary lesion. Other presenting complaints of metastatic breast carcinoma include neurologic symptoms from brain metastases (limb weakness, hemiparesis, headache, personality change, somnolence), gastrointestinal complaints from metastatic carcinoma to the GI tract and particularly the stomach, and chest pain and/or dyspnea caused by malignant pleural effusion. When a woman presents with metastatic adenocarcinoma, a search should be made for an occult breast primary by physical examination and by mammography, because the therapy for advanced breast cancer is highly effective and differs from the treatment of other adenocarcinomas.

There has been controversy in recent years regarding mammorgraphic screening of asymptomatic women to detect subclinical breast carcinoma. Clinical studies have shown that nonpalpable carcinomas detected by mammography are almost always localized and rarely involve axillary lymph nodes. As a consequence, these early lesions usually have an excellent prognosis when resected surgically. However, concern has been expressed with regard to the radiation exposure of healthy women in the screened population. Newer mammographic techniques have substantially reduced radiation exposure; at present, routine mammographic screening is recommended for all women over 50 on a yearly basis. In addition, high risk patients—those with a previous breast cancer, with breast cancer in a close female relative, with severe fibrocystic disease making physical examination difficult, and with substantial previous radiation exposure—should probably be screened more intensively. In symptomatic women mammography is an extremely valuable diagnostic aid and should be employed without hesitation.

Diagnosis, Clinical Evaluation, and Staging

The diagnosis of breast carcinoma is made by biopsy and pathologic examination. In the past standard clinical practice was to do a biopsy and frozen section under general anesthesia and, if the specimen revealed carcinoma, to proceed immediately to a more extensive operation, often a radical mastectomy. More recently, surgeons have often chosen to obtain a biopsy specimen from suspicious breast masses under local anesthesia. This allows discussion of the diagnosis and proposed therapeutic plans with the patient. Mammograms of breast masses are helpful not only to confirm suspicion of malignancy, but also to aid in localization of lesions if biopsy under local anesthesia is selected. However, a negative mammogram does not exclude malignancy, and suspicious palpable lesions require biopsy regardless of mammographic findings.

If a breast mass is highly suspicious for malignancy or if biopsy proof of malignancy has been obtained, the history and physical examination should be repeated. A chest x-ray and screening laboratory evaluation of liver function are also recommended. A bone scan will occasionally reveal subclinical areas of metastatic bone involvement, but this is unusual in asymptomatic patients. If the history and physical examination reveal symptoms or signs of possible skeletal, hepatic, or central nervous system (CNS) metastatic involvement, these organs should be evaluated with appropriate isotope scans or other diagnostic radiologic procedures.

The most important staging information relates to the presence or absence of metastatic carcinoma in the ipsilateral axillary lymph nodes. This information, as well as data on the presence or absence of steroid hormone receptors in the tumor cells, will be obtained at surgery. The clinical staging of breast cancer is presented in Table 10. The importance of determining the presence or absence of metastases in axillary nodes is emphasized in the prognostic data presented in Table 11. Although postmenopausal women do slightly better on the whole than premenopausal women, the major negative prognostic factor is involvement of axillary lymph nodes with metastatic tumor, particularly when many nodes are involved. These data have important implications regarding selection of therapy. Steroid hormone receptor information has a major effect on management decisions and efforts to obtain tissue for analysis of estrogen, and, if possible, progesterone receptor content should be made not only at the time of primary surgical treatment but also if biopsy of subsequent recurrent local or metastatic lesions is undertaken.

Therapy and Complications

Surgery, radiation therapy, and systemic therapy by manipulation of hormones or by means of cytotoxic chemotherapy all offer valuable means of treatment for carcinoma of breast. Selection of therapy depends mainly on the stage of disease. Combinations of local and systemic therapeutic modalities are increasingly employed.

Surgical Therapy

Surgical resection is the most common initial therapy of carcinoma of the breast. Considerable controversy exists over which surgical procedure represents the most definitive therapy. Options vary from simple excisional biopsy to radical surgical procedures. The various operations and their definitions are outlined in Table 12. There is no convincing evidence that any operation listed in this table is superior in prolonging survival. Total mastectomy with axillary dissection is now widely recognized as current standard surgical therapy. Axillary dissection is necesary since the status of the axillary nodes is a highly important prognostic factor and determines, in part, whether additional or adjuvant therapy will be necessary. Extensive local disease may require a radical mastectomy for adequate surgical resection, although combined therapy consisting of more limited surgery followed by radiation offers an alternative. When a subclinical breast mass is found by mammography, a simple excision of the mass or of the quadrant of the breast containing the mass (partial mastectomy) is felt by some authorities to constitute adequate therapy. Newer local therapeutic approaches are directed at reducing the extent of surgery by combining excision of the tumor mass of area of the breast containing the tumor with radiaton therapy to the remaining breast tissue. Plastic surgical procedures have been developed to reconstruct breasts following cancer surgery in cases where cure appears likely.

Table 10. Clinical Staging of Breast Cancer

Stage I	Tumor confined within breast, no skin or muscle involvement; lymph nodes free of metastases
Stage II	Tumor confined within breast; no skin or muscle involvement; lymph nodes contain metastatic tumor
Stage III	Advanced local tumor, skin and/or muscle involved; lymph nodes may or may not contain metastatic tumor
Stage IV	Metastases to distant organs

Table 11. Prognostic Factors Influencing 5-year Disease Free Survival in Breast Cancer, Following Surgical Therapy[a]

Menopausal and Nodal Status	*Disease Free at 5 Years (%)*
All patients	60.3
Negative nodes	82.3
Positive nodes	24.9
1-3 positive	50
⩾ 4 positive	21.1
Premenopausal all patients	52.7
Negative nodes	78.8
Positive nodes	30.0
1-3 positive	54.2
⩾ 4 positive	13.9
Postmenopausal all patients	63.6
Negative nodes	83.6
Positive nodes	37.5
1-3 positive	48.3
⩾ 4 positive	25.9

[a] From data of Fisher (Surg Gyn Obstet 140:528, 1975)

Table 12. Surgical Options for Initial Therapy of Breast Cancer

Operation	*Definition*
Teilectomy or lumpectomy	Removal of malignant area from breast
Partial mastectomy	Removal of quadrant of breast containing tumor
Simple (total) mastectomy	Removal of entire breast
Modified radical mastectomy or simple mastectomy with axillary staging	Removal of entire breast and dissection and removal of ipsilateral axillary nodes
Radical Mastectomy	Removal of entire breast, pectoralis major, pectoralis minor, and dissection and removal of ipsilateral axillary nodes
Superradical mastectomy	Removal of entire breast, pectoralis major, pectoralis minor, and ipsilateral axillary and internal mammary nodes

Complications of surgical therapy relate to the interruption of lymphatics and blood vessels of the ipsilateral arm. Edema of the arm and hand, stiffness and pain in the arm and shoulder, and limitation of motion of the arm and shoulder are most commonly seen. These can be minimized with physical therapy. The more extensive the surgery, the more frequent and severe the complications become.

Radiation Therapy

Radiation therapy may be used as an alternative to surgery for control of local disease. It is particularly valuable in patients who are poor operative risks, who have very advanced local tumor that would require extensive surgery for complete resection, or who have inflammatory carcinoma. Radiation therapy is also helpful in the palliation of localized symptomatic metastatic disease such as skin recurrences, CNS metastases, or painful bone metastases.

Radiation therapy has been widely used for postoperative prophylactic treatment of breast cancer, especially when axillary nodes are found to be involved with metastatic tumor. Although postoperative radiation therapy in such patients does reduce the frequency of local tumor recurrence, survival is not prolonged. If postsurgical breast cancer patients are followed up regularly and local recurrences treated promptly with radiation therapy, control of local disease is as good as in the prophylactically irradiated patients. Routine postoperative radiation of breast cancer patients is unjustified.

Major complications of radiation therapy are similar to those of surgery and include edema, circulatory interference, and limitation of motion in the ipsilateral arm. Areas of lung included in radiation fields may become fibrotic in time; acute radiation pneumonitis is rare. Characteristic atrophic skin changes are universal in the radiated field. These follow an initial erythematous skin reaction, which subsides quickly following completion of therapy. Occasionally, a fibrous reaction to radiation, particularly in patients who have also had surgery, may cause a brachial plexus neuropathy with attendant pain and weakness in the ipsilateral arm and hand.

Systemic Therapy

Many patients with breast cancer will develop widespread metastatic disease requiring systemic therapy. While any organ may be involved with metastatic disease, the most common sites are skin, bone, lung, liver, and brain. Metastatic disease to bone may be widespread and yet compatible with survival for several years. In addition to palliative systemic therapy, local radiation therapy and, occasionally, orthopedic surgery for impending or actual pathologic fractures, may be necessary for good palliative management. Metastatic disease of the lung or liver is a more serious development, although on occasion prolonged survival is possible if response to systemic therapy is good. Brain metastases can be palliated with corticosteroid therapy to reduce symptoms caused by edema, but radiation therapy to the brain is required for good control. Breast cancer may metastasize to the GI tract and produce symptoms mimicking gastritis or ulcer disease. Adrenal metastases may, rarely, be so extensive that adrenal insufficiency results. Malignant pleural effusions produce pain and dyspnea. These are best managed by chest-tube drainage and instillation of agents such as quinacrine (Atabrine) or tetracycline to produce pleural sclerosis and prevent reaccumulation of fluid.

Hormonal Therapy

Hormonal manipulations are the oldest method of systemic therapy for breast cancer. Hormonal therapeutic options are outlined in Table 13. Before analysis of steroid hormone receptors became widely available, response to hormone therapy was difficult to predict; only about one-third of all patients responded to treatment. Steroid hormone receptors, usually measured as estrogen or progesterone receptors, are cytoplasmic proteins that bind to the hormone and facilitate transport of the hormone-receptor complex into the nucleus of the cell where DNA-directed RNA transcription is affected. If tumor tissue is positive for estrogen receptor, response to hormone manipulation will occur in 50-60% of patients; if both estrogen and progesterone receptors are present, response rates approaching 80% are reported. If steroid hormone receptors are absent in tumor tissue, responses to hormone therapy are rare, and systemic therapy with cytotoxic drugs should be employed. Hormonal therapy, either ablative or additive, is most useful in receptor-positive patients with metastatic disease involving mainly bone or soft tissue. Response of metastatic liver disease or lymphangitic pulmonary disease is less satisfactory. Because response to hormone treatment is often slow, cytotoxic drug therapy is preferred for patients with life-

Table 13. Hormonal Therapy Alternatives for Metastatic Breast Cancer in Steroid Hormone Receptor Positive Patients

Method	*Comment*
Premenopausal	
Ablative	
Oophorectomy	Surgery or radiation therapy
Tamoxifen	10 mg bid
Additive	
Androgens	Fluoxymesterone 10 mg tid
Postmenopausal	
Ablative	
Tamoxifen	10 mg bid
Additive	
Estrogen	Diethylstilbesterol 5 mg tid
Androgen	Fluoxymesterone 10 mg tid
Of occasional use at any age if other measures fail	
Adrenalectomy	Requires adrenal hormone replacement
Hypophysectomy	Requires adrenal and thyroid hormone replacement
Glucocorticoids	Prednisone or decadron
Progestins	Megace 40 mg qid
Aminoglutethimide	Chemical adrenalectomy, requires adrenal hormone replacement

threatening metastatic disease involving the liver, bone marrow, or lungs even if tumor tissue is receptor positive.

Newer hormonal agents have increased the available options in hormone therapy for breast cancer. Tamoxifen, a drug that blocks the action of estrogen at the cellular level, offers an alternative to ablative surgical procedures, especially adrenalectomy and hypophysectomy, avoiding the need for replacement adrenal hormone therapy (and thyroid hormone in the case of hypophysectomy) and having the clear advantage of reversibility. Aminoglutethimide, a drug that blocks adrenal steroid hormone synthesis, also is an alternative to ablative surgery but is more difficult to administer, has more side effects than tamoxifen, and also requires adrenal hormone replacement.

Studies of adjuvant hormonal therapy following surgical management of primary breast cancer have not shown a prolongation of survival. However, steroid hormone receptor-positive women may represent a subgroup that might benefit from adjuvant hormonal therapy. Studies of adjuvant hormonal therapy alone or in combination with cytotoxic drugs in receptor-positive patients will be necessary to determine the role of this approach.

Cytotoxic Chemotherapy

A variety of cytotoxic drugs demonstrate activity against breast cancer. The finding by investigators in the 1960s that intermittent combination chemotherapy could produce a high proportion of objective and subjective responses with acceptable toxicity in women with widespread metastatic breast cancer has led to an increasing role for chemotherapy. Introduction of new drugs such as doxorubicin (Adriamycin) and combinations of cytotoxic agents with hormones (androgens, prednisone) or tamoxifen have led to increasingly effective therapeutic regimens. Table 14 lists some of the established combinations of cytotoxic drugs for therapy of metastatic breast cancer as well as some promising but still investigational regimens.

Combination chemotherapy is the most dependable treatment for metastatic breast cancer and is capable of producing responses in 60-70% of patients. It is particularly useful in management of hepatic and pulmonary metastases, which often do not respond well to hormonal manipulations. Responses to chemotherapy are usually rapid, so this treatment is preferred in patients with life-threatening illness or when symptoms are widespread and very severe. It is not yet possible to predict which patients will respond to cytotoxic chemotherapy, and a therapeutic trial is necessary. Responsiveness to cytotoxic chemotherapy does not appear to be influenced by steroid hormone receptor content.

The greatest potential for use of combination chemotherapy lies in the adjuvant therapy of women at high risk (positive axillary nodes) of subclinical metastatic disease following mastectomy. Several studies have shown a survival advantage for premenopausal women treated with adjuvant chemotherapy following mastectomy. No definite benefit has been shown to date for postmenopausal women, although several studies are in progress using both hormonal and cytotoxic adjuvant therapy. Recent reappraisal of data from Milan (Bonadonna et al.) suggest that postmenopausal women may benefit from adjuvant chemotherapy if it is possible to treat them with full doses of cytotoxic drugs. These data need confirmation before adjuvant chemotherapy can be recommended routinely in stage II postmenopausal women. Adjuvant combination chemotherapy appears to be beneficial for women with inflammatory breast carcinoma following local therapy, usually with radiation.

Table 14. Combination Chemotherapeutic Regimens for Treatment of Breast Cancer

Established	
CMF	Cyclophosphamide 100 mg/m² orally day 1 → 14 5-fluorouracil 600 mg/m² IV day 1, day 8 Methotrexate 40 mg/m² IV day 1, day 8 –repeat every 4 weeks
CMFP	Same as CMF with prednisone 40 mg/m² orally day 1 → 14
CAF	Cyclophosphamide 100 mg/m² orally day 1 → 14 Adriamycin 30 mg/m² IV day 1, day 8 5-fluorouracil 500 mg/m² IV day 1, day 8 –repeat every 4 weeks
AV	Adriamycin 60 mg/m² IV day 1 Vincristine 1.2 mg/m² IV day 1 –repeat every 3 weeks
Investigational	
CMF-TAM	CMF regimen (above) with tamoxifen
CAF-TAM	CAF regimen (above) with tamoxifen
AVD-HEX	Adriamycin, vinblastine, DTIC, hexamethylmelamine
HOM	Hexamethylmelamine, vincristine, methotrexate

Side effects and toxicities of combination chemotherapy are usually acceptable but may be severe. Nausea, vomiting, fatigue, and alopecia are usually present to some extent. Myelosuppression represents the major potential toxicity and, if severe, may increase susceptibility to serious or even fatal infectious or bleeding complications. Combination cytotoxic drug therapy should be given by or under the supervision of specialists familiar with these complications and their management.

The advances made in the therapy of breast cancer in the past decade include:

- The introduction of new systemic therapies with hormone and cytotoxic agents
- A better ability to predict the response to hormonal therapy by measurement of steroid hormone receptors
- The ability to identify women at high risk of developing recurrent disease following mastectomy by examining the axillary nodes for the presence or absence of metastases
- Improved early detection by means of mammography
- The use of adjuvant therapeutic techniques combining surgery, radiation therapy, and systemic therapy in women at high risk

Clinical and laboratory studies currently in progress promise further improvements in future years.

CARCINOMA OF THE LUNG

Incidence and Etiology

Carcinoma of the lung represents a major public health problem in the United States, with approximately 117,000 new cases and 101,300 deaths in 1980. It accounts for 22% of all cancers in men and 6% of all cancers in women and is the most common cause of cancer deaths in men. The male/female incidence is about 3:1; however, this difference is narrowing with the increase in smoking by women. Over the past half century, lung cancer incidence and death rates have risen sharply and steadily, in large part related to the increase in cigarette smoking. The peak incidence is in the sixth decade; 90% of cases are diagnosed in patients between ages 40 and 80. Despite sophisticated diagnostic techniques and modern surgical management, the median survival from diagnosis remains less than 6 months; the overall 5-year survival is an appalling 8%.

The relationship of lung cancer to certain occupations and environmental exposures has been recognized since the fifteenth century, when miners in Saxony were noted to develop pulmonary problems. Later, radioactive radon gas encountered in uranium mines was identified as the causative agent. Other occupational exposures associated with an increased risk for lung cancer include arsenic, nickel, iron oxides, chromium, and asbestos. Asbestos increases the risk for bronchogenic carconoma 8-10 times in smokers without appreciably affecting nonsmokers.

Although animal studies and epidemiologic evidence implicate air pollution (with 3,4-benzpyrene, nickel, zinc, coal, and tar fumes) as a carcinogenic factor in lung cancer, without question the most important carcinogen for lung cancer is cigarette smoke. The evidence linking cigarette smoking to lung cancer is overwhelming and includes not only epidemiologic correlation (the incidence of lung cancer is three- to 25-fold greater among smokers than nonsmokers, depending on histologic type) but also induction of animal tumors by application of tobacco tar, the presence of 3,4-benzpyrene and other carcinogens in cigarette smoke and the finding of premalignant changes in the bronchial epithelium of heavy smokers. Emphasis on prevention of lung cancer could result in the saving of thousands of lives every year.

Pathology

Lung cancer is classified into four major pathologic types, as shown in Table 15. The relative incidence figures are only approximate for several reasons: difficulty arises in classifying the very anaplastic or undifferentiated tumors, small biopsies obtained at bronchoscopy or percutaneously pose technical problems and may not be representative of the tumor as a whole, mixed tumors including two or more of the histologic types have been encountered, and surgical series contain more patients with resectable tumors, especially squamous cell carcinomas, while in autopsy series the anaplastic small cell and adenocarcinomas predominate.

Each histologic type of lung cancer has a characteristic clinical and radiologic behavior pattern (Table 15). Squamous cell (or epidermoid) carcinoma arises centrally in the large bronchi, metastasizes late, and is the most common cell type in surgical series because of its relatively high resectability. It produces symptoms within the chest and is usually detected before distant spread has taken place. The 5-year survival rate is better than for any other cell type.

Adenocarcinomas of the lung usually occur as peripheral nodules and therefore may produce no symptoms until hematogenous dissemination has taken place. They may be associated with preexisting pulmonary scars. A subtype, bronchoalveolar carcinoma, may present initially with diffuse pulmonary involvement and copious mucoid secretions. These tumors have an increased incidence in patients with interstitial pulmonary fibrosis, such as occurs in scleroderma. Adenocarcinomas may be resectable if detected early and thus have an intermediate prognosis.

Large-cell carcinoma is a wastebasket category of anaplastic tumors that may represent undifferentiated squamous cell and adenocarcinomas. They tend to invade locally, disseminate widely, and behave in general like poorly differentiated squamous cell and adenocarcinomas.

Small-cell anaplastic (oat cell) carcinomas are probably related to carcinoid tumors and arise from neuroendocrine cells in the bronchial mucosa. These tumors are frequently

Table 15. Histologic and Radiologic Features of Lung Cancer

Histologic Type	*Approximate Frequency (%)*	*Characteristic Radiologic Findings*	*Cavitation*	*Mediastinal Adenopathy*	*Comments*
Squamous cell	40	Large hilar or perihilar mass	8-10%	Occasional	Atelectasis and postobstructive pneumonia; late metastases
Small-cell anaplastic	25	Large hilar mass	Uncommon	Very common	Early hematogenous dissemination, atelectasis and postobstructive pneumonia
Adenocarcinoma	15	Small peripheral nodule	Rare	Uncommon	Early hematogenous dissemination, scar carcinoma
Large-cell anaplastic	20	Large peripheral mass	Uncommon	Occasional	Intermediate propensity for metastasis

associated with hilar and mediastinal node involvement that may be massive at times; early hematogenous dissemination is almost invariable. Small-cell carcinomas are considered unresectable by definition since metastatic disease, even if not detected initially, rapidly follows diagnosis. These tumors have a very short survival but are remarkably sensitive to chemotherapy. For this reason lung cancers are commonly divided for clinical purposes into small-cell and non-small-cell types.

Clinical Features

The clinical manifestations of lung cancers include local effects of the primary tumor, effects due to invasion of adjacent tissues within the chest, symptoms due to distant metastases, and paraneoplastic syndromes. Only about 5% of patients are asymptomatic and thus diagnosed by routine chest x-ray examination. Because of the differing natural histories of the four histologic types it can be predicted, for example, that a patient with extensive local symptoms is likely to have squamous cell carcinoma, while a person with findings of widespread metastatic malignancy at the time of diagnosis is likely to have small-cell carcinoma. These clinicopathologic correlations have important implications for staging and therapy.

Clinical problems produced by the primary lung cancer itself include cough, hemoptysis, and bronchial obstruction with resulting atelectasis and postobstructive pneumonia. Local invasion may cause chest pain, rib destruction, pleural effusion, and dysphagia due to esophageal compression. Pericardial effusion, tamponade, and arrhythmias may indicate cardiac involvement, while superior vena cava syndrome results from invasion or extrinsic compression of the superior vena cava. Vocal cord paralysis with hoarseness follows invasion of the recurrent laryngeal nerve (more commonly on the left) and an elevated hemidiaphragm occurs due to phrenic nerve involvement. Pancoast's syndrome, associated with a tumor in the apex of the lung (squamous cell or adenocarcinoma), includes severe neuritic pain due to invasion of the lower brachial plexus roots, Horner's syndrome (ptosis, miosis, enophthalmos, and decreased sweating on the ipsilateral side of the face) due to involvement of sympathetic nerves, and destruction of the upper ribs and vertebral bodies.

It is important to remember that many patients with lung cancer, especially those with small-cell carcinoma and adenocarcinomas, first present with metastatic tumor without any chest symptoms. Bone pain, jaundice, hepatomegaly or liver failure, pancytopenia with thrombocytopenic hemorrhage, and seizure or other neurologic manifestation may be the initial findings in many patients. Lymphadenopathy, soft tissue masses, or skin lesions occasionally are presenting complaints. In these patients, biopsy of the metastatic lesion yields the diagnosis of cancer and chest x-ray examination suggests the lung as the primary site.

A bewildering variety of remote effects of malignancy or paraneoplastic syndromes occur in association with lung cancers and other tumors and are discussed in a subsequent section. One in particular, hypertrophic pulmonary osteoarthropathy (HPO), is most often associated with intrathoracic neoplasms. This syndrome is characterized by clubbing of the fingers, synovitis, and pain in the distal ends of the long bones due to periosteal new bone formation. The pathogenesis of HPO is not understood. The disease usually responds dramatically to successful treatment of the underlying tumor. Failing this, anti-inflammatory agents may be employed.

Diagnosis and Evaluation

The diagnosis of carcinoma of the lung is usually straightforward and requires pathologic examination of tissue obtained from the primary tumor or a metastatic site. Sputum cytology is a simple noninvasive diagnostic tool with a high degree of accuracy, even for cell-type identification. It is most useful for central lesions. Fiberoptic bronchoscopy with biopsy or bronchial washings yields a diagnosis in a high proportion of patients and has a very low complication rate. Peripheral lung tumors are best approached with percutaneous needle aspiration biopsy under fluoroscopic monitoring. Pneumothorax commonly follows this procedure but usually resolves spontaneously.

If a diagnosis cannot be made using one of the above procedures and if no evidence of metastictic disease is present (which might be readily biopsied), scalene node biopsy, mediastinoscopy, and, ultimately, thoracotomy may be necessary to obtain a tissue diagnosis. These more invasive procedures also yield important information on the presence or absence of lymph node involvement and thus on the feasibility of surgical resection for cure.

Once a diagnosis of lung cancer has been made, three questions must be answered sequentially: are there distant metastases? If not, is the patient operable; and, if so, is the tumor resectable? A thorough history and detailed physical examination will detect most metastases or suggest the need for further studies. Screening blood chemistries and CBC may indicate the need for liver or bone scanning. Computed tomography (CT) of the brain in the absence of neurologic signs or symptoms is rarely rewarding, except perhaps for small-cell carcinoma. Bone marrow aspiration and biopsy reveal a high incidence of bone marrow invasion in small-cell carcinoma but are not indicated for the other histologic types.

If no metastases are detected, the patient is a potential candidate for surgery (except in the case of small-cell carcinoma). Medical operability must be assessed with thorough evaluations, especially of the cardiovascular and respiratory systems. In many lung cancer patients, particularly heavy smokers, the presence of severe chronic obstructive pulmonary disease makes major surgery in general, and pulmonary resection in particular, impossible. Pulmonary function tests and arterial blood gases help determine whether the patient can survive the operation or be rendered a respiratory cripple by it.

Assuming the tumor is localized to the chest and the patient is medically operable, the physician and the surgeon must then decide whether the tumor is resectable. Most authorities state that mediastinal node metastases (except perhaps with certain squamous cell carcinomas), contralateral hilar node metastases, malignant pleural effusion, superior vena cava obstruction, and phrenic or recurrent laryngeal nerve paralysis represent contraindications to surgery. Ipsilateral hilar node involvement undoubtedly worsens the prognosis, but most surgeons recommend resections for these patients. In the past, about 50% of patients coming to thoracotomy were found to have unresectable tumors at the time of surgery. With the use of preoperative mediastinoscopy to reject those patients with mediastinal involvement, the resectability rate at subsequent thoracotomy rises to 85-95%. Scalene node biopsy may be used as an alternative to mediastinoscopy for determination of unresectability when palpable adenopathy is present, but the yield from scalene node biopsy is extremely low when nodes are not palpable.

Treatment

Non-Small-Cell Lung Cancer

Surgery is the treatment of choice for resectable lung cancers. The 5-year survival of all patients who have undergone lung tumor resection is 25% irrespective of the cell type and extent of surgery. Resected patients with lymph node involvement have a 5-year survival (16%), only about one-half that of patients without nodal metastases (34%). Most deaths occur in the first 2 postoperative years, after which the survival curve tends to level off. Most patients die with both local recurrence and distant dissemination. Squamous cell carcinoma has the highest resectability rate and 5-year survival, followed in order by adenocarcinoma and large-cell anaplastic carcinoma.

Because the survival rate following resection is poor, the use of adjuvant radiation therapy and chemotherapy has been explored. Neither preoperative nor postoperative radiotherapy has improved survival when compared with surgery alone in prospective randomized trials. The only exception is in Pancoast's tumors, in which radiation therapy followed by surgery seems to be the optimal approach. In other situations there is no benefit of adjuvant radiation therapy to the resectable patient with non-small-cell lung cancer.

Adjuvant chemotherapy for patients with resectable non-small-cell lung cancer has also proved disappointing to date. In several prospective randomized trials the use of postoperative chemotherapy with various single agents did not improve the survival compared with surgery alone; in some instances, it was actually harmful. Nevertheless, trials of new single agents and combinations in the adjuvant setting continue in the hope of improving the surgical cure rate. Early results with adjuvant BCG immunotherapy in patients with very early stage lung cancer have been encouraging, and additional studies of various types of immunotherapy in lung cancer are in progress.

The treatment of patients with unresectable non-small-cell carcinoma with tumor limited to the chest is a subject of controversy. Radiation therapy has an unquestioned role in these patients for the palliation of disturbing symptoms such as cough, hemoptysis, chest pain, superior vena cava obstruction, and so forth. The controversy arises over the use of immediate radiation therapy in asymptomatic, inoperable patients. Supporters of immediate radiation therapy contend that in selected patients such treatment may result in a prolongation of suvival. Opponents point out, however, that immediate treatment does not seem to prolong survival or delay the onset of symptoms. They suggest that palliation is best accomplished by withholding radiation until required to relieve symptoms caused by progressive tumor. This course would also avoid unnecessary radiation to a large group of patients who die of widespread dissemination without developing local chest symptoms. On balance, the bulk of the evidence favors the second alternative, that is, withholding treatment until symptoms develop, although this question is still open and under continuing investigation.

Radiation therapy is also indicated for palliation of painful bony metastases and for brain metastases. There is no indication for radiation to the primary tumor in patients with distant metastases, unless there are symptoms related to the disease in the chest.

Chemotherapy for non-small-cell lung cancer has a limited role at present. Response rates are relatively low and prolongation of survival only minimal at best. Nevertheless, a trial of chemotherapy is indicated for patients with symptomatic metastatic disease in the hope of achieving a palliative response. A number of single agents, including alkylating agents, methotrexate, Adriamycin, nitrosoureas, cis-platinum, and others, are active against non-small-cell cancer. Combinations of active single agents are also in use, and considerable research effort is being directed toward finding new agents and combinations that may improve the response rate and overall survival for this very large group of patients.

Small-Cell Lung Cancer

Because of its very different biologic behavior and high sensitivity to chemotherapy and radiation therapy, small-cell carcinoma must be considered separately from the other types of lung cancer. The clinical onset of small-cell carcinoma is usually sudden, reflecting the rapid doubling time of this tumor. Early hematogenous dissemination is almost invariable and over 80% of patients have extrathoracic metastases at the time of diagnosis. Even in patients without evidence of metastatic disease who undergo curative resections, 95% of those dying within 30 days of surgery are found to have distant metastases at autopsy. For this reason, a local therapeutic modality, such as surgery or radiation, cannot be expected to cure the disease or even to prolong survival significantly.

The pattern of metastatic spread of small-cell carcinoma has some bearing on its treatment. Over 30% of patients develop brain metastases before death and, in about one-third of these patients, the brain is involved at the time of diagnosis. Many authorities have employed brain irradiation as part of the initial management of patients with small-cell carcinoma (as is done in the treatment of acute lymphocytic leukemia in children) in an attempt to delay or avoid the neurologic complications of CNS metastases.

Liver involvement occurs in over 40% of patients and is often present at diagnosis. Extensive pretreatment staging evaluation including percutaneous liver biopsy and peritoneoscopy have been employed by some groups to detect liver metastases. The use of liver scanning for this purpose is inadvisable because of the numerous false-positive results and the inability of the technique to detect small (<2-3 cm) tumor deposits. Liver involvement is a poor prognostic sign.

Bone marrow involvement, which may be present without

any abnormality in the peripheral blood picture, also occurs in over 40% of these patients. Unlike other solid tumors, small-cell carcinoma in the bone marrow may be detected by bone marrow aspiration as well as by biopsy; both procedures are recommended. Extensive marrow replacement by tumor may compromise the patient's ability to tolerate subsequent myelotoxic chemotherapy.

Bony metastases from small-cell carcinoma may be of either the osteolytic or osteoblastic variety. A pretreatment bone scan is an essential part of the staging evaluation. It is important to recognize vertebral body involvement, which may lead to spinal cord compression by extradural tumor with consequent neurologic deficits. This constitutes a medical emergency and requires immediate myelography and treatment with radiation therapy.

Metastatic involvement with small-cell carcinoma may occur in almost any organ or tissue. Skin and lymph node metastases are frequent. Retroperitoneal lymph node involvement with pancreatic invasion and clinical acute pancreatitis has been reported. Meningeal carcinomatosis may be a late event with severe neurologic consequences. At autopsy, massive widespread tumor involvement is usually found.

Staging is important in terms of prognosis for small-cell carcinoma. Patients with disease limited to the chest (limited disease) have a better prognosis than those with extrathoracic metastases (extensive disease), irrespective of treatment. Performance status (a measure of the degree of general debility the patient suffers) is also an important prognostic variable. Age, sex, and subtle distinctions in tumor histologic type have no influence on prognosis in this disease. The specific pattern of metastatic disease and its extent are undoubtedly important for prognosis. Detailed information on this point is being collected.

Like other rapidly growing tumors such as Burkitt's lymphoma and acute leukemia, small-cell carcinoma is markedly sensitive to multiple chemotherapeutic agents (Table 16). The combination of active single agents (Table 17) results in improved response rates and prolonged survivals in this disease. Currently, combination chemotherapy is the basic element in treatment of both limited and extensive small-cell carcinoma of the lung and has resulted in median survivals of 1 year or more in some series. More importantly, long-term disease-free survival has been achieved in a small proportion of patients, including some with widespread disease, leading to the belief among many oncologists that this disease is potentially curable.

Table 16. Chemotherapeutic Agents with Activity Against Small-Cell Carcinoma of the Lung

Cyclophosphamide
Adriamycin
Methotrexate
Vincristine
VP-16
CCNU
Hexamethylmelamine
Procarbazine

Table 17. Examples of Some Commonly Used Drug Combinations in Small-Cell Carcinomas of the Lung

Regimen	*Response Rate (%)*
Cyclophosphamide, vincristine, methotrexate	68
Cyclophosphamide, vincristine, methotrexate, CCNU	78
Cyclophosphamide, methotrexate, CCNU	75
Cyclophosphamide, vincristine, Adriamycin, methotrexate	83
Cyclophosphamide, vincristine, Adriamycin	75

The role of radiation in the treatment of either limited or extensive small-cell carcinoma has come into question. It is not clear whether the combined modality approach including both radiation therapy and chemotherapy offers any survival advantage over the use of chemotherapy alone; the studies to date have yielded conflicting results. There is little doubt, however, that irradiated patients have a decreased tolerance to chemotherapy and an increased incidence of side effects. The appropriate use of radiotherapy in conjunction with chemotherapy remains to be determined.

Several important points about small-cell carcinoma of the lung are worthy of reemphasis:

1. Small-cell carcinoma of the lung is a highly malignant tumor that is almost invariably metastatic at the time of diagnosis.
2. Surgery is contraindicated if a tissue diagnosis can be made without a thoracotomy.
3. Without treatment the median survival is approximately 6 weeks; with combination chemotherapy, with or without radiation therapy, median survivals in excess of 1 year have been achieved.
4. Long-term disease-free survivals are occasionally obtained, even in patients with widespread disease, suggesting that small-cell carcinoma of the lung is a potentially curable tumor.
5. The incidence of small-cell carcinoma would fall dramatically in only 1-2 decades if cigarette smoking were to cease immediately.

MESOTHELIOMA

Incidence and Etiology

Pleural mesothelioma is a rare tumor originating from the surface lining or mesothelium of the pleura. Mesotheliomas may arise from other serosal surfaces such as the peritoneum or pericardium, but the pleural origin is the most common. The incidence is low, about two to three per million population in the United States and England but appears to be rising, due in part to improved recognition of the disease, and in part to a true increase in frequency, probably related to asbestos exposure. Among persons exposed to asbestos, the incidence of mesothelioma is 300 times greater than that in the general population. The greater the duration and intensity of the exposure, the greater the risk for mesothelioma, usually 25-50 years after first exposure.

Pathology

Mesotheliomas may be either solitary or diffuse. Solitary mesotheliomas are localized, encapsulated, and generally cured with surgery. Diffuse mesotheliomas occur as multiple nodules on the pleura and tend to form a large encasing plaque that, in advanced cases, compresses the entire lung. Microscopically the tumor may have epithelial or mesenchymal (sarcomatous) features or a mixture of the two.

Clinical Features

Dyspnea, weight loss, chest pain, and cough are the most common symptoms of mesothelioma. Eventually intractable chest pain develops in most patients, due to direct infiltration of the chest wall. Marked cachexia and respiratory failure are frequent findings in the terminal stages.

Physical findings include signs of pleural fluid in the involved hemithorax, bulging of intercostal spaces, and displacement of the trachea and mediastinum. Clubbing, Horner's syndrome, and supraclavicular or axillary adenopathy also may occur. Chest x-ray films reveal unilateral pleural effusion, pleural thickening, and often signs of asbestosis. Cytologic examination of aspirated pleural fluid may yield malignant cells, but open thoracotomy is generally required for a definitive diagnosis.

Treatment

Regardless of treatment diffuse mesothelioma is invariably fatal and survival after diagnosis averages only 8-10 months. Surgery is often necessary for diagnosis but has little therapeutic benefit due to the widespread and invasive nature of the tumor. External radiation offers symptomatic palliation in many cases but no survival benefit, although some investigators suggest that very high-dose irradiation may prolong survival. Intrapleural radioactive colloidal gold (^{198}Au) has been used to control pleural effusion with long-term success in a few cases. The role of chemotherapy in mesothelioma has not been studied extensively, but several agents including Adriamycin, alkylating agents, and 5-fluorouracil appear to have activity. Early reports with combination chemotherapy are encouraging, and combined modality treatment including surgical pleurectomy, external radiation, and chemotherapy has had early success.

GASTROINTESTINAL MALIGNANCIES

CANCER OF THE COLON AND RECTUM

Incidence and Etiology

According to American Cancer Society estimates, over 114,000 new cases of colorectal cancer occurred in the United States in 1980; 5% of Americans can be expected to develop the disease. Of all cancers in Americans, 15% are of colorectal origin; this disease is the second most common cause of cancer deaths in both men and women. The overall 5-year survival rate of 25% has not improved over the past 25 years and probably will not improve until methods for earlier detection are available.

The etiology of colon cancer is unknown, but epidemiologic evidence implicates dietary factors. The disease, common in industrialized societies and less frequent in underdeveloped nations, may be related to dietary fat intake. One suggested mechanism to explain the role of dietary fat involves the production of carcinogens from bile acids and other metabolites by the action of gut flora. The level of fat intake affects the type of bile acids produced and the composition of bacterial flora. Animal experiments confirm the role of high-fat diets in producing colon tumors.

A variety of preexisting colonic conditions predispose to the development of cancer. Adenomatous polyps greater than 2 cm in diameter have a significant risk of undergoing malignant degeneration. Over one-half of all villous adenomas contain foci of malignant degeneration and, therefore, require resection when discovered. Both familial colonic polyposis and Gardner's syndrome (colonic polyposis associated with osteomas, fibromas, and lipomas) have essentially a 100% probability of colonic cancer in affected patients; for this reason prophylactic total colectomy is indicated. Both ulcerative colitis and Crohn's colitis predispose to colonic carcinoma that may be very difficult to recognize and to treat.

Pathology

Carcinomas occur more frequently in the distal portion of the colon. Seventy percent involve the rectum, sigmoid, and descending colon; 15% the transverse colon; and 15% the cecum and ascending colon. Over one-half of all colorectal cancers are within reach of the sigmoidoscope. The histology of colorectal cancer is almost always adenocarcinoma, although squamous cell carcinomas occur in the anus.

The gross pathologic appearance of colorectal carcinomas varies and has an important effect on symptoms. Cancers of the cecum and ascending colon tend to be large polypoid masses with little intramural invasion, while tumors of the descending and sigmoid colon generally occur as constricting annular lesions with considerable fibrous tissue. Rectal cancers may be bulky, friable, polypoid lesions or ulcerating, invasive lesions.

Table 18. Dukes Classification of Colon Cancer

	Dukes Stage	*5-Year Survival (%)*
A	Confined to mucosa and submucosa	74-100
B_1	Penetration into muscularis	64
B_2	Extension through serosa	40-60
C	Regional lymph node involvement	~20
D	Involvement of adjacent organs or distant metastases	~5

Dukes, in 1932, observed that the prognosis of colon cancer is dependent on the degree of tumor penetration through the colonic wall; this observation led to a pathologic staging system that bears his name (Table 18). The size of the tumor, presence of vascular invasion, and degree of differentiation seem to have little independent prognostic significance. Mucinous carcinomas, however, have a worse prognosis than the more common nonmucinous variety. At the time of initial surgery 40-70% of patients have regional lymph node metastases (Dukes C) and 15-25% have liver metastases (Dukes D).

Clinical Features

Tumors in the cecum and ascending colon may remain clinically silent for long periods since they rarely cause obstruction or obvious bleeding. Right-sided colon lesions may present with anemia due to occult gastrointestinal blood loss or with a palpable abdominal mass. Pain, often described as cramping or colicky, eventually occurs in the majority of patients with right-sided tumors. Weight loss is also common.

Cancers of the left colon, which tend to be annular and constricting, often present with symptoms related to obstruction, pain, or change in bowel habits. Gross rectal bleeding is common, especially with rectal cancers. Pain with rectal cancers is generally a late phenomenon associated with extensive local infiltration of tumor.

Physical examination of the colon cancer patient usually reveals either gross or occult rectal bleeding, an abdominal mass, or a rectal lesion on digital examination. Evidence of metastatic disease, namely hepatomegaly or supraclavicular adenopathy, may also be detected on physical exam.

Diagnosis

When the history and physical examination suggest carcinoma of the colon, sigmoidoscopy and colonoscopy with biopsy of any suspicious lesion should be the next step. A careful barium enema, with air-contrast examination as well, is important in order to define the location and extent of the lesion and to detect additional synchronous lesions. Before any attempt at curative surgery is undertaken, a chest x-ray examination and liver function tests should be obtained to screen for metastases. Routine use of radionuclide liver scanning for this purpose is unwarranted because of the high false-positive and false-negative rates with this procedure. In patients with normal liver size by physical examination and normal chemical tests of liver function, the liver scan is unlikely to detect metastases that, if present, are probably smaller than the limits of resolution of the technique. In such cases, careful examination of the liver under direct vision and multiple liver biopsies at the time of laparotomy are necessary to determine whether liver metastases are present. Since spread to the bone is uncommon, screening bone scans also are not recommended unless specific symptoms or findings suggest that bony metastases have occurred.

Carcinoembryonic antigen (CEA) is not useful in the diagnosis of colon cancer since a normal level does not exclude the diagnosis, and an elevated level may be encountered with other benign and malignant conditions. Under some circumstances, following the CEA level after treatment may give clinically useful information.

Treatment

Surgery is the only potentially curative treatment for colon cancer and should follow diagnosis as quickly as possible. Even in the presence of metastatic disease, surgery is often advisable for palliation: to relieve or prevent obstruction, to reduce severe pain or bleeding, and to ameliorate disabling diarrhea and tenesmus. Preoperative radiotherapy for cancers of the rectum and rectosigmoid, followed by abdominal-perineal resection, has been shown to increase the 5-year survival when compared with surgery alone. Postoperative radiation for rectal and rectosigmoid lesions also may be effective and is currently under study. Radiation is also indicated for the palliative treatment of locally recurrent tumors and painful bony metastases.

Despite 25 years of intensive study, chemotherapy for advanced colon cancer or for earlier cases in the surgical adjuvant setting has not resulted in a clear prolongation of patient survival. Nevertheless, chemotherapy has a definite role in palliation of advanced symptomatic disease and is undergoing further testing as adjuvant treatment. The most active agent is 5-fluorouracil with a 20% response rate; the nitrosoureas and mitomycin C also have some activity. Combination chemotherapy has achieved improved response rates in some reports, but others indicate no benefit with this approach. Improved survival in advanced colon cancer must await introduction of more effective cytotoxic agents.

Clinical Course

Despite numerous surgical efforts to prevent it, local recurrence remains a major problem in patients with colorectal cancer. Local recurrence may be the only site of relapse, or it may accompany disseminated disease. Distant metastasis without local recurrence also occurs. Locally recurrent tumor generally produces severe pain and bleeding related to invasion of the bladder, vagina, or perineum. Intra-abdominal abscesses may occur and present difficult problems in management.

Metastatic disease involves the liver and lungs most commonly, but bone and brain can also be involved. Liver metastases often produce nausea, vomiting, jaundice, right upper quadrant pain, and ascites. Hepatic failure is not an uncommon cause of death among these patients. Pulmonary metastases appear as multiple macronodules and only occasionally cause respiratory symptoms.

Patients with metastatic or recurrent disease have a median survival of 5-7 months with only 10% surviving more than 18 months. Progression of the disease is generally rapid and inexorable, although transient improvement following chemotherapy may occur.

GASTRIC CARCINOMA

Incidence and Etiology

Gastric carcinoma is one of the leading causes of cancer deaths worldwide and a major public health problem in Japan, where more than 50% of all malignancies in men arise in the stomach.

In the United States, adenocarcinoma of the stomach accounts for about 10% of all cancer deaths; 23,000 new cases were detected in 1980. For reasons entirely unknown, the incidence of gastric cancer in the United States has been declining steadily for the past half century; in 1930, the age-adjusted death rate for gastric cancer was 28.9 per 100,000, and by 1967 it had fallen to 9.7 per 100,000. A similar decline has taken place in Australia, Canada, and England. The incidence in Japan is about 8 times the U.S. rate. Other areas of high incidence include central Europe, Finland, Iceland, West Germany, Chile, and parts of the Soviet Union. Japanese immigrants to the United States have a progressively lower incidence of gastric cancer as their duration of U.S. residence increases, suggesting that environmental rather than hereditary factors are responsible for gastric cancer. Although no definite gastric carcinogen has been identified, a variety of dietary substances have been implicated including smoked meats and fish, saki, moldy soybean products (aflatoxin), smoked tortillas, and so forth.

Several benign gastric conditions are thought to predispose to gastric carcinoma. Pernicious anemia with its associated gastric achlorhydria is a well-known risk factor. Pernicious anemia patients have an incidence of gastric cancer 22 times that of the general population. Benign gastric ulcer, once generally but erroneously accepted as a risk factor, now appears to have no relationship to subsequent gastric malignancy. No conclusive evidence of a cause-and-effect relationship between gastric cancer and chronic atrophic gastritis or gastric adenoma exists, but the issue is unresolved. Diffuse gastric polyposis is definitely a premalignant lesion.

Gastric cancer in the United States is a disease of the elderly. Sixty percent of cases arise in the 60-70 age group and only 5% of patients are younger than 40. Men outnumber women by a ratio of 3:2.

Pathology

Although lymphomas and sarcomas may arise in the stomach and metastases from breast cancer and melanoma occasionally may involve the gastric mucosa, the vast majority of gastric cancers are adenocarcinomas. Most carcinomas occur in the antrum and along the lesser curvature. Seventy-five percent of gastric cancers ulcerate and are often indistinguishable from benign gastric ulcer on inspection; 10% are polypoid, 5% superficially spreading, and 10% scirrhous, characterized by an intense desmoplastic reaction. Scirrhous tumors may be localized or may involve the entire stomach producing a thickened, stiff appearance termed leather bottle or linitis plastica. Microscopically, gastric cancers vary widely in their degree of anaplasia. Some tumors have easily recognizable glands with obvious mucin production. In others, no glands can be identified and mucin is absent. The degree of anaplasia, or grade, is correlated with the prognosis.

Gastric cancer spreads by direct extension into the omentum, pancreas, transverse colon, liver, esophagus, and biliary tree. Regional lymph nodes are involved frequently and distant nodal metastases to the left supraclavicular node (Virchow's node), axillary, and inguinal nodes may also occur. Hematogenous dissemination most often involves the liver and liver metastases are present at the time of surgery in 30% of patients. Lung, bone, brain, bone marrow, and cutaneous metastases also occur. Peritoneal implantation is another mode of spread and may result in malignant ascites, Krukenberg's tumors (ovarian metastases), tumor in the prerectal pouch, and bowel obstruction.

Clinical Features

Abdominal pain is the most common complaint among patients with gastric cancer. In some cases the pain is similar to that of peptic ulcer disease, but more often it is a vague upper abdominal discomfort. Anorexia, nausea, vomiting, and weight loss are also common features. If tumor involves the cardia or extends into the esophagus, dysphagia may be a prominent symptom.

Symptoms related to metastatic disease may be the initial complaint. Jaundice, bone pain, ascites, pelvic pain, bowel obstruction, neurologic problems, respiratory difficulties, or pancytopenia due to marrow involvement may be the first manifestation of gastric cancer or may occur later with disease progression. On examination epigastric tenderness or a mass may be noted and findings related to metastatic spread may be detected. Laboratory findings are nonspecific and rarely helpful in making the diagnosis.

Diagnosis

Roentgenographic examination of the stomach, including fluoroscopy, is the method of diagnosis in most cases and will detect gastric cancer in 90% of symptomatic patients. The distinction between benign and malignant gastric ulcers is particularly difficult, however, and frequently requires further study: either repeat x-ray films showing ulcer healing as evidence of benign disease or gastroscopy with biopsy. All cases of gastric cancer detected radiographically require biopsy confirmation, generally obtained at gastroscopy.

An evaluation for metastatic disease should follow the diagnosis and precede surgery. In most cases, a physical examination and history are sufficient to indicate whether metastases are present. Further workup should include a chest x-ray, liver function tests, bone scan, and careful examination of the peripheral blood smear for evidence of myelophthisic anemia. Routine liver scanning is not recommended for the reasons discussed above.

Treatment

Surgery is the only curative approach to gastric cancer, but, unfortunately, only about one-half of all patients are eligible for potentially curative resections. The 5-year survival rate for this disease is a dismal 5-15% that has not improved in the past 3 decades. Radiation therapy has little role in the treatment of unresectable gastric carcinoma. The use of radiation therapy in this disease is limited to the palliative treatment of painful bony metastases. Patients with unresectable gastric cancer generally progress rapidly to death within 4-6 months on the average.

Several chemotherapeutic agents, including 5-fluorouracil,

mitomycin C, doxorubicin, and lomustine are active in gastric carcinoma. Objective response rates range between 20 and 30%. Combinations of active single agents appear in some reports to give higher response rates, but remissions are generally brief and survival curves unaltered. Trials of chemotherapy in the surgical adjuvant setting have, as yet, yielded no convincing evidence of benefit.

PANCREATIC CARCINOMA

Pancreatic carcinoma is as common as gastric carcinoma in the United States, but its incidence has been steadily and inexplicably increasing. The etiology is unknown, and no clear-cut risk factors have been identified. Most pancreatic cancers are adenocarcinomas; rarely, squamous cell carcinomas and adenoacanthomas are recognized. Islet cell carcinomas of the pancreas are discussed later.

Clinical Features

Abdominal pain, weight loss, and obstructive jaundice are the most common presenting symptoms of pancreatic carcinoma and develop eventually in almost all patients. Pain may precede other signs and symptoms and, especially if radiation to the back is a prominent feature, may be mistaken for intervertebral disk disease. Tumors of the head of the pancreas (75% of cases) cause obstruction of the common bile duct in 75-90% of patients and the resulting jaundice is unrelentingly progressive. Painless jaundice, long described as characteristic of carcinoma of the head of the pancreas, is in fact uncommon; in most patients, pain precedes the first evidence of jaundice. Painless jaundice should suggest carcinoma of the ampulla of Vater or of the bile ducts. Carcinoma of the head of the pancreas may also be responsible for massive gastrointestinal hemorrhage due to tumor erosion into the duodenum, or for the development of steatorrhea secondary to obstruction of the pancreatic duct and consequent impairment of fat digestion.

Carcinomas involving the body and tail of the pancreas generally produce severe pain with radiation to the back. Jaundice is uncommon unless extensive liver metastases have occurred. Gastrointestinal bleeding may result from tumor erosion into the stomach or colon and from esophageal varices secondary to portal hypertension produced by tumor invading the portal vein. Splenomegaly caused by tumor invasion of the splenic vein also may occur.

Physical examination generally reveals evidence of weight loss, jaundice, and severe pain. Hepatomegaly may be detected if liver metastases are extensive, and enlargement of the gallbladder, found at surgery in almost every patient, can be recognized on physical exam in perhaps 30-50% of patients. A palpable upper abdominal mass representing the primary tumor may be noted and splenomegaly may be present. Lymphadenopathy in the cervical and supraclavicular regions is evidence of metastatic spread. Pancreatic carcinoma metastasizes early and widely. In addition to local extension, tumor may involve the lung, liver, bone, brain, and peritoneum producing malignant ascites.

Blood chemical findings frequently are abnormal in patients with pancreatic carcinoma but rarely of diagnostic utility. Although the presence of hyperglycemia and elevated amylase or lipase are suggestive, they are neither invariably observed nor specific for pancreatic cancer.

Diagnosis

When carcinoma of the pancreas is suspected on clinical grounds an abdominal CT scan and ultrasound examination of the pancreas are probably the most useful diagnostic procedures. These methods can confirm the presence of extrahepatic biliary obstruction, detect gallstones (ultrasound), and ascertain whether a pancreatic mass is present (CT is more accurate in assessing the body and tail of the pancreas). Some authorities also recommend percutaneous transhepatic cholangiography to examine the extent of common bile duct involvement, especially if surgery to bypass the biliary obstruction is contemplated. Endoscopic retrograde cholangiopancreatography (ERCP) may be useful especially for small tumors in the head of the pancreas or for carcinomas of the ampulla of Vater and biliary tree. In the past an upper gastrointestinal series, hypotonic duodenography, pancreatic angiography, and selenomethionine pancreatic scanning were widely used for the evaluation of suspected pancreatic malignancies, but these techniques have been largely supplanted by CT and ultrasound in most centers today.

Tissue confirmation of a characteristic radiographic or ultrasound picture is essential. If liver metastases are present, a percutaneous liver biopsy may be the most direct method to obtain a tissue diagnosis. If a pancreatic mass is readily observed by CT or ultrasound, a percutaneous needle aspiration biopsy of the mass under CT or ultrasound guidance is a safe and useful technique that may obviate exploratory surgery. In other cases, exploratory laparotomy may be necessary to obtain a tissue diagnosis.

Treatment

The treatment of pancreatic carcinoma is far from satisfactory; this is reflected in the appalling 5-year survival rate of less than 1%. Curative surgical resections are possible only in about 10-25% of patients with carcinoma of the head of the pancreas who come to exploration; the operative morbidity and mortality of pancreatoduodenectomy (Whipple procedure) may be significant. Carcinomas of the body and tail of the pancreas are rarely, if ever, diagnosed early enough to permit surgical treatment with curative intent.

Although surgical cure is rarely possible, many patients with carcinoma of the head of the pancreas can benefit from surgical palliation by means of biliary diversion and gastroenterostomy. Radiation therapy for unresectable pancreatic tumors appears to be ineffective. Chemotherapy may play a role in palliative treatment. Several agents including 5-fluorouracil, doxorubicin, mitomycin C, and streptozotocin have limited activity; when used singly or in combination they occasionally offer symptomatic relief.

Despite the lack of a definitive treatment modality for most patients, supportive measures must not be ignored. Adequate narcotic analgesics are essential, and liberal doses by parenteral routes if necessary are the cornerstone of effective palliation. Pancreatic insufficiency with resultant steatorrhea can be treated with pancreatic enzyme replacement (e.g., Viokase) and medium-chain triglycerides that provide an absorbable source of nutrition. Pruritus secondary to biliary obstruction is often at least relieved partially with oral cholestyramine, a resin that binds bile salts in the gut reducing circulating levels.

PRIMARY CARCINOMA OF THE LIVER

Incidence and Etiology

Primary hepatic cancers are rare in the West but common in many parts of Africa and the Far East. Approximately 90% arise from liver cells (hepatoma, hepatocellular carcinoma) and 5% arise from bile duct cells (cholangiocarcinoma). Other forms are quite rare. In the United States, hepatomas account for about 0.75% of all cancer deaths. Peak incidence is in the sixth decade of life and men outnumber women by 3:2.

Several risk factors for hepatoma have been identified. Aflatoxin from moldy peanuts, senecio alkaloids from certain plants, liver-fluke infestation, and cirrhosis, especially hemochromatosis and postnecrotic cirrhosis, have been associated with primary hepatic cancer. More than 50% of patients with hepatoma have underlying cirrhosis, and about 4% of cirrhotics will develop hepatoma. An association between vinyl chloride exposure and the extremely rare hepatic angiosarcoma recently has been recognized.

Clinical Features and Diagnosis

Hepatomegaly, right upper quadrant pain, and tenderness are the most common findings of hepatoma but may be masked if the tumor arises in a cirrhotic liver. The sudden appearance of ascites or jaundice or an abrupt increase in liver size or intensity of pain may suggest the development of hepatoma in a patient with underlying cirrhosis. Fever and weight loss are also frequently present. In the patient with a normal liver, the development of hepatoma is usually more obvious. Physical examination may reveal a palpable hepatic mass, hepatic or pleural friction rub, and evidence of ascites.

Laboratory findings may include an elevated alkaline phosphatase, positive α-fetoprotein, and abnormal liver scan (not useful in the cirrhotic patient). These findings require confirmation by tissue diagnosis, which is generally obtained by percutaneous needle biopsy if coagulation parameters permit.

Treatment

Solitary hepatomas occurring in normal livers may be amenable to curative surgical resection. Preoperative angiography is usually recommended to determine whether the lesion is truly solitary. The 5-year survival rate among patients resected for cure is 16%. Most patients, however, have diffuse or multiple hepatomas that cannot be resected. Radiation therapy is ineffective, but there have been some encouraging results with chemotherapy. Doxorubicin, 5-fluorouracil, and methotrexate have some antitumor activity. The use of hepatic artery infusion of chemotherapeutic agents has no established advantage over the less expensive, safer, and the more convenient use of systemic treatment. Regardless of treatment, most patients die from liver failure within a few months of diagnosis.

CARCINOMA OF THE GALLBLADDER

Carcinoma of the gallbladder is a complication of cholelithiasis, albeit an uncommon one. In populations where gallstones are common, such as the American Indians of the Southwest, the incidence of carcinoma of the gallbladder is very high. Among the Bantu, in whom gallstones are rarely encountered, the incidence is negligible. In the United States, about 6,000 cases occur per year; the disease is much more common in women than in men. Peak incidence is around age 60.

Presenting symptoms of the patient with carcinoma of the gallbladder include right upper quadrant pain, anorexia, nausea, weight loss, and jaundice. Physical examination may reveal a right upper quadrant mass and hepatomegaly. The serum level of alkaline phosphatase usually is elevated. Unfortunately, most of the signs and symptoms of gallbladder cancer mimic those of benign gallbladder disease and a preoperative diagnosis of carcinoma of the gallbladder is made in only about 5% of cases.

At surgery, the tumor generally is found to involve most of the gallbladder and to invade the liver as well. Regional nodes are involved frequently and hematogenous spread may also occur. Curative surgery is rarely possible and rapid progression to death within a few months is the typical course. Neither radiation therapy nor chemotherapy has been shown to be beneficial; the 5-year survival is less than 5%.

CARCINOMA OF THE EXTRAHEPATIC BILIARY DUCTS

Bile duct carcinoma is an uncommon tumor, occurring with about one-half the frequency of gallbladder carcinoma. It occurs in association with *Clonorchis sinensis* infestation and with ulcerative colitis but appears to have no relationship to cholelithiasis. The clinical presentation depends largely on the site of origin within the extrahepatic biliary system. Because most of the tumors occur in the common bile duct, jaundice that is usually painless is the most frequent clinical manifestation. Tumors arising in the cystic duct may mimic acute cholecystitis, while those arising in the hepatic ducts may cause only pain, fever, and weight loss without jaundice. On physical examination jaundice, hepatomegaly, and an enlarged gallbladder frequently are detected.

If the diagnosis is suspected preoperatively a transhepatic cholangiogram may demonstrate the tumor. Most cases, however, are discovered at surgery. Curative resection may be attempted but is rarely successful since tumor extension into the liver, portal vein, hepatic artery, pancreas, and duodenum is usually present. Tumors of the distal common duct, however, are occasionally cured by radical pancreatoduodenectomy. Palliative surgery for the relief of biliary obstruction plays an important role. Radiation therapy is ineffective, and, although chemotherapy with 5-fluorouracil may produce responses, they are usually brief.

MALIGNANT NEOPLASMS OF THE URINARY TRACT AND TESTES

RENAL CELL CARCINOMA

Pathology

Adenocarcinoma of renal origin (also called hypernephroma or clear cell carcinoma) arises in adults from tubular cells or from renal cortical adenomas. The frequency of malignant transformation of cortical adenomas is not known. The malignant cells are often well differentiated with abundant clear cytoplasm; hence the term clear cell carcinoma, although 25% of tumors may have a granular cytoplasm. The characteristic clear cell appearance often makes it possible to deduce the site of the primary tumor when biopsy material is obtained from a metastatic site.

Incidence and Etiology

Renal cell carcinomas comprise 1-2% of all malignant tumors. The average age at diagnosis is 50-60 years. Men are affected twice as often as women. The etiology of renal cell carcinoma is not known.

Clinical Features

Renal cell carcinoma may be asymptomatic and discovered by intravenous pyelography (IVP) performed to investigate microscopic hematuria. Symptomatic renal cell carcinoma may present with gross hematuria, flank or groin pain, or with a palpable flank or abdominal mass. Presenting symptoms may relate to metastatic disease involving bone, brain, or other organs. Pulmonary metastases may be asymptomatic, detected by routine chest x-ray; they also may cause cough, hemoptysis, or dyspnea.

Renal cell carcinomas are associated with a variety of systemic syndromes that may precede diagnosis of the underlying tumor by weeks or months. These syndromes include fever, anemia, erythrocytosis, hypercalcemia, amyloidosis, hypertension, neuromyopathy, hepatomegaly unrelated to metastatic disease, and ectopic gonadotropin production. The presence of any one or a combination of these systemic syndromes should alert the clinician to consider renal cell carcinoma in the differential diagnosis.

The natural history of renal cell carcinoma is complex. The growth rate may be extremely variable, and long survivals have been recorded even in the presence of metastatic disease. Furthermore, documented metastases have appeared as long as 30 years after nephrectomy and apparent cure. Despite occasional prolonged survivals in patients with advanced disease, in large series the 5-year survival rate for unresectable renal cell carcinoma is less than 5%. Much has been made of spontaneous regressions of this tumor. While cases of spontaneous regression of the primary tumor or of metastatic foci (usually in the lung) following resection of the primary tumor have been recorded, this phenomenon is extremely rare and expectations of regression should not be allowed to influence therapeutic decisions.

Extension of renal cell carcinoma is both direct, by invasion through the renal capsule into perinephric tissues and growth into the renal vasculature, and metastatic via the bloodstream to distant organs. Death is caused by organ failure due to progressive metastatic disease. Uncontrolled hypercalcemia may also be a cause of death.

Diagnosis, Clinical Evaluation, and Staging

Diagnosis is usually made by IVP. Arteriography may be confirmatory and may be useful in presurgical assessment to determine the presence or absence of involvement of renal vasculature. Material for pathologic examination may be obtained in the course of surgery for primary therapy, but a diagnosis may be made by arteriography alone or supported by needle biopsy. Surgical candidates should be evaluated with chest x-ray films and bone scans. Brain and liver scans should be obtained if the history and physical examination suggest involvement of these organs. Computed tomographic scans of the abdomen may aid in determining the extent of the primary tumor and the presence or absence of intra-abdominal metastatic disease. The clinical staging of renal cell carcinoma is presented in Table 19.

Treatment

Surgery is the only curative therapy for renal cell carcinoma. Early stages have a fairly good prognosis: the 10-year survival for stage I is 75-80%; for stage II, it is 50-60%. The prognosis for more advanced disease is poor. Radical surgery, consisting of nephrectomy with contiguous resection of the renal vein, inferior vena cava, and adjacent lymph nodes, may be employed in selected cases of stage III disease, but the morbidity and mortality of such extensive surgery must be weighed against the limited survival of these patients. Surgical resection of a large symptomatic tumor mass may be worthwhile for palliation of pain or intractable hematuria even if resection is incomplete or if metastases are present.

Radiation therapy may be used to palliate symptoms caused by unresectable local tumor and is very useful in the management of localized symptomatic metastatic lesions, often in bone. Preoperative or postoperative radiation therapy has not been shown to improve surgical survival rates.

At present, there is no consistently effective systemic drug therapy for renal cell carcinoma. Much attention has been

Table 19. Clinical Staging of Renal Cell Carcinoma

Stage I	Tumor confined within the renal capsule
Stage II	Invasion of perinephric fat
Stage III	Involvement of renal vein, inferior vena cava, or lymph nodes
Stage IV	Involvement of adjacent organs or distant metastases

given to hormonal therapy either with progestins or with androgens. Response rates varying from 15-30% have been reported usually involving temporary regression of metastatic pulmonary nodules, although worthwhile clinical improvement occasionally may occur. Progestins have little toxicity and therefore are usually the first choice for symptomatic palliation for a patient with advanced disease. Cytotoxic drug therapy has shown little efficacy. Marginal activity has been reported with alkylating agents, vinca alkaloids, and hydroxyurea, but useful cytotoxic drug therapy awaits the introduction of more effective single agents and combinations.

TRANSITIONAL CELL CARCINOMA OF THE URINARY BLADDER

Pathology

Most carcinomas of the urinary bladder arise in transitional epithelium. Both the histologic grade of the tumor and the degree of invasiveness are important prognostic factors. Low-grade (Broder grades I and II) malignancies, often multifocal, are most commonly papillary carcinomas that tend to remain localized in the bladder epithelium for long periods. High-grade tumors (Broder grades III and IV) have a greater tendency to invade the bladder wall.

Incidence and Etiology

Bladder cancer accounts for about 3% of cancer deaths. It is most common in elderly patients (age 50-70). Men are affected more frequently than women.

An increased risk of bladder cancer has been associated with exposure to a variety of chemical compounds, especially the analine dyes, but a growing list of chemical compounds has been shown to cause bladder cancer in animals and may contribute to the etiology of this disease in man. Other possible bladder carcinogens include tobacco tars excreted in the urine of smokers and chronic bladder infections such as those caused by schistosomes.

Clinical Features

Hematuria is the presenting symptom in 75% of patients with bladder cancer. Frequency, dysuria or other symptoms of bladder irritation may also be present. Occasionally, ureteral obstruction by asymptomatic bladder cancer may cause renal failure of insidious onset, resulting in an initial presentation with uremia.

Repeated local recurrences following local therapy of noninvasive low-grade papillary carcinomas may occur over a period of many years. Eventually, these tumors may become poorly differentiated and invasive. Poorly differentiated tumors spread locally within the pelvis, producing renal and bowel obstruction as well as pain due to invasion of the bony structures and nerve roots. These tumors commonly metastasize to regional lymph nodes, bones, lung, liver, and brain. Renal failure is the most common cause of death unless diversionary surgery has been performed, in which case cachexia and distant organ failure due to progressive metastatic disease are usually fatal.

Table 20. Clinical Staging of Transitional Cell Carcinoma of Bladder

Stage 0	Papillary carcinoma; no invasion of submucosa
Stage A	Invasion of submucosa
Stage B	Invasion of muscle wall of bladder
Stage C	Extension into surrounding fat
Stage D	Extension to adjacent organs or distant metastases

Diagnosis, Clinical Evaluation, and Staging

Diagnosis is made by cystoscopy and transurethral biopsy. Cystography and IVP are useful in tumor localization and in determining ureteral patency. Computed tomography or ultrasound examination of the pelvis may be helpful in determining the extent of tumor. Bone scan and chest x-ray examination are recommended to exclude metastatic disease of these organs. Many authorities also recommend lymphangiography to assess the abdominal and pelvic lymph nodes. The clinical staging of bladder cancer is presented in Table 20.

Treatment

Treatment of low-grade localized (stage 0, A) carcinomas is primarily surgical. Many papillary carcinomas can be resected or fulgurated transurethrally. While local recurrences are common, repeated resections or fulgurations can provide prolonged survival with little morbidity. For more aggressive or extensive lesions partial or total cystectomy with ureteral diversion to an ileal bladder are possible surgical approaches, but many large, invasive, poorly differentiated lesions are unresectable.

Radiation therapy is a useful alternative to surgery for control of advanced local disease and for palliation of symptomatic metastatic lesions. Preoperative and postoperative radiation therapy have not been conclusively shown to prolong survival, although it is reasonable to add radiation therapy to surgery when complete resection of the tumor is not possible.

Cytotoxic chemotherapy has not been extensively explored in the treatment of bladder cancer. Instillation of thiotepa or doxorubicin into the bladder is used in the management of recurrent or multifocal low-grade papillary carcinomas. Systemic chemotherapy is largely investigational. Alkylating agents, 5-fluorouracil, doxorubicin, and *cis*-platinum have shown promising activity as single agents. Experience with combinations of active drugs is needed before the role of chemotherapy can be determined, but early results are encouraging.

ADENOCARCINOMA OF THE PROSTATE

Incidence and Etiology

Adenocarcinoma of the prostate may be the most common malignant tumor of men if microscopic tumors, discovered incidentally in up to 14% of male autopsies, are considered. In terms of clinically significant malignancies, carcinoma of the prostate ranks in frequency after lung and colorectal cancer. The incidence of prostate cancer increases with age. The etiology is not known but the tumors are almost always dependent to some extent on androgenic hormones.

Clinical Features

Prostate cancer is often diagnosed in an asymptomatic individual by palpation of a hard prostatic nodule on routine rectal examination or as an incidental pathologic finding following transurethral prostatic resection for presumed benign prostatic hypertrophy. When local symptoms are present, they almost always relate to bladder obstruction. Bone pain due to metastatic disease is a common presentation. Rarely, bone disease in the spine may be so extensive that symptoms of spinal cord compression may be the presenting complaint.

The biologic behavior of prostate cancer is variable. In some cases, growth is slow and disease remains localized. In most cases, metastases to regional lymph nodes and bone occur. Even in the presence of bone metastases, the disease may follow an indolent course for a time. In younger men (age <70) bony metastases are often rapidly progressive, and metastatic disease of the lungs and liver develops. Death usually results from cachexia and progressive bone disease eventually resulting in bone marrow failure.

Diagnosis, Clinical Evaluation, and Staging

Diagnosis is made by biopsy that can often be done by needle through the rectum. Prostate cancer is frequently, but not invariably, associated with elevations in serum acid phosphatase. As yet a consistent relationship between serum acid phosphatase level and the extent or progression of the disease has not been demonstrated. Bone scans are indicated in all patients with apparently localized prostate cancer and will frequently reveal unsuspected metastases. Lymphangiography or abdominal CT scans may be performed to evaluate the status of abdominal lymph nodes, especially if disease appears localized and radical surgery is contemplated. Bone x-ray films often show the characteristic osteoblastic lesions of metastatic prostate cancer. Osteoblastic bone lesions and an elevated serum acid phosphatase in an elderly man are suggestive but not diagnostic of prostate cancer; histologic confirmation should be obtained. The clinical staging of prostate cancer is outlined in Table 21. Within each stage, poorly differentiated tumors tend to have a more aggressive behavior than well-differentiated tumors, and some staging systems subdivide the stages to take into account the grade of the tumor; however, these staging classifications are not yet widely accepted.

Table 21. Clinical Staging of Adenocarcinoma of Prostate

Stage A	Microscopic disease confined to prostate
Stage B	Palpable disease confined to prostate
Stage C	Spread to adjacent tissues
Stage D	Distant metastases

Treatment

Localized prostate carcinoma (stage A or B) may be managed either surgically or with radiation therapy. Total prostatic resection, the usual operation, is complicated by impotence in 70-80% of cases and incontinence in 10-15%. Radiation therapy to the prostate may also result in impotence, but incontinence is unusual. Surgery and radiation therapy give equivalent results in terms of survival. For locally advanced disease, radiation therapy may be preferable to surgery on the basis of lower complication rates. Assessment of abdominal lymph nodes for metastatic involvement by means of exploratory laparotomy, biopsy, and extension of surgical or radiation therapy to include lymph nodes involved with metastatic disease currently are investigational approaches. Whether survival will be prolonged by these more aggressive local measures remains to be seen.

Therapy of metastatic prostate cancer usually centers around efforts to relieve painful bony disease. When localized, painful lesions may be treated effectively with small radiation fields. Often, however, widespread disease produces multiple symptomatic areas, requiring systemic therapy. Endocrine therapy is effective in palliation of 80% of symptomatic patients. Either castration or estrogen therapy may be used. Both may cause symptomatic improvement and sometimes even objective disease regression, but neither has been shown to prolong survival. When estrogen therapy is given in low doses (diethylstilbestrol, 1 mg per day) therapeutic results are equivalent to those of castration, and major toxic effects such as cardiovascular complaints are minimal. Therefore, castration and estrogen therapy may be regarded as equivalent. Because neither prolongs survival, there is no reason to treat asymptomatic patients. Also, there is no advantage to combined castration and estrogen therapy over either alone.

When symptoms recur after an initial response to hormone therapy, further symptomatic improvement occasionally may be obtained with additional endocrine treatment: initial estrogen therapy followed by castration, or vice versa; corticosteroid therapy; or progesterone therapy. Secondary hormonal respones are neither as complete nor as long-lived as the initial responses. Adrenalectomy and hypophysectomy have been used for palliation, but marginal results and complications limit the usefulness of these procedures. Medical adrenalectomy by administration of aminoglutethimide, a drug that blocks adrenal steroid hormone synthesis, currently is under study.

Cytotoxic drug therapy of advanced prostate carcinoma is a very promising but as yet little-studied therapeutic alternative. Alkylating agents, 5-fluorouracil, doxorubicin, *cis*-platinum, and Estracyt, a drug that combines an alkylating agent with a steroid hormone, each have a fairly high degree of activity. Combinations of individually active agents are under development, and early results are promising. The place of cytotoxic chemotherapy in the treatment of advanced prostate cancer is not yet clear, but chemotherapy should be considered in patients who have brief or incomplete responses to hormonal therapy.

Table 22. Germ Cell Malignancies of the Testes

Histologic Category	*Frequency (%)*
Pure types	
Seminoma	40
Embryonal cell carcinoma	15-20
Choriocarcinoma	Rare
Teratocarcinoma	20-25
Mixed types	15-20

GERM CELL MALIGNANCIES OF THE TESTES

Pathology

Many systems of classification of germ cell carcinomas of the testes have been proposed. Clinically, these tumors are conveniently divided into pure seminomas and other germ cell carcinomas. A listing of the major types and their relative frequencies appears in Table 22. Some classifications include teratoma as a histologic category. While teratomas may appear histologically benign, in adults they should always be regarded as malignant.

Incidence and Etiology

Testicular germ cell carcinomas are the most common malignant tumors of young men and are the fourth leading cause of death in men aged 15-34 years. While these tumors account for only 1% of all cancers, they have a social and economic impact out of proportion to their incidence, since the patient is often the father and breadwinner of a young family.

Germ cell carcinomas occur more frequently in undescended testes, even after these have been surgically placed in the scrotum. A history of trauma or infection frequently precedes the diagnosis of testicular malignancy, but this association may be spurious.

Clinical Features

Testicular germ cell tumors usually present as testicular masses that may be painful. Painful testicular tumors may be hard to distinguish clinically from epididymitis, and antibiotic therapy often is given. Any tender testicular mass that does not resolve promptly and completely with antibiotic therapy requires biopsy. Occasionally, testicular tumors may present as abdominal masses or lymphadenopathy or with symptoms of metastatic disease involving the lungs, liver, bones, or brain. Production of gonadotropins by malignant germ cell tumors may cause painful gynecomastia.

Seminomas have a different clinical behavior than the other germ cell malignancies. They have a greater tendency to remain localized, and when metastases occur, they tend to involve para-aortic lymph nodes first followed by spread to iliac, mediastinal, and supraclavicular nodes. Metastasis via the bloodstream to distant organs occurs late in the disease course. By contrast, nonseminomatous germ cell tumors, particularly those with embryonal or choriocarcinomatous elements, are characterized by early and widespread metastases to regional lymph nodes and distant organs.

Diagnosis, Clinical Evaluation, and Staging

The diagnosis of testicular carcinoma is generally made by testicular biopsy by means of a high inguinal orchiectomy. Germ cell testicular tumors frequently produce α-fetoprotein and/or human chorionic gonadotropin (HCG) that can be detected in the serum. If present, these markers provide a useful tool with which to follow disease activity and response to therapy. All patients with suspected or proven testicular carcinoma should have serum assays of α-fetoprotein and HCG.

The staging workup should include a chest x-ray (with tomograms if there is suspicion of abnormality), bone scan, lymphangiogram, or abdominal CT scan and, if signs or symptoms warrant, a CT brain scan. α-Fetoprotein and HCG determinations should be repeated following orchiectomy if initial values of either were elevated. In nonseminomatous tumors without evidence of distant metastases, a para-aortic lymph node dissection is recommended to determine whether microscopic lymph node metastases are present. The clinical staging of testicular germ cell tumors is shown in Table 23.

Treatment

Because of differences in clinical behavior, treatment of pure seminomas differs considerably from that of other histologies both in selection of the initial therapeutic modality and in the degree of success. For these reasons, therapy for pure seminomas is discussed separately.

Seminomas

Stage I seminomas are treated by high inguinal orchiectomy followed by radiation therapy to the para-aortic and ipsilateral iliac lymph nodes unless these have been resected and found to be free of microscopic tumor. Results of such treatment are excellent with 10-year disease-free survivals ranging from 75% (stage IB) to greater than 95% (stage Ia); For stage II and stage III disease, radiation fields are extended to include mediastinal and left supraclavicular lymphnodes. While stage II disease is often well controlled by such therapy (70-75% 10-year disease-free survival), the outlook for stage III disease is not nearly as good. Fortunately, advanced presentations are unusual in pure seminonmas.

Due to the success of surgery and radiation therapy in the management of most seminomas, there is not a great deal of experience with cytotoxic drug therapy. Available information suggests that this tumor is highly responsive to a variety of cytotoxic drugs including alkylating agents, antimetabolites, and doxorubicin. Recent studies suggest that the combination of *cis*-platinum, vinblastine, and bleomycin is as effective in the therapy of advanced seminoma as it has proven to be in

Table 23. Clinical Staging of Testicular Germ Cell Carcinomas

Stage Ia	Tumor confined to testis
Stage Ib	Microscopic metastases in retroperitoneal lymph nodes
Stage II	Clinically detectable metastases in retroperitoneal lymph nodes
Stage III	Metastases in lymph nodes above the diaphragm or metastases to distant organs

the therapy of nonseminomatous testicular germ cell tumors (vide infra). Cytotoxic drug therapy should be considered for stage III seminomas and for recurrent seminomas following initial surgical or radiation therapy, perhaps combined with radiation therapy to areas of bulk disease when possible. Clinical studies investigating this approach are in progress.

Nonseminomatous germ cell tumors
The treatment of this group of tumors was revolutionized in the 1970s and represents one of the most dramatic areas of therapeutic progress in the past decade. Before 1970, surgery with or without radiation therapy was successful only in the small minority of patients who had stage Ia disease. For stage Ib disease, regardless of the local therapy employed survivals were poor, ranging from 5-50% at 10 years depending on the histologic subtype.

The introduction of highly effective systemic therapy for advanced nonseminomatous testicular tumors marked the beginning of a major change in prognosis. A combination of vinblastine and bleomycin was shown to be capable of inducing a high response rate (70-80%) in a variety of histologic subtypes even in very advanced clinical stages, although the toxicity of this regimen was marked. Many of the responses obtained were, however, complete and prolonged, more than justifying the severe side effects. Recent series of patients with advanced disease treated with a combination of vinblastine, bleomycin, and *cis*-platinum report an 80% complete response rate with a median duration of more than 2 years. The toxicity of this regimen, while appreciable, is usually not so severe as to preclude outpatient treatment. Other drug regimens are under study. Maintenance chemotherapy, initially recommended, has not been shown to add any benefit.

With the availability of highly effective systemic therapy, there is great interest in the use of cytotoxic drug therapy early in high risk situations (stage Ib) since the outlook for patients treated only with local therapy is poor. The success of combination therapy of advanced disease with regimens such as those discussed above is so great, however, that many authorities feel that recurrences can be treated and cured as and when they occur, avoiding the difficult and toxic adjuvant chemotherapy in some patients who are indeed cured by initial surgical intervention.

MALIGNANT NEOPLASMS OF THE FEMALE REPRODUCTIVE ORGANS

OVARIAN CARCINOMA

Pathology

Most malignant ovarian tumors (Table 24) are carcinomas arising from the surface epithelium of the ovary. These are often cystic and if they contain clear fluid they are called serous; when mucin is produced they are termed mucinous. Solid carcinomas, particularly when poorly differentiated, have a more aggressive behavior. Ovarian carcinomas may be graded according to the degree of abnormality of the malignant cells. The more poorly differentiated tumors have a worse prognosis. Very well-differentiated or borderline carcinomas are usually localized and have an excellent prognosis.

Table 24. Malignant Tumors of the Ovary

Type	*Frequency (%)*
Carcinoma	80-85
Serous	40%
Mucinous	10-15
Solid (undifferentiated)	15
Endometrioid	15
Stromal	
Granulosa-theca cell	5%
Arrhenoblastoma	Very rare
Germ cell	
Teratoma (malignant)	1%
Embryonal carcinoma	Very rare
Dysgerminoma	1%
Other	
Clear cell carcinoma	5-10%
Metastatic carcinoma	5%

Incidence and Etiology

Although ovarian cancer is the third most common gynecologic malignancy, it is the most frequently fatal cancer of the female reproductive organs and the fourth most common fatal cancer of women. The death rate from ovarian carcinoma has increased threefold over the last 40 years. Although ovarian carcinoma may occur at any age, the greatest incidence is in middle-aged women (40-60 years). White women are affected more often than black women.

The etiology of ovarian cancer is not known, and no environmental or other predisposing factors have been identified. There are familial associations on occasion. There is also an association of ovarian carcinoma with carcinoma of the breast.

Clinical Features

The onset of ovarian carcinoma is often insidious, probably because the intra-abdominal location of the tumor allows for considerable growth before symptoms occur. A frequent presenting complaint is increasing abdominal girth caused by ascites. Ascitic fluid may be produced by the primary tumor itself but more often is associated with widespread implants of carcinoma on peritoneal and serosal surfaces. Pelvic pain and urinary symptoms caused by pressure of a pelvic mass on the bladder often are the presenting symptoms. A painless pelvic or abdominal mass is a common early sign, noted either by the patient or by the physician in the course of a routine physical examination. Occasionally a patient may complain of dyspnea caused by diaphragmatic elevation due to ascites or by pleural effusion. Pleural effusions may be caused by metastatic pleural implants but more often are reactive and secondary to malignant ascites. Abnormal vaginal bleeding is an occasional complaint. Bowel obstruction rarely occurs early; this is more frequent later in the course of disease.

Most ovarian carcinomas (70%) are disseminated at the time of diagnosis, tending to spread throughout the abdominal cavity and causing implants of tumor on the peritoneum and serosal surfaces of the abdominal organs. Abdominal lymph nodes draining the ovaries may be involved. Dissemination via the bloodstream is less frequent and a late manifestation. Severe impairment of organ function by ovarian carcinomatous metastases is rare. However, bulk effects of peritoneal and serosal tumor implants frequently cause mechanical problems, most commonly bowel obstruction, which is the major cause of death in ovarian carcinoma. Ureteral obstruction and renal failure is another frequent fatal complication. Uncontrolled ascites often associated with pleural effusions commonly occurs in advancing disease, causing pressure symptoms, anorexia, early satiety, and dyspnea.

Diagnosis, Clinical Evaluation, and Staging

Diagnosis of ovarian carcinoma is made by biopsy and histologic examination of tissue. In patients presenting with ascites and massive intra-abdominal disease, paracentesis and cytologic demonstration of malignant adenocarcinoma cells is acceptable for diagnosis. In most cases exploratory laparotomy is necessary to obtain tissue for histologic examination and to obtain staging information. Before surgery, a thorough history, physical and chest x-ray exam, and screening blood chemistries should be obtained. An IVP is useful to check on ureteral patency. Isotopic or radiologic evaluation of bones, liver, and brain is not necessary unless signs or symptoms point directly to problems in these organs. Most staging information is obtained at laparotomy. In patients who are poor risks for major surgery or in whom adequate staging was not done at initial surgery, laparoscopy may provide valuable staging information. The staging system for ovarian carcinoma is given in Table 25. Most carcinomas present in advanced stages. Even with localized disease (stage I and II) a substantial proportion of patients relapse after initial therapy.

Treatment

Treatment of ovarian carcinoma depends on the extent or stage of the tumor. Surgery and radiation therapy are useful for localized disease. Chemotherapy has improved the management of disseminated disease. Studies of combinations of surgery, radiation therapy, and chemotherapy offer promise of better management of all stages of disease in the future.

Table 25. Clinical Staging of Ovarian Carcinoma

Stage	*Definition*	*5-year Survival (%)*
I	Growth limited to ovaries	60%
A	–One ovary, no ascites	60%
B	–Both ovaries, no ascites	60%
C	–One or both ovaries, ascites present	50-55%
II	One or both ovaries involved with pelvic extension	40%
A	–Extension to uterus or tubes only	60%
B	–Extension to other pelvic tissues	40%
III	Peritoneal metastases	5-10%
IV	Distant metastases outside peritoneal cavity	0%

Surgery

Laparotomy is the usual method of diagnosis and the most reliable means of staging. At the time of laparotomy the peritoneum, intra-abdominal organs, and the under surface of the diaphragm should be carefully inspected and any suspicious lesions biopsied. Ascitic fluid should be submitted for cytologic examination. If ovarian carcinoma is confirmed by biopsy and if the tumor seems resectable, a bilateral salpingo-oophorectomy and total abdominal hysterectomy is usually done. Metastatic deposits should be resected when possible. Even if complete removal of tumor is not feasible, many authorities feel that partial removal of masses of tumor or debulking surgery improves symptoms and response to subsequent therapy. In young women with stage Ia disease, unilateral salpingo-oophorectomy with biopsy of the uterus and opposite ovary may be done if future childbearing is desired. Many such patients, however, will have positive biopsy specimens, requiring further surgery.

Surgery is also useful in advanced disease as a palliative measure to relieve symptoms of bowel obstruction or occasionally to relieve pain or pressure caused by single large deposits of tumor. Ascites that cannot be controlled by other means occasionally can be palliated for a time by implantation of devices that deliver ascitic fluid into the venous circulation.

Radiation Therapy

Radiation therapy is often useful for palliation of patients with unresectable tumors and is the standard therapy following surgery for stage II disease. In some centers radiation therapy is used for definitive treatment of stage III disease, although the use of chemotherapy for this stage is more generally accepted. Studies of intra-abdominal radiation with the radionuclide ^{32}P in stage I disease are in progress.

Chemotherapy

A variety of drugs including alkylating agents, doxorubicin, *cis*-platinum, 5-fluorouracil, and hexamethylmelamine are active against ovarian carcinomas. Cytotoxic chemotherapy is used for primary treatment of stages III and IV disease. Single-drug therapy with alkylating agents has been considered standard treatment and will produce responses in 40-50% of patients. In recent years cytotoxic drug combinations have been shown to increase the response rate and the proportion of complete responses. There is as yet no drug combination that can be considered standard.

Complete clinical regression of disease can occur following treatment of even advanced ovarian carcinoma with chemotherapy. In such cases the question of when to stop therapy arises. Second look laparotomy or laparoscopy is the most reliable means of resolving this question.

The use of chemotherapy as an adjunct to surgery in earlier

stage disease (stages I and II) has been investigated, but the ability of such therapy to prolong survival has not been shown.

OVARIAN STROMAL AND GERM CELL TUMORS

Noncarcinomatous malignant tumors of the ovary are listed in Table 24. These include tumors arising from stromal elements (granulosa-theca cell tumors and the very rare arrhenoblastomas) that may produce hormones and associated symptoms. Estrogen production by granulosa-theca cell tumors can cause abnormal uterine bleeding; androgen production by arrhenoblastomas may result in masculinization. Hormone production in children can cause precocious puberty.

Germ cell tumors of the ovary are rare and include counterparts of testicular germ cell tumors in men. Ovarian stromal malignancies and dysgerminomas tend to remain localized to the ovaries but can present problems with local recurrence following initial surgical or radiation treatment. Combination chemotherapy has been employed for refractory local disease or for widespread metastatic disease, but chemotherapy is not as effective for ovarian germ cell tumors as it is for germ cell tumors of the testis.

UTERINE MALIGNANCIES

Endometrial Carcinoma

Pathology

Adenocarcinomas constitute 90% of malignancies of the uterine corpus. These tumors arise from the endometrium. Occasionally, squamoid features are present intermixed with more typical adenocarcinoma, a condition termed adenocanthoma. There is no prognostic significance to this finding, however.

Incidence and Etiology

Endometrial carcinoma increases in frequency with age. As the population of this country has increased in mean age, the proportion of endometrial carcinomas has also increased until at present the incidence of endometrial carcinoma is roughly equal to that of the once much more common cervical carcinoma. Endometrial carcinoma has a clear relationship to hormonal factors. The disease is unusual in women castrated at a young age and occurs with startling frequency in women with estrogen-producing tumors. Although some controversy persists, the weight of evidence shows that administration of estrogens to postmenopausal women increases their risk of endometrial carcinoma.

Clinical Features

Endometrial carcinoma presents most commonly with abnormal vaginal bleeding. This disease should be suspected in any postmenopausal woman who develops vaginal bleeding or spotting. Occasionally, pelvic discomfort caused by an enlarged uterus, abdominal mass, or symptoms caused by bladder or rectal compression are the initial complaints.

Endometrial carcinoma usually remains localized for long periods, especially when the tumor is well differentiated. Direct spread to cervix, vagina, or other pelvic organs may occur, and progressive local growth may cause recurrent vaginal bleeding, gastrointestinal obstructive symptoms, pelvic pain, and rectovaginal or vesicovaginal fistula formation. Metastasis to distant organs is usually a late phenomenon.

Diagnosis, Clinical Evaluation, and Staging

Endometrial carcinoma may be diagnosed by cytologic examination (Pap smear) obtained at pelvic examination, but the accuracy is not as great as in the diagnosis of cervical carcinoma. Dilatation and curettage (D and C) is a highly accurate means of diagnosis. The clinical evaluation should emphasize a thorough pelvic examination with biopsy of any suspicious areas seen in the vagina or cervix. The biopsies are often done in conjunction with the diagnostic D and C.

If a diagnosis of endometrial carcinoma is made and if further surgery is contemplated, careful preoperative medical evaluation may be needed since most patients with endometrial carcinoma are elderly. Preoperative sigmoidoscopy and cystoscopy can be performed to assess the possibility of spread to the rectum or bladder. An IVP may be used to evaluate ureteral patency.

The clinical staging of endometrial carcinoma is outlined in Table 26. Fortunately, most patients present with localized disease.

Treatment

Surgery. If the staging evaluation suggests the disease is localized, total abdominal hysterectomy and bilateral salpingo-oophorectomy is carried out in operable patients. More radical surgery including lymph node dissection has not been shown to prolong survival. Surgical results for treatment of stage I disease are excellent (85-90% 5-year survival). Survival in more advanced stages is less satisfactory (Table 26).

Radiation Therapy. Radiation therapy with external treatment or with internal treatment by insertion of a radioisotope implant into the uterus offers an alternative to surgery in patients who are poor operative risks. Although preoperative radiation therapy is often employed, there is little evidence that this approach improves survival. Radiation therapy is the preferred treatment for unresectable disease localized within the pelvis and may be used in conjunction with surgery when disease cannot be completely resected or when the risk of local recurrence is high.

Table 26. Clinical Staging of Endometrial Carcinoma

Stage	*Definition*	*5-year Survival (%)*
0	Carcinoma in situ	100%
I	Carcinoma confined to uterine corpus	85-90%
II	Involvement of uterine corpus and cervix	50-65%
III	Extension outside uterus but not outside the true pelvis	30%
IV-A	Extension outside true pelvis or involvement of bladder or rectum	<10%
IV-B	Metastases to distant organs	<10%

Systemic Therapy. When endometrial carcinoma is recurrent after local treatment measures with surgery or radiation therapy have failed or in patients who have symptomatic metastatic disease, systemic therapy with hormones or cytotoxic drugs may be helpful. Endometrial carcinoma may respond to therapy with progestational agents in 20-30% of cases. Hormonal responses occasionally may last for several months. Active cytotoxic drugs include alkylating agents and doxorubicin. Combination chemotherapy is still investigational as are combinations of hormonal and cytotoxic therapy, and combined local and systemic therapy for early stage disease.

Uterine Sarcomas

Uterine sarcomas are rare and include endometrial sarcomas (a fibrosarcoma-like malignancy), leiomyosarcomas, and mixed mesodermal sarcomas. All are capable of widespread metastases to distant organs, most often to the lung. When the tumor appears localized, surgical resection is recommended; the ability of additional treatment with radiation therapy or chemotherapy to improve the cure rate after surgery has not yet been fully defined. Combination chemotherapy may be used in advanced metastatic disease in an attempt to relieve symptoms.

Choriocarcinoma

Gestational choriocarcinoma arises from a malignant transformation of the placental chorionic epithelium. Choriocarcinoma rarely arises as a germ cell malignancy of ovarian origin; this tumor is very refractory to treatment and has a much worse prognosis than gestational choriocarcinoma. Choriocarcinomas produce human chorionic gonadotropin (HCG) that, when measured by sensitive assay techniques (β subunit), provides an exquisitely sensitive measure of tumor burden and activity. Gestational choriocarcinoma is of great biologic interest because it arises in fetal tissue and thus represents the only human neoplasm that has HLA incompatibility with its host.

Most choriocarcinomas (50%) follow pregnancies in which a hydatidiform mole is present. Twenty-five percent follow spontaneous abortions and 25% follow normal full-term deliveries. Persistent or invasive moles or choriocarcinomas occur in from 1:12,000-40,000 term deliveries. Any molar pregnancy should raise concern of either persistent molar disease or choriocarcinoma. Molar tissue, either evacuated spontaneously or removed by therapeutic D and C should be examined histologically, but choriocarcinoma may be difficult to diagnose with certainty. A better indication of the presence of choriocarcinoma is the level of the serum HCG. If elevated levels persist for more than 6 weeks after spontaneous or surgical evacuation of a mole or if levels rise after an initial drop, persistent molar disease or choriocarcinoma is present.

Choriocarcinoma may present with signs and symptoms of metastatic disease, especially when there is no history of a molar pregnancy. Cough, hemoptysis, and dyspnea may result from pulmonary involvement. Central nervous system involvement may be reflected by complaints of headache, visual changes, or somnolence. Liver metastases may result in abdominal pain, anorexia, and jaundice. Uncontrolled choriocarcinoma is rapidly fatal, usually due to metastatic disease of the lungs, liver, and brain.

If choriocarcinoma is suspected, either because of a history of molar pregnancy or because a histologic diagnosis has been made from biopsy of metastatic lesions in a young woman, the most important staging information is the serum HCG level. Chest x-ray examination, liver function tests, and, if clinical signs or symptoms warrant, radioisotope or CT scans of the brain, liver, or bone should also be done.

Gestational choriocarcinoma is highly responsive to chemotherapy and, in fact, was the first human malignancy to be cured with chemotherapy. In addition to the treatment of metastatic choriocarcinoma, chemotherapy is the preferred method of treatment for persistent or invasive molar disease, because reproductive function is preserved by this approach. Cytotoxic drugs active against choriocarcinoma are numerous but methotrexate and actinomycin D are most commonly used.

Treatment is guided by the response of serum HCG level and is continued until the level has dropped to zero and remained at zero through two subsequent chemotherapy courses. Patients are then followed with HCG determinations at regular intervals for several months. If the HCG remains zero for 1-2 years, patients may be considered cured.

Choriocarcinomas can be divided into good and poor risk categories on the following basis: good risk patients are those with a history of disease of less than 2 months duration, with HCG levels less than 100,000 IU/ml, and with either pelvic disease only, or pelvic disease and pulmonary metastases only. Such patients (and patients with persistent molar disease or invasive moles) will be cured with chemotherapy in 95-98% of cases. Poor risk patients are those with disease duration greater than 2 months, HCG levels greater than 100,000 IU/ml, and liver or brain metastases. The prognosis of poor risk patients following chemotherapy is not nearly as good as the prognosis of good risk patients. Aggressive therapy with combinations of cytotoxic drugs can, however, induce remissions and even cures in some of these advanced patients. With modern diagnostic and therapeutic techniques, advanced choriocarcinoma is, fortunately, rare.

Cervical Carcinoma

Pathology

Approximately 95% of cervical malignancies are squamous cell carcinomas; the remaining 4-5% are adenocarcinomas. Other malignancies, such as sarcomas, are rare. Most squamous cell carcinomas arise from the squamocolumnar junction of the cervical epithelium. Adenocarcinomas arise from glandular epithelium within the endocervical canal.

Incidence and Etiology

The incidence of cervical carcinoma becomes appreciable in the third decade of life, and peaks in the fourth and fifth decades. The etiology is unknown, but an association with early and frequent sexual activity is well established. Cervical carcinoma is more common in black and Oriental women.

Whether this is a racial difference or related to different patterns of marriage and childbearing in these groups is not known. An association of cervical carcinoma with genital herpesvirus infection has been noted, but definite etiologic evidence is lacking.

Clinical Features

Most cervical carcinomas cause few symptoms, and, in this country, the majority are detected during routine pelvic examinations by means of exfoliative cytology (Pap smear). While some argue that the decline in the death rate from cervical carcinoma in this country may be related to factors other than early detection, there is little doubt that yearly Pap smears, especially in high risk groups such as blacks, can detect cervical carcinoma at an early and highly curable stage of the disease.

The most frequent symptom of cervical carcinoma is contact bleeding from the vagina, usually after mild trauma following coitus or douche. Purulent vaginal discharge may be a presenting symptom. Advanced carcinomas may cause pelvic pain or passage of urine or feces from the vagina due to fistula formation.

Cervical carcinomas tend to spread locally by direct extension to other pelvic organs and tissues. Metastases to the bone and lung are almost always a late manifestation. Para-aortic node involvement with disease extension into and erosion of vertebral bodies or direct extension into pelvic bony structures often produces severe pain as a consequence of nerve root involvement. Death may result from general debility from uncontrolled local disease, from renal failure caused by ureteral obstruction, or from bowel obstruction due to progressive pelvic tumor. Distant organ failure caused by metastatic disease is unusual.

Diagnosis, Clinical Evaluation, and Staging

A thorough pelvic examination is the most important staging procedure. Exfoliative cytology and biopsy of any suspicious cervical lesion is mandatory. Iodine staining (Schiller's test) may reveal suspicious areas when the cervix appears normal. If cytology is positive but no lesion is identifiable, a cone biopsy or a four-quadrant biopsy of the cervix should be done. If invasive carcinoma is found in cervical biopsy specimens an IVP, barium enema, cystoscopy, and sigmoidoscopy are recommended as staging procedures prior to definitive therapy. Lymphangiography or CT of the pelvis and abdomen may also play a role in a complete staging evaluation. Staging of cervical carcinoma is outlined in Table 27. In clinically advanced stages (II, III, IV), exploratory laparotomy with biopsy of the pelvic and para-aortic nodes is sometimes done to assist in planning of the radiation fields.

Treatment

Because of the primarily local nature of cervical carcinomas, surgery and radiation therapy are the major therapeutic modalities. For stage 0 carcinoma, or carcinoma in situ, wide-cone biopsy with careful cytologic follow-up constitutes sufficient therapy if future childbearing is desired. In other cases, total hysterectomy with removal of a wide vaginal cuff is appropriate. The cure rate of carcinoma in situ approaches 100%.

Table 27. Clinical Staging of Cervical Carcinoma

Stage	*Definition*
0	Malignancy confined to epithelium—carcinoma in situ
I	Malignancy confined strictly to cervix
Ia	Microscopic disease
Ib	Clinically overt disease
II	Malignancy extends beyond cervix but not to pelvic wall or to lower one-third of vagina
IIa	Involves upper vagina without extension to parametrium
IIb	Extension to parametrium but not to pelvic wall
III	Malignancy extends to pelvic wall or lower vagina
IIIa	Malignancy involves lower one-third of vagina, no extension to pelvic wall
IIIb	Malignancy extends to pelvic wall
IV	Malignancy extends beyond true pelvis or involves bladder or rectum

Total abdominal hysterectomy with wide vaginal cuff removal is also used for treatment of stage Ia (microscopic invasive) carcinoma. More advanced stages are usually treated primarily with radiation therapy both externally and internally by means of cesium or radium applications. In advanced cervical carcinoma, palliative surgery may be combined with radiation therapy for relief of ureteral or bowel obstruction or correction of fistulas. Patients with localized cervical carcinoma (stages I and II) have a reasonably good prognosis with local therapy (60-70% 5-year survival). Control of more advanced disease is considerably less satisfactory.

For locally recurrent or metastatic cervical carcinoma, cytotoxic chemotherapy has been used but with only marginal results. Recent introduction of new active agents, such as *cis*-platinum, offers hope of improved management in the future.

Unusual Gynecologic Malignancies

Adenocarcinoma of the Fallopian Tubes

These tumors comprise about 1% of all gynecologic malignancies. They are seldom diagnosed preoperatively, and it is often difficult to be certain that they are not in fact metastatic foci from ovarian carcinoma. Therapy is primarily surgical. Radiation therapy and chemotherapy are used to treat recurrent or metastatic disease in a manner similar to that used to treat ovarian carcinoma.

Carcinoma of the Vulva and Vagina

Squamous cell carcinoma of the vulva and vagina comprise 1-2% of gynecologic cancers. They behave much like squamous cell carcinomas arising elsewhere, having a tendency to invade locally and spread to regional lymph nodes. Distant metastases are a late phenomenon; the major clinical problems are created by locally progressive tumor.

Squamous cell carcinomas of the vulva and vagina may present with bleeding, discomfort, discharge, or as an ulcerated lesion found during routine physical examination. Biopsy is required to establish the diagnosis. Vulvar carcinomas are treated surgically. Complete vulvectomy and pelvic lymph node dissection is the conventional procedure. Vaginal carcinomas may be treated either with surgery or radiation therapy.

Adenocarcinomas of the vagina are rare malignancies that occur with increased frequency in young women exposed in utero to diethylstilbestrol. A maternal history of such exposure warrants regular and thorough checkups for early detection of these lesions in women at risk.

MALIGNANT TUMORS OF THE ENDOCRINE GLANDS

THYROID CARCINOMA

Most thyroid malignancies are epithelial in origin and are classified in four major histologic types (Table 28). Approximately 9,100 new cases of thyroid carcinoma were reported, and 1,050 deaths occurred in 1980, according to American Cancer Society figures. The male/female ratio for all thyroid carcinomas is 1:2.

The cause of thyroid carcinoma is unknown in most cases, but previous radiation to the head and neck has recently been recognized as an important risk factor. In the 1920s and 1930s external radiation to the head, neck, and upper chest was commonly used in children for nonmalignant conditions such as tonsillitis, acne, and an enlarged thymus. These patients, as adults, have an increased risk of developing thyroid cancer as well as other thyroid problems.

Most patients with thyroid carcinoma present with a painless mass in the neck. Occasionally, other symptoms, such as neck pressure or difficulty swallowing, or symptoms related to the presence of distant metastases first bring the patient to medical attention. On examination a solitary nodule in an otherwise normal thyroid gland is suggestive of malignancy. In a patient with a multinodular goiter, rapid growth of the goiter, hard consistency of a nodule, and the presence of cervical lymphadenopathy or hoarse voice are highly suspicious. Psammoma bodies, finely stippled calcifications seen on neck x-ray, suggest papillary carcinoma. An ^{131}I scan characteristically reveals a cold nodule in thyroid cancer. A large but functioning nodule within a multinodular goiter may also prove to be cancer, however; If such a nodule enlarges or fails to regress during a course of suppressive therapy with exogenous thyroid hormone, malignancy is suspected.

Surgery is necessary for diagnosis and is the preferred treatment for local disease. Most authorities recommend total or near-total thyroidectomy with exploration of the neck if lymph nodes are involved. Six weeks after surgery when endogenous thyroid hormone has disappeared and TSH levels are high, a dose of ^{131}I should be given to destroy any remaining thyroid tissue and to demonstrate any functioning metastases on scan. If such metastases are seen, a therapeutic dose of ^{131}I is given and the patient is placed on suppressive doses of T_4. At prescribed intervals, the T_4 is withheld to allow TSH levels to rise, and repeat ^{131}I scanning is performed in an attempt to detect further metastases. Suppressive therapy is then resumed and generally continued for life.

Local recurrences can be treated by surgery or external radiation. Distant nonfunctioning metastases that do not respond to suppression may present difficult therapeutic problems. Painful bony lesions usually respond well to external radiation; extensive pulmonary metastases may respond to chemotherapy with adriamycin. Other chemotherapeutic agents have not demonstrated any activity in thyroid carcinomas. Serum thyroglobulin levels may be used as a marker to detect recurrence or metastasis from a differentiated thyroid carcinoma following thyroidectomy. It is expected that in the future this test will play a major role in the management of thyroid cancer patients.

Papillary carcinoma is the most frequent type seen in the United States and occurs in all age groups including children and young adults. Papillary carcinoma tends to have an excellent prognosis. It can metastasize locally to regional lymph nodes, but distant metastases are extremely uncommon. Death is usually due to local infiltration with asphyxiation or hemorrhage.

Follicular carcinomas closely resemble normal thyroid tissue histologically. Follicular or mixed papillary-follicular carcinomas may concentrate ^{131}I, with important diagnostic and therapeutic implications. Patients with follicular carcinomas also tend to have a good prognosis but distant metastases, especially to the lung, are common.

Both follicular and papillary carcinomas may undergo transition to anaplastic carcinoma. More frequently, anaplastic carcinomas arise de novo. These tumors are extremely malignant and respond poorly to both surgery and radiation. They meta-

Table 28. Thyroid Carcinomas

Histologic Type (Frequency)	*M:F Ratio*	*Peak Age at Diagnosis (Decade)*	*Metastases*	*^{131}I Uptake*	*Substances Produced*	*Median Survival (years)*
Papillary (67%)	1:3	3-4	Regional nodes	Uncommon	Rarely T_3, T_4	12-15
Follicular (22%)	1:3	5	Distant, especially lung	Common	Rarely T_3, T_4	10-12
Medullary (10%)	1:2	6	Regional nodes	Never	Calcitonin, ACTH, prostaglandins, serotonin, histaminase	10
Anaplastic (1-5%)	1:1	6-7	Regional nodes	Rare	–	0.5-1

stasize early and widely but usually cause death by local invasion. Experience with chemotherapy is limited but promising.

Medullary carcinoma of the thyroid is a neoplasm of the parafollicular calcitonin-secreting cells; therefore, treatment with exogenous T_4 or ^{131}I is unwarranted. Medullary carcinomas may occur on a familial basis in association with pheochromocytomas, parathyroid adenomas, and mucosal neuromas. This association is referred to as Sipple's syndrome, or multiple endocrine neoplasia type 2. Local invasion and indolent growth are characteristic of medullary carcinomas but distant metastases do occur.

Despite calcitonin production by many medullary carcinomas, hypocalcemia is rare. Calcitonin levels may be used to screen family members or to detect progression or recurrence in a patient previously treated for medullary carcinoma. Other bioactive substances may be produced by medullary carcinomas (Table 28) including prostaglandins, which may be responsible for severe diarrhea in these patients.

ADRENAL CARCINOMA

Adrenocortical carcinoma is rare, occurring with a frequency of one in 500,000 population. It may occur at any age; the mean age at presentation is 38. The etiology is unknown.

Although nonfunctioning adrenocortical carcinomas occur, the majority of cases present with one of four endocrine syndromes: Cushing's syndrome, virilization of female patients, feminization of male patients, and precocious puberty in children. Very rare manifestations include hypoglycemia, polycythemia, inappropriate secretion of antidiuretic hormone, and hypermineralocorticism.

Abnormal steroidogenesis and consequent endocrine syndromes probably arise because of inefficiency in cortisol production by the malignant adrenal tissue. Because of various biosynthetic defects, these tumors can make excessive quantities of weak androgens, estrogens, or glucocorticoid precursors that are secreted into the circulation, causing the recognized endocrine effects. Often there is overlap of the typical syndromes, and Cushing's syndrome with virilization and striking elevations in urinary 17-ketosteroids is highly characteristic of adrenal carcinoma.

The diagnosis of adrenal carcinoma depends on recognizition of the endocrine manifestations and demonstration of an adrenal mass. Differentation from adrenal adenomas is readily accomplished by use of the adrenocorticotropic hormone (ACTH) stimulation and dexamethasone suppression tests that reveal complete autonomy in cases of Cushing's syndrome due to adrenal carcinoma. The presence of metastases (most commonly to liver and lung) or bulky tumor with local invasion is also diagnostic of malignant adrenal tumor. Many patients complain of abdominal pain, and a mass is often palpable at the time of diagnosis.

Intravenous pyelography, arteriography, and CT scanning are used to define the extent of the tumor prior to surgery. Exploratory laparotomy is usually necessary to establish a tissue diagnosis and determine resectability. If at all possible, en bloc resection of the tumor should be performed. Palliative resections may be worthwhile to reduce excessive hormone levels and ameliorate local symptoms. Patients may require corticosteroid replacement therapy intraoperatively and postoperatively because the uninvolved adrenal gland may be atrophic and nonfunctional due to suppression from endogenous hypersecretion by the tumor.

Ortho-para-DDD (*o,p'*DDD), an inhibitor of adrenal steroidogenesis, may cause regression of the tumor and a decrease in hormone secretion in patients with unresectable or metastatic adrenal carcinomas. The toxicity, especially gastrointestinal and neuromuscular, is severe but usually tolerable with dosage adjustments. Approximately one-third of patients demonstrate objective tumor regressions, and twice as many have a reduction in hormone levels and in endocrine symptoms. Some patients, despite a reduction in hormone levels, have progressive tumor while taking *o,p'*DDD. Prophylactic use of *o,p'*DDD following surgery has been advocated by some in the hope of preventing or delaying recurrent disease. Considerable controversy regarding the role of *o,p'*DDD exists, however, and some investigators have found no benefit from its use. Conventional chemotherapy has not as yet had an adequate trial in adrenocortical carcinoma.

Median survival from time of diagnosis is 3-4 years. Death is usually a consequence of massive local tumor invasion or of pulmonary or hepatic failure secondary to metastatic disease.

Pheochromocytoma, a rare tumor of adrenal medullary origin, is even more rarely malignant. Surgical resection is the treatment of choice. In unresectable cases, chronic administration of an α-adrenergic blocking agent may be useful in controlling symptoms due to hypersecretion of catecholamines.

ISLET CELL CARCINOMAS OF THE PANCREAS

Most pancreatic islet cell tumors are benign and cause symptoms by excessive production of one or more hormones including insulin, gastrin, ACTH, melanocyte-stimulating hormone (MSH), glucagon, serotonin, and vasoactive intestinal polypeptide (VIP). Only approximately 10% of such tumors are malignant and add the problems of distant metastases and local invasion to those of endocrine hyperfunction. Islet cell carcinomas can occur at any age but peak between ages 40 and 70. They may involve any portion of the pancreas, but the tail is most commonly involved. Multiple lesions in the pancreas occur in 10-20% of hormone-producing carcinomas but are not seen in nonfunctioning tumors.

Insulin-producing islet cell carcinomas present with symptoms of hypoglycemia. The diagnosis depends on a demonstration of elevated insulin to glucose ratios during fasting. Surgery is indicated unless widespread (usually hepatic) metastases have been demonstrated. In recurrent, metastatic, or unresectable cases diazoxide may be used to counteract hypoglycemia. The tumor can be treated successfully in many cases with streptozotocin, a nitrosourea, either alone or in combination with 5-fluorouracil.

Gastrin-producing islet cell tumors are frequently malignant and about 50% will have metastatic disease (regional nodes, liver) at the time of diagnosis. These tumors are responsible for Zollinger-Ellison syndrome, a constellation of clinical findings including gastric hypersecretion, hypergastrinemia, and severe peptic ulceration. Presenting symptoms include peptic ulcer (often multiple, atypically located, and extremely resistant to antacid management) in most patients, and diarrhea and malabsorption in a minority of them. Surgical excision of the tumor is usually not possible because of the frequency of multiple lesions and of metastatic disease. Total gastrectomy is often necessary to prevent recurrent ulceration. The use of cimetidine, however, may offer an alternative to total gastrectomy in some patients. Antitumor chemotherapy with streptozotocin alone or in combination with 5-fluorouracil may cause tumor regression and improvement in symptoms due to gastric hypersecretion in cases where other measures have failed.

Glucagon-secreting islet cell tumors are usually malignant and present with a bizarre clinical syndrome characterized by a severe skin rash (necrolytic migratory erythema), weight loss, anemia, hyperglycemia, stomatitis, and hepatic metastases. Surgical removal, if possible, is the treatment of choice. Failing this, the use of either streptozotocin or dacarbazine (DTIC) may produce remission.

Pancreatic cholera, a syndrome of profuse watery diarrhea, hypokalemia, and achlorhydria, occurs in patients with non-β islet cell tumors secreting vasoactive intestinal polypeptide and possibly other bioactive substances as well. In those cases in which a malignant islet cell tumor is responsible (about 50%), treatment with streptozotocin and/or 5-fluorouracil may produce dramatic remissions in the severe diarrhea.

MALIGNANT NEOPLASMS OF THE HEAD, NECK, AND ESOPHAGUS

SQUAMOUS CELL CARCINOMAS OF THE HEAD AND NECK

Pathology, Incidence, and Etiology

The great majority of all malignant tumors arising from structures of the head and neck are squamous cell carcinomas. Sites of origin and relative frequencies are presented in Table 29.

As a group, squamous cell carcinomas of the head and neck account for about 5% of all malignant tumors and affect mainly an older population. Their strategic location causes cosmetic and functional problems that give these cancers a clinical prominence out of proportion to their incidence.

Table 29. Squamous Cell Carcinomas of the Head and Neck

Site of Origin	*Proportion of Total Head and Neck Squamous Cell Tumors (%)*
Larynx	15-20
Tongue	10-15
Lip	10-15
Buccal mucosa	10
Oropharynx	10
Floor of mouth	8-10
Hypopharynx	5-10
Nasopharynx	1-5

Squamous cell carcinomas of the head and neck are associated with poor oral hygiene, smoking, and excessive alcohol intake; in Eastern countries, they are associated with the habit of chewing betel nuts, particularly when combined with smoking.

Clinical Features

Presenting signs and symptoms of head and neck carcinomas depend very much on the anatomic site of origin. Early lesions may be asymptomatic in the mouth. They can be suspected by the finding of whitish or erythematous plaques on the oral mucosa during routine physical or dental examinations. Symptomatic lesions of the oral cavity or tongue most often cause pain or bleeding due to ulceration. Lesions in the oropharynx may cause pain or difficulty in swallowing and in breathing due to esophageal or tracheal obstruction. Carcinomas arising in the sinuses may cause pain and bloody nasal discharge. Problems in breathing, unilateral hearing problems, eustachian tube obstruction, and cranial neuropathies are presenting symptoms of carcinomas arising in the nasopharynx. Tumors of the larynx and surrounding tissues often present with hoarseness, cough, and dysphagia. Neck masses due to metastatic carcinoma in cervical lymph nodes from asymptomatic primary lesions elsewhere in the head and neck area are a fairly common mode of presentation. Discovery of the primary tumor may be difficult, requiring sophisticated physical examination and x-ray techniques. Occasionally, a tumor that has been symptomatically silent in its site of origin will cause pain by direct extension into adjacent bony structures. Lymphoepithelioma, a variety of nasopharyngeal carcinoma that is rare in this country, may present with widespread disease of bone and lung.

Squamous cell carcinomas arising in structures of the head and neck tend to be locally invasive. Metastases to regional lymph nodes in the neck are common, but metastases to distant organs occur late in the disease course and are seldom of major clinical significance. Death is usually caused by locally progressive tumor with obstruction of the airway or pharynx. Erosion of tumor into blood vessels and consequent hemorrhage is an occasional terminal event.

Diagnosis, Clinical Evaluation, and Staging

Diagnosis of squamous cell carcinoma of the head and neck is made by biopsy of a suspected lesion. Presenting symptoms or signs will direct attention to a particular anatomic site. Special techniques, such as mirror examination of the oral cavity, pharyngeal areas, and larynx, are necessary for a complete evaluation. Palpation is valuable to determine the full extent of the lesion; hard or firm areas are highly suspicious for involvement by tumor. X-ray studies of the facial bones and sinuses, computed tomography of the sinuses and larynx, and x-ray contrast studies of the pharynx and larynx may all aid in determining the extent of the tumor. Computed tomography is a particularly useful procedure and provides an excellent assessment of the tumor extent and the status of surrounding bony and soft tissue structures.

The initial clinical evaluation should include careful palpation of the neck and submandibular areas to search for lymphadenopathy. A chest x-ray should be obtained, but studies to exclude other sites of metastatic disease are not indicated unless clinical symptoms and signs point directly to problems in these areas. The TNM system is most often employed in clinical staging of head and neck cancers (Table 4).

Treatment

Because of the predominently local nature of squamous cell head and neck cancers, surgery and radiation therapy are the primary modalities of treatment. Proper management of these lesions depends as much on the cosmetic and functional consequences of therapy as on the eradication of disease. Selection of the initial treatment modality depends on the size and location of the lesion and on the presence or absence of regional lymph node involvement. These decisions and the coordination of subsequent therapy are highly specialized undertakings requiring close consultation by specialists in surgery and radiation therapy.

Cytotoxic drug therapy may offer useful palliation for recurrent or metastatic squamous cell carcinomas of the head and neck. Methotrexate is used most frequently. High-dose methotrexate-leucovorin rescue therapy and regional arterial perfusion with methotrexate offer no advantage over conventional treatment with weekly or biweekly intravenous methotrexate. Other active drugs include bleomycin, doxorubicin, and *cis*-platinum. Combination therapy is investigational.

MALIGNANT NEOPLASMS OF THE SALIVARY GLANDS

Most salivary gland tumors are benign. Malignant tumors include adenocarcinomas, mucoepidermoid tumors, squamous cell carcinomas, and mixed tumors. The parotid gland is most often affected. A painless mass in the area of the parotid gland is the most common presenting sign. Facial paralysis due to tumor compression of the facial nerve occurs in one-third of patients with malignant parotid tumors. Growth occurs by local extension into surrounding bony structures of the ear and skull. Metastases to regional lymph nodes and distant metastases, most commonly to the lungs, occur late in the disease course. Treatment is primarily surgical. Radiation therapy may be used to treat unresectable tumors or recurrent disease following surgery. Survival is on the order of 50% at 5 years.

MALIGNANT NEOPLASMS OF THE ESOPHAGUS

Pathology, Incidence, and Etiology

Almost all esophageal cancers are squamous cell carcinomas. Approximately 50% arise in the distal third of the esophagus, 40% in the middle third, and, fortunately, only 10% arise in the upper third.

Esophageal cancer accounts for approximately 1% of all malignancies in this country, but the disease is much more common in the Far East, Middle East, and East Africa. Men are affected more often than women. The disease is more common in elderly people.

While the precise etiology of esophageal carconoma is not known, a variety of associations with environmental factors and with congenital and acquired diseases of the esophagus have been identified. An increased incidence of esophageal cancer is seen in congenital short esophagus, achalasia, esophageal webs, Plummer-Vinson syndrome (esophageal web and iron deficiency anemia), and following lye strictures of the esophagus. The recent striking increase in esophageal cancer among East Africans is thought to be related to the home-brewing of beer in galvanized drums, possibly implicating zinc and other compounds as environmental carcinogens.

Clinical Features

The initial complaint is almost always dysphagia. A complaint of difficulty in swallowing, particularly when progressive, must always be taken seriously and warrants x-ray evaluation. Esophageal carcinomas may perforate the esophagus causing pain, pneumomediastinum, and subcutaneous emphysema in the thorax and neck. Fistula formation to a bronchus or the trachea may cause spasmodic coughing following eating or drinking and recurrent pulmonary infections. Carcinomas in the upper esophagus may cause hoarseness, cough, or respiratory difficulty. Rarely, a tumor may erode into the aorta, resulting in massive hematemesis and death.

Esophageal carcinoma is locally invasive, and death usually is caused by obstruction of the esophagus resulting in inability to eat or drink. In this situation, aspiration of food or liquid commonly occurs, and the resulting pneumonitis is frequently fatal. Metastases to regional lymph nodes and to lung and liver do occur, but seldom present a serious clinical problem.

Diagnosis, Clinical Evaluation, and Staging

Suspicion of esophageal carcinoma may be confirmed by x-ray studies (barium swallow, esophagram). Esophagoscopy with biopsy is usually diagnostic. If major surgical procedures are contemplated, bronchoscopy is advised to exclude the possibility of tumor extension into the trachea or bronchi. Chest x-ray should be obtained to evaluate mediastinal lymph nodes. Computed tomography of the chest may provide valuable information of the extent of the primary tumor. The TNM classification is used for the clinical staging of esophageal carconoma (Table 4).

Treatment

Treatment of esophageal cancer by either surgery or radiation therapy has not had great success. Five-year survival rates are only 5-10%. Radiation therapy is the preferred treatment modality for tumors in the upper third of the esophagus. Lower esophageal carcinomas may be resected if the tumor appears localized. For tumors arising in the lower esophagus, anastomosis of the remaining esophagus and stomach can sometimes be performed. Tumors arising higher in the esophagus may require interposition of a length of bowel to reconstruct the resected area. Obstructing esophageal lesions may be palliated by dilatation or by insertion of an artificial lumen through the obstructing tumor. There is a danger of esophageal perforation with these procedures. Radiation therapy of esophageal cancer gives results equivalent to surgery in most series, and probably represents a more desirable treatment because of a lower moribidity and mortality. Combined surgery and radiation therapy may improve survival rates, but controlled studies are not yet available.

Cytotoxic chemotherapy of esophageal carcinoma has had little success to date. Alkylating agents and bleomycin have shown some anticarcinogenic activity. *Cis*-platinum appears to have appreciable activity in early studies and, in combination with other cytotoxic agents, may provide more effective therapy in the future.

MALIGNANT NEOPLASMS OF THE SKIN

SQUAMOUS CELL CARCINOMA

Incidence and Etiology

Squamous cell carcinomas of the skin are the most common cancers in humans. The incidence of these tumors increases with increasing age. Blacks are affected less often than Caucasians. Several environmental factors have been found to be etiologically significant. The most important of these is exposure to ultraviolet radiation in sunlight or to more energetic radiation in the form of x-rays. Known chemical carcinogens include coal tars and arsenic. Because squamous cell carcinomas of the skin sometimes arise in scars or in severely burned areas, there has long been recognition that severe or repeated trauma is a risk factor. Xeroderma pigmentosa, an autosomal recessive inherited disorder of DNA repair, is associated with an extremely high incidence of skin malignancy, including squamous cell carcinoma.

Clinical Features

Squamous cell carcinomas of the skin usually present as flat or slightly raised ulcerated areas that sometimes bleed. Pain is seldom a prominent symptom. A variety of precancerous skin conditions including actinic keratoses, leukoplakia, and erythroplasia of Queyrat should raise clinical suspicion of a coexistent carcinoma when found on routine physical examination.

Skin cancers spread by direct invasion of surrounding tissue. Metastasis to regional lymph nodes generally occurs late in the disease course, although early widespread dissemination may occur with poorly differentiated tumors, particularly those that arise near mucocutaneous junctions or in previously irradiated skin. Metastasis to visceral organs is unusual.

Diagnosis, Clinical Evaluation, and Staging

A suspicious lesion should be excised and examined histologically. For large lesions or in areas where excisional biopsy might cause functional or cosmetic problems, incisional biopsy is acceptable. The initial examination should include careful palpation to detect lymphadenopathy and thorough examination of the remainder of the skin. Further staging is not usually necessary unless the initial lesion is large or lymph node metastases are suspected. In the case of large invasive lesions, particularly on the face, x-rays of surrounding bony structures or CT is necessary to determine whether invasion of bone has occurred. Squamous cell carcinomas are staged according to the TNM classification (Table 4).

Treatment

The vast majority of squamous cell skin cancers are cured by surgical removal. In areas where excision would cause excessive functional or cosmetic complications, radiation therapy provides an equally satisfactory result. Multiple or recurrent squamous cell carcinomas may respond to topical chemotherapy with 5 fluorouracil cream or ointment, or to immunotherapy by means of sensitization to and subsequent challenge with nonspecific immunostimulants such as dinitrochlorobenzene (DNCB). Invasive or metastatic cutaneous squamous cell tumors may respond transiently to systemic therapy with methotrexate, bleomycin, or *cis*-platinum, but effective combinations have not yet been developed, and worthwhile clinical remissions following systemic chemotherapy are rare.

BASAL CELL CARCINOMA

Basal cell carcinomas are also etiologically related to exposure to ultraviolet radiation in sunlight, to x-ray exposure, and to arsenic. The basal cell nevus syndrome, an autosomal-dominant inherited disorder, is associated with multiple basal cell carcinomas that develop in the second and third decade of life. Basal cell carcinomas present as nonhealing ulcerated lesions, often with a characteristic elevated rolled margin. These tumors progress by local growth and invasion of surrounding structures. Metastases rarely, if ever, occur. Small basal cell carcinomas are cured by surgical excision or, if resection is undesirable for cosmetic or functional reasons, by radiation therapy. Large basal cell carcinomas of the head require careful staging to determine whether adjacent bony or cartilaginous structures are involved so that proper therapeutic planning can be done. Neglected basal cell carcinomas may progress to such an extent that surgical removal is not feasible, and extensive destruction of normal structures may occur. These lesions, often referred to as rodent ulcers, can by palliated by radiation therapy. Multiple basal cell carcinomas may respond to topical chemotherapy or immunotherapy similar to that used to treat squamous cell carcinomas.

MALIGNANT MELANOMA

Pathology

Malignant melanomas derive from melanocytes, derived from neural crest epithelium in the basal layer of the epidermis. Some malignant melanomas are thought to arise from benign nevi (moles), but the frequency of malignant transformation of these ubiquitous lesions is unclear; junctional nevi and blue nevi are thought to have a greater risk of malignant transformation.

Many malignant melanomas can be easily recognized pathologically because of the presence of melanin in the tumor cells. Some undifferentiated melanomas, however, produce no melanin, and may appear histologically as large cell anaplastic tumors. Electron microscopy, by revealing the presence of organelles characteristic of neural crest epithelium, may aid in diagnosis. The histopathology of malignant melanoma is very important prognostically, as the likelihood of regional lymph node involvement and systemic dissemination is correlated with the depth of microscopic invasion of the primary lesion (Table 30).

Incidence and Etiology

Malignant melanomas account for about 1% of all cancers. They are the least common but most frequently fatal skin cancer. Melanomas rarely occur in children; the peak incidence occurs in the fifth to seventh decades of life. Men and women are equally affected, although women have a better prognosis for unknown but possibly hormonal reasons. In this respect, it is interesting, but of uncertain significance, that estrogen receptors have been identified in some malignant melanoma specimens.

Exposure to sunlight is a major risk factor for the development of malignant melanoma. Fair-skinned races and persons are at greater risk; the incidence rises with increasing sun exposure. Although melanocytes are responsive to melanocyte-stimulating hormone (MSH), no relationship between melanoma and high MSH levels (pregnancy, Cushing's disease) has been demonstrated.

Clinical Features

Malignant melanoma may present either as a de novo pigmented skin lesion or as a change in the size and character of an existing mole. Changes that should raise suspicion of malignant transformation include sudden increase in size, change in color, ulceration with oozing or bleeding, surrounding erythema or swelling, and development of tenderness or itching. Malignant melanomas may occasionally present with lymphadenopathy, nonpigmented subcutaneous masses, or with widespread metastatic disease. In some cases of metastatic melanoma no skin primary can be found, although careful questioning occasionally may elicit a history of previous removal of a "benign" mole.

The biologic behavior of malignant melanoma may be quite variable. The tumor may remain localized to skin and regional lymph nodes or recur locally repeatedly over long periods of time. Spontaneous regression of the primary lesion has been reported, but regression of visceral metastases, although described, is rare. Melanomas metastasize widely to lymph nodes, lungs, liver, bone, and brain. Melanomas also may metastasize to the mucosa of the gastrointestinal tract; the resulting polypoid lesions may cause repeated intussusceptions or bleeding. Excess melanin production in advanced metastatic melanoma may cause a slate-gray discoloration of the entire skin (melanosis). The urine and even the cerebrospinal fluid may become black from excess pigment production.

Diagnosis, Clinical Evaluation, and Staging

A suspicious skin lesion should be biopsied promptly. All excised skin lesions should be examined pathologically regardless of clinical impression. When malignant melanoma is suspected, a thorough physical examination with special attention to lymph nodes is mandatory. If malignant melanoma is found in the biopsy specimen, further evaluation should include a chest x-ray and screening evaluation of liver chemistries. If clinical signs or symptoms of liver, bone or brain disease are present, appropriate radionuclide or x-ray studies of these organs are indicated. The clinical staging of malignant melanomas is given in Table 31. It should be noted that regardless of whether lymph nodes are palpable, metastatic disease is likely if the primary tumor invades deeply (Table 31).

Treatment

Excisional biopsy is usually sufficient treatment for small superficial (level 1 or 2) melanomas. Larger lesions and those that have been biopsied incisionally require surgical resection with wide margins around the lesion. Skin grafting is sometimes necessary. If the lesion is located on an extremity and if regional lymph nodes are palpably enlarged, a lymph node dissection should be performed for palliative and cosmetic reasons. There is no evidence that prophylactic lymph node dissection improves survival when lymph nodes are not palpable, even in level 3-5 lesions in which the likelihood of microscopic nodal involvement is high.

Locally recurrent disease presents a difficult management problem. Recurrent tumors or metastatic cutaneous tumors should be removed surgically if possible. Although melanomas are relatively radioresistant, radiation therapy may sometimes provide valuable palliation for locally recurrent symptomatic disease. The therapy of advanced metastatic melanoma is unsatisfactory. Cytotoxic drugs have little activity. The most

Table 30. Level of Invasion and Regional Lymph Node Involvement in Cutaneous Malignant Melanoma

Level	*Definition*	*Positive Nodes (%)*
I	Tumor confined to epidermis	<1
II	Tumor invades papillary dermis	<5
III	Tumor invades to junction of papillary and reticular dermis	20-30
IV	Tumor invades reticular dermis	60-70
V	Tumor invades subcutaneous tissue	60-70

Table 31. Survival of Malignant Melanoma by Clinical Stage

Stage	*Definition*	*5-year Survival (%)*
I	Tumor confined to skin	
Ia	Lesion limited to epidermis	70
Ib	Deeper invasion	45
II	Regional lymph nodes involved	15-20
III	Distant metastases	0

active single agents are DTIC (20% response) and nitrosoureas (15-20% response). Effective combinations of cytotoxic drugs have not yet been developed.

A great deal of attention has been given to immunotherapy of malignant melanoma with nonspecific immunostimulants such as BCG and C-parvum. Direct injection of these agents into cutaneous melanomas will frequently result in regression of the injected lesion and sometimes of adjacent cutaneous lesions as well. Regression of visceral metastases following this therapy is, however, rarely seen. Studies of adjuvant immunotherapy following surgery of high risk patients (level 3-5) who have no clinically overt metastases have been contradictory. At present there is no good evidence that adjuvant immunotherapy is beneficial, although several studies continue to explore this question.

SARCOMAS

Incidence and Etiology

Sarcomas are malignant tumors that arise from connective tissue. A classification of sarcomas is presented in Table 32. As a group, these diseases comprise less than 1% of all human malignancies. Osteogenic sarcoma, liposarcoma, and fibrosarcoma are the most common; other sarcomas are less common and occur with roughly equal incidence. Osteogenic sarcoma and Ewing's sarcoma develop most frequently in children or young adults. Other sarcomas occur mainly in adults but in a slightly younger population than carcinomas.

Table 32. Sarcomas

Cell or Tissue of Origin	*Malignant Tumor*
Bone	Osteosarcoma Parosteal osteogenic sarcoma Malignant giant cell tumor Ewing's sarcoma
Cartilage	Chondrosarcoma
Fat	Liposarcoma
Fibrous tissue	Fibrosarcoma
Muscle	
Smooth	Leiomyosarcoma
Striated	Rhabdomyosarcoma
Mesenchyme	Myxoma Mesenchymoma
Synovium	Synovial cell sarcoma
Vascular and lymphatic tissue	Angiosarcoma Lymphangiosarcoma Hemangiopericytoma Kaposi's sarcoma
Peripheral nerve	Malignant schwannoma Malignant neurilemoma
Unknown origin	Alveolar soft parts sarcoma Malignant fibrous histiocytoma

Sarcomas have been associated with several predisposing factors. A history of trauma or scar in an area where a sarcoma arises is not uncommon, but the association may be merely by chance. Exposure to ionizing radiation is clearly a risk factor. Chemical sarcogens have also been identified including vinyl chloride, associated with the development of hepatic angiosarcoma. Von Recklinghausen's disease is associated with an increased risk of malignant neurilemoma, and Paget's disease of the bone carries an increased risk of osteogenic sarcoma. Viruses clearly produce sarcomas in animals, but no conclusive evidence for a viral etiology of human sarcoma has yet been demonstrated.

OSTEOGENIC SARCOMA

Clinical Features

Osteogenic sarcomas arise in the long bones in over three-fourths of cases, but may also occur in the ilium, vertebrae, or mandible. Local pain and swelling are the usual initial complaints. A history of anorexia, weight loss, and progressive weakness may be obtained. Laboratory evaluation may show anemia, and the alkaline phosphatase is usually elevated. X-ray films of the symptomatic area typically show a destructive bone lesion, often with a surrounding soft tissue mass, and occasionally with a characteristic spiculated pattern of calcification described as a sunburst. When osteogenic sarcoma is suspected, x-ray tomograms of the chest should be obtained to evaluate the possibility of pulmonary metastases. A bone scan and liver function tests are also recommended preoperatively.

Osteogenic sarcomas metastasize early and widely. Metastatic involvement of the lungs is most frequent. The appearance of pulmonary metastases is usually followed by death within a few months, although occasional longer survivals are seen with slowly progressive tumors.

Treatment

If no evidence of metastatic disease is found in the preoperative evaluation, amputation of the entire affected bone is the usual initial therapy. When osteogenic sarcoma arises in bones other than those of the extremities, total resection may be either impossible or associated with such great morbidity that local radiation therapy is preferable as the initial treatment, even though this tumor is relatively radioresistant. The survival following surgery is approximately 20% at 5 years. In most patients metastases appear within 6-12 months after surgery, and the subsequent course of disease is one of relentless progression. Systemic chemotherapy for advanced metastatic disease may occasionally provide temporary palliation. The most active regimens are high-dose methotrexate with leucovorin rescue, adriamycin, or combination therapy including either or both of these agents with vincristine and cyclophosphamide. Early studies suggest that *cis*-platinum will also be useful.

The high frequency of metastatic disease in osteogenic sarcoma has prompted efforts to improve surgical results with adjuvant chemotherapy. Initial reports of such treatment employing either single agents or combination chemotherapy appeared to show a marked prolongation of the disease-free interval following surgery. These studies, however, utilized historical controls, and the results have been questioned. The issue is unclear at present, but remains a focus for continuing clinical research. Another investigational approach for osteogenic sarcoma seeks to avoid amputation of the affected extremity. The affected bone is removed and replaced by an internal prosthesis. The patient is then treated further with local radiation therapy followed by adjuvant chemotherapy. Final results with this approach are not yet available.

PAROSTEAL SARCOMA AND CHONDROSARCOMA

Parosteal sarcoma and chondrosarcoma originate in bone, although chondrosarcoma may also develop in preexisting benign cartilaginous lesions. Both of these sarcomas are slowly progressive local lesions. Metastases are uncommon and occur late in the disease course. These tumors should be completely removed surgically. Amputation, when possible, is advised to prevent local recurrence.

SOFT TISSUE SARCOMAS

All sarcomas except those that arise in bone and cartilage are included in this group (Table 32). The usual initial finding is a painless soft tissue mass. Occasionally the overlying skin may be warm or red. Sarcomas may present with signs or symptoms of metastatic disease in the lymph nodes, lung, liver, or brain. Systemic symptoms, especially fever of unknown origin, may be present and may sometimes precede diagnosis of the underlying disease by several weeks or months. Diagnosis is established by biopsy and microscopic examination. Further work-up should include chest x-ray, bone scan, and liver funtion tests to determine whether metastatic disease is present.

The natural history of soft tissue sarcomas varies greatly depending on the histologic type. Some are indolent diseases; the primary lesion grows slowly and, if it recurs following surgery, may be well controlled with repeated surgical resections. Even in the presence of metastatic disease, prolonged survival with little morbidity is possible. Examples of such slow-growing sarcomas include alveolar soft parts sarcoma and well-differentiated fibrosarcoma and leiomyosarcoma. Other soft tissue sarcomas such as synovial cell sarcoma, rhabdomyosarcoma, and undifferentiated sarcoma typically exhibit very aggressive behavior with early metastatic spread and rapid progression. Prolonged survival is rare with these varieties.

Initial therapy of soft tissue sarcomas is complete surgical resection if possible, or resection followed by radiation therapy if residual disease is present. The response of metastatic sarcomas to systemic cytotoxic chemotherapy is unpredictable, but on occasion excellent regressions of disease with significant symptomatic improvement can be obtained. Drugs active against soft tissue sarcomas include cyclophosphamide, Adriamycin, vincristine, actinomycin D, DTIC, and *cis*-platinum. Combination chemotherapy is more effective than single-agent treatment. One of the more active and widely used combinations incorporates cyclophosphamide, Adriamycin, vincristine, and DTIC (CYVADIC). Adjuvant chemotherapy of sarcomas is under study, but no benefit has yet been demonstrated in prospective randomized trials.

KAPOSI'S SARCOMA

Kaposi's sarcoma is discussed separately because of its unusual clinical behavior and its responsiveness to therapy. The disease usually presents as a tender, often ulcerated, purple skin lesion. Biopsy reveals an extremely vascular sarcomatous tumor. In locally advanced disease multiple sharply circumscribed, deeply pigmented, and sometimes ulcerated skin lesions, typically on a lower extremity, may be seen. The disease may remain localized to skin for several years before visceral metastases develop. Following biopsy and histologic diagnosis a technetium radionuclide scan of the affected area (usually a leg) should be done. This vascular tumor will often be detected by the scan in areas that are not apparent clinically.

Kaposi's sarcoma is very sensitive to radiation therapy. All involved areas including those identified by the technetium scan should be encompassed by the radiation treatment field. Recurrent or metastatic disease is responsive to treatment with chemotherapy. Cyclophosphamide, vincristine, and actinomycin D have been used in combination and provide very good response rates.

EWING'S SARCOMA

Ewing's sarcoma is a malignant small-cell tumor seen in children and young adults. The disease usually presents as a localized bone lesion causing pain or pathologic fracture. Early and widespread metastases to other bones and internal organs occur. Local therapy only, either by amputation or radiation therapy, is not satisfactory since the 5-year survival rate is a dismal 5-15%. Recent trials combining radiation therapy of the primary lesion and systemic chemotherapy with cyclophosphamide, Adriamycin, and vincristine appear to show at least a delay in development of metastatic disease and perhaps a prolongation of survival.

MALIGNANT FIBROUS HISTIOCYTOMA

Malignant fibrous histiocytoma is a soft tissue sarcoma of uncertain origin that has been diagnosed with increasing frequency in the past 5 years. The tumor may present as an isolated lytic lesion of bone often with adjacent soft tissue swelling (either as a reaction or due to actual tumor infiltration), or as a soft tissue mass. Metastases are common. Microscopic examination of biopsy material reveals a large cell anaplastic tumor with marked pleomorphism and multinucleated tumor giant cells. If there is infiltration with granulocytes, the tumor is called an inflammatory fibrous histiocytoma.

Therapy consists of eradication of the primary tumor by surgery, radiation therapy, or both if possible. Chemotherapy of recurrent or metastatic disease has not yet had adequate trials. Brief responses to combinations of drugs used in sarcoma therapy have, however, been reported.

MALIGNANT BRAIN TUMORS

PRIMARY BRAIN TUMORS

Incidence and Etiology

The American Cancer Society data indicate that of 405,000 cancer deaths in the United States in 1980, 9,800 occurred due to malignant brain tumors. Tumors of the brain and central nervous system are the second most common cause of cancer deaths in children under the age of 15, but they are much less common in adults. The etiology of brain tumors in man is entirely unknown, although viral and chemical carcinogens can produce gliomas in experimental animals. No geographic or epidemiologic associations are recognized. Hereditary factors play a role only in rare cases of gliomas associated with neurofibromatosis or tuberous sclerosis.

The pathologic classification of brain tumors is hampered by the existence of numerous systems of nomenclature and by the fact that mixed tumors are common; small biopsy specimens may not adequately reflect the nature of the bulk of the tumor. An abbreviated classification scheme is shown in Table 33. It is worth noting that many of these tumors have benign counterparts that may produce devastating neurologic symptoms. The growth rates, locations, and invasiveness of benign tumors differ from the cancers, however, and will not be discussed further here.

Clinical Features

Malignant brain tumors produce symptoms by invasion or compression of adjacent structures, elevation of intracranial pressure (due to the tumor mass itself, surrounding cerebral edema, or to a secondary obstructive hydrocephalus), and by herniation of uninvolved brain tissue. In some cases minimal or no symptoms are encountered. Most patients with brain tumors, at some time in their course, will have headaches, which may be mild or severe. Headache awakening the patient from sleep or present on first awakening in the morning is typical for brain tumors but not specific. The headache due to elevated intracranial pressure is typically bifrontal or bioccipital and is often accompanied by vomiting. Elevation of intracranial pressure also causes depression in the level of consciousness, initially manifested by drowsiness and lethargy but often progressing to stupor, coma, and death.

Table 33. Classification of Malignant Brain Tumors

Malignant gliomas
Glioblastoma multiforme
Astrocytoma
Ependymoma
Oligodendroglioma
Mixed glioma
Medulloblastoma
Other
Malignant meningiona
Neurofibrosarcoma
Malignant neurilemoma
Sarcoma
Other
Metastatic neoplasms

A vague change in mental function may be the presenting symptom in patients with brain tumor and may be difficult to distinguish from depression, anxiety, or fatigue. Emotional lability, lack of spontaneity, forgetfulness, withdrawal from interpersonal relationships and similar problems are often reported by the patient's family while the patient himself denies the existence of a problem. In later stages obvious intellectual impairment, memory loss, somnolence, confusion, and dementia supervene. Mental symptoms of this nature appear to be related to tumors involving the cerebral white matter in various locations.

Seizures occur in 20-50% of brain tumor patients. The onset of seizures in an adult should always suggest brain tumor, even in the absence of localizing neurologic findings. The location of the tumor frequently may be deduced if focal seizures are observed. Similarly, focal neurologic findings involving motor or sensory function, speech, or cranial nerves may signal the presence of a brain tumor and point to its location.

The diagnosis of brain tumor depends primarily on recognition of suspicious findings on history and thorough neurologic examination. With the advent of computed tomography, brain tumors can be detected in well over 95% of cases. Only infratentorial and suprasellar lesions present any difficulty for this highly accurate and safe technique. As a consequence, skull films, radionuclide brain scans, and pneumoencephalography are now rarely necessary in the evaluation of the patient with a suspected brain tumor. Cerebral angiography provides valuable information to the neurosurgeon but is not often employed for diagnosis.

Treatment

Neurosurgical exploration with maximal removal of tumor is recommended for all patients with malignant brain tumors in order to establish a definite diagnosis and to decompress the brain. Furthermore, by reducing the tumor burden at a time when the patient may be severely compromised, surgery allows time for the subsequent use of chemotherapy and radiation. Randomized trials have shown that both radiation therapy and chemotherapy with nitrosoureas following neurosurgery for malignant gliomas result in prolongation of survival over patients treated by surgery alone. There is suggestive evidence that the addition of both modalities may result in an additive effect on survival. Nevertheless, malignant glioma is a uniformly fatal disease; fewer than 20% of patients survive more than 1 year after surgery even with the addition of radiation therapy and chemotherapy. However, the quality of survival for most patients is improved, as measured by performance status and ability to function at work or at home; thus, radiation and chemotherapy have become standard adjuncts to surgery in the treatment of gliomas. Future progress in the treatment of malignant brain tumors will depend on the development of more effective drugs and drug combinations and on the use of agents (radiosensitizers) that may enhance the effectiveness of radiation against tumors.

METASTATIC BRAIN TUMORS

Intracranial metastases occur in 10-20% of autopsied patients with cancer and are most commonly associated with primary cancers arising in lung, breast, gastrointestinal tract, kidney, and malignant melanoma. The signs and symptoms produced by metastatic tumors are similar to those seen with primary brain tumors. Since metastatic tumors are most often multiple, however, the symptoms and the neurologic deficits may be much more severe.

Computed tomography of the brain is almost invariably diagnostic; additional studies are rarely necessary. Treatment consists of whole-brain irradiation and/or corticosteroids (e.g., dexamethasone 16 mg per day). In the very rare cases in which the metastatic lesion in the brain is solitary and systemic metastases are either absent or stable, consideration may be given to surgical excision followed by radiation. In most cases, however, progressive systemic malignancy or multiple cerebral lesions makes this approach unwise. Chemotherapy, to date, has found little role in the treatment of metastatic cancer to the brain.

Whole-brain irradiation produces symptomatic improvement and prolongation of survival in 60-75% of patients. Many patients return to normal neurologic status. Median survival following whole-brain irradiation for metastatic tumor is approximately 6 months with fewer than 15% surviving for more than 1 year. Many of these patients, however, succumb to widespread systemic tumor without recurrence of neurologic symptoms.

PARANEOPLASTIC SYNDROMES

The paraneoplastic syndromes are a diverse group of medical problems arising in patients with cancer and thought to represent remote or indirect effects of that cancer. Before a diagnosis of paraneoplastic syndrome can be made, the direct effects of the tumor or its metastases, the toxic effects of various therapeutic maneuvers, and the presence of unrelated illnesses must be carefully ruled out. Most of the paraneoplastic syndromes are rare, and other explanations can often be found for what seems to be a remote effect of cancer.

In some cases the paraneoplastic syndrome may precede the diagnosis of cancer by months or even years. It may respond to successful treatment of the tumor, but in many instances it pursues an independent course. Except in the case of the endocrine syndromes, in which specific hormonal mediators secreted by the tumor have been identified, the causes of paraneoplastic syndromes are unknown.

ENDOCRINE SYNDROMES

The endocrine syndromes, in which there is ectopic hormone production by nonendocrine tumors, are the most common of the paraneoplastic syndromes and the most readily diagnosed. Some of the more common tumor-ectopic hormone associations are listed in Table 34. To be certain that the hormone is produced ectopically by the tumor (and not by a simultaneously occurring disorder of the appropriate endocrine gland), one of the following three conditions must be met: the tumor tissue must be shown to contain abnormally high levels of the hormone; an arteriovenous difference in hormone level across the tumor must be demonstrated; or the hormone level and/or its manifestations must decline following successful treatment of the tumor.

Recognition of the ability of certain cancers to produce hormones ectopically is important from several points of view. Often the hormone disorder precedes the diagnosis of cancer and may alert the clinician to consider an underlying neoplasm in the differential diagnosis. For example, erythrocytosis in a patient without a cardiac, pulmonary, or hematologic disorder should be investigated with an intravenous pyelogram in order to detect an otherwise asymptomatic renal cell carcinoma that is secreting erythropoietin. Such early detection of tumors by means of hormone markers may lead to improved surgical cure rates.

Table 34. Tumors Commonly Associated with Ectopic Hormone Production

Hormone	*Tumor*
ACTH	Lung (small cell) Carcinoid (bronchial) Thyroid (medullary) Pancreas (islet cell) Thymus
ADH	Lung (small cell)
PTH	Lung (squamous cell) Kidney Pancreas Ovary Endometrium Squamous cell carcinomas of head and neck
Erythropoietin	Kidney Hepatoma Cerebellar hemangioblastoma Virilizing ovarian and adrenal tumors Pheochromocytoma
TSH	Choriocarcinoma Hydatidiform mole
ILA[a]	Retroperitoneal sarcomas Hepatoma
Calcitonin	Lung (small cell)

[a]Insulin-like activity

Furthermore, the hormone may serve as a marker for recurrence of tumor following initial treatment. The use of hormonal and other markers for screening large populations for cancer has been proposed.

The metabolic and systemic effects of excessive hormone secretion may add further morbidity in a patient already symptomatic from the direct effects of the tumor and from its treatment. Proper management of symptoms produced by the hormone excess may contribute materially to the patient's comfort. For example, a patient with small-cell carcinoma of the lung and hyponatremia due to ectopic production of antidiuretic hormone will benefit from correction of hyponatremia by fluid restriction while chemotherapy and radiation therapy are being employed against the tumor.

NEUROLOGIC SYNDROMES

Neurologic complications of malignancy occur in 20% of cancer patients and at all levels of the nervous system. The vast majority of these complications are related to direct effects of the tumor and its metastases on the nervous system or to side effects of therapy. In addition vascular, infectious, and metabolic disorders commonly develop in these patients and may produce neurologic manifestations. Neuromusucular disorders as a remote effect of cancer on the nervous system are the rarest form of neurologic complication of malignancy.

Table 35 gives a classification scheme for many of the neurologic syndromes described as remote effects of cancer. However, these syndromes are rarely seen in pure form and extensive overlap between them occurs. Several of these syndromes, such as dermatomyositis, atypical myasthenic syndrome, and subacute spinocerebellar degeneration, are highly suggestive of cancer and, when they occur in a patient without known malignancy, should prompt an investigation for underlying tumor. Many of the other neurologic syndromes arise sufficiently often in patients without cancer to make an extensive evaluation for occult neoplasm unrewarding.

Subacute spinocerebellar degeneration characteristically presents with bilaterally symmetric cerebellar ataxia involving arms and legs, progressing rapidly over 1-2 months. The spinal cord findings (extensor plantar responses, weakness) are invariably overshadowed by the severe cerebellar signs: ataxia of gait, intention tremor, and dysarthria. Nystagmus and vertigo are less prominent. The CSF is usually normal, but a mild mononuclear pleocytosis and elevated protein can be seen. The neurologic condition is irreversible, regardless of whether the tumor is managed successfully.

Muscle weakness, particularly myasthenic syndromes, have been reported in cancer patients. Such patients may occasionally resemble those with classic myasthenia gravis but frequently differ from that entity in the following ways: sparing of the bulbar muscles or involvement of the extremities occurring before bulbar symptoms; loss of deep tendon reflexes; variable or poor response to anticholinesterases but marked sensitivity to curare-like drugs; and improvement of muscle strength with time during a sustained contraction. The Eaton-Lambert syndrome refers to this clinical constellation, combined with a characteristic electromyogram (EMG) pattern revealing a block in transmission in rested muscle and facilitation with repetitive stimulation.

Table 35. Remote Effects of Cancer on the Nervous System

Brain
Dementia
Subacute spinocerebellar degeneration
Encephalomyelitis of brainstem and spinal cord
Spinal cord
Necrotizing myelopathy
Chronic myelopathy (ALS)
Peripheral nerve
Sensory-motor neuropathies
Isolated asymmetrical sensory neuritis
Degeneration of dorsal root ganglia
Neuromuscular junction and muscle
Myasthenic syndromes
Dermatomyositis/polymyositis

Patients with this disorder report weakness most marked in proximal muscles, especially in the pelvic girdle and thighs. Muscle aching, dry mouth, and paresthesias may also occur. Strength on muscle testing may be well preserved, but the EMG is definitive. Most cases of the Eaton-Lambert syndrome are associated with lung cancer, especially with the small-cell variety. Classic myasthenia gravis and overlap syndromes including features of both Eaton-Lambert and myasthenia gravis have also been reported with small cell carcinoma. Other tumors are infrequently associated.

Striking remission of the myasthenic syndromes may follow successful treatment of the underlying tumor. Failing this, guanidine, which increases the amount of acetylcholine released from nerve endings, may produce clinical and electrophysiologic improvement. The anticholinesterases, useful in classic myasthenia gravis, rarely elicit responses in the Eaton-Lambert or overlap syndromes.

CONNECTIVE TISSUE SYNDROMES

Dermatomyositis (and polymyositis) arising in adults may be the first indication of an occult neoplasm. Patients with dermatomyositis have 5-7 times the incidence of malignancy as the general population, and various series of patients with dermatomyositis report an incidence of malignancy from 7-34%. Therefore, an extensive investigation for occult tumor is warranted in every adult with dermatomyositis (or polymyositis).

The clinical and pathologic features of dermatomyositis associated with malignancy do not differ from those in uncomplicated dermatomyositis except that patients with malignancies tend to be older than the general dermatomyositis population. The course of the myopathy is not usually affected by tumor remission or progression, although occasional dramatic improvements in dermatomyositis following tumor treatment do occur.

In women, cancers of the breast, ovary, and uterus are most commonly encountered in the dermatomyositis population. In men, the most common tumors arise in the lung, prostate, and stomach. Nasopharyngeal carcinomas seem to be overrepresented as well, compared to their frequency in the general population. The association between dermatomyositis and malignancy has defied explanation to date.

Several connective tissue diseases have been associated with particular malignancies (scleroderma and alveolar cell carcinoma of lung, systemic lupus erythematosus and lymphoma, acute polyarthritis and various neoplasms) but the nature of the association is unclear. In general, these are not considered remote effects of cancer.

DERMATOLOGIC CONDITIONS ASSOCIATED WITH CANCER

A variety of cutaneous changes are associated with underlying malignancies. These include urticaria, erythema multiforme, bullous disorders, ichthyosis, migratory thrombophlebitis, and hypertrichosis lanugosa. The extent to which each of these dermatologic conditions suggests occult cancer varies.

Acanthosis nigricans is an unusual skin condition arising in some patients with neoplasms (especially adenocarcinomas of the stomach) and in other patients with obesity, Cushing's syndrome, adrenal insufficiency, and acromegaly. The cutaneous findings consist of symmetric velvety, verrucuous hyperpigmented areas in the axilla, groin, beneath the breast, and in other skin folds. It has been suggested that acanthosis nigricans is caused by a peptide hormone excessively secreted by an abnormal pituitary gland in obese patients and those with Cushing's syndrome, and ectopically secreted by certain malignant neoplasms. However, there is no direct evidence to support this hypothesis. Whenever acanthosis nigricans develops in an adult without an endocrine disorder, a search for an underlying neoplasm is mandatory. In most cases the course of the skin disorder will parallel that of the tumor and cure of the tumor will result in cure of the acanthosis nigricans.

NEPHROTIC SYNDROME

Nephrotic syndrome secondary to membranous glomerulonephritis or lipoid nephrosis occurs not uncommonly in Hodgkin's disease and in a variety of solid tumors including carcinomas of the lung, colon, stomach, ovary, and kidney. In most, but not all, cases immunofluorescent studies and electron microscopy reveal deposition of antigen-antibody complexes in the basement membrane of the kidney. The antigen represents a tumor product; in several cases of colon cancer carcinoembryonic antigen (CEA) has been identified in the renal basement membrane, supporting the concept that the renal lesion is produced by an immunologic response to the tumor.

The nephrotic syndrome may precede the diagnosis of cancer, and in some series the prevalence of cancer in unselected adults with nephrotic syndrome is a startling 10%. In most instances, the nephrotic syndrome improves or disappears with removal or successful treatment of the tumor. Recurrence of nephrotic syndrome almost invariably implies recurrence of the tumor. Evaluation of an adult with unexplained nephrotic syndrome should include tests for underlying malignancy.

ONCOLOGIC EMERGENCIES

The following section is intended to present the signs and symptoms and discuss the immediate therapy of common emergencies that occur in cancer patients. Severe morbidity or fatality may result without prompt recognition and therapy of these conditions. In addition to the conditions discussed below, cancer patients are also subject to hematologic emergencies such as bleeding and to cardiac emergencies such as pericardial effusion and tamponade. These problems are discussed in detail elsewhere in this book.

INCREASED INTRACRANIAL PRESSURE

Elevated intracranial pressure most frequently occurs as a consequence of metastatic involvement of the brain, but it may also be encountered with primary brain tumors and with meningeal carcinomatosis due to leukemias or solid tumors. Headache is the earliest symptom, followed by nausea, vomiting, and visual blurring. Focal neurologic signs and personality changes may also develop. As the tumor enlarges and brain edema increases, lethargy, somnolence, and ultimately coma supervene.

Physical examination may reveal focal neurologic signs that, in combination with papilledema in a known cancer patient, almost always indicate metastatic brain disease. A fixed and dilated pupil is a late sign reflecting tentorial herniation. Computed tomography of the brain is the most useful examination to confirm the presence of metastatic tumor. If meningeal involvement is suspected, lumbar puncture should be performed and CSF cytology obtained.

Treatment of increased intracranial pressure should include prompt administration of dexamethasone (usually 4 mg q 6 h) followed by neurosurgery in the case of primary brain tumors or radiation therapy in the case of metastatic tumors. Meningeal carcinomatosis may be treated with intrathecal instillation of methotrexate or cytosine arabinoside. Radiation therapy may also be helpful.

SPINAL CORD COMPRESSION

Spinal cord compression usually follows tumor extension from vertebral bodies or the epidural space into the spinal canal. Occasionally, pathologic fractures of vertebral bodies involved with metastatic tumor may cause cord compression. Back pain is almost always an early complaint. Numbness and weakness in the legs, and sometimes also in the arms, follow. Urinary retention and severe leg weakness usually progress to paraplegia or quadraplegia within 1-2 days. The most important physical findings are muscular weakness of the extremities, loss of reflexes, and sensory loss with a sensory level. Suspicion of cord compression requires prompt lumbar myelography to confirm the diagnosis and to localize the level of obstruction. Therapy should begin with steroid administration (dexamethasone 4mg q6h) followed by radiation therapy, laminectomy, or both. When cord compression is caused by malignant lymphoma, appropriate chemotherapy is often the quickest method to relieve pressure and reverse symptoms.

SUPERIOR VENA CAVA SYNDROME

Tumors involving the mediastinum, most often bronchogenic carcinoma, metastatic breast cancer, and malignant lymphoma, may obstruct the superior vena cava resulting in edema of the upper extremities, upper thorax, the neck, and head. Early signs include neck vein distention and periorbital and conjunctival edema. More extensive facial and neck edema, flushing, and eventually cyanosis occur as obstruction worsens. If the process occurs gradually, collateral circulation develops and results in a prominent venous pattern visible on the chest. A chest x-ray will almost invariably show a mediastinal tumor mass. A technitium radionuclide flow study provides a prompt and easy method to confirm the diagnosis and to follow the progress of therapy. If symptoms are severe, diuretics and dexamethasone may be used in an attempt to relieve edema, but recovery depends on prompt institution of radiotherapy to the mediastinal tumor mass. If the obstruction is caused by a malignant lymphoma, appropriate chemotherapy will produce rapid improvement and may be used in conjuntion with radiotherapy.

UPPER AIRWAY COMPRESSION

Compression of the upper airway occurs most often with head and neck cancers, thyroid cancers, and superior mediastinal tumors such as malignant lymphomas. Symptoms include cough and respiratory distress, paticularly when supine. Inspiratory stridor is sometimes heard on physical examination. Chest x-ray examination usually reveals a mediastinal mass and shows the trachea displaced from its normal position. Unless obstruction is high, tracheostomy is not usually helpful or even possible; immediate treatment with radiation therapy to the tumor mass is necessary. If lymphoma is responsible for compressive symptoms, chemotherapy may also be helpful.

URETERAL OBSTRUCTION

Bilateral complete ureteral obstruction may be caused by pelvic tumors of the cervix, ovary, bladder, colorectum, or by malignant lymphomas. The resulting hydronephrosis may result in uremia of insidious onset. Progressive nausea, vomiting, lethargy, and eventually somnolence, coma, and death from metabolic abnormalities and cardiac arrhythmias result. Physical examination may reveal the pelvic tumor mass, the characteristic odor of uremia, and asterixis. A history of oliguria or anuria is often obtained. Retrograde peylography (if possible) will confirm the suspicion of obstruction. Percutaneous or surgical nephrostomies may be placed to relieve obstruction and preserve renal function if subsequent therapy of the underlying disease is feasible.

PNEUMOTHORAX

Pneumothorax in cancer patients may result from tumor erosion from the lung into the pleural space. Sudden chest pain, dyspnea, and tachycardia are the usual symptoms. Small pneumothoraces may resolve spontaneously; larger penumothoraces require the placement of a chest tube. Repeated pneumothoraces may benefit from pleural sclerosis by instillation of atabrine or tetracycline into the pleural space through a chest tube. Tension pneumothorax is a life-threatening condition. The physical examination reveals a hyperresonant hemithorax with absent breath sounds and deviation of the trachea away from the affected side. If a chest tube cannot be inserted immediately, pressure must be released by placing a large-gauge needle into the affected pleural space.

METABOLIC EMERGENCIES

Hypercalcemia

Hypercalcemia caused by metastatic bone involvement occurs most commonly with breast cancer, bronchogenic cancer, and multiple myeloma and may be seen occasionally with metastatic hypernephromas. Hypercalcemia may also result from ectopic tumor production of parathyroid hormone or other mediators such as prostaglandins or osteoclast-activating factor. Early symptoms include urinary frequency, constipation, nausea, and vomiting. Weakness and progressing lethargy may occur, followed by coma, seizures, and death. There are no specific physical signs of hypercalcemia. In cancer patients with unexplained lethargy, vomiting, or coma hypercalcemia should be suspected and the serum calcium measured. Emergency treatment of severe hypercalcemia should begin with intravenous administration of mithramycin, 25 μgm/kg. Because dehydration and azotemia are invariably present, intravenous hydration and diuresis will not only help correct fluid and electrolyte abnormalities but will also aid in calcium excretion. Mithramycin may be repeated every 3-4 days as needed while measures directed against the underlying disease are insituted. Calcitonin is also an effective therapy for acute hypercalcemia. Long-term control of hypercalcemia depends mainly on treatment of the underlying disease. Oral phosphate therapy, corticosteroids, and prostaglandin antagonists may occasionally aid in management while definitive therapeutic measures are in progress.

Hyperuricemia

Very high uric acid levels may precipitate attacks of acute gouty arthritis or, more seriously, may result in acute renal failure. Hyperuricemia is most often encountered in acute leukemia and malignant lymphoma, usually as a result of rapid tumor lysis following therapy. Emergency treatment of hyperuricemia and acute renal failure depends on efforts to induce diuresis with hydration and diuretics. Alkalinization of the urine will aid in uric acid excretion. Dialysis may be necessary. The best therapy is anticipation and prevention, using allopurinol. When high uric acid loads are anticipated, a dose of 600 mg of allopurinol daily is recommended and, if possible, should commence several days before chemotherapy is given.

Hypoglycemia

Confusion, lethargy, anxiety, sweating, tachycardia, and coma may occur as a consequence of hypoglycemia associated with insulin-producing islet cell carcinomas of the pancreas or with large retroperitoneal tumors. The characteristic symptoms should lead to measurement of the blood glucose level and, if islet cell tumor is suspected, to determination of serum insulin levels. Immediate therapy consists of intravenous administration of glucose. Long-term control ultimately depends on therapy of the underlying disease, but hyperglycemic agents such as glucagon and diazoxide may be helpful in controlling symtoms.

Lactic Acidosis

Lactic acidosis may rarely be seen as a consequence of tumor metabolism, particularly with widespread and rapidly progressive malignant lymphomas. Weakness, lethargy, and tachypnea are the usual symptoms. Clinical chemistries will reveal an anion gap and a low blood pH. An elevated serum lactate level is diagnostic. Immediate therapy consists of correction of acidosis with intravenous bicarbonate. Long-term control depends on therapy directed against the underlying disease.

INFECTIOUS EMERGENCIES

Sepsis

Cancer patients are prone to develop severe infections because of the frequency of leukopenia in this group, either as a result of marrow replacement by tumor or as a consequence of myelosuppressive therapy. The danger of sepsis becomes appreciable when the granulocyte count is below 1,000/mm^3 and great when the granulocyte count is below 500/mm^3. A patient with fever, chills, and a low granulocyte count must be hospitalized promptly and immediate cultures of blood, urine, sputum, and any other fluid or tissue suspect as an infection source must be obtained. Pending results of the cultures and antibiotic sensitivities, the severely leukopenic patient with suspected sepsis should be started immediately on broad-spectrum intravenous antibiotic therapy. A combination of an aminoglycoside antibiotic with carbenicillin or a cephalosporin provides good broad-spectrum coverage pending identification of the responsible organism. In leukopenic patients with persistent sepsis despite adequate antibiotic therapy, and in whom leukopenia is likely to be prolonged, transfusions of leukocytes should be considered.

IATROGENIC EMERGENCIES

The Tumor Lysis Syndrome

This syndrome may be seen following intial therapy of large or widely disseminated tumors that are very sensitive to treatment, such as acute leukemias and malignant lymphomas. The problem arises from rapid lysis of malignant cells resulting in a massive systemic load of potassium, phosphate, uric acid, other organic acids, and nitrogen compounds. These loads may be beyond the capacity of the kidneys to excrete; preexisting renal impairment exacerbates the problem. The resulting acidosis, hyperkalemia, and hyperphosphatemia (with consequent hypocalcemia) may be of very rapid onset and can produce fatal cardiac arrhythmias. Hyperuricemia, sometimes despite allopurinol therapy, and azotemia also occur. If the syndrome is recognized fatality can be prevented by prompt correction of acidosis, hyperkalemia, and hypocalcemia and maintenance of a vigorous forced diuresis. Dialysis may be necessary. If the patient can be carried through these initial metabolic difficulties, a good tumor response to therapy usually follows.

QUESTIONS

1. A 26-year-old previously healthy woman has a left cervical mass and a mediastinal mass seen on chest x-ray. She is asymptomatic. No other abnormalities are found on physical exam. Biopsy of the cervical mass shows Hodgkin's disease with nodular sclerosis. Abdominal CT scan and bone marrow biopsy are normal. The patient's stage and proper therapy are
   A. Stage IA–mantle irradiation to 4,500 rads
   B. Stage IIA–mantle irradiation to 4,500 rads
   C. Stage uncertain–staging laparotomy and repositioning of the ovaries
   D. Stage uncertain–treat with 6 courses of MOPP to save patient major surgery
2. A 30-year-old man has had daily fevers for the past 2 months and has lost 25 lb. A right axillary node is palpable; physical exam is otherwise normal. Biopsy of the node shows lymphocyte depleted Hodgkin's disease. CBC shows anemia. Liver function tests are normal. Chest x-ray is normal, but abdominal CT scan shows large abnormal para-aortic lymph nodes. Bone marrow biopsy shows hypercellular marrow with increased myelopoiesis. The patient's stage and management are
   A. Stage indeterminate–should have staging laparotomy; subsequent therapy depends on pathologic results

B. Stage indeterminate—should have liver biopsy

C. Stage IIIB—should have total lymphoid radiation therapy to 4,500 rads

D. At least stage IIIB—should be treated with combination chemotherapy (MOPP) for a minimum of 6 courses.

3. A 25-year-old man complains of nonproductive cough and wheezing. A lymph node is palpable in his neck. A chest x-ray shows a large superior mediastinal mass deviating the tracheal air column. Proper workup and management are

A. Referral to a surgeon for prompt biopsy of the lymph node

B. Schedule abdominal CT scan and bone marrow biopsy

C. Hospitalize and consult surgeon for biopsy; meanwhile obtain abdominal CT scan

D. Hospitalize: emergency consultation for radiation therapy to mediastinum; obtain biopsy specimen of node when stable

4. Unfavorable (poor prognosis) varieties of non-Hodgkin's lymphoma (NHL) are

A. Diffuse poorly differentiated lymphocytic

B. Diffuse well-differentiated lymphocytic

C. Diffuse histiocytic

D. Diffuse undifferentiated (Burkitt's type)

E. Nodular poorly differentiated lymphocytic

5. A staging laparotomy should be done in NHL

A. Always

B. When therapy would be affected by findings

C. For diagnosis

D. To remove the spleen so that subsequent therapy will be better tolerated

6. An asymptomatic 80-year-old woman in otherwise excellent health has a small right cervical lymph node found on routine physical exam. Biopsy shows diffuse well-differentiated lymphocytic lymphoma. Subsequent studies including CBC, liver function tests, chest x-ray, and abdominal CT scan are normal, but bone marrow biopsy shows an increase in normal-appearing lymphocytes. Proper management is

A. Exploratory staging laparotomy

B. Mantle irradiation therapy to 4,500 rads

C. Observation, monthly checkups, treatment if and when disease becomes symptomatic

D. Chemotherapy with an easily tolerated combination (e.g., chlorambucil-prednisone)

7. Renal failure seen in multiple myeloma may be caused by

A. Hypercalcemia

B. Stones

C. Myeloma protein

D. Amyloidosis

E. Tumor infiltration of kidneys

F. All of the above

8. Patients at high risk to develop breast cancer who should receive yearly mammograms are

A. Women who have relatives who have had breast cancer

B. Women who have had irradiation to breasts (e.g., for treatment of fibrocystic disease)

C. Women who have had cancer in one breast

D. Women who have had acute bacterial mastitis

E. All of the above

9. The most important test(s) to aid in subsequent management of breast cancer is (are)

A. Lung scan

B. Estrogen receptor status of the patient's tumor

C. Serum CEA titer

D. Information regarding involvement of axillary nodes with tumor

E. Liver biopsy

10. A 32-year-old woman has had a mastectomy with axillary node exploration. The tumor is estrogen receptor positive; 12 of 12 axillary nodes contain metastatic tumor. Chest x-ray, liver function tests, and bone scan are normal. The best current management is

A. Prophylactic radiation therapy to mastectomy site and adjacent lymph nodes

B. Bilateral oophorectomy

C. Combination chemotherapy (e.g., cyclophosphamide, methotrexate, 5-fluorouracil) for 1 year

D. Immunotherapy with BCG

E. Close follow-up; treatment of further problems if and when they occur.

11. It is important to know the histologic type of lung cancer because

A. This makes it easier to discuss the prognosis with the patient and family.

B. Small-cell carcinomas receive different and potentially very effective treatment.

C. Knowing the histology helps predict where metastases will appear.

D. Small-cell carcinomas are seldom operable and the patient can be saved major surgery.

E. It is not important at all.

12. Criteria for inoperability of lung cancers include

A. Involvement of mediastinal nodes

B. Involvement of pleura and ribs

C. Distant metastases

D. Small-cell anaplastic histology

E. All of the above

13. A 61-year-old man presents with confusion, hepatomegaly, and a right upper lobe mass on his chest x-ray

with hilar adenopathy also visible. Serum sodium is 110. The most likely diagnosis is

A. Squamous cell carcinoma
B. Small-cell anaplastic carcinoma
C. Adenocarcinoma
D. Islet cell carcinoma of pancreas metastatic to liver and lung

14. Patients at high risk to develop colon carcinoma who need close observation are

A. Patients with multiple colonic polyposis
B. Patients with inflammatory bowel disease
C. Patients with Gardner's syndrome
D. Patients with Crohn's disease
E. All of the above

15. Prognosis following surgery for colon cancer depends most on

A. The degree of differentiation of tumor cells
B. The Duke's classification
C. The presence (or absence) of vascular invasion by tumor
D. The patient's age
E. All of the above

16. While gastrointestinal adenocarcinomas are not markedly responsive to chemotherapy, the most responsive tumors are those of

A. Colon
B. Rectum
C. Stomach
D. Pancreas
E. Small bowel
F. Gall bladder and bile ducts

17. A 78-year-old man has a nodule on his prostate gland; needle biopsy shows an adenocarcinoma. Bone scan shows multiple metastatic foci. He is asymptomatic. Correct management is

A. Radical prostatectomy followed by pelvic radiation therapy
B. Bilateral orchiectomy
C. Oral diethylstilbesterol
D. Observation; treatment of problems when they become symptomatic with appropriate therapy
E. Radiation to prostate followed by orchiectomy and oral diethylstilbesterol

18. A 36-year-old man has an enlarged testicle. High inguinal orchiectomy is done. Pathology shows a pure seminoma. He should

A. Have an abdominal CT scan: if negative, receive radiation to mediastinal and para-aortic nodes
B. Have an abdominal CT scan: if positive, receive radiation to para-aortic nodes and iliac nodes on the side of the tumor
C. Have a laparotomy, retroperitoneal lymph node dissection, and whole abdominal radiation therapy
D. Be treated with cyclophosphamide, Adriamycin, and *cis*-platinum

19. A 20-year-old man has an enlarged testicle and tenderness of his nipples. High inguinal orchiectomy is done. Pathology shows teratocarcinoma with embryonal elements. Abdominal CT is positive. Serum HCG and α-fetoprotein are elevated postoperatively. He should

A. Have a retroperitoneal lymph node dissection followed by radiation therapy to the para-aortic area
B. Begin chemotherapy with vinblastine, bleomycin, and *cis*-platinum
C. Have a retroperitoneal lymph node dissection followed by chemotherapy
D. Have para-aortic node irradiation followed by chemotherapy

20. A 45-year-old woman, previously in excellent health, has a 6-week history of enlargement of her abdomen. She has a 6×10 cm pelvic mass, a 6×6 cm mass in the umbilical area, and obvious clinical ascites. Abdominal x-ray shows early small bowel obstruction. Diagnostic paracentesis fluid contains adenocarcinoma cells consistent with an ovarian primary. She should

A. Be admitted to a hospice for terminal care
B. Begin whole abdominal radiation therapy
C. Undergo laparotomy with removal of as much bulk tumor as possible, and begin on chemotherapy
D. Have surgery to bypass obstructed small bowel and being on chemotherapy

21. The most common presenting sign or symptom of endometrial cancer is

A. Abnormal vaginal bleeding
B. Bowel obstruction
C. Foul vaginal discharge
D. Pelvic pain
E. Dysuria

22. Which procedure(s) is (are) useful in diagnosis or staging of cervical cancer?

A. Pap test
B. Schilling test
C. Cone biopsy
D. Brain scan
E. Pelvic CT scan

23. A 22-year-old woman has a D and C for a molar pregnancy. Her serum β-HCG titer falls from 42,000 to 10,000 after 6 weeks but then increases to 12,000. A chest x-ray shows 2 metastatic parenchymal lesions. Therapy and prognosis are

A. Hysterectomy, pelvic radiation, and combination

chemotherapy with a 50% probablitiy of cure

B. Treatment every other week with methotrexate until serum β-HCG titer is 0; 90%+ probability of cure

C. Pelvic radiation therapy followed by methotrexate until serum β-HCG titer is 0; 98% probability of cure

D. Methotrexate treatment until chest x-ray clears with a 70% probablitiy of cure

24. The histologic variety of thyroid cancer most likely to concentrate ^{131}I is

A. Undifferentiated carcinoma

B. Papillary carcinoma

C. Follicular carcinoma

D. Medullary carcinoma

25. Prognosis in malignant melanoma is most dependent on

A. The amount of lymphocyte infiltration of the tumor

B. The depth of invasion (Clark's level) or thickness in millimeters of the primary tumor

C. The ability of the patient to demonstrate an intact delayed hypersensitivity reaction to DNCB

D. The length of time waited before biopsy of a suspicious lesion

E. Whether the patient is male or female

26. A 17-year-old boy complains of pain in his right arm progressive over several weeks. A x-ray shows a lytic bone lesion. Biopsy shows a small round cell malignant tumor. Most likely diagnosis and appropriate therapy is

A. Osteosarcoma–forequarter amputation followed by high dose methotrexate with leucovorin rescue

B. Acute leukemia–intensive antileukemia chemotherapy; brain and spinal cord irradiation

C. Rhabdomyosarcoma–irradiation to lesion followed by amputation

D. Ewing's sarcoma–irradiation to lesion followed by combination chemotherapy

E. Malignant fibrous histiocytoma–irradiation to lesion and adjacent lymph nodes

27. The following syndromes may be associated with lung cancer:

A. Hypertrophic osteoarthropathy

B. Inappropriate ADH

C. Cushing's syndrome

D. Cerebellar degeneration

E. All of the above

28. A patient with breast cancer has been well for 2 years on tamoxifen. Her family calls to tell you she has had back pain for several weeks of increasing severity and now has trouble walking. You should

A. Explain to the family that her condition is terminal and arrange for admission to a nursing home

B. Call a prescription for a narcotic analgesic to the patient's pharmacy

C. Arrange consultation with a radiation therapist next week

D. Admit to the hospital; consult neurosurgeon for an emergency myelogram; notify radiation therapist and medical oncologist of situation

29. The best management of hypercalcemia with CNS depression is

A. Intravenous phosphate

B. Low calcium diet and oral phosphates

C. Indomethacin

D. Vigorous hydration, diuretics if needed, intravenous mithramycin

E. Prednisone

30. A 22-year-old man is hospitalized to evaluate abdominal pain. On physical exam, diffuse adenopathy, pleural effusions, hepatosplenomegaly, and ascites are noted. Abdominal CT scan shows a huge retroperitoneal mass, presumably matted para-aortic nodes. Serum LDH is 8,000. BUN is 35. Uric acid is 12.0 Biopsy of a lymph node shows undifferentiated lymphoma, possibly Burkitt's type. You should

A. Consult with a surgeon to arrange a staging laparotomy

B. Consult with a radiation therapist to arrange treatment

C. Consult with a medical oncologist to start chemotherapy

D. Consult with a nephrologist, insert a shunt in preparation for hemodialysis, then consult with a medical oncologist to start chemotherapy

ANSWERS

1. C
2. D
3. D
4. A, C, D
5. B, C
6. C
7. F
8. A, B, C
9. B, D
10. C
11. B, D
12. E
13. B
14. E
15. B
16. C
17. D
18. B
19. B
20. C
21. A
22. A, B, C, E
23. B
24. C
25. B
26. D
27. E
28. D
29. D
30. D

BIBLIOGRAPHY

Introduction

DeVita VT, Hellaman S, Rosenberg SA (eds): *Cancer: Principles and Practice of Oncology*. Philadelphia, JB Lippincott, 1982.

Schein PS: Cancer chemotherapy: Current concepts and results. In *Current Research in Oncology*. CB Anfinsen (ed), New York, Academic Press Inc, 1973, pp. 167-208.

Shimkin MB: *Contrary to Nature* (DHEW Publication No. [NIH] 76-720). Washington, D.C., U.S. Government Printing Office, 1977.

Skipper HE: Kinetics of mammary tumor cell growth and implications for therapy. *Cancer* 28:1479-1499, 1971.

TNM classification of malignant tumors, International Union Against Cancer (UICC) Committee on TNM Classification. Geneva, UICC, 1974.

Hodgkin's Disease

Arseneau JC, Rosenthal SN: Hodgkin's disease. In *Hematology and Oncology*, MA Lichtman, JW Adamson (eds). New York, Grune & Stratton, Inc, 1980, pp. 180-183.

Glatstein E: Radiotherapy in Hodgkin's disease: Past achievements and future progress. *Cancer* 1977. 39:837-842.

Kaplan HS: *Hodgkin's Disease*, ed. 2. Cambridge, Harvard University Press, 1980.

Lewis BJ, DeVita VT Jr: Combination therapy of the lymphomas. *Semin Hematol* 1978. 15:431-457.

Non-Hodgkin's Lymphoma

Arseneau JC, Rosenthal SN: Non-Hodgkin's lymphomas. In *Hematology and Oncology*, MA Lichtman, JW Adamson (eds). New York, Grune & Stratton, Inc, 1980, pp. 184-188.

Lewis BJ, DeVita VT Jr: Combination therapy of the lymphomas. *Semin Hematol* 15:431-457, 1978.

Lutzner M (Moderator): Cutaneous T-cell lymphomas: The Sézary syndrome, mycocis fungoides, and related disorders. *Ann Intern Med* 83:534-552, 1975.

Neiman RS, Dervan P, Haudenschild C, et al. Angioimmunoblastic lymphadenopathy. *Cancer* 41:507-518, 1978.

Proceedings of the Conference on Non-Hodgkin's Lymphomas. *Cancer Treat Rep* 61:935-1230, 1977.

Multiple Myeloma and Macroglobulinemia

Farhangi M, Osserman EF: The treatment of multiple myeloma. *Semin Hematol* 10:149-161, 1973.

Kyle RA: Multiple myeloma: Review of 869 cases. *Mayo Clin Proc* 59: 29-40, 1975.

Kyle RA, Elveback LR: Management and prognosis of multiple myeloma. *Mayo Clin Proc* 51:751-760, 1976.

McCallister BD, Bayrd ED, Harrison EG, et al.: Primary macroglobulinemia. *Am J Med* 43:394-434, 1967.

Malignant Neoplasms of Breast

Bonadonna G, Grusamolino E, Valagussa P, et al.: Combination chemotherapy as an adjuvant treatment in operable breast cancer. *N Engl J Med* 294:405-410, 1976.

Fisher B: Cooperative clinical trials in primary breast cancer: A critical appraisal. *Cancer* 31:1271-1286, 1973.

Fisher B, Slack NH, Cavanaugh PJ, et al.: Postoperative radiotherapy in the treatment of breast cancer: Results of the NSABP clinical trial. *Ann Surg* 172:711-732, 1970.

Henderson IC, Canellos GP: Cancer of the breast: The past decade. *N Engl J Med* 302:17-30, 78-90, 1980.

Sadowsky NL, Kalisher L, White G, et al.: Radiologic detection of breast cancer: Review and recommendations. *N Engl J Med* 294: 370-373, 1976.

Stoll BA (ed): *Breast Cancer Management: Early and Late*. London, Heineman Books, 1977.

Carcinoma of the Lung

Greco FA, Einhorn LH, Richardson RL, Oldham RK: Small cell lung cancer: Progress and perspectives. *Semin Oncol* 5:323-325, 1978.

Legha SS, Muggia FM: Pleural mesothelioma: Clinical features and therapeutic implications. *Ann Intern Med* 87:613-621, 1977.

Mittman C, Bruderman I: Lung cancer: To operate or not? *Am Rev Resp Dis* 116:477-496, 1977.

Should asymptomatic patients with inoperable bronchogenic carcinoma receive immediate radiotherapy? (Editorial) *Am Rev Resp Dis* 1978. 117:405-414,

Weiss RB: Small-cell carcinoma of the lung: Therapeutic management. *Ann Intern Med* 88:522-531, 1978.

Malignant Tumors of the Gastrointestinal Tract

Gudjonsson B, Livstone EM, Spiro HM: Cancer of the pancreas: Diagnostic accuracy and survival statistics. *Cancer* 42:2494-2506, 1978.

Ihde DC, Sherlock P, Winawer SJ, et al.: Clinical manifestations of hepatoma: A review of 6 years' experience at a cancer hospital. *Am J Med* 56:83-91, 1974.

Moertel CG: Alimentary tract cancer. In *Cancer Medicine*, JF Holland, E Frei (eds). Philadelphia, Lea & Febiger, 1973, pp. 1519-1635.

Moertel CG: Clinical management of advanced gastrointestinal cancer. *Cancer* 36:675-682, 1975.

Piehler JM, Crichlow RW: Primary carcinoma of the gallbladder. *Surg Gynecol Obstet* 147:929-942, 1978.

Malignant Tumors of the Urinary Tract and Testes

Anderson T, Waldmann TA, Javadpour N, Glatstein E: Testicular germ cell neoplasms: Recent advances in diagnosis and therapy. *Ann Intern Med* 90:373-385, 1979.

Byar DP: The Veterans Administration Cooperative Urological Research Group's studies of cancer of the prostate. *Cancer* 32: 1126-1130, 1973.

Holland JM: Cancer of the kidney: Natural history and staging. *Cancer* 1973. 32:1030-1042.

Klein LA: Prostatic carcinoma. *N Engl J Med* 300:824-833, 1979.

Prout GR (ed): Symposium on uroepithelial tumors. *Urol Clin North Am* 3:1-193, 1976.

Malignant Tumors of the Female Reproductive Organs

Bagley CM Jr, Young RC, Canellos GP, et al.: Treatment of ovarian carcinoma: Possibilities for progress. *N Engl J Med* 287:856-862, 1972.

DeVita VT, Wasserman TH, Young RC, et al: Perspectives on research in gynecologic oncology: Treatment protocols. *Cancer* 38:509-525, 1976.

Gusberg SB: The evolution of modern treatment of corpus cancer. *Cancer* 38:602-609, 1976.

Hertz R: Choriocarcinoma and related gestational trophoblastic tumors in Women. New York, Raven Press, 1978.

Wasserman TH, Carter SK: The integration of chemotherapy into combined modality treatment of solic tumors. VIII. Cervical cancer. *Cancer Treat Rev* 4:25-46, 1977.

Malignant Tumors of the Endocrine Glands

Friesen SR: Tumors of the endocrine pancrease. *N Engl J Med* 306:580-590, 1982.

Hutter AM Jr, Kayhoe DE: Adrenal cortical carcinoma: Clinical features of 138 patients. *Am J Med* 41:572-580, 1966.

Regan PT, Maladelada JR: A reappraisal of clinical, roentgenographic, and endoscopic features of the Zollinger-Ellison syndrome. *Mayo Clin Proc* 53:19-23, 1978.

Russell MA, Gilbert EF, Jaeschke WF: Prognostic features of thyroid cancer: A long-term follow-up of 68 cases. *Cancer* 36:553-559, 1975.

Malignant Tumors of the Head, Neck, and Esophagus

Camishion RC, Manuele VJ: The esophagus. In *Management of the Patient with Cancer*, ed. 2., TF Nealon (ed). Philadelphia, WB Saunders Co, 1976, pp. 376-390.

Fletcher GH: Place of irradiation in the management of head and neck cancers. *Semin Oncol* 4:375-385, 1977.

Pratt LL: Workup and staging of patients with head and neck cancer. *Semin Oncol* 4:357-363, 1977.

Malignant Tumors of Skin

Fitzpatrick TB (ed): *Dermatology in General Medicine*, ed. 2. New York, McGraw-Hill Book Co, 1979.

Milton GW: *Malignant Melanoma of the Skin and Mucous Membrane*. New York, Churchill Livingstone, Inc, 1977.

Sarcomas

Jaffe N, Frei E: Osteogenic sarcoma: Advances in treatment. *CA* 26: 351-359, 1976.

Rosen G, Caparros B, Mosende C, et al.: Curability of Ewing's sarcoma and considerations for future therapeutic trials. *Cancer* 41:888-889, 1978.

Wilbur JR, Sutow WW, Sullivan MP, et al.: Chemotherapy of sarcomas. *Cancer* 36:765-769, 1975.

Malignant Tumors of the Brain

Gutin PH: Corticosteroid therapy in patients with cerebral tumors: Benefits, mechanisms, problems, practicalities. *Semin Oncol* 2:49-56, 1975.

Hendrickson FR: Radiation therapy of metastatic tumors. *Semin Oncol* 2:43-46, 1975.

Posner JB, Shapiro WR: Brain tumor: Current status of treatment and its complications. (Editorial) *Arch Neurol* 32:781-784, 1975.

Paraneoplastic Syndromes

International Conference on the Paraneoplastic Syndromes. *Ann NY Acad Sci* 230:1-577, 1974.

Lee JC, Yamauchi H, Hopper J: The association of cancer and the nephrotic syndrome. *Ann Intern Med* 64:41-51, 1966.

Oncologic Emergencies

Oncologic emergencies. *Semin Oncol* 5:123-227, 1978.

CHAPTER 13

PULMONARY DISEASES

Basil Varkey

Kesavan Kutty

DIAGNOSIS OF LUNG DISEASES

Hippocrates believed that the purpose of breathing was to "cool the heart," whose function it was to generate heat and thereby maintain life. An understanding of the functions of the lungs have come a long way. Besides the all-important function of respiration leading to oxygenation of blood and sustenance of life, the lungs have nonrespiratory functions as well. The structure of the lungs is well suited to these functions, but it also predisposes them to various disorders. The vast endothelial area for gas exchange is also exposed to the external environment and may be damaged as a result of infection, atmospheric pollutants, and irritant gases. Similarly, it is the filtering function of the lungs that makes them prone to emboli-septic, bland as well as particulate matter. Even though metabolic functions are discharged by the lungs, to what extent aberrations therein may produce disease is not well known.

A variety of diseases and disorders may affect the lungs primarily or secondarily. Although great strides have been made in diagnostic procedures, (e.g., fiberoptic bronchoscopy, computed tomography) the initial diagnostic approach to a patient with lung disease is still along the traditional lines of history, physical examination, assessment of the roentgenogram, and differential diagnosis of possibilities.

CLINICAL EVALUATION

Presenting Complaints

The chief symptoms of lung disease are cough, sputum production, dyspnea, chest pain, wheezing, and hemoptysis. In evaluating these symptoms, particular attention must be paid to the mode of onset, course of symptoms, and the circumstances under which the symptom(s) appeared.

Cough

Cough is a protective mechanism, designed to keep the tracheobronchial tree clear of sputum or aspirated material. It consists of a rapid sequence of events, that is, a deep inspiration followed by closure of the glottis with contraction of the expiratory muscles to produce sufficient positive airway pressure and then a sudden opening of the glottis, generating a very forceful and rapid air flow with the resultant expulsion of the irritating influence(s). In general, presence of cough implies diseases or disorders that involve the airways. In evaluating cough one must particularly note whether it is productive of sputum or not. Similarly, the mode of onset, acute or chronic, should also be noted. Associated symptoms such as fever commonly denote an infection. The presence of cough in a smoker may either mean evidence of bronchitis or of a bronchogenic neoplasm. A nocturnal cough suggests episodes of bronchospasm or presence of heart failure. Presence of cough during swallowing is characteristic of aspiration either through the glottis or, more commonly, a tracheoesophageal fistula. Bronchial asthma may present with cough as the only symptom.

Sputum Production

Sputum is defined as mucoid tracheobronchial secretion, produced by the mucin-secreting glands of the air passages. Mucus thus secreted is cleared by the ciliary action in the tracheobronchial tree; after it reaches the pharynx, it is swallowed. The expectoration of sputum always indicates an abnormality. Presence of cough and sputum on most days for a period of 3 months in a year for 2 consecutive years is indicative of chronic bronchitis. Yellow sputum is most commonly due to bacterial bronchitis, but sputum loaded with eosinophils in an exacerbation of asthma may have the same apperance. Production of large quantities of mucopurulent sputum is characteristic of bronchiectasis. Foul-smelling sputum is the hallmark of anaerobic lung abscesses. Even though alveolar carcinoma is associated classically with production of voluminous quantities of sputum, this manifestation is rather uncommon.

Dyspnea

Dyspnea has been defined as awareness of breathing. Breathing normally is a subconscious process and, when one becomes aware of it, dyspnea is said to be present. However, to the clinician, dyspnea means presence of respiratory distress. To interpret this symptom meaningfully, it should be taken in the context in which it appears. For example, dyspnea occurring during rest is always abnormal, whereas that occurring during exercise should be interpreted in relationship to the amount of exercise that produces the symptom. If such levels of exertion were previously tolerated well by the subject, then the symptom becomes significant. Dyspnea may be due to disorders that affect the lungs and/or heart or those that involve oxygen delivery to the tissues. Acute onset of dyspnea may suggest acute pulmonary edema, a pneumothorax, or pulmonary embolism as well as acute airway obstruction. Inquiry into the precipitating factors may be useful. A number of pulmonary as well as extrapulmonary disorders may produce dyspnea on a chronic basis. Associated respiratory symptoms such as the presence of cough, sputum production, or hemoptysis are useful clues in elucidation of the cause of dyspnea. In evaluating chronically dyspneic states, an occupational history is also of paramount importance. Occurrence of orthopnea or paroxysmal nocturnal dyspnea suggests the presence of heart failure. Dyspnea occurring in the postoperative state should always arouse the suspicion of either pulmonary embolization or presence of acute pulmonary edema related to fluid overload. In the presence of a normal chest roentgenogram dyspnea may be due to pulmonary embolism, early interstitial lung disease, airway obstruction, chest wall or neuromuscular disorders, or anxiety. Abnormal chest roentgenograms accompany dyspneic states due to heart failure, interstitial lung disease, large pleural effusion, or emphysema. Worsening of preexistent dyspnea in a smoker should always arouse the suspicion of the development of a bronchogenic carcinoma; and a change in the patient's roentgenogram may or may not be present.

Chest Pain

In clinical practice, several types of chest pain are often encountered. Chest pain of cardiac origin tends to be located in the retrosternal or in the precordial area and may be related to myocardial or pericardial processes. In cases of anginal pain, a temporal relationship can often be seen to exertion. The other types of chest pain are pleural, pain of intercostal neuritis, muscular, and costochondral pain. Acute inflammation of the pleura leads to a pleuritic type of chest pain that worsens on deep breathing, coughing, or even with movement of that part of the chest wall. This type of pain may be the initial manifestation of pneumonia, pulmonary infarction, or pleurodynia. Intercostal neuralgia tends to be of a shooting character often coming from the back forwards. The pain is characteristically made worse by coughing or sneezing, but not generally with phases of respiration, and is frequently a pre-eruptive manifestation of herpes zoster. In occasional cases, the pain may persist after the eruptions have subsided. Muscular pain is superficial and may be the aftermath of violent movements of chest wall muscles or from muscle bruising from trauma. The latter may produce rib fractures as well. Costochondral pain is typically located along the anterior portion of the chest and along the costochondral articulations. In Tietze's syndrome, the swelling and pain occur in the costochondral joints of the upper ribs.

Hemoptysis

Hemoptysis by definition refers to the expectoration of frank blood in the sputum. The causes of hemoptysis are listed separately in Table 1. Patients with acute respiratory infections, acute bronchitis, or bacterial pneumonia may have streaks or small clots of blood in their sputum. However, expectoration of larger quantities of frank blood in the sputum signifies a serious underlying disease such as pulmonary thromboembolism, mitral stenosis, bronchiectasis, bronchogenic carcinoma, bronchial adenoma, tuberculosis, or inhaled foreign body. In the history, the following specific points should be noted: whether the present episode is the initial one or whether prior bouts have been present; quantity of bleeding, associated symptoms such as chest pain, fever, weight loss, or dyspnea on exertion; previous history of sputum production, chest trauma, or recent leg swelling or loss of consciousness; and a history of ingestion of medications, especially anticoagulants. Also, one should inquire regarding smoking habits and previous episodes of recurrent pneumonia, especially in the younger patient (the latter is suggestive of bronchiectasis or bronchial adenoma). Recurrent hemoptyses are seen in mitral stenosis, bronchiectasis, an inhaled foreign body, bronchial adenoma, pulmonary hemosiderosis, and arteriovenous malformations of the lung. Massive hemoptysis is defined as expectoration of more than 600 cc of blood per 24 h; the most important causes are active and inactive tuberculosis, bronchiectasis, lung abscess, carcinoma, arteriovenous fistulae, and pulmonary aspergillomas.

Table 1. Causes of Hemoptysis

Infections
Tuberculosis
Lung abscess
Bronchiectasis
Klebsiella pneumonia
Chronic bronchitis
Aspergilloma
Paragonimiasis
Schistosomiasis
Strongyloidiasis
Cardiovascular Disorders
Pulmonary thromboembolism
Mitral stenosis
Arteriovenous fistula
Other vascular malformations of the lung
Neoplasms
Bronchogenic carcinoma
Laryngeal carcinoma
Nasopharyngeal carcinoma
Bronchial adenoma
Autoimmune
Goodpasture's syndrome
Wegener's granulomatosis
Polyarteritis nodosa
Lupus pneumonitis
Miscellaneous
Intralobar sequestration
Idiopathic pulmonary hemosiderosis
Inhaled foreign body
Ingestion of anticoagulants

Wheezing

Wheezing refers to a musical noise produced by passage of air across a narrowed bronchus. Wheezing, the sine qua non of asthma, may also be seen in other forms of airway obstruction. It is also encountered in situations where tenacious secretions obstruct the airways. Unprecedented onset of wheezing in a middle-aged person would suggest left ventricular failure rather than bronchial asthma. Other causes of wheezing are obstructing endobronchial lesions such as a bronchogenic carcinoma or an inhaled foreign body.

Past History

A detailed history of all illnesses, particularly respiratory illnesses, should be obtained. Patients should be asked whether chest roentgenograms were obtained in the past and whether they are available for review. Since the number of drug-induced lung disorders are increasing, a careful history of all current and past medications and drug habits, if any, should be recorded. Enquiry should be directed to other habits: alcohol, tobacco, pets, smoking (quantitate in terms of pack years), and hobbies. Travel history may be important in some instances.

A detailed occupational history is important. This should cover not only the current occupation but all jobs in the past, in chronologic order. A list of specific industries and occupations that may predispose to lung cancer is given in Table 2.

Table 2. Industries/Occupations That May Produce Pulmonary Neoplasia

Asbestos workers
Arsenic exposure
Chromate workers
Coke oven workers
Fluorspar mining
Hematite mining
Mustard gas exposure
Nickel workers
Uranium miners

The fact that many occupations may lead to lung diseases is well known (e.g., silicosis, coal-worker's pneumoconiosis). Less well known is the fact that there may be a long latent period between the time of exposure and the onset of symptoms (e.g., asbestosis). Recent information has also directed attention to occupational asthma and hypersensitivity lung disease.

Physical Examination

A summary of physical findings in various pulmonary disorders is presented in Table 3. Other than findings elicited on examination of the respiratory system, certain physical signs may have relevance to pulmonary disorders. Examples of these are indicated in Table 4.

BASIC LABORATORY TESTS

The most useful basic tests in evaluating a pulmonary disorder are skin tests, sputum examination, examination of pleural fluid if present, and measurement of arterial blood gas tensions. Other ancillary studies include complete blood counts, serologic examinations, and pulmonary function tests. These tests ought to be selectively based on the diagnostic impression.

Skin Tests

Immediate or type 1 skin reactions are useful in evaluating allergy to various agents, especially when interpreted in the proper clinical perspective. Type 3 reactions that manifest erythema and local edema are useful in detecting hypersensitivity to aspergillus antigens. Delayed hypersensitivity or type 4 response is the most clinically useful; it is embodied in tuberculin testing. 0.1 cc of Tween-stabilized purified protein derivative (PPD-S) is injected intradermally to raise a wheal. The extent of induration is carefully assessed at 48 hours; when it is between 0 and 4 mm, the reaction is interpreted as negative; between 5 and 9 mm as doubtful, and 10 mm and above as positive. A positive test indicates infection with *Mycobacterium tuberculosis* in the past or a prior BCG (bacille Calmette Guérin) inoculation. A doubtful reaction signifies infection with *M. tuberculosis* or other mycobacteria and necessitates clinical correlation or retesting. Tuberculin testing should be combined with tests for cutaneous reactivity, using streptokinase/streptodornase, mumps, and Trichophyton antigens. Negative responses to all these antigens indicate anergy. The Kveim test involves intradermal injection of a specially prepared antigen; it is useful in the diagnosis of sarcoidosis. However, the lack of widespread availability of the antigen precludes its frequent clinical use.

Table 3. Typical Physical Findings in the Chest in Common Pulmonary Disorders

Disorder	*Mediastinal Shift*	*Percussion*	*Breath Sounds*	*Adventitious Sounds*	*Vocal Resonance*	*Other*
Atelectasis due to endobronchial obstruction	Present; towards side of lesion	Impaired over affected area	Diminished or absent	None	Diminished or absent	Crowding of ribs, flattening of chest wall over area of lesion and diminished chest wall movement
Consolidation (pneumonia, infarction, etc.)	None	Impaired over affected area	Bronchial	Rales	A to E changes, whispering pectoriloquy	Splinting due to pain may reduce ipsilateral chest wall movement
Cavitation	May be shifted towards side of lesion if fibrosis has occurred	Impaired	Bronchial	Coarse rales	Increased A to E changes	–
Asthma	None	Normal	Normal with prolonged exhalation	High-pitched rhonchi (wheeze) mostly expiratory	Normal	Use of accessory muscles may be apparent
Emphysema	None	Hyperresonant	Decreased with prolonged expiration	Rhonchi may present	Decreased	Purse-lip breathing; cherubic and pink
Chronic bronchitis	None	Normal	Normal with prolonged exhalation	Expiratory rhonchi, coarse rales	Normal	Blue, often obese
Pleural effusion	Shifted to opposite side	Very impaired (dull)	Diminished or absent over effusion	None	Reduced or absent	–
Pneumothorax	Shifted to opposite side	Normal to hyperresonant	Normal to diminished	None	Diminished	Affected side may move less

Table 4. Physical Signs of Significance to Pulmonary Disorders

Physical Sign	*Significance*
Pallor	Anemia, may cause dyspnea
Central cyanosis	Oxygen desaturation; interstitial fibrosis
Plethora	Erythrocytosis; chronic bronchitis with oxygen desaturation
Verrucous eruptions of the nostrils (lupus pernio), maculopapular eruptions, erythema annulare, subcutaneous nodules, hypertrophic scars	Sarcoidosis
Erythema nodosum	Sarcoidosis, histoplasmosis, blastomycosis
Verrucous ulcers with advancing edges and central healing	Blastomycosis
Cutaneous sinuses	Actinomycosis, coccidioidomycosis
Subcutaneous nodules along extensor surfaces	Rheumatoid arthritis
Cafe au lait spots	Von Recklinghausen's disease; may have intrathoracic neurofibromas
Nasal septal perforation	Wegener's granulomatosis, sarcoidosis
Bullous myringitis	Mycoplasma pneumonia
Herpes labialis	Pneumococcal pneumonia
Swelling of face, ruddy complexion, upper extremity swelling (SVC syndrome)	Superior vena cava obstruction, most commonly due to malignant neoplasms
Distended neck veins	Heart failure, emphysema (may be unable to feel the distended veins)
Miosis, ptosis, anhidrosis, enophthalmos on one side of the face (Horner's syndrome)	Superior sulcus tumor (Pancoast's)
Clubbing of fingers	Bronchogenic carcinoma, idiopathic interstitial pulmonary fibrosis, asbestosis, all intrathoracic suppurative processes (empyema, lung abscess, bronchiectasis)
Clubbing with pain, stiffness, and swelling of distal long bones (hypertrophic osteoarthropathy)	Bronchogenic carcinoma
Sclerodactyly and Raynaud's phenomenon	Progressive systemic sclerosis
Generalized lymphadenopathy	Sarcoidosis, lymphoma
Supraclavicular lymphadenopathy	Metastatic bronchogenic carcinoma
Thoracic cage abnormalities (scoliosis, kyphosis, straight back syndrome)	Abnormal chest roentgenogram (e.g., prominent pulmonary artery), restrictive ventilatory impairment, and other physical findings (e.g., systolic murmur)

Sputum Examination

Obtaining a Specimen

In patients who expectorate sputum, the mucus should be collected in a clean, sterile container. For those who do not, induction is needed, either by a 15-minute inhalation of heated aerosol of 15% saline or of an aerosol of physiologic saline produced by an ultrasonic nebulizer. In certain instances, translaryngeal aspiration will be necessary to obtain sputum (see below). Gross characteristics of the specimen should be noted such as viscidity, color, odor, and the presence of blood. For best results, especially those involving bacteriologic or mycologic examination, the specimen should be hand-carried promptly to the laboratory.

Microscopic Examination

The quickest and easiest microscopic examination of the sputum consists of the wet-mount preparation. After placing a small portion of the mucus on a clean microscope slide and teasing it to give a fairly even smear, it is covered with a coverslip. The smear is examined under a microscope, first under low power and then under an oil immersion lens. A good sputum specimen will contain several alveolar macrophages: round, large cells with granular inclusions and an oval, eccentrically placed nucleus. If there are large numbers of squamous cells (large cells, with a flat shape and central nucleus) it indicates significant contamination with oral/pharyngeal secretions and necessitates another sample. The presence of several neutrophils signifies infection, most often bacterial. More than 20% eosinophils (cells with bilobed nuclei and large, refractile granules) mean atopic disease. Charcot-Leyden crystals have the same meaning, as they are disintegration products of the granules from the eosinophils.

The coverslip is then removed, the smear dried, and a Gram stain performed to evaluate the bacteriologic status. Bacteria in the vicinity of the squamous cells are most likely to originate from the mouth flora and should be avoided, but those in and around the pus cells but away from squamous cells should be assessed for their morphology and staining characteristics. Gram-positive cocci in pairs or chains probably represent pneumococci, but if they are in groups they may be staphylococci. *Hemophilus influenzae* appear as small, Gram-negative pleomorphic bacilli, whereas *Klebsiella* are large, Gram-negative rods that may be encapsulated. The distribution of the organism(s) should be noted: if an organism is seen in large numbers, dominant over others, infection with that organism is suggested. The results of the Gram smear should be interpreted in the context of clinical history and culture results, but they also provide a sound guideline for initial management. To visualize *Mycobacterium tuberculosis*, acid-fast staining with Ziehl-Nielsen stain is necessary; pretreatment of sputum with 10% potassium hydroxide is usually needed to demonstrate fungi.

Routine bacterial cultures of the sputum may be useful when interpreted in the context of other findings. Isolation of one organism in pure culture from sputum and/or from blood lends support to that organism being the infective agent. Isolation of the same dominant organism as seen from the Gram smear will also have the same meaning. Besides routine cultures, cultures for fungi and mycobacteria are also useful.

Cytologic Examination

If a delay is expected between collecting sputum and processing it the specimen should be placed in a fixative, which is usually 50% ethyl alcohol. The cells are examined after staining with the Papanicolaou method. Results vary depending on the number of samples submitted and the proficiency of the cytopathologist. In bronchogenic carcinoma, an initial sputum examination has a 50% positivity that rises to 80% with three or more good specimens. In cancers metastatic to the lung, this falls to about 50% with three or more good samples.

Translaryngeal Aspiration

In patients with pneumonia in the presence of immunosuppression, gross oral suppuration, or with poor cough mechanism and total inability to raise secretions, a translaryngeal aspiration is appropriate. With the patient's neck hyperextended, the neck is adequately sterilized with topical antiseptics. The cricothyroid membrane is palpated and after anesthetizing the skin and subcutaneous tissues overlying this membrane, a large-bore needle is inserted through it into the trachea. A sterile plastic catheter is then threaded in and any secretions present in the trachea are suctioned into a sterile syringe. If no secretions are obtained, a few drops of saline are instilled into the trachea that produces a cough, and the secretions are quickly aspirated. The material thus obtained is sent for appropriate studies including anaerobic culture. Inability to hyperextend the neck, bleeding diathesis, an extremely dyspneic patient, or the presence of infected lesions in the neck are contraindications to translaryngeal aspiration. Subcutaneous emphysema and bleeding into the bronchial tree are complications, but, when properly performed, this is a safe procedure.

Examination of Pleural Fluid

This will be discussed subsequently in the section on pleural effusions.

Blood Gas Studies

A sample of arterial blood is obtained in a heparinized syringe with a fine needle (25 gauge) under adequate local anesthesia from the brachial or the radial artery. The syringe should be placed in ice immediately and the sample analyzed for the pH and the tension of P_{O_2} and P_{CO_2}. Normal pH varies between 7.35 and 7.45. Alkalosis exists when it exceeds 7.45 and acidosis when it is below 7.35. Normal ranges for P_{CO_2} vary from laboratory to laboratory but, in general, a level over 44 mm Hg needs careful review. A P_{CO_2} level below 35 mm Hg is produced by hyperventilation, often from the pain of puncture. Normal P_{O_2} at sea level varies between 80 and 105 mm Hg in room air. For every decade after 25-30 years of age, the anticipated P_{O_2} declines by about 4 mm. For most bedside calculations, multiplication of the percentage of ambient oxygen (that the subject is breathing) by a factor of 6 gives a rough estimate of the expected P_{O_2}.

ROENTGENOGRAPHY, SCINTISCAN, AND ULTRASOUND EXAMINATION

Roentgenographic Techniques

Suspicion of any form of lung disease is the prime indication for obtaining a chest roentgenographic examination. For most practical purposes, a posteroanterior (PA) view is adequate. But unless supplemented by a lateral view, processes in the retrosternal and retrocardiac areas as well as a very small pleural effusion in the posterior costophrenic sulcus may be missed. Additional roentgenographic examinations may be necessary depending on circumstances. Penetrated views and left anterior oblique views may be necessary to evaluate lesions in the left lower lobe or lesions in the retrocardiac areas. To visualize the apices of the lung satisfactorily it may be necessary to obtain lordotic views and oblique projections. Similarly, oblique projections may also be indicated when separation of pulmonary infiltrates or masses from the adjoining or superimposed structures is necessary. The commonest manifestation of a small pleural effusion is a blunted costophrenic angle on either side. To distinguish a pleural effusion from pleural fibrosis or thickening in this area, an ipsilateral decubitus view is very helpful. Although inspiration-expiration films have been advocated in the localization of air trapping, subpulmonic effusions, and so forth, the most rewarding application of these views lies in detecting a small pneumothorax. Similarly, radiographs before and after Valsalva's and Müller's maneuvers have been advocated for differentiating vascular from solid lesions, but they have no practical use in most instances. Besides being helpful in detecting left atrial enlargement and in the evaluation of mediastinal lesions, a barium esophagogram may also be helpful in the investigation of unexplained, recurrent lower lobe pneumonia that may be secondary to esophageal stricture and/or achalasia.

Tomography (laminography or planigraphy) is performed to evaluate a slice of lung tissue in a particular plane of the thorax. This method utilizes a reciprocal movement of the x-ray source and the film. By altering the ratio of the distances between the x-ray source and the object, and that between the object and the x-ray film, the level of the cut can be adjusted. Similarly, by adjusting the tube-film excursion, the thickness of the slice also can be regulated. The advantages of tomography are

1. Precise analysis of the morphology of the lesion is made possible, such as cavitation and/or calcification in a pulmonary nodule, or an intracavitary fungus ball. The presence of characteristic patterns of calcification in a pulmonary nodule bespeaks its benignity (see the section on neoplasms of the lung).
2. Apart from delineating a lesion from the surrounding structures, the anatomic plane in which an infiltrate or density is located can be assessed accurately. The latter also helps the

bronchoscopist to brush or biopsy the appropriate segments.

3. Unsuspected associated disease, such as other areas of infiltration or satellite nodules around a pulmonary nodule, may be detected.

Full-lung tomograms are often obtained in the hope that a pulmonary nodule will manifest that is not apparent on a routine roentgenogram. In the authors' experience, this is seldom fruitful.

Bronchography

Bronchography is done by instillation of a contrast medium into the tracheobronchial tree to outline its anatomy. The main indication for bronchography is to diagnose bronchiectasis and to assess its severity and extent. With the advent of fiberoptic bronchoscopy and brushing, it has little role in the diagnosis of bronchial carcinoma. It may delineate a bronchopleural or a tracheoesophageal fistula and aid in the preoperative assessment of decortication of a fibrothorax.

Pulmonary Arteriography

The main indication for pulmonary arteriography is in the investigation of pulmonary thromboembolic disease when other measures give equivocal results, or when a conclusive diagnosis is mandatory, such as before interruption of the vena cava, prior to pulmonary embolectomy or suspected emboli in patients who are at high risk for anticoagulation. Other indications for pulmonary arteriography are in the diagnosis of vascular anomalies of the lung such as arteriovenous fistulae or in an occasional patient with bronchogenic carcinoma who is otherwise operable but in whom neoplastic invasion of the pulmonary vessels is considered a likelihood.

CT (Computed Tomography) Scanning

CT scanning makes it possible to obtain an image of a thin, transverse slice of the thorax. When an x-ray beam emerges through the thorax the rays show different degrees of attenuation as a result of passing through organs of varying tissue density. A computer analyzes the changes in this attenuation and reconstructs an image that is the scan. CT scanning is invaluable in the evaluation of mediastinal lesions. It helps distinguish between vascular, solid, and cystic structures in a noninvasive manner. The areas that are the blind spots of conventional radiographs such as the mediastinum, the posterior costophrenic sulcus, and paravertebral areas are evaluated satisfactorily by computed tomography. However, the facilities are costly and are not available at all institutions. In deciding to order a CT scan of the chest, how the results will affect the decision-making process and its cost-benefit ratio must be considered.

Scintiscans

Scintiscans of the lung depend on the use of various radioactive isotopes. Perfusion, ventilation, and gallium scanning are three categories of commonly performed scintiscans of the lung.

Perfusion scans assess the vasculature of the lung. When administered intravenously, microspheres of radioactive human serum albumin enter the lung circulation and become trapped in pulmonary capillaries. External imaging of the activity produced within the lungs by these trapped particles makes it possible to assess the extent of perfusion in each area. This is done by anterior and posterior as well as left and right lateral imaging. Areas devoid of perfusion are free of radioactivity. In pulmonary embolism, these defects usually have a segmental or subsegmental pattern.

Ventilation scanning is performed by using a radioactive tracer gas that is usually ^{133}Xe. The gas is inhaled to the point of equilibration within the lung, after which it is exhaled; during exhalation the washout is detected by imaging. In areas that have normal ventilation, the radioactivity is cleared after approximately 3 minutes. It is possible to detect areas that have abnormal ventilation patterns such as air trapping by serial imaging.

Comparing perfusion as well as ventilation scans with a chest radiogram done at the time of the scanning procedure, it is possible to assess the probability of pulmonary emboli. A completely normal four-view lung scan excludes pulmonary embolism for all practical purposes. The presence of perfusion defects in areas that are normally ventilated is strongly suggestive of pulmonary embolization. However, in the vast majority of patients with obstructive airway disease or heart failure, diagnosing or excluding pulmonary embolism on the basis of these studies is not easy. In patients with bronchogenic carcinoma who manifest significant hypoxemia, a perfusion lung scan may detect vascular invasion and these patients fare rather poorly if they are operated.

Gallium (^{67}Ga) has an affinity for leukocytes and accumulation of this isotope after parenteral injection is found to occur in inflammatory foci as well as in tumor tissue. ^{67}Ga scanning has been recommended as a staging procedure in cases of bronchogenic carcinoma. It may also be useful in patients who have other types of inflammatory lung disease or pleural disease.

Ultrasonography

The basis of ultrasonography is the use of high-frequency sound waves emitted from a transducer held close to the patient's chest wall. Some of these waves are reflected back, which can be sensed by the transducer, and the image thus produced is available for review. Since the sound beams do not adequately penetrate through the aerated lung tissue, the main use of the technique lies in the detection of very small or loculated pleural effusions or solid densities in the pleural space.

BASICS OF PHYSIOLOGY AND PULMONARY FUNCTION TESTING

Physiology

Ventilation is defined as the intake and distribution of air from the external environment to the alveolus and its return to the exterior. The process of gas exchange in the alveolus is termed diffusion, and it involves passive movement of gases based on concentration gradients. The process of gas exchange is made possible by the maintenance of a constant blood flow from the right ventricle through the pulmonary artery and arterioles into the capillaries and then through pulmonary veins into the left heart. This function is perfusion.

Ventilation

The process of ventilation is controlled by the metabolic needs of the tissues. Tissue demands for oxygen increase substantially during exercise, febrile states, and other metabolic stresses. Impulses from the peripheral and central chemoreceptors as well as from the receptors in the lung are received in the medulla, where the information is assimilated and appropriate changes in ventilation initiated. Stimulation of these receptors occur in pneumonia, asthma, and in various neurologic disorders as well as from ingestion of drugs such as aspirin. Depression of these receptors leads to hypoventilation as seen in obesity, severe chronic bronchitis, severe metabolic alkalosis, and myxedema.

The various compartments of ventilation are schematically represented in Figure 1.

Even in healthy persons, the amount of inhaled air is distributed in a somewhat uneven manner because of variations in intrapleural pressures. In an erect person, the intrapleural pressure tends to be maximally negative at the apices and less negative at the bases. This leads to more distention of the alveoli at the apex than at the bases and, for this reason, a slow breath from the functional residual capacity (FRC) level is distributed preferentially to the lower lobes. But with increasing breathing frequency and increasing rates of flow, the distribution becomes more uniform. Thus, during rest, when the lower lobes get the maximal share of blood supply, ventilation is also preferentially distributed there. During exercise, a more equitable distribution of blood flow occurs; this is matched by a redistribution of ventilation.

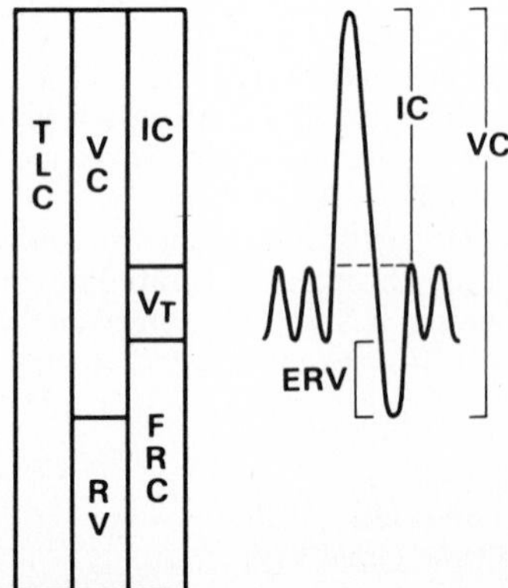

Figure 1. Compartments of ventilation. ERV = expiratory reserve volume; FRC = functional residual capacity; IC = inspiratory capacity; VC = vital capacity; V_T = tidal volume; RV = residual volume; and TLC = total lung capacity.

Abnormal Ventilation

The two major patterns of impaired ventilation are obstruction and restriction. Obstructive impairments are characterized by obstruction to air flow. The diseases in which obstructive impairment may be seen are asthma, chronic bronchitis, emphysema, bronchiectasis, and cystic fibrosis. Restrictive impairments are characterized by limitation of the amount of air contained within the lungs. These disorders lead to diminution of various lung volumes, especially the total lung capacity. Examples are pulmonary fibrosis, fibrothorax, and postoperative states after lung resection.

Diffusion

Diffusion is a passive process of gas transfer based on concentration gradients. The quantity of a gas that diffuses across the alveolar-capillary membrane per unit of time based on differences in pressure of the gas in the alveolus and that in the blood is known as the diffusing capacity (DL) of the lung for that gas. The commonest gas used for measuring this is carbon monoxide (CO). The measurement (DL_{CO}) is expressed as ml/min/mm Hg. It has a membrane (D_m) and capillary blood volume (V_c) components. The values correlate well with lung volume and body size. The single-breath (SB) determination is quick and easy to perform, although it involves breath holding for about 8-10 seconds. A steady state (SS) determination is also possible.

Elevated values for DL_{CO} are often seen in asthmatics, presumably from the augmented intrathoracic blood volume (V_c), due to increased negative intrathoracic pressure. Intrapulmonary hemorrhage can also lead to a high DL_{CO}. Diminutions in DL_{CO} are often seen in anemia and in diseases that affect or destroy pulmonary vasculature, such as pulmonary vasculitis, thromboembolic diseases, interstitial lung diseases, emphysema, and pulmonary resection.

Perfusion

The distribution of blood flow in the lungs is uneven since the low pressure circulation is vulnerable to gravitational influence(s). A progressive difference in blood flow is apparent between the apices, where blood flow is scarce, to the bases, where it is considerable. In the normal person this probably leads to very slight ventilation-perfusion mismatching, but its effects can be considerable in patients with underlying lung disease.

Pulmonary Function Tests

Pulmonary function tests are performed to determine the type and degree of physiologic impairment resulting from a particular disease process. Taken in conjunction with the clinical history and roentgenographic evaluation, they offer a strong clue to the underlying disease. Pulmonary function tests are useful in the following circumstances:

1. Early detection of lung disease
2. Evaluation of the adequacy of pulmonary function prior to surgery
3. Differential diagnosis of dyspneic states

4. Quantitation of pulmonary disability
5. Assessment of the severity and progression of lung disease, and response to specific therapy
6. In the followup of patients who are being treated for other disorders with drugs that may affect the lungs adversely
7. Epidemiologic surveys
8. Screening of people who work in environments that are hazardous to lung function

The rapid advancement in the field of biomedical technology has led to the development of a number of tests of pulmonary function that may be classified as tests in routine use, those used in special situations, and those yet to gain clinical usefulness. Included in the first category are forced spirometry and its subunits, lung-volume studies, diffusion tests, and blood gas tensions. The second category includes the flow-volume loop and its modifications, as well as body plethysmography. Closing volume, frequency dependence of compliance, and so forth, fall in the third category.

Forced Expiratory Spirometry

This consists of a forced, quick, and complete exhalation from a position of maximal inspiration. The exhalation record is obtained on a moving drum. A normal spirogram is depicted in Figure 2. The entire volume constitutes the forced vital capacity (FVC). FVC is reduced in restrictive disorders and often in obstructive disorders as well. The volume of the FVC exhaled in the first second constitutes the 1-second forced expiratory volume ($FEV_{1.0}$). Normally, this exceeds 87% of the FVC and the ratio of $FEV_{1.0}$ to FVC expressed as a percentage should be over 70. Airway obstruction is present when the ratio is below 70. $FEV_{1.0}$ is reduced primarily in airway obstruction (an example is shown in Fig. 3) and secondarily (due to reduction in FVC) in restrictive conditions; the ratio $\left(\frac{FEV_{1.0}}{FVC}\right)$ helps differentiate obstructive and restrictive conditions.

From the forced expiratory spirogram, the rate of flow of the exhaled air may be computed. The standard measurements are the forced expiratory flow between 200 to 1200 cc volume of the FVC ($FEF_{200\text{-}1200}$) and that between 25 and 75% of the FVC ($FEF_{25\text{-}75\%}$). Reduction of the latter is another sensitive guide to the presence of airway obstruction. However, flow rates also may be reduced in restrictive lung disease secondary to a low vital capacity. Review of the spirograms, use of the $FEV_{1.0}$/FVC ratio, and clinical correlation are necessary under such circumstances.

Lung volume measurements are performed while the patient is breathing at ease through a special circuit spirometer, either by the helium dilution or nitrogen washout method. Diffusion capacity is estimated using a nontoxic concentration of carbon monoxide. Blood gas tensions are determined on a sample of heparinized arterial blood. Clinical correlation of abnormal pulmonary function data ideally should be done after review of a current chest radiogram. Table 5 represents the patterns of ventilatory impairments as seen on routine pulmonary function testing.

Specialized Tests of Lung Function

Specialized tests of lung function include flow-volume loops, closing volume, plethysmography, and frequency dependence of compliance. Flow-volume loops are extremely helpful in the

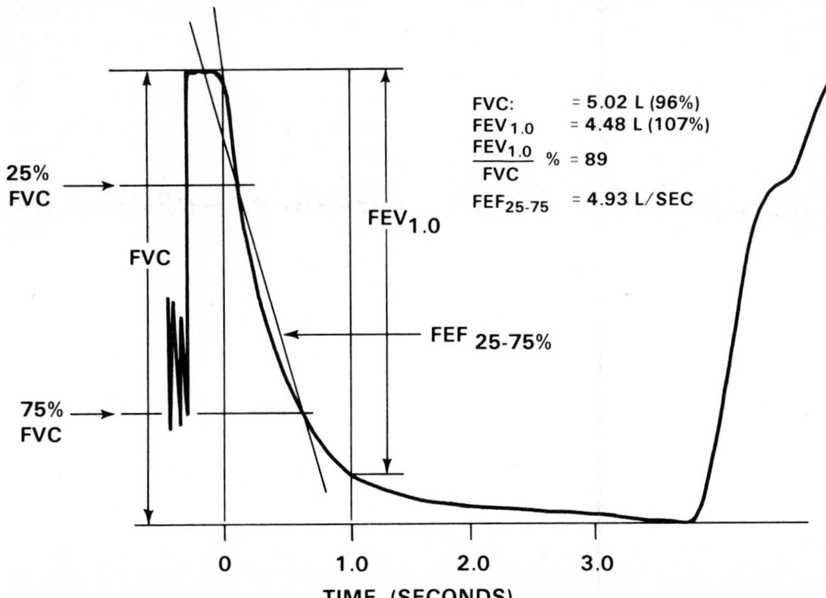

Figure 2. Normal forced expiratory spirometry.

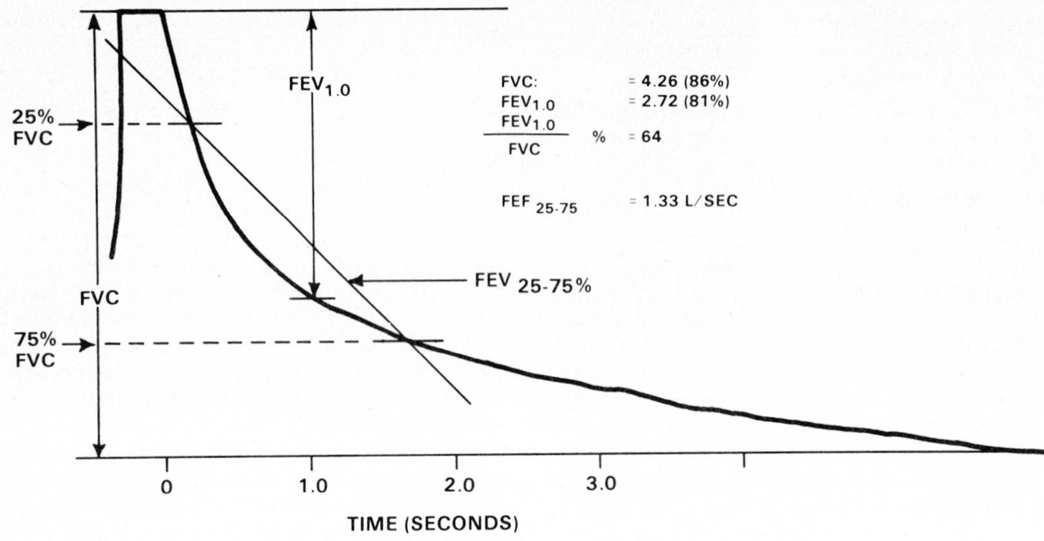

Figure 3. Forced expiratory spirometry in airway obstruction.

early diagnosis of upper-airway obstruction. Closing volume, flow-volume loops, and frequency dependence of compliance may also be helpful in the early diagnosis of obstructive airway disease.

BRONCHOSCOPY AND BIOPSY

Bronchoscopy

The indications for bronchoscopy and the preferred type of bronchoscope in different clinical situations are shown in Tables 6 and 7. Rigid bronchoscopy can be done under local anesthesia, but, in general, most situations would necessitate use of general anesthesia. It also necessitates extension of the neck and for this reason is uncomfortable. With the rigid bronchoscope, visualization is up to the segmental openings. Fiberoptic bronchoscopy can be done transnasally or through an oral endotracheal tube and involves minimal discomfort; general anesthesia is unnecessary and visualization to the sub-subsegmental level is possible.

Fiberoptic Bronchoscopy

The patient is prepared by fasting for at least 6 hours, and premedicated with 50-75 mg demerol and 0.6 mg atropine ½ hour before the procedure. Although fiberoptic bronchoscopy may be done transnasally, the authors prefer bronchoscopy through an indwelling endotracheal tube because patency of the airway is ensured and repeated introduction and withdrawals for brushings and biopsies are possible. After topical anesthesia is applied, a flexible endotracheal tube is placed and securely taped. The fiberoptic bronchoscope is introduced and systematic examination of the entire tracheobronchial tree is carried out segment by segment, and lobe by lobe. Brushings and biopsy specimens are obtained from abnormal areas. In cases of infiltrates or nodules without endobronchial lesions, brushings as well as biopsies are obtained from the lesions after placing the brush or forceps into the area under fluoroscopic control. In addition to the aspirate, brushings, and biopsies, postbronchoscopic sputa are collected when bronchogenic carcinoma is suspected. A positive diagnosis of carcinoma can

Table 5. Typical Pulmonary Function Abnormalities in Obstructive and Restrictive Ventilatory Impairments

Type of Impairment	*Vital Capacity (VC)*	*Forced Vital Capacity (FVC)*	*$FEV_{1.0}$*	*$\frac{FEV_{1.0}}{FVC}$*	*$FEF_{200-1,200}$*	*$FEF_{25-75\%}$*	*FRC and RV*	*TLC*
Obstructive	May be normal or reduced	Generally reduced	Always reduced	<70	Reduced	Reduced	Increased	Normal or high
Restrictive	Reduced	Reduced	May be normal or reduced	>70	Normal	Normal	Normal or low	Always reduced

Table 6. Indications for Bronchoscopy

Diagnostic	*Therapeutic*
Cough of unclear etiology	Foreign body in tracheobronchial tree
Hemoptysis	Tracheobronchial toilet for excessive secretions
Atelectasis	Atelectasis (due to secretions)
Abnormal chest radiograph	Aspiration
Positive sputum cytology	Lavage
Paralysis of diaphragm	
Recurrent laryngeal nerve paralysis	
Acute inhalation injury	
Assessment of tracheal damage during mechanical ventilation with endotracheal tube	

be made by bronchoscopic methods in about 98% of cases when the lesions are visible, and in about 60-70% cases when the lesions are not, depending on size and location of the radiographic abnormality.

Laryngospasm may occur during the procedure and usually reflects inadequate local anesthesia. Bronchospasm is especially likely in asthmatics. Syncope and vasovagal attacks are very unusual. Bleeding may complicate brushing or biopsy procedures and occasionally may be alarming. This tends to occur more in the acutely ill or immunosuppressed patients. Major hemorrhage occurs in less than 1% of procedures. Some degree of hypoxemia during the procedure is usual; baseline blood gas studies should be obtained to determine the need for oxygen during the procedure.

Biopsy Techniques

Tissue for diagnostic purposes may be obtained by biopsy of the pleura (considered in section on disorders of the pleura), lung, mediastinal lymph nodes, and scalene nodes.

Lung Biopsy

Any persistent pulmonary lesions undiagnosed by conventional methods where a specific tissue diagnosis would change the line of management is an indication for lung biopsy. Lung biopsy may be done by percutaneous needle aspiration, a percutaneous cutting or drill technique, transbronchial biopsy, or by open incision. The easiest and the least invasive approach should be tried first, unless circumstances dictate otherwise. The most important considerations in selecting the approach are the severity of the illness, roentgenographic appearance, expertise available, the most likely diagnosis, and the size of the sample needed by the pathologist to come to a definite diagnosis.

Table 7. Bronchoscopy: Procedure of Choice, Rigid vs. Fiberscope

Rigid	*Fiberscope*
Foreign body	Peripheral/upper lobe lesions
Vascular tumors	Slight hemoptysis
Pediatric patient	Mechanical problems in the neck
Suspected large airway obstruction	Airway management during mechanical ventilation
Massive hemoptysis	Transbronchial lung biopsy

Transbronchial Lung Biopsy

This is done through a bronchoscope, usually under fluoroscopic guidance. Special biopsy forceps are placed in the area of the infiltrate and as the patient exhales after a maximal inspiration, a piece of lung tissue is obtained by closing the forceps. The diagnostic accuracy varies from 62-79%. Insufficient tissue is obtained in about one-fifth of cases. Specific diagnosis based on tissue examination alone is possible in about 50-60% of all diffuse pulmonary diseases. In sarcoidosis the yield depends on the presence or absence of interstitial infiltrates; even when absent, about 60% positivity can be anticipated. Pneumothorax occurs in 5-10% of cases and major bleeding in less than 5%, the incidence being higher in acutely ill and immunosuppressed patients.

Open Lung Biopsy

Samples of lung tissue obtained through an intercostal incision offer adequate material for histologic, bacteriologic, and electron microscopic examination. Samples of lung tissue from abnormal areas can also be obtained under direct vision through a thoracoscope, a technique that has been employed successfully in immunosuppressed children with pulmonary infiltrates. In most cases, open lung biopsy reveals a definite pathologic diagnosis, but a definitive etiologic diagnosis may not be obtained in about 20-30% of cases, especially in patients with diffuse infiltrates occurring in the setting of immunosuppression. Presently, however, this appears to be the most definitive method.

Needle Biopsy of the Lung

This technique has been employed in the diagnosis of nodules of the lung. Types of needle biopsy commonly performed are aspiration and cutting or drill biopsy. Aspiration biopsy is the preferred method. In cases of neoplasm the diagnostic yield is as high as 95%, but the accuracy is not as high for benign lesions. Needle biopsy of the solitary pulmonary nodule is generally unnecessary if thoracotomy and resection are considered to be likely procedures in a given case.

ANATOMY AND DEVELOPMENTAL ABNORMALITIES

ANATOMY

From a functional viewpoint, the airways and lung may be considered to consist of two components; conducting airways and the terminal respiratory units. Conducting airways consist of trachea, bronchi, and nonrespiratory bronchioles whose main function is transportation of air. Respiratory units consist of respiratory bronchioles, alveolar ducts, and alveoli that serve the important function of gas exchange.

The trachea divides into the right and left main bronchi at the carina. This angle of bifurcation, although variable from person to person, is less acute on the right, thus favoring gravitational processes to occur more commonly in the right lung. Each lung has several bronchopulmonary segments; each segment is supplied by a segmental bronchus and its corresponding segmental branch of the pulmonary artery. Functionally, each segment is fairly independent, although collateral circulation and ventilation between adjacent segments occur. Knowledge of the anatomy of these bronchopulmonary segments, which are separated by incomplete connective tissue, is not only important to the surgeon and bronchoscopist but also to the primary care physician since certain disease processes have a predilection to affect certain segments. Examples of these are tuberculosis in the apical and posterior segments of the upper lobes and gravitational (aspiration) pneumonia, and lung abscess in the posterior segments of the upper lobes and superior segments of the lower lobes.

The right lung is divided into 10 segments: three in the right upper lobe, two in the middle lobe, and five in the right lower lobe. The segments of the right upper lobe are apical, posterior, and anterior; the middle-lobe segments are lateral and medial; and the lower lobe segments are superior, medial basal, anterior basal, lateral basal, and posterior basal. The left lung has eight segments. The upper division bronchus of the left upper lobe (equivalent to the right upper lobe bronchus) has two divisions and, hence, two segments. These are the apical posterior and anterior segments. The lower division of the upper lobe bronchus leads into superior lingular and inferior lingular segments. The lower lobe has four segments: superior, anteromedial basal, lateral basal, and posterior basal.

The bronchi subdivide into smaller and smaller bronchioles and eventually into terminal respiratory bronchioles. The terminal respiratory bronchioles near the hilum are formed after about ten divisions, whereas to the periphery they are formed only after more divisions. The bronchi and pulmonary arteries are found in close company and share a connective tissue sheath.

The conducting airways have an epithelial lining made of ciliated cells and gland cells that produce mucus. The bronchi are supported by fibrous tissue; they also contain muscle elements that respond to a variety of neurohumoral and chemical stimuli. In the bronchi, the epithelium is pseudostratified and contains submucosal glands, whereas in the bronchiole the epithelium is columnar or ciliated and contains ciliated cells and Clara cells. The bronchial wall is supported by a connective tissue sheath containing plates and cartilage, but cartilage is absent in the bronchiolar wall. The bronchial tree is covered by a watery secretion, sol, that has a more viscid discontinuous gel on its top. The cilia beat in the sol layer and propel inhaled foreign substances towards the larynx for clearance. This two-layered system along with the ciliary apparatus is often referred to as the mucociliary escalator.

Respiratory units (acini or primary lobules in some textbooks) are structures distal to the terminal bronchioles. As the term indicates, the major function of these units are in the exchange of gases: uptake of oxygen and elimination of carbon dioxide. These respiratory units consist of respiratory bronchioles, alveolar ducts, and alveoli. After two to five generations of respiratory bronchioles, a further two to five generations of alveolar ducts are formed. Each of these alveolar ducts leads to 10-16 alveoli. Thus, one can visualize the enormous number of alveoli, estimated to be about 300 million, within the lungs. The surface area covered by these alveoli approximates 70 square meters, or larger than a tennis court. About 90% of this alveolar surface is also covered by capillaries.

Embryology

The lung originates from the primitive foregut and is recognizable even in a 3-week-old embryo. By the seventh week (14 mm-size embryo), the major bronchi and the segmental bronchi are developing; these developing bronchi encroach on a mass of mesenchyme and expand into the pleural cavities. During this encroachment, they become covered with a mesothelial lining that eventually forms the visceral and parietal pleura. Segmental bronchi further branch and form respiratory bronchioles. From about the twenty-fourth week until full term, there is a progressive increase in the number of alveoli and blood vessels. At full term, the infant's tracheobronchial system is comparable to an adult's, except the alveoli number only about one-tenth of that of the adult.

DEVELOPMENTAL ABNORMALITIES

Only some of the more important congenital abnormalities of the airways, lungs, and the pulmonary blood vessels will be considered here. For a more comprehensive review of congenital abnormalities, the reader is referred to the review article by Landing. Genetically-induced pulmonary disorders are not included in this section.

Anomalies of The Airways and Lung Parenchyma

Tracheoesophageal Fistula

Tracheoesophageal fistulae, which may be of different types, are usually associated with atresia in some part of the esophagus. In the most common type, type A, there is atresia of the proximal exophagus; the distal trachea communicates with the distal esophagus through a fistula.

The first manifestation in the neonatal period is bubbles forming at the mouth because of accumulated secretions. If this goes unnoticed, choking and gagging because of aspiration occur at the first feeding. Diagnosis can be promptly made by inability to insert a soft catheter into the stomach and roentgenographic demonstration of air in the stomach. Tracheoesophageal fistulae are amenable to surgery and the mortality is low if there is no diagnostic delay, low birth weight, or concomitant disease.

Bronchogenic Cysts

Bronchogenic cysts are formed by separation of small buds during development of the airways and lung. These cysts are often solitary; they have a ciliated epithelial lining and are filled with fluid. They may not cause any symptoms and may be discovered as a smooth-bordered, usually homogenous, central roentgenographic density. Bronchogenic cysts may get infected through a poorly communicating airway or from infection in a contiguous lung segment. The clinical and roentgenographic manifestations of an infected bronchogenic cyst simulates a lung abscess. Bronchogenic cysts causing symptoms are best dealt with by surgical resection.

Congenital Lobar Emphysema

Despite the name, there is no destruction of alveoli in congenital emphysema. However, there is marked overinflation of alveoli. The primary defect in congenital lobar emphysema is probably in the bronchus. A deficiency in the cartilage of the bronchial wall may cause bronchial narrowing on expiration and consequent air trapping and overdistention. Partial bronchial obstruction due to other causes (stenosis, inflammatory exudate, aspirated mucus, tumor) may produce the pattern of congenital lobar emphysema.

Congenital lobar emphysema is seen predominantly in male infants. Congenital cardiac anomalies coexist in about 50% of the infants with this disorder. The usual location is in the upper lobe, most often in the left side. Physical findings depend on the area and the extent of overdistention. Hyperresonance to percussion and wheezing may be detected. In severe cases, chest-wall retraction, mediastinal shift, and cyanosis may be evident. Chest roentgenogram shows the affected area to be overdistended and devoid of lung markings; mediastinal displacement and herniation to the other side may be present. Persistent hyperlucency from air trapping may be expected in inspiration and expiration roentgenograms.

Surgical resection of the overinflated lobe was the common procedure adopted in the past. Presently, there is a trend to treat these infants conservatively by using a bronchial catheter or a bronchoscope. Passing a catheter endobronchially into the overdistended area may deflate the lobar emphysema. Bronchoscopy may be diagnostic (e.g., stricture) and also therapeutic (e.g., removal of inspissated mucus).

Pulmonary Sequestration

As the name implies, pulmonary sequestration is an area set apart from the lung and tracheobronchial tree. It derives its arterial blood supply from the systemic circulation. Two types of sequestrations, intralobar and extralobar, are recognized. Intralobar refers to a sequestration that is in continuity with the normal lung and shares the same pleural investment. The venous drainage of such an intralobar sequestration is usually through the pulmonary veins. In distrinction to this, in an extralobar sequestration there is a separate pleural lining and the venous drainage is usually to the systemic vein. Some sequestrations may share characteristics of both types.

The pathogenetic theories of a sequestration include development of an additional tracheobronchial bud, development of an anomalous systemic vessel that may cause traction and separation of a part of the developing lung bud, and retention of systemic blood supply secondary to impairment in the pulmonary arterial circulation.

A sequestration may not produce symptoms and may be first noted roentgenographically as a solitary pulmonary nodule. The sequestered area may get infected through a bronchial communication; symptoms of pulmonary infection (fever, chills, cough, purulent sputum) may ensue. Hemoptysis may also be a feature. Sequestrations have a predilection for the lower lobe, particularly the left posterior basal area. Roentgenographically, they present as a solid mass or as a mass with an air-fluid level. The latter presentation usually occurs in association with an infection. Diagnosis may be established by demonstration of systemic arterial blood supply by aortography.

If a sequestration causes symptoms, is subject to repeated infections, or when distinction from a malignant neoplasm cannot be made, surgical resection is recommended. For a safe and well-planned surgery, it is imperative to perform a preoperative aortography to study the location and anatomic relationship of the systemic blood supply.

Anomalies of the Pulmonary Vessels

Pulmonary Arteriovenous Fistula

Pulmonary arteriovenous (A-V) fistulas may be single or multiple, asymptomatic or symptomatic, and may be of different sizes. One of the symptoms that is distressing is recurrent hemoptysis, which may be massive. Since these are areas of right-to-left shunting, hypoxemia and secondary polycythemia may be present. On physical examination, cyanosis may be manifest. Auscultation of the chest over a peripherally located A-V fistula may reveal a murmur. One clue to the presence of pulmonary A-V fistulas is the finding of telangiectasia in other parts of the body, particularly skin and mucous membranes (Rendu-Osler-Weber disease). Roentgenographically, these are rounded densities that simulate metastatic neoplasms. Fluoroscopic examination while changing intrathoracic pressures (Valsalva's and Müller's maneuvers) may demonstrate shrinking and enlarging of the densities. From a physiologic standpoint, the demonstration of hypoxemia even when supplemented with 100% oxygen, confirms the presence of a large right-to-left shunt. Surgery is the treatment of choice but may present difficulties because of the multiplicity of lesions. Accurate localization by angiography and determination of the relative size of the A-V fistula are important for planning surgical resection.

Pulmonary Artery Aneurysm

This is usually manifest as an abnormal roentgenogram. The roentgenographic findings include a prominent hilum showing a figure eight outline, hilar mass, and curvilinear calcification in the wall of the pulmonary artery. Pulmonary artery aneurysms are associated with other cardiac abnormalities, particularly an atrial septal defect.

Anomalous Pulmonary Venous Return
This term is used when, instead of the four pulmonary veins emptying into the left atrium, one or more of them empty into the right atrium or vena cavae. When anomalous pulmonary venous return is detected, the presence of other disorders, especially an atrial septal defect, should be suspected. One type of anomalous pulmonary venous return, the scimitar syndrome, has a characteristic roentgenographic picture. The venous return in this condition is to the inferior vena cava below the diaphragm. Scimitar syndrome is associated with other congenital abnormalities (e.g., agenesis or hypoplasia of the lung).

Unilateral Hyperlucent Lung
Swyer-James and Macleod's syndromes are synonyms for unilateral hyperlucent lung. This syndrome was originally defined as hyperlucency due to a hypoplastic pulmonary artery and its branches but since has been redefined as due to obliterative bronchitis or bronchiolitis associated with hypoplasia of the pulmonary artery. Whether the vascular hypoplasia or the obstructive bronchiolitis is the primary event cannot be ascertained in most cases. It is a moot point, however, since this does not affect the presentation and management of this disorder. Most patients with this condition may have a history of a viral respiratory infection, adenovirus, rubeola, or respiratory syncytial virus in childhood. The affected lung may appear small and, on bronchography, the bronchi look dilated and beaded (pruned-tree appearance). This is often discovered on an incidental chest roentgenogram since most often a hyperlucent lung does not cause symptoms.

The roentgenographic diagnosis of unilateral hyperlucent lung requires that the affected lung be normal or smaller than the contralateral lung. This requirement distinguishes this syndrome from compensatory, congenital lobar, or obstructive emphysema. In most cases, no treatment is necessary. If bronchiectasis is present in the affected lung and repeated infections occur, surgical resection may be appropriate.

PULMONARY MYCOSES

Infections due to a variety of organisms affecting the lungs and respiratory tract are discussed in the chapter on infectious diseases. Since pulmonary involvement is the most important and most frequent manifestation of systemic deep mycoses, these are discussed in this section.
Discussions here will be confined to histoplasmosis, coccidioidomycosis, blastomycosis, and pulmonary diseases caused by aspergillus. The first three are the most important systemic mycoses in the United States. Diseases caused by aspergillus are included for two reasons: the variety of clinical forms in which they present and the increasing frequency of life-threatening infections in immunosuppressed patients, particularly in those undergoing chemotherapy for various malignancies.

HISTOPLASMOSIS

Histoplasmosis is caused by a dimorphic (mycelial form in nature and yeast form in tissue) fungus, *Histoplasma capsulatum*. The main endemic areas of histoplasmosis are the Mississippi and Ohio River valleys. However, it has been recognized in many countries within the temperate and tropical zones. The fungus grows in the soil and its growth is favored by blackbird, chicken, or bat droppings. The infectious microconidia (<5 microns) become airborne when the soil becomes dry or is disturbed and may be inhaled. In the respiratory units of the lung, the organisms convert into parasitic yeast forms.

The clinical expressions and the course of the infection are varied, dependent on many factors (e.g., size of the inoculum, previous exposure to the fungus, age, immunocompetence, preexisting chronic lung disease). The primary infection is usually asymptomatic; symptomatic primary infection may occur in infants and young children. A large inoculum (heavy exposure to microconida) leads to acute histoplasmosis. This is the type usually associated with epidemics. Chronic pulmonary histoplasmosis is an expression of the disease usually seen in persons with underlying emphysema. Disseminated histoplasmosis should be considered an opportunistic infection occurring in patients with immunoincompetence (the immune defect may not be apparent in some). Histoplasmoma is a nodular mass that develops around a primary focus of infection and presents as a solitary pulmonary nodule. Although growth may occur, the nonmalignant nature of the mass is confirmed if concentric calcifications are noted within (see Fig. 26). Mediastinal granuloma and mediastinal fibrosis are two rare expressions of histoplasmosis and are discussed in the section on disorders of the pleura, mediastinum, and diaphragm.

Clinical Features

Primary infection is not usually detected clinically. Residual pulmonary nodules, calcifications within the lung, hilar or mediastinal lymph nodes, or in the spleen and positive histoplasmin skin tests are the imprints left behind in some cases and are of no clinical consequence. Primary infection in children may present with brassy cough and fever.

Acute histoplasmosis clinically manifests 1-3 weeks after a heavy exposure. Influenza-like symptoms such as fever, headache, myalgia, diaphoresis, chills, cough, pleuritic pain, nausea, vomiting, and malaise are present in varying combinations and intensity. Symptoms are more severe in persons with no previous exposure (primary type) compared to those who have been infected previously (reinfection type). Hilar and mediastinal lymphadenopathy and pleural involvement with or without effusion are more common in acute histoplasmosis of the primary type. Physical findings are usually sparse. Fever, rales, and hepatosplenomegaly may be present. Erythema nodosum has also been described. In most cases, symptoms spontaneously abate in approximately 10 days.

Chronic pulmonary histoplasmosis mimics tuberculosis. Productive cough, fever, malaise, and weight loss are the usual symptoms. Unlike acute histoplasmosis that almost always is a self-limiting illness, chronic pulmonary histoplasmosis is progressive. Cavitary disease, progressive enlargement of cavities, infiltrates progressing to fibrotic changes in the dependent segments (possibly due to antigenic spillage), and worsening pulmonary function are the consequences of untreated chronic pulmonary histoplasmosis.

Disseminated histoplasmosis may have an acute, a subacute, or a chronic presentation dependent to a large extent on the degree of immunologic impairment of the host. The symptoms are similar to that of acute histoplasmosis but are more severe and persistent. Examination is likely to reveal pallor, hepatosplenomegaly, and generalized lymphadenopathy. Untreated acute disseminated histoplasmosis is uniformly fatal. Subacute and chronic disseminated histoplasmosis may present with fever that may be intermittent, malaise, and weight loss. Splenomegaly and oropharyngeal ulcers may be present. The latter should be particularly sought on physical examination since they are frequent (estimated 25-75%) and are readily accessible for a biopsy. These lesions start as a plaque or nodule and later ulcerate. The ulcer has thickened edges and may appear in the pharynx, nose, lips, tongue, gingiva, or buccal mucosa. Because of its propensity to involve the meninges, heart, and adrenals, disseminated histoplasmosis should be considered in the differential diagnosis of chronic meningitis, endocarditis, and adrenal insufficiency.

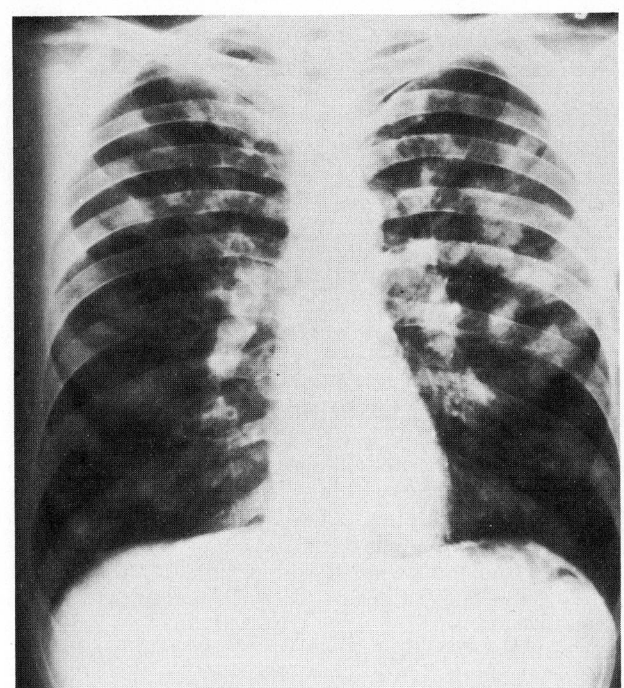

Figure 4. Primary histoplasmosis; multiple nodular infiltrates and hilar adenopathy.

Roentgenographic Features

The roentgenographic sequelae of primary histoplasmosis have already been described. Diffuse bilateral pulmonary nodular infiltrates (poorly or well defined) with hilar/mediastinal adenopathy is the usual finding in acute histoplasmosis (Fig. 4). These nodules may heal with calcifications. Large mediastinal lymph nodes may occasionally cause bronchial obstruction and atelectasis. Pleural effusions are infrequent.

Reticulonodular infiltrates in the apical and posterior segments of the upper lobes that simulate tuberculosis are the early findings in chronic pulmonary histoplasmosis. Previous chest roentgenograms, if available, are likely to reveal emphysema, particularly bullae or cysts in the apical areas. Later cavitation, progressive enlargement of the cavity, interstitial infiltrates in the lower lobes, and eventually volume loss due to fibrosis are manifest.

Chest roentgenographic findings are variable in disseminated histoplasmosis. Examples are interstitial infiltrates, localized pneumonic infiltrates, miliary infiltrates, and residual features of a previous infection. However, the more important point to keep in mind is that disseminated histoplasmosis may be present with an apparently normal chest roentgenogram.

Diagnosis

Confirmation of the diagnosis of histoplasmosis is by isolation of the organism from tissue or biologic material. However, the clinical setting, roentgenogram, serology, and microscopy are all helpful in arriving at a diagnosis.

Sputum, urine, and blood cultures are not usually done and are considered of low diagnostic yield in primary and acute histoplasmosis. Although skin test and serologic conversion happens after a primary infection, this is rarely useful in actual practice. Diagnosis is based mainly on the clinical and roentgenographic findings. The roentgenographic findings in acute histoplasmosis are fairly characteristic. A strong presumptive diagnosis can be made if, in addition to the roentgenographic findings, there is also a history of exposure (e.g., bulldozing a starling roost), similar illness in other exposed persons, and consistent clinical features.

In chronic pulmonary histoplasmosis, skin tests and serology (complement fixation test) are not useful. A negative histoplasmin skin test or a negative serology does not rule out the diagnosis. The findings of a high titer (>1:32) occasionally may be helpful but is not specific enough for a confident diagnosis. Clinical and roentgenographic findings (previously described) allow a presumptive diagnosis. Efforts should be concentrated in obtaining mycologic confirmation by repeated sputum smears and cultures. This may be negative in pneumonic infiltrates and thin-walled cavities. When thick-walled cavities are present, the diagnostic yield of sputum is about 50%.

The histoplasmin skin test has no place in the diagnosis of disseminated histoplamosis. Complement fixation titer over 1:32 in the presence of consistent clinical features suggests the diagnosis. Hematologic abnormalities (anemia, leukopenia, thrombocytopenia) and liver function abnormalities (increased transaminase, alkaline phosphatase, bilirubin) are frequently encountered. Because of the very serious nature of the disease, an aggressive diagnostic approach is warranted. Cultures from different sources such as bone marrow, blood, sputum, bronchial brushings, urine, ulcers, liver biopsy, and histopathologic study of these as well as any other aspirated or resected tissue, should be done. If consistent morphologic findings of the yeast are noted by periodic acid-Shiff (PAS) or Gomori methenamine silver (GMS) stain, treatment may be started since the culture results may take 2 or more weeks.

Treatment

Treatment with amphotericin B (total dose of 2 g) is indicated in all cases of chronic pulmonary and disseminated histoplasmosis. Primary and acute histoplasmosis generally do not need amphotericin-B treatment. Severe or prolonged symptoms or massive adenitis in infants and children and prolonged symptoms (more than 1 week) in adults, or progressive hypoxia or full-blown adult respiratory distress syndrome (ARDS), are reasons to treat with amphotericin B. For these conditions some physicians have successfully used an abbreviated (1 g) course of amphotericin B. Concomitant corticosteroid administration may be beneficial in rare occasions (e.g., pericarditis, ARDS).

Since intravenous amphotericin B is the drug of choice in deep mycoses, a few comments on its use and side effects are appropriate. The authors prefer to start with a test dose of 1 mg followed by daily increments of 10 mg (a more rapid increment is indicated in life-threatening illness) to attain a dose of 40 mg (or 0.6 mg/kg), which is then administered as an intravenous drip over 2-6 hours daily until the appropriate total dose (usually 2 g) is reached. Serum creatinine levels are monitored (at least every other day), and if the creatinine level exceeds 3 mg %, the drug should be temporarily withheld. After the clinical course has stabilized, amphotericin B may be given as outpatient treatment on alternate days. Besides serum creatinine, periodic measurements of hematocrit, serum potassium, and magnesium are advisable. Amphotericin B is a nephrotoxic drug with its major effect on the distal tubule. Azotemia, hypokalemia, hypomagnesemia, and anemia are recognized complications of amphotericin B therapy. Other side effects include nausea, vomiting, febrile reactions, and local phlebitis, which may be minimized by appropriate medications (e.g., antiemetics, antipyretics, corticosteroids). A new orally administered antifungal agent, ketoconazole (Nizoral), may be effective in histoplasmosis.

COCCIDIOIDOMYCOSIS

Coccidioidomycosis is caused by *Coccidioides immitis*, a fungus that grows in soil. The mycelial forms proliferate during the rainy season; they mature and form arthrospores during the dry season. The arthrospores become airborne and inhalation of these spores causes the infection. In a rare instance infection may be acquired by cutaneous inoculation. The main endemic regions are the southwestern United States and adjacent areas of northern Mexico.

Primary infections are usually asymptomatic. Symptomatic primary infections are usually self-limited; symptoms do not last more than 3 weeks. When symptoms and signs do not abate in 6 weeks, it indicates persistent coccidioidomycosis. Persistant coccidioidomycosis has different clinical and roentgenographic expressions, namely, pneumonia (acute, persistent, chronic progressive), cavity (acute, chronic), nodules, and disseminated (miliary pattern, extrapulmonary manifestations).

Clinical Features

Symptoms of primary infection (manifest in less than one-half of those infected) are fever, cough, chest pain, and headache. Other manifestations include sore throat, malaise, erythema nodosum, and erythema marginatum.

These symptoms are more intense in acute coccidioidal pneumonia. High fever, cough productive of copious purulent sputum, and occasional hemoptysis may be present. Chronicity of the symptoms (>6 weeks) is characteristic of persistent pneumonia. In chronic progressive pneumonia, a rare category, the symptoms slowly progress over many years. When this is associated with cavitary disease, hemoptysis is more frequent and more severe.

Cavities may develop acutely as a result of parenchymal necrosis during an acute coccidioidal pneumonia. Pneumonic symptoms, described earlier, and hemoptysis are the usual features. Enlarging cavities may rupture into the pleural space and cause a bronchopleural fistula. Chronic cavities usually do not cause symptoms and are recognized roentgenographically.

Another residual lesion of a previous infection is a coccidioidal nodule that is quite obviously a roentgenographic diagnosis. On occasion, the soft center of the nodule may shell out and leave behind a cavity.

Miliary coccidioidomycosis indicates hematogenous dissemination and is a serious development because of increased mortality. The clinical presentation may be acute (fever, dyspnea) or more commonly chronic with low-grade fever and weight loss. Extrapulmonary dissemination may occur to any organ but there is a predilection for skin, bone, lymph nodes, and meninges.

Roentgenographic Features

The usual roentgenographic findings of primary infections (symptomatic or asymptomatic) are single or multiple segmental patchy infiltrates. This characteristically, but not invariably, is associated with hilar lymphadenopathy. Other findings include hilar, mediastinal, and paratracheal lymphadenopathy, varying degrees of atelectasis, and pleural effusion.

In acute coccidioidal pneumonia the infiltrate is usually dense and may be lobar in distribution. Radiolucent areas within the infiltrate (cavities) may be seen. Associated hilar lymphadenopathy is not uncommon; paratracheal lymphadenopathy may herald dissemination. The roentgenographic appearance of chronic progressive pneumonia simulates tuberculosis and histoplasmosis with apical fibronodular infiltrates.

Characteristically residual cavities of coccidioidomycosis are single, less than 4 cm in diameter, located in the upper zones, and have thin walls. Exceptions, particularly thick, shaggy-walled cavities, however, are not infrequent. Sequelae of residual cavities, such as infection and mycetoma formation, are recognized by air-fluid levels and intracavitary densities.

Coccidioidal nodules are often single and are of the same size as residual cavities. Nodules and cavities may coexist (Fig. 5). The appearance of miliary coccidioidomycosis is the same as that of miliary tuberculosis, that is, diffuse, discrete pinpoint nodules.

Diagnosis

The clinical and roentgenographic features are not specific enough for a diagnosis. The usual laboratory tests are also nonspecific (e.g., leukocytosis and elevated erythrocyte sedimentation rate). Eosinophilia, when present, is a helpful clue. Skin test with coccidioidin or with the more sensitive antigen, spherulin, is not diagnostic by itself. However, skin test conversion (negative to positive) in the presence of clinical infection is strongly suggestive of the diagnosis. A negative skin test does not rule out the diagnosis.

Serologic tests in the appropriate geographic, historic, and clinical setting provide a diagnosis in many instances. IgM antibodies that appear early in the disease may be detected by a tube precipitin test or by its improved variations, namely, the latex particle agglutination (LPA) test and immunodiffusion (ID) test. The LPA test is very sensitive but is not very specific. The ID test has increased specificity when set up with appropriate controls. IgG antibodies, which appear later than the IgM antibodies, may be detected by complement fixation (CF) test or ID test. The titer of CF antibody in disseminated disease usually exceeds 1:16. Determination of CF titer is important in the diagnosis and prognosis and in assessing the efficacy of treatment.

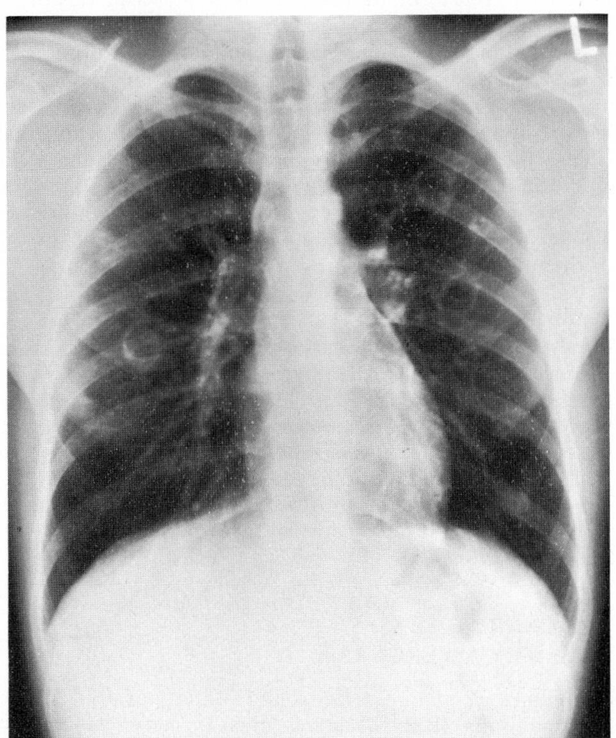

Figure 5. Multiple thin-walled cavities and nodules.

The spherules may be identified on direct microscopic examination of body secretions but there is the possibility of a false-positive reading caused by contaminants. Confirmation of the diagnosis of coccidioidomycosis is by recovery of the fungus from culture of tissue or biologic fluids. Closed-hood systems are strongly recommended to avoid accidental infection of laboratory personnel.

Treatment

Primary infections with *C. immitis* generally do not require treatment. Primary infections in certain situations call for treatment. Examples of such situations are an immunosuppressed state (e.g., lymphoma), pregnancy, uncontrolled diabetes, dark-skinned races (blacks, Asiatics), loss of skin reactivity to coccidioidin or spherulin, high titer of CF antibodies, or toxicity with fever and weight loss, particularly if it is persistent (more than 3 weeks).

Other indications for treatment are necrotizing pneumonia, progressive pneumonia, extrapulmonary disease, and miliary disease. Amphotericin B is the drug used for treatment (see under treatment for histoplasmosis). In coccidioidal meningitis intrathecal or intracisternal amphotericin-B therapy is recommended. Other drugs that have had limited use and success are miconazole and methyl ester of amphotericin B. Human transfer factor has also been tried in some cases. Early results of ketoconazole therapy are promising but further work needs to be done regarding optimal dose, duration of therapy, and the problem of remissions.

Surgical therapy has had applications in incision and drainage of subcutaneous abscess, excision of cutaneous lesion, biopsies, removal of dead bone in osteomyelitis, and arthrodesis. In pulmonary coccidioidomycosis the indications for surgical treatment are a coccidioidal nodule (not diagnosed by any other means) presenting as a solitary nodule thus mimicking bronchogenic carcinoma, a rapidly expanding cavity if considered to be in imminent danger of rupturing, a cavity with serious hemorrhage, and a bronchopleural fistula.

BLASTOMYCOSIS

Blastomycosis is caused by a dimorphic fungus, *Blastomyces dermatitidis*. At room temperature, the fungus grows in the mycelial phase and at body temperature it grows as a yeast. The yeast has a diameter of 5-15 μ and has a characteristic appearance (Fig. 6): spherical, multinucleated, double contoured, and refractile displaying a single broad-based bud. The major endemic areas of blastomycosis are the southeastern United States and Mississippi Valley area including the midwestern states. The distribution of canine blastomycosis is similar supporting the endemic nature of the infection. The

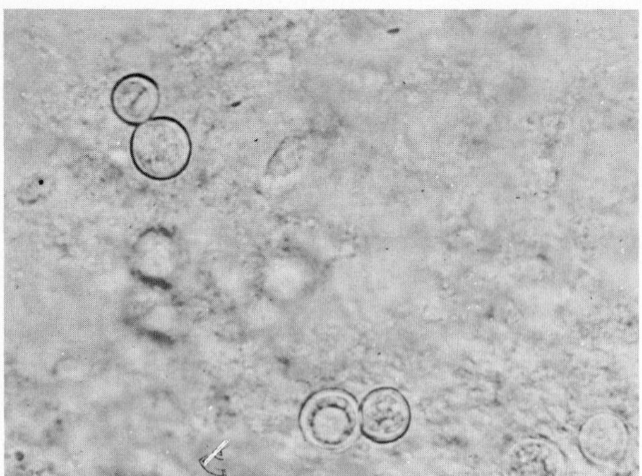

Figure 6. Yeast forms of *Blastomyces dermatitidis*. (Reprinted with permission from *Chest* 77:789, 1980.)

natural habitat of this organism is unknown but is suspected to be the soil.

Infection almost always (in a few cases direct skin inoculation has been reported) is a result of inhalation of spores. In the lower respiratory tract, the spores convert to yeast forms, proliferate, and establish a primary focus of infection. The primary focus may cause no symptoms and may clear spontaneously. An acute form of blastomycosis has been recognized 33-44 days after exposure in epidemics (a cluster of cases suggesting a common source). Acute blastomycosis may subside without any sequelae or it may cause progressive pulmonary infection or an endogenous reactivation after initial resolution. However, the most common form of blastomycosis is the chronic pulmonary form with or without extrapulmonary involvement.

Clinical Features

Acute blastomycosis may present like a bacterial or nonbacterial pneumonia with fever and productive cough. Pleuritic chest pain may be present, but pleural effusion is uncommon. Acute blastomycosis may resolve without specific treatment.

Chronic blastomycosis has a striking predilection for men, particularly those over 40 years of age. Cough and chest pain are the usual symptoms; hemoptysis may be an initial symptom in about 20% of patients. Systemic symptoms such as weight loss, night sweats, and malaise are common. Among the extrapulmonary manifestations, skin lesions are the most frequent and may be present in 25-35% of patients with chronic blastomycosis. The face and trunk appear to be the favored sites. The characteristic lesion of blastomycosis is an ulcer with heaped up edges containing microabscesses that is sharply demarcated from the surrounding normal skin. Blastomycosis may involve virtually every organ in the body. However, the genitourinary system, bones and joints, and central nervous system are more prone to be involved and to cause symptoms (e.g., dysuria, painful bones and joints). It is important to bear in mind that these symptoms may manifest without concomitant respiratory symptoms.

Roentgenographic Features

The common roentgenographic findings of acute blastomycosis are infiltrates or parenchymal consolidation. These may be bilateral and nodular simulating metastatic neoplasms or acute mycotic infections. Cavitation is an uncommon feature.

In chronic blastomycosis the roentgenographic findings are very variable. Pulmonary infiltrates are the most common finding. This may vary from segmental to lobar to bilateral infiltrates. Cavitation is present in about 25% of cases. Other presentations include nodules, miliary nodules, and masslike densities. Hilar or mediastinal enlargement is uncommon and pleural effusion is infrequent.

Diagnosis

The clinical and roentgenographic features are nonspecific and simulate a variety of diseases. The diagnosis is confirmed only by the isolation of *Blastomyces dermatitidis* from cultures of biologic fluids or tissue. However, since the morphology of the organism is distinctive and the culture takes several days, microscopic examination of all biologic material is important. This is best done by preparing a smear of the material mixed with an equal amount of 10% potassium hydroxide. Gomori and PAS stains may also be helpful. Morphologic identification is sufficient for presumptive diagnosis and permits early institution of therapy. Sputum is the most convenient material; multiple deep-coughed, fresh sputa should be smeared, examined under the microscope, and cultured. Microscopy and culture of other material such as aspirates of skin lesions, prostatic fluid, and urine voided after prostatic massage should be pursued. If pulmonary infiltrates are present, fiberoptic bronchoscopy with aspiration of secretions, bronchial brushings, and possible transbronchoscopic lung biopsy should be considered. Other sources depend on the clinical presentations (e.g., biopsy of a lytic bone lesion, aspiration of a swollen joint). Presently skin tests and serologic tests are not useful in diagnosis. Further refinement in serologic tests, particularly immunodiffusion tests, hold promise for the future.

Treatment

All cases of chronic pulmonary and extrapulmonary blastomycosis should be treated intravenously with amphotericin B (total dose of 2 g). In acute blastomycosis there are a few reported instances where recovery has occurred without treatment. However, since the clinical course of acute blastomycosis cannot be predicted it is advisable to treat symptomatic cases with amphotericin B. Ketoconazole may prove to be useful, but at this time there is inadequate data for firm recommendations.

PULMONARY DISEASES CAUSED BY ASPERGILLUS

Aspergilli (*Aspergillus fumigatus* and a variety of other species) are ubiquitous (soil, decaying organic matter, etc.) fungi responsible for a variety of illnesses in humans. The starting point of these illnesses is inhalation of aspergillus spores or conidia. Whether clinical disease develops, and in which form it is expressed, depend on the intensity and frequency of exposure as well as on host factors (atopy, preexisting cavitary disease, immunosuppressed state). Although an extensive literature has developed on various forms of aspergillus lung disease, difficulties in definition and classification of these have not been entirely overcome. The distinct clinical forms of the disease caused by aspergilli include extrinsic asthma, extrinsic allergic alveolitis (malt worker's lung), allergic bronchopulmonary aspergillosis (ABPA), aspergilloma (mycetoma), and invasive aspergillosis.

In persons with extrinsic asthma, aspergillus may act as a specific allergen; inhalation of aspergillus spores may result in release of mediators from mast cells and provoke bronchospasm. Extrinsic allergic alveolitis may result from inhalation of aspergillus organisms present in moldy barley, oats, corn, or hay. Like other hypersensitivity pneumonitides, this occurs primarily in nonatopic individuals. Clinical, roentgenographic, and laboratory findings and diagnosis and principles of treatment are similar to other hypersensitivity pneumonitides (see the section on diffuse infiltrative diseases of the lung).

The three most commonly recognized forms of aspergillus lung disease, namely, allergic bronchopulmonary aspergillosis, aspergilloma, and invasive aspergillosis merit further discussion.

Allergic Bronchopulmonary Aspergillosis

In atopic individuals, aspergillus inhaled from the environment may continue to reside in the bronchi and the consequent antigenic stimulation elicits formation of IgE and IgG antibodies against the fungus. These antibodies react against aspergillus antigens, (type 1 and type 3 reactions), causing bronchospasm and probably immune-complex injury to the bronchi. Proximal saccular bronchiectasis is a serious complication of ABPA.

Wheezing, recurrent fevers, and cough productive of thick, brownish sputum are the clinical features of this disease. Eosinophilia of the sputum and blood are common findings. Roentgenographic findings are varied: transient pulmonary infiltrates, bandlike densities, and atelectasis secondary to mucus plugging of the bronchi. In later stages, contraction of lobes, pulmonary fibrosis, and extensive bronchiectasis may be seen. The results of pulmonary function studies depend on the stage of the disease. Obstructive ventilatory impairment is a common feature. In later stages, restricitve impairment and diminished diffusing capacity may be seen.

Diagnosis

The major criteria for the diagnosis of ABPA are asthma, eosinophilia of sputum and blood, recurrent pulmonary infiltrates, and allergy to antigens of aspergillus by skin test (immediate wheal and flare reaction and late reaction). Other criteria include elevated IgE, aspergillus in sputum, aspergillus precipitins in serum, a history of recurrent fever or pneumonia, and a history of coughing up of sputum plugs. An inhalational challenge test with *A. fumigatus* antigen produces a characteristic dual response (immediate and late), and is usually correlated with increased symptoms. This test is rarely, if ever, needed to make a diagnosis.

Treatment

Antifungal agents are not useful in the treatment of this disorder. Glucocorticosteroids are effective in reducing the symptoms. Along with this, a reduction of the serum IgE level is also observed and is, therefore, a useful parameter for adjustment of steroid dose. Long-term treatment is usually necessary.

Pulmonary Aspergilloma

Aspergilloma is a mycelial mass formed by colonization and growth of aspergilli within an area of destroyed lung. Thus, diseases that cause parenchymal necrosis, namely, tuberculosis, sarcoidosis, pulmonary infarct, bronchiectasis, lung abscess, neoplasm, ankylosing spondilitis, and various pulmonary mycoses predispose to the development of aspergilloma. In a large followup study by the British Tuberculosis Association of patients with healed tuberculosis and residual cavities, 11% developed aspergilloma in 3-4 years. Patients who had a positive precipitin test by immunodiffusion were twice as likely to acquire an aspergilloma as those who did not have precipitins against aspergillus. One of the first roentgenographic changes of aspergillus colonization of a cavity is adjacent pleural thickening; intracavity fluid is less frequently observed.

The most common symptom of a well-established aspergilloma is hemoptysis, which occurs in more than one-half of the patients. This is usually minimal in amount and recurrent. However, severe, gross hemoptysis may occur. The cause of hemoptysis is unclear. Explanations include friction of the mycetoma on the cavitary wall, an endotoxin and/or an anticoagulant liberated by aspergillus, and possible local vascular invasion. Other symptoms include chronic cough and shortness of breath.

The natural history of an aspergilloma is very variable. They may remain stable, increase in size gradually, or spontaneously lyse. Spontaneous lysis has been reported in about 10% of cases.

Diagnosis

The definition makes it clear that the diagnosis of aspergilloma is mainly roentgenographic. The typical roentgenographic appearance is of an intracavitary oval, round, or irregular density that is surrounded by a crescent of air (Fig. 7). Aspergilloma is usually single and located in the upper lobe. The roentgenographic appearance, although typical, is not pathognomic since intracavitary hematoma, lung necrosis, neoplasm, and other mycoses infrequently may cause an intracavitary density. The diagnosis of aspergilloma is further supported by either finding aspergilli in the sputum or by a positive precipitin test. However, the absence of aspergillus in the sputum does not rule out the diagnosis. The presence of multiple precipitin lines on immunodiffusion in a patient with typical roentgenographic appearance makes the diagnosis of aspergilloma certain. A negative precipitin test virtually rules out the diagnosis. Skin test with aspergillus antigen is positive only in a minority of patients with aspergilloma.

Treatment

Systemic antifungal therapy has not been shown to be effective in the treatment of pulmonary aspergilloma. Intracavitary

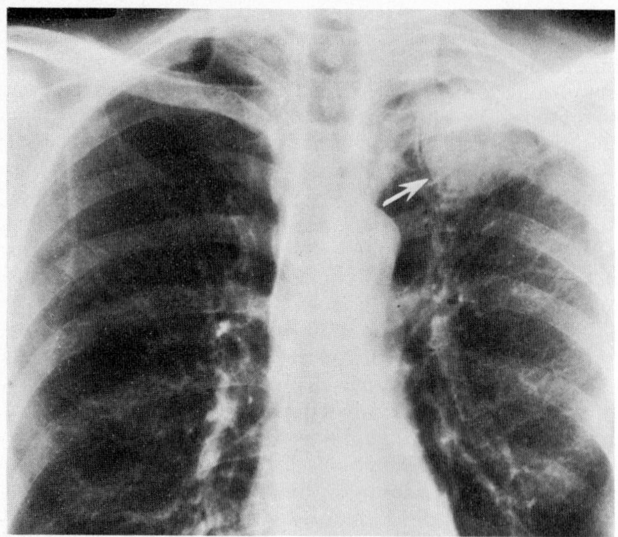

Figure 7. Aspergilloma; intracavitary density and typical crescent (arrow).

instillation of antifungal agents has been tried in a few cases, but these are too few to be conclusive. Long-term prospective studies of aspergilloma have shown that the prognosis and eventual outcome of aspergilloma is dependent on the severity of the underlying diseases rather than on the aspergilloma itself. Routine surgical resection of all aspergillomas is not indicated. Patients with mild or intermittent hemoptysis should be carefully observed; usually these episodes are self-limiting. Massive or life-threatening hemoptysis calls for localization of the site of bleeding and surgical resection.

Invasive Aspergillosis

Invasive aspergillosis is an acute, severe, rapidly progressive infection of the lung that has a tendency to disseminate to various organs. Invasive aspergillosis almost always occurs in a patient who is immunosuppressed or myelosuppressed; the usual setting is a neutropenic patient with a hematogenous malignancy undergoing to cytotoxic chemotherapy. Patients with acute leukemia are particularly susceptible to this infection. Corticosteroids and immunosuppressive drugs predispose to aspergillosis.

Acute onset of fever and dyspnea are the most common symptoms. Cough and pleuritic chest pain may be present. The latter is usually associated with a pleural friction rub.

The roentgenographic features are usually that of a bronchopneumonia and the infiltrates may be miliary, patchy, or dense. Followup roentgenograms are likely to reveal progressive infiltrates and cavity formation. Mycetoma formation within the cavity may be seen. Since aspergillus has a propensity to invade vessels causing thrombosis, the clinical and roentgenographic presentation may be that of a pulmonary embolism and infarction.

The clinical course is one of progressive worsening and usually ends in death in 1-2 weeks. Early institution of therapy (medical and surgical) has been successful in some cases.

Diagnosis

A successful diagnostic approach to invasive aspergillosis demands a high degree of suspicion. In an immunocompromised patient (particularly in one with hematogenous malignancy), if a presumed bacterial pneumonia does not respond to antibacterial therapy, aspergillosis should be considered as a possibility. However, proving this diagnosis is often difficult for many reasons. Fever and pulmonary infiltrates may be due to a variety of causes (infections, extension of primary disease, drug-induced, etc.). Sputum may not be available for examination and absence of aspergilli in the sputum does not rule out the diagnosis of aspergillosis. Invasive procedures aimed at obtaining lung tissue should be performed without delay. An open lung biopsy is the preferred method. The finding of septate, acutely branching hyphae of aspergilli (Fig. 8) in tissue is diagnostic. In a patient whose condition does not permit lung biopsy, presumptive treatment is justified when consistent clinical and roentgenographic findings are present. In this context, finding of aspergilli in sputum is sufficient reason to institute treatment with amphotericin B. Recently attention has been focused on early diagnosis by serologic tests (immunodiffusion) and by nasal cultures. Nasal cultures done as a routine monitoring procedure in immunocompromised patients holds promise as an early diagnostic method.

Treatment

Without specific treatment, invasive aspergillosis is a fatal disease. Even with treatment the mortality is greater than 80%. The drug of choice is amphotericin B. Because of the life-threatening nature of the disease, the increments of dose should be made much more rapidly than described in the section on histoplasmosis. The dose and duration of therapy, although not established, are similar to that employed in other

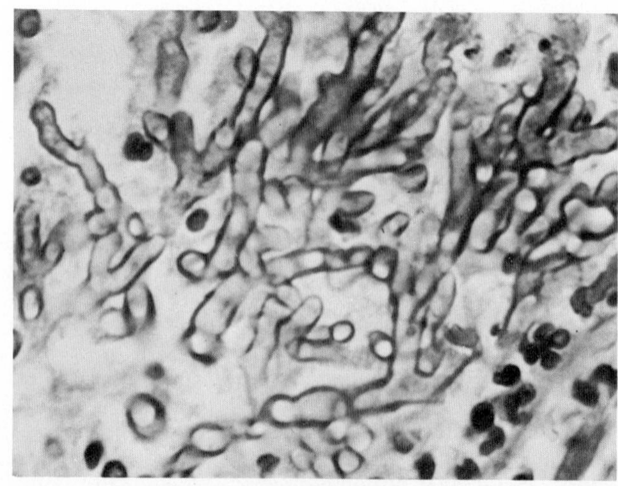

Figure 8. Aspergillus hyphae in tissue.

deep mycoses. Granulocyte transfusions (in neutropenic patients), may be helpful as adjunctive therapy. The role of other drugs (e.g., 5-fluorocytosine, miconazole, ketoconazole) are not well known yet.

OBSTRUCTIVE DISORDERS OF THE AIRWAYS

The term chronic obstructive pulmonary disease (COPD) encompasses several disorders that have certain common features, albeit different etiology and pathogenesis, such as asthma, chronic bronchitis, emphysema, cystic fibrosis, and bronchiectasis. The most important factor that these disorders may have in common is the slowing of expiratory airflow, which is a prerequisite for the diagnosis of chronic obstructive pulmonary disease. The term COPD is far from satisfactory since it does not take into account the etiology, pathogenesis, and the prognosis of the individual diseases in the group; frequently there is an overlap of diseases. COPD may be best viewed as a spectrum of diseases ranging from intrinsic diseases of the airways (chronic bronchitis) to parenchymal disease (emphysema).

Asthma represents hyperresponsiveness of the airways with widespread reversible airway narrowing. Chronic bronchitis exists when cough and expectoration are present on most days for at least 3 months in a year for 2 successive years with other causes, such as tuberculosis and bronchiectasis, having been excluded. When asthmatic symptoms, particularly wheezing, coexist with chronic bronchitis, the condition may be called asthmatic bronchitis. Such overlaps may also exist between bronchitis and bronchiectasis. Two further subclasses exist among the chronic bronchitis population, namely, simple and obstructive. Production of small amounts of mucus alone is the feature of simple chronic bronchitis, whereas significant airway obstruction, hypoxemia, and sometimes hypercapnia denote the often disabling obstructive bronchitis. Emphysema denotes the presence of overinflation of air spaces in addition to destruction of the alveolar septa. Emphysema and chronic bronchitis frequently coexist. Cystic fibrosis is a genetic disorder, characterized by exocrine pancreatic insufficiency, chronic bronchopulmonary disease, infertility, and elevated concentrations of sodium and chloride in the sweat. Bronchiectasis is defined as an abnormal, permanent dilatation of the bronchi with destruction of the bronchial walls.

Discussion will be limited to chronic bronchitis, emphysema, cystic fibrosis, and bronchiectasis. Asthma has been discussed in the chapter on allergies. The differences in the symptomatology, physical findings, and physiologic features between chronic bronchitis and emphysema have led to the development of the concepts of the blue bloater and the pink puffer. These have been summarized in Table 8. While these differences may be an oversimplification if applied to rigidly, they can be helpful in the evaluation of the patient as well as in prognosis.

CHRONIC BRONCHITIS

Etiology and Pathogenesis

In the vast majority of cases of chronic bronchitis, tobacco smoke is the major causative factor. Smoking leads to chronic bronchitis by stimulating mucus secretion from the mucus glands of the bronchi and by impairing mucociliary clearance. Tobacco smoke affects alveolar macrophage function with resultant vulnerability to respiratory infections, consequent

Table 8. Differences Between Blue Bloaters and Pink Puffers

Feature	*Blue Bloater*	*Pink Puffer*
Clinical		
Symptoms	Late onset of dyspnea; sputum production early, cardinal symptom	Early dyspnea and virtually no sputum
Examination	Obese, plethoric, and often cyanotic	Asthenic, pink
	Normal percussion note, generally normal breath sounds with rhonchi and rales	Hyperresonant percussion note and decreased breath sounds
	Cor pulmonale frequent	Cor pulmonale infrequent
Laboratory	Markedly low Pa_{O_2} and often high Pa_{CO_2}	Normal or slightly decreased Pa_{O_2} and Pa_{CO_2}
	Elevated RV and FRC with generally normal TLC and and DLCO	Elevated RV, FRC, and TLC; low DL_{CO}
	Static compliance normal	Static compliance increased
Roentgenographic	Normal A-P diameter and diaphragms, normal or increased heart size	Increased A-P diameter, low diaphragms, small heart (Figs. 9 and 10)

bronchial damage, and further impairment of ciliary mechanisms. Chronic bronchitis may also result from exposure to environmental pollutants and irritants. The combined effects of tobacco smoke and pollutants may be additive.

Pathology

Hypertrophy of the mucus glands of the airways is apparent on microscopic examination. The ratio of the thickness of the mucus glands to the thickness of the mucosal wall (basement membrane to perichondrium) is known as the Reid index (normal <0.4) and is usually increased in chronic bronchitis. In addition, there is increased size of the acini of the glands. Smooth-muscle hyperplasia, edema, and congestion of the bronchial wall with chronic inflammatory cell infiltration, goblet-cell hyperplasia, and intrabronchial mucus plugging are other findings. Distension of respiratory bronchioles with destruction of the wall (centrilobular emphysema) is usually present as well.

Clinical Features

Cough and expectoration are the cardinal features of chronic bronchitis. In the early phases of the disease, these symptoms are dismissed by the patient and often by the physician as smoker's cough. Cough and sputum tend to be present maximally in the morning and reflect pooling of secretions overnight. Symptoms are intermittent at first and are generally manifest on most days of the year as the disease progresses. Sputum is clear and mucoid unless bacterial respiratory infection has supervened, when it may become thick, tenacious, and yellow. Blood-streaking of sputum may also be manifest. With progression of the disease, there is increase in cough and sputum production along with wheezing. Dyspnea is usually not seen in chronic, simple bronchitis and is generally a feature of chronic obstructive bronchitis. The development of the latter occurs over a period of years and is characterized by dyspnea, heart failure, cyanosis, and marked wheezing. Physical examination, which is generally normal in simple chronic bronchitis, reveals expiratory prolongation, rhonchi, and, less commonly, basilar rales in the obstructive type.

Laboratory Findings

Erythrocytosis occurs, particularly in chronic obstructive bronchitis. Roentgenograms may be normal or they may show increased lung markings or present a "dirty lung" appearance. The cardiac silhouette may be normal or enlarged. Pulmonary function studies may be normal in chronic bronchitis. However, in chronic obstructive bronchitis, evidence of airway obstruction (reduced $FEV_{1.0}$/FVC ratio, diminished vital capacity, increased FRC, and RV) is seen. Pa_{O_2} is generally decreased because of ventilation-perfusion mismatching (continued perfusion of nonventilating alveoli). Pa_{CO_2} levels are generally normal although, with advancing disease, hypercapnia may be evident. Sputum examination may show a mixed bacterial population.

Course, Complications, and Prognosis

Symptoms of chronic bronchitis continue unabated with continued exposure to cigarette smoke and/or environmental pollutants. With cessation of such exposure, symptoms generally improve. Conflicting evidence has accumulated regarding the decline in pulmonary function in chronic bronchitics who continue to smoke versus those who do not. On the basis of current evidence, long-term decline in pulmonary function appears to be less in those who stop smoking.

The main complications of chronic bronchitis are respiratory infections, respiratory failure, erythrocytosis, and cor pulmonale. Bacterial colonization of the lower respiratory tract is common in chronic bronchitics, and most respiratory infections, although initially viral, soon evolve into bacterial bronchitis. Increased cough with thick, tenacious, yellow sputum laden with numerous bacteria and polymorphonuclear cells and worsening of respiratory status characterize these bacterial infections. The usual cause of respiratory failure in chronic bronchitis is a respiratory infection. Other factors that may produce respiratory failure are heart failure, uncontrolled oxygen therapy, sedation, surgery involving general anesthesia, and pulmonary thromboembolic disease. Mechanisms of the development of cor pulmonale in the bronchitic are discussed elsewhere in detail but include hypoxemia, hypercapnia, and increased blood viscosity from erythrocytosis in addition to the destruction of the pulmonary vascular bed.

Hypoxemia is the reason for the erythrocytosis in bronchitic patients. Increase in red cell mass is apparent, but characteristically no leukocytosis nor thrombocytosis accompanies this event. This complication in the bronchitics responds to oxygen administration and phlebotomies.

Treatment

All patients with a diagnosis of chronic obstructive pulmonary disease should be given a trial of bronchodilators whether or not spirometric tests show improvement after bronchodilation. Repeat spirometry and review of symptoms after several weeks of treatment may be used as criteria in deciding whether to continue or discontinue therapy. The major drugs used for this purpose are theophylline, theophylline derivatives, and sympathomimetic drugs, usually of the β-2 type. Bronchodilator dosages are represented in Table 9.

Secretions can be reduced considerably in most cases by cessation of exposure to tobacco smoke and other bronchial irritants. Change in occupation or use of filter masks may be necessary to reduce exposure to pollutants and irritants. Expectorants such as glyceryl guaiacolate, potassium iodide, and so on have no proven benefit. Adequate hydration is important in aiding ease of expectoration of sputum. Physical therapy with chest clapping and postural drainage is helpful when bronchiectasis is coexistent.

At the very first symptom of a respiratory infection, patients should be advised to start taking antibiotics, usually tetracycline or ampicillin (divided doses of 1.0 g and 2.0 g daily, respectively). Combinations of sulfamethoxazole and trimethoprim (400 μg and 160 μg, respectively) are also useful in doses of one tablet twice daily for a period of 10 days. Antibiotics are also indicated if change in color of the sputum is noted. In special situations with recurrent respiratory infections, 2-3 weekly courses of antibiotics every month have been recommended.

Table 9. Bronchodilators

Agent	*Mechanism of Action*	*Dosage*	*Route of Administration*	*Side Effects*	*Remarks*
Aminophylline	Inhibition of phosphodiesterase	200 mg qid generally	Oral, rectal, IV	Nausea, vomiting, irritability, palpitations, insomnia, cardiac arrhythmias, and convulsions	Reduce dose by $\frac{1}{2}$ in liver failure, $\frac{1}{3}$ in renal failure. Half-life prolonged smokers and possibly with erythromycin use. Phenobarbital reduces half-life
Ephedrine	α and β adrenergic activity	50 mg tid	Oral	Central nervous system stimulation, insomnia, hypertention, urinary retention	Interacts with MAO inhibitors, guanethidine, and tricyclic antidepressants Tolerance develops when given more than tid.
Isoproterenol	β adrenergic agent	1-2 whiffs q 4 h	Mistometers	Cardiac arrhythmias	Whiffs available in 0.03 to 0.11 mg drug base/dose
			Via IPPB		Aerosol solution available as 1:200
Terbutaline	Selective β_2 agent	2.5 mg qid to 5.0 mg qid	Oral	Muscular tremor, occasional cardiac stimulation	Muscular tremor generally avoidable by gradual increase in dose. Solution for aerosol administration not currently available in United States
		0.25 mg subcutaneously q 4-6 h	Parenteral	Muscular tremor, occasional cardiac stimulation	
Isoetharine	Selective β_2 agent	1-2 puffs q 4 h 0.25 to 0.5 ml in 4 cc saline q 4 h	Aerosol Mistometer aerosol for IPPB	Occasional cardiac stimulation, nausea	
Albuterol	Selective β_2 agent	2 puffs q 6 h (180 μg q 6 h)	Mistometer	Occasional cardiac stimulation, tremor nausea	

Use of intermittent positive-pressure breathing devices (IPPB) to clear airways of secretions or to administer bronchodilator medications have no essential role in the routine management of the bronchitic. Administration of aerosolized medications can be achieved quite satisfactorily with less expensive hand-held nebulizers and patients should be properly educated in their use. Similarly, prophylactic vaccinations against influenza every year and pneumonia (by pneumococcal vaccine) every 3 years are extremely useful.

PULMONARY EMPHYSEMA

Etiology and Pathogenesis

Emphysema is predominantly a disease of men. Cigarette smoke, by mechanisms that are unclear, has been linked to the production of human emphysema by strong circumstantial and epidemiologic data. In response to bacterial respiratory infection and tobacco smoke, the alveolar macrophages and leukocytes release elastase that induces damage to the connective tissues of the lung, particularly in the absence of α_1-antitrypsin. While lung injury is predictable in the absence or a deficiency of the latter, occurrence of emphysema in the presence of normal levels indicates that other as yet unknown mechanisms are operative.

Pathology

In pathologic terms, emphysema represents a permanent, abnormal increase in size of the acinus distal to the terminal bronchiole with destruction of alveolar septa. There are four main pathologic types:

1. Centrilobular (centriacinar): this is defined as emphysematous changes occurring in the respiratory bronchioles. It is particularly associated with chronic bronchitis, tends to be localized, and more severe in the apices.
2. Panlobular (panacinar): in contrast to centrilobular, the involvement is more distal, tends to be localized, more pronounced in the bases, and there is associated bronchiolar destruction. It also produces obliteration of the capillary bed of the alveolus.
3. Irregular (paracicatricial): this type demonstrates irregular involvement of the air spaces and is seen in association with previous scarring. It is essentially a pathologic diagnosis and seldom leads to symptoms.
4. Paraseptal (distal acinar): commonly associated with bullous disease, the involvement is in the periphery of the air space, usually present in subpleural locations, and may lead to bullous disease and spontaneous pneumothorax.

Emphysema, as seen in clinical practice is usually a mixture of centrilobular and panacinar types. The panacinar type alone is seen generally in obliterative bronchiolitis, and α_1-antitrypsin deficiency.

The mechanism of airway obstruction in emphysema deserves mention. Airway obstruction in chronic bronchitis results primarily from changes in airway structure whereas in emphysema, airway obstruction is the secondary effect of involvement of the parenchyma surrounding the airway. Loss of elastic recoil and the compressibility of large airways all predispose to expiratory obstruction and diminished expiratory air flow in emphysema.

Clinical Features

Men are more commonly afflicted by this disease. The onset of symptoms is generally in the fifth decade of life. Dyspnea is the main feature of the disease, although cough and sputum production may be associated due to the accompanying chronic bronchitis. Physical examination in advanced emphysema usually discloses an asthenic individual using accessory muscles during inspiration. Pursing of the lips is often seen during exhalation, which is often a self-discovered technique that prevents premature collapse of the airway. The chest is barrel-shaped and usually shows hyperresonance to percussion, often with obliteration of the cardiac and hepatic dullnesses. Breath sounds appear markedly diminished and exhalation is prolonged, often with a wheeze, particularly in a forced expiration after maximal inspiration. There is muffling of the precordial heart sounds. However, in most cases heart sounds are well heard in the epigastric area.

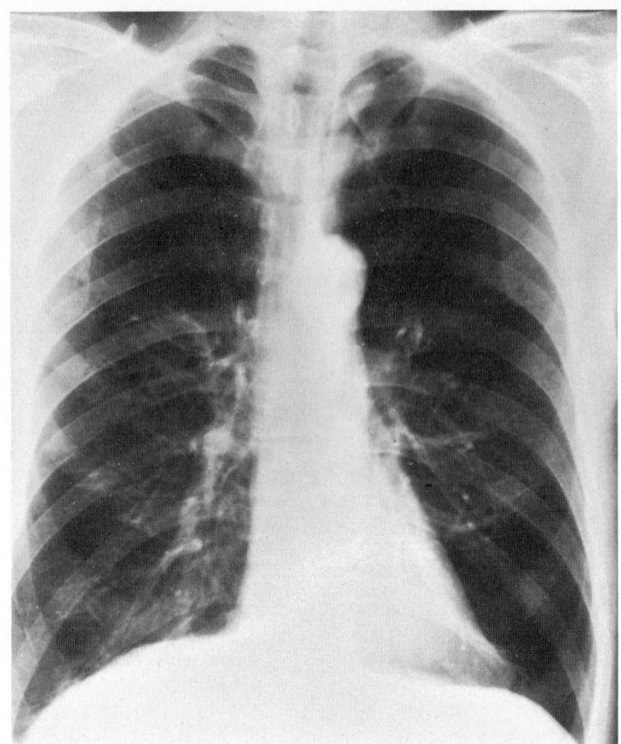

Figure 9. Pulmonary emphysema: hyperinflated lungs, flattened diaphragms.

Laboratory Findings

Roentgenograms of the chest are a good adjunct to the clinical evaluation of emphysema. However, it must be emphasized that in early disease, they may be entirely normal and hence are not recommended for screening for emphysema. Posteroanterior and lateral inspiration views are sufficient. Illustrative roentgenograms are represented in Figures 9 and 10. The most accepted criteria for radiographic diagnosis of emphysema are: overinflation of the lungs manifested by low, flat diaphragms and a large retrosternal air space greater than 3.0 cm, an increase in the anteroposterior diameter of the chest and often kyphosis, and a vertical, narrow heart secondary to elongation of the cardiomediastinal shadow. The pulmonary vasculature in many cases tends to be attenuated towards the periphery of the lungs with prominence of the central pulmonary arteries, which produces a pruned tree appearance; however, this finding is not constant.

Pulmonary function abnormalities are those of expiratory airway obstruction. $FEV_{1.0}$, $FEV_{1.0}/FVC$ ratio and $FEF_{25\text{-}75}$ are decreased. Due to expiratory airway obstruction, progressive air trapping and hyperinflation develop, which are manifested by elevations in residual volume (RV), functional residual capacity (FRC), total lung capacity (TLC), and the ratio of RV to TLC. Diffusing capacity to carbon monoxide (DL_{CO}) is reduced and reflects the loss of vasculature that invariably accompanies acinar destruction. Arterial gas tensions are relatively well-preserved, since destruction of the vasculature parallels that of acini. Other tests such as compliance or measurement of airway resistance are not needed routinely.

Course and Prognosis

Most patients show decline in their respiratory function with time. In general, the average yearly loss in $FEV_{1.0}$ may be between 50 and 100 cc, but it is hard to predict this in a given patient. Marked limitation in activity occurs when the $FEV_{1.0}$ is about 1.0 L. With values of one-half this amount, dyspnea may even limit conversation. Median survival may be as long as 10 years with an $FEV_{1.0}$ over 1.2 L; 5 years with $FEV_{1.0}$ around 1.0 L and around 2 years with an $FEV_{1.0}$ less than 700 cc. Hypercapnia, resting tachycardia, and the presence of cor pulmonale also indicate a poor prognosis.

Treatment

The treatment of pulmonary emphysema can be considered along the same lines as that of chronic bronchitis. Since many of the patients have associated chronic bronchitis, bronchodilator therapy for relief of any reversible bronchospasm will be indicated. Prevention and treatment of bacterial pulmonary infections are important. Presence of severe hypoxemia (Pa_{O_2} of 50 mm Hg or less) either at rest or during exercise would

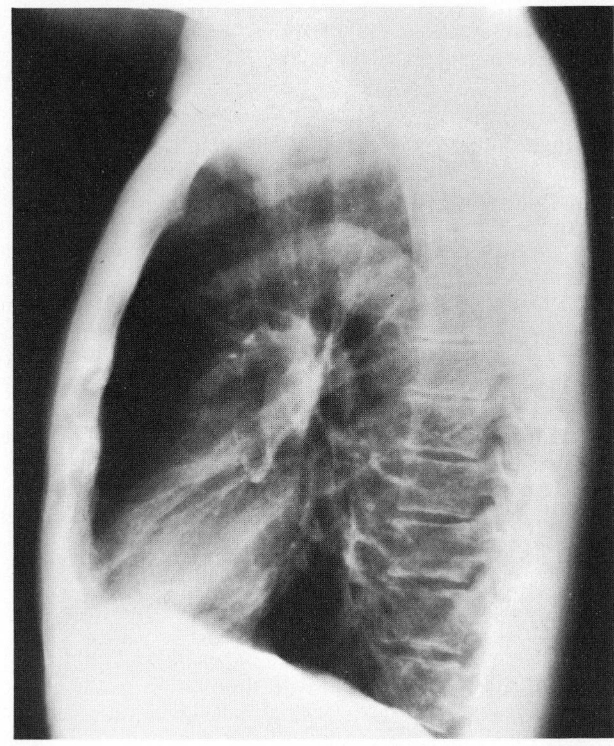

Figure 10. Pulmonary emphysema: attenuated vasculature and increased retrosternal airspace.

dictate a need for appropriate oxygen therapy. A comprehensive process involving bronchodilator therapy, exercise reconditioning, and oxygen therapy as well as psychosocial rehabilitation will be beneficial when it is tailored to the needs of the individual patient. In general, such rehabilitative programs do not lead to improvement in pulmonary function or increased longevity but they improve the quality of life and reduce the frequency of hospitalization.

Alpha$_1$-Antitrypsin Deficiency (AATD)

Emphysema due to this etiology has certain characteristics that help distinguish it from the more usual variety that is not associated with AATD. The majority of patients have symptomatic emphysema before the age of 50. Women are affected as well as men, and a family history of emphysema is often present. The duration of smoking is shorter, usually less than 20 pack years. Emphysema involves predominantly the lower zones, with early loss of basal perfusion and reversal of apex-to-base perfusion characteristics. Serum α_1-globulin levels are reduced or absent. Definitive diagnosis depends on quantitative determination of serum α_1-antitrypsin levels (AAT). Levels of AAT may be elevated transiently during respiratory infections, estrogen therapy, and pregnancy, factors to be reckoned with in evaluating results of AAT determination.

AAT is a protease inhibitor that protects the lungs from leukocyte proteases. Several subgroups of the protease inhibitor (Pi) system of the body are known, and, hence, several phenotypes are present. The normal phenotype is PiM, and the deficient phenotype PiZ. AATD is a genetic autosomal, codominantly inherited disease. In homozygotes (PiZZ), the serum ATT levels are 10-20% of normal; and in heterozygotes (PiMZ, PiSZ, etc.), 50-60%. The relationship between heterozygotes and pulmonary emphysema is controversial, even though faster rates of decline in lung function have been noted in heterozygote smokers.

Apart from the management of pulmonary emphysema, no other specific treatment is available. Cessation of smoking, avoidance of exposure to environmental irritants, and genetic counseling are the most important factors in management.

Bullous Emphysema

Bullous emphysema is defined as a subpleural emphysematous space of 1 cm or larger. It may occur with or without concomitant obstructive airway disease. These lesions may rupture, leading to pneumothorax, or may become infected. Hemorrhage may occur into the bullous lesions. Enlargement of these air spaces may occur with time. Specific surgical management will be indicated under the following circumstances:

1. Large bullous lesions, no more than one or two
2. Progressive enlargement of these bullous lesions, with compromise in function of the rest of the lung and serious limitation of activity in spite of full medical treatment of the associated airway obstruction
3. Occasional case of recurrent pneumothorax in the presence of paraseptal emphysema

No definite criteria or opinion regarding timing of surgical intervention can be made. Specific consideration should be given to the history, review of previous roentgenograms, and pulmonary function studies if these are available, and follow-up for a period of time for a better assessment. Size of the bullous lesions and the state of the remainder of the lungs should be the guiding factors. In general, the more severe and generalized the emphysema, the less is the likelihood of benefit from surgery. The tests that may be of value in assessing the response are the diffusion capacity, static recoil pressure of the lungs at 100% vital capacity, and compliance measurements as well as tests of V/Q mismatching. Resection of bullous lesions should be minimal if any; only plication and oversewing are needed.

CYSTIC FIBROSIS

Cystic fibrosis is a genetic disorder characterized by chronic bronchopulmonary suppuration, exocrine pancreatic insufficiency, and elevated levels of sodium and chloride in the sweat. It is probably transmitted as an autosomal recessive type; however, its exact biochemical defect is unknown. The life expectancy of the disease is longer so that internists are likely to see more patients with this disease.

Pathology and Pathogenesis

Elevated sodium and chloride levels in the sweat and saliva presumably result from defective sodium reabsorption in the gland ducts. Mucous secretions from the exocrine glands have abnormal viscoelastic properties, with potential for inspissation and ductal obstruction. Obstruction in the bronchioles leads to chronic infection. Bronchial obstruction may be aggravated by defects in mucociliary transport. Defects in alveolar macrophage function may explain the propensity for repeated pseudomonas infections. Pancreatic fibrosis is common. Focal biliary cirrhosis, seen in one-fourth of the cases at autopsy, generally does not lead to hypersplenism or portal hypertension.

Clinical Features

The age of presentation is variable, with about two-thirds of patients 10 years old or less, one-fourth of these being infants. Intestinal obstruction secondary to meconium ileus develops among some of these infants (about 10%). Pancreatic insufficiency usually becomes apparent by 2 years of age, characterized by bulky, greasy, foul-smelling stools as well as failure to thrive. In the remainder of the patients, cough, sputum production, repeated respiratory infections, and asthmatic symptoms develop. Digital clubbing is frequent. Blood-streaked sputum and frank hemoptysis become frequent with increasing severity of bronchiectasis. Recurrent pneumothoraces and/or repeated respiratory infections with mucoid *Pseudomonas aeruginosa* or *Staphylococcus aureus* are clues to underlying cystic fibrosis. More than 98% of men with this disease are sterile. Cor pulmonale eventually develops and cardiac or respiratory failure is the usual cause of death.

Laboratory Studies

The diagnostic feature is a sweat chloride level greater than 60 mEq/L in infants and greater than 80 mEq/L in adults after pilocarpine iontophoresis. Abnormal values may also be obtained in hereditary nephrogenic diabetes insipidus, glucose-6-phosphate dehydrogenase deficiency, and untreated adrenal insufficiency. Since laboratory errors are frequent, a laboratory with adequate experience should be chosen and elevated values should also be rechecked. Pulmonary function testing shows airway obstruction in the vast majority of patients. If pancreatic involvement is suspected, pancreatic function tests may be performed. Serum pancreatic isoamylase levels may be low or absent altogether. Secretin-pancreozymin stimulation tests are useful. Aspermia is usual. Microbiologic studies of sputum are necessary. Chest roentgenograms show peribronchial thickening, cystic and bullous lesions, and branching linear densities indicative of fluid-filled bronchi. Unresolved pneumonitis, atelectasis, and apical lesions mimicking tuberculosis are frequent.

Prognosis

About 50% of patients without meconium ileus can be expected to reach 19 years of age. The survival has been related to the abnormalities in the chest roentgenograms, partly by observation and partly by life-table analysis: the worse the roentgenogram, the poorer the survival.

Treatment

Psychologic support is extremely important. Specific respiratory treatment involves segmental postural drainage with chest clapping performed about four times per day, as well as mist therapy to humidify the inhaled air. Intermittent aerosol therapy with *N*-acetylcysteine (Mucomyst) to loosen secretions and 0.125% phenylephrine to reduce mucosal edema are useful. Bronchodilators are indicated when airway obstruction is demonstrated by pulmonary function testing. Antibiotics must be given for respiratory infections in full therapeutic doses for 3-4 weeks. Such therapy, along with adequate respiratory therapy, may help eradicate staphylococcal infection, but pseudomonas is generally refractory. Prophylactic antibiotics are not recommended. Pregnancy carries a 15% mortality, and contraception with barrier methods is preferred since oral contraceptives may worsen airway obstruction and produce cervicitis.

BRONCHIECTASIS

Bronchiectasis is defined as localized or generalized permanent abnormal dilatation of bronchi with destruction of the elastic and muscular layers of the bronchial wall. Three varieties have been described: saccular, tubular, and fusiform. The most notable observation about bronchiectasis is its declining incidence in the postantibiotic era.

Pathology and Pathogenesis

Purulent secretions are usually seen in the abnormal bronchial lumen. Dilated bronchial mucous glands, squamous metaplasia of the bronchial epithelium with ulcerations and fibrosis, and destruction of the elastic and muscular layers of the bronchus are the chief pathologic findings. Extensive bronchial-pulmonary artery anastomoses may be present in the involved areas.

Bronchiectasis may be acquired or congenital. Adenoviral respiratory infection, allergic bronchopulmonary aspergillosis, cystic fibrosis, and chronic bronchitis account for most acquired cases. Measles, whooping cough, primary or secondary staphylococcal or *Klebsiella* infections are infrequent causes. Scarring and fibrosis due to pulmonary tuberculosis cause fewer cases of bronchiectasis. Developmental abnormalities such as bronchogenic cysts, immunodeficiency states, and the recently described immotile-cilia syndrome (ICS) are congenital causes of bronchiectasis. Dysfunction of the ciliary microtubules in ICS not only leads to impaired mucociliary clearance in the airways, but also to immotile spermatozoa. Affected men are infertile. The syndrome of situs inversus, sinusitis, and bronchiectasis (Kartagener's triad) is a subgroup of ICS. Electron microscopy of nasal mucosal smear or of spermatozoa can be of help in diagnosis.

Clinical Features

Chief symptoms of bronchiectasis are cough with production

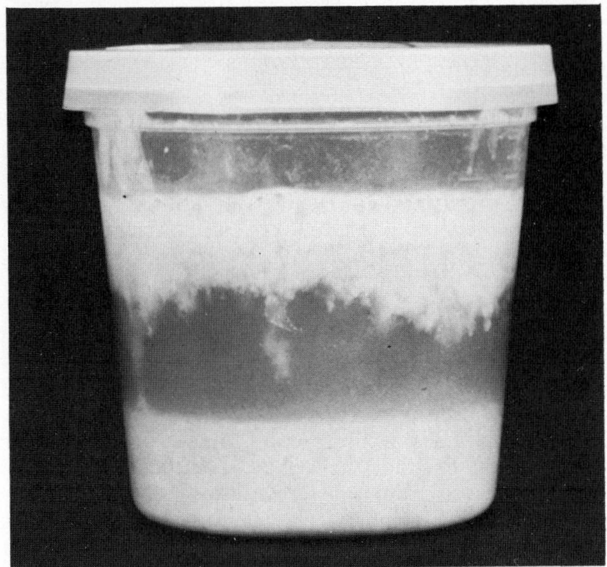

Figure 11. Sputum from a patient with bronchiectasis showing characteristic three layers.

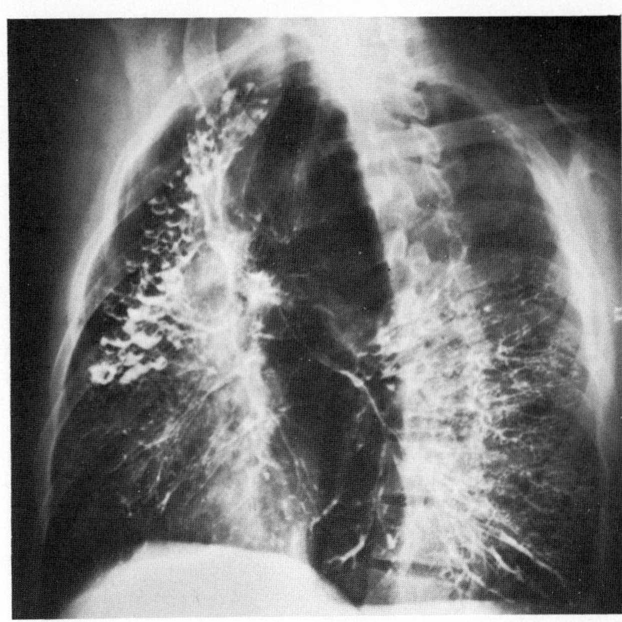

Figure 12. Bronchogram showing cystic bronchiectasis.

of large quantities of mucopurulent or purulent sputum, often from the first decade of life, generally traceable to a bad bout of respiratory infection. In severe cases, the expectorated sputum may settle into three layers: a top mucoid, middle salivary, and bottom layer of purulent debris (Fig. 11). Hemoptysis from rupture of the bronchial-pulmonary anastomoses is common. Recurrent pneumonias involving localized areas often occur. Physical examination may disclose finger clubbing, wheezing, and coarse, bubbling rales in many cases. Lung abscess and empyema may complicate the picture, although amyloidosis and brain abscess are unusual.

Diagnosis

Clinical history and physical examination often provide strong presumptive evidence for bronchiectasis. Chest roentgenograms may be normal; more typically increased bronchial markings, tram-line shadows, and cystic areas are seen. Other findings include air-fluid levels in cavities and branching shadows representing fluid-filled bronchi. Serum immunoglobulin levels may be low when immunodeficiencies are the underlying etiology. Positive diagnosis depends on demonstration of abnormally dilated bronchi by bronchography. A representative bronchogram is shown in Figure 12. Indications for bronchography are recurrent hemoptysis and consideration of surgery. Pneumonia within the preceding 6-8 weeks, evidence of active respiratory infection, and consideration of only medical management are contraindications to bronchography.

Pulmonary function varies with the severity of disease, ranging from normal to obstructive and/or restrictive patterns. Arterial hypoxemia is common and is the result of ventilation-perfusion mismatch.

Treatment

Dependent postural drainage with chest clapping should be performed daily, about 3-4 times if possible, preceding meals. Positioning during postural drainage should be appropriate for the segment(s) to be drained.

Evidence of respiratory infection is the indication for antibiotics. In the presence of purulent sputum, the pathogenic organisms are generally pneumococci or *H. influenzae*; even though cultures may not yield these, empiric therapy with ampicillin or tetracycline is indicated. Prompt therapy and good bronchial hygiene together prevent further bronchial damage. Smoking is strictly forbidden. Exposure to irritating fumes and agents should be avoided as far as possible. Influenza vaccine should be given yearly, and pneumonia vaccination every 3 years.

Severe, localized, disabling disease or severe recurrent hemoptysis are the usual indications for surgery. The role for resectional surgery has dwindled in recent years, mainly because medical management is effective and the disease process is generalized in most cases.

BRONCHIAL OBSTRUCTION, ATELECTASIS, AND UPPER AIRWAY OBSTRUCTION

Bronchial Obstruction

Obstruction of a bronchus, apart from obstructive airway disease, may be the result of three broad classes of pathologic processes: lesions in the lumen such as a mucous plug or inhaled foreign body; lesions in the bronchial wall, such as neoplasms (benign and malignant); and compression or involvement of a bronchus from without, as happens with hilar or mediastinal lymph node enlargement, mediastinal tumors, and aortic aneurysms. Bronchial obstruction is always a result of another pathologic process and the symptoms and signs are due to the primary disease and the mechanical as well as physiologic effects of obstruction.

The most common cause of bronchial obstruction is neoplasm, and this subject will be considered separately. Obstruction may lead to distal atelectasis, bronchiectasis, and with distal infection, to pneumonia and/or lung abscess. Obstruction of a large bronchus may lead to dyspnea, cough, and wheezing. Physical signs include mediastinal shift if there is significant atelectasis, and localized wheezing. Poor or delayed resolution of pneumonia or development of a lung abscess in the absence of predisposing factors should make bronchial obstruction suspect. Apart from volume loss, localized hyperinflation from air trapping is another manifestation of obstruction and is demonstrable by inspiration-expiration films. Tomographic studies may be of value, but diagnosis is confirmed by bronchoscopy. Treatment should be directed toward the etiology.

Atelectasis

Absorption of air in the lobe or segment distal to an endobronchial obstruction leads to atelectasis, a process known as absorption atelectasis; compression of lung tissue from a pneumothorax or large pleural effusion is known as compression atelectasis. Absorption atelectasis is essentially a reflection of bronchial obstruction and should be managed appropriately.

Middle-lobe syndrome represents a special type of atelectasis. An initial episode of mucosal edema or extrinsic compression of the middle-lobe bronchus, not necessarily with complete occlusion of the lumen, can lead to middle-lobe atelectasis. The reason for this is the paucity of collateral ventilation in the right middle lobe as well as the development of full-fledged fissures that tend to isolate the lobe and prevent collateral aeration. In the past, the majority of cases were due to tuberculosis; but now, most cases are secondary to neoplastic enlargement of the lymph nodes surrounding the middle-lobe bronchus. Tuberculosis, however, still accounts for about 4-10% of cases.

Upper Airway Obstruction

Obstruction of the large airways such as the larynx and trachea up to the point of bifurcation will be considered in this section.

Obstruction of the Larynx

Characteristically, obstruction of the larynx occurs due to an inhaled foreign body, mostly food. Laryngeal obstruction may also occur in angioneurotic edema, croup, and following extubation of an indwelling endotracheal tube. Laryngospasm is seen occasionally during anesthetization of the larynx during fiberoptic bronchoscopy. Bilateral vocal cord paralysis and laryngeal tumors may also produce obstruction. Stridor is the key feature of laryngeal obstruction.

In acute laryngeal obstruction due to hereditary angioedema, parenteral administration of epinephrine is the treatment of choice. The victim with impaction of a foreign body in the larynx is unable to cough, speak, or breathe. Blows to the posterior chest wall along the upper thoracic spine followed, if necessary, by Heimlich's maneuver (sudden, firm pressure with the fist in the area between xiphoid and umbilicus) may help dislodge the obstruction. Digital extraction of the foreign body may be attempted as well. Emergency tracheostomy will be lifesaving if other measures fail.

Tracheal Obstruction

Primary tracheal tumors are uncommon. Involvement of the trachea may occur secondarily from local extension of esophageal or bronchogenic carcinoma. Impaction of food in the esophagus may compress the posterior tracheal wall and result in sudden upper airway obstruction, as seen in the cafe coronary. Tracheal obstruction on a more chronic basis may be seen in tracheal stricture following endotracheal intubation.

A characteristic feature of tracheal obstruction is wheezing when the obstruction is within the thorax; stridor accompanies it when the obstruction is above this level. In more chronic cases, diagnosis can be established by tomography and flow-volume loop analysis. Maximal flow at 50% vital capacity ($\dot{V}_{max\ 50}$) is compared during both phases of respiration. (Normally, the expiratory:inspiratory ratio is 0.9 for $\dot{V}_{max 50}$.) This ratio increases in variable extrathoracic obstruction (i.e., inspiratory $\dot{V}_{max 50}$ is reduced). In variable intrathoracic obstruction there is significant reduction in expiratory $\dot{V}_{max 50}$, the ratio is reduced, and a plateau is seen in the expiratory phase. When the obstruction is fixed, flows in both phases are reduced, whether the obstruction is intrathoracic or extrathoracic. Representative flow-volume loops in various types of airway obstruction are shown in Fig. 13.

Management of tracheal obstruction depends upon the acuteness of onset. Emergency intubation, rigid bronchoscopy, and tracheostomy are options; these should ideally be performed at the surgical suite. More chronic cases can be evaluated with ease and be appropriately managed. In suspected upper airway obstruction, fiberoptic bronchoscopy is contraindicated.

DISORDERS OF LUNG CIRCULATION

PULMONARY EDEMA

Pulmonary edema is defined as a pathologic state in which the extravascular water content in the lung is increased. Normally there is a small, constant leak of fluid from the microvasculature of the lung into the lung interstitium, and this fluid is skimmed off by the lymphatics of the lung. Pulmonary edema represents a dynamic extension of this process, wherein excessive filtration or excessive permeability of the microvasculature leads to a fluid load that is above and beyond the clearance capacity of the lymphatic vessels.

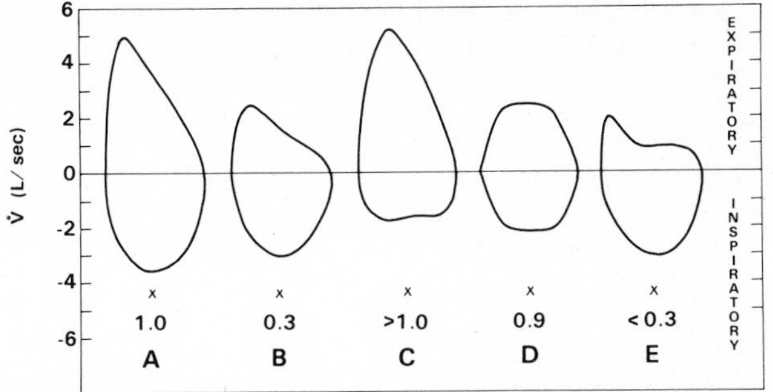

Figure 13. Flow volume loops in various types of airway obstruction: V - flow rate. Figures below each tracing represent ratios of expiratory flow to inspiratory flow at midvital capacity point (x). A = normal; B = airway obstruction in asthma or COPD; C = variable extrathoracic obstruction; D = fixed intrathoracic obstruction; E = varaible intrathoracic obstruction (note the plateau in the expiratory phase).

The dynamics of this fluid filtration are governed by Starling's equation. Four major forces (also called Starling's forces) govern the transvascular fluid flow: a pair of hydrostatic forces (microvascular and perimicrovascular) and a pair of osmotic forces (microvascular and perimicrovascular). The components of each pair operate in opposite directions, and the hydrostatic and osmotic forces within the same compartment are also oriented in opposite directions. The fluid flux thus produced is also dependent on the filtration coefficient of the capillary endothelium. The normal orientation of Starling's forces is in such a way that there is a net efflux of fluid from the capillary lumen into the pericapillary interstitial space, estimated to be about 10-20 cc per hour in humans, which is then cleared by the lymphatics.

The pulmonary capillary endothelium is restrictive in its permeability for various molecules depending on their molecular weights. Its conductivity for fluid itself is low. The permeability of the alveolar epithelium is perhaps even more limited, mainly because of its intricate structure with tight intercellular junctions.

From this physiologic background, it becomes apparent that pulmonary edema may result from excessive fluid filtration (from increased hydrostatic pressure) or from increased permeability of the capillary endothelium. Among the former category are cardiogenic pulmonary edema, (due to arteriosclerotic heart disease, mitral stenosis, left ventricular failure, and fluid overload), high-altitude pulmonary edema, and reexpansion pulmonary edema. In the latter category are adult respiratory distress syndrome, drug-induced pulmonary edema, and neurogenic pulmonary edema. Cardiogenic pulmonary edema is discussed elsewhere and the present review will cover other forms of pulmonary edema.

High-Altitude Pulmonary Edema

Epidemiologic data disclose two classes of people who develop high-altitude pulmonary edema (HAPE): sea-level residents who visit a high altitude area and undertake heavy exertion, such as skiing or military exercises, and high altitude residents who reascend to the high altitude area after a sojourn to sea level, which is generally 10 days or longer. The exact incidence is unknown. Young children are more vulnerable than adults and recurrences are not uncommon especially among those under 21 years. The higher and the faster the ascent, the more probable and more severe the episode of HAPE.

The pathogenesis of HAPE is speculative. Disturbances in pulmonary blood flow secondary to widespread, patchy, hypoxemic vasoconstriction in some areas with overperfusion of others, has been proposed as one mechanism. Another mechanism involves transarterial leakage of plasma and blood. Autopsy studies in persons who have died of HAPE have demonstrated dilatation of the right ventricle, lung lymphatics and larger arteries along with congestion, perivascular hemorrhages, alveolar edema, and thromboses in small- and medium-sized muscular pulmonary arteries. These latter changes are noteworthy for their irregular distribution.

Clinical features of high-altitude pulmonary edema include cough, shortness of breath, and fatigue developing generally within 1-2 days after arrival at high altitude, usually following exertion. These symptoms generally progress once they appear, leading to hospitalization. Other features of high altitude illness such as headache, confusion, and somnolence may be associated. Cyanosis may be evident and auscultation of the lungs may reveal diffuse rales. Purulent sputum or other features of respiratory infection are absent. Chest radiographs show patchy infiltrates that may be unilateral or bilateral with large central pulmonary arteries and normal cardiac size. Perihilar infiltrates may also be seen. Response to bed rest and oxygen is excellent. If symptoms persist after this line of management, transfer to sea level should be strongly considered. It has been suggested that acetazolamide in doses of 500 mg twice daily for 3 days before and 2 days after ascent may prevent HAPE.

Reexpansion Pulmonary Edema

When a chronically collapsed lung (by a pneumothorax or pleural effusion) is rapidly reexpanded, pulmonary edema may develop in that lung. Proposed causes include loss of surfactant due to chronic atelectasis, damage to capillaries of the collapsed lung with alteration in their permeability characteristics, and creation of a significantly negative interstitial hydrostatic pressure from the rapid evacuation of pleural space. The pulmonary edema is usually transient and supportive care is all that is needed.

Adult Respiratory Distress Syndrome (ARDS)

ARDS represents a constellation of clinical, radiographic, physiologic, and pathologic changes that follow diffuse pulmonary injury from a variety of causes, generally sepsis, surgical procedures, trauma, and major medical illnesses. The diffuse pulmonary injury is produced by several mechanism(s) and the common feature is the enhanced capillary permeability. Physiologic disturbances include widening of the alveolar-arterial oxygen gradient, decreased lung compliance, and progressive, refractory hypoxemia. Untreated, the condition is fatal. Further information on ARDS may be found in the section on respiratory failure.

Drug-Induced Pulmonary Edema

The best known among the drugs that may cause pulmonary edema are the opiates. Opiate pulmonary edema classically results from heroin use but may happen after use of codeine or methadone as well. Presence of pulmonary edema with miotic pupils should arouse suspicion of this entity, especially in persons with a background of drug abuse. Presence of milk in the oral cavity and ice around the testicles may be other findings, both being measures adopted by the victim's cohorts to resuscitate the patient from the comatose state. Diagnosis of pulmonary edema is confirmed by chest radiographs. Opiate-induced pulmonary edema is believed to be due to enhanced capillary permeability secondary to hypoxia, to contaminant products in the administered heroin, or to opiate-induced histamine release. Endotracheal intubation may be needed to manage respiratory failure and pulmonary edema. Naloxone intravenously in doses of 0.4 mg every 3-5 minutes is the specific antidote for opiate intoxication. Drug screens of urine and blood are useful since multiple drug poisonings are quite common. Physicians should also be aware of the other less well-known drugs and chemicals that may cause pulmonary edema that are listed in Tables 10 and 11.

Neurogenic Pulmonary Edema

The cause of neurogenic pulmonary edema is believed to be sequestration of blood in the pulmonary circulation secondary to peripheral vasoconstriction following massive sympathetic discharge. Changes in left ventricular performance and active pulmonary venous constriction along with sudden increase in pulmonary blood volume result in pulmonary capillary damage and enhanced permeability. Treatment of the systemic hypertension that often accompanies this syndrome and respiratory support are necessary.

Table 10. Drugs and Chemicals Producing Pulmonary Edema

Narcotics
Heroin
Methadone
Codeine
Analgesics
Propoxyphene
Salicylates
Phenylbutazone
Sedatives-hypnotics
Ethchlorvynol
Barbiturates
Meprobamate
Antineoplastic agents
Nitrogen mustard
Methotrexate
Busulfan
Miscellaneous agents
Nitrofurantoin
Hydrochlorothiazide
Propranolol
Fluorescein
Radiographic contrast media
Herbicides, insecticides, and poisons
Paraquat
Organophosphorus compounds
Cyanide
Blood, blood products, volume expanders
Blood transfusions
Cryoprecipitate
Plasma
Dextran-40
Replacement of blood loss with crystalloid infusions
Industrial Agents, toxic gases, etc. summarized in Table 11

PULMONARY THROMBOEMBOLISM

It has been estimated that pulmonary embolism is the cause of death in the U.S. in over 67,000 instances per year and that clinically serious cases may exceed 630,000 per year. More than 90% of all pulmonary emboli occur in the hospitalized population.

Ninety percent of all pulmonary emboli are secondary to deep venous thrombi in the lower extremities, which originate in the deep veins of the leg and propagate into the popliteal or femoral veins. Superficial venous thrombosis is an uncommon source of pulmonary emboli. Other sources for emboli are the prostatic veins, pelvic veins, and mural thrombi in the right atrium and right ventricle that form in the presence of long-standing heart failure, often accompanied by atrial fibrillation. The most important factors that predispose to deep-vein thrombosis in the lower extremities are: postoperative states (most frequent after hip surgery and prostatectomy, and frequent after thoracic and/or abdominal surgery), trauma (pelvis, spine, or legs, all requiring casts or immobilization), and prolonged bed rest (stroke, respiratory failure, myocardial infarction, quadriplegia, and/or paraplegia). More than one-fourth to one-third of all myocardial infarctions are complicated by development of leg thrombi during the course of hospitalization. Conditions such as obesity, peripheal vascular disease, and malignancies are general predisposing factors. Evidence regarding the role of oral contraceptives is conflicting.

Consequences of Pulmonary Embolism

Obstruction of a pulmonary artery by an embolus may lead to the syndrome of pulmonary embolism or to pulmonary infarction. The sequelae of pulmonary embolism are quite variable and depend upon several factors such as the site, extent, and hemodynamic impact of the embolic obstruction, as well as the presence of prior lung disease and its severity. Obstruction

Table 11. Industrial Agents and Toxic Gases that Produce Pulmonary Edema

Agent	*Circumstances of Exposure*
Oxides of nitrogen	Silage Explosive use in coal mining Oxyacetylene flames in closed areas Chemists Rocket propellant
Phosgene	Herbicide manufacture Gassing (World War I) Chemical industry uses phosgene in chlorination
Ammonia	Refrigeration industry Oil refineries Explosive industry
Ozone	Welding in poorly ventilated areas Smog
Borons	High energy rocket fuel
Methyliodide	Fumigant Fire extinguisher
Chlorine	Alkali manufacture Bleaches Household mixing of cleansing agents Mercury and mercury chloride manufacture
Hydrogen sulfide	Coal mines Gas works Tanneries Fishmeal industry
Sulfurdioxide	Oil refining Paper industry Refrigeration industry
Carbon monoxide	Smoke inhalation Automobile exhaust
Mercury vapor	Confined tanks where mercury vapor exposure occurs
PTFE	Fluon or teflon
Cadmium oxide	Alloy making

of the main pulmonary artery, generally at its bifurcation, may lead to sudden death with or without preceding shock. Acute cor pulmonale, hypotension, and frank right ventricular failure follow when the extent of occlusion exceeds 50% of the cross-sectional area of the pulmonary vasculature.

The physiologic disturbances that follow pulmonary embolism are ventilation of nonperfused alveoli, leading to increase in wasted ventilation (increased physiologic dead space). Increased total ventilation is an attempt to overcome this disturbance and is manifested as tachypnea; airway constriction in the embolized area, to minimize dead-space ventilation; increase in pulmonary vascular resistance and pulmonary hypertension, which are the result of mechanical vascular obstruction, release of pharmacologically active materials from the clot and perhaps reflex mechanisms; and, decreased surfactant synthesis in the embolized area, predisposing to the development of atelectasis and fluid exudation into the alveoli.

Pulmonary infarction, defined as necrosis of lung tissue, is an uncommon consequence of pulmonary embolism (5-10% of cases) and is always the result of occlusion of the peripheral branches of the pulmonary artery. Since total cessation of blood supply is a prerequisite for necrosis, it presupposes disease in the bronchial arteries. Congestive atelectasis, an entity more common than pulmonary infarction mimics the latter clinically and radiographically but differs from it in that necrosis does not take place and that resolution is quick and complete.

Clinical Features

The most common symptom of pulmonary embolism is dyspnea, which may be present in about 80% of cases, and is characteristically sudden in onset although its severity and duration may be variable. Cough and apprehension may be seen in about two-thirds of the cases. Symptoms are variable, and syncope and chest pain are infrequent. Substernal chest pain indistinguishable from myocardial infarction may occur and may be related to sudden pulmonic hypertension. In many cases, a predisposing factor to deep-vein thrombosis is identifiable in the history.

Physical examination usually discloses tachypnea in more than 90% of cases. Fever may be present in more than one-half and usually is low grade, rarely exceeding 104°F. Evidence of pulmonary hypertension (increased intensity of the pulmonary component of the second heart sound, right ventricular heave, right-sided third or fourth heart sound), and/or rales may be present in one-half the affected population, although the latter finding is nonspecific. Evidence of thrombophlebitis may be present in one-third of cases. With massive embolizations (more than 50% occlusion) significant elevations of right-sided pressures are the rule on cardiac catheterization.

By contrast, pulmonary infarction is accompanied by more dramatic symptoms, such as hemoptysis and pleuritic chest pain. Fever is generally present and physical examination discloses splinting of the chest wall, with findings of consolidation in some cases as well as evidence of pleural effusion, all on the affected side. Pleural friction rub is generally present, at least in the early phases.

Diagnosis

Pulmonary angiography is the gold standard for the diagnosis of pulmonary embolism. But the lack of easy availability and invasive nature of this technique necessitates correlation of the clinical data with the available laboratory studies in arriving at a diagnosis. Elevated leukocyte count is usual, but it seldom exceeds 15,000/mm^3. The classic triad of elevated bilirubin and LDH with normal SGOT occurs in a small percentage of cases. Electrocardiograms may reveal sinus tachycardia, P pulmonale, S wave in lead I, and a Q wave with T wave inversions in lead III, but the main advantage of an electrocardiogram is that it helps rule out a myocardial infarction as the cause of the patient's symptoms. Changes from the previous electrocardiogram are more important than observing abnormal findings. Arrhythmias such as atrial flutter and fibrillation, and varying degrees of A-V block that accompany pulmonary embolism may also be demonstrated.

Arterial blood gas analysis generally discloses hypoxemia and hypocapnia (hyperventilation produces low Pa_{CO_2}), findings that are not specific for pulmonary embolism. An arterial Pa_{O_2} greater than 85 mm Hg with the patient breathing room air makes pulmonary embolism less likely. In patients on mechanical ventilators, the same sequence of hypoxemia and hypocapnia is usually seen, but in those receiving mechanical ventilation and muscle relaxants (curariform agents), a paradoxical hypercapnia may be seen along with hypoxemia. The hypercapnia is secondary to increases in dead space in the face of limited minute ventilation.

Chest roentgenograms are usually normal. Elevated hemidiaphragms, localized oligemias, Westermark's sign (abrupt cutoff of a vessel), and Hampton's hump (convex, peripherally located posterior density) have all been emphasized in the radiology literature; but these cannot be depended upon for definitive diagnosis. In pulmonary infarction, the classic finding is a wedge-shaped opacity with ipsilateral pleural effusion, but an infarct may assume any shape. Effusions may be seen without apparent infiltrate and are generally unilateral.

Perfusion (Q) scanning using technitium (^{99m}Tc) macroaggregated albumin is the most frequently employed method for detecting pulmonary emboli. A perfusion lung scan is a sensitive test for pulmonary embolism and a normal six-view lung scan (negative scan) rules out clinically significant pulmonary embolism. A positive scan, that is, large, multiple perfusion defects accompanied by a normal chest roentgenogram in the absence of preexistent lung disease, is indicative of pulmonary embolism (Figs. 14 and 15). However, perfusion defects are not specific for pulmonary emboli. In obstructive airway disease, atelectasis, bullous disease, congestive heart failure, carcinoma of the lung, and respiratory failure, perfusion defects are usual. In such situations, the accuracy of the perfusion defects are usual. In such situations, the accuracy of the fusion scans may be augmented by ventilation (V) scanning. Normal ventilation in the areas of perfusion defects have a good correlation with pulmonary emboli (ventilation-perfusion mismatch) and can be considered as a positive scan. Scans that show areas of match and mismatch on V/Q study are to be considered equivocal in diagnosing or excluding pulmonary emboli.

The arteriographic findings in pulmonary embolism include intraluminal filling defects and vessel cut-offs. Other findings such as localized avascularity or sluggish blood flow are not diagnostic.

The main indications for pulmonary angiography are the presence of lung disease, heart failure, or respiratory failure where V/Q scans are unreliable in the diagnosis of pulmonary embolism; shock with massive pulmonary embolization where either embolectomy or fibrinolytic therapy is being strongly considered; where substantial risk from anticoagulation (bleeding diathesis, recent stroke) mandates a positive diagnosis; where pulmonary embolism cannot be differentiated from other conditions that cause similar picture (pneumonia versus pulmonary infarction); in recurrent pulmonary embolization prior to inferior vena cava interruption. It is strongly recommended that, if possible, a perfusion scan precede the angiogram so that the angiographer may concentrate on the areas of perfusion defects. Pulmonary angiography is a safe procedure in experienced hands. In the National Heart and Lung Institute study, the mortality from pulmonary angiography was less than 0.5% and the morbidity less than 1%.

Apart from these studies, studies that add support to the diagnosis of pulmonary embolism are tests addressed to the diagnosis of deep venous thrombosis. In the presence of deep venous thrombosis, a positive perfusion scan along with a compatible clinical picture strongly suggests pulmonary embolism, no matter how large or how small the perfusion defects are. Although venograms of the leg are the gold standard for diagnosing deep-vein thrombosis, other noninvasive tests are available. Impedance or ultrasonic plethysmography are good noninvasive techniques, but the drawbacks are that previous phlebitis makes the examination difficult and small thrombi may be missed. Uptake of isotope-labelled fibrinogen into actively forming thrombi results in a well-defined target-to-background ratio of radioactivity in areas of phlebothrombosis, and this is the principle of ^{125}I fibrinogen scanning. Disadvantages of this method are that the test takes about 24 hours, old clots are missed, and sensitivity is poor for clots in the upper thigh and pelvis because of significant background radioactivity from local vasculature.

Pleural effusions in association with pulmonary embolism may show a wide spectrum in their characteristics. This wide range probably has to do with the different pathogenetic mechanisms in producing such effusions (atelectasis, associated heart failure, etc). In pulmonary infarction, the fluid is almost always an exudate and tends to be bloody or blood stained, resolving over time. Lack of resolution or intercurrent increase in size denotes coincident complications such as infection and/or reinfarction or heart failure if other factors support that diagnosis. The extent of tests undertaken to confirm the diagnosis of pulmonary embolism is dependent upon the strength of clinical suspicion as well as the condition of the patient. In patients presenting with shock in whom pulmonary embolism is considered a possibility, pulmonary angiography should be undertaken after the first dose of anticoagulant has been administered. In those devoid of shock or hypotension, a four-view perfusion lung scan is a good screening test, along with a ventilation scan if associated heart failure or lung disease is present. If the perfusion scan is negative, it rules out clinically and/or hemodynamically significant pulmonary embolism. If the scan is positive and a compatible clinical picture is present (e.g., an episode of chest pain, diaphoresis, and dyspnea in a person who has been recently immobilized in a cast), or the scan is positive and the chest roentgenogram is normal (Figs. 14 and 15) evidence for pulmonary emboli is adequate and pulmonary angiography need not be done. Equivocal findings on lung scan in the presence of reasonable or strong suspicion of pulmonary embolism or presence of

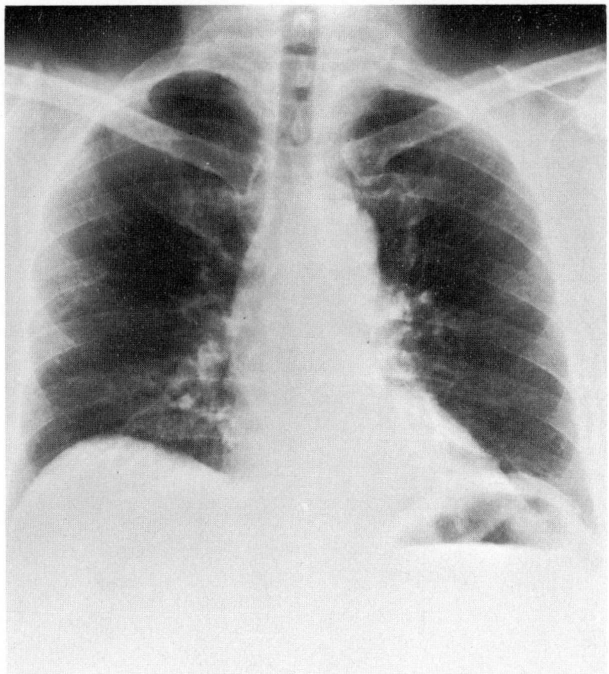

Figure 14. Pulmonary embolism; normal lung fields.

other factors that necessitate angiography indicate that pulmonary angiograms should be obtained. If the suspicion is only slight and the scan is equivocal, the patient's history and clinical features should be reassessed. The diagnostic approach is outlined in Figure 16.

Treatment

The mainstay of treatment of pulmonary embolism is heparin. In cases of massive or submassive embolization, as soon as a clinical diagnosis is made heparin is administered intravenously and then attempts are made to confirm the diagnosis under this heparin cover. The drug is preferably given by continuous infusion, and the activated partial thromboplastin time (APTT) is used as a control for the dosage. Prolongation of APTT by 2-2½ times over the baseline will be adequate and this may take anywhere between 20-30,000 units of heparin daily. Heparin may also be given in bolus doses every 4 hours; but, after such doses, the clotting factors are markedly inhibited for 2-3 hours and the risk of bleeding during this unprotected period is high. Heparin therapy is continued for about 7-10 days. After this period, change to an oral anticoagulant, such as coumarin or dicumarol, is made using prothrombin times as control. The exact duration of further treatment is subject to debate. In cases where a definite correctable precipitating factor is identifiable, the duration of therapy coincides with elimination of the precipitating factor. In other instances, the duration is a matter of clinical judgement. A 3- to 6-month period of oral anticoagulation is employed by many physicians.

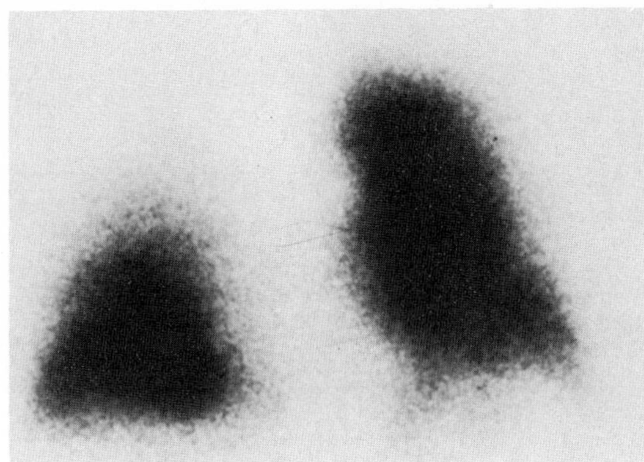

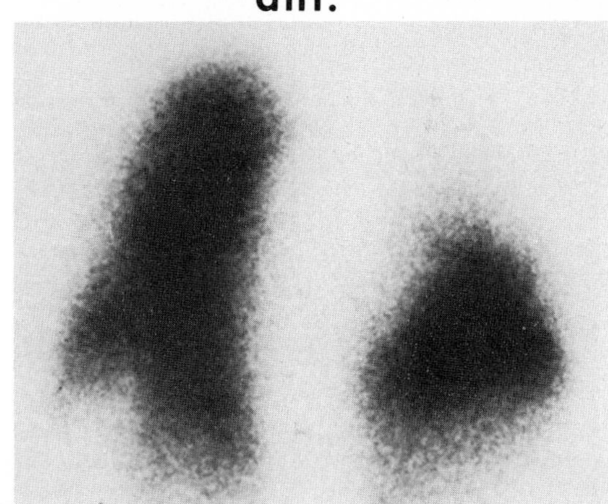

(a)

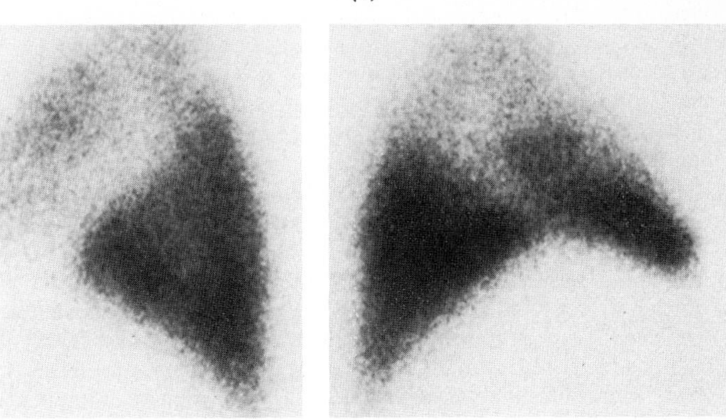

(b)

Figure 15*a* and *b*. Four-view lung scan showing perfusion defects. Angiography showed emboli.

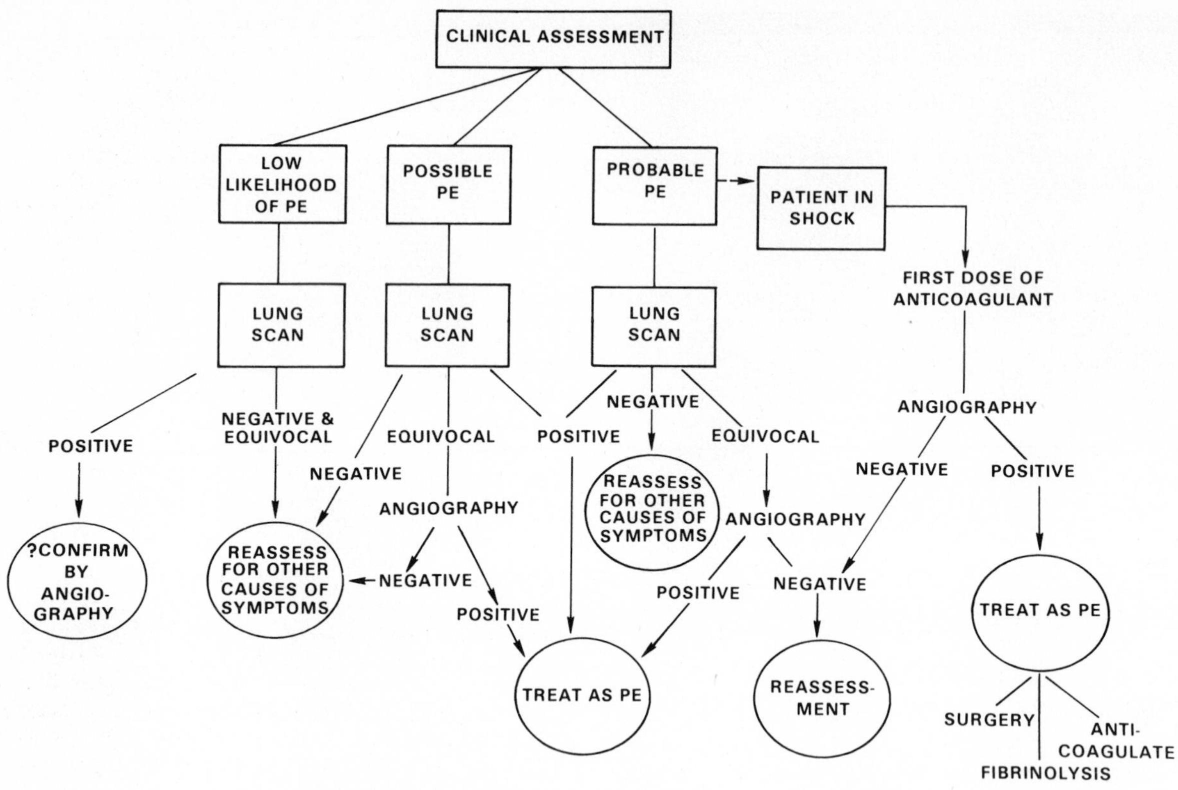

Figure 16. Suggested diagnostic approach to pulmonary embolism.

The main indications of thrombolytic agents (streptokinase and urokinase) are in patients with massive pulmonary embolism and in those with submassive embolism with hypotension and shock. Confirmation of diagnosis is necessary by angiography. The dosage for streptokinase is 250,000 IU given as a loading dose intravenously in normal saline or 5% dextrose in water over a period of 30 minutes. Maintenance therapy with 100,000 IU per hour for 24-72 hours will be needed depending on clinical status. Urokinase is given in an initial loading dose of 4400 IU per kg body weight over a 10-minute period. Maintenance dose of 4400 IU/kg/h for 12 hours will be needed. Heparin has to be continued in therapeutic doses after initial therapy with fibrinolytic agents. The main difference between streptokinase and urokinase is that urokinase is more expensive. Streptokinase is antigenic in humans; urokinase is not. Refractoriness to streptokinase may be seen after a recent streptococcal infection. Active internal bleeding, recent cerebrovascular accident (within the preceding 2 months), or other active intracranial process with the potential for bleeding are absolute contraindications for fibrinolytic therapy. A major surgical procedure within the last 10 days, recent serious gastrointestinal bleeding, recent serious trauma, and severe arterial hypertension are other major but relative contraindications. Recent minor trauma including cardiopulmonary resuscitation, and hemostatic defects constitute some other minor contraindications. Even though thrombolytic therapy leads to rapid resolution of emboli and quicker stabilization of hemodynamic alterations of pulmonary embolism compared to heparin, it has not been demonstrated that they decrease mortality.

Emergency pulmonary embolectomy dictates two prerequisites: angiographic evidence of massive or submassive emboli with refractory stock, and availability of a cardiopulmonary surgical team and bypass facilities. Mortality from the procedure is in the range of 40-100%.

Inferior Vena Cava Interruption

Interruption of the inferior vena cava (IVC) may be performed by plication in patients who can withstand this operation and by use of Mobin-Uddin umbrella or Hunter balloon in those with contraindications to general anesthesia. The following are the indications: contraindication to anticoagulation, chronic predisposition to recurrent pulmonary emboli, recurrence of pulmonary emboli under adequate heparin therapy, during pulmonary embolectomy, and septic pelvic thrombophlebitis.

Prognosis and Prevention

Dalen and associates have pointed out that, out of the 630,000 estimated cases of pulmonary embolism per year, about 67,000 (11%) may die within 1 hour of the episode. Among the survivors, diagnosis is probably not made in nearly 400,000 (71%), of which 120,000 (30%) die and 280,000 (70%) survive. Among those with an established diagnosis (163,000), 13,000 (8%) die and 150,000 survive (92%). Thus, in the undiagnosed group, a clear-cut increase in mortality is apparent. The main determinant for recurrent pulmonary emboli among the survivors is the precipitating factor for the initial pulmonary embolism. Where this influence is transient, a good prognosis can be anticipated. Long-term survival after pulmonary embolism appears to be adversely affected by pre-existing heart disease, especially left ventricular failure and coronary artery disease.

Early ambulation following surgery, trauma, and other illnesses that lead to confinement in bed will prevent venous stasis and help reduce the incidence of deep-vein thrombosis. Low-dose, prophylactic heparin therapy in doses of 5000 units subcutaneously twice daily has been shown to be effective in reducing the incidence of postoperative pulmonary embolism. In patients with eye, head, hip, or prostatic surgery or those with bleeding diathesis or recent or chronic aspirin therapy, low-dose heparin therapy should be avoided.

PULMONARY HYPERTENSION AND COR PULMONALE

Despite the fact that the entire cardiac output passes through the lungs, the pulmonary circulation operates as a low-pressure system. The features that help maintain this low-pressure status are: sparsity of musculature in the precapillary resistance vessels; a large cross-sectional area of the pulmonary vascular bed; and the existence of vessels with little or no blood flow that can be recruited on demand, such as seen during increased pulmonary blood flow that accompanies exercise.

The normal resting pulmonary artery pressures are 25 mm Hg during systole and 10 mm Hg during diastole. The resting mean pulmonary artery pressure is about 15 mm Hg. Little change occurs in the systolic pressure during exercise, whereas the diastolic may rise to 15 mm Hg and the mean may rise to 20 mm Hg. Elevation of the pulmonary artery pressures above these levels indicates pulmonary hypertension. The end-diastolic pressure in the pulmonary artery reflects the left ventricular end-diastolic pressure in persons without underlying lung disease, and the pressure recorded after a catheter has been wedged into a small pulmonary artery (occluding its lumen) represents the pulmonary capillary wedge pressure (PCW), which is the left atrial pressure (normally 5-12 mm Hg). In the early phases of pulmonary hypertension, resting arterial pressures are often normal and only exercise may unmask its existence. Elevation of mean pulmonary artery pressure above 20 mm Hg indicates definite pulmonary hypertension. Clinical states where pulmonary hypertension is encountered may be more common secondary to an underlying disease process or much less commonly as a primary or idiopathic event.

Primary Pulmonary Hypertension

The World Health Organization classifies this disease into three types: plexogenic pulmonary arteriopathy, recurrent pulmonary thromboembolism, and pulmonary veno-occlusive disease. The basis for this classification appears to be related to the prognosis in each of these varieties. The thromboembolic form is the more benign of these and is attended by a longer survival than the other two (about 7 years), the survival in the plexogenic variety being around 3 years, and in the veno-occlusive type, a few months to 2 years.

Primary pulmonary hypertension as it was originally described is predominantly a disease of young women. Autopsy findings of the pulmonary vasculature in this disease consist of organized microemboli, intimal fibrosis, and medial hypertrophy with well-developed and hypertrophied longitudinal muscles. Intraluminal angiomatoid changes, adventitial vascularization, and perivascular lymphocytic collections are other changes. Whether recurrent thromboembolism is the cause or effect of these changes is uncertain.

The main symptoms are dyspnea and syncope on effort. Chest pain indistinguishable from that of coronary insufficiency may occur and may be effort related. Associated Raynaud's phenomenon may be present. Clinical examination discloses evidence of pulmonary hypertension (a loud P_2, systolic murmur in the pulmonary area, a right ventricular heave, and, in late stages, pulmonary regurgitation, etc.). In early cases, however, examination may show only an accentuated P_2. Evidence of right-sided heart failure may be seen in advanced cases. Chest radiographs may demonstrate right ventricular enlargement and prominent central pulmonary artery. In a few cases, dilatation of the main pulmonary artery may occur. Pulmonary angiography and even perfusion lung scans carry a significant risk in these patients.

The prognosis is considered to be poor, but there are occasional cases of prolonged survival and spontaneous remissions. Recently, oral hydralazine and diazoxide have been successfully employed to produce sustained reduction in pulmonary vascular resistance.

Secondary Pulmonary Hypertension

The most common causes of secondary pulmonary hypertension are

1. *Left-sided heart disease.* Left-sided heart disease may be left ventricular (cardiomyopathy; severe aortic or mitral regurgitation) or left atrial (mitral stenosis, cor triatriatum). In these disorders, there is elevation of the left ventricular end-diastolic pressure and/or the left atrial pressure.
2. *Pulmonary vasoconstriction.* Hypoxemia and acidemia result in constriction of the pulmonary vasculature. Reduction in alveolar oxygen tension is the rule at high altitudes, with ensuing pulmonary vasoconstriction and hypertension. Because of the increased prevalence of hypoxemia in chronic bronchitis, these patients are most prone to the development of pulmonary hypertension. Alveolar hypoventilation characterized by hypoxemia and CO_2 retention occurs in neuromuscular respiratory failure, chest wall deformities (kyphoscoliosis), and massive obesity. The

acidemia of CO_2 retention augments the vasoconstrictive response to hypoxemia under these circumstances.

3. *Excessive blood flow.* Pulmonary hypertension follows conditions such as atrial septal defect, ventricular septal defect, and patent ductus arteriosus due to excessive pulmonary blood flow.
4. *Obliteration of the pulmonary vasculature.* It has been estimated that the extent of obliteration of the pulmonary capillary bed must exceed 50% to produce significant pulmonary hypertension. Recurrent pulmonary thromboembolism, interstitial lung disease (progressive systemic sclerosis and sarcoidosis), and late stages of pulmonary emphysema produce pulmonary hypertension by this mechanism. In most varieties of pneumoconiosis with fibrosis, clinically significant pulmonary hypertension is generally not seen unless hypoxemia due to associated chronic bronchitis is present.

Diagnosis

Diagnosis of pulmonary hypertension can be confirmed only by right heart catheterization. The measurements that are of value in establishing the cause of pulmonary hypertension are pulmonary artery pressures, pulmonary capillary wedge pressure, cardiac output, and the response to oxygen and exercise.

Treatment Prognosis

Treatment of pulmonary hypertension depends upon the underlying mechanism. In situations where hypoxia is the factor in the production of pulmonary hypertension, oxygen therapy will be followed by substantial improvement. In left-sided valvular heart disease, replacement of the diseased valve is often followed by significant reductions in pulmonary vascular pressures. Some degree of pulmonary hypertension will persist if secondary changes have occurred in the vasculature.

Cor Pulmonale

The criteria committee of the New York Heart Association has defined cor pulmonale as the occurrence of right ventricular enlargement or failure in the presence of a disease process that primarily involves the lungs, pulmonary vasculature, or respiratory gas exchange, and results in pulmonary hypertension. The right ventricular enlargement may be hypertrophy, dilatation, or both. Similarly, the cor pulmonale may be acute, as in massive pulmonary embolism, or chronic, as in chronic obstructive pulmonary disease.

Etiology and Pathogenesis

The initial event in cor pulmonale is pulmonary vasoconstriction that leads to pulmonary hypertension. This is usually brought about by hypoxemia and hypercapnia. Hypoxemia is the mechanism whereby the process is initiated in natives of high altitudes and in early chronic obstructive pulmonary disease, whereas both factors may be operative in alveolar hypoventilation (chest-wall abnormalities, neuromuscular respiratory failure, or central or obstructive sleep apnea states). Obliteration of the pulmonary capillary bed occurs in recurrent pulmonary thromboembolism, schistosomiasis, advanced pulmonary emphysema, interstitial lung disease, and sickle cell disease. Often the hypoxemia and obliterative factors operate simultaneously to produce pulmonary hypertension. Increases in pulmonary vascular resistance may also be brought about by the secondary effects of hypoxemia such as erythrocytosis and increased blood volume. These factors and their interrelationships are outlined in Figure 17.

Independent left ventricular dysfunction may develop in the midst of these events, and whether the cor pulmonale itself predisposes to this complication is uncertain. Concomitant coronary artery disease, hypoxemia, and erythrocytosis with increasing blood viscosity may all lead to this complication.

Clinical Features

There are no symptoms that are specific to cor pulmonale. Dyspnea, weakness, and changes in cerebral function may be observed; but the roles of underlying lung disease and the attendant hypoxia in producing these symptoms are factors to reckon with. Chest pain due to pulmonary hypertension may occur. Symptoms of the underlying lung disease such as cough, sputum, wheezing, or hemoptysis may be evident as well.

Physical signs that indicate pulmonary hypertension include large *a* waves in the jugular venous pulse, a left parasternal heave due to a prominent right ventricular impulse, a loud P_2, a right ventricular gallop, ankle edema, and pulsatile and often tender hepatomegaly if tricuspid insufficiency has supervened due to right ventricular dilatation. Pleural effusion does not occur as a result of cor pulmonale, and seldom does ascites.

Diagnosis

Presence of a disease with the potential for cor pulmonale and the clinical evidence of pulmonary hypertension, as discussed in the preceding paragraphs, together lead to the diagnosis of cor pulmonale. Electrocardiographic and roentgenographic manifestations of cor pulmonale are listed in Table 12. Differentiation from left heart failure secondary to arteriosclerotic heart disease is important. Unless the patient has asso-

Table 12. Electrocardiographic and Radiographic Manifestations of Cor Pulmonale

Electrocardiographic[a]
Right axis deviation of QRS complex, +110° or greater
R wave to S wave ratio >1 in V_1 [b]
R wave to S wave ratio <1 in V_6
P pulmonale
S_1, S_2, S_3, or S_1Q_3 pattern
Clockwise rotation of electrical axis[b]
Incomplete right bundle-branch block pattern[b]
Radiographic
Cardiomegaly with right ventricular and often right atrial enlargement
Prominent central pulmonary artery with attenuated peripheral branches
Radiographic features of the associated lung disease that leads to cor pulmonale[b]

[a] Any two of first six would confirm the presence of cor pulmonale
[b] Most characteristic when associated airway obstruction is present

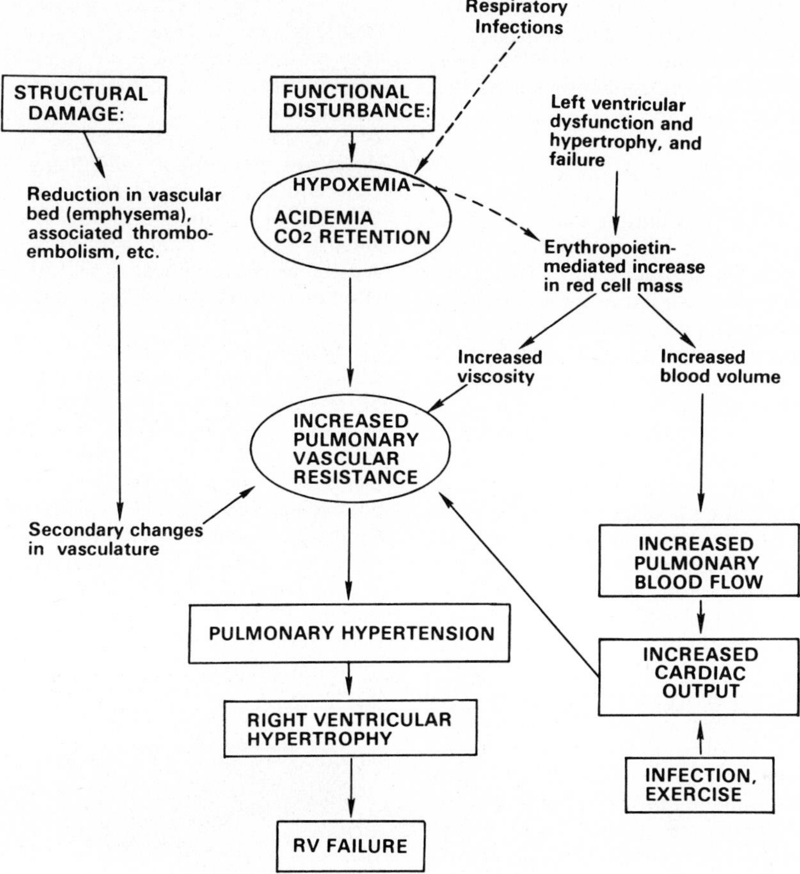

Figure 17. Pathogenetic factors in cor pulmonale.

ciated pulmonary edema, the presence of significant arterial hypoxemia (Pa_{O_2} less than 60) and CO_2 retention would favor the diagnosis of cor pulmonale. Laboratory studies may demonstrate associated erythrocytosis. Pulmonary function tests would generally reflect the underlying lung disease. In patients with normal lungs, nocturnal hypoxemia may be the cause of cor pulmonale, and sleep studies may be needed to establish the diagnosis.

Treatment and Prognosis

Besides appropriate treatment of the underlying disease, the following are important in the management of cor pulmonale.

1. *Oxygen.* Clinical studies have shown that long-term controlled oxygen administration to hypoxemic patients with cor pulmonale has resulted in diminution of pulmonary artery pressures.
2. *Phlebotomy.* When the hematocrit exceeds 55%, the increased blood viscosity seriously impairs myocardial performance and worsens the pulmonary hypertension. Phlebotomies are indicated to keep the hematocrit below this level.
3. *Digitalis.* Since digitalis raises the cardiac output, the resultant increase in pulmonary blood flow may worsen cor pulmonale in some patients. There is also an enhanced risk of arrhythmias due to this drug in the presence of hypoxemia. However, left ventricular dysfunction and failure, which may co-exist with cor pulmonale, improves with digitalis. Hence, the use of digitalis should be selective.
4. *Diuretics.* Fluid overload often complicates cor pulmonale, especially with frank right ventricular failure. Bed rest and improved oxygenation in most cases lead to prompt diuresis. Diuretics, if needed, should be used in small doses with close monitoring of electrolyte status.

Prognosis is essentially dependent on the underlying lung disease and how effectively it is being managed.

PULMONARY DISEASES DUE TO PHYSICAL AND CHEMICAL AGENTS

Pneumoconiosis is the general term applied to occupational lung disease caused by inhalation and permanent retention of dusts that elicit a tissue reaction. Many specific diseases are included in this broad category. Examples are silicosis, asbestosis, coal workers' pneumoconiosis, and pneumoconioses from nonasbestos silicates, graphite, aluminum, iron, and tin. Only the "big 3" (in terms of prevalence and medicosocioeconomic implications) will be considered here.

SILICOSIS

Silicon is a common and widely distributed element; one of the most common forms in which silicon exists is silicon dioxide. Silicon dioxide is commonly referred to as silica and is responsible for the disease silicosis. Exposure to silica can occur in a variety of occupations (e.g., mining or tunneling, quarrying, chipping, grinding, sandblasting, grinding or polishing in pottery and in foundry work, and cutting or manufacturing of heat-resistant bricks).

Inhaled silica particles of 1-5 μ in size reach the respiratory units of the lung. They are ingested by the alveolar macrophages that eventually succumb to the cytotoxic effects of silica. The liberated silica particles are again ingested by other macrophages. Such a cycle of macrophage ingestion and death continues. The death of macrophages results in release of lysosomal enzymes that play a key role in the formation of collagen, which in turn leads to fibrosis. The silica particles are carried by the lymphatics to the lymph nodes in the hilum. Less frequently they reach the mediastinal nodes and, rarely, even to the supraclavicular nodes. The parenchymal reaction elicited by silica and lysosomal enzymes of the macrophages develops into fibrotic nodules. These are typically small, less than a few millimeters in diameter, and are scattered throughout the lungs but are more numerous in the upper lung lobes. This form of silicosis is termed simple silicosis. These nodules may become calcified. In some cases, progression into complicated silicosis occurs. Complicated silicosis refers to large confluent masses of fibrotic tissue with or without cavitation. The factors responsible for the progression of simple silicosis to complicated silicosis are not well-understood; infection is generally considered an important factor. This infection may be due to *M. tuberculosis*, as has been recognized for many years, or due to atypical mycobacteriae, fungi, or bacteriae. Another form of silicosis is acute silicosis that develops after a relatively brief exposure (months to 3 years). A subset of acute silicosis is silicoproteinosis, the roentgenographic appearance of which is one of homogenous alveolar infiltrates similar to that of pulmonary alveolar proteinosis. Finer particle size and intense exposure are recognized as the main factors in the pathogenesis of silicoproteinosis.

Clinical Features

Patients with simple silicosis may be asymptomatic. Roentgenographic manifestations of simple silicosis usually take about 20 years after initial exposure. Shortness of breath on exertion may be an initial symptom. Cough and sputum production are frequent. Often these symptoms take many years to develop and are difficult to evaluate because of the coexistence of another factor, cigarette smoking. In complicated silicosis, in addition to dyspnea and cough, generalized symptoms (malaise, weight loss) are also usually present. Physical findings vary with the extent of the disease. Expiratory prolongation, rales, and rhonchi may be present. Clubbing is not a usual feature. Pulmonary function tests may reveal an obstructive ventilatory impairment, less commonly restriction, or a combined defect may be seen. Other findings include decreased pulmonary compliance, decreased diffusing capacity, and hypoxemia at rest or induced by exercise. As mentioned earlier, infection should be suspected when complicated silicosis occurs. Another association that increases the morbidity of complicated silicosis is collagen vascular disease (rheumatoid arthritis, scleroderma, lupus erythematosus).

Roentgenographic Features

Clinically significant disease is almost never seen in the absence of roentgenographic abnormalities. Simple silicosis manifests as multiple nodules, several millimeters in diameter, scattered throughout but more noticeable in the upper lung fields. These nodules may infrequently calcify; associated hilar node enlargement and egg shell calcification may be seen (Fig. 18). Complicated silicosis manifests as bilateral upper lobe confluent masses that may be necrotic in the center. As these masses retract towards the hilum because of the fibrosis, the nodules present in the lower lung fields become less obvious because of compensatory emphysema (Fig. 19). Caplan's syndrome is pulmonary nodules (0.5-5 cm) occurring in patients

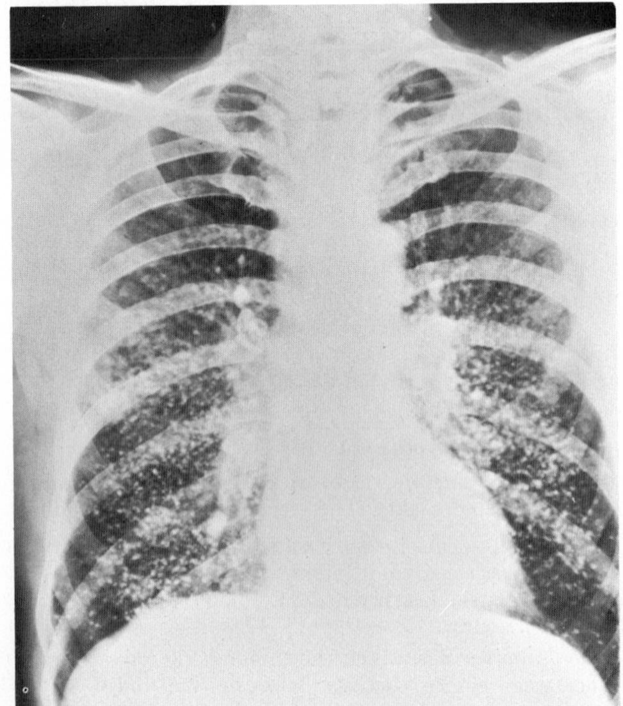

Figure 18. Simple silicosis; diffuse calcified nodules and prominent calcified (eggshell) hilar nodes.

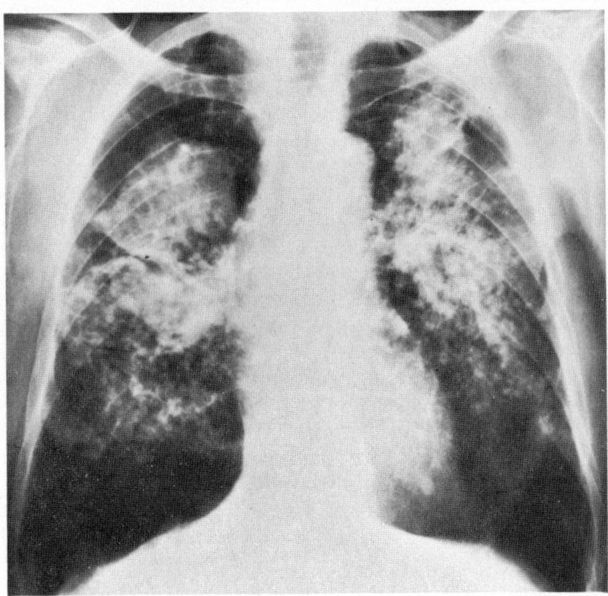

Figure 19. Complicated silicosis.

with rheumatoid arthritis and pneumoconioses (silicosis, coal workers' pneumoconiosis).

Diagnosis

Diagnosis of silicosis is based on the history of exposure and chest roentgenographic appearance. When discordant clinical or roentgenographic features are present a lung biopsy may be necessary for diagnosis. Open lung biopsy is the preferred procedure. The excised lung tissue is examined for silica. This can be done by different methods: microscopy with polarized light, scanning electron microscopy, or energy dispersive x-ray analysis.

There is no specific treatment for silicosis. Efforts should be aimed at prevention of the disease, prevention of complications, and treatment of complications. The main complications are infections (particularly mycobacterial), progressive respiratory insufficiency, cor pulmonale, and respiratory failure.

ASBESTOSIS

Asbestos is the general term used for a group of heat-resistant fibrous minerals. Chrysotile, crocidolite, amosite, and anthrophyllite are four of the more important forms of asbestos. Because asbestos has thousands of industrial uses, occupational exposure to asbestos can occur in a wide variety of occupations. Examples are boilermaker, brake-lining maker or worker, construction worker, docker, filter worker, insulation worker, lagger, gasket maker, pipe coverer or cutter, plumber, rock miner, shipbuilder, or braker and steam fitter.

Fibrosis of the lung caused by inhalation of asbestos is called asbestosis. There is usually a long latent period of 20 years or more from the time of exposure to the appearance of clinical or roentgenographic manifestations of asbestosis and other asbestos-related diseases. In one study exposure to asbestos in concentrations near 5 million particles per cubic foot caused asbestosis after 20 years in 38% of the persons exposed. In addition to the amount and duration of exposure, individual factors may also influence the development of asbestosis. Although the exact mechanism by which asbestos fibers cause asbestosis is unknown physical effects, chemical effects, and host factors are all implicated. Respiratory bronchioles are involved early with peribronchiolar fibrosis and eventually this proceeds to diffuse interstitial fibrosis.

Clinical Features

The most common symptom is dyspnea on exertion that usually manifests after 10 years or more of asbestos exposure. Cough may also be present, but is not as frequent a symptom as dyspnea. It is usually nonproductive and may be paroxysmal. In some, particularly in advanced cases, tightness or pain in the chest wall may be present. The most important physical findings are basilar cellophane rales on inspiration and clubbing of the fingers. Pulmonary function tests typically show a restrictive ventilatory impairment with reduced lung volumes, decreased diffusing capacity, and hypoxemia at rest or on exercise.

Roentgenographic Features

The major roentgenographic features are depicted in Figure 20. The following findings help differentiate asbestosis from silicosis and other diffuse interstitial disease: the predominantly lower-zone location of the infiltrates, the rarity of hilar node enlargement or calcification, and pleural thickening and hyaline or calcified pleural plaques. Pleural thickening is typically seen in the axillary areas and calcified pleural plaques are typically seen over the diaphragm.

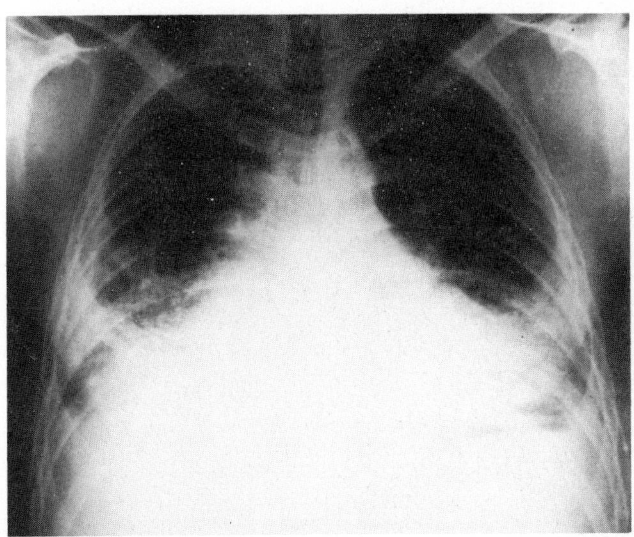

Figure 20. Asbestosis. (Reprinted with permission from *Postgraduate Medicine* 63:48, 1978.)

Diagnosis

The diagnosis of asbestosis is made by the history of exposure to asbestos, exertional dyspnea, basilar rales with or without clubbing, and typical roentgenographic features mentioned in the preceding paragraph. Pulmonary function impairment as described earlier lends further support to the diagnosis. As in any other disease, if discordant features are present, more proof is necessary for the diagnosis. Thus, in an occasional case, a lung biopsy may be needed. Asbestos bodies (Fig. 21) and interstitial fibrosis are the hallmarks of asbestosis. Electron microscopy aids in the detection of smaller uncoated fibers.

Complications of asbestosis are progressive fibrosis leading to cor pulmonale and respiratory failure. There is no specific treatment for asbestosis. Efforts should be directed at prevention of asbestosis as well as in prompt treatment of respiratory infections since infections may accelerate the fibrosis.

Other Asbestos-Related Pleuropulmonary Disease

The association of pleural plaques with occupational and environmental exposure to asbestos has been established. Pleural plaques are multiple, usually bilateral, discrete thickenings of the parietal pleura. They appear grossly as shiny white areas and have the consistency of cartilage. The favored locations are in the lower half of the chest close to the ribs and over the diaphragm. Calcific deposition in the plaques are common, but may not always be detected on roentgenograms. Bilateral diaphragmatic calcification is an almost sure sign of previous asbestos exposure. Pleural plaques rarely cause symptoms and do not require any treatment. These are benign lesions and no predisposition towards malignancy has been demonstrated.

An exudative, serosanguineous pleural effusion may result from occupational or paraoccupational exposure to asbestos.

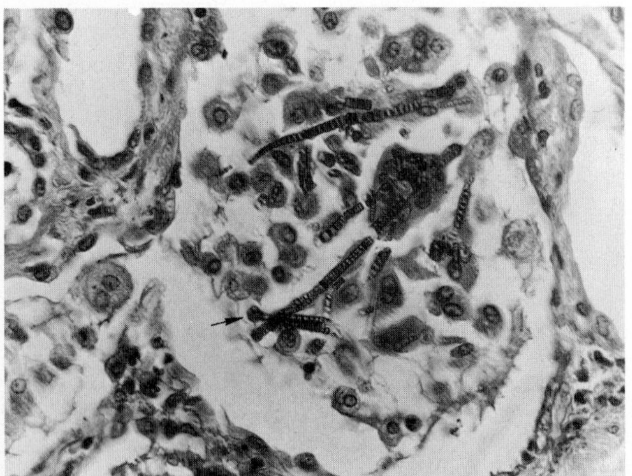

Figure 21. Asbestos bodies; asbestos fibers with an acid mucopolysaccharide and iron coating seen as elongated beaded bodies with clubbed ends. (Reprinted with permission from *Postgraduate Medicine* 63:48, 1978.)

Unlike asbestosis, prolonged exposure is not necessary for the development of asbestos pleural effusion. The usual symptoms are pleuritic chest pain and dyspnea. The course of benign asbestos pleural effusion is self-limited; occasionally it may cause chronic pleural thickening and restrictive pulmonary impairment. The diagnosis is mainly a diagnosis of exclusion of other causes of pleural effusion. Pleural fluid findings as well as needle biopsy of the pleura are likely to be nonspecific and nondiagnostic. Open biopsy of the pleura and adjacent lung may be needed in an occasional case; asbestos bodies may be seen in the lung tissue close to the pleura.

The relationship of malignant pleural mesothelioma to asbestos exposure has been clearly established. This neoplasm is discussed in the section on disorders of the pleura, mediastinum, and diaphragm.

Several epidemiologic studies have established the fact that bronchogenic carcinoma is increased in persons exposed to asbestos. This increase is much more striking in those asbestos workers who also smoke. Cigarette smoking and asbestos exposure work synergistically as cocarcinogens.

COAL WORKERS' PNEUMOCONIOSIS

Coal workers' pneumoconiosis (CWP) results from deposition of coal dust in the lungs. This disease is confined to those who actually work in underground coal mines. The degree of exposure to coal dust in the mine, however, varies with the location and type of job. The workers who work (cutting, blasting) at the coal face have the greatest exposure to coal dust. Those involved in transportation of coal do not have as much exposure. A heavy and prolonged exposure is usually required for clinically and roentgenographically manifest disease. There are a variety of clinical expressions of the damage done by coal dust. These are chronic bronchitis, simple CWP, complicated CWP (also referred to as progressive massive fibrosis) and Caplan's syndrome.

Coal dust of respirable size reach the respiratory units and are ingested by alveolar macrophages. These macrophages then move toward the terminal bronchiole and are swept up by the mucociliary escalator. When the exposure is heavy and/or the clearance mechanisms are ineffective, macrophages containing coal are retained in the respiratory bronchioles. Proteolytic enzymes are released when macrophages lyse. Fibrin deposition also occurs and gradually a coal macule consisting of an aggregate of coal dust, dying macrophages, fibroblasts, and connective tissue forms in the area of the respiratory bronchiole. It is not clear why some patients develop complicated CWP (progressive massive fibrosis) while others remain as simple CWP. Some of the postulated mechanisms in the development of complicated CWP are: action of silica contained in the coal, effect of pulmonary infection by bacteria or mycobacteria, and altered immunologic responses of the host.

Clinical Features

Simple CWP may cause no symptoms; in some, cough with sputum production and wheezing may be present. Complicated CWP is usually manifested by dyspnea on effort. In addition, severe bronchitic symptoms including the striking finding of black sputum (melanoptysis) may be seen. In simple CWP, pulmonary function tests are generally normal in nonsmokers; in some, mild abnormalities such as slight decreases in total lung capacity, vital capacity, 1-second expiratory volume, or evidence of small airway disease may be seen. In those with complicated CWP, evidence of obstructive and restrictive impairment are striking.

Roentgenographic Features

Simple CWP is indicated by the presence of roentgenographic densities of a diameter of 1 cm or less throughout the lung fields. Complicated CWP refers to one or more opacities of more than 1 cm in diameter.

Diagnosis

Like in other pneumoconioses, diagnosis is based on the history and chest roentgenogram. Diffuse small nodules or larger (>1 cm) nodules in a coal miner is virtually diagnostic of the disease and no further diagnostic workup is necessary.

There is no specific treatment for the disease. Symptomatic bronchitis and bronchospasm are treated with bronchodilators; complicating infections should be promptly treated with appropriate antimicrobial agents. In those with associated collagen vascular disease, corticosteroids should be considered. As in other pneumoconioses, the major thrust should be toward prevention of the disease and its complications.

OCCUPATIONAL ASTHMA AND BRONCHITIS

Occupational Asthma

Asthma may be brought on by a variety of occupational exposures. Chemical irritation (e.g., sulfur dioxide, nitrogen dioxide), pharmacologic modulation (e.g., cotton bract), and immunologic reaction (e.g., toluene diisocyanate) are the pathogenetic mechanisms, acting singly or in combination, that are responsible for occupational asthma.

Byssinosis was originally described in cotton workers but now has been recognized also in flax, hemp, and sisal workers. A particular feature of byssinosis is the increase in severity of the symptoms noted when reexposure occurs after an absence. One possible explanation for this is the replenishment of histamine in the mast cells during the period of avoidance. Cotton bract is considered responsible for stimulating the release of histamine and consequent asthma.

Toluene diisocyanate (TDI) asthma results from sensitization to TDI vapor; this may occur due to an acute exposure to a high concentration of TDI or a chronic exposure to a low concentration of the vapor. Once sensitized, bronchial constriction and asthma occur even with inhalation of a very low concentration of TDI.

The clinical features, diagnosis, and treatment of occupational asthma in general will now be considered.

Clinical Features

Although wheezing is the most characteristic symptom of asthma, in some it may be absent. Other symptoms such as tightness in the chest, cough, and breathlessness may be present. In the early stages, symptoms occur during, or a variable period after, exposure and subside when away from work. In later stages, symptoms become recurrent and persistent. Chest roentgenogram may be normal or may show hyperinflation.

Diagnosis

Diagnosis may be considered in two parts; diagnosis of asthma brought on by occupational exposure and diagnosis of the specific offending agent. Awareness of the variability of symptoms, particularly symptoms other than wheezing, is essential. Some patients may have a history of atopy, asthma, or a family history of asthma. A carefully taken history with emphasis on the sequence of events in terms of exposure and symptoms is the most important factor in arriving at the correct diagnosis. Identifying the offending agent may be quite difficult. If reaginic antibodies against the offending antigen are present in the serum, a positive skin test (wheal-and-flare) and a positive radioallergosorbent test (RAST) are expected. However, the absence of reaginic antibodies in some cases and the unavailability of specific antigens limit the diagnostic usefulness of these tests. Bronchial provocation tests are being increasingly used in diagnosis. This involves an inhalational challenge with a small, accurately measured amount of the suspected antigen. Spirometric values, especially 1-second espiratory volume ($FEV_{1.0}$) before and sequentially after the challenge are obtained. The dose of the antigen is increased if there is no response after the initial challenge. A positive test is one in which significant decline in $FEV_{1.0}$ is observed after inhalation of the antigen. There are three types of positive responses: immediate (minutes to 2 hours), delayed (4-8 hours or more), and dual (combination of immediate and delayed) are recognized. The immediate reaction can be reversed by inhalation of β-adrenergic drugs and can be blocked by pretreatment with cromolyn sodium but not by corticosteroids. The late reaction is more refractory to inhalational treatment with β-adrenergic drugs but can be blocked by pretreatment with corticosteroids. Bronchial provocation tests should be done only in specialized laboratories under constant physician supervision.

Treatment

Asthmatic symptoms due to occupational exposure are relieved by the use of bronchodilators, as in the treatment of bronchial asthma. A crucial aspect of the treatment is prevention of further exposure to the offending agent. If this is impossible because of economic or other factors, blocking drugs (cromolyn sodium, corticosteroids) are recommended.

Occupational Bronchitis

Occupational bronchitis as an entity is not as well-delineated as occupational asthma. This is mainly because the effects of exposure to occupational dusts, cigarette smoke, and other environmental factors are difficult to separate. However, some recent studies suggest an increased prevelance of cough with expectoration (chronic bronchitis) in coal miners that is out of proportion to what one expects with cigarette smoking alone. This industrial bronchitis has also been suspected in grain handlers. However, in this group the factor of hypersensitivity and occupational asthma clouds the issue.

CHEMICAL, THERMAL, RADIATION, AND ASPIRATION INJURIES

Chemical Injury

Industrial progress and proliferation of chemicals go hand in hand. Exposure to these chemicals often, but not invariably, occurs in an occupational setting (see Table 13). The most notable nonoccupational exposure (by just breathing) is exposure to polluted air.

Air pollution may be considered to be of three different types based on products and sources. These are: products of reaction between solar radiation and the components of motor-vehicle emission (hydrocarbons, oxides of nitrogen, etc.), a sulfur oxide and particulate complex liberated with the burning of coal and crude oil, and varied substances (arsenic, cadmium, hydrogen sulfide, lead, and mercury) released from smelters, refineries, and manufacturing plants. Type 2 (a sulfur oxide-particulate complex) air pollution has been found in some early studies to cause increased mortality in elderly persons with chronic lung or heart disease. Air pollution increases the incidence and morbidity of lower respiratory tract infections, worsens asthma, and adversely affects the course of chronic obstructive pulmonary disease (COPD). Air pollution is also suspected to be a pathogenetic factor in COPD.

Besides air pollution, a large number of gases and fumes have a direct toxic effect on the respiratory tract. Others may cause severe systemic abnormalities (e.g., cyanide, metal fume), asphyxia (e.g., carbon dioxide, methane), or hypoxia (e.g., carbon monoxide). Direct respiratory tract injury may result from exposure to ammonia, cadmium, chlorine, ozone, sulfur dioxide, and oxides of nitrogen.

Table 13. Chemicals and Their Common Occupational Sources

Chemicals	*Common Occupational Sources*
Ammonia	Manufacture of fertilizer, refrigeration units
Cadmium	Smelting of ores, welding
Chlorine	Manufacture of bleaches, disinfectants, alkalies
Oxides of nitrogen	Handling fresh silage, arc welding
Sulfur dioxide	Oil refining, manufacture of paper, refrigeration units
Ozone	Flying high-altitude supersonic airplanes, arc welding
Cyanide	Manufacture of synthetic rubber, electroplating, gold extraction
Carbon monoxide	Fire fighting, burning of organic materials
Zinc, copper, and magnesium oxides	Galvanizing, smelting
Nitrogen, carbon dioxide	Mining, diving
Methane	Mining

One of the oxides of nitrogen, nitrogen dioxide, is responsible for silo-filler's disease, a disease affecting farmers who handle fresh silage. This disease characteristically has acute, delayed, and chronic effects. The immediate reaction to the nitrogen dioxide exposure is coughing, chest tightness, and choking. Hours later, severe dyspnea due to noncardiac pulmonary edema develops and may be fatal. Weeks later, increased shortness of breath, cough, and progressive hypoxemia may develop (pathologically, bronchiolitis obliterans) and may proceed to progressive respiratory failure.

Diagnosis

The diagnosis of respiratory tract injury due to local action of chemical irritants is self-evident in most cases since symptoms are manifest immediately after exposure. However, in some cases symptoms may follow only after a latent period of 1-8 hours or more. Hence, persons who are exposed to a chemical irritant but are asymptomatic should be closely observed for many hours. Serial measurements of arterial blood gases are particularly useful in this group since a drop in arterial oxygen tension (Po_2) almost invariably happens before symptoms or roentgenographic abnormalities (atelectasis, noncardiac pulmonary edema).

Treatment

The general principles are to maintain adequate ventilation and oxygenation and to prevent (when possible) or treat complications. Tracheostomy is indicated if respiration is impaired because of laryngospasm or edema of the upper respiratory tract. Tracheobronchial clearance (respiratory therapy and fiberoptic bronchoscopy may be helpful) should be optimized to prevent atelectasis. Oxygen should be administered as needed to correct hypoxia. Corticosteroids in large doses (methyl prednisolone 30 mg/kg/24 h intravenously) is recommended by some experts. Complications of adult respiratory distress syndrome should be anticipated.

Some specific chemical injuries require specific modalities of treatment. In cyanide poisoning immediate inhalation of amyl nitrite and intravenous administration of 3% sodium nitrite (0.39 ml/kg) followed by 25% sodium thiosulfate (1.95 ml/kg) are indicated. In symptomatic carbon monoxide poisoning, 100% oxygen by a tight-fitting mask is recommended; hyperbaric oxygenation may be lifesaving.

Thermal Injury

The upper respiratory tract above the larynx is the site of thermal injury. With the exception of steam inhalation, direct injury to the lungs does not occur. Survivors of fires may have direct thermal injury but more significant clinically are the respiratory effects of inhalation of smoke (products of combustion). Chemical injuries (discussed in the preceding section) due to carbon monoxide, oxides of nitrogen, and other chemicals may lead to acute pulmonary edema and ARDS. Early clinical manifestations of thermal injuries are stridor because of laryngeal edema and bronchospasm. Cough productive of bloody, frothy sputum is indicative of pulmonary edema. Thermal injuries presenting with minimal or no symptoms but with findings of facial burns or singed nasal hairs calls for continued close observation in a hospital.

Radiation Injury

The effects of radiation injury depend on the amount of lung exposed to radiation, the total dose, the energy of the beam, the potentiating effect of some cytotoxic drugs, and unknown host factors. Two different reactions are recognized; radiation pneumonitis, an acute or subacute response that appears 6-12 weeks after completion of the course of radiation, and radiation fibrosis, a chronic response that takes 6 months or more to develop.

Common symptoms of radiation pneumonitis are a dry cough and increased dyspnea. Pain in the chest wall or pleuritic in nature is an infrequent feature. Fever may be present. New infiltrates are found in the chest roentgenogram. Roentgenographic findings of infiltrates sharply confined to the region of the lung incorporated in the radiation port along with a consistent time course and symptoms are diagnostic. Early pathologic reactions are pulmonary vascular congestion, alveolar edema, and hyaline membrane formation. These are followed by desquamation of the bronchial and alveolar epithelium and thrombosis of the small blood vessels. In addition to symptomatic treatment corticosteroids are indicated as soon as the diagnosis is made.

Radiation fibrosis is a sequela of radiation pneumonitis. This progression from pneumonitis to fibrosis is almost invariable. Progressive dyspnea is the symptom. Chest roentgenogram typically shows, in addition to the infiltrates in the irradiated area, volume loss in the ipsilateral lung. Pleural thickening is frequent and pleural effusions may also be present. Pathologically there is interstitial fibrosis and fibrous pleuritis.

There is no specific treatment for radiation fibrosis and treatment with corticosteroids is generally ineffective.

Aspiration Injury

The sequelae of aspiration vary with volume, character, and the presence or absence of bacteria in the aspirated material. Hence different clinical syndromes may result. These include chemical pneumonia due to aspiration of gastric contents of a low pH, lipoid pneumonia due to aspiration of lipid material (commonly mineral oil), anaerobic pneumonia and abscess due to aspiration (gravitation) of infected material from the oral cavity (usually gingivitis is present), and a superimposed bacterial infection following aspiration of gastric contents. Further discussion in this section will be confined to chemical pneumonia.

Chemical (aspiration) pneumonia results from aspiration of acidic gastric contents (pH 2.5 or less). Pathologically, the acidic aspirate causes damage to the bronchial mucosa and alveolar epithelium; the consequent inflammation results in exudation of fluid and neutrophils into the airways and alveoli.

Cough, wheezing, and dyspnea are the common symptoms and are acute in onset. Fever may be present. The usual roentgenographic finding (which may take a few hours after the aspiration to develop) is mottled lower-lobe infiltrates. Hypoxia is invariably seen and worsening hypoxia is a poor prognostic sign.

Diagnosis

The diagnosis is based on the presence of predisposing factors (altered consciousness, esophageal dysfunction, advanced age), witnessing the aspiration or finding food particles on tracheobronchial suctioning, consistent clinical and roentgenographic features, and hypoxia.

The most important complication is ARDS, which usually develops 24-48 hours after aspiration. The other complication is infection (Gram-negative bacteria and anaerobes).

Treatment

The principles consist of adequate clearance of tracheobronchial secretions, correction of hypoxia, and maintenance of optimal intravascular volume. The clinical status, arterial blood gases, and chest roentgenogram should be assessed periodically. If progressive worsening occurs, intubation and mechanical ventilation along with positive end expiratory pressure are indicated. Although controversial, the authors prefer corticosteroids (as discussed in chemical injury), if the diagnosis is made within a few hours after the aspiration. Antimicrobials are not indicated unless there is a clear indication of a superimposed bacterial pneumonia.

DROWNING, TRAUMA AND DRUG-INDUCED DISEASE

Drowning

From a pathophysiologic standpoint saltwater drowning and freshwater drowning are different. In saltwater drowning, water passes from the pulmonary capillaries into the alveoli causing hemoconcentration, whereas in freshwater drowning, water passes into the capillaries from the alveoli causing intravascular hemolysis. However, in actual clinical situations this distinction serves little purpose. The immediate cause of death in drowning is neither hemoconcentration nor hemolysis but, rather, asphyxia secondary to reflex laryngospasm.

Symptoms and signs of nervous system dysfunction, restlessness, confusion, delirium, convulsions, and coma are common following resuscitation. Cardiovascular findings (tachycardia, gallop) and respiratory symptoms (tachypynea, laryngospasm, bronchospasm, cough) frequently coexist. A low-grade fever is not unexpected but hyperthermia is infrequent and ominous.

Chest roentgenogram may be normal initially. The characteristic pattern of pulmonary edema usually takes a few hours to manifest. Hypoxia is invariable; the level of carbon dioxide tension is dependent on the level of alveolar ventilation. Leukocytosis and electrolyte disturbances are commonly seen; sodium and chloride concentrations may be increased in some cases of saltwater drowning. Other infrequent laboratory findings include albuminuria, microscopic hematuria, and hemoglobinuria.

The immediate treatment consists of clearing debris and

secretions from the airway and instituting mouth-to-mouth respiration. External cardiac massage should be started, if necessary. If spontaneous breathing does not resume, endotracheal intubation and mechanical ventilation are indicated. Supplemental oxygen should be administered. Nasogastric suctioning aids in removing food, water, and air from the stomach. Corticosteroids may be used in large doses. Respiratory complications of drowning include atelectasis, aspiration pneumonia, bacterial infections, and ARDS.

Thoracic Trauma

Thoracic trauma, blunt or penetrating, may occur in industrial and automobile accidents, cardiac resuscitation, or knife and gunshot wounds. Blunt trauma to the chest, usually caused by direct impact of the steering wheel, is one of the important causes of morbidity and mortality in automobile accidents. Injuries to the chest wall commonly causes rib fractures; if these are multiple, the stability of the chest wall may be affected causing a flail chest. Other consequences of chest wall trauma include pneumothorax, pneumomediastinum, hemothorax, hemomediastinum, lung hematoma, contusion, compression syndrome, bronchial rupture, and aortic rupture. Posttraumatic pulmonary insufficiency (ARDS) is a serious complication of thoracic trauma.

Localized trauma causing a localized area of bleeding in the lung is a hematoma; a more diffuse injury and consequent widespread hemorrhage is called a lung contusion. In both hematoma and contusion there may be a considerable latent period before roentgenographic findings manifest; hematoma may simulate a pulmonary infarction and contusion may simulate a pneumonia. Clinical manifestations include cough, hemoptysis, and fever (usually low grade). Clearance of tracheobronchial secretions, correction of hypoxia, and treatment of infections (if present) are to be emphasized.

An anterior chest-wall crush injury may cause compression of the heart against the vertebrae (compression syndrome). Because of the compression there is retrograde emptying of the heart; this raises venous pressures in the superior vena cava system. Thus, findings of conjunctival and mucosal bleeding, swelling of the eye lids, proptosis, and purplish discoloration of the face, shoulders, and arms may be seen. If the compression is relieved spontaneous recovery follows.

Partial or complete rupture of the trachea or a bronchus may follow a sudden anteroposterior compression. These are usually manifested by dyspnea, pneumothorax, pneumomediastinum, and subcutaneous emphysema. Localization of the injury and definitive repair are indicated. A partial rupture may go unrecognized and may cause late sequelae of bronchial stricture and atelectasis.

Thoracic injury may also affect the heart or the aorta. The former usually manifests as a hemopericardium or a pneumopericardium. Aortic rupture usually occurs a few centimeters distal to the origin of the left subclavin artery. This area is particularly vulnerable to sudden deceleration injury because the area immediately above it is relatively fixed. A complete rupture is fatal within minutes. Usually the rupture is a partial one and physical findings may be absent; disparity in blood pressures of the upper and lower extremities may provide a clue in a minority of patients. The most important findings in the diagnosis are roentgenographic, that is, mediastinal widening and blurring of the aortic area. When this diagnosis is suspected an aortogram should be done; if the diagnosis is confirmed surgical repair should be carried out as soon as possible. A late sequela of undetected partial aortic rupture is chronic traumatic aneurysm.

Drug-Induced Pulmonary Disease

The most important factor in the diagnosis of drug-induced pulmonary disease is a comprehensive history. The clinical presentation of drug induced pulmonary disease has a very wide spectrum; consider the life-threatening anaphylaxis due to penicillin, perhaps less dramatic, but serious illness of acute pulmonary edema due to heroin, and the insidious pulmonary fibrosis caused by bleomycin. It would not be possible here, to cover in detail every drug known to cause a pulmonary disease or disorder. The reader will find Table 14 helpful in approaching the problem of drug-induced pulmonary disease. A number of drugs not included in the table cause pleural or mediastinal disorders. Nitrofurantoin may cause a pleural effusion. Procainamide, hydralazine, phenytoin, and isoniazid are recognized causes of systemic lupus erythematosis and consequent pleural effusions. Mediastinal and hilar prominences on roentgenograms may be due to corticosteroids (mediastinal lipomatosis) or diphylhydantoin (lymphadenopathy).

Besides a careful history, an assessment of the time relationship from exposure to development of syptoms and roentgenographic findings is very helpful in the diagnosis. The physical findings are clearly dependent on the types of pulmonary reactions (see column 1 of Table 14). Roentgenographic findings also vary with the types of reactions and sites of injury. There are no specific diagnostic tests for drug-induced pulmonary disease.

Rarely, a rechallenge with the suspected drug under physician supervision may prove the diagnosis. An open lung biopsy is helpful in selected situations (e.g., newly developing infiltrates in a leukemic patient receiving cytotoxic therapy). The advantage of a biopsy in these situations is twofold: to exclude infections or other causes, and to possibly find a characteristic histologic picture to confirm the diagnosis of drug-induced pulmonary disease.

The general principle of treatment is further avoidance of the drug; specific treatments vary with the type and severity of the disease.

DIFFUSE INFILTRATIVE DISEASES OF THE LUNG

Disease processes that affect the lung parenchyma may predominantly involve the alveoli or the layer of connective tissue between the epithelial layers of the alveoli, namely, the lung interstitium. Several pathologic processes lead to infiltrations in these areas, most of them involving the interstitium

Table 14. Drug-Induced Pulmonary Disease

Type/Location of Reaction	*Class of Drug*	*Specific Drugs (Partial List)*
Pulmonary edema (noncardiac)	Narcotics	Heroin, methadone, morphine
	Analgesics	Aspirin, D-propoxyphene
	Others	Ethchlorvynol, hydrochlorothiazide
Pulmonary infiltrates with eosinophilia	Chemotherapeutic agents	Nitrofurantoin, p-aminosalicylic acid, Methotrexate, penicillin, sulfonamides, Procarbazine
	Others	Imipramine, cromolyn sodium
Diffuse alveolar/interstitial infiltrates	Chemotherapeutic agents	Bleomycin, busulfan, nitrofurantoin, cyclophosphamide, methotrexate, chlorambucil, azathioprine, gold, chloroquine,
	Antihypertensives	hexamethonium, mecamylamine, pentolinium
	Vasoconstrictors	methylsergide, oxygen
	Others	Marijuana smoke, mineral oil, talc
Pulmonary thromboembolism	Estrogens	Diethylstilbesterol, progesterone
Bronchospasm	Chemotherapeutic agents	Penicillin, ampicillin
	Parasympathomimetics	Mecholyl, neostigmine
	β-adrenergic blocker	Propanolol
	Analgesics	Aspirin, indomethacin
	Anesthetics	Ethylether, althesin
	Hormones	Pituitary snuff, pancreatin
	Others	Piperazine, tartrazine
Respiratory muscle paralysis	Chemotherapeutic agents	Kanamycin, streptomycin, neomycin, gentamicin, polymyxin B
	Neuromuscular blockers	Tubocurarine, succinylcholine
Respiratory depression/acute respiratory failure	Narcotics	Heroin, methadone, morphine, cocaine
	Sedatives	Barbiturates
	Tranquilizers	Diazepam, chlordiazepoxide, nitrazepam

either selectively or predominantly. A few disorders such as alveolar proteinosis and alveolar microlithiasis involve the alveoli selectively.

Infiltrations of the interstitium may be due to disorders that primarily affect the lungs or from systemic diseases. In either event, the commonest symptom referable to such infiltration is dyspnea, but the systemic manifestations of the primary disease may overshadow the pulmonary symptoms in the latter instance. The earliest clinical sign is tachypnea. Depending upon the disease entity, finger clubbing and/or end-inspiratory rales on chest auscultation may be present. Chest roentgenograms may demonstrate findings characteristic of each disease but, in general, may vary from normal lung fields to small lung to diffuse interstitial (nodular, reticular, or reticulonodular) infiltration. Interstitial lung disease characteristically leads to diminution of vital capacity, total lung capacity, and DL_{CO}. Hypoxemia may be present at rest or may become manifest after exercise, indicating concomitant involvement of the pulmonary vasculature.

Infiltrative diseases of the lungs may be classified as:

1. Infiltration due to systemic diseases
   Sarcoidosis
   Collagen-vascular disease
   Hematologic disorders
   Histiocytosis X
2. Infiltrative diseases due to inhaled organic substances
   Hypersensitivity pneumonitides
3. Infiltrative diseases due to inhaled inorganic substances
   Occupational pneumoconiosis
4. Diffuse infiltrative diseases of unknown origin
   Diffuse interstitial pulmonary fibrosis
   Other miscellaneous entities

Diseases under categories 1, 2, and 4 will be considered in this chapter. Pulmonary infiltration due to inhaled inorganic substances (occupational pneumoconiosis) is discussed separately in another chapter.

PULMONARY INFILTRATION DUE TO SYSTEMIC DISORDERS

Sarcoidosis

Mitchell and Scadding have defined sarcoidosis as a disease characterized by the presence in several affected organs and tissues of noncaseating epithelioid cell granulomas, proceeding either to resolution or to conversion into featureless hyaline connective tissue. The etiology of this systemic disorder is not known. It affects predominantly younger age groups (90%

between 20 and 40 years of age) and is more prevalent in blacks in the United States, with an estimated prevalence of about 60 cases per 100,000 population.

The hallmark of sarcoidosis is the noncaseating granuloma, which contains epithelioid cells (large, 20 μ in size, mononuclear, derived from macrophages) and giant cells (several times larger than epithelioid cells, multinucleated, and containing asteroid, Schaumann's, and residual inclusion bodies) with lymphocytes and plasma cells in the peripheral areas and variable degrees of fibrosis and hyalinization.

Among the immunologic disturbances noted in sarcoidosis, the most important are depressed T-lymphocyte function, decreased peripheral T-cell and increased peripheral B-cell populations, and increased numbers of total and activated T lymphocytes in the lung. Circulating immune complexes may be present. Recently, a monocyte chemotactic factor has been identified from the T lymphocytes of sarcoid lung that leads to local aggregation of monocytes, indicating its potential for the creation and maintenance of the granulomata of this disease.

Clinical Features

The most frequent mode of presentation of sarcoidosis is an abnormal chest roentgenogram, obtained generally as part of a pre-employment physical examination or as part of a routine evaluation of other illnesses. Symptoms referable to pulmonary involvement do, however, occur in a variable number of cases such as dyspnea and cough in about 30-35% and chest pain in about 20% of cases. Cough is generally dry; sputum production and hemoptysis are infrequent. In about 15-30% of patients, constitutional symptoms occur such as malaise, fatigue, and weight loss, thus underscoring the systemic nature of the disease. Weakness, lethargy, easy fatigability, and fever are other symptoms. The incidence of extrapulmonary involvement varies depending upon the criteria employed (symptomatic versus asymptomatic, gross versus microscopic), the intensity with which such involvement is looked for, and the specialty of the investigator (pathologist, ophthalmologist, dermatologist, etc.). A fair assessment of the frequency of extrapulmonary involvement is probably peripheral lymphadenopathy, skin lesions, eye lesions, salivary gland involvement, nervous system lesions, and nasal and oral involvement, in that order. Cardiac involvement leading to symptomatic heart disease is infrequent. Tables 15 and 16 represent the frequency of extrapulmonary involvement. Such involvement is suggested by signs and symptoms that denote dysfunction of the affected organs in the course of an established diagnosis of sarcoidosis. Even though hepatic granulomata can be demonstrated in most cases, clinical dysfunction related to this is uncommon.

Table 15. Extrapulmonary manifestations of Sarcoidosis and Their Frequency[a]

Peripheral lymphadenopathy	73%
Skin lesions	32%
Eye lesions	21%
Salivary gland enlargement	6%
Nervous system involvement	5%
Nose and oral cavity	3.5%

[a](Source: Mayock et al)

Laboratory Features

Cutaneous anergy reflects the disturbed T-cell function. Leukopenia is a frequent manifestation as well as elevated serum globulin and immunoglobulins. Hypercalcemia, hyperuricemia, and hypercalciuria may be evident. Elevated levels of serum angiotensin-converting enzyme (ACE) and lysozyme have been found. ACE may be elevated in about 80% of cases of sarcoidosis and in other diseases such as Gaucher's disease, leprosy, and coccidioidomycosis; but, since these conditions are clinically distinguishable from sarcoidosis an elevated value adds further support to the clinical diagnosis of sarcoidosis.

Roentgenographic Features

The most characteristic roentgenographic manifestations of sarcoidosis is bilateral hilar adenopathy (BHL) in association with paratracheal adenopathy. Parenchymal infiltrates may be present with or without lymphadenopathy. Based on this variable picture, certain groups can be identified. Group 1 consists of BHL alone (Fig. 22); group 2 consists of BHL with parenchymal infiltration; and group 3, parenchymal infiltrates alone. Roentgenographic appearance in advanced cases of group 3 is indistinguishable from that of pulmonary fibrosis. The term group rather than stage is preferable since the latter

Table 16. Patterns of Cutaneous, Ocular, and Neurologic Lesions in Sarcoidosis[ab]

Cutaneous Lesions		Ocular Lesions		Neurologic Lesions	
Maculopapular lesions	46%	Uveitis	37%	Extremity paresis	16%
Subcutaneous nodules	14%	Blindness	8%	Facial paralysis	12%
Hypo- or depigmentation	12%	Blurred vision	3%	Paresthesias	12%
Alopecia	7%	Scotoma	3%		
E. nodosum	6%	Conjunctivitis	3%		
Lupus pernio	1% or less				

[a](Source: Mayock et al)
[b]Figures represent percentages of those having cutaneous, ocular, and neurologic lesions.

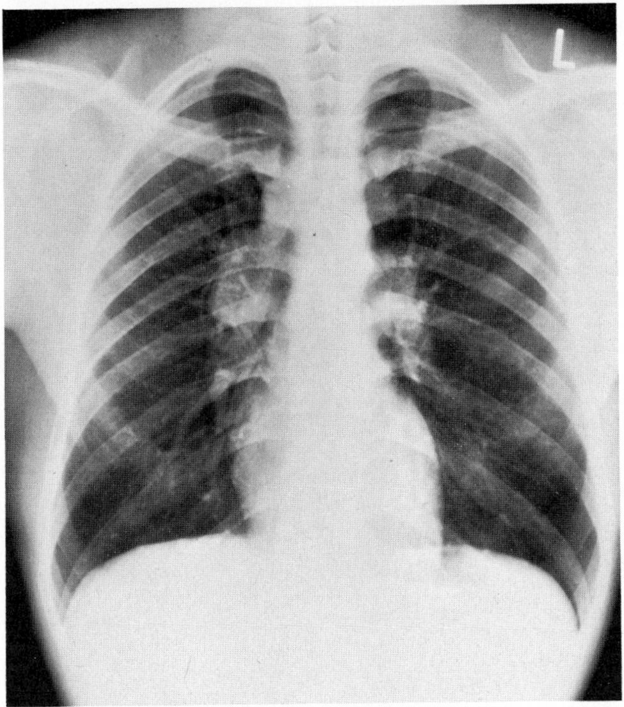

Figure 22. Sarcoidosis with bilateral hilar and right paratracheal lymph node enlargement (group 1).

imparts the mistaken impression that one necessarily progresses to the next. Uncommon patterns of sarcoidosis are anterior and/or posterior mediastinal lymphadenopathy, unilateral hilar adenopathy, multiple nodules, and miliary densities.

Diagnosis

Differential diagnosis is mainly from lymphoproliferative disorders as well as other causes of mediastinal adenopathy. In the authors' opinion, tissue confirmation is needed in all cases; the initial procedure of choice is transbronchial lung biopsy via a fiberoptic bronchoscope. In group I sarcoidosis, 60-100% positivity can be expected, depending on the number of biopsies performed. The positivity clearly approaches 95-100% when biopsy specimens are obtained from areas of pulmonary infiltration. Palpable lymph nodes in the scalene group or enlarged mediastinal or paratracheal nodes, skin lesions, or conjunctival lesions are other sites from where tissue may be obtained for diagnosis. The extent of such procedures employed depends mainly on the confidence with which sarcoidosis is diagnosed from a chest roentgenogram. The more atypical the manifestation, the more invasive the diagnostic procedure. However, the advent of the transbronchoscopic biopsy technique has improved the approach in that it is a safe, uniformly applicable, low morbidity procedure with a satisfactory yield.

Treatment

Corticosteroids are used in the treatment of sarcoidosis. There is no uniformity of opinion regarding their efficacy, nor are there any clear directions regarding the dosage and duration of such treatment. Due to the high probability of spontaneous resolution in group 1 cases, there is general agreement that observation until resolution or progression into another group is all that is needed. Vital organ involvement (e.g., eye, heart) and disfiguring skin lesions are indications for steroid therapy. Progressive pulmonary disease (best demonstrated by deteriorating pulmonary function studies) is also another indication. The authors prefer prednisone at a dose of 60 mg daily for 8-12 weeks. If there is improvement or if worsening has been halted, prednisone is continued and the dosage tapered by 10 mg every 8-12 weeks with clinical, physiologic, and roentgenographic monitoring. The minimum steroid dose needed to maintain improvement is then continued, preferably on an alternate-day schedule. Treatment is discontinued after 2 years with further observation for possible relapse. Some authorities have recommended that serial levels of serum angiotensin-converting enzyme be used to monitor progression of the disease and its response to therapy.

The rate of spontaneous resolution in group 1 cases approaches 80%; in Lofgren's syndrome (acute onset, arthralgia, erythema nodosum, and BHL), the rate of resolution is almost 100%. In group 2 or Group 3 cases, the rate of spontaneous resolution may vary from 30-50%. Irreversible pulmonary fibrosis occurs in some cases. This predisposes to cor pulmonale. Cystic areas within the fibrosed lungs may be the sites of aspergilloma formation. Progressive respiratory insufficiency and hemoptysis from the aspergillomas together account for the 5-10% mortality in this disease.

Collagen-Vascular Disorders

The extent of pulmonary involvement in collagen vascular disorders may vary considerably depending upon the criteria employed (clinical, roentgenographic, or histopathologic). Since these disorders involve connective tissue and blood vessels all over the body, the involvement of other systems may precede that of the lungs and dominate the clinical picture. In addition to the lung involvement that may result in varying degrees of lung dysfunction, associated pleural disease may also be present, depending on the type of disease. Pleuropulmonary manifestations of collagen vascular disorders are presented in Table 17. Even though the various disorders are represented here as pure entities, overlaps in the clinical picture of various collagen vascular disorders are common.

Hematologic Disorders

Involvement of the lungs occurs in a variety of hematologic disorders such as sickle cell disease, various types of leukemias and lymphomas, multiple myeloma, extramedullary hematopoeisis, Waldenström's macroglobulinemia, and mycosis fungoides. Sickle cell hemoglobinopathy may lead to intravascular thrombosis in the pulmonary arteries, arterioles, and capillaries, producing pulmonary infarction. In advanced cases,

Table 17. Clinical, Physiologic, and Radiographic Aspects of Pulmonary Involvement in Collagen Vascular Disorders

	Pertinent clinical, physiologic, and pathologic data	Radiographic Features		Therapy
		Lungs	*Pleura*	
I. "Rheumatoid Disease" 1) Diffuse interstitial fibrosis*	Exertional dyspnea, cough, pleuritic pain, clubbing, and cor pulmonale Frequency of pulmonary fibrosis greater with the presence of subcutaneous nodules. Less frequent with milder disease. End-inspiratory rales may be present. Restrictive ventilatory impairment; resting or exercise-induced hypoxemia. Nonspecific interstitial pneumonitis with lymphocysts, plasma cells, macrophages, polymorphs and eosinophils.	Small nodular or punctate lesions in early stages; later stages show medium to coarse reticulation and progressive loss of lung volume. Actual "honeycombing" is uncommon.	Pleural effusion or pleural thickening may coexist.	Mild disease needs only observation. Progressive worsening may dictate need for corticosteroids
2) Pleuritis with/without effusion	Remarkable predilection for males. Asymptomatic and an incidental finding in many cases. May antedate RA symptoms. Exudative, generally unilateral effusion with low sugar and high neutrophil count, Restrictive ventilatory impairment generally found.		Pleural thickening and/or effusion. May remain unchanged for months to years	No definite data available. Repeated aspirations, corticosteroids decortication, have all been tried.
3) Rheumatoid non-pneumoconiotic nodule	Relatively uncommon. Associated rheumatoid nodules may be present in the other parts of the body. No symptoms unless nodules enlarge or infection supervenes or nodules cavitate. Eosinophilia may occur. Restrictive ventilatory impairment may be found. Central zone of fibrinoid necrosis surrounded by a palisading layer of fibroblasts arranged perpendicular to the area of necrosis, and a layer of cellular or sclerotic granulation tissue surrounding the palisading layer.	Well-circumscribed, multiple, 2-7 cm in diameter, generally peripheral. Often cavitate leaving thick walls. Nodules may ebb and progress.	Pleural effusion and spontaneous pneumothorax may coexist.	Treatment not indicated unless complications occur. Steroids of limited value.
4) Caplan's syndrome	History of coal mining, silica, or asbestos exposure present. Other features same as 3. Central necrosis with peripheral fibroblasts arranged vertical to necrotic zone, with mononuclear, polymorphonuclear or giant cell infiltration. Necrotic zone contains the inorganic dust. A dark concentric ring surrounds the central core.	Well-circumscribed round, peripheral, 0.5-5.0 cm in size, cavitation usual, calcification and fibrosis, as well as rapid development in "crops".		No definite treatment needed.
5) Pulmonary hypertension and arteritis	Symptoms of precordial pain and dyspnea.	No features referable to pulmonary hypertension as such.		Uncertain.
6) Airway obstruction	Obstructive ventilatory impairment. Histopathologically,	Slight Hyperinflation.		Uncertain.

Table 17. Continued.

	Pertinent clinical, physiologic, and pathologic data	Radiographic Features: Lungs	Radiographic Features: Pleura	Therapy
	obliterative bronchiolitis may be present.			
II. Systemic lupus erythematosus[ab]	Lung and pleural involvement may vary from 50 to 70 percent of cases. Renal and CNS are other features.			
1) Pleurisy with or without effusion	Most common manifestation. Pleuritic type of pain may be an early symptom. Effusions are frequently small, bilateral or may be massive. Pericardial effusion and cardiomegaly may coexist. Exudative effusion, low glucose levels may be seen. LE cells may be seen in effusion. Pleural biopsy may show immunofluorescence to IgG and C_3.		Effusion may be seen.	Corticosteroids.
2) Infiltrates	Dyspnea. Cough with or without sputum. Significant restrictive lung disease may be present.	Resemble disc atelectasis.		
3) Acute lupus pneumonitis	Dyspnea and fever; cough, sputum. Evidence of infection absent. Severely ill. Biopsy may show alveolar wall thickening and mononuclear cell infiltration. Immunologic studies show granular IgG and C_3 immunofluorescence. Evidence of vasculitis may be seen.	Nonhomogenous infiltrate, localized or diffuse. Diagnosis is one of exclusion. Cardiomegaly may be present.		Corticosteroids with or without azathioprine.
4) Diffuse interstitial pneumonitis/ fibrosis	Much less common. Incidence varies from 0-3 percent. Dyspnea may be a symptom. Restrictive impairment on pulmonary function testing.	Diffuse reticulonodular infiltrates.		May respond to corticosteroids.
5) Diaphragmatic dysfunction	Dyspnea. Restrictive ventilatory impairment.	Elevated diaphragms. Fluoroscopy may show very little movement of the domes of diaphragms. Lungs appear small as a consequence.		Unknown.
III. Polymyositis-dermatomyositis	Dyspnea and cough may be present in a small number of cases. Aspiration pneumonia may occur secondary to pharyngeal muscle weakness. Pulmonary function tests show restrictive impairment when interstitial lung disease is present.	Reticulonodular infiltrate, or diffuse reticular infiltrate more at bases. Generally radiographs are normal.	No known cases of pleural involvement.	Corticosteroids.
IV. Progressive systemic sclerosis	Progressive dyspnea, cough may be productive. Pulmonary function tests generally show restrictive ventilatory defects and decreased DL_{CO} even when chest radiographs are normal. Aspiration pneumonia may occur because of esophageal dysfunction.	Reticular or reticulonodular infiltrates, predominantly lower zones, with little upper zone changes. Cystic lesions may occur in the late stages. Changes	Pneumothorax may occur. Other than slight basal pleural thickening, pleural involvement is uncommon.	Steroids generally ineffective.

Table 17. Continued.

	Pertinent clinical, physiologic, and pathologic data	Radiographic Features: Lungs	Radiographic Features: Pleura	Therapy
	Increased incidence of bronchio-alveolar carcinoma. Biopsy may show interstitial lung disease & vasculitis, sclerosis of the vessels or intimal proliferation.	due to aspiration pneumonia may be superadded.		
V. Sjögren's syndrome	Extent of pulmonary involvement varies between 1.5-9 percent. Chief symptoms are cough, pleuritic pain, dyspnea and recurrent pneumonias. Pleural effusions may occur. Interstitial disease, with lymphoid follicles may be observed. Pseudolymphomas occur with the potential for progression into malignant lymphoma. Diaphragmatic myopathy is very rare.	Diffuse interstitial infiltrates with reticular or reticulonodular pattern, diffuse air space infiltration, or bibasilar infiltrates.	Pleural effusion unilateral or bilateral.	Bronchodilator therapy may be needed, as well as humidification. Corticosteroids are useful in some cases. Corticosteroid or cytotoxic drugs or radiation may prevent progression into malignant lymphoma. The latter developing in Sjögren's syndrome is generally resistant to therapy.
VI. Ankylosing spondylitis	Incidence of pulmonary involvement is 1.3-30%. Chest wall restriction occurs more commonly but it does not lead to any clinical problems, although pulmonary function studies may show diminished vital capacity, and total lung capacity and increased residual volume and functional residual capacity. Apical fibrobullous lesions occur, initially unilateral and then bilateral. Colonization of these lesions with aspergillus may occur.	Initially one-sided but later bilateral, fibrobullous lesions that may have thin or thick walls. There may be formation of aspergillomas in these abnormal air spaces. "Bamboospine" is characteristic.	Apical pleural thickening. Rare cases of pleural effusion have been recorded. Diffuse pleural thickening has been reported.	Aspergillomas generally do not need surgical management unless life-threatening hemoptysis occurs.
VII. Goodpasture's syndrome	Rare disease, primary in young men. Hemoptysis is the leading symptom. Associated renal disease may be present and may be characterized by proteinuria, hematuria, red cell casts and azotemia. Pulmonary manifestations may precede renal disease by weeks to 1 year. Linear deposits of IgG in the renal basement membrane and antiglomerular basement membrane antibodies in the serum.	Bilateral, diffuse, pulmonary infiltrates.	No known pleural manifestations.	Bilateral nephrectomy.
VIII. Necrotizing vasculitis of the polyarteritis nodosa type. (PAN)	Classic PAN usually does not affect lungs. In allergic angiitis with granulomatosis (Churg-Strauss) lung lesions may be seen in the background of asthma. Eosinophilia may be present. Cough, wheezing, and hemoptysis may occur.	Fleeting pulmonary infiltrates, diffuse interstitial lung disease, or nodularity with cavitation. The radiographs may be normal.	Pleural effusion may occur rarely.	Corticosteroids or low dose cyclophosphamide.
IX. Wegener's granulomatosis (Fig. 23)	Involves upper and/or lower respiratory tract and/or kidneys. Extent of lung involvement approaches 95%,	Bilateral nodular infiltrative lesions that cavitate. Mass densities or airway	Pleural thickening and pleural effusions are uncommon.	1) In patients without renal failure, cyclophosphamide is

Table 17. Continued.

	Pertinent clinical, physiologic, and pathologic data	Radiographic Features: Lungs	Radiographic Features: Pleura	Therapy
	followed by paranasal sinuses (90%), kidneys (85%), nasopharynx (70%) and eyes (60%). A limited form involving only the lungs is well known. Presenting symptoms refer to upper respiratory tract and include nasal discharge, sinusitis, otitis media and nasal ulcerative lesions. Cough, hemoptysis and chest pain are symptoms of lung involvement. Pathologically the lesions are necrotizing granulomatous vasculitides.	obstruction from endobronchial lesions are uncommon patterns.		started in 1-2 mg/kg body weight and continued for 2 weeks. If needed. dose may be raised by 25 mg increments, keeping WBC count over 3,000/mm³. 2) In patients with renal failure, cyclophosphamide is started IV in 4 mg/kg × 3 days with reduction in dose thereafter to 1-2 mg/kg per day. Associated steroid therapy may be needed in both instances.
X. Lymphomatoid granulomatosis	Sinus and upper airway involvement unusual. Lung involvement is 100%. Leukopenia and anergy common. Skin and kidneys are involved (45%). ESR may be normal. Spleen, lymph node and bone marrow are generally not involved. Tendency to develop into lymphoma. Lesions are angiocentric and angiodestructive, with atypical lymphocytoid cellular infiltration.	Bilateral, hazy, multiple densities, which may later coalesce or become better defined. Cavitation uncommon.	Pleural effusion may occur.	Cyclophosphamide therapy is useful when started early.

[a] More than one type of manifestation or roentgenographic feature may be present at one time.

[b] Most common cause of pulmonary processes in SLE is infection. Diligent search should be made to document an infectious ailment in these patients, especially in the presence of pulmonary infiltrates and pleural effusions.

cor pulmonale may ensue. In addition, this disease predisposes to pneumococcal, salmonella, and mycoplasma infections of the lung.

Leukemias

Symptoms of lung involvement in the leukemias are nonspecific and include cough, fever, bloody sputum, chest pain, and dyspnea. Pulmonary involvement is generally seen later in the course of the established disease, but a relatively infrequent initial presentation with diffuse lung involvement is well known and may be characterized by respiratory distress, oxygenation failure, and poor prognosis. Roentgenographic features are nonspecific and include reticulonodular or nodular densities. Large solitary or multiple mass lesions due to chloroma formation are rare. A pattern of diffuse pulmonary infiltration secondary to alveolar proteinosis has been reported in various types of leukemias. Pulmonary infiltrates in the leukemias are often due to infections. However, differentiation from intrapulmonary hemorrhage, drug-induced lung disease, and leukemic infiltration is difficult. Definitive diagnosis of these lesions is possible only by lung biopsy, the need for which must be dictated by clinical circumstances.

Lymphomas

The vast majority of cases of lymphoma (over 99%) that involve the lung are of either Hodgkin's or non-Hodgkin's type, with primary pulmonary lymphoma accounting for the remainder. Constitutional symptoms referable to the primary disease such as weight loss, night sweats, and pruritus may be manifest. In the primary type as well as in a very small fraction of non-Hodgkin's type, pulmonary manifestations may be the sole presenting feature. Cough, dyspnea, sputum production, chest pain, and bloody sputum are symptoms indicative of pulmonary involvement. Clinical examination generally shows evidence of extrathoracic disease. Pleural effusions may be present in about 30% of cases. Superior vena cava obstruction is another mode of presentation.

Pathologically, Hodgkin's lymphoma may be either lympho-

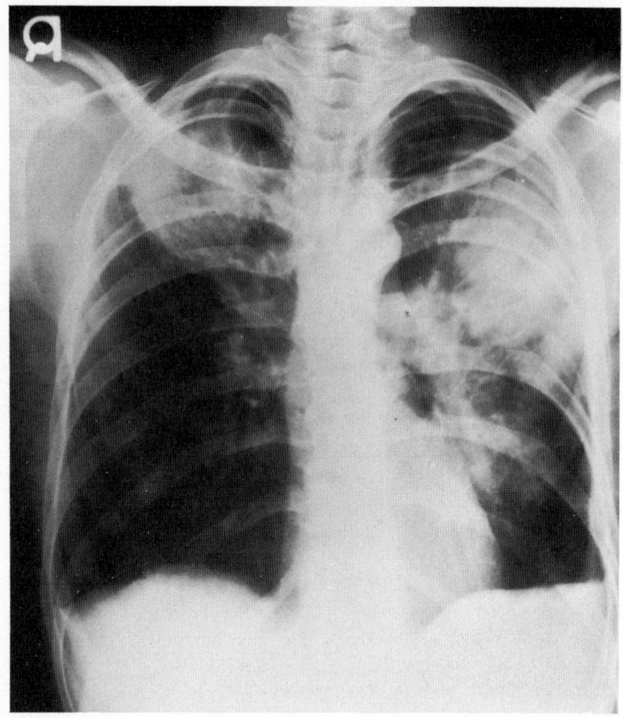

Figure 23. Wegener's granulomatosis. Bilateral opacities are present. Right upper zone density is cavitated.

cyte predominant, nodular sclerosing, or the mixed cellular type. Another variety, lymphocyte depletion type, tends to be predominantly subdiaphragmatic. Non-Hodgkin's lymphoma may be a nodular or diffuse type. Primary pulmonary lymphoma is usually lymphocytic or, less commonly, histiocytic.

Most common intrathoracic roentgenographic manifestation of a lymphoma is mediastinal lymphadenopathy. Approximately 40-50% of patients manifest this feature on initial presentation. Characteristically, the lymphadenopathy is bilateral and asymmetric. Enlargement of the anterior mediastinal nodes may cause sternal erosion, and posterior mediastinal lymphadenopathy may manifest as a paravertebral masses. Calcification of these nodes may occur after radiotherapy. Parenchymal lesions are seen in about one-third of the cases in association with mediastinal lymphadenopathy (mediastinal lymphadenopathy may be absent in cases that have undergone prior mediastinal irradiation). These lesions may be nodular, reticulonodular, or lobar densities and atelectasis secondary to endobronchial involvement. Cavitation may occur in Hodgkin's lymphoma. Pleural effusions occur in 10-15% of cases. These may be serous, serosanguineous, or chylous and are usually secondary to mediastinal lymph node involvement.

Diagnosis is made by lung or mediastinal node biopsy obtained by an appropriate route. Fiberoptic bronchoscopy, mediastinoscopy, Chamberlain's procedure, or full throacotomy are available options. Accessible extrapulmonary lesions, if present, should be biopsied first.

The reader is referred to the section on lymphomas for management. Primary pulmonary lymphoma managed by resectional surgery in one series resulted in a 57% 5-year survival.

Multiple Myeloma

In a retrospective review of 958 cases of multiple myeloma, 46% had thoracic involvement during the course of the illness. These were classified as thoracic skeletal abnormalities in 28%, pulmonary infiltrates in 10%, plasmacytomas in 12%, and pleural effusions in 6%. The most frequent cause of pulmonary infiltrates was pneumonia; the most common cause of pleural effusion was congestive heart failure secondary to amyloidosis. Pleural effusions secondary to myelomatous pleural involvement also occurred. In the past, the majority of the cases of pneumonia were secondary to *Diplococcus (Streptococcus) pneumoniae*; but an increasing role of Gram-negative bacteria and opportunistic organisms is becoming apparent. Pulmonary thromboembolic disease was diagnosed in 1.5% of cases and was the cause of death in six cases.

Waldenström's Macroglobulinemia

Pleuropulmonary manifestations were judged to be on the order of 0-3% in cases of Waldenström's macroglobulinemia, but this low incidence is said to be due to infrequent recognition of the pulmonary abnormalities. The major symptoms of lung involvement are cough and dyspnea. Roentgenologic appearances of these pulmonary abnormalities include mass lesions, pleural effusions often with high protein content and monoclonal gammopathy in the fluid, diffuse pulmonary infiltrates, and hilar enlargement. Lung involvement is sometimes the sole feature of the disease, and clinical recognition is important since therapy with chlorambucil is generally followed by improvement.

Mycosis Fungoides

Although necropsy studies show that lung involvement is common in mycosis fungoides, there are no specific symptoms or roentgenologic features. Roentgenographically, these may manifest as nodules, infiltrates, pleural effusion, or mediastinal adenopathy.

Histiocytosis X

Eosinophilic granuloma, Letterer-Siwe disease, and Hand-Schüller-Christian disease together are referred to as histiocytosis X. Lung involvement in histiocytosis X may occur in conjunction with the systemic disease or as isolated lung disease. Pathologically, there is severe interstitial fibrosis with collections of histiocytes, lymphocytes, and eosinophils.

Histiocytosis X is predominantly a disease of young adults with a distinct male preponderance. Symptoms of lung involvement include cough, sputum production, dyspnea, chest pain, recurrent pneumothorax, and hemoptysis. Systemic manifestations such as weight loss and fever may be present. In the presence of systemic disease lymphadenopathy, splenomegaly, and diabetes insipidus may occur. Peripheral eosinophilia is not seen. Most common roentgenographic manifestations are miliary nodulation with a reticular pattern; less frequent are cystic lesions and honeycombing. Pulmonary physiologic data show generally restrictive ventilatory impairment, but airway obstruction and the development of pulmonary emphysema are not rare. No treatment regimen has been found to be effective. Thoracotomy and pleurodesis may be needed for recurrent pneumothoraces. Spontaneous improvement may occur; but with extremes of age, diffuse extrapulmonary disease, recurrent pneumothoraces, or extensive initial lung involvement with cyst formations and low DL_{CO}, a poor outcome is likely.

INFILTRATIVE DISEASES DUE TO INHALED ORGANIC SUBSTANCES (HYPERSENSITIVITY PNEUMONITIDES)

Hypersensitivity pneumonitis is defined as an immunologically mediated lung inflammation secondary to inhalation of a variety of organic dusts. These dusts contain proteinaceous antigens, many of fungal origin. Various agents leading to hypersensitivity pneumonitides and the occupations predisposed to them are outlined in Table 18.

Hypersensitivity pneumonitis may occur in both atopic and nonatopic people. The immunologic reactivity of the host is a key factor since the disease develops in only a small fraction of exposed persons. It has been suggested that the basic pathogenetic mechanism is Arthus (type 3) reaction involving the lung. The response may vary depending on the atopic status of the individual, with the atopic person showing an immediate airway obstruction-type response followed later by a parenchymal reaction, wheras nonatopic people show generally only the late reaction. Precipitating antibodies to the specific agents, belonging to the IgG type, are often detected in the serum.

Early hypersensitivity pneumonitis is characterized by granulomatous interstitial pneumonitis. There is infiltration of the pulmonary interstitium with lymphocytes and some plasma cells. Central areas of necrosis, Langhan's giant cells, epithelioid cells, and foreign body giant cells are seen in the interstitium. In the alveoli, foamy histiocytes and plasma cells may be present. In the chronic type, there is interstitial and focal peribronchial fibrosis, with thickened alveolar septa and lymphocytic infiltration.

Clinical Features

Hypersensitivity pneumonitis may present in an acute or chronic form. In the acute form symptoms of myalgia, fevers, chills, chest tightness, cough, and dyspnea occur about 4-6 hours after exposure to the offending organic dust. Wheezing is notable for its absence. These manifestations subside in

Table 18. The Hypersensitivity Pneumonitides

Disease	*Source of Exposure*	*Specific Agent*
Aspergillosis	Aspergillus spores	*Aspergillus fumigatus*
Bagassosis	Moldy bagasse	*Thermoactinomyces vulgaris*
Chicken raiser's disease	Chicken protein	Feathers, serum, and droppings
Cheese worker's lung	Moldy cheese	*Penicillium casei*
Coffee worker's lung	Coffee bean dust	Coffee dust
Detergent worker's lung	Detergent making	*Bacillus subtilis*
Dog house disease	Moldy straw	*Aspergillus versicolor*
Furrier's lung	Animal hair dust	None known
Humidifier lung	Fungal spores	Thermophilic actinomycetes
Maple bark stripper's lung	Moldy maple bark	*Cryptostroma corticale*
Malt worker's lung	Moldy barley	*Aspergillus clavatus* *Aspergillus fumigatus*
Mushroom worker's lung	Mushroom compost	*Micropolyspora faeni* *Thermoactinomyces vulgaris*
New Guinea lung (Papuan lung)	Moldy thatch dust	None known
Paprika splitter's lung	Paprika	Mucor stolonifer
Pituitary snuff taker's lung	Pituitary snuff	Bovine and porcine proteins
Sequoiosis	Redwood sawdust	Graphium, *Aurobasidium pullulans*
Suberosis	Cork dust	*Penicillium frequentans*
Wheat weavil disease	Wheat flour	*Sitophilus granarius*
Wood pulp worker's disease	Moldy wood pulp	*Alternaria*
Pigeon breeder's lung	Avian protein	None known

about 12-18 hours. Spontaneous recovery follows, and symptoms recur on re-exposure. Physical examination may disclose an acutely ill patient with tachypnea, tachycardia, and late inspiratory basilar rales. Leukocytosis is generally present as well as elevated levels of serum IgG, IgM, and IgA. Elevated IgE levels indicate concomitant allergic diathesis (asthma or rhinitis). Precipitins to the offending organic material are often found in the serum, but these are only of limited help in establishing a diagnosis. Roentgenograms of the chest may be normal or may show a patchy, diffuse infiltrate or fine nodular pattern with a symmetrical distribution. Pulmonary function studies show diminished vital capacity, the total lung capacity, diminished lung compliance, and low DL_{CO}. Diminution in $FEV_{1.0}$ and expiratory flow rates may be observed as well.

Prolonged exposure to organic dust, irrespective of quantity, may lead to the chronic form of hypersensitivity pneumonitis characterized by chronic, progressive dyspnea and interstitial fibrosis. Chest roentgenograms show diffuse fibrotic disease, often with honeycombing. Pulmonary physiologic derangements include progressive restrictive ventilatory impairment with hypoxemia and low DL_{CO}.

Diagnosis

Diagnosis depends upon a thorough clinical history and on pulmonary function testing following careful exposure to the offending antigen. Other ancillary methods are precipitins and chest roentgenograms, although these by themselves are not diagnostic and should be taken in conjunction with the entire picture. A search of the work environment or home may be necessary to obtain the antigenic material from the dusts or molds. Lung biopsy may be useful and the findings should be correlated with the clinical picture.

Treatment

Identification and avoidance of the responsible antigen are the principal factors in management. In the acute phase, these alone may be sufficient. In selected cases, corticosteroids may be administered to hasten recovery. In the chronic stage, corticosteroids may be useful; but, once irreversible fibrosis has occurred, the benefits of steroid therapy may only be minimal.

DIFFUSE INFILTRATIVE DISEASES OF UNKNOWN ORIGIN

Diffuse Interstitial Pulmonary Fibrosis

Diffuse interstitial pulmonary fibrosis (DIPF) is a disease of unknown etiology characterized by inflammation and fibrosis of the pulmonary interstitium. This disease has been described under several synonyms and is largely a disease of exclusion even though it has certain distinct clinical, histologic, and roentgenographic aspects. Classification of this entity continues to be controversial. The major reason for the controversy is the fact that the disease essentially represents a spectrum in terms of clinical, roentgenographic, histologic, and immunologic features.

Although the triggering mechanism is unknown, it is believed that the interstitial collagen becomes recognized as antigenic and "nonself" leading to its disruption, rearrangement, and replacement by abnormal collagen. Recent demonstration of increased collagenase in the lower respiratory tract of patients with DIPF is in keeping with the central theme of collagen destruction and supports the concept of sustained lysis and disordered resynthesis. The initial influenza-like illness that characterizes the onset of DIPF, in many cases suggests that a viral infection may initiate this process, whereas the familial clustering of some cases may denote a hereditary/familial predisposition.

Histologic features include alveolar septal fibrosis and interstitial infiltration by lymphocytes, macrophages, plasma cells, neutrophils, and eosinophils. Cuboidalization of the alveolar lining cells and desquamation of cells into the alveolar space are other findings. Granulomas, arteritis, and mineral deposits are absent. Based on cellular characteristics, a system of classification was proposed (giant cell, lymphoid, desquamative, usual, etc.) for the interstitial pneumonias, indicating prognosis and guiding therapy; but the only usefulness of this classification may be in predicting to some extent the responsiveness to therapy. Differences between usual (UIP) and desquamative interstitial pneumonias (DIP) are represented in Table 19. Although DIPF is considered a progressive and uniformly fatal disease, there are occasional long-term survivors. However, average survival in this disease is only 47 months from the onset of symptoms. DeRemee et al. have suggested that patients without rales and clubbing run a relatively benign course. There is also evidence that the histologic features influence survival, namely, better with DIP and worse with UIP.

Clinical Features

The disease has been described in infancy and old age, but the peak incidence is in the fifth and sixth decades of life, without predilection for either sex. Exertional dyspnea is the most frequent symptom. Nonproductive cough is a late manifestation. As many as one-half the patients relate an influenza-like illness prior to the onset of dyspnea. Constitutional symptoms such as weight loss, fever, myalgias, and arthralgias may be present. Roughly three-fourths of the patients may manifest clubbing and, in a few, clubbing may be the presenting symptom. Hypertrophic osteoarthropathy rarely accompanies clubbing. Tachypnea is the earliest physical sign. Rales of an end-inspiratory type (resembling the tearing apart of the Velcro adhesive in blood pressure cuffs, called "Velcro rales," also called cellophane rales) may be heard. Cardiac exam may be normal, but an accentuated pulmonic component of the second sound is frequently present. With significant arterial desaturation, central cyanosis may appear.

Laboratory Features

Erythrocytosis is uncommon, although it may occur in the very late stages of the disease. Sedimentation rate may be increased. Many patients with DIPF exhibit immunologic abnormalities that include cryoimmunoglobulins, rheumatoid factor, antinuclear antibodies, positive lupus erythematosus (LE) cell phenomenon, and elevated serum immunoglobulins. Circulating immune complexes have also been found and

Table 19. Histologic Features of Usual and Desquamative Interstitial Pneumonia (UIP and DIP)

	UIP	*DIP*
Fibrosis	Marked	Minimal
Necrosis	None to mild	None
Hyaline membranes	Moderate	None
Exudate (type)	Pleomorphic and dense	Mononuclear cells
Exudate (site)	Predominantly interstitial	Predominantly alveolar, sparse interstitial
Lymphoid follicles	None to very mild	Moderate
Alveolar wall thickening	Marked	None to slight
Uniformity of lesions	Highly variegated	Monotonously uniform

correlate well with cellular infiltration of the biopsied lung specimen.

Arterial hypoxemia at rest or on exercise occurs in the large majority of patients and is due to ventilation-perfusion mismatching. Pulmonary function studies show findings typical of a restrictive ventilatory impairment including low vital capacity, reduced lung volumes, and reduced DL_{CO}. The reduced DL_{CO} is due to ventilation-perfusion mismatching as well as attenuation of the vascular bed.

Roentgenographic Features

Chest roentgenograms may be normal in about 15% of the cases. The other abnormal patterns are small lungs and/or lungs with infiltrates. These infiltrates may be reticular, reticulonodular, nodular, or of a ground glass appearance. Air bronchograms may be seen with diffuse disease. In advanced cases, honeycombing may occur (Fig. 24).

Diagnosis

As proposed by DeRemee et al., a definitive diagnosis of DIPF may be made in the presence of rales, finger clubbing, and altered immune activity. In the absence of altered immunity, the diagnosis becomes probable and, when only histologic evidence with or without immune abnormalities is present, the diagnosis becomes possible. The entire phenomena, taken together, make the clinical picture quite characteristic.

The final diagnosis, however, depends upon open lung biopsy. Arguments against lung biopsy are often made on the grounds that functional deterioration would necessitate steroid therapy, notwithstanding the findings of the biopsy. No doubt this is true; but the degree of cellularity and the extent of fibrosis (UIP versus DIP) give a clue as to the outcome of therapy as well as help grade the severity and, to some extent, the prognosis in a given case. Also, differentiation from vasculitis and pneumoconiosis is possible only on the basis of a lung biopsy. Analysis of bronchoalveolar lavage fluid for immunoglobulins, lymphocytes, and neutrophils may help distinguish between various interstitial lung diseases, but the usefulness of this method is not yet established.

Treatment

Corticosteroids are the drugs currently employed for treatment of DIPF. In general, the more cellular and less fibrotic the findings on lung biopsy, the more the likelihood of steroid responsiveness. In an analysis of 20 patients treated with prednisone-azathioprine regimen, Winterbauer et al. found that the degree of fibrosis as well as the duration of the disease were factors in judging responsiveness to treatment. This is explained by the fact that the shorter the history, the less the likelihood of extensive fibrosis.

Prednisone is started in a dose of 1 mg/kg body weight although, in Winterbauer's series, a large dose of 100 mg per day was employed initially. The dosage should be gradually tapered using pulmonary physiologic testing as the control. Use of gallium-67 scintiscanning and exercise pulmonary func-

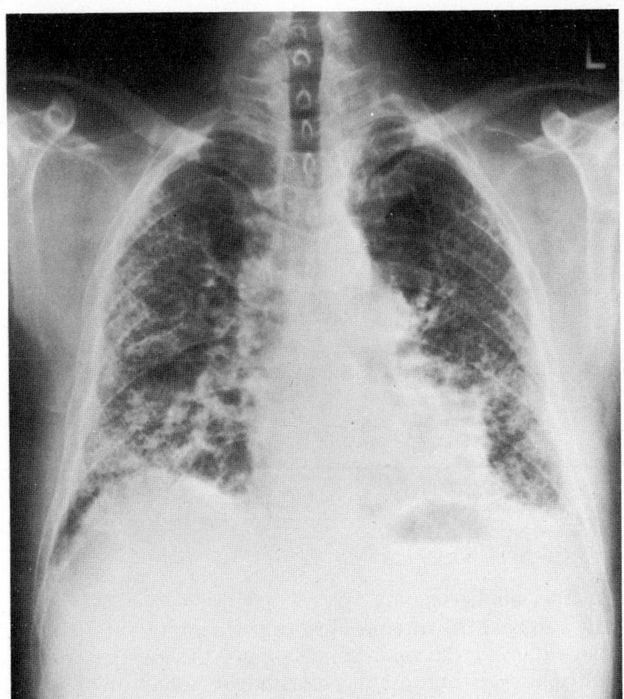

Figure 24. Diffuse interstitial pulmonary fibrosis. Widespread interstitial infiltration with honeycombing.

tion studies have both been advocated as criteria to judge dosage reductions. The minimal amount of steroid that maintains the improvement is continued. Withdrawal of steroids or abrupt reductions in dosage have both been followed by severe worsening in status. The duration of steroid therapy is indeterminate. Oxygen therapy may be needed if resting hypoxemia (Pa_{O_2} less than 50 mm Hg) is present or if it develops on exercise.

Other Miscellaneous Entities

Pulmonary Alveolar Proteinosis

This disease is characterized by widespread alveolar filling with a proteinaceous, lipid-rich, PAS-positive material. The disease may occur as a primary disorder or it may occur in association with various types of leukemias, paraproteinemias, and silicosis. Presenting symptoms are exertional dyspnea, productive cough, and often constitutional symptoms such as weight loss. Finger clubbing may be observed and bibasilar rales may be heard. Roentgenographically it appears as a diffuse, bilateral, air-space infiltration. Diagnosis is made by lung biopsy. Complications include progressive respiratory insufficiency and pulmonary infections with *Nocardia*, *Candida*, *Aspergillus*, and *Staphylococcus*. Lobar lavage is the accepted method of treatment, although aerosolized trypsin administered via IPPB has been employed successfully.

Idiopathic Pulmonary Hemosiderosis

This is a rare disease of the young. Recurrent hemoptysis, iron deficiency anemia, and fleeting pulmonary infiltrates characterize its clinical course. Men are affected twice as frequently as women. Generalized lymphadenopathy and hepatosplenomegaly may be associated. Transient pulmonary infiltrates of bibasilar and perihilar distribution may be seen on chest roentgenograms during active hemorrhage. Diagnosis is made by lung biopsy and by exclusion of Goodpasture's syndrome with appropriate studies.

Pulmonary Lymphangioleiomyomatosis

This rare disorder occurs exclusively in women of child-bearing age and is generally believed to be a hamartomatous process with proliferation of smooth-muscle cells along the lymphatics, bronchioles, and alveoli characterizing its pathology. Clinical features are progressive dyspnea, recurrent pneumothoraces, and chylous pleural effusions. No curative treatment is available.

NEOPLASMS OF THE LUNG

MALIGNANT NEOPLASMS

Bronchogenic Carcinoma

Since a substantial amount of information in this area has been provided in the section on oncology, the focus here is on the diagnostic workup and preoperative evaluation of primary malignant lung neoplasms and the management of a solitary pulmonary nodule.

Diagnostic Evaluation

Even at the time of initial presentation, only about one-fifth of the patients with bronchogenic carcinoma have a neoplasm localized to the chest. Clinical history and thorough physical examination along with various laboratory screening tests may help identify those with metastases. Although an intelligent assessment of the likely cell type is possible based on presenting features and roentgenographic characteristics, the final arbiter is the tissue diagnosis.

Cytologic examination of an induced or expectorated sample of sputum should be uniformly employed in all instances where a lung carcinoma is suspected. The likelihood of a positive diagnosis by this method varies from 50% for peripheral lesions to almost 90% for central lesions. The results may be even better with repeated samples. In many instances, identification of the cell type is possible. If small cell carcinoma is unequivocally diagnosed by this method, surgical therapy or staging mediastinoscopy are contraindicated.

Flexible fiberoptic bronchoscopy (FFB) is indicated under the following circumstances: when lung cancer is suspected and sputum examination is either unrevealing or yields equivocal results, and when sputum examination discloses malignant cells other than a small cell type to assess the feasibility of resection from the standpoint of tracheobronchial anatomy. During FFB, it is possible not only to visualize endobronchial lesions if present, but also to obtain tissue by direct biopsy and/or brushing/biopsy under fluoroscopic guidance of localized nodules or infiltrates. When endobronchial lesions are visualized by the endoscopist, the likelihood of a positive diagnosis exceeds 95% but drops to around 70% when such lesions are not visualized. Postbronchoscopy sputa should be collected for cytologic evaluation.

If sputum cytologic examinations and FFB have been unrewarding, further diagnostic approaches should be tailored to suit the clinical setting. If palpable lymph nodes are present, these should be biopsied, especially those in the scalene group. Mediastinoscopy is useful for diagnosis and staging purposes. Diagnostic yield of mediastinoscopy is higher in the presence of abnormality in the mediastinal area demonstrated by chest roentgenogram, computed tomography (CT) or gallium 67 scintiscan, and when large proximal densities are present in the chest roentgenograms. Metastatic involvement of scalene nodes or contralateral mediastinal nodes are contraindications to resectional surgery. Ipsilateral mediastinal node involvement with carcinoma other than squamous cell type and ipsilateral nodal involvement in patients with poor pulmonary reserve would obviate resectional surgery. If mediastinal or palpable peripheral nodes are absent, thoracotomy, frozen-section examination, and resection can be considered if cardiovascular/pulmonary function is adequate. If, on the other hand, general anesthesia and surgery are considered risky on these grounds, further attempts to obtain tissue should be made only if it is necessary to carry out a treatment plan. In accessible lesions, transthoracic needle aspiration may be attempted. The risk of pneumothorax from this procedure is about 20-30%, and that of bleeding around 20%; positive results may be obtained in 80-90% of cases depending on the expertise of the operator. Transthoracic needle aspiration is inadvisable if the patient is otherwise a candidate for surgery and/or if the lesion is close to the heart or major vessels.

Preoperative Evaluation

Surgical resection offers the best cure rate for bronchogenic carcinoma. Contraindications to thoracotomy and resection are outlined in Table 20. Routine brain, bone, or liver scanning is generally nonproductive; these should be reserved for cases with abnormal neurologic findings, bone pain, or abnormal liver function tests, respectively. The role of clinical assessment, pulmonary function testing, and of avoidance of smoking once surgery is decided upon, cannot be overemphasized. The best index of pulmonary function is the $FEV_{1.0}$. Pulmonary resection for pneumonectomy is inadvisable if $FEV_{1.0}$ is less than 2.0 L, particularly for a right pneumonectomy. Similarly, lobectomy is inadvisable if the $FEV_{1.0}$ is less than 1.3 L.

Prognosis of Non-Small-Cell Lung Cancer

Prognosis depends on the stage of the disease. Staging, based on the TNM classification, is outlined in Table 21. In Stage 0, (usually epidermoid carcinoma), the 5-year survival is approximately 70%, which drops to 30-40 percent for Stage I. A dismal 10-15% characterizes Stage II and the 5-year survival is only 1% in Stage III.

Carcinoids and Bronchial Gland Tumors

In the past, these tumors were collectively called bronchial adenomas. Except for the rare mucous gland adenomas, (see classification in Table 22), these are considered low-grade carcinomas that lead to local invasion, with local lymphatic and widespread metastases. Together they account for 5% of all lung neoplasms. Among these, carcinoids are the most frequent, comprising 80%.

Table 20. Contraindications to Thoracotomy and Resection in Bronchogenic Carcinoma

Operability
Poor cardiac reserve (recent myocardial infarction, etc.)[a]
Poor pulmonary reserve[a]
Age over 70[b]
Small cell carcinoma[a]
Resectability
Distant metastases[a]
Superior vena cava obstruction[a]
Pericardial/esophageal/phrenic nerve involvement[a]
Recurrent laryngeal nerve involvement[a]
Contralateral mediastinal lymph node involvement[a]
Involvement of trachea, carina, or lesion within 2.0 cm from carina[a]
Malignant pleural effusion[a]
Pleural effusion[a]
Chest wall involvement except in Pancoast's tumor[a]

[a] Absolute
[b] Relative

The location of carcinoids may be central or peripheral in the bronchial tree, originating from Kultchitsky's cells of the bronchial mucous glands or those of the bronchial mucosa, respectively. Typical carcinoids have a more uniform pattern of cellularity and do not generally metastasize, whereas atypical types are more pleomorphic on histology and generally

Table 21. Staging of Lung Cancer (TNM)

(T) Primary tumors

- To–No evidence of primary tumor
- Tx–Positive cytology of sputum/bronchial secretion with negative chest x-ray and bronchoscopy
- T_1 –Tumor <3.0 cm in diameter, with surrounding aerated lung tissue, bronchial invasion at bronchoscopy not proximal to lobar bronchus
- T_2 –Tumor >3.0 cm; extends to hilum; proximal extent at least 2.0 cm from main carina; if atelectasis/obstructive pneumonitis present, entire lung is not involved; no pleural effusion
- T_3 –Tumor size immaterial; extension into contiguous structures, such as chest wall, mediastinum, or diaphragm, proximal extension to within 2.0 cm of carina; atelectasis/obstructive pneumonitis of entire lung; pleural effusion

(N) Regional lymph nodes

- N_0 –No metastases to regional lymph node
- N_1 –Regional lymph node metastases
- N_2 –Mediastinal lymph node metastases

(M) Distant metastases

- M_0 –No distant metastases
- M_1 –Distant metastasis(es) present

Stage	*TNM*
0	Tx N_0 M_0
I	T_1 N_0 M_0
	T_1 N_1 M_0
	T_2 N_0 M_0
II	T_2 N_1 M_0
III	T_3, any N or M
	N_2, any T or M
	M_1, any T or N

Table 22. Carcinoids and Bronchial Gland Tumors

Carcinoids[a]
Central
Peripheral
Bronchial gland tumors
Cylindromas (adenoid cystic carcinomas)
Mucoepidermoid carcinomas
Mucous gland adenomas
Benign mixed tumors
Acinic cell tumors
Oncocytomas

[a] Typical and atypical, based on histology.

metastasize. Carcinoids appear as endobronchial lesions and lead to a wide variety of symptoms: cough, recurrent post-obstructive pneumonias, and hemoptyses are local effects, whereas carcinoid syndrome represents the systemic manifestation. The latter is characterized by flushing episodes, wheezing, lacrimation, periorbital edema, and (in cases of bronchial carcinoids as opposed to intestinal carcinoids) left-sided cardiac valvular lesions. Carcinoid syndrome reflects widespread metastases and is confirmed by increased urinary excretion of 5-hydroxyindoleacetic acid. Occasionally, the carcinoids may be elaborate ectopic ACTH or growth hormone resulting in Cushing's syndrome or acromegaly, respectively.

Diagnosis depends on the clinical history, occurrence in younger age groups, and by bronchoscopy. Treatment is thoracotomy and resection that may need bilobectomy or even pneumonectomy depending on tumor location. Mediastinoscopy is indicated if mediastinal widening is apparent on chest roentgenogram. Prognosis is good in nonmetastatic typical carcinoids (94% 5-year survival), fair in metastatic (71% 5-year survival); and worse in atypical cases (30-50% mortality within 5 years of diagnosis).

In the order of frequency, bronchial gland tumors are cylindromas (also called adenoid cystic carcinomas) mucoepidermoid carcinomas, and mucous gland adenomas. Cylindromas involve major bronchi or the trachea and show a tendency for early metastases, manifest local symptoms, and carry a prognosis similar to that of atypical carcinoids. Mucoepidermoid carcinoma is uncommon. Mucous gland adenoma is rare, benign, and similar in histology to mixed salivary gland tumors.

Other Malignant Tumors of the Lung (Metastatic)

Almost all tumor metastases to the lungs occur via a hematogenous route, whereas some tend to spread via the lymphatics. Approximately 50% of patients dying with tumor metastases have lung involvement and in the vast majority of cases, the primary tumor is in the colorectum, genitourinary tract, breast, or skeletal tissue. Ipsilateral or contralateral metastases from a primary cancer in the lung are also known to occur.

In the hematogenous type, the roentgenograms generally show a nodular pattern without lymph node enlargement. Presence of reticulonodular infiltrates, hilar-mediastinal adenopathy, and/or pleural effusion characterizes the lymphatic spread (or lymphangitis carcinomatosa). Neoplasms that produce the latter pattern originate in the breast, lung, prostate, and gastrointestinal tract. Whereas most neoplasms produce multiple metastases sarcomas, testicular and breast cancers, left colon, rectal, and renal carcinomas may produce solitary metastases. If such metastases are truly solitary (computed tomography may be very helpful here) resection is followed by 5-year survival in more than 30% of cases, particularly when the primary neoplasm is osteogenic sarcoma, fibrosarcoma, hypernephroma, or breast carcinoma.

Endobronchial metastases to a major airway occur in less than 2% of patients with a solid tumor, mostly from renal and colorectal carcinomas and occasionally from melanomas and sarcomas. Characteristic histologic appearance and previous history of these extrapulmonary neoplasms in a given case may help differentiate these lesions from bronchogenic carcinoma.

BENIGN TUMORS

The most frequent benign tumor in the lung is a hamartoma, which is a benign neoplasm of connective tissue, often showing a prominent cartilage component. They are more frequent in men and are found in the peripheral lung fields, generally on a routine chest roentgenogram. Presence of stippled calcification (popcorn type, Fig. 25) indicative of a benign process is present in about one-fifth of cases but is not diagnostic of hamartoma. In other cases, no calcification may be evident. Slow enlargement occurs over time. Thoracotomy and resection may be needed for definitive diagnosis and for differentiation from carcinoma if the benign nature of the solitary nodule cannot otherwise be confirmed.

Other benign tumors of the lungs are mixed tumors, lipomas, hemangiomas, and sugar (clear cell) tumors.

SOLITARY PULMONARY NODULE

Solitary pulmonary nodule (SPN) is a roentgenographic diagnosis defined as a single, well-circumscribed (surrounded by aerated lung tissue), nodular pulmonary density less than 6.0 cm in diameter. In most cases the patient remains asymptomatic. In resected cases of SPN, a histologic diagnosis of bronchogenic carcinoma may be obtained in anywhere between 17 to 63%, the incidence correlating with advancing age. Solitary metastatic tumors, mycotic and other granulomas, hamartomas, and miscellaneous entities including intrapulmonary lymph nodes, pulmonary infarction, and pulmonary fibrosis comprise the remainder.

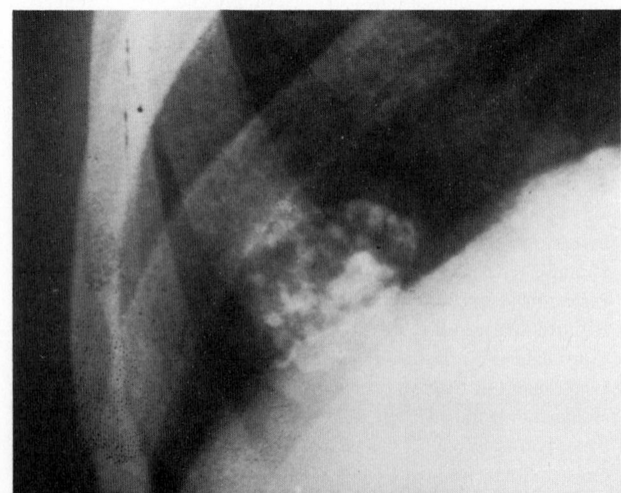

Figure 25. Popcorn calcification in a benign lung nodule (harmartoma in this case).

An organized approach to the management of solitary pulmonary nodule is essential since a significant number of them are bronchogenic carcinomas, and since a favorable prognosis (40-80% 5-year survival) can be expected in such cases if they are properly managed.

Adequate clinical history including review of systems, thorough physical examination, and review of old roentgenograms if available, are the essentials in decision-making. Other factors entering into consideration are the presence of coexistent lung disease, age, history of smoking, and tomographic appearances of the nodule. The correct management approach to solitary pulmonary nodule is resection, unless the following conditions prevail: younger age (<35), prohibitive impairment of pulmonary/cardiovascular function, absence of smoking history, stability of the lesion as demonstrated by old roentgenograms, and characteristic benign calcifications such as popcorn (Fig. 25) or concentric patterns (Fig. 26). The author's approach to SPN is schematically shown in Fig. 27.

Differences exist among physicians with reference to extent of the workup of a solitary pulmonary nodule prior to its resection. In the authors' opinion search for an extrapulmonary neoplasm producing a metastatic SPN is indicated only when review of systems or clinical examination suggest that possibility (e.g., change in bowel habits, presence of occult blood in stools). Similarly, metastases should be looked for only when clinical features (pain and tenderness in the long bones, an enlarged nodular liver, localizing neurologic findings, etc.) or basic laboratory studies (complete blood counts, urinalysis, liver function tests, and serum calcium) suggest that

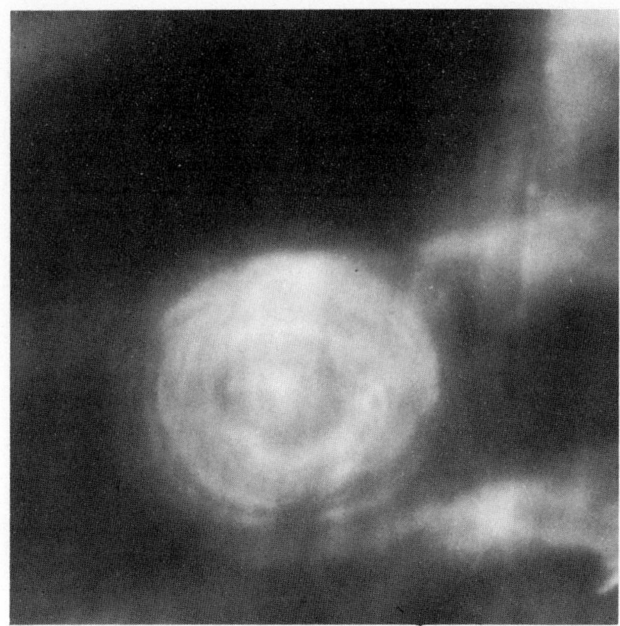

Figure 26. Concentric calcification in a histoplasmoma.

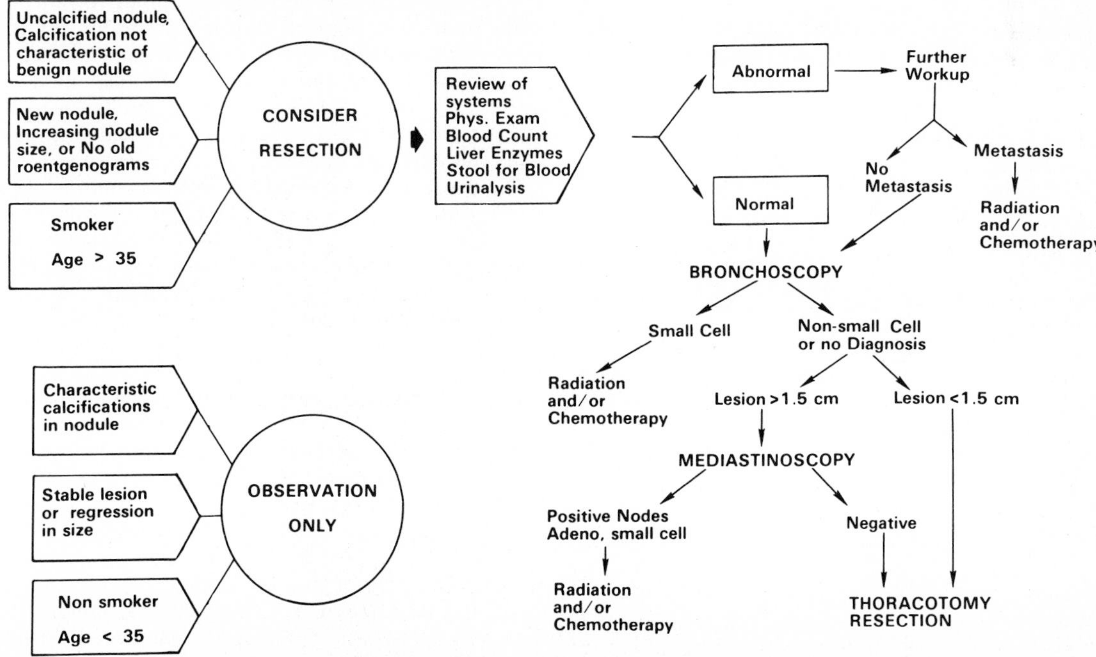

Figure 27. Suggested management approach to solitary pulmonary nodule.

likelihood. Even though bronchoscopy and brushing are low-yield procedures (less than 60% positive results for malignancy) in SPN they should nevertheless be undertaken, mainly to rule out more proximal endobronchial lesions and also to assess tracheobronchial anatomy. Mediastinoscopy is indicated if the lesion exceeds 1.5 cm in diameter. A positive mediastinoscopy (unless the nodes are low and ipsilateral) or a diagnosis of adenocarcinoma or small cell carcinoma by mediastinoscopy obviates thorocotomy. When the resected nodule demonstrates bronchogenic carcinoma, postoperative lifelong followup is necessary. Postoperative irradiation may be necessary depending on the clinical circumstances.

Needle biopsy of SPN yields a greater than 90% positive result for malignancy when the nodule is malignant. A definitive diagnosis of benign disease is made by this technique in only a smaller number of instances (30-40%). Thus the outcome of this procedure does not shift the major emphasis in the management of SPN, namely, resection. In the authors' opinion, needle biopsy is indicated when resection is not feasible and a diagnosis is essential. Other possible indications include a patient whose pulmonary function is borderline and in whom a definitive diagnosis of malignancy would tilt the decision in favor of thoracotomy and resection.

DISORDERS OF THE PLEURA, MEDIASTINUM, AND DIAPHRAGM

DISORDERS OF THE PLEURA

Pneumothorax

Pneumothorax, the presence of air in the pleural space, may be classified into three types: induced, traumatic, and spontaneous. Induced pneumothorax (deliberate introduction of air into the pleural cavity) was once used as a therapeutic modality to collapse tuberculous cavities. Now it has limited use in diagnosis, to define the relationship of a peripheral lesion to the pleura. Traumatic pneumothorax may be caused by penetrating or blunt injury or by surgical procedures (e.g., thoracentesis, subclavian vein catheterization, needle biopsy of lung). Spontaneous pneumothorax may be either primary (no known cause) or secondary (associated with an underlying disease).

Primary spontaneous pneumothorax occurs more commonly in men than in women. Most often it occurs in young, tall, asthenic men. Although the pathogenesis is not well understood, one reasonable theory is that of rupture of subpleurally located blebs. The configuration of the thoracic cage and traction pressures exerted onto the alveolar walls are considered the predisposing factors.

Secondary spontaneous pneumothorax is usually caused by underlying lung disease. Table 23 lists the more common causes of secondary spontaneous pneumothorax.

Table 23. Causes of Spontaneous Pneumothorax

Obstructive disorders
Emphysema
Bronchial asthma
Infections
Tuberculosis
Necrotizing pneumonia
Lung abscess
Diffuse infiltrative diseases
Histiocytosis X
Sarcoidosis
Complicating ventilator management
Associated with PEEP
High airway pressures
Airway obstruction
Rare causes
Malignant neoplasm of lung or pleura
Pulmonary infarction
Marfan's syndrome
Ehlers-Danlos syndrome
Tuberous sclerosis
Catamenial (associated with menstrual periods)

Clinical Features

The clinical features depend on the volume of air in the pleural cavity and the nature and degree of underlying lung disease. A few patients may even be completely asymptomatic. The most common symptoms are chest pain and dyspnea. The chest pain is usually sudden in origin; the degree of dyspnea depends on the severity of the pneumothorax and the underlying disease. The interposed air between the examining finger or the stethoscope and, the collapsed lung is responsible for the physical signs in the affected side, namely, hyperresonance on percussion, diminished to absent tactile fremitus, and absent breath sounds. In the presence of severe emphysema, particularly bullous emphysema, the diagnosis of pneumothorax by these signs could be very difficult.

The chest roentgenogram shows the margin of the lung separated from parietal pleura by air (Fig. 28). An air-fluid level in the pleural cavity is not an uncommon associated finding. When a small pneumothorax is suspected (e.g., after a transbronchoscopic lung biopsy), an expiratory chest roentgenogram is helpful in delineating the pneumothorax.

Treatment

Primary spontaneous pneumothorax often needs no treatment. If the patient is dyspneic or if a tension pneumothorax is present, the air is evacuated by aspiration or by an intercostal tube under waterseal. The authors prefer the latter. However, a flutter valve attached to the chest tube may obviate the necessity for hospitalization. It is unusual for the air leak to persist more than a few days. In the rare instance where air leak persists more than a week, thoracotomy and obliteration of the pleural space by inducing pleural symphysis (mechanical abrasion, talc, decortication) is recommended. With this procedure, cysts or bullae can also be removed. In most patients, primary pneumothorax does not recur; hence, preventive

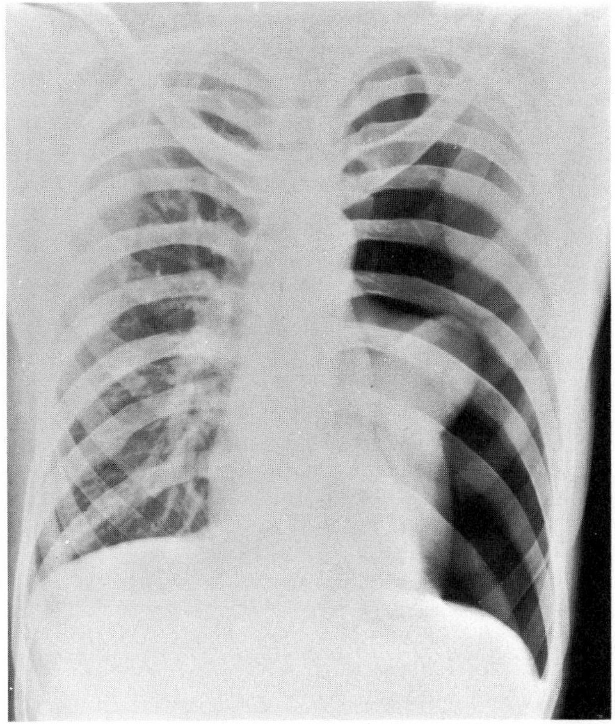

Figure 28. Spontaneous pneumothorax; entire left lung is collapsed.

operative procedures are not necessary. However, the operative procedures mentioned earlier are recommended for ipsilateral recurrence.

Pneumothorax secondary to lung disease is more serious because of further impairment of lung function caused by the pneumothorax. Hospitalization is required, and the patient should be closely observed for respiratory distress and respiratory failure. Arterial blood gases are particularly helpful in following these patients. If the pneumothorax is large or respiratory distress is present, evacuation of air by intercostal tube under waterseal should be promptly undertaken. Continued air leak for more than a week calls for thoracotomy if the patient is an acceptable surgical risk.

Complications

Tension pneumothorax, with mediastinal displacement and compromised venous return to the heart, is a medical emergency. Prompt intervention, by aspiration of air, preferably intercostal tube under waterseal, is indicated. Other complications of pneumothorax include hemopneumothorax (occurring in about 25% of patients), pyopneumothorax (usually secondary to a lung abscess or necrotizing pneumonia), pneumomediastinum, and chronic pneumothorax.

Pleural Disease and Pleural Effusion

The distinctive symptom of pleural disease is pain, and the most common clinical expression of pleural disease is pleural effusion. Pleuritic pain is typically sharp and stabbing and is made worse on inspiration. The pain is usually located over the chest wall; however, it may be referred and be felt in the shoulder or the abdominal wall. The presence of fluid in the pleural cavity provides a good opportunity for the physician to establish a definitive diagnosis.

Pathophysiology

The dynamics of pleural fluid formation and absorption depends upon the opposing hydrostatic and oncotic pressures acting on the parietal and visceral layers of the pleura. Since oncotic pressures exerted on the parietal and visceral pleura are equal, the difference in forces is due to the inequality of hydrostatic pressures. The parietal pleura has increased hydrostatic pressure because it is supplied by the systemic circulation. In normal persons, a balance of these forces is maintained and about 10 ml of low protein fluid remains in the pleural cavity. In disease conditions, abnormal amounts of pleural fluid accumulate. Basic mechanisms that promote pleural fluid accumulation are an increase in hydrostatic pressure (e.g., congestive heart failure), a decrease in oncotic pressure of the blood (e.g., severe hypoalbuminemia), an increase in capillary permeability (e.g., pneumonia), a decrease in lymphatic drainage and reabsorption of fluid (e.g., involvement of the lymph nodes by malignant neoplasms), and, rarely, an increase in intrapleural negative pressure (e.g., atelectasis). A number of these mechanisms may be operative in combination also.

Clinical Features

Pleural effusions may present with dyspnea at rest, particularly in patients with compromised lung function. Often the underlying disease causing the pleural effusion is responsible for the presenting symptoms. The physical findings may be normal when there is less than 300 ml of fluid in the pleural space. In larger pleural effusions, the percussion note is dull and breath sounds are strikingly diminished or absent on auscultation. In addition to these findings, in massive ($>$1,000 ml) effusions, a contralateral mediastinal shift is usually present.

Roentgenographic Features

Free pleural fluid has a characteristic roentgenographic appearance: a meniscus in the costophrenic angle in the posteroanterior view and blunting of the posterior gutter in the lateral view. Approximately 300 ml of fluid is needed for this roentgenographic appearance. When the amount of fluid is less or when it is located between the inferior part of the lung and the diaphragm (infrapulmonary effusion), a lateral decubitus view is useful in demonstrating the presence of pleural effusion. Pleural fluid may assume other appearances including that of a pseudotumor or tumors (Fig. 29). Absence of contralateral mediastinal shift in the presence of a massive effusion suggests fixation of the mediastinum due to malignancy.

Diagnosis

Pleural fluid is accessible and examination of the aspirated pleural fluid is most valuable in diagnosis. In all cases, except when the clinical diagnosis is certain (e.g., uncomplicated con-

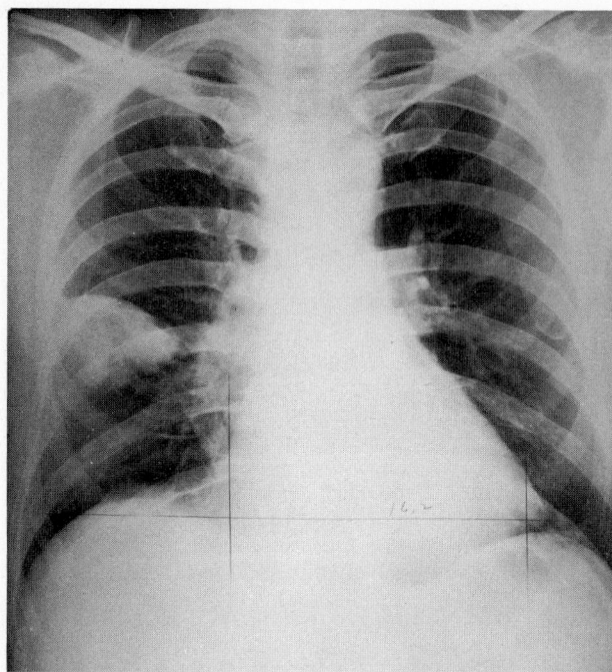

Figure 29. Intralobar effusion (pseudotumor).

Table 24. Causes of Transudates and Exudates

Transudates
Common
Congestive heart failure
Cirrhosis
Less Common
Peritoneal dialysis
Nephrotic syndrome
Myxedema
Exudates
Common
Neoplasm
Parapneumonic effusion
Pulmonary infarction
Uncommon
Tuberculosis
Fungal disease
Parasitic disease
Viral disease
Collagen vascular disease
Pancreatitis
Asbestos effusion
Uremic effusion
Chylothorax
Meigs syndrome
Dressler's syndrome
Sarcoidosis

gestive cardiac failure), thoracentesis should be done. The aspirated pleural fluid should be first observed for gross characteristics. A red tinge indicates blood; milky color suggests a chylothorax; and a putrid smell suggests anaerobic infection. The most useful tests are total protein, lactate dehydrogenase, blood cell counts and differential, cytologic examination, microscopic examination after appropriate staining for bacteria and acid-fast bacilli, and appropriate cultures. Other selectively useful tests include pleural fluid amylase, glucose, and pH determinations.

The first objective is to determine whether the fluid represents a transudate or an exudate. No further diagnostic investigation is usually necessary for transudates. Table 24 lists the more common causes of transudates and exudates. The distinction between transudate and exudate is made by determining protein and LDH in the pleural fluid and serum. The presence of any one or more of the following criteria would indicate the fluid to be an exudate: pleural fluid to serum total protein ratio greater than 0.5, pleural fluid LDH of greater than 200 IU, and pleural fluid serum LDH ratio of greater than 0.6.

Pleural fluids with a leucocyte count greater than 1,000/ml are likely to be exudates. A predominance of neutrophils would suggest a parapneumonic effusion or an acute inflammation (e.g., pulmonary infarction, pancreatitis, and lupus pleuritis). Several days after the acute event, the effusion is likely to show mononuclear cells. Predominantly mononuclear cells suggest effusions secondary to tuberculosis, carcinoma, or chronic effusion. Pleural fluid eosinophilia has no specificity. Presence of red blood cells over 10,000/mm^3 will cause the fluid to appear hemorrhagic. When pleural fluid appears grossly hemorrhagic in the absence of trauma, malignancy is the first diagnosis to be considered. A bloody effusion in the setting of congestive heart failure, particularly if it has neutrophilic predominance, should suggest a concomitant pulmonary infarction.

Cytologic examination of the fluid as soon as possible after aspiration is likely to yield best results. In cases of documented neoplastic involvement of the pleura, cytologic examination has a diagnostic yield as high as 60%. The false positives and false negatives vary from one laboratory to the other, depending on specimen handling, processing, and the expertise of the cytologist.

The pleural fluid glucose should be compared with the serum glucose; a reduced pleural fluid glucose is associated with rheumatoid effusion, empyema, carcinoma, tuberculosis, and esophageal rupture. Pleural fluid amylase is higher than normal serum values in acute pancreatitis, pancreatitic pseudocyst, esophageal rupture, and primary or metastatic tumor of the lung. Chylothorax (chylous effusion) occurs when the thoracic duct empties into the pleural space and is most commonly caused by lymphoma or malignancy. It may also follow external or surgical trauma. Analysis of a chylous effusion will show a high concentration of triglycerides, whereas a cholesterol (chyliform) effusion, which appears grossly similar to chylothorax, shows a high concentration of cholesterol and does not stain positively with Sudan III. Cholesterol effusions have no specificity and may be found in any long-standing effusion (e.g., tuberculous pleurisy and rheumatoid disease).

A Gram-stain examination of the centrifuged pleural fluid should be performed in every parapneumonic effusion. In suspected tuberculous pleural effusion, the centrifuged specimen should be stained with acid-fast stain; but the diagnostic yield of microscopic examination of the pleural fluid in tuberculous pleurisy is only approximately 20%. Depending on the clinical circumstances, appropriate cultures of the pleural fluid should be undertaken: aerobic and anaerobic cultures, cultures for tuberculosis, and fungal organisms.

Pleural fluid pH is helpful when it is done in a parapneumonic effusion. The pleural fluid should be collected, as one collects an arterial blood gas sample, in a heparinized syringe without air bubbles and examined as quickly as possible. The finding of a low pleural fluid pH, that is less than 7.3 in the context of a parapneumonic effusion indicates that the fluid is either already an empyema or will behave like an empyema. This finding usually requires institution of closed chest-tube drainage.

Percutaneous pleural biopsy with a needle (preferably Abrams' needle) is indicated when an exudative pleural effusion remains undiagnosed and carcinoma and tuberculosis remain high in the list of possible diagnoses. The diagnostic yield of pleural biopsy in carcinoma is better than 60% when multiple biopsies are done; in tuberculous pleural effusion, the rate is even higher, 80-85%.

Treatment

Treatment should be directed to the cause of the pleural effusion. Malignant pleural effusions, regardless of the type of malignancy, are usually massive and recurrent. Dyspnea caused by these effusions can be relieved by repeated thoracetesis. Rather than subject the patient to the discomfort of repeated aspirations, measures to obliterate the pleural space should be attempted. A number of drugs (nitrogen mustard, bleomycin, radioactive isotopes, antimalarial drugs) and operative procedures have been used in the past. The authors try to achieve pleural symphysis in a recurrent massive malignant pleural effusion by complete drainage of the pleural fluid under negative pressure by an intercostal tube followed by instillation of tetracycline 500-1,000 mg in 50-100 ml normal saline. The tube is then clamped, the patient is rotated into different positions, and left in these positions for 15-30 minutes each. After approximately 1-2 hours, the clamp is removed and drainage resumed under water seal for 1-2 days.

Pleural Neoplasms

The vast majority of pleural malignancies are metastatic rather than primary. Carcinoma of the breast and lung commonly metastasize to the pleura. Hodgkin's and non-Hodgkin's lymphoma and carcinomas of the ovary, stomach, and colon may also metastasize to the pleura. The presence of pleural effusion with an established diagnosis of one of these malignancies need not necessarily mean that the pleura is directly involved with the tumor; the pleural effusion in such instances may be due to other causes (e.g., obstruction of lymphatic drainage by involvement of lymph nodes, infection, hypoproteinemia).

Primary neoplasms of the pleura may be benign or malignant. The great majority of these primary pleural tumors are mesotheliomas that arise from mesothelial lining cells. These mesotheliomas may be local or diffuse, benign or malignant. In histology, they may appear epithelial, fibrous, or of mixed types.

Local Fibrous Mesothelioma

This is a rare neoplasm that usually presents as an incidental finding, a rounded density, in a chest roentgenogram. The peak incidence seems to be in the fifth and sixth decades of life. Some patients may have a vague, dull chest pain. Pleural effusion is uncommon. According to some reports, there is a high incidence of associated hypertrophic pulmonary osteoarthropy. Some have also reported associated hypoglycemia. Surgical resection affords complete cure in most cases.

Diffuse Malignant Mesothelioma

This is a rare, highly malignant neoplasm with a well-established relationship with exposure to asbestos fibers. The incidence may be as high as 10% in workers exposed to crociodolite asbestos fibers. Malignant mesothelioma is more frequent in men and invariably causes symptoms. Chest pain that may be dull or pleuritic in nature is a common symptom. Dyspnea, cough, and weight loss are frequently associated. Pleural effusion is the most common physical finding. Roentgenographic evidence of pleural fluid is common; pleural nodules are seen less frequently. The pleural fluid is usually hemorrhagic, viscous, and exudative and may have an increased hyaluronic acid content. Cytologic examination, sputum examination, and bronchoscopy are likely to be nondiagnostic. Needle biopsy of the pleura may be diagnostic only in a minority of cases. In most cases, the diagnosis is made only after thoracotomy. The course of malignant mesothelioma is one of rapid progression and the average survival time from the onset of symptoms is less than 1 year. Although excisional surgery has been attempted, results are very poor. Chemotherapy may afford palliation.

DISORDERS OF THE MEDIASTINUM

Pneumomediastinum

Pneumomediastinum indicates the presence of air in the mediastinum. This may be of no clinical consequence or could indicate a serious disease (e.g., rupture of the esophagus or bronchus). The causes are many: coughing, straining, traumatic compression of the chest, asthma, pneumonia, miliary tuberculosis, diabetic ketoacidosis, and as a complication of mechanical ventilation (particularly when used with positive end-expiratory pressure). Pneumomediastinum has been also described as a very rare consequence of marijuana smoking and pulmonary function testing. All of these causes have one factor in common, that is, a change in the pressure relationship between intra-alveolar and surrounding interstitial pressures.

This alveolar-interstitial pressure gradient is considered to be the basic pathogenetic mechanism of a pneumomediastinum. This pressure gradient results in shearing of alveolar walls; the free air moves along the perivascular sheaths into the mediastinum and then along the great vessels and vascular sheaths into the subcutaneous tissues of the neck.

Diagnosis

Typically, there is a sudden onset of substernal chest pain that may follow an episode of cough or straining. This pain may at times radiate to the neck and arm. There is often associated dyspnea that may be aggravated by swallowing. Diagnosis is made by the characteristic feel of crepitus in the subcutaneous tissues of the neck. Although Hamman's sign (a crunching sound synchronous with the heart beat) is described as a finding of pneumomediastinum, it may be absent and, when present, is not specific. Roentgenographic demonstration of air in the mediastinal tissues is characteristic. The mediastinal structures, particularly the heart border and the aortic knob, are often outlined with unusual clarity. On a lateral view, free air is seen anterior to the cardiac opacity.

Treatment

No treatment is necessary in most cases since decompression occurs by the dissection of air in the subcutaneous tissues and the air is absorbed eventually. However, if large amounts of air progressively accumulate, this may diminish the venous return to the heart. Treatment recommended is subcutaneous incision in the neck or a tracheostomy. If the cause of pneumomediastinum is rupture of an esophagus or bronchus, treatment should be directed to surgical correction of the rupture.

Mediastinitis, Adenitis, Granuloma, and Fibrosis

Mediastinitis

Mediastinal infection may occur due to different causes. The most important one is a rupture or perforation of the esophagus that may follow esophageal endoscopy, foreign body, trauma, neoplasm, and violent vomiting. Other causes include rupture or perforation of the trachea or major airways, bronchoscopy, bronchogenic carcinoma, and as a complication of thoracic surgery (e.g., mediastinoscopy). Mediastinal infection may be an extension of infection of another area; nasopharynx, oropharynx, lung, pleural space, sternum, and vertebrae.

Clinical Features. Acute mediastinitis usually presents with the signs of an acute infection such as chills, high fever, and tachycardia. Pain on swallowing and difficulty in breathing may be present. Retrosternal pain may be severe and may be made worse by swallowing or breathing. On examination, there may be fullness and tenderness in the supraclavicular notch and tenderness over the sternum or crepitus. Depending on the localization of the infection, there may be signs of compression of mediastinal structures. Helpful clues to look for in the chest roentgenogram are mediastinal widening, pneumomediastinum, and an air-fluid level. Prompt surgical exploration, closure of the perforated area, drainage of abscesses (if present), and appropriate antimicrobials are indicated.

Mediastinal Adenitis, Granuloma, and Fibrosis

Mediastinal adenopathy and adenitis are features of primary infection with tuberculosis and fungal infections. In most of these cases, healing occurs spontaneously with residual calcification but no significant sequelae. An occasional patient may have large lymph nodes with adenitis and periadenitis that may cause compressive symptoms. These include brassy cough, bronchial obstruction, and distal obstructive pneumonitis. The latter, if recurrent and associated with atelectasis of the middle lobe, is referred to as middle lobe syndrome. Calcified lymph nodes may press and erode a bronchus, causing cough and hemoptysis; stones (broncholiths) may then be expectorated.

Mediastinal granuloma is a mass formed by a coalescence of lymph nodes affected by a granulomatous infection. These heal by fibrous encapsulation and usually do not affect contiguous structures. However, a few, particularly granulomas due to histoplasmosis and tuberculosis, may cause problems such as traction diverticula of the esophagus, superior venal cava obstruction, or bronchial obstruction.

Rarely, instead of forming an encapsulated mass, caseating mediastinal lymph nodes may produce exuberant fibrosis without a distinct capsule; this is referred to as mediastinal fibrosis. Although the reason for this continued fibrosis is unknown, the presence of lymphocytes at the periphery of the enlarging lesions suggest that this could be a hypersensitivity response to the antigenic substances of the causative organisms (often *H. capsulatum*). The consequence of mediastinal fibrosis, compressive syndromes, is again similar to any other enlarging mediastinal lesion.

Primary Neoplasms and Cysts

Primary neoplasms and cysts of the mediastinum may occur at any age. Their manifestations are variable from asymptomatic to nonspecific symptoms to chronic symptoms and even to acute life-threatening cardiorespiratory emergencies. The diagnosis and appropriate treatment of these neoplasms and cysts require the best efforts of many talents; primary care physicians, radiologists, surgeons, pathologists, radiotherapists, oncologists, and so forth.

The mediastinum may be divided into three compartments: anterior, middle, and posterior. This division is based on anatomic landmarks and is useful in the roentgenographic localization of mediastinal masses. The importance of this classification is that certain masses have a predilection to be localized in a particular compartment. The anterior mediastinum lies between the sternum anteriorly and the pericardium and brachiocephalic vessels posteriorly. Thymomas are the most important tumors arising in this compartment. Other thymus-originating masses such as thymic cyst and carcinoid tumors are less common. Other tumors to consider in this compartment are germ cell neoplasms, thyroid, parathyroid adenoma, malignant lymphoma, primary carcinoma, and mesenchymal tumors. The middle mediastinum is between the anterior compartment and the anterior spinal ligament. Congenital cystic lesions (pericardial, bronchogenic, enteric, thymic, etc.) have a predilection to manifest in this compartment. The posterior mediastinum extends from the anterior spinal ligament to the posterior chest wall, medial to the pulmonary sulci. Neurogenic tumors are the most common type of tumors arising from the posterior mediastinum.

Approximately 75% of all mediastinal masses are benign. However, the incidence of malignancy is higher in children and is in the range of 40-50%. The combined results of a number of studies show that the most common tumor in adults is thymoma and represents 21% of all lesions. Next in the order are neurogenic tumors, 20%; congenital cysts, 19%; lymphomas, 13%; and germ cell neoplasms, 11%. In children, the relative frequency of these lesions are different: neurogenic tumors, 38%; lymphoma, 19%; and mesenchymal tumors, 10%.

Clinical Features

In adults, most often primary neoplasms and cysts are asymptomatic and are unexpectedly discovered on a chest roentgenogram. The presence of symptoms increases the probability of malignancy. Previous reports indicate that 95% of patients who were asymptomatic had benign lesions, whereas, among those with symptoms, 50% had benign lesions. The symptoms are those caused by direct invasion or compression of adjacent mediastinal structures by the mass: chest pain, cough, dyspnea, dysphagia, hoarseness, stridor, respiratory infection, and hemoptysis. Other manifestations include obstruction of pulmonary outflow tract, pericardial effusion, cardiac tamponade, superior vena cava syndrome, vocal cord paralysis, Horner's syndrome, chylothorax, and chylopericardium.

Systemic manifestations secondary to hormonal products of the mediastinal tumors may be prominent features. Examples are hypercalcemia induced by a parathyroid adenoma, thyrotoxicosis produced by an intrathoracic goiter, and arterial hypertension produced by a pheochromocytoma. Other endocrine abnormalities include hypoglycemia and Cushing's disease. In addition to these, some other associations that are worth remembering are thymoma and myasthenia gravis, neurogenic tumors and osteoarthropathy, Hodgkin's disease and Pel-Ebstein fever, and neurofibroma and von Recklinghausen's disease.

Diagnosis

Rarely does a history and physical provide a definitive diagnosis in mediastinal masses. However, it lays the groundwork for an orderly diagnostic evaluation. The major steps to arrive at the correct diagnosis of a mediastinal mass are localization, ruling out a mass of vascular origin, and definitive histologic diagnosis. Chest roentgenograms, particularly a lateral projection, help in localization. Comparison with previous roentgenograms, if available, is very helpful. Clearly, increasing size of the mass is more indicative of a neoplasm. Roentgenograms also help in defining the density of the mass whether cystic, solid, or calcified. This can be further clarified by the use of laminographic studies. A barium swallow would detect the presence of intrinsic or extrinsic compression or communication with the esophagus. Fluoroscopy is only of limited use. Computed tomography is a very good tool in delineating a mediastinal mass as well as in characterizing the nature of the mass. Angiography has a role in defining the relationship of a mediastinal mass to adjacent vascular structures. This is particularly indicated when the density cannot be definitely separated from the aorta. Pneumomediastinography, by introduction of CO_2, is a rarely used method to differentiate mediastinal masses from thymic hyperplasia. Myelography is used to detect invasion of the intervertebral foramen by a posterior mediastinal lesion. Ultrasound is of limited help in differentiating cystic and solid mediastinal lesions. Radioisotope scanning is helpful in identifying intrathoracic goiter; it also has some application in identifying parathyroid adenoma and lymphoma. Other tests include radioimmunoassay for measurement of parathyroid hormone in suspected cases of parathyroid adenoma and measurement of alpha fetoprotein and carcinoembryonic antigen when germ cell neoplasms and primary carcinomas are suspected.

The preceeding discussion is not intended to convey the idea that all these procedures are necessary; selective use should be made depending on the localization, presentation, and, most importantly, the probable diagnosis considered in a particular patient. A definitive histiologic diagnosis is needed in most cases. Anterior mediastinoscopy and mediastinotomy are the most useful procedures in obtaining a specific tissue diagnosis. Exploratory thoracotomy may be needed in some cases.

Treatment

Specific treatment depends on the nature of the mediastinal neoplasm or cyst. Surgical treatment, excision of the mass, is recommended in many; the operative mortality for all mediastinal tumors ranges from 0-4%. Complications such as infections, hemorrhage, and injury to the phrenic or recurrent laryngeal nerve may occur in 4-11% of patients. Radiation therapy is useful in certain situations (e.g., seminoma and Hodgkin's disease). The extent of the disease plays a large role in determining the type of treatment. Chemotherapy either alone or combined with other modalities is used in the treatment of some neoplasms. For a more detailed discussion of specific tumors arising from the mediastinum, the reader is referred to the chapter on oncology.

DISORDERS OF THE DIAPHRAGM

Although uncommon, there are many disorders that primarily affect the diaphragm. Here, comments are directed to two entities; diaphragmatic hernias and diaphragmatic neoplasms.

Diaphragmatic Hernias

Hernias of the diaphragm may be congenital or acquired. There are three major types of congenital hernias: Bochdalek's, Morgagni's, and esophageal hiatal hernia. Of these, hernia through the foramen of Bochdalek, posterolaterally situated, is the most common. The incidence is estimated to be 1 in 4,000 live births with a male predominance. Most often it occurs through the left leaf of the diaphragm. Sometimes these hernias are associated with congenital abnormalities of the lung (decreased number of bronchial divisions or partial agenesis). The symptoms that the infant experiences are related to the presence of abdominal viscera in the pleural cavity. Dyspnea and cyanosis may occur in a newborn infant and may progressively worsen. A chest roentgenogram will reveal the presence of abdominal viscera in the thorax. It may not be possible to distinguish an eventration of the diaphragm from a congenital hernia, but this differentiation is not of any importance since both conditions are treated by surgery. Rarely Bochdalek's hernias occur in older children and even in adults. In contrast to the neonatal Bochdalek's hernia, these are usually right-sided suggesting that the liver may have exerted a protective effect in early life.

Hernia through the foramen of Morgagni, which is situated just behind the xyphoid process, most often occurs in the right side. The hernia is a direct type with a membranous sac. This type of hernia is rarely clinically significant and is usually an incidental finding in a chest radiograph.

Hernia through the esophageal hiatus is less common than Bochdalek's hernia in infants and children and may present as repeated regurgitation of ingested food. Regurgitation may cause esophagitis and eventually stricture. Some children may get better as they grow older, but in others surgery may be needed to reduce or prevent the gastroesophageal reflex.

Acquired diaphragmatic hernia through the esophageal hiatus is usually secondary to trauma. The left leaf of the diaphragm is more susceptible to injury and hernia formation probably because the liver protects the right leaf. Increased intra-abdominal pressure resulting from injury that is not countered by an appropriate intrathoracic pressure is considered the pathogenetic mechanism of traumatic hernia. The treatment is directed towards surgical correction. Rare causes of perforation of the diaphragm include extension of an abscess from the liver or from the pleural cavity.

Diaphragmatic Neoplasms

Primary tumors of the diaphragm are very rare. The benign tumors in this category include lipoma, mesothelioma, fibroma, and neurofibroma. The diaphragm is also a recognized site for endometrial implants and may be associated with catamenial pneumothorax. Of the tumors, the most common one is lipoma. Of the malignant primary tumors, the most common are sarcoma and malignant mesothelioma.

ACUTE RESPIRATORY FAILURE

Acute respiratory failure indicates a sudden inability of the lungs and heart to maintain adequate arterial oxygenation and/or adequate carbon dioxide elimination. Arterial blood gas analysis is used to determine the adequacy of oxygenation and carbon dioxide elimination. Hence, the appropriate definition of acute respiratory failure is a state in which the arterial oxygen tension (Pa_{O_2}) is below the predicted normal range for the patient's age at the prevalent barometric pressure (in the absence of intracardiac right-to-left shunting), or the arterial carbon dioxide tension (Pa_{CO_2}) is above 50 mm Hg (not due to respiratory compensation for metabolic alkalemia).

A more practical and simple definition of acute respiratory failure is the sudden development of Pa_{O_2} of less than 50 mm Hg with or without CO_2 retention. An acute increase of $PaCO_2$ to more than 50 mm Hg is called acute ventilatory failure; an acute decrease of Pa_{O_2} to less than 50 mm Hg without CO_2 retention is designated acute oxygenation failure. This distinction has important pathogenetic and therapeutic implications. Table 25 shows this classification and lists a number of causes of respiratory failure. Of these, acute ventilatory failure occurring in chronic obstructive pulmonary disease, neuromuscular diseases, and acute oxygenation failure occurring in ARDS will be highlighted in the latter part of this chapter.

Clinical Features

Although the clinical features of acute respiratory failure may be obvious and striking in some instances (e.g., dyspnea and tachypnea following chest trauma), in many others it may be subtle (e.g., acute ventilatory failure superimposed on chronic respiratory failure due to COPD) and escape detection. The usual symptoms and signs are restlessness, headache, confusion, and tachycardia. Drowsiness leading to loss of consciousness may occur in later stages. Cyanosis is a finding that is often missed. Besides these manifestations, which are all due to the blood gas abnormalities (hypoxemia and/or hypercap-

Table 25. Respiratory Failure: Classification and Causes[a]

- Ventilatory failure
  - Thoracic diseases
    - Lung and airway diseases: Chronic obstructive pulmonary disease, asthma, bronchiolitis, epiglottitis, laryngeal edema, foreign body
    - Pleural diseases: Pleural effusion, pneumothorax, fibrothorax
    - Chest wall disorders: Kyphoscoliosis, thoracoplasty, flail chest
  - Neuromuscular diseases/disorders
    - Brain disorders: Infections, cerebrovascular disease, drugs (sedatives, tranquilizers, analgesics, anesthetic agents), myxedema, primary alveolar hypoventilation
    - Muscular and myoneural junction disorders: Muscular dystrophy, myotonia, drugs (curariform drugs, aminoglycosides), myasthenia gravis, tetanus
    - Neural and spinal cord disorders: Guillain-Barré syndrome, poliomyelitis, amyotrophic lateral sclerosis, peripheral neuritis, cervical cord transection
- Oxygenation failure
  - Diffuse interstitial diseases
    - Interstitial pneumonitis, fibrosis, sarcoidosis, pneumoconioses, lymphangitis carcinomatosa, interstitial pulmonary edema
  - Alveolar diseases
    - Pneumonias, pulmonary edema, diseases with increased alveolar capillary permeability (see ARDS)
  - Vascular diseases
    - Pulmonary embolism, fat embolism, vasculitis
  - Adult respiratory distress syndrome
    - (Table 28)

[a]This is not a complete list of diseases/disorders that cause respiratory failure.

nia), features of the underlying disease (Table 25) would also be present.

Diagnosis

It is obvious from the above discussion that there are no pathognomonic clinical features and the diagnosis of acute respiratory failure could be difficult. Awareness of the conditions that may lead to respiratory failure, is the first requisite for diagnosis. The diagnosis is made by a simple test, that is, arterial puncture and analysis of the blood to determine oxygen and carbon dioxide tensions and pH. These values should be interpreted in the light of clinical circumstances and in comparison to results (if available) of previous arterial gas analyses. In addition to the diagnosis of acute respiratory failure, which by definition is a laboratory diagnosis, the clinician should make an assessment of the underlying disease and precipitating cause(s) of the acute respiratory failure.

Principles of Treatment

Conceptually the principles of treatment of acute respiratory failure are not different from that of acute failure of other systems, that is, to support the failed system while maintaining function of all other systems until the failure is corrected or repaired to functional stability. The treatment can be considered in two phases: support of respiration and circulation, and treatment of precipitating factors and complications.

ACUTE VENTILATORY FAILURE IN COPD

A major cause of hypoxemia in COPD is ventilation-perfusion mismatching. However, with advanced COPD alveolar ventilation is diminished and is manifested by hypercapnia and hypoxemia. Because of renal compensatory mechanisms (retention of bicarbonate), this state, namely, chronic respiratory failure, is not incompatible with life. Acute ventilatory failure develops in patients with COPD (who may or may not have chronic respiratory failure) due to conditions that further decrease alveolar ventilation. The most important precipitating condition is infection. Others include bronchospasm (due to a variety of reasons), congestive cardiac failure, pulmonary embolism, and pneumothorax.

Treatment

The priorities are to assure adequate oxygenation and ventilation. Controlled oxygen therapy is the cornerstone of management of ventilatory failure in COPD. Oxygen should be used as a drug in the appropriate dose. Too little oxygen places the patient at risk for vital organ dysfunction, damage, and death while too much oxygen may cause progressive hypercapnia, CO_2 narcosis, and acidosis. The correct dose of oxygen is the dose that satisfies the oxygen needs of the tissues. There are many variables (e.g., hemoglobin, cardiac output, shifts in oxygen-dissociation curves, etc.) affecting tissue oxygen delivery. Since direct measurement of tissue oxygenation is not possible, determination of arterial oxygen tension (PaO_2) remains the most useful measure.

Because of the shape of the oxyhemoglobin dissociation curve, that is, oxygen tension/saturation relationship, relatively small increases in PaO_2 from initial values in the 40's results in a substantial increase in oxygen saturation and thereby oxygen content. An acceptable PaO_2 to aim for in patients with COPD is one between 50 and 60mm Hg. This may be achieved by using a Venturi mask or a nasal cannula. Venturi masks are capable of delivering oxygen at a concentration of 24 to 35%. Oxygen can also be given by nasal cannula at a low rate of 1-2 L/min. Although nasal cannula has an advantage over the mask of providing uninterrupted oxygen delivery even when eating or conversing, it has a disadvantage that the exact concentration of oxygen cannot be adjusted as precisely as in the Venturi mask. A moderate increase in $paCO_2$ often follows oxygen treatment but is neither a cause for discontinuing oxygen treatment nor a cause for intubation.

Endotracheal intubation and mechanical ventilation should be avoided in this group of patients because of the complications associated with intubation and mechanical ventilation and because of the difficulty in weaning off the ventilator. However, when oxygen is given in an uncontrolled manner or in some cases even with controlled oxygen therapy, progressively worsening hypercapnia and acidosis may occur. Failure of controlled oxygen therapy usually happens in a setting of depressed ventilatory drive (e.g., CNS depressants) or in patients who are initially severely hypoxic and acidotic. Although a variety of criteria for intubation and mechanical ventilation have been developed (Table 26) it is best to base the decision on the patient's clinical status as well as results of arterial blood gases. Evaluation over a period of time of changes in mental status (confusion, restlessness), ineffective cough, and changes in arterial blood gases is more helpful than single measurements in arriving at a decision.

For mechanical ventilatory assistance, a volume-cycled ventilator is preferred over a pressure-cycled ventilator. A tidal volume of 8-10 ml/kg and inspiratory/expiratory time ratio of 1:2 or 1:3 is satisfactory in most instances. The respiratory rate should be adjusted to maintain an appropriate inspiratory/expiratory ratio. In making any adjustment in the ventilator setting (inspired oxygen concentration, tidal volume, respiratory rate), the goal of ventilatory management is to attain arterial blood gas volumes that existed at a previous stable state (if known, this information is of immense help) and not normal arterial gases. Failure to follow this may result in rapid

Table 26. Criteria for Mechanical Ventilatory Assistance[a]

Respiratory rate	>35
Vital capacity (ml/kg)	<10
Inspiratory Force (cm H_2O)	<25
Pa_{O_2} mm Hg	<50 room air
	<70 on mask oxygen
P(A–a O_2) (mm Hg)	>450 on 100% oxygen
Pa_{CO_2} (mm Hg)	>55 (with acidosis)
V_D/V_T	>0.60

[a]Reverse of these criteria may be used for eligibility for weaning.

changes in pH in blood and consequent chances of cardiac arrhythmias and seizures. With the availability of low pressure cuffed tubes, there is no longer a need to follow strict deadlines for performance of a tracheostomy. However, it is appropriate to evaluate the need for tracheostomy, one week after intubation. Table 27 is a list of monitoring aids in respiratory failure.

Attention should be focussed on treatment of the precipitating factor(s) and in correcting all reversible components. Thus, bronchospasm (wheezing) should be treated with bronchodilators (e.g., isoproterenol, isoetharine, terbutaline sulfate, theophylline, etc.). Suggested intravenous aminophylline dose is a loading dose of 5-6 mg/kg and a maintenance dose of 0.5 mg/kg/h. Since corticosteroids potentiate the action of bronchodilators, the authors prefer to use them in all cases of respiratory failure where wheezing is present. Optimal tracheobronchial secretion clearance should be achieved by frequent nasotracheal suctioning. Antibiotics (e.g., ampicillin or tetracycline) is administered if infection is present or suspected. Adequate nutritional support and progressively increasing sitting periods and early ambulation are important but generally are not stressed enough.

In addition to the criteria for weaning (Table 26), bedside assessment is necessary. The patient should be alert and responsive, clinical condition must be improved and stabilized, and oxygenation should be adequate at an inspired oxygen concentration of less than 40%. A trial of T-tube breathing or intermittent mandatory ventilation (IMV) may be used for weaning. Several hours of T-tube trial should precede the extubation. In the immediate postextubation period, feeding should be avoided because of the danger of aspiration. Intensive respiratory care, more specifically attention to clearing of secretions by cough and postural drainage, are of paramount importance in the first 24-48 hours after extubation.

ACUTE VENTILATORY FAILURE IN NEUROMUSCULAR DISEASES

Ventilatory failure occurs despite normal lungs and airways in neuromuscular diseases. Often this is due to weakness of inspiratory muscles and poor cough mechanism. Chronic hypoxemia and cor pulmonale are generally not seen in neuromuscular respiratory failure. Acute, chronic, or periodic bouts of ventilatory failure may be seen in spinal cord and myoneural junction diseases. The common causes of neuromuscular respiratory failure are Guillain-Barré syndrome, myasthenia gravis, and demyelinating degenerative and infectious neuromuscular diseases.

Table 27. Monitoring Aids in Patients with Respiratory Failure

Arterial blood gases—Pa_{O_2}, Pa_{CO_2}, $P(A-a\ O_2)$
Shunt fraction (Qs/Qt)
Hematocrit and hemoglobin
Electrolyte status, intake and output, daily weight
Tidal volume, minute ventilation
Vital capacity
PI max (inspiratory force)
Compliance
Chest radiographs
Mixed venous oxygen tension ($P\bar{v}O_2$)
Swan-Ganz catheterization
Electrocardiogram

Treatment

In contrast to ventilatory failure in COPD, clinical assessment and arterial blood gas results cannot be solely relied upon for a decision regarding intubation and mechanical ventilation. Respiratory muscle paralysis may be very subtle, yet has the potential to progress fast and culminate in a respiratory arrest. Hence, measurements that can assess respiratory muscle function are important. With increasing weakness of respiratory muscles the vital capacity (VC) and maximum inspiratory pressure (P_I max) are progressively reduced. Intubation and mechanical ventilation are indicated when the VC falls to twice the predicted tidal volume or P_I max falls to less than −20 cm H_2O (measured by a pressure manometer). Dysphagia, maximum expiratory pressure (PE max) of less than 40 cm H_2O, and hypercapnia are also indications for mechanical ventilatory support.

Ventilator management is fairly similar to that of a COPD patient in ventilatory failure except that ventilation is more easily achieved, complications are less common, and tracheostomy is more often necessary. In every case where recovery is not expected in 1-2 weeks, tracheostomy is recommended. Physical therapy plays an important role in the management of these patients. Noninvasive measures (iron lung, chest cuirass, rocking bed) and electrophrenic respirator, although useful in chronic neuromuscular respiratory failure, should not be the mainstay in acute ventilatory failure.

ADULT RESPIRATORY DISTRESS SYNDROME (ARDS)

ARDS is a catastrophic form of respiratory failure that follows a major medical or surgical illness or trauma characterized by progressive respiratory distress, refractory hypoxemia, and pulmonary edema secondary to enhanced capillary permeability. This entity differs from the respiratory failure in COPD in that the major therapeutic problem here is oxygenation failure, and also in that most cases if not all, require early mechanical ventilatory support. Whereas the long-term prognosis for COPD with respiratory failure is poor, the prognosis for ARDS is good if the patient recovers from the catastrophe.

Clinical states that lead to ARDS are summarized in Table 28. The central theme in its pathogenesis is enhanced pulmonary capillary permeability. This may be brought on by several mechanisms: the underlying illness may lead to metabolic events that lead to release of vasoactive materials (kinins and amines), decreased pulmonary blood flow in some of these states may lead to decreased surfactant synthesis, and platelet

Table 28. Causes of Adult Respiratory Distress Syndrome

Infections
Pneumonias from viral, bacterial, or fungal agents
Miliary tuberculosis
Inhalation injury
Smoke inhalation
Oxygen toxicity
Hydrocarbon ingestion
Aspiration of gastric acid
Near drowning
Trauma
Shock
Hemorrhagic or septic
Fat embolism
Narcotic and illicit drug overdose
Pancreatitis
Neurogenic pulmonary edema
Postcardiopulmonary bypass

and leukocyte aggregates that accompany hypotensive states may migrate into pulmonary capillaries, leading to disruption of the capillary integrity. Physiologically, there is increased extravascular lung water, decreased lung compliance and right-to-left intrapulmonary shunting of blood flow. Pulmonary edema, congestion, hemorrhage, microatelectasis, and hyaline membrane formation are the chief pathologic findings in the lungs.

A background of a serious medical or surgical illness (sepsis, shock, or trauma) is frequently identifiable in the history. In instances where trauma is the underlying illness, a history of shock and resuscitation followed by a latent period of stability is often present before respiratory failure sets in rather dramatically. During this latent period, although the patient is asymptomatic from a respiratory standpoint, fever, and tachypnea are usually present. Normal chest roentgenograms generally characterize this period although, on analysis of arterial blood gases, respiratory alkalosis and a widening of the alveolar arterial oxygen gradient are evident. Further on in the course of ARDS, progressive dyspnea, intercostal retractions, rhonchi, and rales are present. Progressive diffuse pulmonary infiltration is seen in the radiographs. Refractory hypoxemia is evident during this phase with low $PaCO_2$ levels. In the advanced stages of the illness, CO_2 retention and a combined metabolic and respiratory acidosis are present. These signs are ominous and if untreated, the illness is generally fatal.

The key point in diagnosis of ARDS is suspicion. Recognition of a disease that holds the potential for ARDS should alert the physician to the likelihood of this complication. Presence of hypoxemia and/or widening of the alveolar arterial oxygen gradient in the setting of a severe medical or surgical illness is the harbinger of early illness, and should be pursued with serial blood gas measurements, roentgenographs, and oxygen administration. Differentiation from cardiogenic pulmonary edema cannot be made confidently on clinical or on roentgenographic grounds, which bespeaks the need for Swan-Ganz catheterization in these cases.

Treatment

The major objectives are to ensure adequate oxygenation at the tissue level while adequately treating the underlying process responsible for ARDS. Since refractory hypoxemia is a characteristic of this condition, often progressively increasing oxygen concentrations are necessary to achieve a satisfactory PaO_2. The most useful criteria to follow regarding the adequacy of tissue oxygenation are the arterial as well as mixed venous oxygen tensions (PaO_2 and $P\bar{v}O_2$, respectively). The aim should be to maintain the PaO_2 above 60 mm Hg and the $P\bar{v}O_2$ between 30 and 40 mm Hg. In almost all cases, there is an element of overhydration, which should be treated with judicious, small doses of a rapid-acting diuretic (furosemide, for example) given intravenously. This, combined with supplemental oxygen therapy may help maintain oxygenation in the required range. The effect of these modalities of therapy on hemodynamic values should be frequently reassessed by a Swan-Ganz catheter. Both overhydration and underhydration should be avoided.

Indications for mechanical ventilatory assistance are outlined in Table 26. It should be noted that one need not wait for these values to develop in every given case; one may choose mechanical ventilatory assistance even earlier if the serial values show a clearly deteriorating trend, despite adequate therapy.

It is customary to set a large tidal volume (e.g., 15 ml/kg body weight) in a volume-cycled ventilator to ventilate patients with ARDS. One drawback of such a large tidal volume is the development of severe hypocapnia. This should be corrected by adding dead space to the ventilator tubing or by blending 3% carbon dioxide to the inhaled air oxygen mixture. Patients with ARDS are very tachypneic and it is generally necessary to use sedation and/or muscle relaxants to achieve synchronization with the ventilator, to provide between 10-12 breaths/min. After placing the patient on these ventilator settings and on 60% oxygen for ½ hour, a blood gas analysis is done. Under such conditions, it serves a twofold purpose: to measure the shunt and to provide a guideline regarding necessity for positive end-expiratory pressure (PEEP). The criteria used for PEEP is a PaO_2 of less than 60 on 60% inspired oxygen (FiO_2).

PEEP is started at an initial level of 5 cm H_2O and is increased in increments of 3-5 cm H_2O until a desired response (by arterial and mixed venous blood gas tensions) is obtained. Serial responses of the effective compliance and changes in mixed venous oxygen tensions to increments in PEEP have been used to determine the optimal PEEP. Once an effective level of PEEP has been achieved, the FiO_2 should be brought down gradually using the FiO_2 to keep the PaO_2 above 60 mm Hg in order to avoid the risk of oxygen toxicity.

Ancillary measures to be employed in caring for a patient with ARDS are: meticulous control of fluid and electrolyte status, skilled nursing care, control of infection when present, treatment of underlying conditions, and corticosteroids when the inciting factors are gastric acid aspiration, fat embolism, respiratory burns, drowning, and viral pneumonia.

The reverse of the criteria for mechanical ventilation may be used for determining the appropriate time for weaning. Steady levels of PaO_2, decreasing $P(A - a)_{O_2}$ gradient, and decreasing shunt fraction are good guidelines. The techniques of weaning are similar to the ones described earlier for respiratory failure in COPD. The authors prefer to continue PEEP in conjunction with the IMV and to eliminate PEEP in successive stages. It is felt that PEEP probably should be removed last of all. A period of observation of 6-12 hours is appropriate after removal of PEEP and before extubating the patient.

The prognosis for satisfactory recovery of lung function is excellent in survivors of ARDS. In long-term studies, victims of ARDS showed recovery of normal lung function within 1 year of the episode. However, some disturbances in gas transfer, manifested by a low diffusing capacity, may persist.

QUESTIONS

(More than one answer may be correct)

1. Physical findings in a large pleural effusion include
   A. Mediastinal shift to the same side as the effusion
   B. Dullness to percussion over the affected side
   C. Presence of a localized wheeze over the effusion
   D. Diminished breath sounds and diminished vocal resonance over the effusion itself
2. Tuberculin skin testing
   A. Is performed by subcutaneous injection of 0.1 cc of Tween-stabilized purified protein derivative (PPD-S).
   B. A positive skin test indicates active pulmonary tuberculosis.
   C. A positive response is manifested by 10 mm of local erythema.
   D. Depends upon delayed hypersensitivity or type 4 response.
3. On microscopic examination of sputum
   A. Specimen with numerous squamous cells is adequate.
   B. Specimen with alveolar macrophages represents a good sample.
   C. *H. influenzae* appears as large, Gram-negative encapsulated rods and *Klebsiella* pneumoniae appears as small, Gram-negative pleomorphic bacilli.
   D. Cells with bilobed nuclei and large refractile granules, may be seen in large numbers in asthmatics during an exacerbation.
4. An obstructive ventilatory impairment is present when
   A. $FEV_{1.0}/FVC$ ratio is below 70%
   B. $FEF_{25\text{-}75}$ is reduced
   C. FRC, RV, and possibly TLC are elevated
   D. Total lung capacity is reduced
5. The following statements regarding various compartments of the lung volume are correct:
   A. Vital capacity is the amount of air exhaled from a maximal inspiratory position to the point of maximal exhalation.
   B. Expiratory reserve volume is the amount of air exhaled from the end of a tidal exhalation to the point of maximal exhalation.
   C. Residual volume is the amount of air present in the lung at the end of a maximal exhalation.
   D. Functional residual capacity is the sum of expiratory reserve volume and the residual volume.
6. Which of the following complications usually follow fiberoptic bronchoscopy?
   A. Laryngospasm
   B. Pneumothorax
   C. Hemorrhage
   D. Hypoxemia
7. True statements concerning the conducting airways include which of the following?
   A. Bronchial epithelium is pseudostratified, and bronchiolar epithelium is columnar or ciliated.
   B. Bronchial walls contain goblet cells that form submucosal glands that secrete mucus.
   C. Bronchial smooth muscle responds to a variety of neurohumoral and chemical stimuli.
   D. Bronchial and bronchiolar walls have cartilages to maintain their patency.
8. Pulmonary sequestration
   A. Has a predilection to occur in the upper lobes
   B. May present as a solitary pulmonary nodule
   C. Predisposes to the development of a malignant neoplasm
   D. May be diagnosed by aortography
9. Disseminated histoplasmosis
   A. Usually occurs in immunologically impaired hosts
   B. May present with pallor, hepatosplenomegaly, lymphadenopathy, and oropharyngeal ulcers
   C. Has the propensity to involve the meninges, heart, and adrenals
   D. Can be ruled out as the diagnosis if the histoplasmin skin test and complement fixation tests are negative
10. In primary infections with *Coccidioides immitis*
    A. Symptoms are usually absent.
    B. Eosinophilia may be present.
    C. Patchy infiltrates, often with hilar adenopathy, are found in roentgenograms.
    D. Treatment with amphotericin-B is indicated.

11. In patients with blastomycosis
    A. Infection is usually acquired through cutaneous inoculation.
    B. Hemoptysis may be present.
    C. Hilar adenopathy is a common roentgenographic feature.
    D. Dissemination of infection to bones, joints, genitourinary system, and central nervous system may occur.
12. Allergic bronchopulmonary aspergillosis
    A. Is a disease occurring in atopic patients
    B. Presents with progressive cavitary pulmonary infiltrates
    C. Is associated with eosinophilia of sputum and blood
    D. Is treated with amphotericin-B
13. Adverse effects of therapy with amphotericin-B include
    A. Azotemia
    B. Anemia
    C. Hypokalemia
    D. Hypomagnesemia
14. The following are of paramount importance in the management of a patient with chronic bronchitis:
    A. Adequate doses of theophylline and β-2 adrenergic agents
    B. Cessation of smoking and avoidance of atmospheric irritants
    C. Antibiotic therapy when sputum changes or when symptoms indicate respiratory infection
    D. Regular treatment with mucolytics such as acetylcysteine, and expectorants like glyceryl guaiacolate and potassium iodide
15. At the end of a long evaluation of progressive exertional dyspnea, a 58-year-old man is found to have severe pulmonary emphysema. His $FEV_{1.0}$ is 1.2 L. Lung volume studies show significant overinflation. A pulmonary consultant has recommended an exercise reconditioning and rehabilitation program. Which of the following is (are) correct?
    A. General exercise reconditioning would lead to improvement of his $FEV_{1.0}$.
    B. General exercise reconditioning will lead to improved exercise tolerance.
    C. The entire program can be expected to improve his longevity substantially.
    D. The program will improve the quality of life, reduce hospitalizations, and will tend to provide a positive outlook on life.
16. Features that help distinguish between pink puffers and blue bloaters include
    A. Abnormal pulmonary function studies that demonstrate airway obstruction
    B. Body habitus, frequency of cor pulmonale, and disturbances in lung compliance
    C. Extent of exposure to cigarette smoke and atmospheric/environmental pollutants
    D. Presence or absence of sputum production as well as dyspnea
17. In patients with chronic obstructive pulmonary disease, long-term oxygen therapy is generally indicated in the following clinical situations:
    A. In an emphysematous patient, who demonstrates a drop in Pa O_2 from 72 mm Hg to 69 mm Hg on exercise
    B. In a patient with long-standing chronic bronchitis with a hemoglobin of 18.5 g and a hematocrit of 58%
    C. In far-advanced pulmonary emphysema when a patient demonstrates weight loss and chronic muscle wasting
    D. When hypoxemia coexists with evidence of pulmonary hypertension and/or cor pulmonale
18. Which of the following statements about cystic fibrosis is true?
    A. Survival into adult age is possible.
    B. The standard method of contraception is an estrogen-progesterone combination.
    C. Extent of chest roentgenographic abnormalities does have an influence on prognosis.
    D. Sweat chloride levels greater than 60 mEq/L in infants and over 80 mEq/L in adults are specific for this disorder.
19. In the course of a routine examination, a 58-year-old businessman is found to have a hematocrit of 61% and hemaglobin of 20.0 g. He has a long history of cough with expectoration of mucoid sputum. He has a long history of cigarette smoking, quantified as 60 pack/years. Which of the following data would match his clinical situation?

	Pulmonary artery pressure (mm Hg)	*Pulmonary Capillary Wedge Pressure (mm Hg)*	*PaO_2 (mm Hg)*	*$PaCO_2$ (mm Hg)*	*pH*
A.	48/30	18	76	38	7.48
B.	58/30	12	55	55	7.36
C.	52/28	22	70	28	7.52
D.	50/28	8	50	48	7.34

20. What would be the recommendations for his management?
    A. Furosemide 40 mg daily, digoxin 0.25 mg daily, long-acting theophylline 300 mg every 12 h
    B. Furosemide 40 mg daily, digoxin 0.25 mg daily, long-acting theophylline 300 mg every 12 h, and oxygen 4 L/min by nasal cannula
    C. Furosemide 40 mg daily, digoxin 0.25 mg daily, long-acting theophylline 300 mg every 12 h, terbutaline 2.5 mg qid

D. Long-acting theophylline 300 mg every 12 h, terbutaline 2-5 mg qid and oxygen by nasal cannula at 2 L/min

21. A 20-year-old pharmacy student has had episodic wheezing, expectoration, and fever for the last several years. He has noted worsening of his symptoms during the last 18 months. He received a course of tetracycline and bronchodilators in appropriate doses without significant improvement. Chest roentgenogram shows a left upper lobe infiltrate with cystic lucencies and a nonhomogeneous right lower zone infiltrate. Remainder of the lung fields are normal. The patient is a nonsmoker, and there is a family history of atopic disease. Which of the following studies would be most helpful?

A. Sweat chloride level

B. Tuberculin skin test

C. An aspergillus skin test

D. Serum alpha-1 antitrypsin level

22. Indications for fiberoptic bronchoscopy include

A. A 45-year smoker whose chest roentgenogram shows a right upper lobe 5-cm mass density

B. A 60-year-old man who has inspiratory stridor and, on flow volume loop analysis, a ratio of expiratory to inspiratory $\dot{V}max_{50}$ that exceeds 1.5

C. A 46-year-old postoperative patient who demonstrates complete atelectasis of the right lower lobe that has poorly responded to chest physical therapy and suctioning

D. Active, massive hemoptysis in a 50-year-old man

23. A 25-year-old man is brought in a comatose state to the emergency room. He has a past history of intravenous drug abuse. Chest radiographs show pulmonary edema. The emergency room physician suspects opiate-induced pulmonary edema. Which of the following would support this diagnosis?

A. Pupillary size of 2 mm bilaterally

B. Ice around the testicles

C. Milk droplets in the oral cavity

D. Rapid clearing of consciousness following intravenous administration of naloxone

24. The content of protein in the pulmonary edema fluid is increased in which of the following?

A. Pulmonary edema accompanying sepsis

B. Hemorrhagic pancreatitis

C. Gastric hydrochloric acid aspiration

D. Acute papillary muscle rupture

25. Which of the following factors are most commonly associated with increased risk for deep venous thrombosis?

A. Congestive heart failure

B. Recent trauma to the lower extremities leading to an immobilization cast

C. Prolonged bed rest

D. Superficial venous thrombosis

26. A 52-year-old man with chronic bronchitis and emphysema is admitted with the diagnosis of respiratory failure. His initial chest radiograph was free of any infiltrates. Worsening of his condition led to endotracheal intubation and mechanical ventilation. On the fourth day on a mechanical ventilator, the nurse reports he has a fever of 102° F. Heart rate has risen by 35 beats/min. Chest radiographs reveal a right lower lobe infiltrate. On 30% oxygen, his PaO_2 has dropped by 25 mm Hg to 50, and $PaCO_2$ has dropped by 18 mm to 28. Which of the following is (are) now indicated?

A. Ventilation-perfusion scanning to look for areas of mismatch

B. Fibrin-split products

C. ^{125}I fibrinogen scanning

D. Pulmonary angiography

27. Pulmonary angiographic findings diagnostic of pulmonary embolism are

A. Localized oligemia involving multiple areas of the lung

B. Delayed filling of one or more of the branches of the pulmonary artery

C. Delayed filling, sluggish blood flow, and localized oligemias

D. Intraluminal filling defects and sharp vessel cutoffs

28. Which of the following statement(s) concerning the use of fibrinolytic agents in pulmonary thromboembolic disease is (are) true?

A. Fibrinolytic agents lead to rapid resolution of emboli.

B. Use of fibrinolytic agents is accompanied by significant reduction in mortality from pulmonary embolism.

C. Fibrinolytic agents lead to faster stabilization of disturbances in hemodynamic status following massive pulmonary embolism.

D. They can be used even in patients who have had a cerebrovascular accident within the preceding 5 weeks, and follow-up administration of other anticoagulants is unnecessary.

29. In which of the following situations will you prescribe mini (low) dose herparin therapy to prevent development of deep venous thrombosis?

A. Intraocular surgery

B. Elective upper abdominal or thoracic surgical procedures

C. Hip replacements with a Moore prosthesis

D. Congestive heart failure being treated in the hospital by digitalis, diuretics, and bed rest

30. Which of the following roentgenographic findings are characteristic of asbestosis and differentiate it from silicosis?

A. Lower lobe fibrosis

B. Upper lobe fibrosis

C. Pleural thickening and fibrosis

D. Hilar lymphadenopathy

31. Which of the following findings may be related to an occupational history of insulation work for 25 years?

A. Reduced 1-second forced expiratory volume (FEV_1) and increased residual volume

B. Roentgenographic finding of circumscribed mass and malignant appearing cells on sputum cytology

C. Roentgenographic finding of egg-shell calcifications

D. Encasement of left lung with thickened pleura and pleural effusion

32. The effects of radiation injury depend on

A. Volume of lung exposed to radiation

B. Total dose of radiation

C. The energy of the beam

D. Concurrent administration of cytotoxic drugs

33. A 25-year-old black man is seen in the emergency room for complaints of redness and swelling involving the shins bilaterally. He has had febrile episodes and some dry cough, as well as arthralgias. A chest roentgenogram was obtained that shows bilateral hilar and paratracheal lymphadenopathy. Which of the following abnormalities can be found on laboratory assessment of this patient?

A. Increased sedimentation rate and depressed peripheral T-lymphocyte function

B. Increased peripheral B-lymphocyte population and increased total T lymphocytes in the lung

C. Increased levels of serum angiotensin converting enzyme (ACE)

D. Epithelioid cells, giant cells, lymphocytes, and plasma cells may be seen on appropriate tissue biopsy with varying degrees of fibrosis

34. What is the most appropriate plan of management for this patient?

A. Hospitalization, mediastinoscopy, and biopsy

B. Hospitalization, open lung biopsy

C. Hospitalization, bronchoscopy, and corticosteroids

D. Hospitalization, transbronchial lung biopsy; no corticosteroids

35. A patient is admitted to the hospital with far-advanced rheumatoid arthritis. Which of the following complications may be part of his/her rheumatoid disease?

A. Chest radiographs show coarse reticulation, with well-circumscribed, multiple nodules

B. Restrictive ventilatory impairment on pulmonary function testing

C. Pulmonary arterial pressures 50/28 mm Hg, pulmonary capillary wedge pressure 10 mm Hg, PaO_2:72, $PaCO_2$:36, pH: 7.42

D. Left-sided, unilateral pleural effusion, with protein 1.5 g/dl, LDH of 55 U/ml, and fluid to serum protein ratio and LDH ratio 0.3 and 0.4, respectively

36. A 58-year-old man was found to have a right upper lobe solitary pulmonary nodule on a routine chest roentgenogram obtained prior to an inguinal herniorrhaphy. He has a 40 pack/year history of cigarette smoking. Review of systems and physical examination discloses no abnormalities. Which of the following are now indicated?

A. Sputum examination for malignant cells and acid-fast bacilli

B. A tuberculin skin test with 5 TU PPD

C. Obtain a prior chest radiograph obtained during a routine insurance physical examination 3 years ago

D. Recommend thoracotomy

37. A 55-year-old steam fitter is found to have a left upper lobe solitary pulmonary nodule on routine 2-yearly employment physical examination. He is a cigarette smoker with a 50 pack/year history of smoking. Review of systems discloses no abnormality. The nodule is new and is free of calcification on tomography; it measures 2 cm in diameter. A PPD skin test shows 13 mm induration at 48 hours. Urinalysis, liver function tests, and complete blood count are normal. The most appropriate management for this patient is

A. Workup for a primary extrathoracic neoplasm by intravenous pyelogram, barium enema, and upper gastrointestinal series, in that order

B. Careful follow-up every 3 months with repeated chest radiographs

C. One year's course of isoniazid with pyridoxine

D. Thoracotomy and resection of nodule

38. A reduced pleural fluid glucose concentration of 30 mg/100 ml (serum glucose 105 mg/100 ml) is consistent with a diagnosis of effusion caused by

A. Hepatic cirrhosis

B. Pancreatitis

C. Nephrotic syndrome

D. Rheumatoid arthritis

39. In which of the following patients would you perform a percutaneous needle biopsy of the pleura?

A. A 22-year-old woman with low-grade fever, malaise, pleuritic chest pain, and right-sided pleural effusion. Pleural fluid findings: straw colored, protein 4.8 g/100 ml; lactic dehydrogenase 370 U/ml; white cells $-5900/mm^3$ with 90% lymphocytes (Serum values—protein 6.9 g/100 ml; LDH 200 U/ml).

B. A 65-year-old foundry worker with dyspnea, wheezing, cardiomegaly, hepatomegaly, ankle edema, bibasilar rales, and right-sided effusion. Pleural fluid findings: straw colored; protein 3 g/100 ml; lactic dehydrogenase 108 U/ml; white cells $200/mm^3$ with 90% lymphocytes (serum values: protein 7.2 g/100 ml, LDH 280 U/ml).

C. A 40-year-old shipyard worker with gradual onset dyspnea and right-sided pleural effusion. Pleural fluid findings: serosanguinous; protein 3.5 g/100 ml; lactic dehydrogenase 450 U/ml; glucose 60 mg/100 ml; white cells 200/mm^3 with 95% mononuclear cells (serum values: protein 6.2 g/100 ml; LDH 200 U/ml; glucose 110 mg/100 ml).

D. A 30-year-old man who had multiple thoracenteses to evacuate fluid from a left-sided hydropneumothorax due to rib fractures resulting from a fall, returns 2 months later with fever, left-sided chest pain, and a small loculated left-sided effusion. Pleural fluid findings: cloudy and malodorous, protein 5.5 g/100 ml; lactic dehydrogenase—not obtained; glucose 40 mg/100 ml; white cells 50,000/mm^3 with 100% neutrophils; pH 6.9 (serum values: protein 6.5 g/100 ml; glucose 100 mg/100 ml).

40. Which of the following statements regarding malignant pleural mesothelioma is/are true?

A. Increased incidence occurs in asbestos workers.

B. Chest pain and pleural effusion are the usual presenting manifestations.

C. Pleural fluid is usually a hemorrhagic exudate.

D. Although sputum cytology is unrewarding, bronchoscopic brushings and biopsy combined with percutaneous needle biopsy of the pleura are frequently diagnostic.

41. Which of the following statements regarding mediastinal masses is/are true?

A. Most mediastinal masses diagnosed in the asymptomatic adult are malignant.

B. They may manifest as superior vena cava obstruction.

C. Thyroid tumors are the commonest cause of masses arising from the anterior mediastinum.

D. Neurogenic tumors are the commonest cause of masses arising from the posterior mediastinum.

42. In a patient with chronic obstructive pulmonary disease who develops acute ventilatory failure, an increase in arterial P_{CO_2} during oxygen administration is

A. An indication to stop oxygen

B. An indication to evaluate the dosage of oxygen the patient is receiving

C. An indication for endotracheal intubation

D. An indication for bronchodilator therapy and clearance of tracheobronchial secretions by suctioning and physiotherapy

43. In a patient with myasthenia gravis and an acute viral respiratory infection, which of the following measurements help in deciding when to intubate and use mechanical ventilatory assistance?

A. Vital capacity

B. Total lung capacity

C. Maximum inspiratory pressure

D. Lung compliance

44. Which of the following is/are often required in the management of adult respiratory distress syndrome?

A. Oxygen supplementation and mechanical ventilatory assistance

B. Positive end-expiratory pressure (PEEP)

C. Assessment of hemodynamic values by Swan-Ganz catheter

D. Bronchodilators

45. Causes of adult respiratory distress syndrome (ARDS) include

A. Severe emphysema

B. Pancreatitis

C. Bilateral cavitary tuberculosis

D. Viral pneumonia

ANSWERS

1. B, D
2. D
3. B, D
4. A, B, C
5. All correct
6. D
7. A, B, C
8. B, D
9. A, B, C
10. A, B, C
11. B, D
12. A, C
13. All correct
14. A, B, C
15. B, D
16. B, D
17. B, D
18. A
19. D
20. D
21. A, B, C
22. A, C
23. All correct
24. A, B, C
25. A, B, C
26. D
27. D
28. A, C
29. B, D
30. A, C
31. B, D
32. All correct
33. All correct
34. D
35. A, B, C
36. A, B, C
37. D
38. D
39. A, C
40. A, B, C
41. B, D
42. B, D
43. A, C
44. A, B, C
45. B, D

BIBLIOGRAPHY

TEXTBOOKS AND MONOGRAPHS

Baum GL (ed): *Textbook of Pulmonary Diseases*, ed. 2. Boston, Little, Brown & Co, 1974.

Fishman AP (ed): *Pulmonary Diseases and Disorders*. New York, McGraw-Hill Book Co, 1980.

Fraser RG, Pare JAP: *Diagnosis of Diseases of the Chest,* ed. 2. (four volumes). Philadelphia, W B Saunders Co, 1977.

Hatano S, Strasser T (eds): *Primary Pulmonary Hypertension*. Report on a WHO meeting held in Geneva, Switzerland, October 15-17, 1973. Geneva: World Health Organization, 1975.

Hodgkin JE: *Chronic Obstructive Pulmonary Disease: Current Concepts in Diagnosis and Comprehensive Care*. Park Ridge, Illinois, American College of Chest Physicians, 1979.

Petty TL (ed): *Pulmonary Diagnostic Techniques*. Philadelphia, Lea & Febiger, 1975.

Pontoppidan H, Geffin B, Lowenstein E: *Acute Respiratory Failure in the Adult*. Boston, Little, Brown & Co, 1973.

West JB: *Pulmonary Pathophysiology–The Essentials*. Baltimore, Williams & Wilkins, 1977.

ARTICLES

Diagnosis of Lung Diseases

Bartlett JA: Diagnostic accuracy of transtracheal aspiration bacteriologic studies. *Am Rev Resp Dis* 115:777-782, 1977.

Davidson M, Tempest B, Palmer DL: Bacteriologic diagnosis of acute pneumonia: Comparison of sputum, transtracheal aspirates, and lung aspirates. *JAMA* 235:158-163, 1976.

Light RW, MacGregor MI, Ball WC Jr, et al.: Diagnostic significance of pleural fluid pH and pCO_2. *Chest* 64:591-596, 1973.

Sackner MA: Bronchofiberscopy: State of the art. *Am Rev Resp Dis* 111:62-88, 1975.

Anatomy and Developmental Abnormalities

Dines DE, Arms RA, Bernatz PE, Gomes MR: Pulmonary arteriovenous fistulas. *Mayo Clin Proc* 49:460-465, 1974.

Landing BH, Dixon LG: Congenital malformation and genetic disorders of the respiratory tract (larynx, trachea, bronchi, and lungs). *Am Rev Resp Dis* 120:151-185, 1979.

Zumbro GL, Treasure RL, Seitter G, et al.: Pulmonary sequestration: A broad spectrum of bronchopulmonary foregut abnormalities. *Ann Thorac Surg* 20:161-169, 1975.

Pulmonary Mycoses

Catanzaro A: Pulmonary coccidioidomycosis. *Med Clin North Am* 64: 461-473, 1980.

Goodwin RA Jr, Des Prez RM: Histoplasmosis: State of the art. *Am Rev Resp Dis* 117:929-956, 1978.

Kumar UN, Varkey B, Landis FB: Allergic bronchopulmonary aspergillosis: An increasing clinical problem. *Postgrad Med* 58(6):141-145, 1975.

Varkey B, Rose HD, Lohaus G, et al.: Blastomycosis: Clinical and immunologic aspects. Clinical Conference in Pulmonary Disease from Wood Veterans Administration Medical Center and Medical College of Wisconsin, Milwaukee. *Chest* 77:789-795, 1980.

Varkey B, Rose HD: Pulmonary aspergilloma: A rational approach to treatment. *Am J Med* 61:626-631, 1976.

Obstructive Disorders of the Airways

Eliasson R, Mossberg B, Cramner P, et al.: The immotile-cilia syndrome: A congenital ciliary abnormality as an etiologic factor in chronic airway infections and male sterility. *N Engl J Med* 297: 1-6, 1977.

Kryger M, Bode F, Artic R, et al.: Diagnosis of obstruction of the upper and central airways. *Am J Med* 1:85-93, 1976.

Lertzman MM, Cherniack RM: Rehabilitation of patients with chronic obstructive pulmonary disease. *Am Rev Resp Dis* 114:1145-1165, 1976.

Wood RE, Boat TF, Doershuk CF; Cystic fibrosis: State of the art. *Am Rev Resp Dis* 113:833-878, 1976.

Disorders of Lung Circulation

Dalen JE, Alpert JS: Natural history of pulmonary embolism. *Prog Cardiovasc Dis* 17:257-270, 1975.

Fishman AP: Chronic cor pulmonale: State of the art. *Am Rev Resp Dis* 114:775-794, 1976.

Houston CS: High altitude illness: Disease with protean manifestations. *JAMA* 236:2193-2195, 1976.

Moser KM: Pulmonary embolism. *Am Rev Resp Dis*115:829-852, 1977.

Staub NC: Pulmonary edema: Physiologic approaches to management. *Chest* 74:559-564, 1978.

Pulmonary Diseases Due to Physical and Chemical Agents

Gross NJ: Pulmonary effects of radiation therapy. *Ann Intern Med* 86:81-92, 1977.

Karr RM, Davies RJ, Butcher BT, et al.: Occupational asthma. *J Allergy Clin Immunol* 61:54-65, 1978.

Morgan WKC, Lapp NL: Respiratory disease in coal miners. *Am Rev Resp Dis* 113:531-559, 1976.

Varkey B, Kumar UN: Asbestos-related diseases of lung and pleura: Clinical picture and illustrative cases. *Postgrad Med* 63:48-66, 1978.

Ziskind M, Jones RN, Weill H: Silicosis. *Am Rev Resp Dis* 113:643-665, 1976.

Diffuse Infiltrative Diseases of the Lung

Bartlett JG, Gorbach SL: The triple threat of aspiration pneumonia. *Chest* 68:560-566, 1975.

Basset F, Corrin B, Spencer H, et al.: Pulmonary histiocytosis X. *Am Rev Resp Dis* 118:811-820, 1978.

Carrington CB, Gaensler EA, Coutu RE, et al.: Natural history and treated course of usual and desquamative interstitial pneumonia. *N Engl J Med* 298:801-809, 1978.

DeRemee RA, Harrison EG Jr, Andersen HA: The concept of classic interstitial pneumonitis: Fibrosis (CIP-F) as a clinicopathologic syndrome. *Chest* 61:213-220, 1972.

Hunninghake GW, Fauci AS: Pulmonary involvement in the collagen vascular diseases. *Am Rev Resp Dis* 119:471-503, 1979.

Israel HL, Atkinson GW: Sarcoidosis. *Basics of Resp Dis* 7:1-6, 1978.

Kintzer JS Jr, Rosenow EC III, Kyle RA: Thoracic and pulmonary abnormalities in multiple myeloma: A review of 958 cases. *Arch Intern Med* 138:727-730, 1978.

Mayock RL, Bertrans P, Morrison CE, et al.: Manifestations of sarcoidosis: Analysis of 145 patients, with a review of 9 series selected from the literature. *Am J Med* 35:67-89, 1963.

Schlueter DP: Response of the lung to inhaled antigens. *Am J Med* 57:476-492, 1974.

Winterbauer RH, Hammar SP, Hallman KO, et al.: Diffuse interstitial pneumonitis: Clinicopathologic correlations in 20 patients treated with prednisone/azathioprine. *Am J Med* 65:661-672, 1978.

Neoplasms of the Lung

Neff TA: When the x-ray shows a spot in the lung. *Resident and Staff Physician* 24 (11):89-101, 1978.

Ramming KP: Surgery for pulmonary metastases. *Surg Clin North Am* 60 (4):815-824, 1980.

Salyer DC, Salyer WR, Eggleston JC: Bronchial carcinoid tumors. *Cancer* 36:1522-1537, 1975.

Disorders of the Pleura, Mediastinum, and Diaphragm

Light RW, MacGregor MI, Luchsinger PC, et al.: Pleural effusions: The diagnostic separation of transudates and exudates. *Ann Intern Med* 77-507-513, 1972.

Silverman NA, Sabiston DC Jr: Primary tumors and cysts of the mediastinum *Curr Probl Cancer* 2(5):1-55, 1977.

Taryle DA, Lakshiminarayan S, Sahn SA: Pleural mesotheliomas: An analysis of 18 cases and review of the literature. *Medicine* 55: 153-162, 1976.

Acute Respiratory Failure

Bone RC: Treatment of respiratory failure due to advanced chronic osbtructive lung disease. *Arch Intern Med* 140:1018-1021, 1980.

O'Donohue WJ Jr, Baker JP, et al.: Respiratory failure in neuromuscular disease: Management in a respiratory intensive care unit. *JAMA* 235:733-735, 1976.

Petty TL, Ashbaugh DG: The adult respiratory distress syndrome: Clinical features, factors influencing prognosis, and principles of management. *Chest* 60:233-239, 1971.

Suter PM, Fairley HB, Isenberg MD: Optimum end-expiratory pressure in patients with acute pulmonary failure. *N Engl J Med* 292:284-289, 1975.

CHAPTER 14
RHEUMATOLOGY

Edward J. Pisko
Carlos A. Agudelo
Robert A. Turner

AN APPROACH TO THE RHEUMATOLOGIC PATIENT

HISTORY

The medical history as it relates to rheumatic disease is not appreciably different from the standard history; however, it is worthwhile to emphasize a few points that are useful in evaluating patients and to help distinguish organic disease from funtional (psychogenic) disease.

Pain is the major rheumatologic complaint, and relief of pain is the stated objective of most patient visits. However, patients with this complaint may have other objectives in coming to see a physician. Among these are worry that rheumatic diseases are familial, an abnormal screening test for such things as rheumatoid factor, and inquiry as to the latest miracle cure for arthritis, a desire to obtain disability, or to be transferred to a less-stressful job. A knowledge of patient objectives will facilitate the interview and help fulfill patient expectations.

When pain is the major complaint, it is important to ascertain whether the pain is localized or diffuse as localized conditions are often self-limited or responsive to conservative therapy. Further questioning may reveal that the localized process is part of a systemic disorder. "Hurting all over" may be a common initial complaint; however, with further questioning, most patients with organic disease can localize it to various joints and the inability to do this makes a functional illness more likely. Patients often need careful guidance in delineating complaints such as hand pain, and it is often necessary to point to individual structures in order to localize the discomfort. It is important to ascertain if pain is present on motion, weight-bearing, rest, or at night.

Stiffness, particularly in the morning, is an important complaint. The duration of morning stiffness is an excellent measure of inflammation and has proved to be a good means of measuring the response to therapy in rheumatoid arthritis. Once stiffness has been differentiated from pain, it is relatively easy to determine its duration by asking when the patient arises from bed and when the stiffness starts to improve. The difference in hours should be recorded. Another useful measure of inflammation is the duration of time from arising to the onset of fatigue. The shorter the duration, the more severe the inflammation. Patients should be asked when they feel so tired they can't go on or when they feel "all played out." Patients with functional illness will often awake with fatigue, and this may not vary throughout the day. Also, patients with functional illness may be stiff in the morning.

Weakness is another important complaint in individuals with rheumatic disease. Patients will often confuse weakness with fatigue, particularly if functional illness is present. Organic disease is suggested when patients have difficulty with specific tasks such as arising from a chair, climbing a stepstool, or loosening jar lids. Upper extremity clumsiness may also be due to weakness.

PHYSICAL EXAMINATION

A careful and thorough general physical examination is important in evaluating patients with rheumatic complaints. Skin abnormalities may provide important clues to the diagnosis of such disorders as Reiter's syndrome or vasculitis. A careful physical may reveal a pericardial friction rub providing a clue to an extra-articular manifestation of rheumatoid arthritis. However, careful joint examination remains the most important means of diagnosing rheumatic disease and assessing disease activity. An assessment of the degree of inflammation is the major goal of examination. Inflammation is heralded by heat, pain, redness, and swelling; however, especially with chronic conditions, these signs may not be obvious and joint tenderness is the most useful sign that inflammation is present. Patients with functional illness are often diffusely tender; this helps distinguish them from patients with organic disease. Joint swelling is also an important sign of inflammation. Swelling is often visible, but usually is detected by palpation. Both fluid accumulation and synovial proliferation are responsible for swelling. A knowledge of the location, thickness, and consistency of the normal synovial reflection of joints is necessary for the detection of synovial thickening.

All joints should be moved through a normal range of motion. Pain on motion and limitation of motion are important clues to disease; their absence makes it unlikely that disease is present in the joint being examined. Careful joint examination also requires that supporting tendons be palpated for tenderness.

LABORATORY TESTS

The laboratory is often quite helpful in making diagnoses, but laboratory testing should never supplant a careful history and physical examination. Much useful information can be learned from simple tests such as the complete blood count and urinalysis. The following tests are especially important in evaluating patients with rheumatic diseases.

Synovianalysis

Synovial fluid analysis, or synovianalysis, is an often neglected but very important means of evaluating the patient with joint disease. Most importantly, this is the means for diagnosing two highly treatable disorders, crystalline joint disease and septic arthritis. In other disorders, synovianalysis can be an important adjunct to diagnosis or to assessment of disease activity.

Synovial fluid is obtained after preparing the skin with antiseptics, usually iodine and alcohol. Sterile drapes or gloves are usually not needed; in fact, the talc crystals contained in the gloves can cause confusion with pathologic crystals. Careful skin preparation is most important and can usually prevent culture contamination or the introduction of pathogens into the joint.

Synovianalysis begins as the fluid is withdrawn; it is important to ascertain if any blood observed is thoroughly mixed with the fluid or appears suddenly as occurs with a traumatic tap. Two tests give immediate useful information. Clarity is evaluated by reading newsprint through the fluid. Synovial fluid is normally clear, and turbidity implies inflammation. Viscosity is evaluated by letting the fluid drip from the syringe. Normal fluid is viscous and forms a string several inches in length. Inflammatory fluid forms drops that readily fall from the needle.

The synovial fluid should be observed for clotting. Normal fluid is essentially an ultrafiltrate of plasma with the exception that fibrinogen and several clotting factors are not present. When clotting is observed, joint inflammation is present.

Hyaluronic acid is the major constituent of joint fluid that is not present in plasma and is responsible for the fluid's viscosity. Hyaluronic acid is present in a polymerized form in normal fluid. Depolymerization, which occurs with inflammation, is roughly measured by the mucin clot test. This test is performed by adding synovial fluid to weak acetic acid and observing whether there is a tight clot (normal fluid) or clouds and shreds (inflammatory fluid).

The white blood cell count of the fluid also yields useful information. Heparin is used as the anticoagulant instead of calcium citrate since the latter can form crystals that can confuse the interpretation. It is important to dilute the fluid with saline since acetic acid, the usual diluent, will clot the fluid and give false readings. The values for normal fluid and the fluid in various conditions are given in Table 1. For convenience, the fluids have been divided into three groups: noninflammatory (group 1), inflammatory (group 2), and inflammatory infectious (group 3). Overlap in the white count and other measures of inflammation occur between the groups, emphasizing the importance of culture in distinguishing group 2 and group 3 fluids. Wright's stain and differential count are sometimes useful. With acute infection, the white blood cells are predominantly polymorphonuclear. In osteoarthritis and in normal fluid, the cells are predominantly mononuclear. Occasionally the synovial fluid will be

Table 1. Synovianalysis

	Clarity	*Viscosity*	*Mucin Clot*	*WBC/mm²*	*Glucose*	*Other*
Normal	Transparent	Normal	Good	<200	Normal[a]	
Noninflammatory						
Osteoarthritis	Transparent	Normal	Good	<1,500	Normal	
Trauma	Transp. turbid	Normal or ↓	Good or ↓	<2,000 RBC	Normal	May be cloudy
Inflammatory						
SLE	Transparent Sl. turbid	Normal	Good	<5,000	Normal	LE cells
Rheumatic fever	Sl. cloudy	↓	Good-Poor	<15,000	Normal	
Gout	Turbid	Poor	Poor	5,000 to 40,000	Normal	Urate crystals
Pseudogout	Turbid	Poor	Poor	<20,000	Normal	Calcium pyrophosphate crystals
Rheumetoid arthritis	Turbid	Poor	Poor	5,000 to 40,000	↓	Ragocytes
Reiter's disease	Turbid	Poor	Poor	10,000 to 100,000	Normal	Pekin cell
Infectious						
Septic	Turbid Purulent	Poor	Poor	50,000 to 200,000	↓	Positive culture
Tuberculous	Cloudy	↓	Poor	5,000 to 20,000	↓	Positive culture
Viral	Cloudy	↓	↓	5,000 to 15,000	?	Positive or negative culture
Fungous	Cloudy	↓	↓	5,000 to 25,000	?	Positive culture

[a] A normal synovial glucose is about two-thirds the blood glucose if the patient has been fasting.

bloody, or red blood cells will predominate on the smear. The differential diagnosis of bloody synovial fluid includes trauma, villonodular synovitis, and tumors such as a synovial sarcoma.

Culture is most important, and all fluid obtained for diagnoses should be cultured for bacteria, tuberculosis, and fungus. Special handling may facilitate the growth of gonococcus. Viral cultures, although not readily available, may be useful.

Examination of the fluid with polarizing microscopy for crystals is also very important. The diagnosis of gout is made only with the identification of monosodium urate crystals. This disease is treatable and preventable; however, the diagnosis should be firm before subjecting patients to possibly toxic therapies. Ragocytes are polymorphonuclear leukocytes that have ingested particles consisting primarily of immunoglobulin. These are most commonly found in rheumatoid arthritis; however, they also may be seen in other type 2 and 3 fluids. The Pekin cell consists of a macrophage that has ingested several polymorphonuclear cells. It is found most frequently in Reiter's disease, but can be present in a variety of other disorders.

Sedimentation Rate

The erythrocyte sedimentation rate is the oldest measure of inflammation; it remains a valuable tool for evaluating patients with rheumatic diseases. This test is reported as the distance in millimeters that a column of anticoagulated blood falls in 1 hour. The rate of fall is related to the concentration of acute phase reactants in the blood. A variety of proteins such as ceruloplasmin and haptoglobin comprise the acute phase reactants; however, fibrinogen is by far the most important contributor to an abnormal sedimentation rate. Globulins may also increase the rate. Disorders that deform red cells, such as sickle cell anemia, will cause falsely low sedimentation rates. Congestive heart failure may also do this.

Several methods have been utilized to perform this test; however, the method as described by Westergren remains the most useful. The normal value is 1-7 mm, although there is a tendency for values to rise with age; values in the 20-35 mm range are considered only mild elevations, 35-55 mm are moderate, and values above 55 mm are considered marked elevations.

An elevated sedimentation rate is a good indication that inflammation is present. Conversely, a normal sedimentation rate is often reassuring. However, there are exceptions to this; for example, the sedimentation rate is often normal in polymyositis. In rheumatoid arthritis, the sedimentation rate only roughly parallels disease activity.

The sedimentation rate may be very valuable in certain diseases. An elevated sedimentation rate is the sine qua non of polymyalgia rheumatica. In systemic lupus erythematosus, an elevated sedimentation rate implies a worse prognosis. In evaluating an elevated sedimentation rate, it is important to remember that nonrheumatoid diseases such as malignancies, particularly of the hematopoietic system, can often be responsible.

Rheumatoid Factor

Rheumatoid factors are antibodies to immunoglobulin G (IgG). They were first described by Waaler in 1940 and named because of their association with rheumatoid arthritis. Subsequent study has found rheumatoid factor in a variety of infectious, connective tissue, and idiopathic disorders. Rheumatoid factors may belong to the IgM, IgA, or IgG classes. The significance of IgG rheumatoid factor is still under study, and IgA rheumatoid factors are rare. Conventional tests measure primarily IgM rheumatoid factor.

The most common test for detection of rheumatoid factor is the latex agglutination test (RA-Latex). Latex beads are coated with pooled IgG containing some IgG aggregates. Test sera are positive if the particles agglutinate. A value of 1:160 or greater is considered positive, and 5% of the normal population will be positive when this value is used. The prevalence rises with age, and one-third of elderly individuals may be positive. About 75% of patients with rheumatoid arthritis are positive; statistically, these individuals have a worse prognosis. The test is often negative during the first year of the disease. Positive tests also occur in a variety of infections such as subacute bacterial endocarditis, trypanosomiasis, and tuberculosis. Interstitial pulmonary disease is frequently associated with rheumatoid factor. Other connective tissue disorders such as systemic lupus erythematosus (SLE), progressive systemic sclerosis, or polyarteritis nodosa may have a positive rheumatoid factor.

The sensitized sheep cell agglutination test (SCAT) is the oldest test for the detection of rheumatoid factor. Test sera agglutinate sheep cells coated with rabbit antisheep red cell antibody. The rheumatoid factor thus combines with rabbit IgG. Heterophil antibodies must be absorbed first. This test is much less likely to be positive in conditions other than rheumatoid arthritis and is more specific for this disease. It is positive in about one-half of all patients with rheumatoid arthritis.

Antinuclear Antibodies

The detection of antinuclear antibodies has greatly aided the diagnosis of connective tissue disorders. They are detected primarily by indirect immunofluorescence, in which a tissue section such as rat liver or kidney is incubated with the test sera. Antibodies that have combined with nuclear consituents are then detected by first adding a fluoresceinated antiimmunoglobulin and then detecting these antibodies with a fluorescence microscope. Antinuclear antibodies may belong to the IgG, IgM, or IgA classes; however, the most useful information is obtained when fluoresceinated anti-IgG antibodies are used to detect IgG antinuclear antibodies.

Various patterns of nuclear fluorescence are seen. The most common pattern is homogeneous; this pattern is also the most nonspecific. It can be found in low titers in a variety of connective tissue disorders such as rheumatoid arthritis. At high titers, a homogeneous pattern is fairly specific for systemic lupus erythematosus. Two antigens are responsible for this pattern: deoxynucleoprotein and nuclear histones. Antibodies to deoxynucleoprotein are also responsible for the LE cell phenomenon. The peripheral pattern of nuclear fluorescence also detects antibodies to deoxynucleoprotein but in addition detects antibodies to native (double-stranded) DNA. This pattern, also called the rim or shaggy pattern, is highly specific for SLE.

Antibodies to native DNA may also be detected using a variety of other techniques, most of which involve the precipitation of complexes of antibody and DNA. High titers of these antibodies are specific for SLE.

A speckled pattern of nuclear fluorescence is due to antibodies to acidic nuclear proteins, primarily ribonucleoprotein (RNP) and the Sm antigen. These two antigens make up extractable nuclear antigen (ENA) which, when digested with ribonuclease, leaves the Sm antigen. These antigens are detected by immunodiffusion or hemagglutination techniques. Sm antibody is highly specific for SLE. High titers of antibody to RNP are specific for mixed connective tissue disease, but low titers are also found in SLE and other connective tissue disorders.

Speckled fluorescent antinuclear antibodies may also be seen in Sjögren's syndrome, and antibodies to specific acid nuclear proteins have been detected by immunodiffusion in this disease. Speckled fluorescent antinuclear antibodies are also seen in progressive systemic sclerosis; at high titers, fluorescent antinucleolar antibodies are quite specific for this disease. The antigen is RNA.

The detection of antinuclear antibodies is currently under intense investigation, and new antibodies and associations for old antibodies are being found at a rapid rate.

RHEUMATOID ARTHRITIS

Pathogenesis

Both cellular and humoral mechanisms may be involved in the pathogenesis of rheumatoid arthritis. Rheumatoid factors of the immunoglobulin G and M varieties form complexes that interact with cellular components and perpetuate acute and chronic inflammatory processes. Neutrophils are found predominantly in the synovial fluid and many contain phagocytosed complexes; mononuclear cell infiltration is present in the synovium with synovial hypertrophy and invasion of cartilage.

Clinical Features

Rheumatoid arthritis is a common medical problem with estimates of prevalence of approximately 1-3% of the population, depending on the criteria used for making the diagnosis. The standard criteria over the past several years have been those

Table 2. Criteria for Rheumatoid Arthritis

Stiffness	X-ray changes
Pain or tenderness	Rheumatoid factor
Swelling	Inflammatory synovial fluid
Polyarticularity	Synovial membrane histologic changes
Symmetry	Characteristic nodule histology
Clinical nodularity	

devised by a committee of the American Rheumatism Association. A summary of these criteria is shown in Table 2.

This disease is characterized by morning stiffness that should, in keeping with the criteria, last for over 1 hour but that may or may not be present in a given patient at some stage in the disease. There is characteristically pain or tenderness along with swelling for at least 6 weeks in one joint for criteria 2 and 3, but usually multiple joints are involved as noted in criterion 4. For criterion 4, at least two joints must be involved within 3 months. All of the joints in the body may be affected, although the disease involves characteristically the proximal joints of the hands and feet with the metacarpophalangeal and metatarsophalangeal joints being those most commonly affected. Rheumatoid arthritis is a symmetrical disease, and subcutaneous nodules occur over bony prominences and on extensor surfaces as noted in criterion 6. Roentgenograms of the joints show periarticular osteoporosis early, with joint space narrowing and erosion occurring later. As discussed in an earlier section, rheumatoid factor is an anti-immunoglobulin G that is classically measured as IgM directed against the Fc, complement fixing, portion of IgG. Of the patients with rheumatoid arthritis, 60-80% will have a positive test for rheumatoid factor by a standard method.

The synovial fluid in rheumatoid arthritis shows evidence of inflammation with an elevated white blood cell count, a decreased glucose and, as noted in criterion 9, poor mucin precipitate formed from the synovial fluid. This is thought to be due to degradation of the hyaluronic acid in the chronic inflammatory process. If a biopsy of the synovial membrane is performed, chracteristic histologic changes occur showing synovial hypertrophy, palisading of lymphocytes, and infiltration of the synovium with mononuclear cells. Deposition of fibrin detected by immunofluorescence, on the synovial surface and interstitially is also one of the histologic characteristics. If rheumatoid nodules are biopsied from either a subcutaneous site or from other sites in the body, they may show characteristic histologic changes with granulomatous foci, central necrosis, chronic inflammatory cell infiltration, and peripheral fibrosis.

The criteria noted above emphasize the articular involvement that is the hallmark of this disease. This articular involvement is highly variable since many patients exhibiting three of the criteria fall into the category of probable rheumatoid arthritis; many patients exhibiting seven or more of the criteria fall into the category of classic rheumatoid arthritis. The spectrum of joint involvement ranges from involvement of the hands and feet to involvement of the large peripheral joints and spine. Characteristically, cervical spine involvement is more common than lumbar spine involvement. As with clinical joint involvement, the appearance of extra-articular problems is a highly variable phenomenon. Systemic problems such as fever, malaise, and easy fatiguability are sometimes present. The major extraarticular involvement in rheumatoid arthritis can be considered under the cardiopulmonary, hematologic, neurovascular, and miscellaneous categories.

The most common cardiopulmonary manifestation of rheumatoid arthritis is inflammation of the serosal surfaces, which may occur in up to 50% of patients depending on the sensitivity of the test utilized to demonstrate this abnormality. The high prevalence may be related to the similarity between the pericardium, pleura, and synovium. Autopsy studies and echocardiography demonstrate a prevalence in this range for pericardial involvement although clinically apparent pericarditis may occur in only 1-2% of patients. Pleuritis by history or chest x-ray evidence may occur in 20% of patients. Rheumatoid nodules may occur in the myocardial tissue giving rise to atrioventricular conduction delays; when other areas of the conducting system are involved, clinically important arrhythmias may occur. Rheumatoid nodules occasionally may also involve the heart valves or valve rings. Rheumatoid nodules may occur in the lungs either as solitary lesions that require serial chest x-rays or biopsy for diagnosis. There is an equally prevalent (1%) occurrence of confluent irregular, pulmonary nodularity associated with pneumoconiosis in patients with so-called Caplan's syndrome. Interstitial involvement of the lungs may occur with 30-40% of patients on careful study showing abnormal diffusing capacities. Smoking seems to enhance the development of interstitial pulmonary abnormalities and should be discouraged in patients with rheumatoid arthritis. The occurrence of clinical interstitial fibrosis is uncommon, however, in patients with rheumatoid arthritis. Myocarditis may occur, although this is an uncommon lesion. Rarely, arteritis of the coronary vessels may lead to myocardial infarction or other problems; uncommonly, arteritis of the pulmonary vasculature may occur and lead to pulmonary hypertension.

Rheumatoid arthritis patients occasionally may develop a fulminating vasculitis. These patients exhibit classic skin lesions of vasculitis with digital pulp nodules, purpuric skin lesions, or areas of necrosis on the fingertips. The most common extra-articular lesion associated with diffuse vasculitis is a peripheral neuropathy that may involve both motor and sensory nerve components. Entrapment neuropathies of the median or ulnar nerves in the upper extremity and peroneal or saphenous nerves of the lower extremity may also occur in patients without clinically demonstrated vasculitis. The most common neurologic finding in rheumatoid arthritis patients is a digital neuropathy that is sensory and may be clinically unimpressive. About 20-30% of patients may develop atlantoaxial joint involvement and 1 percent may develop neurologic complications involving the cervical cord, requiring orthopedic or neurosurgical correction. Careful x-rays prior to surgical intervention are indicated in all rheumatoid arthritis patients suspected of having this problem.

Hematologic abnormalities include a hypochromic microcytic anemia that may be the result of intestinal blood loss related to anti-inflammatory agent therapy or normochromic normocytic anemia with a low iron-binding capacity related to the chronic disease process involving the reticuloendothelial system in rheumatoid arthritis. Anemia, splenomegaly, and leukopenia may occur as an entity called Felty's syndrome. This may be seen in up to 5% of rheumatoid arthritis patients coming to medical attention. These patients may be highly seropositive with minimal joint involvement and may have neutrophil specific, antinuclear antibodies detectable in the peripheral blood. Lymphadenopathy may occur in rheumatoid arthritis patients with biopsy findings suggesting giant follicular lymphoma. However, there is no progression and the lymphadenopathy resolves along with the total inflammatory picture under antirheumatic therapy or spontaneous remission. Megaloblastic anemia has been described secondary to a vitamin B_{12} or (more commonly) folic acid deficiency in patients with chronically active rheumatoid arthritis. Cryoglobulinemia related to circulating immune complexes also may occur; some patients may develop a hyperviscosity syndrome due to high titers of IgG-IgM rheumatoid factor complexes circulating in the peripheral blood.

Other organ systems may be involved in rheumatoid arthritis. In some patients with rheumatoid nodule involvement of the sclera, there may be striking eye lesions of scleromalacia perforans. Dry eyes from Sjögren's syndrome may occur with other ocular lesions including conjunctivitis, deep iritis, or uveitis (less common than in other rheumatologic diseases like ankylosing spondilitis), or corneal ulcers occuring in some patients. Cricoarytenoid joint involvement with laryngeal stridor may occur, along with a polymyositis-type picture from diffuse inflammatory myopathy.

Treatment

Medical therapy is designed to decrease the inflammatory aspects and/or cause a remission of the disease with a decrease in joint deformities and erosions. General management is important with counseling of the patient and family concerning the variable and remittable nature of the disease. Physical therapy and occupational therapy programs available for decreasing pain and increasing mobility and function are also important aspects of the overall management of this disease. Surgical therapy of chronic deformities has been rewarding. Recent advances in surgical procedures allow total joint replacement when pain and deformities require this therapy.

Anti-inflammatory agents should be the first line of medical treatment for patients with rheumatoid arthritis. Of the salicylates, aspirin (ASA) is the most frequently used, being the least expensive and most effective of the available preparations. Most patients can tolerate 12-16 aspirin tablets a day, and this dose usually provides effective anti-inflammatory activity. An occasional patient may require up to 24 tablets a day to achieve the therapeutic blood level of approximately 30 mg/dl. One of the most predictable but least serious side effects of aspirin is tinnitus that can be accompanied by a high-frequency hearing loss usually reversible when the aspirin dosage is decreased. Hematologic side effects such as decreased platelet adhesiveness and/or increased prothrombin time may occur but are clinically important only in patients with predisposing hematologic problems. A potentially serious side effect is the occurrence of asthma and anaphylactic shock in some patients. This seems to be related to the inhibition of prostaglandin synthesis and may occur with other oral anti-inflammatory agents that exhibit this activity. The most consistently troublesome major side effects produced by aspirin involve the gastrointestinal tract; the most serious problem is the development of peptic ulcer disease. Aspirin is, therefore, given after meals and at bedtime with either milk or an antacid. In high doses it can produce elevated levels of liver enzymes, although serious liver damage with aspirin therapy in rheumatoid arthritis has not been a major problem. Although aspirin is relatively safe and inexpensive, a continuing search for new agents has produced numerous alternatives that should be considered, especially when aspirin is poorly tolerated. These drugs are listed in Table 3.

Like ASA, these agents inhibit prostaglandins and can produce anaphylaxis in patients with aspirin allergy. At maximum doses, they probably cause less gastrointestinal side effects and ulcers than aspirin and are effective agents in patients who do not tolerate aspirin. The daily cost to the patient of maximal dose therapy with these newer agents ranges from 5-10 times that of aspirin. However, their greater potential safety makes them very useful in treating this disease. Indomethacin is a useful agent in doses of 50-100 mg before bedtime in conjunction with daytime doses of other nonsteroidal anti-inflammatory agents for patients having moderate inflammation despite maximal therapy with other nonsteroidal drugs.

Of the older drugs, one of the most potent is phenylbutazone. The drug is useful in short-term therapy, but is used infrequently for longer periods because of the rare but potentially devastating side effect of marrow suppression. Agranulocytosis may be seen in younger people in the early stages of

Table 3. Nonsteroid Anti-Inflammatory Agents

Drugs	*Tablet Size (mg)*	*Maximum Dosage Mg Per Day*
Salicylates		
Aspirin	325	6,500
Propionic acid derivatives		
Ibuprofen (Motrin)	300, 400, 600	2,400
Fenoprofen (Nalfon)	300, 600	3,000
Naproxen (Naprosyn)	250, 375, 500	1,000
Indole derivatives		
Indomethacin (Indocin)	25, 50	200
Tolmetin (Tolectin)	200, 400	1,800
Miscellaneous agents		
Phenylbutazone (Azolid, Butazolidin)	100	400
Sulindac (Clinoril)	150, 200	200
Piroxicam (Feldene)	20	20

treatment and aplastic anemia may occur in the elderly, usually after a prolonged period of treatment. A newer agent with much less frequent gastrointestinal side effects than phenylbutazone is the indene derivative sulindac (Clinoril), whose long half-life makes it effective in a dose of two 200 mg tablets per day. The first agent approved for once a day use is piroxicam (Feldene) which appears to offer good efficacy and an acceptably low side effect incidence when used in the 20 mg/day recommended dosage.

Patients developing severe extra-articular manifestations such as severe pleuritis or pericarditis may be treated with systemic corticosteroids. Local intra-articular corticosteroid injection therapy is fairly well accepted, and its infrequent use may allow control of the inflammatory process that would be unobtainable otherwise without utilizing more potentially toxic and long-term approaches to antiarthritic therapy. None of the nonsteroidal or steroidal anti-inflammatory agents have been shown to slow the progression of this disease.

The major long-acting agents presently approved for the treatment of rheumatoid arthritis are shown in Table 4. Antimalarial agents have long been utilized for the treatment of this disease. The onset of effect is subtle, occuring between 3 and 6 months after the beginning of therapy. Selective accumulation in the retina occurs and retinal toxicity may progress despite discontinuation of therapy. This side effect necessitates care in not exceeding the maximal dose per day and attempted withdrawal of the drug at various periods during therapy.

Other devastating side effects of antimalarial agents are: exfoliative dermatitis, severe leukopenia, peripheral neuropathy, and myopathy. With the development of other long-acting agents, the use of this class of drugs may decline in the future.

Gold salts are available as gold sodium thiomalate (Myochrysine) or gold thioglucose (Solganol). Injections are required each week for approximately the first 6 months and maintenance therapy is usually then continued for up to many years. On such regimens, up to 80% of patients may respond, and there is convincing evidence that this drug slows the radiographic progression of rheumatoid arthritis. Side effects are relatively common, with 10% of patients developing rashes.

Table 4. Long-Acting Agents Used in Treatment of Rheumatoid Arthritis

Drugs	*Tablet Size (mg)*	*Maximum No. of Tablets Per Day*
Antimalarials		
Hydroxychloroquine (Plaquenil)	200	2
Gold salts		
Aurothiomalate (Myochrysine)	Injectable	50 mg per week or per month
Aurothioglucose (Solganal)	Ampules	
Miscellaneous		
D-Penicillamine (Cuprimine)	125, 250	4

Potentially serious side effects, such as bone marrow suppression and nephrotic syndrome, require close monitoring of white blood cell counts and urinalyses during therapy. Intramuscular therapy is initiated with 10 mg the first week, 25 mg the second week, and 50 mg weekly thereafter until toxic reactions appear, the response is adequate, or a total dose of 1-2 g has been given. If the response is good, maintenance therapy is continued with 50 mg every 2-4 weeks.

Penicillamine is the latest addition to the treatment regimens for rheumatoid arthritis. It is now available in 125- and 250-milligram tablets. Therapy is usually begun with one tablet and increased at bimonthly or greater intervals to doses no greater than 1 g per day. As with gold, the onset of clinical response is slow, and side effects requiring withdrawal of the drug may occur in up to 30% of patients. Taste impairment is common but not serious and symptoms may range from mild anorexia to intractable vomiting necessitating cessation of therapy. A morbilliform rash with pruritus and ocular and lingular ulcerations may occur early in treatment. Pemphigoid eruptions may occur infrequently. Late skin rashes require withdrawal of the drug but early rashes may resolve with decreased dosages. One of the most dangerous side effects is marrow aplasia that tends to occur in the middle or late phases of treatment and requires immediate cessation of the drug. Proteinuria may resolve on continued treatment but increasing proteinuria requires discontinuation of the drug in some patients. A lupus-like syndrome produced by unknown immunologic mechanisms may also occur and is accompanied by antinuclear antibodies detectable by the usual methods.

OSTEOARTHRITIS

Osteoarthritis is the most common form of arthritis, its incidence increasing with age until almost all individuals have roentgenographic evidence of this disease. There is disparity between the roentgenographic findings and symptoms; however, the high prevalence ensures that this disease will be a major cause of disability. The terms degenerative joint disease and osteoarthrosis have gained favor because they avoid suggesting that this disease is primarily an inflammatory arthritis.

Etiology

Osteoarthritis is essentially the final common pathway of bone remodeling in joints damaged by trauma, inflammation, or metabolic diseases, although often an underlying disorder is not found and the disease has been considered an essential concomitant of aging. However, disease susceptibility is so variable that it is likely that as yet unknown metabolic or mechanical factors are responsible for this disease in patients without documented trauma or underlying disease. Hereditary factors are important as distal interphalangeal joint disease is often familial and has a female preponderance.

When osteoarthritis occurs in individuals without underlying joint disease it is called primary osteoarthritis. Among the diseases that cause secondary osteoarthritis by damaging joints are the inflammatory arthritides: rheumatoid arthritis, gout, and septic arthritis. Osteoarthritis may also be related to the metabolic diseases ochronosis or chondrocalcinosis. In the hip, congenital changes or aseptic necrosis may lead to disease. Occasionally, a single episode of trauma precedes osteoarthritis; however, repeated stress or trauma is more likely to cause the disease. Activities as diverse as ballet dancing or operating a jackhammer have been implicated. A variant of osteoarthritis is the neurotrophic joint (Charcot's joint), in which denervation leads to repeated trauma and often severe osteoarthritic changes. Tabes dorsalis is the classic cause; however, many diseases, of which diabetes mellitus is the most common, are responsible.

Pathogenesis

Osteoarthritis is a disease in which there is both destruction of cartilage and new bone formation. Cartilage is made up primarily of proteoglycan aggregates joined to a hyaluronic acid core and a collagen framework. The earliest change is a loss of glycosaminoglycan, a constituent of proteoglycan. There is also cartilage swelling. Fibrillation, or small breaks in the cartilage, occurs next and may progress to vertical clefts or cysts. With cartilage loss, the underlying bone becomes worn and resembles ivory (eburnation). New bone formation occurs and there is increased bone density (sclerosis). The new bone also frequently forms osteophytes (bony outgrowths), usually at the joint margins. New cartilage may also form in these areas.

Clinical Features

Osteoarthritis is manifested primarily by pain, that is usually present on motion or weight bearing. The pain is often relieved by rest, although with severe disease resting pain does occur and night pain may be a prominent feature. Morning stiffness frequently occurs, but usually lasts for less than one-half hour. Stiffness (gelling) may also occur after inactivity. Usually only a few joints are affected and patients may be grouped by whether the distal and proximal interphalangeal joints, knees and hips, or the spine are prominently involved.

Distal interphalangeal joint involvement is heralded by firm swellings about the joints known as Herberden's nodes. The same swelling in the proximal interphalangeal joint is known as Bouchard's node. The swelling is due to fibrous tissue as well as new bone and cartilage formation. Gelatinous cysts may occur in these joints and inflammation may be present intermittently. Lateral deviation of these joints is a frequent late finding. The metacarpophalangeal joints are usually spared, which differentiates this disease from rheumatoid arthritis that often has metacarpophalangeal synovitis. The involvement of the first carpometacarpal joint is rather specific for osteoarthritis. Disease of the first metatarsophalangeal joint is also quite common.

Osteoarthritis of the knee is manifested by pain on motion or weight bearing. Patients may complain of joint creaking and on examination fine crepitus may be palpated with joint motion. Muscle wasting and flexion contracture may accompany severe disease. The osteophytes are easily palpable and synovial thickening also may be detected. Synovial effusions may occur, and the fluid is usually noninflammatory.

Hip disease is usually manifested by weight-bearing pain over the groin or laterally over the joint. Occasionally, buttock or low-back pain may mimic spine disease; pain may also be referred to the knee. Flexion contracture may occur and the hip may be adducted and externally rotated, causing functional shortening of the leg, a compensating scoliosis, and pelvic tilt. This disarray of mechanical forces can cause pain in many areas.

The midportions of the cervical, thoracic, and lumbar spines are frequently involved in osteoarthritis. Symptoms may be localized or radiate in a radicular fashion when nerve-root irritation or compression occurs. Nerve-root compression may be secondary to the mild protrusion of a degenerating disk. Vertebral body osteophytes that project posteriorly into the foramen or osteophytes that arise from the apophyseal joints may cause nerve-root symptoms. Anterior vertebral osteophytes are common, but are usually not the cause of symptoms except during the rare compression of vertebral arteries. Osteoarthritis of the acromioclavicular joint occurs; however, shoulder pain is more likely to be due to inflammation of supporting structures. Other joints such as the elbow and ankle are rarely involved in the absence of repeated stress.

Osteoarthritis usually involves only a few joints; however, occasionally patients, usually women, will have simultaneous involvement of the proximal and distal interphalangeal, carpometacarpal, knee, first metatarsophalangeal and spinal apophyseal joints. This has been called generalized osteoarthritis. This most likely is a variant of osteoarthritis. Erosive osteoarthritis primarily involves the distal and proximal interphalangeal joints. Inflammation is more prominent and roentgenograms reveal more cystic and erosive changes. This represents a more severe variant of osteoarthritis.

The clinical course of osteoarthritis is variable, although the roentgenographic findings are stable or progressive. Pain is often related to injury or inflammation in adjacent tendons, ligaments, or muscles. These structures may become quiescent and long asymptomatic periods may intervene. Episodic synovitis also may occur and is often related to trauma, although concomitant crystalline or inflammatory joint disease should be ruled out. The pain of osteoarthritis is also closely related to associated factors such as emotional stress or depression. Patients with similar roentgenographic findings may have widely disparate degrees of pain, emphasizing the variability in individual pain thresholds.

Laboratory Manifestations

The laboratory is primarily helpful in eliminating other diagnoses. Rheumatoid factor occurs no more frequently than would be expected in normal people in this age group. Complete blood counts are normal. Sedimentation rates are sometimes slightly elevated in erosive or generalized osteoarthritis, but they are usually normal. Synovianalysis is helpful in ruling out inflammatory disorders such as crystalline joint disease that may occur concomitantly. Joint fluid usually has less than

$1500/mm^3$ cells, predominantly mononuclear. Synovial biopsy may reveal fibrous tissue and only rarely shows significant mononuclear cell infiltrates.

Roentgenographic Manifestations

Roentgenograms parallel the pathologic findings. Cartilage destruction is manifested by joint space narrowing that is often asymmetrical, unlike inflammatory disorders. Increased bone density or sclerosis parallels new bone growth. Cysts are frequently found. Osteophytes represent new bone growth at joint margins or at the tibial spines of the knee. Osteoporosis is not a feature of this disease.

Differential Diagnosis

When several joints are involved, confusion may occur with rheumatoid arthritis. The pattern of joint involvement is different, with osteoarthritis being more likely to involve the distal interphalangeal joints and rheumatoid arthritis involving the metacarpophalangeal joints. An elevated sedimentation rate, mild anemia, and inflammatory joint fluid support the diagnosis of rheumatoid arthritis. Polymyalgia rheumatica also affects older patients; however, fatigue and stiffness are much more prominent and the sedimentation rate is characteristically high. In an individual joint it is important to remember that degenerative changes on roentgenogram do not always mean that osteoarthritis is the cause of pain, as trauma or tendonitis may be responsible and the osteoarthritis may be incidental.

Treatment

Treatment consists of patient education, altering daily activities, physical therapy, analgesics, and the nonsteroidal antiinflammatory agents. Patient reassurance that this is a noncrippling disease is important. Patients need to be cautioned not to stress their joints repeatedly, for which a new job may be helpful. It is important to emphasize the overuse of a joint may hasten rather than delay the disease process. Rest is important and a specific program may be necessary. Heat, either moist or dry, is often helpful. Physical therapy consists of range-of-motion exercises to maintain mobility. Strengthening exercises, such as quadricep strengthening exercises for the knee, are helpful in maintaining and improving function. Cervical traction may benefit cervical spine disease and complete bed rest for brief periods may benefit lumbar spine disease. The nonsteroidal antiinflammatory agents are useful in providing pain relief and improving function. Occasionally, full anti-inflammatory dosages may be necessary; however, often smaller dosages such as 650 mg of aspirin q.i.d. or fenoprofen, 300 mg q.i.d., suffice. The lowest dose that relieves symptoms should be used. Indomethacin at dosages of 75-150 mg per day is particularly valuable in hip or knee disease, and may benefit other osteoarthritic disease as well. This drug is more toxic and should be used with caution particularly when employed long term. Patients often do not require medicine for long periods, particularly when their daily activity has been altered. Intra-articular corticosteroids have been used but are probably no more efficacious than a placebo. Since inflammation is minimal, the rationale for their usage is less strong than in rheumatoid arthritis. Experimental evidence suggests that corticosteroids have harmful effects on cartilage.

Total hip replacement has proved to be a very effective therapy for severe hip disease. Pain is almost always relieved and function is often improved. Knee replacement usually relieves pain although function may not be improved. A totally satisfactory prosthesis has not been developed and slippage or infection may result in a fused knee joint. Other joint prostheses are still experimental. Osteotomy may be helpful in selected patients.

THE SERONEGATIVE SPONDYLOARTHROPATHIES

The spondyloarthropathies are often familial with a male predominance. The entire group of diseases is characterized by arthritis of the sacroiliac and spinal joints, although peripheral arthritis also occurs. There is also involvement of the aortic root, uveal tract, skin, and urethra. The specific entities such as ankylosing spondylitis, Reiter's disease, psoriatic arthritis, and the arthritis of inflammatory bowel disease are discussed in subsequent sections. An overlap between these diseases sometimes occurs making patient classification difficult. Rheumatoid factor is characteristically absent; hence, these diseases have been called the seronegative spondyloarthropathies or polyarthropathies. They also have been called the rheumatoid variants; however, there are more differences than similarities between spondyloarthropathies and rheumatoid arthritis.

The presence of HLA-B27 antigen in a high percentage of spondyloarthropathic patients has fascinated students of these diseases. HLA-B27 is one of the histocompatibility antigens on cell surfaces. Currently four groups of antigen (A,B,C,D) have been described and one antigen from each group is inherited from each parent. The A, B, and C antigens are defined by reacting specific antisera from multiparous women with the subject's lymphocytes; a positive reaction occurs with complement activation and cytotoxicity. The D locus antigens are defined by mixed-lymphocyte culture. Since not all people with the HLA-B27 antigen develop disease and not all patients with a spondyloarthropathy have the HLA-B27 antigen, it has been postulated that an immune response gene near the HLA-B27 gene on the sixth chromosome that is in linkage disequilibrium with HLA-B27, might be responsible for the disease manifestations. Evidence for this theory comes from animal studies. The environmental factors that might stimulate the immune response gene or interact with the HLA-B27 antigen remain unknown.

In the United States 7% of whites and 4% of blacks have the HLA-B27 antigen and their risk for developing ankylosing spondylitis is 20%. The male-female ratio of these patients identified by screening HLA-B27 inidividuals is approximately equal, unlike the marked male predominance of ankylosing spondylitis. The HLA-B27 antigen is also associated with uveitis alone, some forms of juvenile chronic polyarthritis, and a reactive arthritis that occurs after *Salmonella* and *Yersinia enterocolitica* infections.

ANKYLOSING SPONDYLITIS

Approximately one in every 1,000 people in the population have ankylosing spondylitis, which is a chronic, progressive, inflammatory form of arthritis that primarily involves the sacroiliac joints and spine. It is usually a disease of young adult men. The inflammation results in new bone formation and eventually there is ossification of the involved joints (bony ankylosis). It is a systemic disease that may involve the heart and eyes.

Clinical Features

Men are affected nine times more frequently than women and the disease commonly occurs during the teenage years through the twenties, although it rarely begins after the age of 40.

Patients almost invariably have low back pain. The onset is insidious, and it is common for the pain to have been present for several months before medical attention is sought. The pain is usually nonradiating, but may radiate in a sciatic distribution. A neurologic examination can distinguish the disease from a herniated nucleus pulposus.

Especially during the early stages of the disease, the back pain tends to be exacerbated by rest and relieved in part by mild exercise. Morning stiffness is common and may also be helped by exercise. Although low back pain is the major complaint, weight loss, fatigue, and fever may be present; occasionally these systemic symptoms are the presenting complaints.

Peripheral joint involvement may be the presenting complaint and one-half of all patients have peripheral joint disease, usually affecting the knees and ankles. These joints may also be involved later in the course of the disease and there may also be synovitis of the wrists and small joints of the hands and feet. Synovitis is usually transient. Although not present initially, hip and shoulder disease is the most common form of peripheral joint involvement and a major cause of disability.

Patients frequently have chest pain that can mimic cardiac disease. This is usually due to costovertebral joint involvement. True heart disease is a rare and late manifestation of this disease. The primary lesion is aortic insufficiency that may lead to secondary congestive heart failure. Conduction abnormalities may also be present. Iritis occurs in 20% of patients and may be the presenting complaint. This may manifest itself as ocular pain, redness, or decreased vision. Ophthalmologic consultation and slit-lamp examination is mandatory when iritis is suspected. Asymptomatic fibrocavitary lesions of the upper lobes of the lungs may be present; however, symptoms may occur on the rare occasion when there is colonization of these lesions with aspergilli.

Early in this illness, physical examination may be normal or only reveal paravertebral muscle spasm. As the disease progresses, lumbosacral spine motion is limited. This should be evaluated in flexion, extension, and with lateral bending. Lumbosacral spine motion can be quantitated by placing a mark at L-5 and another 10 cm higher. On full flexion, the distance between the two lines should increase by at least 5 cm. Similarly, chest expansion is often decreased and the difference between inspiration and expiration should be measured at T-4. A value of less than 2.5 cm is considered abnormal. These values are useful guides; however, normal values are related to age, sex, and obesity. The often used finger-to-floor distance is not a useful guide to lumbosacral spine flexion as hip flexion is involved in this maneuver.

As the disease progresses, patients acquire a characteristic posture. There is a loss of normal lumbar lordosis and dorsal kyphosis occurs frequently. Patients often become round-shouldered. With advanced disease muscle wasting occurs most notably in the buttocks. Hip flexion contractures cause a compensatory flexion of the knees. Flexion deformities of the cervical spine combined with other deformities may lead to a reduction in forward vision. Decreased chest expansion leads to abdominal breathing, which manifests as abdominal distention.

Laboratory Manifestations

HLA-B27 testing is positive in approximately 80-90% of patients. The erythrocyte sedimentation rate is elevated at some time during the course of the disease in 80% of patients, but it may be normal in the presence of active disease; Tests for rheumatoid factor are characteristically negative.

Roentgenographic Manifestations

Roentgenograms are essential to making the diagnosis. The sacroiliac joints are characteristically abnormal with the early findings occuring on the iliac side of the joint. There are subchondral cortical erosions that appear as irregularities of the joint margins. These changes may be accompanied by sclerosis (increased bone density). With disease progression, bony ankylosis occurs so that the joint space is obliterated. The changes are almost always bilateral. The characteristic radiologic finding in the spine are the syndesmophytes that are bony bridges between two vertebral bodies. A syndesmophyte begins as an ossification of the outer portion of the annulus fibrosus. They usually occur laterally, although anterior syndesmophytes also occur. The dorsolumbar spine is the earliest area involved. The syndesmophytes extend cephalad with eventual cervical spine involvement. By contrast, osteophytes, which occur in degenerative arthritis, are horizontal outgrowths of bone. Syndesmophytes are symmetrical and when they are extensive, the resultant roentgenographic picture is called a bamboo spine. Destructive lesions of the upper and lower anterior vertebral surfaces cause a loss of the normal vertebral contour and a characteristic squaring of the vertebral body. Osteoporosis is a frequent finding. Interspinous ossification and disk ossification also may occur along with apophyseal joint fusions.

Pathology

Early synovial changes resemble those in rheumatoid arthritis; however, joint fibrosis and bony ankylosis are much more common in this illness. Inflammation also occurs at points of ligamentous attachment to bone such as the intervertebral disk and iliac crest. This inflammation may be associated with an erosive defect on cortical bone. Periostitis also occurs frequently. New bone formation is characteristic of this disease. The aortic pathology consists of fibrosis and necrosis of the media.

Diagnosis

In the presence of chronic low back pain and roentgenographic evidence of sacroiliitis at least one of the following objective criteria should be present: decreased lumbosacral spine flexion, decreased chest expansion, documented iritis, and aortic insufficiency. In patients with roentgenographic evidence of sacroiliitis who do not have back pain, two of the above criteria are sufficient for the diagnosis. In early disease, roentgenograms of the sacroiliac joints may be normal and a presumptive diagnosis can be made when other disease criteria are met and bone scan shows increased uptake over the sacroiliac joints. With follow-up, the sacroiliac joints should become abnormal or another diagnosis should be entertained. Presence of the HLA-B27 antigen is also helpful.

The differential diagnosis includes all other causes of low back pain. The roentgenographic findings in ankylosing spondylitis are characteristic and the diagnosis is not difficult. However, it can be difficult to decide which patients to evaluate for this disease. In this regard, it is important to remember that the typical patient is a young male with insidious onset of low back pain and stiffness that subsides with exercise and is exacerbated by rest.

Treatment

The most important aspect of treatment is a proper exercise program that encourages erect posture and proper breathing. The exercise program should be instituted by a physical therapist and reviewed by the physician on each visit. Patient compliance is facilitated by having a close working relationship between the patient and physician.

Nonsteroidal anti-inflammatory agents are beneficial in reducing inflammation and relieving pain so that proper posture and exercise programs can be maintained. Aspirin, in anti-inflammatory doses, is beneficial. Although indomethacin is not as well tolerated, in the presence of a severe flare-up it may be more effective in a dose of 150-200 mg/day. Phenylbutazone is a very efficacious drug; however, its usefulness is limited due to its toxicity, which includes aplastic anemia. While dosages of 400 mg a day in four divided doses may be needed initially, patients can often be maintained on 100 mg a day. The newer nonsteroidal anti-inflammatory agents should also prove to be efficacious. Medications need not be given continuously and may be discontinued when little inflammation or pain is present. Patients who respond poorly to aspirin initially may do well on this drug later when the disease is less severe. With proper treatment, severe deformities can be prevented and a relatively normal existence maintained. Most patients can continue to work for many years, particularly if the work is sedentary. However, life expectancy may be decreased because of mortality due to complications such as aortic insufficiency.

REITER'S DISEASE

Reiter's disease is a distinct clinical entity that is characterized by arthritis, conjunctivitis, and nonspecific urethritis. These features are the classic triad of Reiter's syndrome. Mucocutaneous lesions are also highly characteristic of this illness and include keratoderma blennorrhagicum, circinate balanitis, and painless oral ulcerations. This illness is a common form of arthritis in young adult men. The association with the HLA-B27 antigen has aided the recognition of cases that do not have all the clinical features. An infectious etiology has long been suspected. Most recently, chlamydiae have been cultured. However, the presence of these organisms in normal people makes interpretation of their significance difficult.

Clinical Features

The age at onset is usually between 16 and 45, although childhood cases and disease in elderly patients have been described. The disease is very rare in women, particularly if the classic triad is adhered to for diagnosis. There are two major presentations of this disease. In North America and the United Kingdom, the disease usually begins with urethritis, and a history of promiscuous sexual activity is often obtained. In the remainder of Europe, Asia, and North Africa, the disease usually follows an episode of dysentery due to a variety of organisms of which *Shigella dysenteriae* is by far the most frequent. When the disease follows an episode of diarrhea, the typical clinical features, including urethritis, appear in 1-3 weeks.

The mode of onset and clinical course of disease are very variable. Approximately one-half the patients have an acute onset. Weight loss, fatigue, and fever are common at the time of presentation; however, patients may not complain of these symptoms unless questioned.

The arthritis most commonly affects the knees and ankles. Joint disease is often asymmetrical and the shoulders, wrists, and elbows may also be involved. Large effusions may occur in the lower extremities. The small joints of the hands are occasionally involved. The findings in the foot include not only ankle effusions, but also plantar fasciitis, achilles tendonitis, and calcaneal bursitis. Periarticular tenderness, particularly of the heel, is common. The metatarsophalangeal joints may be involved, and when the small joints of the toes are involved there is often diffuse swelling or sausage digits. Nail changes, similar to those found in psoriatic arthritis, also occur. Patients often complain of back pain; however, radiographic evidence of spondylitis or sacroiliitis may not be present initially. The arthritis resolves within 3 weeks to several months in most patients; however, about 5% of patients will have persistent arthritis and about 60% will have recurrent episodes. These are usually accompanied by the other disease features such as urethritis and conjunctivitis. It is not uncommon for a patient who did not have all disease features initially to manifest with them in subsequent disease episodes. Sacroiliac joint involvement is more common with prolonged disease and one-half of patients develop sacroiliitis after 5 years of disease. These patients are more likely to be HLA-B27 positive. Spondylitis also occurs; however, decreased chest expansion is rare.

The major genitourinary disease manifestation is a urethritis that usually has a mucoid discharge, although frankly purulent or watery discharge may occur. Urethral cultures are usually sterile, but occasionally show gonococcus, reflecting for the most part promiscuous sexual activity. The urethritis usually clears spontaneously in 1-3 weeks. Prostatitis, urethral stricture, and prostatic ulceration may accompany this disease.

Conjunctivitis may be severe and purulent or may be clinically missed unless searched for. It also clears in several weeks without specific therapy. Uveitis may be present in 10-30% of patients initially; however, it occurs more frequently with subsequent disease episodes, particularly in patients with the HLA-B27 antigen.

About one-third of patients develop mucocutaneous disease. Painless oral ulcers that can become confluent are often missed unless a careful examination is made. *Keratoderma blennorrhagicum* is a rash that primarily occurs on the soles and palms. The lesions begin as erythematous pustules made up of hyperkeratotic tissue, expand, and become confluent. Eventually there are large, circumscribed, scaly lesions on an erythematous base. Histologically, these lesions resemble pustular psoriasis. In circumcised males, the lesions are similar, occurring over the corona and glans penis. Uncircumcised men develop ulcerated lesions that resemble the mouth ulcers. The lesions tend to become confluent giving rise to the name *circinate balanitis*. Histologically, all the lesions are similar. Aortic insufficiency is a rare complication of the disease.

Laboratory Manifestations

The sedimentation rate is elevated and often remains high despite clinical improvement. A polymophonuclear leukocytosis is frequent and the count may reach 20,000/mm^3. Joint fluid is inflammatory and may appear purulent with acute disease. The cell count ranges from 10,000-100,000 and there is often a preponderance of neutrophils. Joint fluid complement may be elevated. Synovianalysis may reveal a macrophage that has ingested one or several polymorphonuclear leukocytes. This is known as a Pekin or Reiter cell and may also occur in other disorders. The HLA-B27 antigen is present in about 80% of cases.

Roentgenographic Manifestations

Roentgenograms are often normal with early disease. Later juxta-articular erosions may occur. Periostitis is frequently found particularly at the insertion of the Achilles' tendon, where it may have a fluffy appearance. Periostitis occurs over other areas such as the phalanges. Calcaneal spurs may be present. Unilateral sacroiliitis may occur in about 17% of the patients. Joint ankylosis is rare. Syndesmophytes may be found with chronic or recurrent disease, but they are thicker and asymmetrical when compared to ankylosing spondylitis.

Diagnosis

The diagnosis can usually be made if two disease manifestations of the classic triad are present. The mucocutaneous lesions are characteristic and can be weighted equally. Occasionally, patients have only the typical arthritis. In this instance, if the patient is a young adult man and the HLA-B27 is positive, a presumptive diagnosis of incomplete Reiter's syndrome can be made. These patients should, however, be watched closely for additional disease features that confirm the diagnosis or suggest another.

The greatest confusion in diagnosis involves the differentiation of Reiter's disease from septic arthritis, particularly gonorrheal arthritis. All acutely inflamed joints should be cultured and urethral cultures should be obtained.

Treatment and Prognosis

Bed rest is indicated for acutely ill patients and splinting may occasionally be helpful. Anti-inflammatory dosages of aspirin are useful; however, indomethacin and phenylbutazone are usually more efficacious. The latter drug's usefulness is limited by its potential toxicity. Patients who cannot tolerate these drugs should benefit from the newer nonsteroidal anti-inflammatory agents. Corticosteroids are occasionally given to patients with severe systemic illness but are not always effective. A 5- to 7-day course of tetacycline is usually given for urethritis; however, there is no clear-cut evidence that the disease course is altered. Patients with spondylitis and sacroiliitis may need physical therapy as in ankylosing spondylitis. Cutaneous lesions may benefit from topical corticosteroid creams. Uveitis should be treated with topical steroids and atropine. Conjunctivitis usually requires no therapy.

Reiter's disease has been thought to have an excellent prognosis; however, patients with spondylitis or chronic arthritis may become disabled.

PSORIATIC ARTHRITIS

Psoriatic arthritis is a chronic disease that occurs in 6% of patients with psoriasis. It has certain characteristic features that distinguish it from the other arthritides.

Clinical Features

Women are more likely to develop psoriatic arthritis than men. The age of onset is similar to that found in rheumatoid arthritis. The skin lesions almost always antedate the onset of arthritis. Occasionally, only a small area of psoriasis is found in the scalp, skin creases, or elbows. The severity of the skin disease parallels that of the arthritis in only a small number of patients. Nail changes occur in about 80% of patients, although these changes are not specific for psoriatic arthritis and they may occur less frequently in uncomplicated psoriasis and other inflammatory arthritides. The nail changes consist of pitting, transverse ridging, thickening (keratosis), and the nail may be lifted off its bed (onycholysis). There are five basic patterns of disease, as shown in Table 5.

Laboratory Manifestations

There are no distinctive laboratory features. Rheumatoid factor is characteristically absent. Its presence in high titer suggests the coexistence of two common diseases, rheuma-

Table 5. Patterns of Psoriatic Arthritis

Patterns	*Features*
Mild asymmetrical oligoarthritis	Tends to affect the DIP, PIP, MCP, wrist, and lower extremity joints.
Symmetrical polyarthritis	Resembles rheumatoid arthritis, but rheumatoid factor and subcutaneous nodules are absent.
Extensive DIP joint disease	Considered classic, but found only in 5% patients.
Primarily sacroiliitis and spondylitis	Higher incidence of HLA-B27. More often have uveitis and aortic insufficiency. Whole digit may be swollen and inflamed—sausage toe.
Arthritis mutilans	Rare—extensive joint destruction (osteolysis), deformities, and ankylosis.

toid arthritis and psoriasis. The sedimentation rate is frequently elevated in active disease. The HLA-B27 antigen is found in one-third of patients and is associated with the roentgenographic finding of sacroiliitis. Joint fluid is inflammatory, and is similar to that found in rheumatoid arthritis.

Roentgenographic Manifestations

Roentgenograms may be normal early in the disease or in the presence of mild disease. However, in advanced disease, roentgenograms are characteristic. The most common finding is asymmetrical soft tissue swelling that involves only a few joints including the DIP joints. This mirrors the clinical picture. In more advanced disease there may be erosions of the terminal tufts; these may become totally resorbed (acro-osteolysis). Entire joints may be resorbed (arthritis mutilans). Whittling of the distal phalanges occurs and when this is accompanied by erosions of the proximal portion of the adjacent phalanx, the pencil in a cup deformity occurs. Periostitis and joint ankylosis also occur. Sacroiliitis may be present and occasionally will be unilateral. Spondylitis resembling that found in ankylosing spondylitis occurs. However, the spondylitis is more likely to resemble that found in Reiter's disease, that is the syndesmophytes are often asymmetrical and nonmarginal.

Diagnosis

Psoriatic arthritis should be suspected in any patient with psoriasis and arthritis that lasts for more than 3 weeks and is recurrent. Synovitis of the distal interphalangeal joints, particularly with nail changes, suggests the diagnosis. The absence of rheumatoid factor is helpful diagnostically. Roentgenograms are quite helpful when characteristic lesions such as acro-osteolysis are found.

The differential diagnosis includes rheumatoid arthritis. The pattern of joint involvement in psoriatic arthritis, particularly with distal interphalangeal joint disease, is the major differential point. However, occasionally only the absence of rheumatoid factor and subcutaneous nodules distinguishes this illness from rheumatoid arthritis. Osteoarthritis and erosive osteoarthritis frequently involve the distal interphalangeal joints. When these patients have psoriasis the differential diagnosis may depend upon roentgenographic findings. Psoriatic arthritis may closely resemble ankylosing spondylitis or Reiter's disease. The cutaneous lesions of Reiter's disease are similar clinically and identical histologically to psoriatic lesions; however, urethritis and conjunctivitis are rare in psoriatic arthritis. Gout may occur concomitantly with psoriatic arthritis and synovianalysis should be performed on acutely inflamed joints in order to search for urate crystals. Patients may be misdiagnosed as having gout on the basis of hyperuricemia, which occurs in approximately 15% of psoriasis patients.

Treatment

Many patients with oligoarticular or classic disease require only intermittent nonsteroidal anti-inflammatory therapy. With active inflammation, full anti-inflammatory dosages of aspirin should be used. Indomethacin is occasionally more effective than aspirin. The newer anti-inflammatory agents are also effective. Patients are occasionally systemically ill with fever and malaise and benefit from rest. In those patients whose skin disease activity parallels the arthritis, the psoriasis should be treated vigorously. Gold salt therapy may be useful with severe peripheral joint disease, particularly if the disease resembles rheumatoid arthritis. Antimalarial agents are contraindicated since they may cause severe skin reactions. Methotrexate and other cytotoxic agents have been used for patients with severe disease; however, because of severe side effects, these drugs should be used only rarely and by those skilled in their employment.

ARTHRITIS ASSOCIATED WITH INFLAMMATORY BOWEL DISEASE

Approximately 20% of patients with ulcerative colitis develop arthritis. These patients generally have more severe gastrointestinal disease and are more likely to develop uveitis, pyoderma, and mouth ulcerations. About 50% of these patients develop a peripheral arthritis and the other 50% develop an arthritis that is indistinguishable from ankylosing spondylitis.

The peripheral arthritis usually occurs with an exacerbation of the bowel disease and when the disease is eliminated by colectomy, arthritis subsides. The large joints are most commonly affected and the lower extremities are more likely to be involved. Active synovitis is present on examination; however, erosions are rare on roentgenograms. This arthritis usually clears within several weeks to a few months and recurrences are rare.

Unlike the peripheral arthritis, which always occurs after the onset of bowel disease, the form of the arthritis that resembles ankylosing spondylitis is as likely to antedate the bowel disease as follow it. This arthritis follows a clinical course similar to that of ankylosing spondylitis, and the severity of the arthritis is unrelated to the severity of the bowel disease. Colectomy has no effect on this arthritis. There is a high incidence (approximately 75%) of HLA-B27 antigen in this group of patients.

The arthritis of regional enteritis is similar. The percentage of patients with peripheral arthritis may be greater in regional enteritis than with ulcerative colitis. The peripheral arthritis rarely precedes bowel symptoms. Surgery is not as effective as in ulcerative colitis, reflecting the difficulty of removing all diseased bowel in regional enteritis. The patients with regional enteritis and arthritis resembling ankylosing spondylitis also frequently have the HLA-B27 antigen and the course of their arthritis does not parallel the course of their bowel disease.

INFECTIOUS ARTHRITIS

Infectious (septic) arthritis is a highly treatable condition that occurs in all age groups and both sexes. Prompt therapy is important to prevent joint destruction. The diagnosis is facilitated by the prompt performance of synovianalysis and culture and institution of appropriate antimicrobial therapy.

Clinical Features

The septic joint is usually inflamed, and with acute infection, the redness, heat, swelling, and tenderness is often marked. Limitation of motion may be striking. Any joint may become infected, but the large joints, especially the knees, hips, and shoulders are most commonly affected. Patients are often febrile and may experience shaking chills.

A careful history and physical examination may reveal a nidus of infection. The skin, cervix, pharynx, lungs, sinuses, and rectum are all possible sources of infection. Typical skin lesions commonly occur in gonococcal septic arthritis, and are a reflection of septicemia. The lesions are erythematous macules which may contain a vesicle or pustule and a central necrotic area; they may yield positive cultures. Gonococcal arthritis is also more likely to be polyarticular, although this sometimes occurs with other organisms. Septic arthritis may occur in healthy individuals with normal joints; however, often the infected joint is abnormal or the patient is immunocompromised. Other factors that may predispose to septic arthritis include trauma and coexistent arthritis, such as rheumatoid arthritis or occasionally gout. Chronic illnesses such as diabetes mellitus and debilitating conditions also increase susceptibility. Intravenous drug abuse may lead to unusual sites of infection such as the sacroiliac and sternoclavicular joints as well as the intervertebral disk. In patients who have an underlying arthritis and in those receiving immunosuppressive therapy, a high index of suspicion coupled with synovianalysis and culture is essential in establishing the correct diagnosis.

Laboratory Manifestations

A polymorphonuclear leukocytosis and an elevated sedimentation rate are frequently found, but their absence does not rule out septic arthritis. Synovianalysis and culture should always be performed in any patient suspected of having arthritis. The joint fluid is usually turbid or cloudy, viscosity is decreased, and the mucin clot is poor. White blood cell counts range from 5000-200,000/ mm^3 with the higher counts occurring in acute bacterial infections. Polymorphonuclear leukocytes usually predominate. The synovial fluid glucose is frequently decreased to 40-50% or less of the simultaneous blood value.

Gram stain and culture are essential to a correct diagnosis and appropriate therapy. Cultures should routinely be plated on blood agar and also chocolate agar if *Neisseria gonorrhoeae* or *Hemophilus influenzae* infections are suspected. If suspected, fungal and mycobacterial cultures must be performed on special media. Anerobic infections are rare, but thioglycollate broth should be used if this is suspected.

The organisms cultured consist mainly of Gram-positive and Gram-negative cocci. Gram-negative bacilli are most often seen in immunocompromised or elderly individuals. *Staphylococcus aureus*, *Streptococcus pneumoniae*, and *S. pyogenes* occur frequently. *N. gonorrhoeae* makes up almost all of the Gram-negative cocci and is responsible for about 50% of all septic arthritis. Gonococcal arthritis is common in younger adults, but all ages are affected. *H. influenzae* infection occurs rarely in adults and is more common in children.

Roentgenographic Manifestations

Roentgenograms may only reveal soft tissue swelling for the first 1 or 2 weeks; however, they should be performed initially for future comparison to ascertain if there is underlying disease such as arthritis or osteomyelitis. The roentgenograms are valuable in following the disease, and contralateral roentgenograms may facilitate the recognition of subtle changes. The abnormal findings consist of bone rarefaction and later erosion and joint space narrowing secondary to loss of cartilage. Radioisotope scanning techniques are not specific for infection; however, they may help to distinguish abscess from joint sepsis. Counter immunoelectrophoresis and gas-liquid chromatography seem to be promising methods of rapidly determining the presence of bacterial antigens in the joint fluid.

Treatment

Septic arthritis should be treated with intravenous antibiotics; the Gram stain is the guide to selection of initial treatment. When Gram-positive cocci are seen on smear, nafcillin is the drug of choice; if streptococcal infection such as that due to *S. pneumoniae* is strongly suspected, penicillin G is appropriate therapy. *N. gonorrhoeae* accounts for nearly all the Gram-negative cocci and should be treated with penicillin G. Gonococcal arthritis is responsible for about one-half of all septic arthritis and may affect all ages, although it is most common in young adults. In children, Gram-negative bacilli are usually *H. influenzae* and ampicillin should be given; in adults a variety of Gram-negative bacilli may be responsible and gentamicin should be administered, and with more severe infection, carbenicillin should be added. Gram stain is often negative in patients with gonococcal arthritis; penicillin G should be administered to a young adult who has septic arthritis with a negative Gram stain. In older patients or immunocompromised hosts, both staphylococci and Gram-negative bacteria should be covered when Gram stains are negative. Antibiotics may be altered as sensitivities are available.

Joint aspiration is an important part of the management of septic arthritis. Joint destruction is secondary to such factors as enzymes from polymorphonuclear leukocytes and activated complement components, their removal protects the joint from more severe destruction. In addition, fluid removal facilitates killing by bactericidal antibiotics, since the inflammatory fluid in the joint may inhibit bacterial growth. Joint fluid antibiotic concentrations are adequate if serum levels are maintained; the instillation of antibiotics into the joint is unnecessary and may itself cause synovitis. Inflammation promotes the entry of antibiotics into the joint. With clinical improvement, joint fluid antibiotic levels may fall, thus dosages should not be decreased with clinical improvement.

All fluid aspirated should be cultured and synovianalysis performed. In addition, an assessment of bactericidal activity against the cultured organism should be performed on synovial fluid as well as on serum. Joints should be aspirated daily or more often with severe inflammation. Aspiration should be continued until cultures are negative and joint fluid white counts are significantly lower. The fall in white blood cell count may take up to a week. If fluid can not be aspirated or if significant improvement does not occur in a week, surgical drainage should be performed. Splinting reduces pain and inflammation and bed rest is helpful for acutely ill patients. Treatment should be continued for 2 weeks in gonococcal or streptococcal infections. Staphylococcal and Gram-negative infections may require 4-6 weeks of therapy.

TUBERCULOUS ARTHRITIS

Since the incidence of tuberculous arthritis has fallen, there is danger in missing this treatable disease if it is not considered in the differential diagnosis of joint or spine pain. The mycobacteria may enter the joint from the blood or adjacent bone. Active tuberculosis is often not present and bone may harbor the mycobacteria as a result of previous hematogenous disease or spread from contiguous sites of infection. About half the cases of tuberculous arthritis will have involvement of the spine (Pott's disease); disease also occurs in the large joints (knee, hip, shoulder), and occasionally the wrist and ankle. The major readiographic manifestation of Pott's disease is disk space narrowing; frequently there is involvement of adjacent vertebrae and visible paraspinous abscesses. When other joints are involved, soft tissue swelling may be the only radiographic finding. Cartilage may be preserved, although destructive changes occur with advanced disease. Joint fluid should be aspirated when tuberculous arthritis is suspected. A polymorphonuclear leukocytosis occurs and the sugar may be low. Acid-fast smears may be positive in 20% of cases and culture in 80%. Synovial biopsy may be helpful, revealing typical caseating and noncaseating granulomata. Using the combination of synovianalysis, synovial fluid stain, and culture, 95% of cases of tuberculous arthritis may be diagnosed. The intermediate strength PPD is positive in 90% of cases. Treatment is the same as for active pulmonary disease. Atypical mycobacterial infections may also occur, and have a predilection for the tendons of the hand and wrist. Culture and sensitivity testing is especially important with the atypical mycobacteria, since drug resistance is often a problem. Surgical drainage is sometimes necessary in these infections.

SJÖGREN'S SYNDROME

Henrik Sjögren described the syndrome of keratoconjunctivitis sicca (dry eyes), xerostomia (dry mouth), and parotid gland enlargement, often in association with rheumatoid arthritis in 1933. There is a higher incidence of HLA-B8 in the affected patients. Other diseases such as progressive systemic sclerosis, systemic lupus erythematosus, primary biliary cirrhosis, and chronic active hepatitis have also been associated with Sjögren's syndrome.

Pathology

Salivary gland biopsy reveals an infiltration of the gland with lymphocytes and to a lesser extent plasma cells. The structure may be distorted in severe disease and germinal follicles may be present. Secretory acini may atrophy and duct lining cells may become hyperplastic and proliferate leading to epimyoepithelial islands. Any salivary gland may be biopsied; however, the lip salivary glands yield useful information and lip biopsy, a relatively benign procedure, is preferred.

Disease is usually confined to the salivary glands; however, changes occasionally occur in lymph nodes. There is a spectrum of findings from benign lymphocytic infiltration to pseudolymphoma (lymphocytic proliferation that resembles but does not fulfill the criteria for lymphoma) to frank reticulum cell sarcoma or undifferentiated stem cell lymphoma. Lymphocytic proliferation occurs in lung and kidney where it may be responsible for renal tubular acidosis.

Clinical Features

The typical patient with Sjögren's syndrome is a middle-aged or elderly woman, although men and women of all ages may be affected. Symptoms may begin insidiously or may have a dramatic onset. Patients with keratoconjunctivitis sicca, which is due to decreased lacrimal gland flow, often complain of dry eyes or a gritty sensation in their eyes, particularly in the morning. A variety of other symptoms occur, including redness or irritation. Dry mouth is a common symptom, particularly among anxious patients. Xerostomia secondary to decreased salivary gland flow is associated with difficulty in swallowing dry crackers, drinking copious amounts of liquids with meals, and frequent snacking on hard candy. Rampant dental caries may also occur. Patients may present with acute parotitis, or painless salivary gland or lymph node enlargement.

The eyes may be inflamed or appear normal. The tongue appears dry or fissured and saliva may be absent from the sublingual vestibule. Parotid gland enlargement may be dramatic and the facial appearance altered. Salivary glands are usually firm and nontender. Lymphadenopathy and hepatosplenomegaly may be present. Nonthrombocytopenic purpura may occur over the lower extremities, and its healing leaves hyperpigmented areas.

Investigation of keratoconjunctivitis begins with Schirmer's test, in which a standard piece of filter paper is placed in the conjunctival sac. Fifteen mm of wetting is normal at 5 minutes, and 5 mm or less is suggestive of this syndrome. Staining of devitalized tissue over the bulbar conjunctive and cornea with rose bengal is a more specific finding. Slit lamp examination may reveal debris and devitalized epithelium in filaments (filamentary keratitis).

Xerostomia is evaluated by several measures including salivary flow from the parotid ducts. Sialography is performed by injecting dye into the parotid ducts. The abnormal findings consist of duct distortion and delayed emptying. The uptake of ^{99m}Tc-labeled pertechnetate is a good measure of parotid gland function.

Laboratory Manifestations

The ESR is usually elevated. The anemia of chronic disease, leukopenia, and eosinophilia sometimes occur. A variety of serologic immune abnormalities occur, including antisalivary duct antibodies, antithyroglobulin antibodies, rheumatoid factor, and antinuclear antibodies. The immunofluorescence pattern is often homogeneous or speckled, although all patterns occur. Many patients have a diffuse hyperglobulinemia. Immune complexes such as mixed cryoglobulins may be responsible for some abnormalities, particularly the rare occurence of glomerulonephritis. Waldenstrom's macroglobulinemia also occurs.

Treatment

Sjögren's syndrome is usually benign, and tear replacement is the mainstay of therapy. Patients should also drink copious amounts of liquid with their meals. The therapy of associated disorders such as rheumatoid arthritis is not altered by the presence of this syndrome. More vigorous therapy may be necessary when organs become infiltrated with lymphocytes, and preliminary evidence suggests that corticosteroids and cyclophosphamide may be useful in these situations. Patients should be watched for the development of lymphoma.

SYSTEMIC LUPUS ERYTHEMATOSUS

The first recognition of systemic lupus erythematosus (SLE) is credited to Kaposi in 1872. Osler emphasized the systemic nature of the disease, which has skin, articular, cardiovascular, and renal manifestations. Pathologic descriptions followed, but the next major advance was the description of the LE-cell phenomenon by Hargraves and coworkers in 1948. Since then, numerous circulating antibodies have been reported, their interaction with complement and different tissues have been investigated, and an antigen-antibody complex-mediated tissue injury has been proposed. Systemic lupus erythematosus is a multisystem disease of unknown etiology and variable course. It may be acute and fulminating, slowly progressive with remissions and exacerbations, or mild illness. The disease may affect the skin, joints, kidneys, nervous sytem, serous membranes, lungs, heart, and blood. The laboratory features are highlighted by immunologic abnormalities, especially the presence of a variety of circulating antibodies to nuclear and other tissue antigens. The disease is more frequent in young women between the ages of 15 and 40, but children and older individuals are often affected. The sex ratio varies in different studies from 7-10 females to 1 male and its incidence is higher in blacks. A prevalence of 1 in 245 black women aged 15-64 has been reported. An increased incidence of SLE, other connective tissue diseases, and serologic abnormalities have been reported in relatives of patients with SLE.

Animal models for SLE, the New Zealand Black (NZB) and NZB/NZW F_{one}, hybrid mouse, and the canine lupus model have contributed significantly to the understanding of pathogenetic mechanisms involved in SLE. Multiple factors such as genetic, immunologic, and viral influences may play a role.

The most characteristic histologic findings include hematoxylin bodies consisting of homogeneous masses of nuclear material that stain bluish purple with hematoxylin. These are identical with the inclusion body of the LE cell and fibrinoid necrosis affecting especially small arteries, arterioles, and capillaries. Vascular lesions in the spleen take the form of concentric periarterial fibrosis, the so-called onion skin lesions.

Diagnostic Criteria

In 1971, the American Rheumatism Association proposed a preliminary criteria for the diagnosis of SLE. At least four of the criteria listed below must be present serially or simultaneously, during any interval of observation.

1. Facial erythema (butterfly rash). Diffuse erythema, flat or raised, over the malar eminence(s) and/or bridge of the nose; may be unilateral
2. Discoid lupus. Erythematous raised patches with adherent keratotic scaling and follicular plugging; atrophic scarring may occur in older lesions; may be present anywhere in the body
3. Raynaud's phenomenon. Requires a two-phase color reaction, by patient's history or physician's observation
4. Alopecia. Rapid loss of a large amount of the scalp hair, by patient's history or physician's observation
5. Photosensitivity. Unusual skin reaction from exposure to sunlight, by patient's history or physician's observation
6. Oral or nasopharyngeal ulceration
7. Arthritis without deformity. One or more peripheral joints involved with any of the following in the absence of deformity: pain on motion, tenderness, or effusion

or periarticular soft tissue swelling. (Peripheral joints, as defined for this purpose, are the feet, ankles, knees, hips, shoulders, elbows, wrists, metacarpophalangeal, proximal interphalangeal and temporomandibular joints.)

8. LE cells. Two or more classic LE cells seen on one occasion or one cell seen on two or more occasions, using an accepted published method[a]
9. Chronic false-positive serologic test for syphilis, known to be present for at least 6 months and confirmed by TPI or Reiter's tests
10. Profuse proteniuria, greater than 3.5 g/day
11. Cellular casts. May be red cell, hemoglobin, granular, tubular, or mixed
12. One or both of the following
    A. Pleuritis, good history of pleuritic pain; or rub heard by a physician; or x-ray evidence of both pleural thickening and fluid
    B. Pericarditis, documented by a rub, ECG or echocardiography
13. One or both of the following
    A. Psychosis
    B. Convulsions, by patient's history or physician's observation in the absence of uremia or offending drugs
14. One or more of the following
    A. Hemolytic anemia
    B. Leukopenia, WBC less than $4{,}000/mm^3$ on two or more occasions
    C. Thrombocytopenia, platelet count less than $100{,}000/mm^3$

The clinical presentation of SLE may be quite protean. The disease may have a sudden onset, sometimes after sun or drug exposure, with high fever, multisystem involvement, polyserositis, CNS manifestations, may run a chronic course with remissions and exacerbations, or have a benign course with minimal arthralgias, arthritis, and immunologic abnormalities.

Clinical Features

Skin

The dermatologic manifestations of SLE are numerous. The classic butterfly rash is seen in about 25% of the patients. Malar rash, discoid lesions, and maculopapular eruptions are common. About 30% of the patients give a history of photosensitivity. Urticaria, periungual erythema, nail changes with pitting, ridging, and onycholysis may occur. Mucosal lesions with painful or painless oral or nasal ulcerations, leading to perforation of the septum in some patients, are usually associated with active disease.

Alopecia is an important manifestation occurring in up to 65% of patients. The distribution is usually patchy and new hair growth alternates with alopecia, which also may be total.

[a]A positive test for antinuclear antibodies at a significant titer may be used instead of a positive LE cell.

Rheumatoid-like subcutaneous nodules have been noted in a small percentage of patients. They are usually smaller than the nodules in rheumatoid arthritis and are often of short duration. Characteristic Raynaud's phenomenon is found in up to 15% of the patients with SLE; it may be the first sign of the disease, persisting for several years before other manifestations occur. Occasionally, the vascular changes may result in ulceration and necrosis with loss of finger tips.

Musculoskeletal

Polyarthralgias and/or polyarthritis are the most common manifestations of SLE and arthritis occurs in 90-100% of patients. The small joints of the hands and the knees are most commonly involved and the disease is usually symmetrical. The arthritis is typically nondeforming and erosions are not seen; however, a few patients develop ulnar deviation and swan neck deformities. Morning stiffness is frequently present and joint symptoms may be severe; however, the clinical findings often do not correlate with the symptomatology.

Synovial fluid shows less than $3{,}000\ cells/mm^3$ with a good to fair mucin clot and LE cells may be present. Aseptic necrosis of the joints in SLE is frequently associated with long-term corticosteroid therapy.

An inflammatory myopathy, manifested by pain and tenderness of muscles and proximal weakness, occurs. This should be differentiated from a steroid-induced myopathy.

Cardiovascular

Cardiac involvement may occur, especially in the form of pericarditis, in about 25% of patients. It may be transitory, short lasting, easily missed, and rarely may lead to tamponade. Vasculitis leading to myocardial ischemia and infarction occurs. Arrhythmias are very uncommon. Involvement of the valves occurs and aortic insufficiency has been described. Verrucous endocarditis is a common pathologic finding that does not correlate with clinical manifestations. Hypertension is commonly related to renal involvement and/or corticosteroid therapy.

Pulmonary

Pleuritis occurs in about 30% of the patients. A small, unilateral pleural effusion is the rule and LE cells may be found in the pleural fluid. In most instances the effusions resolve spontaneously. A lupus pneumonitis with plate-like atelectasis may occur and in severe cases the occurrence of bilateral pulmonary hemorrhages is of poor prognosis.

Central Nervous System

Neurologic disease is one of the most serious manifestations of SLE. Central nervous system dysfunction is a common, difficult, and frequently emergent problem in systemic lupus erythematosus. The clinical variability and the lack of specific diagnostic laboratory criteria may complicate the distinction between the manifestations of SLE and the neurologic sequelae of secondary metabolic disturbances, drug treatment, or incidental illness. A wide variety of neurologic manifestations have been described in SLE and involvement of the nervous system is now recognized in at least 50% of the cases. Aberrant behavior in the form of psychosis or depression are the most common manifestations but convulsions, chorea, cerebral vascular accidents leading to focal neurologic abnormalities, cranial nerve disorders, transverse myelopathy, and peripheral neuropathy can occur. Central nervous system manifestations usually correlate with highly active severe disease and a worse prognosis. Twenty-seven percent of the patients who present with neurologic symptoms may succumb.

Papilledema has occasionally been reported. Retinal lesions, in the form of a small, ovoid or circular, white, exudate-like spots, in the absence of hypertension or diabetes mellitus, are so called cytoid bodies. They consist of aggregates of swollen nerve fibers and the products of proliferating and degenerating axonal structures. The cytoid bodies are found in less than 10% of SLE patients but their presence is highly suggestive of systemic lupus erythematosus.

Renal

The incidence of clinically serious renal involvement in SLE is about 50%. Virtually all patients with systemic lupus erythematosus whose renal tissue is studied by light microscopy, immunofluorescence, and electron microscopy prove to have some evidence of involvement. Four renal lesions are now recognized: minimal or mesangial proliferative lupus nephritis, focal proliferative lupus nephritis, diffuse proliferative lupus nephritis, and membranous nephropathy. A common mechanism, the glomerular deposition of immune complexes containing nuclear antigens, apparently mediates the proliferative lesions. Renal involvement is a serious feature of SLE, accounting for approximately 50% of all fatalities. Diffuse proliferative lupus nephritis has the worse prognosis with about 30% 5-year survival in those patients presenting with this lesion. Renal manifestations usually appear early in the course of the disease and include microscopic hematuria, proteinuria, and cylindruria (including red cell casts). Patients may present with nephrotic syndrome and this is more frequently associated with diffuse proliferative lupus nephritis or membranous lupus nephropathy. Focal lupus nephropathy is present in the majority of patients and may be a mild, nonprogressive form of lupus nephritis.

Several patterns of immunofluorescent staining have been described with IgG, IgM, and C3 deposits. Electron microscopy may reveal electron dense deposits (either mesangial or subendothelial), and virus-like particles. Serious, active renal disease correlates best with abnormal urinary sediment, anti-DNA antibodies, and low complement levels.

Gastrointestinal

Nonspecific gastrointestinal (GI) manifestations during active disease are frequent in systemic lupus erythematosus. Episodes of nausea, vomiting, and abdominal pain may occur. Sterile peritonitis or vasculitis of the small vessels leading to lesions in the GI tract and pancreatitis may also occur. Colonic perforations have been reported. Hepatic enlargement occurs, but jaundice is rare. Aspirin-induced hepatitis has been reported.

Hematologic

Anemia is the most common hematologic abnormality seen in systemic lupus erythematosus, occurring in 75% of patients. Most patients have a mild form of anemia, normocytic and normochromic with normal bone marrow iron stores, decreased plasma iron, decreased total iron-binding capacity, and poor or no response to iron therapy, the so-called anemia of chronic disease. This form of anemia usually does not require any special therapy, and improves during remissions or with control of the systemic manifestations of the disease with corticosteroids. Iron deficiency anemia may occur secondary to chronic blood loss. A Coombs-positive autoimmune hemolytic anemia occurs in about 5% of patients. Other causes of anemia include renal disease, drug-induced, and rarely pure red cell aplasia.

Leukopenia is found during the course of the disease in about 50% of the patients. Granulocytopenia as well as lymphopenia may occur. The total white blood cell count in these patients usually ranges between 2,000 and 4,000 cells/mm^3. Leukocytosis is rare in the absence of infection or steroid therapy.

Thrombocytopenia occurs in about 30% of the patients and is usually mild with values ranging from 100,000 to 150,000/mm^3. In 5% of patients, severe thrombocytopenia occurs and acute thrombocytopenic purpura may be the first manifestation of systemic lupus erythematosus. The thrombocytopenia of SLE is usually due to peripheral destruction secondary to antibodies directed against platelets. Occasionally, autoimmune hemolytic anemia and thrombocytopenia occur in the same patient.

Laboratory Manifestations

Multiple laboratory abnormalities have been described in SLE. As previously discussed, most patients will present with a mild form of anemia, that of chronic disease. Leukopenia is common. The erythrocyte sedimentation rate is elevated and may remain high in clinically apparent remissions. About 60% of patients have an abnormal urinalysis with proteinuria, microscopic hematuria, and cylindruria.

The characteristic feature of SLE is the presence of numerous serum protein and serologic abnormalities, including a variety of autoantibodies. Hypergammaglobulinemia is very common. Multiple antibodies directed against nuclear and cytoplasmic constituents have been found including antibodies against native and single-stranded DNA, DNA-histone and nuclear RNA-protein. Recently antineuronal antibodies have been described and they may correlate with central nervous system disease. Virtually all patients during active disease have a positive test for antinuclear antibodies by immunofluorescence technique. The presence of antinuclear antibodies lacks diagnostic specificity and has to be correlated with the clinical findings. Antinuclear antibodies by immunofluorescence may be reported in several patterns, with a homogenous or diffuse pattern being the most frequent. A peripheral, rim or shaggy pattern is less common, but is quite specific for SLE. A speckled pattern in SLE, correlates best with anti-SM or anti-RNP antibodies (ribonucleoprotein) in low titers. High titers of anti-RNP antibodies are suggestive of mixed connective tissue disease.

Antibodies against native (double-stranded) DNA are important markers of disease and are part of the DNA-anti-DNA immune complex involved in the pathogenesis of the renal lesion. High levels of DNA antibodies correlate well with serious, active renal disease.

Positive LE cells are found in 60-80% of the patients during active disease. This test detects antibody directed against deoxiribonucleoprotein. Positive LE cells may be present as well in synovial and pleural fluids. This test has been largely replaced by the antinuclear antibodies (ANA).

A positive rheumatoid factor occurs in 30% of the patients with SLE. Both IgG and IgM rheumatoid factors have been found. A false-positive serologic test for syphillis occurs in 10-20% of the patients, and these patients may have a circulating anticoagulant.

Activation of the complement system either through the classic or an alternative pathway occurs. Low complement levels, CH50, C3, and C4 correlate best with active renal disease. Inherited deficiencies of components of the complement system have been reported and these patients may be more susceptible to connective tissue diseases. Patients with inherited deficiency of C2 are at increased risk for SLE.

Immunofluorescence of skin reveals immunoglobulin and complement deposits at the dermoepidermal junction in about 50% of uninvolved skin and in almost 100% of patients with skin lesions.

Treatment

Proper management depends on an appreciation of the enormous variability of the potential course of the illness in any one patient. General measures include proper rest during periods of active disease, avoidance of drugs such as oral contraceptives, penicillin, and sulfonamide that may potentiate or bring about flares of the disease. Patients should be advised to avoid excessive sunlight, particularly those with photosensitivity. Sunscreen creams may be helpful.

Many patients have a benign, mild form of disease predominantly with joint symptoms and can be controlled with salicylate therapy or other nonsteroidal anti-inflammatory agents. In a few patients aspirin can induce hepatic toxicity that improves after discontinuation of the drug. Some SLE patients may be more sensitive to ibuprofen and serious side effects may occur.

Antimalarials are helpful in patients with skin and articular manifestations. Hydroxychloroquine, 200-400 mg daily, is the drug of choice. Its usefulness is limited due to retinal toxicity, with potential blindness. Opthalmologic evaluations every 4-6 months are necessary. Although the mechanism of action is unknown, it probably acts by reducing light sensitivity of the skin.

Corticosteroids benefit many patients with SLE. Clear indications for their use include severe multisystem involvement, autoimmune hemolytic anemia, or thrombocytopenic purpura. Starting dosages range from 40-80 mg daily with slow tapering as the patient improves. In some patients control of the disease is achieved with alternate-day therapy. Most patients with severe central nervous sytem or renal disease are treated with corticosteroids in very high dosages; but the benefit in these situations is not always clear. Infection is a frequent complication and cause of death.

Several immunosuppressive drugs including azathioprine, cyclophosphamide, and chlorambucil have been used in patients with SLE mainly for severe central nervous system manifestations and diffuse proliferative glomerulonephritis. A few controlled trials in diffuse proliferative nephritis treated with combination therapy using azathioprine or cyclophosphamide with concomitant prednisone give conflicting results. Severe side effects including bone marrow depression, hemorrhagic cystitis, infection, and the possibility of increased risk for developing neoplasms, primarily of the lymphoid system, limit their potential usefulness.

Recently, plasmapheresis has been tried with some success in patients with immune-complex mediated renal disease. Its value in the management of diffuse lupus nephritis is not known.

DRUG-INDUCED SLE

Since hydralazine-induced SLE was first described in 1954, numerous drugs have been associated with the induction of SLE (Table 6).

Drug-induced SLE differs from naturally occurring SLE in several aspects including rarity of renal involvement, normal complement levels, and clinical improvement in a few days after discontinuation of the offending drug. Immunologic abnormalities may persist for up to 2 years. Up to 80% of patients on procainamide may develop antinuclear antibodies without developing clinical symptoms. Since not all patients on these drugs develop drug-induced lupus, a poorly understood underlying susceptibility may be present.

Table 6. Lupus-Inducing Drugs

Chlorpromazine
Contraceptives
D-Penicillamine
Griseofulvin
Hydralazine
Isoniazid
Mephenytoin
Methyldopa
Methylthiouracil
Penicillin
Phenytoin
Practolol
Procainamide
Propylthiouracil
Sulphonamides
Tetracycline

PROGRESSIVE SYSTEMIC SCLEROSIS

Progressive systemic sclerosis belongs to a group of disorders characterized by sclerodermatous skin changes consisting of swelling, thickening, and/or tightening of the skin. The older term for this disorder is scleroderma; however, it is common now to refer to the various disorders with sclerodermatous skin changes as the scleroderma syndromes that also include localized scleroderma (morphea) and eosinophillic fasciitis. Progressive systemic sclerosis is a systemic disorder characterized by degeneration of tissue and chronic inflammatory changes that result in fibrosis. The disease involves the skin, esophagus, and lungs. The joints, heart, small intestine, large intestine, and kidneys are less frequently involved. Not only is the etiology unknown, but there is debate over which abnormalities are important in the pathogenesis of this disease. The vascular abnormalities have been considered to be primary. Skin fibroblasts produce increased amounts of collagen, and it has been thought that disordered collagen synthesis may be the etiology. Immune abnormalities are frequently found in these patients and an autoimmune etiology has been suggested.

The incidence of this disease is approximately 1 in 370,000. The disease occurs twice as frequently in women as in men and commonly presents between the ages of 30 and 50, although it can occur at any age and is found frequently over the age of 65. The disease is more commonly found in coal miners and in people exposed to silica dust. The course can be variable and rare spontaneous remissions have occurred.

Clinical Features

Skin is involved in essentially all patients, although extremely rare patients have been described with the typical visceral lesions and no skin findings. Diagnosis can be made when the skin findings include more than the hands and forearms. The skin of the face, lower extremities, proximal extremities, upper trunk, and back is frequently involved. Initially, the skin may be diffusely swollen, giving the digits a sausage-shaped appearance. Later, the skin appears thickened and there is a loss of folds, giving a tight appearance to the skin. With time, the skin may become thinned and ulcerations may occur over the distal digits and joint surfaces. Skin thickening is the most typical lesion and patients may never develop swelling or thinning. The hand changes frequently give rise to flexion contractures. The changes in the face cause a decrease in the oral aperture.

Histologically, the skin changes include epidermal thinning, a loss of rete pegs, and a loss of sebaceous and sweat glands. Dermal collagen is increased in the subcutis. Unfortunately, these classic changes are usually only present in patients in whom the diagnosis is not in doubt, and the biopsy is usually not helpful in patients with early disease. A homogenization of dermal collagen may be the only early finding.

Raynaud's phenomenon occurs in virtually all patients. Classically, there is a triphasic color change, although all patients do not experience all three phases. With exposure to cold or with emotional change, the hands may first turn white or ashen; this represents tissue anoxia. The hands then turn blue (cyanosis) and finally red, due to hyperemia, (increased blood flow in vessels that are no longer occluded). The color changes may be accompanied by pain, paresthesias, or a feeling of fullness as blood flow returns. Raynaud's phenomenon is the most common presenting complaint in this disease and this symptom may antedate skin changes by several years. With angiography, there is narrowing of the lumen of the digital arteries. Histologically, the most marked finding in these vessels is intimal proliferation.

Myalgias, arthralgias, and arthritis are the presenting complaints in approximately one-third of patients. These patients are often labeled as having rheumatoid arthritis initially. The early changes on synovial biopsy resemble rheumatoid arthritis; however, with chronic disease, fibrosis ensues. Synovial fluid usually contains less than 2,000 cells, mostly lymphocytes.

The esophagus is involved in 90% of patients. Early satiety and epigastric or chest burning are the most frequent complaints, although dysphagia frequently occurs. Abnormalities are frequent on manometric studies and there is a loss of normal peristalsis that is also found when the esophagus is studied roentgenographically after a barium meal. With advanced disease, the esophagus becomes dilated. The gastroesophageal sphincter is often incompetent, allowing gastric acid to reflux into the esophagus. This may lead to esophaeal ulceration and stricture, although perforation is rare. Histologically, there is thinning of the mucosa, atrophy of the muscularis, and fibrous tissue proliferation in the lamina propia.

Pulmonary involvement occurs in about 75% of patients. The most common symptom is dyspnea on exertion, although patients may develop a chronic dry cough. Functional abnormalities often antedate symptoms. (This is mainly due to decreased activity). The roentgenographic findings consist of diffuse reticular changes in the lower two-thirds of the lungs. On pulmonary function testing there is usually a decrease in the single breath carbon monoxide diffusing capacity. Initially, this may be the only finding; however, patients usually progress to a restrictive pattern on pulmonary function testing. Patients may also develop obstructive pulmonary disease. Histologically, the major findings are interstitial and alveolar fibrosis. Patients with interstitial lung disease may develop alveolar or broncial carcinoma, the only malignancies that occur with an increased frequency in this disease.

The small intestine is frequently involved, and this may lead to malabsorption and profound weight loss. Clinically, patients develop bloating and intermittent diarrhea and constipation. Adynamic ileus with intestinal obstruction may occur. Histologically, the small intestine changes look similar to those in the esophagus. As in the esophagus, there is hypomotility and this may lead to an overgrowth of bacteria. Hypomotility may be noted on roentgenogram after a barium meal, which may be retained in the second and third portions of the duodenum and this area may become widely dilated. Flocculation, hypersegmentation, and dilatation may occur in other areas of the small bowel. Patients may develop severe cachexia late in their disease course.

Asymptomatic large-mouth sacculations may occur in the large bowel secondary to atrophy of the muscularis. Rarely, they perforate and there may be resulting air in the wall of the large bowel (pneumatosis intestinalis). A small number of patients develop kidney involvement. This complication usually results in death within a few months. Renal involvement is usually heralded by the onset of malignant hypertension, proteinuria, and rapidly progressive renal failure. Histologically, the glomeruli are usually spared; the major lesions are arterial fibrinoid necrosis and hyperplasia of the intima. These changes closely resemble the findings in malignant nephrosclerosis; however, in progressive systemic sclerosis there may be collagen surrounding the adventitial tissues of the blood vessels. Congestive heart failure may accompany the severe renal disease and hypertension. Congestive heart failure may also occur secondary to pulmonary disease. A primary cardiomyopathy with myocardial fibrosis occurs and may be associated with conduction defects or heart block.

It is not unusual for patients with progressive systemic sclerosis to have an associated myopathy. There is a well-recognized overlap with polymyositis that is called sclerodermatomyositis. However, it is typical for patients to have less florid muscle disease with mild elevations of muscle enzymes and mild muscle weakness. Progressive systemic sclerosis may also be associated with Sjögren's syndrome and rarely with Hashimoto's thyroiditis.

Laboratory Manifestations

About 50% of the patients have an elevation of ESR and immunoglobulins. Rheumatoid factor is present in about 25% and antinuclear antibodies are present in 75% of patients. Immunofluorescent antinucleolar antibodies, when present in high titer, are very suggestive of progressive systemic sclerosis. However, speckled antinuclear antibodies are most commonly reported. Some of those patients with speckled antinuclear antibodies may have had mixed connective tissue disease. With severe malabsorption, patients may develop anemia of chronic disease and with severe renal disease, patients may develop a microangiopathic hemolytic anemia. Muscle enzymes are sometimes elevated.

Roentgenographic Manifestations

Hand roentgenographs often show diffuse osteoporosis. Dissolution of the distal tufts of the phalanx and soft tissue calcification around the digits and over large joints are typical late lesions. In the presence of these lesions, the diagnosis is not usually in doubt.

Diagnosis

The diagnosis of progressive systemic sclerosis can be made when the typical skin changes involve more than the hands and forearms. The diagnosis is definite if two of the following three are present: typical pulmonary disease, esophageal involvement, and Raynaud's phenomenon. Progressive systemic sclerosis may share features with systemic lupus erthematosus and rheumatoid arthritis and these diseases should be diagnostically excluded. In addition, patients should not have serologic evidence of mixed connective tissue disease.

Treatment

There is no evidence that any treatment alters the course of this disease. However, much can be done to make these patients more comfortable. In particular, psychologic support is very important in this disfiguring and frightening illness. It is important that patients avoid trauma, particularly to their hands. The avoidance of cold is extremely important and the patient should be instructed to wear warm gloves and stockings. It is not clear that there is any therapy that decreases the severity of Raynaud's phenomenon better than avoidance of cold; however, the vasoactive drugs, phenoxybenzamine, guanethidine, methyldopa, reserpine, and prazosin have been used. The nonsteroidal anti-inflammatory agents may help joint symptoms. Postprandial antacids may help esophageal symptoms and it is often advisable to elevate the head of the bed to avoid reflux. Patients with malabsorption often respond to broad-spectrum antibiotics such as tetracycline. In the presence of congestive heart failure, digitalis should be used sparingly if a cardiomyopathy or cor pulmonale is suspected. Nephrectomy and dialysis or transplantation have been suggested for patients with renal involvement. A few cases have had the reversal of renal disease after vigorous antihypertensive therapy. Physical therapy may help modify joint contractures from skin disease, and emollients help pruritis that is secondary to sebaceous gland atrophy.

Systemic involvement, especially renal involvement, is associated with a much worse prognosis. The 10-year survival is excellent with only skin disease and Raynaud's phenomenon.

OTHER SCLERODERMA SYNDROMES

CREST syndrome refers to a constellation of findings: calcinosis, often more severe than that found in progressive systemic sclerosis, Raynaud's phenomenon, esophageal disease as in progressive systemic sclerosis, sclerodactyly (sclerodermatous skin changes confined to the fingers, but by convention also generally the hands, wrists, and face), and telangiectasia (usually more prominent than in progressive systemic sclerosis). The principle value in separating these patients from those with progressive systemic sclerosis is in the identification of a group of patients with sclerodermatous skin changes who have a better prognosis, often having their disease for 10-15 years. Interstitial pulmonary disease is rare as is cor pulmonale, but primary pulmonary hypertension from vessel changes in the pulmonary arteries may be a late disease complication.

Morphea or localized scleroderma is a benign lesion without systemic manifestations that consists of waxy-appearing, white-yellow, sclerotic plaques surrounded by a violaceous halo of inflammation. The lesions usually heal over months to years leaving atrophic areas of incresased or decreased pigmentation.

Linear scleroderma, another form of nonsystemic localized scleroderma, often affects the extremities or the frontoparietal area of the face. The lesions may run the entire length of an extremity and hemiatrophy and joint contractures may occur, requiring physical therapy.

Eosinophilic fasciitis is a newly described entity characterized by diffuse swelling of the skin and underlying tissues of the hands, feet, and extremities; occasionally the trunk is involved. The skin takes on an orange peel-like puckered appearance and contractures may occur. The disease sometimes follows heavy physical exertion. Eosinophilia and hyperglobulinemia are usually present with early disease. The diagnosis is made by full thickness biopsy of skin down to muscle. Inflammation may be diffuse but it is most marked in the fascia that is greatly thickened and infiltrated with mononuclear cells and also often eosinophils. This entity responds well to corticosteroids and is usually self-limited after several years; however, thrombocytopenic purpura and aplastic anemia are not uncommon complications.

POLYMYOSITIS AND DERMATOMYOSITIS

Polymyositis and dermatomyositis are inflammatory disorders of skeletal muscle that are characteristically manifested by symmetrical, proximal muscle weakness. Clinically and pathologically, these disorders are similar and are distinguished primarily by the presence of a rash in dermatomyositis. This discussion will refer to both disorders unless either entity is specifically mentioned. These diseases are often associated with malignancy and may overlap with other connective tissue disorders such as progressive systemic sclerosis (scleroderma), systemic lupus erythematosus, mixed connective tissue disease, rheumatoid arthritis, Sjögrens syndrome, and polyarteritis nodosa.

Clinical Features

The incidence is about four per million. The average age of onset is about 40, although disease occurs in children and in older people. The sex ratio in polymyositis is two females to one male. Cases associated with another connective tissue disorder are predominantly in women. The sex ratio in dermatomyositis is approximately equal.

About 75% of patients present with proximal muscle weakness and virtually all develop this during their illness. Some complain of difficulty arising from a low chair or getting up a high step, while others develop a waddling gait with severe weakness. Dysphagia occurs in 15% of patients and is due to weakness of the posterior pharyngeal muscles and involvement of the proximal third of the esophogus, which is made of skeletal muscle. A small number of patients may develop dyspnea due to intercostal muscle weakness. Distal muscles are weak in 20%. Muscle pain and tenderness are present at some time in two-thirds of patients. Particularly with dermatomyositis, there may be soft tissue swelling over involved muscles. Joint contractures and profound muscle atrophy may be found in late disease.

Arthralgias and/or arthritis may be found in one-quarter of patients. Not surprisingly, these individuals are more likely to have an associated connective tissue disease. Interstitial pulmonary fibrosis, primarily at the bases, is a rare disease complication. These patients may also have alveolar infiltrates. Aspiration pneumonia due to a weakened swallowing mechanism is a rare complication, as is cardiomyopathy. About one-third of patients have an abnormal electrocardiogram. The findings are usually minor; however, conduction abnormalities may occur. Hypomotility of the distal esophogus is present in 50% of patients when carefully searched for; however, it is not usually clinically significant. Small bowel hypomotility also occurs. About 20% of patients have Raynaud's phenomenon and these are more likely to have an associated connective tissue disorder.

The classic rash of dermatomyositis occurs in 40% of all patients with myositis. Characteristically, there is a dusky red eruption of the face, which commonly affects the malar and periorbital areas. This eruption may also occur over the neck, shoulders, and upper part of the chest. The eyelids may also be lilac colored giving rise to the classic heliotrope rash, which is highly suggestive of dermatomyositis. These patients may also have periorbital edema and telangiectasia. Nail fold capillaries may be prominent and ecchymoses or telanglectasia may occur in the periungual area. These nail changes are often associated with other connective tissue diseases such as progressive systemic sclerosis and SLE. A patchy red eruption may also occur over the extensor surfaces of the joints such as the small joints of the hand, knees, elbows, and the medial malleoli of the ankles. This lesion is often smooth and slightly scaley; when long-standing there may be areas of atrophy. Eczematoid eruptions and sclerodactyly also occur.

The childhood form of myositis is associated with a vasculitis that may result in gastrointestinal perforation and a secondary mediastinitis or peritonitis. Soft-tissue calcification, particularly of muscle, also occurs. These lesions are now less common as the disease is treated vigorously.

About 10-17% of patients with myositis have an associated malignancy. The spectrum of malignancies roughly parallels the distribution in the general population. Men over 50 years of age and patients with dermatomyositis are more likely to have a malignancy. Patients with an associated connective tissue disorder are much less likely to have a malignancy. The myositis antedates the malignancy in about two-thirds of cases. A careful search for a malignancy is warranted, especially in high-risk patients. Patients occasionally respond dramatically to tumor resection; however, these patients are usually receiving concomitant corticosteroids. The minimal search for a malignancy should include a careful history and physical, serial stools for blood, a careful urinalysis for red cells, mammography, intravenous pyelography, sigmoidoscopy, and roentgenograms of the upper and lower gastrointestinal tracts.

Laboratory Manifestations

Elevation of muscle enzymes secondary to muscle damage is a characteristic feature. The creatine phosphokinase (CPK), aldolase, serum glutamic oxaloacetic transaminase (SGOT), serum glutamic pyruvic transaminase (SGPT), and the lactic dehydrogenase (LDH) may be elevated. Of these, the CPK and aldolase are highly sensitive and relatively specific for muscle damage. The CPK is most widely used and is elevated initially in about 70% of patients and eventually is elevated in about 95%. Only a very rare patient does not have an elevation during the disease course, and the disease should be diagnosed with extreme caution when this occurs.

About 50% of patients have an elevated sedimentation rate; however, it is not a good guide to disease activity. About 40% of patients have a positive rheumatoid factor, and 20% have antinuclear antibodies. These patients are more likely to have an associated connective tissue disorder.

The muscle biopsy is abnormal in 75-90% of patients. It is important to select a muscle for biopsy that is weakened but not atrophied. The EMG may be useful in selecting a biopsy site; however, because of electrode-induced changes, the biopsy should be performed rapidly. The quadriceps and deltoid muscles are biopsied most frequently. A normal biopsy may reflect the patchy nature of the disease and if clinically warranted, a second biopsy should be performed. The muscle biopsy may show degeneration, fibrosis, or necrosis of fibers. Phagocytosis of fibers by macrophages occurs. Regeneration of muscle is manifested by finding fibers of variable size, basophilia, central nuclei, and prominent nucleoli. While findings consistent with degeneration are most commonly found, the characteristic lesion is inflammatory and is present in 75% of biopsies. The cellular infiltrate is primarily lymphocytic, although plasma cells are also found. The infiltrate is often perivascular.

The electromyogram is abnormal in about 90% of patients. The most characteristic lesion is a short-duration, low-amplitude, polyphasic action potential. Spontaneous fibrillations, positive sawtooth potentials, insertional irritability, and bizarre potentials occur.

Diagnosis

The following criteria are adapted from Bohan: symmetrical proximal muscle weakness, characteristic electromyography, elevated muscle enzymes, abnormal muscle biopsy, and the typical skin rash of dermatomyositis. Polymyositis is definite if the first four criteria are met and probable with three of the first four. Dermatomyositis is definite when the skin rash is accompanied by three of the first four criteria and probable with two of the first four criteria.

Sarcoidosis may have an associated myositis that is only distinguishable due to the presence of granulomata on biopsy. Polymyalgia rheumatica is dintinguishable because the EMG and biopsy are normal and proximal muscle weakness is not found on physical. Endocrinopathies such as Addison's disease, Cushing's disease, thyrotoxicosis, and hypothyroidism may mimic an inflammatory myopathy. Hypothyroidism may be associated with very high levels of CPK. Drugs such as clofibrate, hydroxychloroquine, penicillamine, and particularly ethanol may cause a toxic myopathy.

Treatment

The initial treatment consists of 50-100 mg of prednisone per day in four divided doses. The most important parameter to follow is muscle strength and dosages should only be reduced with improvement. The CPK may be lower in 2-6 weeks and usually heralds muscle strength improvement; however, muscle strength may not improve for 1-3 months. As strength testing returns to normal, prednisone may be tapered slowly. About 75% of patients respond to prednisone. Relapses are usually associated with a too rapid dosage reduction and a prompt increase in dosage is important when this occurs. The CPK should be performed on each visit; a rise indicates that a relapse will occur over the next month and the prednisone dosage should be increased. Only in a rare instance can prednisone be discontinued.

If no improvement in muscle strength occurs after 3 months of therapy, cytotoxic therapy is a consideration. Methotrexate, cyclophosphamide, azathioprine, and chlorambucil have been used with moderate success. Methotrexate has been used most widely; however, no study has clearly demonstrated its superiority over the other agents. It is administered intraveneously on a weekly basis. Because their efficacy has not clearly been demonstrated and because of their toxicities, these drugs should be administered cautiously by physicians skilled in their usage.

Prognosis

About 50% of patients will be alive after 7 years of disease. The prognosis is better with younger age and worse if there is an associated malignancy. Occasionally, as with severe systemic lupus erythematosus, the prognosis is related to an associated connective tissue disease. Patients most commonly die of malignancy; sepsis is the next most common cause of mortality. Profound weakness and associated dyspnea is occasionally the cause of death.

MIXED CONNECTIVE TISSUE DISEASE

Mixed connective tissue disease was described by Sharp and coworkers in 1972 and is a clinical entity with features of progressive systemic sclerosis (PSS), systemic lupus erythematosus (SLE), and polymyositis. Early cases may have only Raynaud's phenomenon or the picture may resemble rheumatoid arthritis (RA). The disease is serologically defined and high titers of antibody to nuclear ribonucleoprotein are invariable present.

Clinical Features

The average age of onset is 37; however, the range is wide and children and elderly people have had typical disease. The female to male ratio is 4:1. The presenting complaint is often Raynaud's phenomenon or swelling of the hands. Proximal muscle weakness, pleuritic or pericardial pain, and the typical symptoms of rheumatoid arthritis are less common. Malaise, fatigue, and low-grade fever may be present initially and occasionally are the only symptoms. The characteristic skin lesion, which occurs in about two-thirds of patients, is diffuse swelling of the hands. Digital swelling is most prominent and the digits may appear sausage shaped and tapered. Digital ulcerations are rare. As in PSS, biopsy reveals an increase in dermal collagen. Rashes that closely resemble those seen in dermatomyositis and SLE occur and telangiectasia are common. Almost all patients have arthralgias, and two-thirds have arthritis. As with SLE, the arthritis is usually nondeforming (nonerosive); however, erosive disease may occur that is indistinguishable from rheumatoid arthritis. These patients often subsequently develop more typical features of MCTD. Proximal muscle weakness is common and patients may have a myopathy that is indistinguishable from polymyositis. The EMG, biopsy, or muscle enzyme elevations are not appreciably different from those seen in polymyositis. Esophageal dysfunction resembling that seen in PSS is found in 80% of patients when carefully searched for. Similarly, lung disease resembling that seen in PSS occurs in two-thirds of patients. Heart disease is rare with pericarditis being most frequent although other lesions occur. Kidney disease is rare, occurring in 10% of patients, and is much less severe than that found in SLE. Death from renal disease is rare. Histologically, the renal lesions have features of both SLE and PSS. Neurologic lesions also occur in about 10% of patients and are milder than those found in SLE. Trigeminal neuropathy occurs most frequently, although a variety of lesions have been described. Lymphadenopathy and hepatosplenomegaly are frequently found.

Laboratory Manifestations

An elevated sedimentation rate, mild leukopenia, and the anemia of chronic disease are common in active disease. Muscle enzymes such as the CPK and aldolase are frequently elevated. Hemolytic anemia and thrombocytopenia are rarely present.

The characteristic laboratory feature of MCTD is a high titer of antibodies to nuclear ribonucleoprotein (RNP). Patients with MCTD were first found to have antibodies to extractable nuclear antigen (ENA), an acid-extractable nuclear antigen. Although their titers were lower, patients with SLE also often had antibodies to ENA. It was subsequently found that if ENA was digested with ribonuclease (destroying the RNP) the antibody titer to ENA dropped dramatically in MCTD and remained high in SLE. The antigen in MCTD is therefore RNP and the antigen in SLE has been named the Sm antigen. Antibodies to RNP and Sm are found using both hemagglutination and immunodiffusion techniques. Low titers of anti-RNP antibodies are sometimes seen in SLE, these may be detected by hemagglutination but not by immunodiffusion. Antibodies to Sm are extremely rare in MCTD. Conventional fluorescent antinuclear antibody (FANA) testing reveals a high titer (≥1:1800) speckled pattern. Patients with SLE, who have antibodies to Sm will have identical patterns, although the titers tend to be lower. Only a minority of SLE patients have speckled FANA and antibodies to Sm. A homogeneous FANA is most common in SLE. Antibodies to native DNA and hypocomplementemia, frequent features of SLE, are rarely found in MCTD.

Diagnosis

MCTD should be considered as a possibility in any patient with features of SLE, PSS, polymyositis, or rheumatoid arthritis. A FANA should be obtained and if the pattern is speckled in a high titer, then testing for RNP and Sm antibodies should be obtained. The diagnosis depends upon finding high titers of anti-RNP antibodies by hemagglutination or immunodiffusion.

Treatment

Patients with MCTD respond well to corticosteroids. High dosages (60-80 mg a day) should be reserved for patients with severe organ system involvement such as myositis or renal disease. Many patients need only nonsteroidal anti-inflammatory agents such as aspirin. With mild systemic disease and organ involvement, small doses of prednisone (5-10 mg a day) may suffice. Although the pulmonary and esophageal lesions resemble those found in PSS, which is not responsive to corticosteroids, preliminary evidence suggests that MCTD patients with lung and esophageal involvement may respond to corticosteroids. These findings should be viewed cautiously until they are confirmed. Skin disease and Raynaud's phenomenon respond poorly to corticosteroids.

The prognosis of MCTD is much better than that of SLE, PSS, or polymyositis and deaths have been rare. The disease tends to change over time and at times the disease will closely resemble SLE or RA; much later the clinical picture will resemble scleroderma. Patients may have only vague systemic complaints and Raynaud's phenomenon for several years.

VASCULITIS

The term vasculitis refers to inflammation and necrosis of the blood vessels. The primary vasculitides are diseases in which the characteristic lesion is inflammation of the vessel wall, although vasculitis may also be a prominent feature of diseases such as rheumatoid arthritis, systemic lupus erythematosis, and acute rheumatic fever. In this section only the primary vasculitides will be discussed. The classification of this group of disorders is confusing and has been based on pathologic, clinical, and pathogenetic criteria. Despite difficulties in classification, it is important to attempt a definite diagnosis as treatment and prognosis of individual entities are variable. The following sections describe the entities that account for the majority of cases of primary vasculitis; however, it is not inclusive as almost a hundred entities have been described.

POLYARTERITIS NODOSA

Polyarteritis nodosa (PN) is a multisystem disorder, in which the characteristic lesion is necrotizing inflammation of medium and small muscular arteries. The older term, periarteritis, has been replaced, as it is now recognized that a panarteritis occurs. The classic disease is now rare as milder and earlier cases are seen and the disease is altered by therapy. The classic nodose lesions occur when there is weakening of the vessel wall from inflammation and subsequent aneurysmal dilation of the artery. These are now rarely palpated in the skin; however, these lesions are usually seen on abdominal and renal angiography.

The etiology is unknown, but 30-50% of cases are positive for the hepatitis-B antigen. An altered immune response to this virus has been suggested. The hepatitis-B antigen is also often found in mixed cryoglobulinemia, which also gives rise to a vasculitis. This antigen may be responsible for a variety of clinical syndromes including the serum sickness-like prodrome of hepatitis B.

Clinical Features

The disease occurs at all ages, but is most common in midlife and occurs more frequently in men. The onset of disease may be sudden or even explosive. Systemic symptoms such as fever, malaise, and weight loss are frequently present. The presenting complaints are quite variable and are related to the major organ system involved. Hematuria, hypertensive encephalopathy, or congestive heart failure may be the presenting features. More insidious disease may present with mononeuritis multiplex or myalgias and arthralgias. The kidney is involved in about 80% of cases; of these, the majority have a vasculitis on kidney biopsy, although about one-third of cases have glomerulitis. The urine sediment shows red cells, white cells, and a variety of casts. Proteinuria is common. Hypertension is frequently present and may be severe. About two-thirds of patients succumb to renal disease. Cardiac disease may be secondary to hypertension, although a primary coronary vasculitis occurs.

A variety of neurologic manifestations have been described, although mononeuritis multiplex is the most common and characteristic lesion. Abdominal pain with bowel infarction and bleeding also occurs. Arthralgias are common, but frank arthritis is rare. Skin involvement is also rare. Livedo reticularis and splinter hemorrhages occur. Myalgias and weakness are frequent complaints, and an occasional patient has the clinical features of polymyositis. The degree of pulmonary involvement in PN depends on the classification of vasculitis used. In this discussion, patients with eosinophilia, asthma, and pulmonary infiltrates are discussed under Churg-Strauss syndrome (allergic granulomatosis). However, overlap between classic polyarteritis nodosa and Churg-Strauss syndrome occurs; therefore, patients may have typical polyarteritis nodosa and pulmonary infiltrates. A vasculitis of the pulmonary or bronchial arteries may occur in polyarteritis nodosa.

Laboratory Manifestations

Laboratory abnormalities are frequent, but not specific. A leukocytosis and the anemia of chronic disease are common and the Westergren sedimentation rate is usually elevated in active disease. Rheumatoid factor is found in over one-half the patients and increased levels of immunoglobulin are sometimes detected.

The pathologic findings are the basis for making the diagnosis and the diagnosis should be made with extreme caution in the absence of a positive biopsy, the exception being the typical angiographic features described below. Skin and muscle biopsies are most frequently abnormal; however, the yield in blind biopsy is low. Because the vasculitis frequently skips large areas of vessel, numerous serial sections may be required. Lesions are also found in various stages of development, with early lesions showing a polymorphonuclear leukocyte predominance and late lesions showing mononuclear cells. Fibrosis and intimal proliferation occur and may lead to vessel occlusion. Liver and kidney biopsies may be helpful, but they are hazardous. Renal arteriography may be helpful in identifying hazards to biopsy, such as perinephric hematomas, and in diagnosis. Renal, celiac, or mesenteric angiography usually reveal microaneurysms of medium-sized arteries. This lesion is highly characteristic of polyarteritis nodosa, but has also been found in rare cases of SLE and Wegener's granulomatosis. In the presence of classic disease features, the typical angiographic findings confirm the diagnosis. Testicular biopsy may be helpful and biopsies of the vasonervorum in patients with mononeuritis multiplex may yield positive findings.

Treatment

Polyarteritis nodosa was a catastrophic disease prior to treatment with corticosteroids. Although good, controlled studies have not been performed, the available evidence suggests that corticosteroids are helpful in treating this illness and promoting survival. Dosages such as 80 mg per day of prednisone in divided doses should be utilized in acutely ill patients and the dose should be tapered to the lowest level that controls disease activity. Recently, the success in treating Wegener's granulomatosis with cyclophosphamide has promted its usage in PN. Preliminary reports are favorable; however, this drug should be used only by those skilled in its administration.

CHURG-STRAUSS SYNDROME (ALLERGIC GRANULOMATOSIS AND EOSINOPHILIA)

This entity, also known as polyarteritis with lung involvement, was described in 1951. Like polyarteritis nodosa, the classic syndrome is rarely seen; it is more common to see an overlap between this syndrome and polyarteritis nodosa. As first described, this illness is characterized by fever, eosinophilia (often greater than 1500/mm^3), and asthma. The asthma may precede the onset of vasculitis by weeks to many years, although some patients have a simultaneous onset of asthma and vasculitis. The asthma is of variable severity and occasionally improves with the onset of vasculitis. The characteristic histologic finding is the necrotizing extravascular granuloma. Recently cases have been described that are typical in all respects except that granulomata are not seen, perhaps reflecting an earlier stage of the disease. The vessel changes are similar to those found in polyarteritis nodosa, except that eosinophils are more prominent.

Renal disease is less common than in polyarteritis nodosa and is usually much less severe. There is a spectrum of pulmonary findings but evanescent pulmonary infiltrates are most commonly seen. The gastrointestinal tract may be involved and cardiomyopathy occurs. Mononeuritis multiplex is frequently seen as are arthralgias and myalgias. The treatment is similar to that of polyarteritis nodosa.

WEGENER'S GRANULOMATOSIS

This well-defined clinical entity is characterized by a granulomatous, necrotizing vasculitis of the upper and lower respiratory tracts. The lung is usually involved and the characteristic lesion consists of multiple nodular infiltrates that may cavitate, although other lesions occur. Nasopharyngeal lesions are common and severe tissue destruction from necrotizing granulomata may give rise to a saddle nose deformity. Sinusitis is common and may be the presenting complaint.

The kidney is involved in about 85% of cases. The characteristic renal lesion is a glomerulitis that may progress to a necrotizing glomerulonephritis, often with granuloma formation. The absence of eosinophilia helps to distinguish this disease from Churg-Strauss syndrome (allergic granulomatosis and eosinophilia) and the predominant pulmonary disease helps distinguish this entity from polyartritis nodosa.

The prognosis is extremely poor, and steroids have not been efficacious. Recently, uncontrolled studies have indicated that cytotoxic agents, particularly cyclophosphamide, are very efficacious. Steroids are usually also needed acutely for control of disease activity.

HYPERSENSITIVITY ANGIITIS AND LEUKOCYTOCLASTIC VASCULITIS

Classic hypersensitivity angiitis is characterized by inflammation of small arteries; it is distinguishable from polyarteritis nodosa because of its propensity for the lesions to all be of the same age. Cutaneous lesions are prominent and the disease is usually associated with exposure to an antigen such as a drug. As in other forms of vasculitis, the classic picture is rarely seen. This form of vasculitis is now being subsumed under the heading leukocytoclastic vasculitis, which also involves small arteries; however, the postcapillary venule is most characteristically involved. Biopsy reveals infiltration of vessels with polymorphonuclear leukocytes and nuclear debris. The characteristic skin lesion is palpable purpura or urticaria. Leukocytoclastic vasculitis includes various forms of vasculitis associated with connective tissue disorders. Henoch-Schönlein purpura also falls under this heading. Henoch-Schönlein purpura is a disease of young adults characterized by nonthrombocytopenic purpura, arthralgias, abdominal pain with occasional hemorrhage, and glomerulitis. The illness is usually self-limited, but may become chronic. Another rare form of vasculitis that falls under this heading is essential mixed cryoglobulinemia. The cryoglobulin is an immune complex, usually of rheumatoid factor and IgG, which precipitates in the cold. It is called essential since the cryoglobulins are not associated with an infectious disease or connective tissue disorder as they sometimes are. In addition to the typical skin changes glomerulonephritis, hepatosplenomegaly, and lymphadenopathy are frequently present.

GIANT CELL ARTERITIS

Giant cell arteritis is an inflammatory necrotizing vasculitis of the aortic root arteries. There is a female preponderance, and the disease affects those over the age of 55. The disease is also known as temporal arteritis, as clinical involvement of this artery is easier to recognize. There is a well-recognized overlap with polymyalgia rheumatica as the patients with giant cell arteritis may have the polymyalgia rheumatica symptom complex. Conversely, patients with polymyalgia rheumatica may occasionally develop giant cell arteritis.

Giant cell arteritis is a systemic illness commonly associated with fever, malaise, anorexia, weight loss, and arthralgias. Temporal artery involvement is manifested by headache that often is unilateral. The artery may be tender, particularly if rubbed by eyeglasses. Opthalmic artery involvement is manifested by loss of vision. Jaw claudication and scalp tenderness are less common disease manifestations. Cerebral vascular accident and myocardial infarction are rare complications of this disease. Physical examination may reveal swollen, tender temporal arteries. Pulsation of the temporal and other arteries may be decreased and vascular occlusion occurs. Arterial bruits may be heard over the large vessels.

An elevated sedimentation rate is the major consistent abnormal laboratory finding, and values are usually greater than 60 mm/hr. Cases have been found with a normal sedimentation rate. The anemia of chronic disease is often present. Biopsy is diagnostic. A large section of temporal artery should be obtained and multiple sections evaluated as the inflammation may skip segments. Biopsy reveals round-cell inflammation and giant cells. The diagnosis is occasionally made with a normal biopsy and a typical clinical picture since to delay treatment is to risk blindness.

Treatment consists of at least 60 mg of prednisone a day. Higher doses occasionally are necessary. Prednisone may be gradually tapered as symptoms improve and the sedimentation rate returns to normal. The maintenance dose of prednisone, or that which normalizes the sedimentation rate and alleviates symptoms, is variable. Treatment is usually necessary for 2-4 years. Unilateral blindness occurs, and vigorous corticosteroid therapy is usually necessary to prevent bilateral blindness.

POLYMYALGIA RHEUMATICA

Polymyalgia rheumatica (PMR) affects people over the age of 50 and is included with the vasculitides because of the frequent overlap with giant cell arteritis. Disease symptoms are usually quite dramatic and consist of shoulder and hip girdle pain, severe morning stiffness, and fatigue. Fever, weight loss, anorexia, and depression may also be present. The symptoms may be explosive or insidious and several weeks may intervene before medical attention is sought.

Patients often appear ill, in pain, and depressed. Shoulder and hip motion may be limited by pain and occasionally a mild synovitis, particularly of the knees, may be present. The major laboratory abnormality is an elevated sedimentation rate, which is often quite high and values above 60mm/h are common. The anemia of chronic disease is often present and minor hepatic enzyme abnormalities, particularly of the alkaline phosphatase, occur.

Differential diagnosis includes giant cell arteritis. Temporal artery biopsy should be performed if any symptoms or signs of this disease are present. Even in the absence of specific findings suggestive of giant cell arteritis, 20% of biopsies may be positive. Polymyositis is ruled out easily as muscle-strength testing, electromyogram, muscle biopsy, and muscle enzymes are normal. Occult malignancies, particularly of the hematopoietic system, are often responsible for high sedimentation rates and systemic symptoms and therefore should be considered in the differential diagnosis. A rapid response to treatment favors the diagnosis of polymyalgia rheumatica, although caution is warranted as malignancies are more common in this age group.

Treatment consists of 10-20 mg of prednisone a day. The response to therapy is dramatic, and symptoms are greatly improved within a week. The absence of such a response suggests another diagnosis, in which case temporal artery biopsy should be performed and a search for occult malignancy undertaken. The dosage of prednisone can usually be tapered to 5-10 mg per day with a normal sedimentation rate. The disease is self-limited, and therapy can usually be discontinued after 2-3 years.

CRYSTAL-INDUCED SYNOVITIS

Certain crystals have been found to induce an acute synovitis in humans. Monosodium urate, calcium pyrophosphate dihydrate, hydroxyapatite, and depot adrenocorticosteroid preparations for intra-articular injections are crystals shown to be associated with synovial inflammation.

The pathophysiology of crystal-induced synovitis is not completely understood. The presence of a particular crystal in a joint effusion is not enough to explain the events associated with such synovitis since in some instances the crystal may be found, when all inflammation has subsided, in quiescent joints.

The most common forms of crystalline synovitis are those associated with sodium urate and with calcium pyrophosphate as an acute form of arthritis, but chronic joint disease may also result. The acute arthritis induced by crystals have similar characteristics with rapid onset, a self-limited nature, phagocytosis of the crystal by polymorphonuclear leukocytes with subsequent release of lysosomal enzymes, and other inflammatory mediators. Differences in crystal morphology and clinical presentation are helpful in diagnosis.

GOUT

The term gout is traced to the Latin word *gutta*, a drop, and reflects the ancient belief that the disease was caused by a poison, falling drop by drop into the joint. Gout is a heterogenous group of diseases in which characteristic manifestations include an increased serum urate level, deposits of monosodium urate in or around the joints, and recurrent attacks of acute arthritis. In some patients uric acid urolithiases and/or renal disease involving glomerular, tubular, and interstitial tissues may occur.

Hyperuricemia

Hyperuricemia is a biochemical abnormality defined solely by the serum urate concentration. Uric acid is the final degradation product in the purine metabolism as the humans lack the enzyme uricase that in other animals splits uric acid into alantoin and CO_2. Multiple conditions are associated with hyperuricemia (Table 7).

Increased uric acid production that is seen in enzyme defects, myeloproliferative diseases, and other disorders of increased cell turnover and diminished uric acid excretion by the kidneys, singly or in combination, account for the production of hyperuricemia.

Using an enzymatic method (uricase method) for the determination of uric acid it is accepted that the upper limit of normal for serum urate is 7.0 mg/dl in men and 6.0 mg/dl in premenopausal women. The plasma concentration is maintained at a constant level during adulthood and results from

Table 7. Common Conditions Associated with Hyperuricemia

Primary Gout
Myeloproliferative diseases
Lymphoproliferative diseases
Chronic hemolytic anemias
Sarcoidosis
Psoriasis
Renal insufficiency
Drugs: Diuretics; low dose salicylates; pyrazinamide
Lead toxicity
Alcoholism
Ketoacidosis
Starvation
Obesity
Glycogen storage disease
Toxemia of pregnancy

stable and nearly equal rates of uric acid synthesis and renal excretion. Urate is almost completely filtered by the glomerulus and then subsequent steps of reabsorption-secretion-reabsorption-secretion occur in the tubules. Between 400 and 600 mg of uric acid is excreted by the kidney daily. Approximately 150 mg urate is secreted into the gastrointestinal tract, where it is degraded by bacteria. This intestinal process does not influence serum levels.

Plasma solution is saturated with urate at 6.4-6.8 mg/100 ml at 37° C. At greater concentrations urate precipitates as monosodium urate crystals. This precipitation is influenced by urate concentration, pH, and temperature, but not all factors involved in precipitation are known and it is puzzling that some people may tolerate high levels of plasma urate without ever demonstrating urate deposits and/or gouty attacks.

Acute Gout

Acute gouty attacks are characterized by dramatic acute inflammation, usually monoarticular and more frequently involving lower extremity joints. In about 60% of patients the first attack involves the first metatarsophalangeal joint. Within a few hours the affected joint becomes red, swollen, warm, and very tender; the acute attack resolves spontaneously in a few days and leaves no apparent sequelae. Fever and modest leucocytosis may occur. In some patients the initial episode may be polyarticular. Rarely tophaceous deposits may be found at the time of the first attack. Although hyperuricemia is characteristic of gout, normal serum urate values may be seen during the acute attack. As the disease evolves into a chronic state, if untreated large tophi may develop and the acute episodes may become polyarticular, leading to a destructive type of arthritis with tophaceous deposits in joints and surrounding tissues. In this stage, confusion with rheumatoid arthritis is possible as the physical findings may mimic a rheumatoid process. A high sedimentation rate and a positive rheumatoid factor may be present. Gout occurs primarily in men; in women, it is more likely to occur after menopause.

McCarty and Hollander in 1961 demonstrated monosodium urate monohydrate (MSU) crystals in synovial fluids of patients with acute gouty arthritis; thus, gout became the first of the crystal-induced arthritides in which a crystal was identified in joint fluids. Proper identification of these urate crystals requires the use of a compensated polarizing microscope but often they may be seen under regular light microscopy. By compensated polarizing microscope, monosodium urate crystals are typically strongly negatively birefringent (Figure 1A). Most standard microscopes can be modified to identify crystals using two polarizing disks and a color compensator. Cellophane tape in association with polarizing disks can readily turn an ordinary light microscope into a polarizing one.

Synovial effusions in acute gout are typically inflammatory with most effusions having 5,000-25,000 WBC/mm^3 mostly polymorphonuclear leukocytes. Monosodium urate crystals can be seen either intracellularly or extracellularly. Acute gouty effusions without detectable crystals have been reported, but such fluids may contain crystals visible only by electron microscopy.

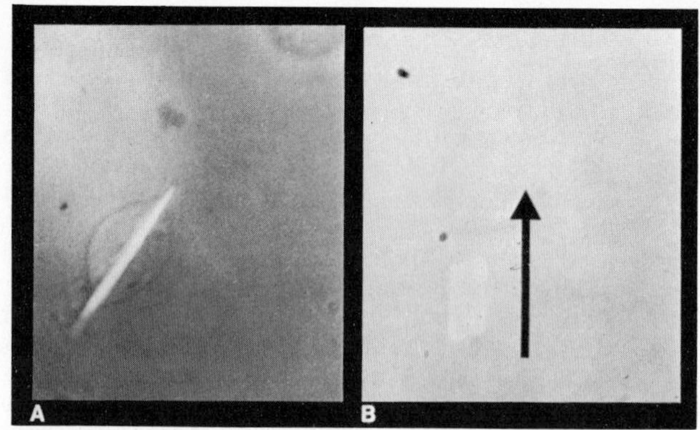

Figure 1. Synovial fluid viewed under polarizing microscope. (A) Urate crystal phagocytosed by a WBC; the needlelike crystal appears intensely negatively birefringent (diagnosis, gout). (B) Calcium pyrophosphate crystal that appears rectangular, 2 to 25 μ in length, blue, and weakly positively birefringent (diagnosis, pseudogout). (Photos from *Gout: A Clinical Comprehensive*, New York, MEDCOM Inc., 1971. By permission of the publisher.)

As the acute attack subsides, the patient becomes asymptomatic until a new attack occurs. This intervening period is variable and may last up to several years. During this interim period, the diagnosis of gout is based on the previous history of acute arthritis with clinical response to colchicine, hyperuricemia, and identification of monosodium urate crystals from a visible tophus or asymptomatic first metatarsophalangeal joints. Tophaceous deposits are often seen on the helix of the ear and over extensor surfaces of the elbows; these deposits are usually firm and when needled a chalky white material is obtained that reveals the typical monosodium urate crystals under the compensated polarizing microscope. If biopsy is obtained, the sample should be fixed in absolute alcohol as formalin fixatives contain water that dissolves urate crystals.

During the acute attack, the only radiographic abnormality may be swelling of the soft tissues. In chronic gout, destructive lesions with a punched-out appearance may occur in the subchondral bone at the bases or heads of phalanges. The most common location of these punched-out lesions is at the medial aspect of the head of the first metatarsophalangeal joint and their edge may characteristically show a thin, shell-like configuration continuous with adjacent bone contour or the overhanging margin as described by Martel. Significant osteoporosis is absent.

Gouty Renal Disease

Deposition of sodium urate crystals in the renal interstitial tissue and the resulting inflammatory reaction leads to parenchymal renal damage or urate nephropathy. Chronic renal disease with progressive renal failure may occur. Significant urate nephropathy is associated with chronic hyperuricemia and is rare in the absence of gout. Hypertension is often found in the gouty population and contributes to the renal damage. Renal stones composed of uric acid are found in about 10-25%

of gouty patients; however, most patients with uric acid stones do not have hyperuricemia or gouty arthritis. The cause of the renal stones is a persistently acid urine that favors precipitation of uric acid, associated in some patients with an increased uric acid concentration.

Treatment of Acute Gout

The treatment of gout involves several phases. Once the diagnosis of the acute attack is confirmed, rest and anti-inflammatory drugs are necessary. When the acute attack subsides, definitive therapy requires anti-inflammatory prophylaxis and management of the underlying hyperuricemia to prevent recurrent attacks, joint damage, and uric acid nephropathy.

For the management of acute gout, several drugs are available. Colchicine has been considered quite specific, if given at the onset of the attack. It can be administered either by mouth or intravenously. Oral colchicine is given as 0.5-0.6 mg tablets, one or two, every 1-2 hours until either improvement, gastrointestinal side effects with nausea, vomiting or diarrhea occur, or 14 tablets have been given. Significant relief is common after a few hours, and the dosage may be tapered to one tablet, two or three times daily. Intravenously, 2 mg of colchicine is given in 10-20 ml of normal saline. Another 1 mg dose may be given once or twice at 4-6 hour intervals up to a total of 4 mg in a 24-hour period. Inadvertent extravenous infiltration may be very irritating. As the patient improves, oral maintenance therapy of 2-3 tablets daily is instituted. The major advantages of intravenous colchicine are the avoidance of gastrointestinal toxicity associated with the oral route, and rapidity of response. Rarely, in large doses, colchicine may produce bone marrow depression, leukopenia, and renal or hepatic toxicity. The mechanism of colchicine's action in so specifically relieving the acute gouty attack is not completely understood. It may involve the inhibition of a chemotactic factor produced by phagocytizing leukocytes; this chemotactic factor may be a major mediator of the acute monosodium urate-induced synovitis. Other possible mechanisms include the interference with microtubular subunit protein aggregation in polymorphonuclear leucocytes, inhibition of lysosomal degranulation, and release of lysosomal enzymes during phagocytosis of urate crystals.

Phenylbutazone (Butazolidin) is a very effective drug in the treatment of acute gout; 600-800 mg/daily in divided doses are given for 2-3 days, tapering the dosage to 300 mg/daily as the patient improves. Rare but serious toxic manifestations limit its usefulness. Gastric or duodenal ulceration may occur and their presence is a contraindication to phenylbutazone therapy; fluid retention is frequent, and the disadvantages of giving this drug to a patient with congestive heart failure must be considered. The most serious side effect is marrow depression, but is rare during brief therapy. Phenylbutazone potentiates the effects of warfarin and tolbutamide. Indomethacin, in doses up to 200 mg/day in divided doses, is very effective as well. At these large dosages, the drug is often not well tolerated, producing central nervous sytem and gastrointestinal side effects. Sulindac (Clinoril), in doses of 200 mg twice daily, may have the advantages of twice-daily dosage and probably less gastrointestinal irritation. Other nonsteroidal antiinflammatory agents are presently being tested for their use and effectiveness in acute gout. In an occasional patient with acute attack of a large joint such as the knee, local intra-articular depot corticosteroid injection may be indicated.

Recurrent attacks can be prevented by control of hyperuricemia that may take several months to achieve. Effective prophylaxis during this period is accomplished by adding small doses of colchicine, indomethacin, or another nonsteroidal anti-inflammatory drug.

Control of Hyperuricemia

Effective control of the hyperuricemia is achieved pharmacologically by increasing the renal excretion of uric acid or by decreasing its synthesis. Uricosuric drugs include probenecid (Benemid), and sulfinpyrazone (Anturane). Synthesis is decreased by the xanthine oxidase inhibitor allopurinol (Zyloprim). Uricosurics are indicated if the patient excretes less than 600 mg of uric acid in 24 hours or if allergic to allopurinol. Probenecid is administered in dosages of 0.5-3.0 g daily. Possible side effects include dermatitis and gastrointestinal complaints. Sulfinpyrazone is given in dosages from 200-400 mg daily in divided doses. Toxicity is similar to probenecid. Ticrynafen is a uricosuric that is also a diuretic. It was found to cause severe liver damage and obstructive nephropathy and has been withdrawn from clinical use.

Inhibition of xanthine oxidase by allopurinol decreases uric acid synthesis. This enzyme catalyzes the final two steps in the degradation pathway of purine nucleotides ending in uric acid. Allopurinol is converted to oxipurinol and both are strong inhibitors of xanthine-oxidase. Allopurinol is administered in dosages of 200-600 mg daily in one dose. It is indicated for patients who excrete more than 600-800 mg of uric acid in 24 hours, those with severe tophaceous gout or chronic renal insufficiency and who are allergic to uricosurics. Toxic reactions are usually related to skin rashes; rarely, serious side effects such as vasculitis, granulomatous hepatitis, or agranulocytosis may occur. In the presence of chronic renal failure, allopurinol dosage should be lowered.

There is no consensus regarding the management of asymptomatic hyperuricemia. Treatment of patients with renal uric acid calculi is directed at increasing urine production by increasing fluid intake, maintenance of alkaline urine, and the reduction of total uric acid excretion.

PSEUDOGOUT (CPPD CRYSTAL DEPOSITION DISEASE)

McCarty, Kohn, and Faires in 1962 described an acute synovitis similar to gout but induced by a different crystal, calcium pyrophosphate dihydrate (CPPD). Because of the clinical resemblance to gout, it was named pseudogout. This disease tends to involve large joints such as the knees, wrists, and shoulders but rarely may involve the first metatarsophalangeal joint. Calcification visible by x-ray in cartilage or menisci is often but not invariably present. As with gout, attacks are self-limited and usually monoarticular, but polyarticular involvement and chronic arthritis with joint destruction may occur. This disease has been associated with a number of degenerative and metabolic diseases such as hyperparathyroidism, ochronosis and hemochromatosis.

Diagnosis is based on clinical presentation, x-ray findings, and demonstration of characteristic weakly positive, birefringent, rhomboid, or rod-like crystals by compensated polarized light microscopy (Figure 1B). The reasons for the precipitation of CPPD are not known. Synovial fluid during the acute attack is characteristically inflammatory with 4,000 to 20,000 WBC/mm^3, mostly polymorphonuclear leucocytes. Asymptomatic calcific deposits may occur.

Nonsteroidal anti-inflammatory drugs, including salicylates, are effective in controlling the acute attacks of pseudogout. Colchicine may be of benefit as well. In some patients, aspiration of the involved joint seems effective in controlling acute symptoms.

HYDROXYAPATITE-ASSOCIATED SYNOVITIS

Hydroxyapatite crystals have been identified by electron microscopy in synovial fluids of patients with acute arthritis, exacerbations of osteoarthritis, and in renal dialysis patients. These crystals are not seen by light microscopy but they appear to form clumps with shiny globules on wet smears, and on Wright's stain they appear as purple cytoplasmic inclusion bodies. Synovial fluids from the affected joints have shown leukocyte counts ranging from normal to 50,000/mm^3. Patients with chronic renal failure on dialysis treatment may develop attacks of acute arthritis, involving multiple joints, of short duration. Radiographs of involved joints may be normal or reveal subcutaneous calcifications assumed to be hydroxyapatite or amorphous calcium phosphate. Treatment with aspirin or nonsteroidal anti-inflammatory drugs is generally helpful.

STEROID CRYSTAL-INDUCED SYNOVITIS

Intra-articular injection of steroids may induce, in about 2% of the patients, an acute synovitis. This acute inflammatory reaction begins several hours after the injection and subsides over 1-3 days. Its early occurrence after injection helps in differentiation from infection introduced by the injection. The crystalline, but not the soluble, steroids are responsible for this synovitis; they can be seen as positive and negative birefrigent chunks, rods, or globular material by compensated polarized light.

QUESTIONS

1. Which of the following may be hematologic manifestations of systemic lupus erythematosus?
   A. Coombs' positive hemolytic anemia
   B. Leukopenia
   C. Anemia of chronic disease
   D. Thrombocytopenia
   E. Red cell aplasia
2. Features of Sjögren's syndrome may include
   A. Dry eyes
   B. Dry mouth (xerostomia)
   C. Salivary gland enlargement
   D. Lymph node enlargement
   E. Renal tubular acidosis
3. Ankylosing spondylitis
   A. Clinically is usually a disease of young adult men
   B. May affect the eye, heart, and lungs
   C. Unlike rheumatoid arthritis, inflammation is not a prominent feature in this disease
   D. May affect the costovertebral joints resulting in chest pain
   E. May involve nonspinal joints such as the hips, knees, and shoulders
4. Which of the following are predisposing conditions for the development of osteoarthritis?
   A. Trauma
   B. Thyrotoxicosis
   C. Repeated joint popping
   D. Gout
   E. Congenital hip disease
   F. Malnutrition
   G. Infectious arthritis
   H. Ochronosis
5. Nonsteroid anti-inflammatory agents may
   A. Precipitate asthma in susceptible patients
   B. May cause peptic ulcer disease, bowel perforation, and gastrointestinal bleeding
   C. Are effective analgesics at low doses
   D. May reduce joint inflammation in a majority of patients with rheumatoid arthritis
6. Which of the following may be manifestations of extra-articular rheumatoid arthritis?
   A. Pleuritis
   B. Nodular lung disease
   C. Pericarditis
   D. Hepatitis
   E. Scleritis
7. Which of the following are true of gold salt and penicillamine therapy for rheumatoid arthritis?
   A. About 80% of rheumatoid arthritis patients may respond to these drugs
   B. Significant side effects necessitate their discontinuation in 10-30% of patients

C. Late malignancy may result from the usage of these drugs
D. Rash, oral ulceration, proteinuria, and aplastic anemia are potential side effects
E. Six weeks of therapy should determine if a person will respond to these drugs

8. Which of the following are features of inflammatory joint fluid?
A. Viscous joint fluid
B. Poor mucin clot
C. Spontaneous clotting of the fluid
D. White cell count greater than $5000/mm^3$
E. Predominance of lymphocytes in the fluid

9. Laboratory abnormalities often seen in active systemic lupus erythematosus include
A. High titer fluorescent antinuclear antibodies
B. Increased levels of antinative DNA antibodies
C. Low C3 and C4 complement levels
D. Elevated sedimentation rate
E. Antinucleolar antibodies

10. Progressive systemic sclerosis may involve the following organs:
A. Esophagus
B. Joints
C. Small bowel
D. Heart
E. Lungs

11. Which of the following factors increases the possibility of myositis being associated with a malignancy?
A. Old age
B. Positive antinuclear antibody test
C. Skin lesions of dermatomyositis
D. Male sex
E. Elevated sedimentation rate

12. Which of the following are true about the treatment of polymyositis dermatomyositis?
A. All patients are treated with corticosteroids initially.
B. The dose of corticosteroids should be lowered with a fall in the CPK.
C. The dose of corticosteroids should be increased with a rise in the CPK.
D. Muscle strength testing is the most important guide to therapy.
E. Most patients are tapered off prednisone after 1 year of therapy.
F. Cytotoxic therapy should be considered if the patient does not respond to 3 months of high-dose corticosteroids.

13. Which of the following may be causes of myopathy?
A. Sarcoidosis
B. Thyrotoxicosis
C. Chronic ethanol ingestion
D; Hydroxychloroquine therapy
E. Byssinosis

14. Patients with mixed connective tissue disease
A. Have high titers of antinative DNA antibodies
B. Have high titers of speckled fluorescent antinuclear antibodies
C. Have high titers of antibodies to ribonucleoprotein
D. May resemble scleroderma patients
E. May have an arthritis resembling rheumatoid arthritis
F. May have a myositis

15. Which of the following statements are true?
A. Wegener's granulomatosis frequently responds to cyclophosphamide therapy.
B. Churg-Strauss vasculitis is associated with asthma.
C. Cryoglobulinemia may be associated with a leukocytoclastic vasculitis.
D. Polyarteritis nodosa is a form of leukocytoclastic vasculitis.
E. Microaneurysms of medium and small arteries on renal arteriography are characteristic of polyarteritis nodosa.

16. Giant cell arteritis and polymyalgia rheumatica
A. Usually occur in older people
B. May overlap clinically
C. Are associated with high sedimentation rates
D. Are associated with an increased chance of malignancy
E. Are treated with corticosteroids

17. The treatment of acute gout may include
A. Probenecid
B. Allopurinol
C. Colchicine
D. Indomethacin
E. Phenylbutazone

18. Pseudogout
A. Is caused by calcium oxalate crystals
B. May resemble rheumatoid arthritis
C. Is often associated with chondrocalcinosis
D. May resemble gout clinically
E. May be associated with hyperparathyroidism
F. Is caused by negatively birefringent crystals

ANSWERS

1. A,B,C,D,E
2. A,B,C,D,E
3. A,B,D,E
4. A,D,E,G,H
5. A,B,C,D
6. A,B,C,E

7. A,B,D
8. B,C,D
9. A,B,C,D
10. A,B,C,D,E
11. A,C,D
12. A,C,D,F
13. A,B,C,D
14. B,C,D,E,F
15. A,B,C,E
16. A,B,C,E,F
17. C,D,E
18. B,C,D,E

BIBLIOGRAPHY

TEXTBOOKS AND MONOGRAPHS

Cohen AS: *Laboratory Diagnositic Procedures in the Rheumatic Diseases*, ed. 2. Boston; Little, Brown & Co, 1975.

Fries JF, Holman HR: Systemic Lupus Erythematosus: A Clinical Analysis. In *Major Problems in Internal Medicine, Vol. 6*. Philadelphia; W B Saunders Co, 1975.

Katz WA (ed): *Rheumatic Diseases: Diagnosis and Management*. Philadelphia; J B Lippincott Co, 1977.

Kelley WN, Harris ED, Ruddy S, et al (eds): *Textbook of Rheumatology,* Philadelphia, WB Saunders Co, 1981.

McCarty DJ (ed): *Arthritis and Allied Conditions*, ed. 9. Philadelphia; Lea & Febiger, 1979.

Polley HF, Hunder GG: *Rheumatologic Interviewing and Physical Examinaton of the Joints*, ed. 2. Philadephia; W B Saunders Co, 1978.

Samter M (ed): *Immunologic Diseases*, ed. 3. Boston; Little, Brown & Co, 1978.

Scott JT (ed): *Copeman's Testbook of the Rheumatic Diseases*, ed. 5. New York; Churchill Livingstone, Inc, 1978.

Shearn MA: Sjögren's Syndrome. In *Major Problems in Internal Medicine*, Vol. 2. Philadelphia; W B Saunders Co, 1971.

Williams RC Jr: Rheumatoid Arthritis as a Systemic Disease. In *Major Problems in Internal Medicine*, Vol. 4. Philadelphia; W B Saunders Co, 1974.

Wright V, Moll JMH: *Seronegative Polyarthritis*. New York; Elsevier North-Holland Publishing Co, 1976.

Wyngaarden JB, Kelley WN: *Gout and Hyperuricemia*. New York; Grune & Stratton, Inc, 1976.

ARTICLES

Rheumatoid Arthritis

Jensen PS, Steinbach HL: Roentgen features of the rheumatic diseases. *Med Clin North Am* 61:389-404, 1977.

Turner R: Aspirin and newer anti-inflammatory agents in rheumatoid arthritis. *Am Fam Physician* 16:1111-1115, 1977.

Turner R, Collins R, Nomeir AN: Extra-articular manifestations of rheumatoid arthritis. *Bull Rheum Dis* 28:186-199, 1979.

Osteoarthritis

Howell DS, Moskowitz RW: Introduction: Symposium on osteoarthritis: A brief review of research and investigations. *Arthritis Rheuma* 20 (Suppl): S96-S103, 1977.

Moskowitz RW: Cartilage and osteoarthritis: Current concepts (editorial). *J Rheumatol* 4:329-331, 1977.

Resnick D, Shapiro RF, Wiesner KB, et al.: Diffuse idiopathic skeletal hyperostosis (DISH) (ankylosing hyperostosis of Forestier and Rotes-Querol). *Semin Arthritis Rheum* 7:153-187, 1978.

Solomon L: Patterns of osteoarthritis of the hip. *J Bone Joint Surg* (Br) 58B:176-183, 1976.

Ankylosing Spondylitis

Calin A, Porta J, Fried JF, et al.: Clinical history as a screening test for ankylosing spondylitis. *JAMA* 237:2613-2614, 1977.

Kemple K, Bluestone R: The histocompatibility complex and rheumatic diseases. *Med Clin North Am* 61:331-346, 1977.

Khan MA, Kushner I, Braun WE: Comparison of clinical features in HLA-B27 positive and negative patients with ankylosing spondylitis. *Arthritis Rheum* 20:909-912, 1977.

Infectious Arthritis

Goldenberg DL, Cohen AS: Acute infectious arthritis: A review of patients with nongonococcal joint infections (with emphasis on therapy and prognosis. *Am J Med* 60:369-377, 1976.

Handsfield HH, Wiesner PJ, Holmes KK: Treatment of the gonococcal arthritic-dermatitis syndrome. *Ann Intern Med* 84:661-667, 1976.

Mitchell WS, Brooke PM, Stevenson RD, et al.: Septic arthritis in patients with rheumatoid disease: A still underdiagnosed complication. *J Rheumatol* 3:124-133, 1976.

Systemic Lupus Erythematosus

Baldwin DS, Gluck MC, Lowenstein J, et al.: Lupus nephritis: Clinical course as related to morphologic forms and their transitions. *Am J Med* 62:12-30, 1977.

Budman DR, Steinberg AD: Hematologic aspects of systemic lupus erythematosus. *Ann Intern Med* 86:220-229, 1977.

Donadio JV Jr, Holley KE, Ferguson RH, et al.: Treatment of diffuse proliferative lupus nephritis with prednisone and combined prednisone and cyclophosphamide. *N Engl J Med* 299:1151-1155, 1978.

Gibson T, Myers AR: Nervous system involvement in systemic lupus erythematosus. *Ann Intern Med* 89:660-676, 1978.

Rossen RD, Hersh EM, Sharp JT, et al.: Effect of plasma exchange on circulating immune complexes and antibody formation in patients treated with cyclophosphamide and prednisone. *Am J Med* 63: 674-682, 1977.

Systemic Sclerosis (Scleroderma)

Kovalchik MT, Guggenheim SJ, Silverman MH, et al.: The kidney in progressive systemic sclerosis: A prospective study. *Ann Intern Med* 89:881-887, 1978.

Lam M, Ricanati, ES, Khan MA, et al.: Reversal of severe renal failure in systemic sclerosis. *Ann Intern Med* 89:642-643, 1978.

Rowell NR: The prognosis of systemic sclerosis. *Br J Dermatol* 95: 57-60, 1976.

Polymyositis and Dermatomyositis

Bohan A, Peter JB, Bowman RL, et al.: A computer-assisted analysis of 153 patients with polymyositis and dermatomyositis. *Medicine* (Baltimore) 56:255-286, 1977.

Barnes BE: Dermatomyositis and malignancy: A review of the literature. *Ann Intern Med* 84:68-76, 1976.

Mixed Connective Tissue Disease

Sharp GC: Mixed connective tissue disease. *Bull Rheum Dis* 25:828-831, 1974-1975.

Vasculitis

Gilliam JN, Siley JD: Cutaneous necrotizing vasculitis and related disorders. *Ann Allergy* 37:328-339, 1976.

Crystal-Induced Synovitis

Boss GR, Seegmiller JE: Hyperuricemia and gout: Classification, complications, and management. *N Engl J Med* 300:1459-1468, 1979.

Fox IH: Hypouricemic agents in the treatment of gout. *Clin Rheum Dis* 3:145-158, 1977.

McCarty DJ: Calcium pyrophosphate dihydrate crystal deposition disease (pseudogout syndrome): Clinical aspects. *Clin Rheum Dis* 3:61-89, 1977.

CHAPTER 15
TOXICOLOGY

Richard D. Stewart

BASIC PRINCIPLES OF DIAGNOSIS AND TREATMENT

The diagnosis and treatment of acute poisoning is a demanding task because of the sheer number of compounds and possible combinations of compounds that have the potential for injuring man. Fortunately for the physician, recent analytical techniques have revolutionized the speed with which a diagnosis can be confirmed so that effective antidotes, useful in 10-30% of poison cases, can be promptly combined with good supportive treatment to achieve a more favorable outcome than was possible in the 1970's.

EMERGENCY MANAGEMENT

Life Support

The key to successful treatment of the poisoned patient is life support. An adequate airway must be established and a tidal volume of 10-15 ml/kg maintained while the preparation for definitive diagnosis and treatment are carried out.

If the victim is in shock or is hypotensive, vasopressor therapy should be avoided initially and fluids, plasma, or blood administered while monitoring the central venous pressure.

Cardiac arrhythmia or arrest must be promptly and appropriately treated.

Clinical Evaluation

The clinical evaluation of a patient suspected to be poisoned includes the usual history and physical examination with the appropriate laboratory studies. The purpose of the clinical evaluation is to establish a firm baseline against which to measure the progression or course of the illness. The physician should obtain the best history of the intoxication that is possible in an emergency room setting with the full knowledge that in only one-third of the cases will that history be sufficiently accurate to permit the institution of all appropriate antidotal and therapeutic measures.

During the physical examination of the patient, the physician should carefully observe whether the confirmatory signs and symptoms of intoxication of the suspected poison are present. If coma, hyperactivity, or withdrawal are present, it is useful to classify the stage that the patient exhibits. Such classifications are valuable adjuncts in following the course of the illness and advancing a prognosis once the identity of the toxic agent has been confirmed by the laboratory.

CLASSIFICATION OF COMA

Stage	*Features*
0	Asleep, but can be aroused and can answer questions
1	Comatose; withdraws from painful stimuli; reflexes intact
2	Comatose; does not withdraw from painful stimuli; most reflexes intact; no respiratory or circulatory depression
3	Comatose; most or all reflexes absent; no respiratory or circulatory depression
4	Comatose; reflexes absent; respiratory depression or circulatory failure or shock

CLASSIFICATION OF HYPERACTIVITY

Stage	*Features*
1+	Restlessness, irritability, insominia, tremor, hyperreflexia, sweating, mydriasis, flushing
2+	Confusion, hyperactivity, hypertension, tachypnea, tachycardia, extrasystoles, sweating, mydriasis, flushing, mild hyperpyrexia
3+	Delirium, mania, marked hypertension, tachycardia, arrhythmias, hyperpyrexia
4+	Above plus: convulsions, coma, circulatory collapse.

CLASSIFICATION OF WITHDRAWAL

Score	*Features*
0-2	Diarrhea, dilated pupils, goose flesh, hyperactive bowel

sounds, hypertension, insomnia, lacrimation, muscle cramps, restlessness, tachycardia, yawning (each of these features is given a score of 0-2 points)

Total
1-5 Mild withdrawal
6-10 Moderate withdrawal
11-15 Severe withdrawal

The presence of seizures indicates severe withdrawal regardless of the rest of the score.

Laboratory Studies

Until there is laboratory confirmation that a sufficient quantity of a toxic agent has been absorbed and has produced an illness compatible with the signs and symptoms manifested by the patient, the physician should proceed in the care of his patient as though the illness he is attempting to diagnose and treat were due to another cause. Frequently, histories are incomplete, and head trauma and metabolic intoxications are overlooked. Thus, the initial laboratory studies should be selected carefully to avoid an undue loss of time should the illness subsequently prove not to be due to a toxic substance.

In the evaluation of the intoxicated patient, it is generally prudent to include the following laboratory studies: arterial PO_2, PCO_2, and pH; complete blood count; urinalysis; serum electrolytes, blood urea nitrogen, blood sugar, serum bilirubin, and liver enzymes; 12-lead electrocardiogram; and chest x-ray.

The biologic samples submitted to the laboratory for identification of the toxic agent should include an aliquot of emesis or first lavage specimen, urine specimen, clotted blood specimen, heparinized blood sample, contaminated clothing where indicated, and the bottle or container of suspected toxic substance.

Analysis of the postingestion emesis or the first lavage specimen frequently contains a high concentration of the toxic agent, which facilitates laboratory identification. Amount of the toxic agent in these specimens, when correlated with the amount present in urine or blood, often permits an accurate reconstruction of the sequence of events leading to the accidental or deliberate ingestion of a toxic agent.

Because of the frequency of multiple drug ingestion in cases of attempted suicide, a urine specimen (60-100 ml) should be screened for a battery of commonly used therapeutic agents as well as illicit drugs. This can be accomplished in 3-4 hours using thin-layer chromatographic techniques available in most major medical centers or, more rapidly, by using the computerized, gas chromatographic/mass spectrometric instrumentation available in centers specializing in the treatment of the intoxicated patient.

The quantification of the amount of toxic agent present in the blood specimen is indicative of the amount of agent absorbed and is of significant prognostic value. In those instances where it is documented that a potentially lethal quantity of an agent has been absorbed, consideration of procedures such as exchange transfusion, hemoperfusion, and hemodialysis can be entertained.

TREATMENT OF POISONING

Ingested Poisons

The absorption of ingested poisons can be reduced significantly by emesis, gastric lavage, adsorption on activated charcoal, use of cathartics, and, on rare occasions, surgical removal.

Emesis

The simplest procedure to remove the unabsorbed poison is to induce vomiting. The specific contraindications to emesis are semiconsciousness, a comatose state, convulsions, loss of normal gag reflexes, ingestion of a strong alkali, mineral acid, or petroleum solvent, and severe heart disease or advanced pregnancy.

If fully conscious, the patient should drink as much tap water, warm salt water (2-3 teaspoonsful of table salt/glass), or milk as possible. Vomiting can then be induced by stroking the back of the patient's throat with a finger or tongue blade. This procedure should be repeated if indicated. An aliquot of the vomitus should be saved for analysis.

Syrup of ipecac is the most readily available drug for the induction of vomiting. This drug can be administered at home, and many pediatricians routinely dispense this drug to mothers at the baby's 6-month or 1-year checkup along with a poison prevention discussion. The pediatric dose is 10-15 ml orally, repeated one time if necessary. The adult dose is 30 ml (1 oz) orally, repeated one time if necessary. Following the administration of syrup of ipecac, the patient should be given large amounts of fluid and should remain ambulatory. Fifteen minutes later, the patient's throat may be stimulated to induce emesis. In the majority of instances, syrup of ipecac will induce vomiting in 20-30 minutes.

Apomorphine will induce vomiting more rapidly than syrup of ipecac; but, since it must be administered by medical personnel, it is not used in the home as an emetic agent. Apomorphine also produces respiratory depression, but, fortunately, this can be promptly negated with the use of naloxone (Narcan) as soon as adequate emesis has occurred. The usual dose is 0.1 mg/kg intravenously (IV) or subcutaneously. The usual adult dose is 6 mg subcutaneously while children 1-2 years of age receive 1-2 mg subcutaneously. Apomorphine comes as a 6 mg tablet to which 3 cc of diluent is added to achieve a final concentration of 2 mg/ml. Large quantities of oral fluid should be given following the administration of apomorphine; emesis usually ensues in 5-15 minutes.

Naloxone (Narcan) 0.005 mg/kg should be given as soon as adequate emesis has occurred to reverse the central nervous system depressant effect of the narcotic apomorphine. The usual adult dose is 0.4 mg IV; the usual pediatric dose is 0.1 mg IV.

Other emetics such as copper sulfate has a long history as a highly successful emetic agent. However, in those rare instances where emesis has not occurred, toxic amounts of copper sulfate have been absorbed and fatalities have occurred. Sodium chloride is a less effective emetic than is copper sulfate and also is very dangerous. Fatalities due to hypernatremia have occurred. Solutions of sodium chloride or copper sulfate are not recommended as emetic agents.

Gastric Lavage
Removal of the unabsorbed toxic agent by gastric lavage is often the first therapeutic measure to be employed where there is a contraindication to emesis. Obviously, severe respiratory distress and circulatory collapse must be corrected before gastric lavage can be commenced. Generally, gastric lavage is a reasonable procedure to be used within 3 hours after ingestion of a toxic agent.

Gastric lavage can be used in patients who are not completely conscious, who have lost their gag reflex, or who are experiencing convulsive seizures. Ideally, the airway should be protected through the use of a cuffed endotracheal or nasotracheal tube. When this is not possible, the patient should be placed in a head down position and turned on the left side. Lavage is carried out using a large orogastric tube whenever possible. In combative adults, the lavage procedure may have to be compromised with the use of a nasogastric tube. As large a stomach tube as possible is chosen. In an adult, a 28-French Ewald or larger tube should be used.

The preferred lavage fluid is physiologic saline that should be warmed to body temperature to avoid lowering the patient's temperature. The fluid is forced down the tube using a volume of approximately 300 ml in an adult and 10 ml/kg in children. Fluid and gastric contents are aspirated and the initial washings are saved for toxicologic analysis. The lavage procedure is repeated 10-15 times until the washings are clear. In adults, a total of 3 L of wash fluid are used.

Activated Charcoal
Upon the completion of emesis and/or gastric lavage, USP activated powdered charcoal is administered in those instances where the suspected toxic agent is adsorbed on its surface. The dose is 5-10 times the estimated weight of the drug or chemical ingested. Usually, 10-30 g of charcoal in a water slurry is administered orally.

There are no known contraindications to the adminstration of activated charcoal. Since it adsorbs and inactivates ipecac, it is best to administer the charcoal after emesis. If the suspected toxic agent is adsorbed by charcoal, the activated charcoal may be administered orally prior to gastric lavage. Charcoal will also serve as a marker of intestinal transit time so that its appearance in the stool will indicate that absorption of the toxic agent by the gastrointestinal (GI) tract is completed.

Table 1 lists some of the toxic compounds that are well adsorbed by activated charcoal. Recent evidence indicates that activated charcoal not only inhibits drug absorption from the gastrointestinal tract but also increases the clearance of drugs that have already been absorbed and are in the systemic circulation. Drugs are not only absorbed from the gastrointestinal tract but can diffuse from the general circulation into the gastrointestinal lumen. Activated charcoal enhances the rate of drug diffusion from the body into the gastrointestinal tract by efficiently adsorbing the drug from the gastrointestinal fluids.

Table 1. Toxic Compounds Adsorbed by Activated Charcoal

Alcohol	Iodine	Phenol
Amphetamines	Ipecac	Phenolphthalein
Antimony	Malathion	Phenothiazine
Antipyrene	Mercuric chloride	Phosphorus
Atropine	Methylene blue	Potassium permangenate
Arsenic	Morphine	Quinine
Barbiturates	Muscarine	Salicylates
Camphor	Nicotine	Selenium
Cantharides	Opium	Silver
Cocaine	Oxalates	Stramonium
Digitalis	Parathion	Strychnine
Glutethimide	Penicillin	Sulfonamides

Cathartics
Cathartics are useful agents to decrease drug absorption by decreasing GI tract transit time. There are no contraindications to the use of the cathartic agents listed below:

1. Magnesium sulfate (Epsom salt): usual adult dose is 5 g or 50 ml of 10% solution; the usual pediatric dose is 250 mg/kg. One tablespoon (5 g) mixed with a sweet liquid generally produces an effect in 2-4 hours. The dose may be repeated every 2-4 hours until catharsis with a charcoal-marker is observed.
2. Fleet's phosphosoda: 15-30 ml diluted 1:4.
3. Sodium sulfate: 250 mg/kg diluted 1:2 or 1:4.

Antidotes
Effective antidotes are available for some of the commonly encountered agents. A listing of the antidotes is presented in Table 2. Except for the four intoxications listed below, antidotes should not be administered until there has been laboratory confirmation that the absorption of a toxic quantity of an agent has occurred. However, in the case of carbon monoxide poisoning, cyanide poisoning, nitrite or nitrate poisoning, and poisoning with organophosphate insecticides, the antidote should be administered as soon as there is suspicion of the diagnosis.

Forced Diuresis
Forced diuresis is useful in serious poisonings if the toxic agent is excreted in part by the kidneys. This technique should not be used unless specifically indicated because of its potential to exacerbate cerebral edema or circulatory failure. Excretion of alcohol, amphetamine, and strychnine is increased by forced acid diuresis; and of bromides, phenobarbital and salicylates by forced alkaline diuresis. Hypertonic or pharmacologic diuretics should be administered along with adequate fluids to increase the usual urine flow from 0.5-2 ml/kg/h to 3-6 ml/kg/h. Alkaline or acid diuresis should be chosen on the basis of the drug's pK_a. Table 3 lists the therapeutic agents and their dosages.

Table 2. Antidotes

Specific Indications	*Antidote*	*Adolescent and Adult Dose*	*Pediatric Dose*
Amphetamine-induced hyperactivity and psychosis	Chlorpromazine (Thorazine)	25 mg IV q 6 h; reduce dose if barbiturate ingested; titrate subsequent doses to desired response	1 mg/kg IV q 6 h reduce dose if barbiturate ingested; titrate subsequent doses to desired response
Anticholinergics	Physostigmine salicylate (Antrilirium)	2 mg slowly over 2-3 min IV with repeat in 2-5 min if no effect; then lowest effective dose slowly q 30-60 min with recurrence of symptoms	0.5 mg slowly over 2-3 min IV with repeat in 2-5 min if no effect; then lowest effective dose q 30-60 min slowly with recurrence of symptoms.
Carbon monoxide	Oxygen	100% oxygen by inhalation	Same as adult
Cyanide	Amyl nitrite	Inhalation for 30 s of every min; new ampule q 3 min	Same as adult
	Sodium nitrite	10-20 cc of 3% solution, 2.5-5 cc/min IV; may be repeated once with persistence or recurrence of symptoms	0.33 ml/kg of 3% solution, 2.5-5 cc/min IV; may be repeated once with persistence or recurrence of symptoms
	Sodium thiosulfate	50 cc of 25% solution, 2.5-5 cc/min IV, 15 min after sodium nitrite; may be repeated once	1.65 cc/kg of 25% solution, 2.5-5 cc/min IV, 15 min after sodium nitrite; may be repeated once
Heavy metals Arsenic, mercury lead, gold	Dimercaprol	3 mg/kg IM at 4-6 h intervals for 5 days and then 3 mg/kg q 12 h for 5-9 days	3-4 mg/kg IM at 4-6 h intervals for 5 days and then 3-4 mg/kg q 12 h for 5-9 days
Iron	Deferoxamine	1-2 g IM q 6-8 h; for severe intoxication, IV dose not to exceed 15 mg/kg/h; maximal dose per day 6 g	50 mg/kg or 1-2 g IM q 6 h for severe intoxication, IV dose not to exceed 15 mg/kg/h; maximal dose per day 6 g
Lead	Calcium disodium ethylenediamine tetra-acetate (calcium disodium versenate) (CaEDTA)	1 g IV or IV over 1 h twice a day for 5-7 days; repeat course after rest period; add procaine for IM use	20-75 mg/kg/day IM or IV divided into 2-3 doses for 5-7 days; repeat course at 50 mg/kg/day after rest period; add procaine for IM use
Mercury, lead	D-penicillamine (Cuprimine)	250-500 mg orally q 6-8 h depending on severity	For acute therapy, 100 mg/kg/day in 4 divided doses orally for 5 days; for chronic therapy 30-50 mg/kg/day in 4 divided doses orally, maximal dose per day of 1 g
Insecticides Organophosphate anticholinesterase	Pyridine-2-aldoxime-methochloride (2 PAM or pralidoxime)	0.5-1 g given slowly, IV, 500 mg/min after initial treatment with atropine; repeat q 8-12 h as needed	25 mg/kg given slowly IV after initial treatment with atropine; repeat q 8-12 h as needed
Organophosphate and carbamate anticholinesterase	Atropine sulfate	2-3 mg in solution, 0.4 mg/ml IV q 2-5 min until fully atropinized, then as needed to maintain atropinization	0.05 mg/kg in solution, 0.4 mg/ml IV q 2-5 min until fully atropinized, then as needed to maintain atropinization
Methanol and ethylene glycol	Ethanol	ethanol given as a 50% solution IV 0.5-1.5 ml/kg q 2-4 h to maintain a blood level between 100-150 mg%; in mild cases, 3-4 oz of whiskey q 4 h orally	Same as adult
Methemoglobinemia	Methylene blue	1% solution, 10 mg IV, given	1% solution, 1-2 mg/kg IV,

Table 2. Continued

Specific Indications	*Antidote*	*Adolescent and Adult Dose*	*Pediatric Dose*
		slowly over 5-10 min; repeat in 4 h if needed	given slowly over 5-10 min; repeat in 4 h if needed
Narcotic depression	Naloxone HCl	0.4 mg IV repeated q 2-3 min for 2 or 3 doses for initial effect; repeat as needed	0.01 mg/kg IV repeated q 2-3 min for 2 or 3 doses for initial effect; repeat as needed
Phenothiazine extrapyramidal reaction	Diphenhydramine (Benedryl)	10-50 mg IV slowly and then q 6 h orally or IV for maintenance	1-2 mg/kg IV slowly and then q 6 h orally or IV for maintenance
Tricyclic antidepressants	Physostigmine salicylate (Antilirium)	2 mg slowly over 2-3 min IV with repeat in 2-5 min if no effect; then lowest effective dose slowly q 30-60 min with recurrence of symptoms	0.5 mg slowly over 2-3 min IV with repeat in 2-5 min if no effect; then lowest effective dose q 30-60 min slowly with recurrence of symptoms

Dialysis and Hemoperfusion

Hemodialysis, peritoneal dialysis, or hemoperfusion can be considered for those patients in stage 3 or 4 coma (due to a dialyzable or removable drug) who have not responded to adequate supportive treatment. Dialysis is also useful in poisoned patients exhibiting marked hypothermia or hyperthermia, patients with severe electrolyte disturbances not responding to therapy, and patients with hypotension; that is, impaired renal or hepatic function not corrected by the adjustment of circulating blood volume.

The decision whether to employ hemodialysis or hemoperfusion in drug overdose cases may be guided by the following criteria:

1. Severe clinical intoxication with abnormal vital signs. Often this will include hypotension despite fluid replacement, apnea or severe hypothermia, or a combination of these findings.
2. Ingestion and probable absorption of a potentially lethal dose.
3. A blood level that is in the potentially lethal dose range.
4. A degree of intoxication that impairs the normal route of excretion of the drug or an underlying disease in the patient that impairs the function of a major metabolic or excretory organ for that particular drug. An example of such a situation would be when a cirrhotic patient has ingested an overdose of ethchlorvynol.
5. The presence of a significant quantity of a circulating toxin that is metabolized to a more noxious substance. The metabolic conversions of methanol to formaldehyde and ethylene glycol to oxalic acid are typical examples.
6. Progressive clinical deterioration while the patient is under careful medical management.
7. Prolonged coma with its potential hazards, such as aspira-

Table 3. Therapeutic Agents for Forced Diuresis

Urinary Excretion	*Therapeutic Agent*	*Adolescent and Adult Dose*	*Pediatric Dose*
Diuresis	Ethacrynic acid (Edecrin)	50 mg or 0.5-1 mg/kg IV q 8 h	0.5-1 mg/kg IV q 8 h
	Furosemide (Lasix)	20-40 mg IM or IV over 1-2 min q 8-12 h	1-3 mg/kg IM or IV over 1-2 min q 8-12 h
Acidic compounds by alkalinization	Sodium bicarbonate	2 mgEq/kg IV for first h, then sufficient to keep pH >7.5 (usually 2 mEq/kg q 6-8 h); additional potassium	2-4 mEq/kg IV for first h, then sufficient to keep pH>7.5 (usually 2 mEq/kg q 6 h); additional potassium (3-4 mEq/kg/day)
Basic compounds by acidification	Ammonium chloride	1.5 g IV q 6 h up to 6 g/day or orally 8-12 g/day	75 mg/kg IV or orally 6 h up to 2-6 g/day
By osmotic diuresis	Mannitol	25-50 g in 20% solution IV over 30 min q 4-6 h up to 200 g/day	1-2 g/kg in 20% solution IV over 30 min q 4-6 h up to 100 g/day

tion pneumonia, septicemia from infected IV sites, and peripheral neuropathy secondary to pressure ischemia.

8. The presence of an underlying disease such as chronic bronchitis or emphysema, which would increase the hazards of coma.
9. The development of a significant complication, such as aspiration pneumonitis.
10. Poisoning by agents known to produce delayed toxicity. Examples include paraquat, diquat, amanita phalloids, and acetaminophen.

Tables 4 and 5 list the toxic substances whose elimination can be increased by dialysis or hemoperfusion.

Exchange Transfusion

Exchange transfusion can be used to reduce the amount of poison circulating in the blood, and this modality can be lifesaving, particularly when the toxin is nondialyzable. However, the procedure is laborious and carries the risk of transfusion reactions. In infants, it is probably the procedure of choice over dialysis because of the latter's fluctuation in blood volume.

Inhaled Toxic Gas or Vapor

The patient should be removed immediately from the contaminated environment and respiration assisted if the respiratory center is depressed sufficiently to have resulted in

Table 4. Currently Known Dialyzable Poisons and Drugs[a]

- Barbiturates[b]
  - Amobarbital
  - Barbital
  - Butabarbital
  - Butalbital
  - Cyclobarbital
  - Pentobarbital
  - Phenobarbital
  - Quinalbital
  - Secobarbital
- Nonbarbiturate hypnotics, sedatives, and tranquilizers
  - Ethchlorvynol[b]
  - Glutethimide[b]
  - Methaqualone
  - Methyprylon
  - Dipenhylhydantoin
  - Methsuximide
  - Paraldehyde
  - Primidone
  - Diazepam
  - Chloral hydrate
  - Carbromal
  - Chlordiazepoxide
  - Diphenylhydramine
  - Ethianamate
  - Gallamine triethiodide
  - Heroin
  - Meprobamate
- Antidepressants
  - Amphetamine
  - Methamphetamine
  - Monoamine oxidase inhibitors
  - Pargyline
  - Tranylcypromine
  - Isocarboxazid
  - Tricyclic secondary amines
  - Tricyclic tertiary amines
  - Amitryptiline
  - Imipramine
  - Phenelzine
- Alcohols
  - Ethanol[b]
  - Methanol[b]
  - Ethylene glycol
  - Isopropanol
  - Dichloroethane
- Analgesics
  - Acetylsalicylic acid[b]
  - Salicylic acid
  - Methylsalicylate[b]
  - Acetophenetidin
  - Acetaminophen or paracetamol
  - D-Propoxyphene
- Antimicrobials/anticancer agents
  - Gentamicin
  - Kanamycin
  - Neomycin
  - Streptomycin
  - Tobramycin
  - Vancomycin
  - Amikacin
  - Bacitracin
  - Colistin
  - Polymyxin
  - Ampicillin
  - Penicillin
  - Nafcillin
  - Carbenicillin
  - Cephalothin
  - Cephaloridine
  - Cefamandole
  - Sulfonamides
  - Chloramphenicol
  - Tetracycline
  - Nitrofurantoin
  - Fosfomycin

Table 4. Continued

Isoniazid
Cycloserine
Ethambutol
Flucytosine

Chloroquine
Quinine

Azathioprine
Cyclophosphamide
5-fluorouracil
Methotrexate
Colchicine

Metals/inorganics
- Aluminum
- Arsenic[b]
- Iron
- Lead
- Lithium[b]
- Magnesium
- Mercury
- Potassium[b]
- Phosphate[b]
- Sodium[b]
- Strontium
- Tin
- Zinc

- Bromides[b]
- Carbromal
- Chloride[b]
- Iodide
- Fluoride[b]

Plant/animal toxins, herbicides, insecticides
- *Amanita phalloides*
- Amanitin

- Diquat
- Paraquat

- Organophosphates
- Alkyl phosphate
- Demeton-s-methylsulfoxide
- Dimethoate
- Sodium chlorate
- Potassium chlorate
- Methyl mercury complex
- Snake venom

Solvents/gases
- Carbon monoxide
- Camphor
- Carbon tetrachloride
- Eucalyptus oil
- Thiols
- Trichloroethylene
- Toluene

Cardiovascular agents
- Digoxin
- Ouabain

- Chloroquine
- Procainamide
- N-acetyl-procainamide
- Quinine
- Quinidine
- Practolol
- Sotalol
- Diazoxide
- Methyldopa

Endogenous toxins
- Amino acids[b]
- Ammonia
- Uric acid[b]
- Creatinine[b]
- Urea[b]
- Tritium[b]
- Bilirubin
- Lactic acid

- Methyl mercaptans
- Free fatty acids

- Uremic toxins[b]
- Hepatic failure
- Hyperosmolar state[b]
- Metabolic alkalosis[b]
- Water intoxication
- Porphyria
- Peritonitis

Miscellaneous
- Mannitol
- Thiocyanate[b]
- Aniline
- Boric acid
- Potassium dichromate
- Chromic acid
- Sodium citrate
- Dinitro-ortho-cresol
- Chlorpropamide
- Borates
- Folic acid
- Methylprednisolone
- Nitrates

[a] *Trans. Am. Soc. Artif. Int. Organs*, 23:766, 1977
[b] Extensively studied in vivo.

Table 5. Drugs and Poisons Removable with Hemoperfusion[a]

Barbiturates[b]	Chlorinated insecticides
Amobarbital	Polychlorinated biphenyls
Butabarbital	Methyl parathion
Medinal (Russian)	Demeton-s-methyl sulfoxide[b]
Pentobarbital	Dimethoate[b]
Phenobarbital	Nitrostigmine
Quinalbital	Paraquat[b]
Secobarbital	
	Solvents/gases
Nonbarbiturate hypnotics,	Carbon tetrachloride
sedatives, and tranquilizers	Ethylene oxide
Ethchlorvynol[b]	
Glutethimide[b]	Cardiovascular agents
Methyprylon[b]	Digoxin[b]
Methaqualone[b]	Procainamide
	N-acetylprocainamide
Chloral hydrate	
Carbromal	Endogenous toxins
Chlorpromazine	Amino acids
Promazine	Uric acid
Promethazine	Creatinine
Meprobamate	Cholic acid
	Polyamino acids
Antidepressants	Polypeptides
Amitryptiline	
Clomipramine	Uremic toxins
Desipramine	
	Indicans
Alcohols	Phenolic compounds
Ethyl alcohol	Organic acids
	Middle molecules
Analgesics	
Acetyl salicylic acid[b]	Thyroxine
Methyl salicylate[b]	Triiodothyronine
Acetaminophen (Paracetamol)[b]	Immune proteins
Antimicrobials/anticancer agents	Miscellaneous
Methotrexate[b]	Epinephrine
	Norepinephrine
Plant/animal toxins,	L-dopamine
herbicides/insecticides	Methoxamine
Amanita phalloides[b]	Serotonin
Amanitin	Nucleotides
Phalloidin	Cholic acid
	Vitamin B_{12}
	Folic acid
	Bromosulphthalein
	Insulin
	Sucrose dilaurate

[a] *Trans. Am. Soc. Artif. Intern. Organs*, 23:768, 1977.
[b] Extensively studied in vivo.

hypoventilation. The administration of epinephrine-like drugs should be in cases of severe hypotension following overexposure to organic solent vapors because of the danger of inducing life-threatening arrhythmias.

A breath sample for infrared spectrographic or gas chromatographic analysis should be obtained. All absorbed gases and organic compounds that are volatile at body temperatures are excreted in part via the lungs and can be identified rapidly in breath samples. Serial breath analyses allow the construction of excretion, or decay, curves from which the magnitude of the exposure can be estimated.

Skin Contamination

Contamination of the skin with a toxic compound that is able to penetrate the skin barrier should be promptly treated by washing the contaminated area with copious amounts of water. This is often best accomplished in a shower. The use of tincture of green soap in conjunction with copious amounts of water is advantageous since hydrocarbons are more soluble in alcohol and the alkalinity of the solution will hydrolyze the organophosphates. The use of substances that will neutralize the toxic agent is not warranted. Experience has proved that the prompt flushing of an area with large amounts of water is the most efficacious method for the rapid decontamination of skin.

The person doing the decontamination should take care not to inadvertently expose himself. The use of disposable gloves, apron, and shoe covers is advisable.

Eye Contamination

Immediately following contamination, the eyes should be rinsed with copious amounts of water. After the initial first aid flush, a drop of tetracaine (Pontocaine), 0.5% solution, can be placed in the outer canthus to achieve topical anesthesia. Then the eye, lids, and so forth can be thoroughly irrigated with isotonic saline. For the majority of chemicals, a 5-minute irrigation is sufficient; but, in the case of a strong alkali, a 20-minute irrigation is mandatory.

In the home setting, the initial irrigation should be commenced immediately using tap water. This can be accomplished by pouring water from a pitcher held 6-8 inches above the open eye while the head is held back over a sink. The objective is to dilute and remove the toxic agent quickly. Permanent injury to the cornea can occur in the few minutes required to reach an emergency room, hence the necessity for commencing immediate decontamination.

Following irrigation, the eye should be examined by an ophthalmologist or a physician trained in the treatment of eye injuries.

Injected Posions

The application of a loose tourniquet proximal to the point of injection can slow the rate of absorption. Cold compresses may also prove efficacious in reducing the rate of absorption. Quantities of unabsorbed toxic agents may be amenable to removal by surgery or by means of suction similar to the procedure commonly advised for the treatment of snake bite.

TOXIC AGENTS

SEDATIVE-HYPNOTIC CENTRAL NERVOUS SYSTEM DEPRESSANTS

The general central nervous system (CNS) despressants include a large variety of agents of diverse chemical structure. These agents have in common the ability to depress overall activity of the CNS. Acute overdosage with a general CNS depressant results in a behavioral continuum that ranges from initial mild sedation and continues through deep sedation, hypnosis, general anesthesia, coma, and death. On occasion, a phase of ataxia coupled with varying degrees of excitation and euphoria may be exhibited following the onset of sedation. The proximal cause of death in most instances is respiratory failure, a result of respiratory center depression. The rate at which a given individual progresses through this continuum of CNS depression depends upon the agent involved, the route of administration, the dose, the physical condition of the individual, and the use of other pharmacologic agents that may potentiate or inhibit the action of the general CNS depressant in question.

When these agents are used on a regular basis and in sufficient dosage, a certain degree of tolerance coupled with physical dependence typically develops. The withdrawal symptoms associated with physical dependence to the general CNS depressants can be life threatening. It should be noted that the symptoms exhibited during withdrawal are almost diametrically opposite to the symptoms of acute overdosage. Withdrawal symptoms begin with subjective feelings of mild agitation and apprehension that intensify and progress through increasing hyperexcitability, hyperreflexia, and often terminate in generalized convulsions of varying severity. If the individual survives the grand mal seizure, a period of psychotic agitation lasting at least a few days ensues.

Barbiturates

The barbiturates are responsible for a large percentage of drug overdose cases, being surpassed in number only by the benzodiazepine class of drugs. However, they still account for the major proportion of deaths and morbidity in suicides with an overall mortality of 3.5%.

Pharmacology

In isolated organ preparations, the barbiturates have been shown to depress the activity of virtually all biologic tissues. Nerve, striated, smooth, and cardiac muscle activity are depressed. Oxygen consumption of most tissues is depressed. Respiration at the mitochondrial level is depressed. To demonstrate these effects, however, very high concentrations of barbiturates are required. The CNS appears to be unique in its sensitivity to the barbituates and, as a consequence, doses adequate to produce substantial depression of the CNS have only minimal or no effect on peripheral structures.

A primary determinant controlling the absorption, excretion, and metabolism of the barbiturates is the pK of the various agents (the degree of dissociation or ionization at a given pH). In the nonionized form, the barbiturates tend to be lipid soluble and, as a consequence, they pass though cell membranes (which are highly lipid in character) with relative ease. The very lipid-soluble thiobarbiturates concentrate initially in the brain because of its high lipid content and high volume of blood flow. As the blood levels drop, the barbiturate leave the CNS and is redistributed to other tissues. This redistribution is the primary mechanism for termination of the action of the ultrashort barbiturates. CNS uptake of the oxybarbiturates, which are less lipid soluble (and therefore less apt to pass through cell membranes) is less rapid. This class of barbiturates are largely metabolized by the liver and excreted via the kidneys.

In the case of the intermediate and long-acting agents, which have a longer sojourn in the blood stream, significant amounts of unmetabolized barbiturate enter the glomerular filtrate in the kidney. If the pH of the urine is shifted to the alkaline side by judicious use of bicarbonate or carbonic anhydrase inhibitors, it is possible to maintain a large part of the filtered barbiturate in the ionized state and prevent its reabsorption by the renal tubules. Renal excretion of the barbiturates can be markedly enhanced by means of this strategem.

Toxicology

With increasing barbiturate dosage, the electroencephalogram (EEG) shifts to high-amplitude slow waves similar to those occurring in stages 3-4 of normal sleep. The subject is no longer conscious and can be aroused only with great difficulty for a few seconds at a time. Respiratory rate is depressed. Deep tendon reflexes tend to be sluggish. Corneal and pupil reflexes are intact.

As the level of barbiturate intoxication increases, the subject is comatose and is no longer able to be aroused. The amplitude of the slow waves decreases and periods of electrical silence are seen. Respiration is markedly depressed, irregular, and shallow. Signs of cyanosis may be evident. Deep tendon reflexes are usually absent. The pupils, however, remain reactive to light in most cases. Blood pressure is low and the heart rate rapid. Hypothermia is almost always present at this level of intoxication.

Diagnosis

The diagnosis of suspected barbiturate poisoning is confirmed by the laboratory determination of the barbiturate in the blood. In many clinical laboratories, only a serum barbiturate measurement is performed; this does not permit identification of the type of barbiturate ingested, that is, long-acting or short-acting. Thus, a single measurement is of little value except to confirm that a barbiturate is present in the blood.

In clinical toxicology laboratories, the specific barbiturate can be quantitatively identified by rapid gas chromatographic methods. These measurements can be of prognostic value. An initial plasma concentration of 3.5 mg/dl for short-acting drugs and 8.0 mg/dl for long-acting drugs should be regarded as potentially fatal in an otherwise healthy, nonaddicted patient. These high blood concentrations occur after the ingestion of total doses of approximately 3.0 g for short-acting drugs or 5.0 g for long-acting drugs. Serial measurements of the barbiturate concentration are a valuable guide to the adequacy of therapy.

It is critically important in the evaluation of the unconscious patient and in all cases of attempted suicide where multiple drugs are commonly ingested to identify all circulating drugs. The simultaneous ingestion of imipramine (Tofranil) and certain hydrazine derivatives can inhibit the metabolism of the barbiturate by the liver and markedly prolong the biologic half-life. It is recommended that the initial urine of each patient suspected of having ingested a toxic quantity of drug be immediately screened for other drugs. This screening can be readily accomplished in less than 4 hours using thin-layer chromatography techniques and in approximately 1 hour using gas chromatographic mass spectrometric analysis.

Mangement of Intoxication

The management of the patient with barbiturate intoxication must support respiratory and circulatory function, prevent continued drug absorption, and promote drug excretion.

Initial Evaluation of the Patient. The initial evaluation should include an assessment of the vital signs, the respiratory depression, and the depth of coma. An accurate history regarding the type of barbiturate, the amount ingested, and the time lapsed since ingestion should be obtained. Attention should be focused on information regarding possible trauma, previous psychiatric illnesses, attempts at suicide, occupation, and the drugs used by the patient in the treatment of preexisting diseases such as diabetes mellitus, hypertension, and anxiety states. Evidence for the presence of lung, kidney, or liver disease should be sought.

In severe barbiturate intoxication manifesting shock, the following findings are charcteristically observed: corneal and deep tendon reflexes are absent, pupillary response to light is minimal; skin of earlobes, nose, and fingers is often cyanotic; heart rate is increased; electrocardiogram (ECG) often shows nonspecific S-T-stegment and T-wave changes; SGOT and LDH are frequently elevated; hypothermia is present; cutaneous bullae are often present in the interdigital clefts.

The clinical laboratory determinations obtained at the time of the first examination should include: arterial blood gases and pH, serum electrolytes, blood urea nitrogen or creatinine, complete blood count, routine urinalysis, chest and skull x-rays, electrocardiogram, and blood for quantitative barbiturate measurement. Blood should be obtained for typing and cross-matching, and an aliquot of serum should be saved for possible future drug analysis.

Gastric Lavage. Gastric lavage is efficacious if performed within 4 hours of ingestion of a barbiturate. In an unconscious patient, intubation with a cuffed endotracheal tube is strongly recommended before lavage to prevent aspiration of gastric contents should emesis ensue. Induced emesis is recommended only if the patient is seen early and is alert.

In those patients in whom gastric lavage is carried out, 30-60 ml of either 50% magnesium sulfate, Fleet's phosphosoda, or 50% sodium sulfate solution is administered by way of the nasogastric tube immediately after lavage has been completed. The tube is then clamped off for approximately 1 hour after the administration of the cathartic.

Ventilation. An adequate airway with the maintenance of adequate ventilation is essential if respiratory depression is present. An oropharyngeal airway is adequate if respiratory depression is not severe. If respiration is not spontaneous, endotracheal intubation with a cuffed tube should be carried out immediately. This facilitates the regular removal of bronchial secretions in severely comatose patients. A tracheostomy should be performed if assisted ventilation via an endotracheal tube in required for more than 48-72 hours. Serial measurements in the arterial blood gases are desirable to prevent the occurrence of either hyper- or hypoventilation.

Circulatory Depression. In addition to arterial hypotension, severely intoxicated patients manifest low cardiac output, increased peripheral vascular resistance, a prolonged circulation time, and relative hypovolemia. Volume expansion often results in substantial improvement. Serial monitoring of the central venous pressure is mandatory to prevent undue plasma volume expansion and congestive heart failure. Vasopressor drugs have proved efficacious in patients whose blood pressure is unresponsive to adequate hydration and volume expansion.

Forced Alkaline Diuresis. Forced diuresis should be reserved for the treatment of intoxications due to long-acting barbiturates. This method of therapy has little efficacy in the treatment of short-acting barbiturate poisonings. The short-acting barbiturates with high partition coefficients and high pK values passively diffuse through cell membranes depending primarily on their rate of delivery to that membrane. In addition, short-acting barbiturates have a high degree of plasma protein binding. Therefore, forced alkaline diuresis can only minimally increase the renal clearance.

By contrast, the relatively low pK value of phenobarbital permits renal clearance values as high as 17 ml/min with forced alkaline diuresis. In addition, alkalinization converts phenobarbital to the nonionized form, which results in an outflow of the drug from intracellular sites in the CNS to extracellular sites with improvement in cerebral function.

Nursing Care. Severely intoxicated patients should be cared for in an intensive care unit because of the demands required by frequent monitoring of fluid balance, respiratory care, and and vital signs. Care of the eyes to prevent corneal injury, proper removal of secretions, and hourly turning of the patient are of critical importance.

Hemodialysis and Hemoperfusion. These modalities should be considered when a potentially lethal dose has been ingested (3 g for short-acting and 5 g for long-acting barbiturates) or when the blood barbiturate level has reached a potentially lethal concentration (see criteria for use of dialysis and hemoperfusion). Dialysis can shorten the duration of coma by a factor of 4 or more. In simultaneous studies of hemodialysis and forced diuresis for barbiturate intoxication, hemodialysis was found to nine times more efficient for removal of the long-acting drugs and six times more efficient for the removal of short-acting drugs.

Nonbarbiturate Sedatives and Hypnotics

The effects produced by these sedative-hypnotics are qualitatively equivalent to the effects produced by the barbiturates. Sedation, coupled with decreased responsiveness to ongoing environmental stimuli, follows administration of low doses. The sedation is often accompanied by a sense of well-being, euphoria, and relief of anxiety. With increased dosage, ataxia and nystagmus are detectable. When intoxicating doses are ingested, the subject becomes comatose and presents a clinical picture similar to that produced by barbiturate intoxication. Differences in the symptomatology associated with individual sedative-hypnotic agents may, however, be present and can provide valuable clinical clues to help pinpoint a specific causative agent.

Chloral Hydrate

A number of halogenated aliphatic alcohols are utilized as sedative-hypnotic agents, the most important of which is chloral hydrate. Its CNS depressant action is due to the metabolite, trichloroethanol, which has also been utilized as a general hypnotic agent.

Recent studies indicate that chloral hydrate does not suppress rapid eye movement sleep (REM). In other respects, the effects produced by this agent are similar to those produced by the barbiturates. In acute intoxication (4-10 g orally), vomiting due to gastric mucosa irritation may occur. In some subjects, the pupils may be constricted (pinpoint pupil) suggesting morphine overdosage. Individuals who survive massive overdosage commonly exhibit hepatic and renal damage.

Ethchlorovynol (Placidyl)

This agent has a rapid onset and a relatively short duration of action. Its effects are similar to those produced by the barbiturates in almost all respects.

Paraldehyde

Paraldehyde is used principally in an institutional setting and, as a consequence, poisoning with this agent is not too common. Acute intoxication results in signs of CNS depression similar to those produced by the barbiturates. Respiration is rapid and labored. The breath has a characteristic disagreeable odor, and the subject is usually acidotic. After recovery from toxic doses, hepatic, renal, and pulmonary damage are frequent findings.

Piperidinedione Derivatives

Methyprylon (Noludar). In hypnotic doses, this drug produces CNS depressant effects that are essentially the same as those produced by the barbiturates. Acute intoxication with this agent is also imilar to barbiturate overdosage.

Glutethimide (Doridan). Glutethimide produces CNS depressant effects similar to those produced by the barbiturates. In addition, however, glutethimide has atropine-like actions that include mydriasis, suppression of salivary secretions, and depressed gut motility.

Hypotension and mydriasis are characteristic symptoms of glutethimide toxicity. Muscular twitching and frank convulsions have also been reported. The mechanism involved in the production of convulsive activity with toxic levels of this agent remains unexplained.

Methaqualone (Quāālude)

The sedative-hypnotic effects of methaqualone are very similar to those produced by the barbiturates. This agent has become a commonly abused drug in recent years. Its popularity is due to the euphoria that is experienced by many users during the onset of sedation. In intoxicating doses, methaqualone produces hypotension, apparently caused by a direct action of the myocardium. Experimental studies have also demonstrated depression of polysynaptic reflexes at the spinal level.

Diagnosis. The diagnosis of suspected intoxication due to ingestion of the nonbarbiturate sedatives and hypnotics is confirmed by the laboratory determination of their presence in the blood. In clinical toxicology laboratories, the specific drug can be quantitatively identified by rapid gas chromatographic/mass spectrometric or thin layer chromatography methods.

The concentration of the drug in the blood can be used as a prognostic index. The potentially lethal concentrations of these compounds in blood are: chloral hydrate, 25 mg%; paraldehyde, 50 mg%; methyprylon, 10 mg%; ethchlorvynol, 15 mg%; glutethimide, 3-10 mg%; and methaqualone, >3 mg%.

Treatment. The key to survival is high quality supportive management (see the discussion under barbiturates). This includes the following: frequent painstaking observation with careful attention to subtle changes in vital signs, depth of CNS depression, and fluid and electrolyte balance; maintenance of airway with the use of endotracheal and tracheostomy tubes with mechanical assistance in order to maintain adequate ventilation as measured by blood gases; prevention of respiratory infection with frequent turning and suctioning to remove secretions, and early treatment of respiratory tract infection guided by gram stains and cultures of tracheal aspirates; managment of hypotension with electrolyte solution replacement monitored with central venous pressure or pulmonary wedge pressure measurements and dopamine, if necessary, to maintian renal perfusion and the systolic pressure above 90 mm Hg; avoidance of analeptics; prevention of pressure necrosis with frequent turning of the patient, attention to proper eye care, and maintenance of sterile indwelling catheter.

Most of the nonbarbiturate sedatives and hypnotics are removable by dialysis or hemoperfusion and, in selected cases, these modalities may be lifesaving.

Minor Tranquilizers

The minor tranquilizers are utilized therapeutically for the treatment of simple anxiety states and anxiety neurosis. They are of little or no value in the treatment of frank psychotic states. As a group, the minor tranquilizers produce variable degrees of sedation. Some authorities claim that the effects of minor tranquilizers are equivalent to those produced by the older general CNS depressants, particularly the barbiturates. While many similarities do exist, it is possible pharmacologically to differentiate the minor tranquilizers from the barbiturates. In any case, the minor tranquilizers tend to produce less sedation at any given level of calming or antianxiety effect. They also tend to have a higher therapeutic index when compared to the barbiturates.

The minor tranquilizers fall mainly into two chemical groups: the propanediols, which include carisprodol (Soma), meprobamate (Miltown, Equanil), phenaglycodol (Ultran), and tybamate (Tybatran); and the benzodiazepines, which include chlordiazepoxide (Librium), chlorzepate (Tranxene), diazepam (Valium), flurazepam (Dalmane), lorazepam (Ativan), oxazepam (Serax), and prazepam (Verstan, Centrax).

In therapeutic doses, meprobamate and other propanediol derivatives tend to suppress anxiety and induce sedation. Some muscle relaxant activity, which may be in part a function of sedation, is also present. With increasing doses (2 g), sedation becomes more prominent. The EEG is in the high β frequency range (20-25 Hz). This fast activity tends to disappear in sleep. Experimental evidence suggests that meprobamate has some specificity of action at the thalamus, reticular formation, and limbic systems. In laboratory animals, polysnaptic spinal reflexes are depressed to a greater extent than are monosynaptic reflexes. Acute intoxication results in coma, respiratory depression, and death. However, due to its low potency, death from meprobamate is relatively rare.

The benzodizepines are used principally for the treatment of anxiety. They also have been widely utilized as muscle relaxants. Dose-dependent sedation is produced by these agents. Therapeutic doses of benzodiazepines produce EEG effects that differ from the EEG patterns produced by agents such as meprobamate. With benzodiazepines, the frequency of the EEG is reduced with the dominant activity in the α range (8-12 Hz) while the amplitude is increased. The electrical pattern is similar to that produced by phenothiazine tranquilizers such as chlorpromazine. As with meprobamate, the benzodiazepines have a relatively high therapeutic index (this ratio is not quite so good in the case of diazepam); as a consequence, fatalities from acute intoxication are not common.

Diagnosis

The diagnosis of suspected intoxicaiton with the minor tranquilizers is confirmed by the laboratory determination of the drug in the urine followed by quantitation in the blood stream. The therapeutic blood concentration of meprobamate is approximately 1 mg%, while 10 mg% produces toxicity, and 20 mg% is a potentially lethal concentration. The therapeutic blood concentration of chlordiazepoxide ranges from 0.1-0.3 mg/dl; the toxic level is 0.55 mg%, and 2 mg% can be lethal. The therapeutic range for blood diazepam is 0.05-0.25 mg%; the toxic range is 0.5-2.0 mg%, and the potentially lethal concentration is above 2.0 mg%.

Treatment

The keystones of successful therapy and survival in the case of severe intoxications with this group of minor tranquilizing agents is intensive supportive therapy as detailed in the discussion of the barbiturates. A few comments regarding the significant clinical differences between these compounds are in order.

Meprobamate overdose can result in coma, hypotension, shock, respiratory depression, and death. The major clinical difficulty is the hypotension that may be unresponsive to volume replacement and is usually out of proportion to the degree of CNS depression. The use of vasopressor agents has proved most efficacious. Forced diuresis significantly increases the renal excretion of meprobamate. In cases of massive overdose, this drug can be successfully removed from the body with the use of either dialysis or hemoperfusion.

Alcohols

Ethanol

Ingestion of excessive amounts of ethanol is probably the most frequent cause of acute intoxication in humans. In suicide attempts, it is frequently taken in addition to other drugs and is present in significant amount in approximately 30% of overdose cases. In these instances, it potentiates the effects of the sedative-hypnotic agents, it increases the rate of absorption of drugs such as diazepam and, through the induction of hepatic enzymes, it may potentiate the hepatotoxic effects of such drugs as acetaminophen.

Ethanol is rapidly absorbed from the upper gastrointestinal tract and is distributed throughout the tissues of the body proportional to their water content. Its primary pharmacologic effect is that of a central nervous system depressant featuring a broad spectrum of clinical features ranging from inebriation, muscular incoordination, impaired judgement, excitement due to loss of inhibitions, to coma.

A blood alcohol concentration of 80 mg% (0.08 g%) will produce the classic features of alcohol inebriation in the majority of people. A concentration above 300 mg% (0.3 g%) will result in coma and respiratory center depression in the majority of patients. Blood alcohol concentrations above 500 mg% (0.5 g%) are potentially lethal. This concentration can result from the consumption of 500 ml of pure ethanol in 1 hour.

Good supportive care is the cornerstone of effective therapy for the acutely intoxicated patient. In children, severe hypoglycemia and convulsions may occur. In severe poisonings, hemodialysis has proved extremely effective in promptly lowering blood alcohol levels.

Methanol

Methanol (methyl alcohol, wood alcohol) is less inebriating than ethanol. It is readily absorbed through the gastrointestinal tract and rapidly distributed throughout the body tissues. It is metabolized by oxydation to formic acid and formaldehyde, with resultant metabolic acidosis. The metabolite, formaldehyde, is responsible for the damage to the retina resulting in partial or complete blindness.

As little as 10 ml is considered toxic if ingested, and the potentially lethal dose in adults is in the 200-250 ml range. The current permissible breathing zone exposure limit in industry is 200 ppm.

Initial symptoms consists of mild inebriation and drowsiness which is often followed by an asymptomatic period lasting 6-24 hours. Then, if a sufficiently toxic amount has been absorbed, the patient experiences the rapid development of symptoms featuring central nervous system depression, metabolic acidosis, and impairment of vision.

The diagnosis is established by measuring the blood methanol concentration; 20 mg% is a toxic level, while concentrations above 50 mg% may result in visual impairment and death.

Treatment consists of intensive supportive care, the prompt

correction of metabolic acidosis and, most importantly, the inhibition of the metabolism of methanol to its toxic metabolites by means of ethanol administration. Initially, ethanol may be administered at a dose of 0.75 ml/kg IV followed by 0.5 ml/kg every 4 hours. Once the metabolic acidosis has been corrected, the ethanol may be administered orally every 3-4 hours in amounts sufficient to maintain a blood alcohol concentration of 100 mg% (0.1 g%). This therapy should be continued until methanol in the blood is no longer detectable.

When methanol blood concentrations are in excess of 50 mg%, hemodialysis should be seriously considered because of its proved efficacy. Hemodialysis results in prompt reduction of methanol blood levels while at the same time effectively removing the toxic metabolites.

Isopropanol (Isopropyl Alcohol)

Isopropanol is absorbed rapidly through the gastrointestinal tract and then distributed throughout the body in a manner similar to ethanol. The primary effect of this alcohol is central nervous system depression. The rapid metabolism of the alcohol to acetone and the resultant metabolic acidosis can lead to an erroneous diagnosis of diabetic ketoacidosis.

The diagnosis is established by measuring the blood concentration of isopropanol and its metabolite, acetone. In cases of serious intoxication, hemodialysis has proved to be a very effective treatment.

Ethylene Glycol

Ethylene glycol, a major ingredient in radiator antifreeze, is rapidly absorbed through the gastrointestinal tract, and in toxic amounts it can produce prolonged central nervous system depression, pulmonary edema, severe metabolic acidosis, vision impairment that may be permanent, and renal injury secondary to the deposition of oxalic acid crystals. The LD_{50} in humans is estimated to be approximately 1.4 ml/kg. As little as 100 ml can lead to death.

The diagnosis is established by measuring the ethylene glycol concentration in blood. In the emergency room setting, the detection of brilliant birefringent oxalic acid crystals in the urine can serve to establish a presumptive diagnosis.

The prompt administration of ethanol in the manner described above for methanol poisoning can block the metabolism of ethylene glycol to oxalic acid. This therapy, maintaining a blood alcohol level of 100 mg%, should be continued until ethylene glycol is no longer detectable in blood. Good supportive therapy with prompt correction of metabolic acidosis is, of course, indicated. Hemodialysis has proved to be an extremely effective method for the prompt removal of ethylene glycol from the blood stream.

Nonnarcotic Analgesics

Salicylates

Salicylate intoxication continues to increase in the adult population; currently, 20% of the reported cases of salicylate poisoning occur in persons 25 years of age or older. While the majority of adult cases are recognized as suicide attempts, there is a growing awareness that a significant number of patients are unintentionally intoxicated when attempting to take a salicylate on a chronic basis. This latter group can present with such a diverse array of signs and symptoms that the physician must be cognizant of the clinical picture of chronic salicylate intoxication in order to protect the more susceptible patients with significant cardiovascular, pulmonary, liver, or renal disease.

Absorption and Metabolism of Salicylates. Salicylates are administered most frequently as sodium salicylate or acetylsalicylic acid (aspirin). These salts are rapidly absorbed intact from the gastrointestinal tract with appreciable serum concentrations achieved in 30 minutes. In the majority of patients, two-thirds of an ingested dose is absorbed in 1 hour, while peak blood levels are achieved in 2-4 hours.

In the blood, salicylates are hydrolyzed rapidly to salicylic acid that is reversibly bound to serum protein, mainly albumin. The tissue distribution and renal excretion of a salicylate is dependent upon hydrogen ion concentration gradients. The nonionized salicylate penetrates a lipid biologic membrane readily, while the ionized salicylate ion diffuses poorly. At the normal pH of blood, salicylic acid is almost completely ionized (99.996% at a pH of 7.4). Therefore, the respiratory alkalosis frequently seen in salicylate intoxication in adults retards the entrance of salicylate into body tissues. Acidosis promotes the entry of the salicylate from the blood stream and extracellular fluid into the body cells, greatly enhancing the toxic effect of the drug. Thus, avoidance of systemic acidosis becomes a primary therapeutic goal in the treatment of salicylate intoxication.

Toxicity. Toxic effects can be anticipated when 10 g or more of any salicylate is ingested in single or divided doses over 23-24 hours, or when the blood salicylate concentration exceeds 35 mg%. The mean lethal dose of sodium salicylate or of acetyl salicylic acid is 20-30 g in an adult; however, the lethal dose range is very wide. Methyl salicylate is considered slightly more toxic than acetyl salicylate.

The major toxic effects of salicylate are local gastrointestinal irritation, CNS excitation and depression, increased metabolic rate, interference with carbohydrate metabolism, interference with normal blood coagulation mechanisms, noncardiac pulmonary edema, ototoxicity, precipitation of sickle cell crisis, hepatotoxicity, and idiosyncratic or hypersensitivity response.

Salicylates stimulate the medullary respiratory center producing an inappropriate hyperpnea. This increased alveolar ventilation produces a respiratory alkalosis. A single dose of 12 g of aspirin in a 70 kg adult may be expected to produce a serum salicylate level in excess of 35 mg% and mild hyperventilation.

Toxic doses of salicylates cause an altered state of consciousness. Agitation, confusion, memory loss, paranoid and hallucinatory behavior, stupor, and coma are commonly observed. Tremor or movement disorders along with papilledema are other neurologic findings not infrequently observed.

Many of the central nervous systemic toxic effects are due to or aggravated by a severe disturbance in acid-base balance. In the majority of adult salicylate intoxications, the chief cause of the acid-base imbalance is prolonged hyperventilation that results in respiratory alkalosis. In contrast to salicylate poisoning in children, alkalosis in the poisoned adult commonly persists until the stage of terminal respiratory failure. However, in a small number of adults, a metabolic acidosis similar to that seen in children can develop.

Diagnosis. The definitive diagnosis of salicylate intoxication is established by the demonstration of elevated blood levels of salicylates. Current analytical methods are both specific and rapid and the results should be available immediately in all community hospitals with emergency room facilities. Blood salicylate levels as high as 35 mg% are nearly always associated with mild hyperventilation due to the direct stimulation of the respiratory center in the medulla, and severe hyperpnea occurs when the level reaches 50 mg%. Serum salicylate levels in excess of 100 mg% are associated with exceedingly high mortality.

The possibility of salicylate poisoning should be considered in any patient who presents with unexplained hyperpnea in association with vomiting, confusion, lethargy, fever, coma, and convulsions. It must be emphasized that the hyperpnea of salicylate poisoning features an increased depth of respiration without a commensurate increase in rate. Unless specifically sought for, this key though subtle symptom may be missed.

Treatment. Excellent treatises on the treatment of salicylate poisoning are available and are listed at the end of this chapter. With the Done nomogram, it is possible to prognosticate regarding the expected severity of the intoxication provided that the interval since ingestion is known.

Following acute ingestion of a salicylate, early emptying of the stomach is essential. This should be accomplished within four hours of aspirin ingestion or within 6-8 hours following oil of wintergreen ingestion. Vomiting has been demonstrated to be more efficient in evacuating salicylate from the stomach than has gastric lavage. A cathartic is used to facilitate the passage of salicylate through the gastrointestinal tract. The oral administration of sodium bicarbonate in the first hours following ingestion is contraindicated because it may facilitate the absorption of salicylate.

Precise evaluation of the acid-base status is essential for optimal treatment. While the anticipated sequence of acid-base disturbance in severe intoxications is respiratory alkalosis followed by metabolic acidosis and occasionally respiratory acidosis, mixed acid-base disturbance is the rule in the adult. The initial phase of respiratory alkalosis seldom requires specific treatment. However, metabolic acidosis secondary to the ingestion of large amounts of salicylate can be dangerous. Arterial blood pH and gases should be determined frequently, and sodium bicarbonate should be administered at a rate sufficient to correct acidemia. Because salicylic acid may interfere with brain glucose metabolism, glucose should be included in the intravenous solutions. The severity of the potassium deficit may be difficult to estimate because of potassium shifts in and out of body cells with changing arterial pH. Therefore, potassium replacement must be guided by frequent measurements of serum electrolytes and arterial blood pH.

Acetaminophen

Acetaminophen has gained popularity in the United States as an analgesic-antipyretic agent. The compound is rapidly and nearly completely absorbed from the GI tract with peak plasma concentrations being attained in 30-60 minutes following a therapeutic dose. The normal biologic half-life in plasma is 1-2 hours.

The minimum toxic dose is 200-250 mg/kg and the absorption of 25 g is potentially lethal. Overdose amounts of acetaminophen do not produce serious symptoms in the immediate post absorption period. In the first 24 hours, nausea, vomiting, anorexia and abdominal pain predominate. After 24-48 hours, most patients sustain hepatic damage as indicated by elevated levels of serum transaminases and lactic dehydrogenase. In some cases, this may progress to hepatic necrosis and liver failure.

The diagnosis is established by measuring the circulating concentrations of the drug. Blood concentrations of 300 μg/ml 4 hours after ingestion is indicative of a grave prognosis. A blood concentration above 225 μg/ml at 4 hours, or 50 μg/ml at 12 hours, is an indication for the administration of cysteamine or acetylcysteine (Mucomyst) to protect against the development of severe liver disease.

Treatment involves emptying the gastrointestinal tract followed by the administration of activated charcoal and a cathartic agent as described above. Acetylcysteine (Mucomyst) gives promise of being an effective antidote. The drug is currently approved as an investigational new drug so the physician is required to register the patient with the Rocky Mountain Poison Control Center and is then obliged to follow a prescribed protocol. Acetylcysteine is administered orally in a dose of 140 mg/kg diluted in 5 volumes of a soft drink, followed by additional doses of 70 mg/kg every 6-8 hours for a period of 3 days. A prolongation of the biological life of acetaminophen beyond 4 hours is indicative of significant hepatic injury.

Tricyclic Antidepressants

Tricyclic antidepressant intoxication is one of the more serious types of acute drug poisoning encountered today. A dose exceeding 20 mg/kg results in severe intoxication that can feature a triad of life-threatening problems: profound respiratory depression, tonic-clonic convulsions, and life-threatening cardiac arrhythmias. When the drug intake has been less than 10 mg/kg, the clinical picture generally features a vigil coma, mydriasis, hyperactive deep tendon reflexes, moderate sinus tachycardia, elevated blood pressure, and a disturbance of the cardiac conduction system.

Signs and symptoms of tricyclic antidepressant intoxication fall into three categories: atropine-like, neurologic, and cardiovascular (Table 6). The diagnosis is confirmed by a laboratory determination of excessive amounts of the drug in vomitus, lavage fluid, urine, or blood.

Successful treatment features intensive supportive care that ideally should be carried out in an intensive care unit where continuous cardiac monitoring is available. Physostigmine salicylate is the antidote of choice when there is evidence of cardiac or central nervous system toxicity. The recommended initial adult dose is 2 mg given by slow intravenous injection (0.5 mg is the initial pediatric dose). If there is no response, an additional 2 mg dose may be given in 15-20 minutes. If there is

Table 6. Signs and Symptoms of Tricyclic Antidepressant Intoxication[a]

Atropine-like
- *Mydriasis*
- *Sinus tachycardia*
- Dry mouth
- Blurred vision
- Ileus
- Bladder paralysis

Neurologic
- Vigil coma
- *Twitching and jerking of the extremities*
- *Convulsions of short duration, occurring every 5 minutes*
- Chorea, athetosis
- *Hyperactive deep tendon reflexes*
- Agitation, delirium, hallucinations
- Respiratory depression
- *Severe sweating*
- Hyperpyrexia

Cardiovascular
- Conduction and rhythm abnormalities[b]
  - *Intraventricular conduction defects* progressing to complete bundle block
  - Atrioventricular block
  - Arrhythmias
    - *Sinus tachycardia*, atrial tachycardia, atrial fibrillation, atrial flutter, ventricular tachycardia, ventricular flutter
  - ECG changes
    - *Widening of QRS* complexes, prolongation of QT interval, ST-T wave abnormalities
- *Hypertension* or hypotension

[a] Diagnostically most useful signs are italicized
[b] May occur up to 6 days after ingestion

a positive response, repeated doses of 1-4 mg may be given every 30-60 minutes as needed. The experience with continuous intravenous infusions of physostigmine, 0.5-1.0 mg per hour until the patient has been alert and free from all toxic manifestations for at least 12 hours, has been good. After physostigmine has been discontinued, the patient is carefully monitored for an additional 12-24 hours with the reinstitution of physostigmine should signs of tricyclic intoxication reappear.

The response to physostigmine is considered therapeutic if any of the following occur within 10-15 minutes of the initial bolus therapy: reversion of the electrocardiogram toward normal, a significant reduction in hypertension accompanied by a reduction in tachycardia, amelioration of central nervous system depression, or control of seizure activity, and abnormal muscle movement. Because physostigmine itself may be toxic, it is not recommended for routine use.

Street Drugs

Marijuana, Hashish, and THC

Marijuana, hashish, and tetrahydrocannabinol (THC) are derived from *Cannabis sativa*, an annual weed commonly known as hemp or Indian hemp. The psychopotency parallels the content of THC that varies widely from plant to plant depending upon a variety of growing conditions. Marijuana generally consists of a mixture of cut, dried, and ground flowers, leaves, and stems of the *Cannibus*. When a marijuana cigarette is smoked, approximately 25% of the THC is delivered in the smoke. Three to 5 mg of THC is required to produce an enjoyable psychic effect and is generally obtained by smoking 1-2 joints of good quality. Inhaled doses of more than 15 mg and oral doses exceeding 35 mg are said to induce undesirable distortions of mood and perception.

The symptoms of heavy use of marijuana (3-5 times average) are listed below. Hashish and THC cause the same symptoms following the absorption of much smaller quantities. The acute physical effects of heavy usage include nausea, vertigo, rapid and impaired speech, a pressure sensation in the head, restlessness, ataxia, tremors, anxiety, panic, precordial distress, and possible elevation of blood pressure. The acute psychologic effects include sensory novelty, increased awareness of stimuli, vivid images, hallucinations, altered reality testing, decreased concentration and attention span, altered sense of identity, temporal disorganization, and anxiety reaction. True paranoia and toxic psychosis have been reported. Acute adverse reactions lasting 5-8 hours may occur and feature unexpected disorientation, anxiety, panic, depression, paranoia, and fear of dying. When these acute adverse symptoms last longer than 8 hours, they are classified as prolonged and, during this period, flashbacks of unusual hallucinations and feelings originally experienced at the time of use may occur.

Treatment is symptomatic and supportive. Talking down is the recommended approach, preferably without the aid of medication. Should this approach prove unsuccessful, one of the phenothiazines or diazepam may be employed. With severe symptoms, gentle restraint may be required for extreme restlessness and hyperactivity.

The measurement of THC in the plasma provides a laboratory confirmatory test. THC persists in the plasma for approximately 3 days following a single injection.

Hallucinogens

This group of drugs include LSD (lysergic acid diethylamide), PCP (phencyclidine), mescaline, psilocybin, STP (2,5-dimethoxy-4-methylamphetamine), and DMT (dimethyltryptamine).

A patient acutely intoxicated with one of these agents may show the following signs and symptoms: the pupils may be dilated; blood pressure is often elevated; heart rate is increased; tendon reflexes are hyperactive; temperature is elevated; face is flushed; and euphoria, anxiety, or panic are present; paranoid thought disorder; illusions; time and visual distortions; hallucinations; depersonalization; and derealization.

No withdrawal syndrome has been reported with this group of agents.

The hallucinogens induce a state of hypersuggestability that can be used to therapeutic advantage by talking the patient down in a quiet place. Strong reassurance that the drug effects are transient and that the patient will be protected from harm is most effective. When sedation is required, diazepam or barbiturate should be given. Phenothiazines are effective but should be used with caution since there is a possibility that anticholinergic substances might also have been ingested with a resultant increase in anticholinergic toxicity.

Tests for the presence of hallucinogenic agents in biologic fluids are done only in special toxicology laboratories so the diagnosis of acute intoxication must often be made and treatment commenced on the basis of clinical findings alone. Since street drugs are routinely adulterated with a variety of other drugs, the physician should be alert for the signs and symptoms of multiple ingestion.

Severe cases of phencyclidine (PCP) intoxication can be benefited by urine acidification that enhances the excretion of the compound. Ammonium chloride in a dose of 2.75 mEq/kg dissolved in 60 ml of saline can be administered via a gastric tube which is then clamped for 1 hour. This dose is repeated at 6-hour intervals until the urine pH is reduced to a level below 5. This usually requires two doses of ammonium chloride. In addition, ascorbic acid can be administered as intravenous infusion of 2 g dissolved in 500 ml of fluid given over 6 hours and repeated as necessary. After the urine pH is less than 5, furosemide-induced diuresis will greatly enhance the renal excretion of the drug. In emergency situations such as profound coma or intractable seizures, the ammonium chloride can be administered intravenously as a 1-2% solution in saline.

Central Nervous System Stimulants

This group of drugs of abuse includes the amphetamines, most antiobesity drugs, cocaine, methylphenidate (Ritalin), and phenmetrazine (Preludin).

High doses of any of these CNS stimulants results in a fairly characteristic toxic state: the pupils are usually dilated and reactive; respiration is shallow; blood pressure is elevated; heart rate is increased; deep tendon reflexes are hyperactive; temperature is elevated; tremor and sweating may be present along with a hyperactive, paranoid, compulsive, repetitious behavior pattern. Convulsions and frank psychosis may occur.

With the exception of cocaine, a characteristic withdrawal syndrome has been described for this group of agents. It features muscular aches, abdominal pain, voracious hunger, prolonged sleep, lack of energy, and profound psychologic depression that sometimes becomes suicidal. A true physical dependence is not seen with cocaine usage, but there is a strong psychic dependence.

The phenothiazines can be used to control the physical, mental, and autonomic disturbances associated with amphetamine-like intoxications.

Anticholinergics

Included in this category are atropine, belladonna, henbane, and scopolamine.

The signs of acute intoxication include dilated and fixed pupils, increased heart rate, temperature elevation, drowsiness or coma, flushed-dry skin and mucous membranes, sensorium clouding, amnesia, disorientation, and visual hallucinations.

Intoxication can be dramatically reversed with intravenous physostigmine, which has a shorter duration of action than most of the anticholinergic agents and therefore must be given repeatedly (see Table 2).

Narcotics

The narcotics include morphine, codeine, heroin, meperidine (Demerol), methadone, opium, pentazocine, and propoxyphene (Darvon).

Acute intoxication with any one of the narcotic agents results in depressed or absent respiration. The pupils are usually constricted and fixed, except in the case of meperidine and extreme hypoxia which produce dilated pupils. Blood pressure is generally decreased and deep tendon reflexes are slow to absent. Other features of acute intoxication are drowsiness or coma and pulmonary edema. With overdose of propoxyphene, convulsions may be prominent.

Assisted ventilation is indicated if breathing has ceased or is significantly depressed. Shock is treated with plasma expanders and pressor drugs, while pulmonary edema generally responds to positive pressure oxygen.

The narcotic antagonist naloxone (Narcan), 0.01 mg/kg I.V., I.M., or S.C., is the treatment of choice. It is effective in combating any degree of narcotic-induced respiratory depression, including that produced by pentazocine overdosage. An adult may be given a dose of 0.4 mg (1 ml) intravenously every 3 minutes. Failure to obtain significant improvement after 3 or 4 doses suggests that the condition may be due partly or completely to other disease processes or nonopioid drugs. Since the duration of action of some narcotics may exceed that of naloxone, the patient should be kept under continued surveillance, and repeated doses of naloxone should be administered as necessary.

Withdrawal symptoms following the sudden discontinuance or narcotics results in a cluster of signs and symptoms resembling a flu-like illness and may include dilated pupils, rapid pulse, rhinorrhea, lacrimation, vomiting, gooseflesh, multiple aches, pains, and tremulousness. These abstinence symptoms usually begin within 12 hours following cessation of narcotic administration or 36-72 hours after the last dose of methadone.

In the treatment of severe withdrawal syndrome, a single dose of 10-20 mg of intramuscular methadone will render most patients comfortable. Twenty mg of oral methadone is effective treatment for patients with only moderately distressing symptoms.

METALS

Lead

Most cases of lead poisoning in children occur by the ingestion of white lead paint scales (pica); by the ingestion of soluble lead salts in foods, wines, and distilled liquors; and by the use of pewter dishes. In the industrial setting, the use of 1.1 million tons of lead per year in the U.S. sets the stage for accidental overexposure of workers to lead vapor, mist, or dust.

The signs and symptoms of lead poisoning fall into several categories. In the adult, lead colic, the result of spasm of the bowel, is a common presenting symptom. This colic is intermittent and often severe. The adult form also features asymmetrical, painless motor neuropathy usually involving the extensor muscules of the upper extremity. Encephlopathy occurs primarily in children. Antecedent irritability, insomnia, loss of memory, and confusion may progress to seizures, delirium, and coma. In the usual case of chronic overexposure to inorganic lead, hypochromic anemia with basophilic stippling of the red cells along with the development of a lead line, a lead sulfide punctate deposit along the gingival margin of some of the teeth, may occur.

The determination of an abnormal amount of lead in the blood is the definitive diagnostic test. Lead levels less than 40 μg/dl of whole blood are considered within the normal range. Levels greater than 40 μg/dl indicate excessive lead absorption. Levels of 50-80 μg/dl are usually associated with anemia and some symptoms of lead poisoning. Level of 80-100 μg/dl are indicative of serious intoxication. Other useful laboratory tests are 24-hour quantitative urine lead excretion; serum δ-aminolevulinic acid; and CBC with peripheral blood smear for basophilic stipling.

Chelation therapy should be instituted in all symptomatic patients with blood lead levels of 50-60 μg/dl or greater. Calcium EDTA and dimercaprol (British antilewisite) are the agents of choice (see Table 2). Calcium gluconate, 100 mg intravenously in a 10% solution, will dramatically suppress the abdominal colic. In children with signs of encephalopathy, careful treatment of cerebral edema using mannitol and dexamethasone is indicated. Diazepam is effective in controlling seizures.

Arsenic

Within hours following overexposure to arsenic, abdominal pain followed by vomiting and diarrhea commence. Pain in the extremities with muscle weakness and flushing of the skin are often present. Three to 4 days following the onset of symptoms, asymmetrical peripheral neuropathy may occur.

In the acute intoxication, dimercaprol is the chelating agent of choice (see Table 2). Arsenic inactivates sulfhydryl-containing enzymes, thereby producing its toxic effect. Competition for sulfhydryl binding by dimercaprol reverses arsenic poisoning.

The diagnosis can be established by measuring the arsenic in a 24-hour urine specimen. Normal persons excrete an average of 15 μg/day with a range of 5-40 μg/day. Most patients with arsenic poisoning excrete more than 100 μg/day. A blood level of arsenic below 10 μg/dl is in the normal range, but blood levels are highly variable and treacherous from a diagnostic standpoint.

Hair and nails store arsenic so analysis for arsenic content can be of diagnostic value for extended periods after exposure. Four to 6 weeks following exposure, Mees' lines, which are white transverse lines, may be seen on the nails of the hands and feet.

Chronic poisoning from repeated ingestion of small amounts of arsenic is the usual method for homicide by arsenic poisoning. Weight loss, diarrhea alternating with constipation, symmetrical peripheral neuropathy, headache, confusion, dermatitis, and bone marrow damage are important manifestations.

Mercury

Acute inorganic mercury poisoning results from ingestion of soluble mercuric salts and is characterized by corrosive effects on the gastrointestinal tract and renal tubular cell injury. Metalic mercury is relatively nontoxic unless it is converted to an ionized form by acids or strong oxidants. Ethyl and methyl mercury compounds have the potential for damaging the central nervous system.

Ingestion of a corrosive mercurial salt is followed by profuse salivation and intense burning of the mouth and esophagus. Injury of the upper gastrointestinal tract results in abdominal pain, hemorrhage, vomiting, and diarrhea. A few days to weeks later, ulceration of the lower gastrointestinal tract may occur. Damage to the glomerulus can result in the nephrotic syndrome and acute renal failure. Muscle tremor, mild peripheral paresthesia, and liver necrosis may be present. The diagnosis is confirmed by demonstrating an elevation of blood mercury levels from the normal upper level of 10 μg/dl to ranges of 25-50 μg/dl. In chronic cases of poisoning, 24-hour urine excretion exceeds the upper limits of normal, 15 μg/24 hrs., at a time when the blood mercury may be normal.

In severe poisonings when orally ingested mercurial compounds may still be in the gastrointestinal tract, activated charcoal and cathartics are indicated. The use of oral chelating agents should not be instituted until charcoal stools are seen since orally administered chelators may increase absorption of the metal. BAL and D-penicillamine are the chelating agents of choice. Hemodialysis is ineffective in removing the chelated or free metal, however, it may be necessary for treatment of acute renal failure.

TOXIC GASES AND SOLVENTS

A clinical classification of toxic gases is presented in Table 7. The gases are separated into four categories: simple aphyxiants, chemical asphyxiants, irritants, and systemic poisons. When a physician knows to which category a gas belongs, he can predict its toxic effect.

The simple asphyxiants exert their toxic effect by replacement or dilution of atmospheric oxygen. The resultant toxic effect is directly related to the reduction of oxygen concentration. When oxygen concentration falls below 17% at sea level, no physiologic effect is noted, but a candle flame will go out. When the concentration drops to 12%, respiratory effort deepens, coordination is impaired, and dizziness is noted. Below 8%, respiration is labored and is accompanied by cyanosis, nausea, and vomiting. Exposure to 4% oxygen for 40 seconds will produce unconsciousness. As an example of the clinical usefulness of this classification, consider the question of the toxic effect of the inhalation of 10% methane gas in air. Since the oxygen concentration would still be adequate, the physiologic impact would be negligible.

Chemical asphixiants interfere with the normal utilization of oxygen via a chemical reaction. The three gases in this category most commonly encountered are carbon monoxide, hydrogen sulfide, and hydrogen cyanide.

Table 7. Clinical Classification of Toxic Gases

Simple asphyxiants		
Methane	Carbon dioxide	Nitrogen
Ethane	Nitrous oxide	Helium
Acetylene	Hydrogen	Neon
Argon	Fluorocarbon gases	
Chemical asphyxiants		
Carbon monoxide		
Hydrogen sulfide		
Hydrogen cyanide		
Lung irritants		
Simple		
Ammonia	Sulfur dioxide	Formaldehyde
Acrolein	Hydrogen fluoride	Chlorine
Pulmonary edema producing		
Ozone	Phosgene	Nitrogen dioxide
Systemic poisons		
Arsine	Hydrogen selenide	Nickel carbonyl
Phosphine	Carbon disulfide	Stibine

Carbon Monoxide

Carbon monoxide (CO) is man's oldest and most commonly encountered toxic gas. The product of incomplete combustion, it is found in high concentrations in automobile exhaust, in the combustion gases of organic materials, and may be formed endogenously in toxic amounts following the absorption and metabolism of methylene chloride. Carbon monoxide is rapidly absorbed via the lungs in an amount proportional to the minute respiratory volume. Because it has an affinity for hemoglobin 200-250 times that of oxygen, it readily accumulates in the blood as carboxyhemoglobin (COHb), preventing the normal transport of both oxygen and carbon dioxide. In addition, COHb diminishes the oxygen-releasing ability of the remaining hemoglobin, shifting the oxygen disociation curve to the left.

Less than 1% of absorbed CO is oxidized to CO_2 and the rest of the gas is excreted unchanged via the lungs. In the sedentary adult at sea level, the biologic half-life of CO is 4-5 hours. Breathing 100% oxygen by mask reduces the half-life to 40-80 minutes. In a hyperbaric chamber, 100% oxygen at 3 atmospheres further reduces the half-life to 23.5 minutes.

In the healthy adult who is free of cardiovascular disease, the first signs and symptoms of CO poisoning occur at a blood stream saturation of 16-20% COHb. The individual experiences tightness across the forehead progressing to a typical fronto-occipital tension headache. At 30-40% COHb, the headache is severe and accompanied by nausea and vomiting. With exertion, syncope may occur. At 60-70% COHb, convulsions, coma, and death may occur.

The EPA ambient air quality standard for carbon monoxide is 9 ppm for 8 hours, not to be exceeded more than once per year. At sea level, this will result in a maximal COHb saturation of 1.55%. The permissible exposure limit in industry is 50 ppm (time-weighted average) for a normal workday. This will result in a COHb saturation of 7.4%. (A one-pack-a-day cigarette smoker will have an average COHb saturation of 5%.) A concentration of 1,500 ppm for 30 minutes is immediately dangerous to life.

Patients with heart disease, anemia, impaired circulation, and increased metabolic rate are much more susceptible to the hypoxic effects of elevated COHb. It has been demonstrated that patients with severe angina pectoris are adversely affected by COHb saturations in the 2-10% range.

The diagnosis of CO poisoning is established by measuring COHb in blood. This is reported as a percentage saturation of hemoglobin. Thus, a 5% COHb saturation means that 5% of the hemoglobin available for oxygen transport is combined with CO. Analysis of breath for expired CO offers a rapid, alternative method for estimating the COHb body burden.

Mild CO intoxication is treated with 100% oxygen by mask. Patients with significant underlying cardiovascular disease or with COHb saturations in excess of 40% are candidates for hyperbaric oxygen therapy. Patients with severe intoxication should be under medical surveillance for a minimum of 48 hours, during which time serial electrocardiograms (ECGs) and serum enzymes should be obtained.

Hydrogen Sulfide

Exposure to high concentrations of hydrogen sulfide can result in sudden respiratory center paralysis, collapse, and death from asphyxia. Exposure to sublethal doses results in irritation of mucous membranes and eyes resulting in painful conjunctivitis, cough, nausea, vomiting, and CNS depression with depressed respirations. In addition to acting directly on the respiratory center, this gas causes inhibition of oxydative enzyme systems leading to anoxic damage of the cells.

The permissible occupational exposure limit is 10 ppm (time-weighted average) for a normal workday. At a concentration of 0.3 ppm, the distinct rotten egg odor is detectable. Exposure to 70-150 ppm will produce lacrimation, conjunctivitis, and throat and nose irritation after several hours. The concentration immediately dangerous to life is 300 ppm for 30 minutes. Exposures to concentrations above 500 ppm produces loss of consciousness, depressed respirations, and death in 30-60 minutes.

The prompt establishment of adequate respiration is the key to successful therapy. In serious intoxications, the administration of nitrite to form methemoglobin and subsequently sulfmethemoglobin to prevent sulfide from damaging the oxidative enzyme systems is useful. To achieve this, the cyanide treatment schedule in Table 2 should be used, omitting the sodium thiosulfate.

Hydrogen Cyanide

The cyanides are among the most toxic of all industrial chemical compounds, and, although they are produced in large quantity, they are responsible for very few illnesses or deaths because workmen have been properly educated in safe handling of these materials. When hydrogen cyanide gas is absorbed through the lungs, it is rapidly distributed to all organs in the body where it forms stable complexes with the ferric iron in the enzyme ferric cytochrome oxidase. The inhibition of this enzyme blocks aerobic metabolism and hypoxic injury ensues.

The permissible occupational exposure limit is 10 ppm, time weighted for a normal workday. The concentration immediately dangerous to life is 50 ppm.

Since the onset of toxic action is so rapid, therapy to combat the hypoxia must be immediate (see Table 2).

Lung Irritants

The lung irritants are divided into two groups. The gases that are highly water soluble attack the upper respiratory tract and commence their toxic action immediately. A human being will not voluntarily subject himself to a harmful concentration of one of these gases. Therefore, unless a person is trapped in an atmosphere containing a toxic concentration of one of these agents, significant lung injury is not anticipated.

Those gases in the second category are relatively water insoluble and do reach the lower respiratory tract. Exposure to toxic concentrations of these agents results in a delayed pulmonary edema secondary to the extravasation of plasma from the capillaries into the alveoli.

ORGANIC SOLVENTS

The majority of the organic solvents encountered in the workplace and in commercial products are CNS depressants. The magnitude of this depression is proportional to the amount of the solvent absorbed and is not dissimilar from ethanol intoxication. Each of these solvents has a different potential for inducing dermatitis, liver injury, kidney injury, epinephrine sensitization of the heart, or bone marrow injury. However, when properly used, no untoward health effects are to be anticipated.

Table 8 summarizes permissible exposure limits and potential toxic effects of the more commonly encountered solvents.

The diagnosis of exposure to any gas or volatile solvent circulating in the blood stream can be made by measuring either the blood or the breath concentration. The latter technique has proved to be a very useful method in the industrial setting.

INSECTICIDES

Organic Phosphate Insecticides

These agents are rapidly absorbed through the respiratory and gastrointestinal tracts. Some are absorbed through the skin. They all exert their toxic action via permanent inhibition of the cholinesterase enzyme systems.

The two cardinal signs of cholinesterase inhibition are myosis and muscle fasciculations. Other symptoms include headache, giddiness, nervousness, blurred vision, weakness, nausea, cramps, diarrhea, and discomfort. Signs of intoxication include sweating, myosis, tearing, salivation, bradycardia, excessive respiratory tract secretions, vomiting, convulsions, and coma. While death may occur rapidly following ingestion of these agents, symptoms beginning more than 12 hours following suspected ingestion are probably due to some other cause.

The most available diagnostic tests of exposure are the red blood cell and plasma cholinesterase determinations. In significant intoxications, the cholinesterase levels are always markedly reduced. Since the inhibition of the red blood cell cholinesterase is biologically irreversible, 3 months are required for complete restoration of normal enzyme concentrations.

The detection of a specific urinary metabolite of one of the organophosphates provides the physician with a second diagnostic test of exposure.

Prompt treatment of the intoxicated patient who manifests pinpoint pupils and muscular fasciculations is first directed at establishing an adequate airway and reversing any cyanosis. Then atropine sulfate, 2-4 mg, is administered intravenously. This dose is repeated at 5 to 10-minute intervals until signs of atropinization appear (pupil response, dry, flushed skin, tachycardia). In the severely intoxicated patient, massive amounts of atropine may be required.

Pralidoxime (2-PAM chloride) is available as a specific antidote for many of the organophosphate insecticides. It can

Table 8. Organic Solvents

	Permissible Exposure Limit	Dangerous Concentration for 30 Min	Target Organ Injury					
			CNS	*Skin*	*Liver*	*Kidney*	*Blood*	*Heart*
Benzene	1 ppm	2,000 ppm	+	+	–	–	4+	±
Carbon tetrachloride	10 ppm	300 ppm	2+	+	4+	4+	–	2+
Chloroform	50 ppm	1,000 ppm	2+	+	3+	3+	–	2+
Methyl chloroform	350 ppm	1,000 ppm	2+	+	±	±	–	2+
Methylene chloride	200 ppm	5,000 ppm	+	+	±	±	–	2+
Perchloroethylene	100 ppm	500 ppm	+	+	+	±	–	+
Styrene	100 ppm	5,000 ppm	+	+	±	–	–	+
Toluene	200 ppm	2,000 ppm	+	+	±	–	–	±
Trichloroethylene	100 ppm	1,000 ppm	+	+	+	±	–	+
Xylene	100 ppm	10,000 ppm	+	+	±	–	–	±

rejuvenate the phosphorylated enzyme. Instructions for its administration are detailed in its package insert.

Carbamates

The carbamates are reversible cholinesterase inhibitors. The inhibited, carbamylated cholinesterases are rejuvenated by hydrolysis, a process requiring 6-12 hours in the average case. The signs and symptoms of intoxication are similar to those of organophosphate poisoning and feature the cardinal signs of cholinesterase inhibition: pinpoint pupils and muscular fasciculations.

The diagnosis of intoxication can be confirmed by demonstrating a depressed red blood cell and plasma cholinesterase activity. Since this is a biologically reversible cholinesterase inhibition, the blood sample must be drawn early in the course of intoxication.

The treatment is the same as that outlined for the organophosphate insecticide with the exception that pralidoxime chloride is not used.

The number of potentially toxic agents the physician may be required to deal with is encyclopedic. One valuable reference aid is the Poisindex microfiche compilation available in the majority of Poison Control Centers. This reference work is updated every 3 months and, in addition to its most valuable treatment regimens, it contains a carefully selected bibliography dealing with diagnosis and treatment of toxicologic medical problems.

QUESTIONS

(More than one answer may be correct)

1. Stage 3 coma is characterized by
   A. Coma, absent reflexes, respiratory depression, and shock
   B. Coma, withdrawal from painful stimuli, and intact reflexes
   C. Coma, absent reflexes, no response to painful stimuli but no respiratory or circulatory depression
   D. Restlessness, irritability, insomnia, and tremors
   E. Coma with intermittent convulsions
2. Contraindications to the induction of emesis include
   A. Coma, convulsions, or loss of the normal gag reflex
   B. Ingestion of strong alkali, mineral acid, or a petroleum solvent
   C. Severe heart disease or advanced pregnancy
   D. Ingestion of aspirin or barbiturates
   E. Diabetes or renal failure
3. Match the antidote to the poison

Poisons	*Antidotes*
i. Ethylene glycol	A. Ethanol
ii. Tricyclic antidepressants	B. Phenothiazines
iii. Amphetamine	C. Methylene blue
iv. Methanol	D. Physostigmine salicylate
v. Anticholinergics	E. D-Penicillamine
vi. Methemoglobinemia	F. 2 PAM

4. Indications for hemodialysis/hemoperfusion in a case of overdose include
   A. Severe clinical intoxication with abnormal vital signs
   B. Blood level in the potentially lethal range
   C. Need of the overdose patient's ICU bed for other patients in a busy hospital
   D. Potential for conversion of the toxin into a more noxious substance
   E. Poisoning by agents known to produce delayed toxicity
5. Which of the following statements regarding barbiturate intoxication are true?
   A. The long-acting barbiturates are more efficiently cleared by the kidney.
   B. The potentially lethal level for phenobarbital is 3 mg/dl.
   C. Forced alkaline diuresis is very efficacious in treatment of short-acting barbiturates.
   D. Almost all cases of overdose with phenobarbital should be treated immediately with hemoperfusion.
   E. Circulatory depression is a contraindication to hemodialysis and hemoperfusion.
6. Match the potentially lethal blood concentration to the drug.

i. Butabarbital	A. 25 mg/dl
ii. Phenobarbital	B. 10 mg/dl
iii. Chloral hydrate	C. 15 mg/dl
iv. Methypyrlon (Noludar)	D. 3.5 mg/dl
v. Methaqualone (Quāālude)	E. 4 mg/dl
vi. Ethchlorvynol (Placidyl)	F. 8 mg/dl

7. Which of the following statements regarding methanol poisoning is/are true?
   A. Ingestion of as little as 10 ml may prove toxic.
   B. 20 mg/dl is a toxic level; 50 mg/dl may result in visual impairment and death.
   C. Metabolic alkalosis is a prominent feature.
   D. Ethanol is a very effective treatment.
   E. Hemodialysis should be seriously considered when the blood level is in excess of 50 mg/dl.
8. Which of the following statement(s) regarding ethylene glycol poisoning is (are) true?
   A. It is a major ingredient in radiator antifreeze.
   B. As little as 100 ml can cause death.
   C. Renal injury secondary to the deposition of oxalic acid crystals is a prominent feature.

D. Correction of metabolic acidosis and ethanol administration are the mainstays of treatment.

E. Hemodialysis is ineffective in removal of ethylene glycol from the blood stream.

9. Which of the following statement(s) regarding salicylate poisoning is (are) true?

   A. Toxic effects can be anticipated whenever the blood salicylate concentration exceeds 35 mg/dl.

   B. The mean lethal dose of aspirin is 20-30 g in an adult.

   C. Tachypnea produces respiratory alkalosis.

   D. Blood gases and serum K^+ should be closely monitored.

   E. Glucose should not be included in the intravenous solutions.

10. Which of the following statement(s) regarding tricyclic antidepressants is (are) true?

    A. A dose exceeding 20 mg/kg is life threatening.

    B. A dose of ⩽10 mg/kg causes vigil coma.

    C. Hyperventilation is a characteristic feature.

    D. Intravenous physostigmine is the antidote of choice.

    E. Conduction and rhythm abnormalities are uncommon.

11. Which of the following statement(s) regarding lead poisoning is (are) true?

    A. In children, lead colic is a common presenting symptom.

    B. In the adult form, motor neuropathy is often a prominent feature.

    C. Encephalopathy occurs primarily in children.

    D. Levels greater than 40 mg/dl indicate excessive lead absorption.

    E. Treatment with calcium EDTA or dimercaprol is indicated in all symptomatic patients with blood lead levels exceeding 50 mg/dl.

ANSWERS

1. C
2. A, B, C
3. i-A, ii-D, iii-B, iv-A, v-D, vi-C
4. A, B, D, E
5. A
6. i-D, ii-F, iii-A, iv-B, v-E, vi-C
7. A, B, D, E
8. A, B, C, D
9. A, B, D
10. A, B, D
11. B, C, D, E

BIBLIOGRAPHY

Basic Principles of Toxicology

Collins JV, Goulding R: Treatment of acute poisoning at Guy's Hospital: October 1969 to September 1970. *Guy Hosp Rep* 120:31-46, 1971.

Exaire E, Trevino-Becerra A, Monteon F: An overview of treatment with peritoneal dialysis in drug poisoning. *Contrib Nephrol* 17:39-43, 1979.

Mackison FW (ed): NIOSH/OSHA Pocket Guide to Chemical Hazards. DHEW (NIOSH) Publication No 78-210, 1978.

Pond S, Rosenberg J, Benowitz NL, et al: Pharmacokinetics of haemoperfusion for drug overdose. *Clin Pharmacokinet* 4(5):329-354, 1979.

Winchester JF, Gelfand MC, Knepshield JH, et al.: Dialysis and hemoperfusion of poisons and drugs: Update. *Trans Am Soc Artif Intern Organs* 23:762-842, 1977.

Barbiturate and Sedative Poisoning

Berman LB, Jeghers HJ, Schreiner GE, et al: Hemodialysis: Effective therapy for acute barbiturate poisoning. *JAMA* 161:820-827, 1956.

Gumpert NF: Criteria for the use of specific forms of therapy for barbiturate overdose. *Am J Hosp Pharm* 29:428-433, 1972.

Henderson LW, Merrill JP: Treatment of barbiturate intoxication with a report of recent experience at Peter Bent Brigham Hospital. *Ann Intern Med* 64:867-891, 1966.

Mann JB, Sandberg DH: Therapy of sedative overdosage. *Pediatr Clin North Am* 17:617-628, 1970.

Alcohol Poisoning

Elliott RW, Hunter PR: Acute ethanol poisoning treated by hemodialysis. *Postgrad Med J* 50:515-517, 1974.

Setter JG, Singh R, Brackett NC Jr, et al.: Studies on the dialysis of methanol. *Trans Am Soc Artif Intern Organs* 13:178-182, 1967.

Salicylate and Acetaminophen Poisoning

Done AK, Temple AR: Treatment of salicylate poisoning. *Mod Treat* 8:528-551, 1971.

Peterson RG, Rumack BH: Treating acute acetaminophen poisoning with acetylcysteine. *JAMA* 237:2406-2407, 1977.

Winchester JF, Gelfand MC, Helliwell M, et al.: Extracorporeal treatment of salicylate or acetaminophen poisoning: Is there a role? *Arch Intern Med* 141:370-374, 1981.

Tricyclic Antidepressant Poisoning

Stewart RD: Tricyclic antidepressant poisoning. *Am Fam Physician* 19: 136-144, 1979.

Toxic Gases and Solvent Poisoning

Aronow WS, Isbell MW: Carbon monoxide effect on exercise-induced angina pectoris. *Ann Intern Med* 79:392-395, 1973.

Stewart RD, Dodd HC, Erley DS, et al.: Diagnosis of solvent poisoning. *JAMA* 193:1097-1100, 1965.

Stewart RD, Stewart RS, Stamm W, et al.: Rapid estimation of carboxyhemoglobin level in fire fighters. *JAMA* 235:390-392, 1976.

INDEX